Clinical Cardiology

FOURTH EDITION

Clinical Cardiology

Maurice Sokolow, MD

*Professor of Medicine Emeritus
Senior Staff Member, Cardiovascular Research Institute;
formerly Chief of Cardiology and Program Director of
the USPHS Clinical Cardiology Training Program,
University of California, San Francisco*

Malcolm B. McIlroy, MD

*Professor of Medicine
Senior Staff Member, Cardiovascular Research Institute,
University of California, San Francisco*

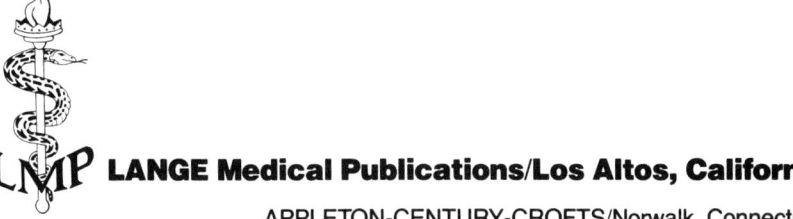

LANGE Medical Publications/Los Altos, California

APPLETON-CENTURY-CROFTS/Norwalk, Connecticut

Notice: The author(s) and publisher of this volume have taken care that the information and recommendations contained herein are accurate and compatible with the standards generally accepted at the time of publication.

Copyright © 1986 by Appleton-Century-Crofts
A Publishing Division of Prentice-Hall
Copyright © 1981, 1979, 1977 by Lange Medical Publications

Spanish Edition: *Editorial El Manual Moderno, S.A. de C.V.,*
Av. Sonora 206, Col. Hipodromo, 06100-Mexico, D.F.
Italian Edition: *Piccin Nuova Libraria, S.p.A., Via Altinate, 107, 35121 Padua, Italy*
Greek Edition: *Paschalidis Medical Publications, 14 Tetrapoleos Street, Ambelokipi,*
Athens, 617, Greece
German Edition: *Springer-Verlag GmbH & Co. KG, Postfach 10 52 80,*
6900 Heidelberg 1, West Germany

All rights reserved. This book, or any parts thereof, may not be used or reproduced in any manner without written permission. For information, address Appleton-Century-Crofts, 25 Van Zant Street, East Norwalk, Connecticut 06855.

87 88 89 90 / 10 9 8 7 6 5 4 3

Prentice-Hall of Australia, Pty. Ltd., Sydney
Prentice-Hall Canada, Inc.
Prentice-Hall Hispanoamericana, S.A., Mexico
Prentice-Hall of India Private Limited, New Delhi
Prentice-Hall International (UK) Limited, London
Prentice-Hall of Japan Inc., Tokyo
Prentice-Hall of Southeast Asia (Pte.) Ltd., Singapore
Whitehall Books Ltd., Wellington, New Zealand
Editora Prentice-Hall do Brasil Ltda., Rio de Janeiro

ISBN: 0-8385-0023-4

PRINTED IN THE UNITED STATES OF AMERICA

*This book is dedicated to
Margaret McIlroy and the memory of Ethel Sokolow*

Table of Contents

Preface	ix
1. Anatomy & Physiology of the Circulatory System	1
2. History Taking	34
3. Physical Examination	42
4. Clinical Physiology	64
5. Special Investigations: Noninvasive	80
6. Special Investigations: Invasive	105
7. Therapeutic Procedures	121
8. Coronary Disease	132
9. Systemic Hypertension	209
10. Cardiac Failure	287
11. Congenital Heart Disease (With Special Reference to Adult Cardiology)	324
12. Valvular Heart Disease; Mitral Valve Disease	368
13. Aortic Valve Disease; Combined Valve Disease	400
14. Conduction Defects	432
15. Cardiac Arrhythmias	466
16. Infective Endocarditis	510
17. Myocardial Disease (Myocarditis & Cardiomyopathy)	527
18. Pericarditis	573
19. Pulmonary Heart Disease	586
20. Diseases of the Aorta & Systemic Arteries	599
21. Miscellaneous Forms of Heart Disease: Cardiac Tumors, Hypotension, Neurocirculatory Asthenia, & Traumatic Heart Disease	609
22. Heart Disease in Pregnancy	617
23. Cardiac Disease & the Surgical Patient	626
Index	633
Equations & Normal Values	Inside Back Cover

Preface

Progress in cardiology research throughout the world remains rapid. In this fourth edition we have tried to include the important clinical advances of the last 5 years and their scientific bases. We found that our book was becoming too large and unwieldy to serve its main purpose. We therefore revised and shortened each chapter by approximately 15%. The only new section is in Chapter 21 on traumatic heart disease.

New developments that have been included involve cardiovascular physiology, special investigations, therapeutic procedures, coronary disease, systemic hypertension, cardiac failure, and myocardial disease. The chapters dealing with these subjects have been more extensively revised. The descriptions of newer therapeutic agents, such as calcium entry–blocking drugs, and procedures, such as coronary thrombolysis and percutaneous coronary transluminal angioplasty, have been expanded, and new ideas on hemodynamics and cardiac function are presented.

To accommodate the many new references to work of the last 5 years, we have deleted a number of older references. The references in most chapters are now arranged under subheadings related to the subjects discussed, so that the reader can find original sources more readily. Although the book is primarily intended for students, house staff, practitioners, and internists, we hope that the extensive lists of up-to-date references will be helpful to cardiologists as well.

We again wish to thank our colleagues, Dr Elias Botvinick, Dr Bruce Brundage, Dr Eric Carlsson, Dr Dai Ru-ping, Dr Gordon Gamsu, Dr Mervin Goldman, Dr Robert Grover, Dr Arthur Hollman, Dr Martin Lipton, Dr Thomas Ports, Dr Nelson Schiller, and Dr Norman Silverman for providing angiograms, echocardiograms, electrocardiograms, radioisotope studies, and x-rays from their files.

We wish to thank our publisher, Dr Jack Lange, and editorial consultant Dr Ernest Jawetz for valuable advice and help with preparation of this book. We also wish to thank Lynn Duncan and Lorraine Matthews for their organizational and secretarial assistance.

Translations of *Clinical Cardiology* into Spanish, German, Italian, and Greek have been published, and French, Polish, and Portuguese translations are in preparation.

Maurice Sokolow
Malcolm B. McIlroy

San Francisco
June, 1986

Notice

The authors have been careful to recommend drug dosages that are in agreement with current official pharmacologic standards and the medical literature. Even so, it is recommended that the physician review drug manufacturers' product information (eg, package inserts) before prescribing. One must be thoroughly conversant with any drugs used in order to advise the patient about signs and symptoms of potential adverse reactions and incompatibilities.

Anatomy & Physiology of the Circulatory System

ANATOMY OF THE HEART

The normal heart lies within its pericardial sac in the middle of the thorax slightly to the left of the midline. The low-pressure right atrium and right ventricle occupy the anterior portion of the heart and the higher-pressure left ventricle and atrium lie posteriorly. The long axis of the heart, from the apex of the left ventricle to the root of the aorta, runs upward and backward at an angle of about 30 degrees from the horizontal plane and 45 degrees from the sagittal plane of the body (Fig 1–1). The apex of the heart rests on the upper surface of the diaphragm, which lies close to the posterior and inferior surfaces of the heart. The lie of the heart varies with the build of the patient and with respiration. It assumes a more vertical position during inspiration and in tall, thin persons, and a more horizontal position during expiration and in persons of heavier build.

EXTERNAL APPEARANCE

Anterior Aspect

As viewed from the front (Fig 1–1), the largest area of the surface of the heart is formed by the triangle-shaped right ventricle, with the pulmonary trunk arising from the apex of the triangle. Above and to the right of the right ventricle, one can see the right atrium—or, more specifically, the right atrial appendage—as an ear-shaped structure overlying the root of the aorta. The groove between the right atrium and ventricle (coronary sulcus) is often filled with fat and is occupied by the right coronary artery. Above the right atrium, the superior vena cava is seen entering the right atrium through the pericardium. The inferior vena cava lies on the diaphragmatic surface of the heart and enters the right atrium from the back. The anterior aspect of the heart reveals only a small part of the left ventricle, lying to the left of the right ventricle and forming the apex of the heart. The anterior

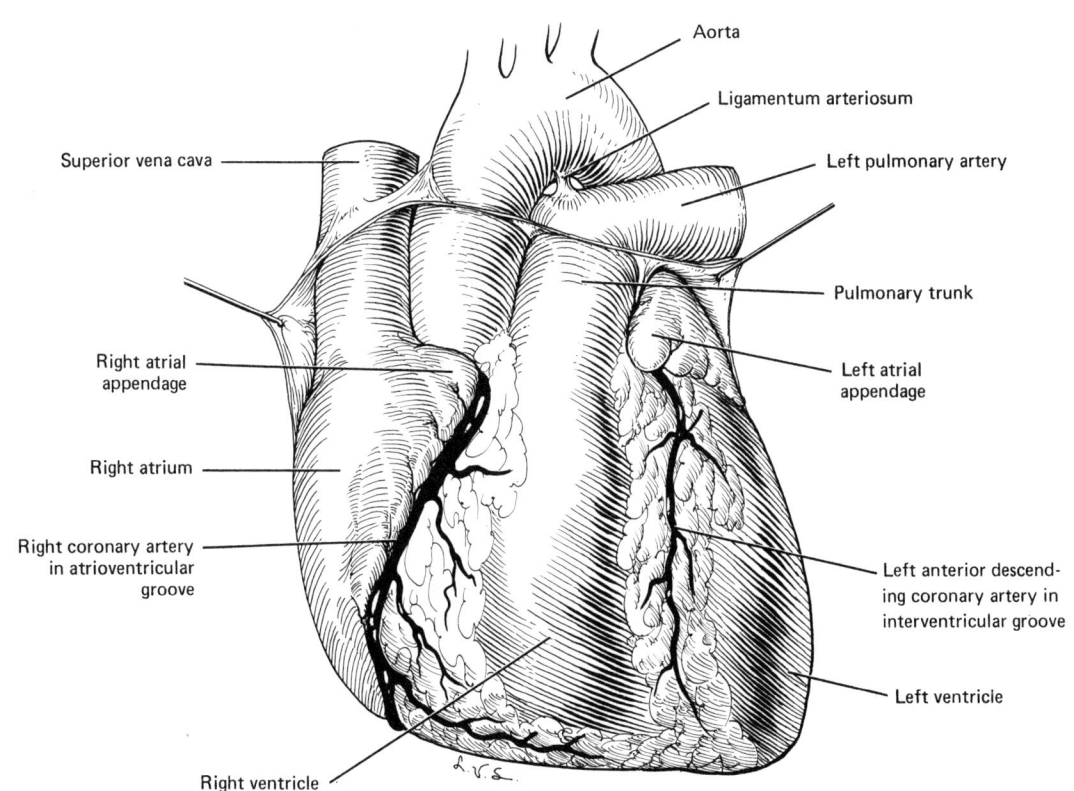

Figure 1–1. Anterior view of the heart.

interventricular sulcus often contains fat and is occupied by the anterior descending branch of the left coronary artery. The only portion of the left atrium visible from the front is the left atrial appendage, which lies above the ventricle and curves around the left side of the origin of the pulmonary trunk. The lungs normally cover most of the anterior surface of the heart, especially during inspiration, leaving only a small area apposed to the back of the sternum and left ribs.

Left-Sided Aspect

As viewed from the left side (Fig 1–2), the left ventricle and left atrium occupy most of the surface of the heart. The posterior interventricular groove separates the left ventricle above from the right ventricle below. The posterior descending branch of the right coronary artery lies in this groove. The atrioventricular groove runs almost vertically in this view, separating the left ventricle from the left atrium. The coronary sinus and the circumflex branch of the left coronary artery lie in this groove and complete the ring of blood vessels forming the base of the corona (crown) after which the blood vessels supplying the heart are named.

Posterior Aspect

The back of the heart mainly rests on the diaphragm and is largely occupied by the left atrium and ventricle plus portions of the right atrium and ventricle, as shown in Fig 1–3. The point at which all 4 chambers meet posteriorly is called the crux of the heart because of the cross-shaped pattern of blood vessels lying at the junction of the posterior interventricular groove and the atrioventricular groove. The vessels forming the cross are the coronary sinus and the posterior descending coronary artery. This latter vessel may be a branch of either the right or the circumflex branch of the left coronary artery depending on whether the right or left coronary artery is the larger (dominant) vessel. The pulmonary veins enter the back of the left atrium. The pattern may vary, but 2 right and 2 left pulmonary veins are normally present.

Right-Sided Aspect

When viewed from the right side, the right atrium and ventricle occupy most of the surface, as shown in Fig 1–4. The superior and inferior venae cavae enter the atrium at the back, and the aorta runs upward from the middle of the heart. The outflow tract of the right ventricle and the pulmonary trunk form the upper border of the heart in this view.

The Great Vessels

The main **pulmonary artery (pulmonary trunk)** runs upward and to the left in front of the aorta and leaves the pericardial sac before dividing into its right and left branches. The left pulmonary artery continues to arch backward in the same line as the main trunk,

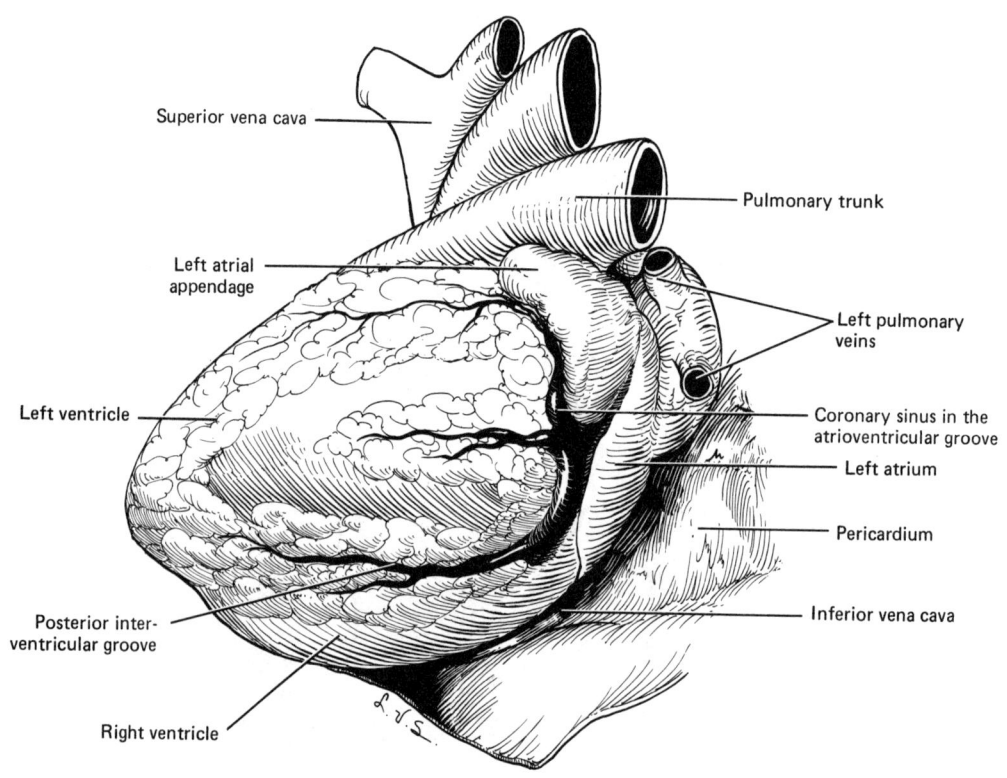

Figure 1–2. The heart viewed from the left side with the apex raised.

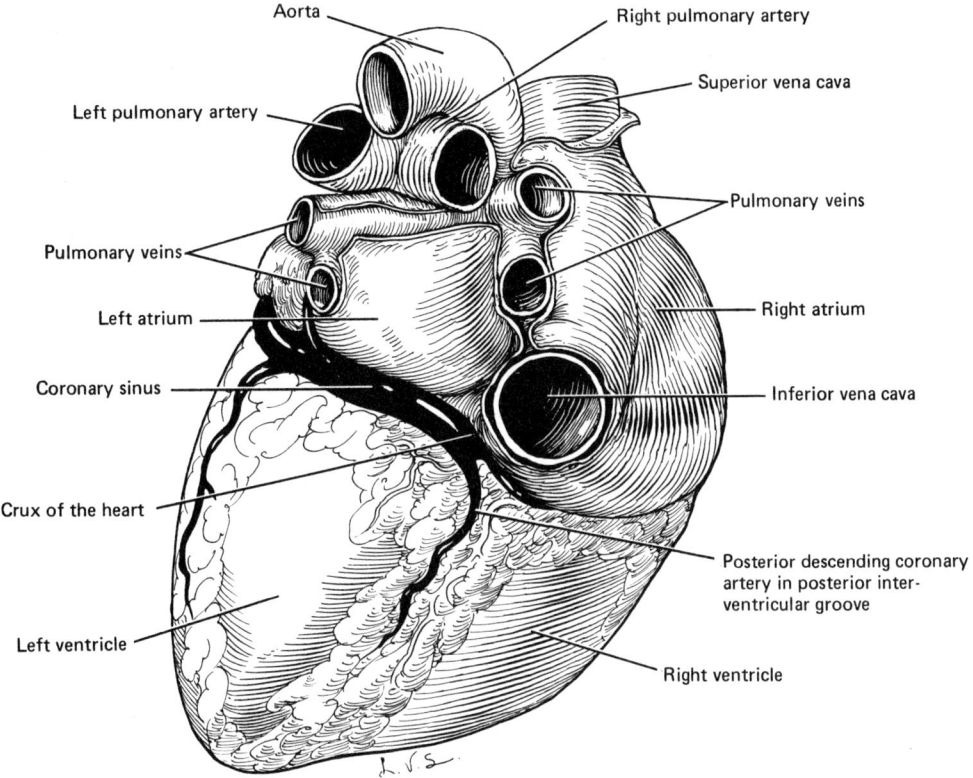

Figure 1-3. The heart viewed from below and behind.

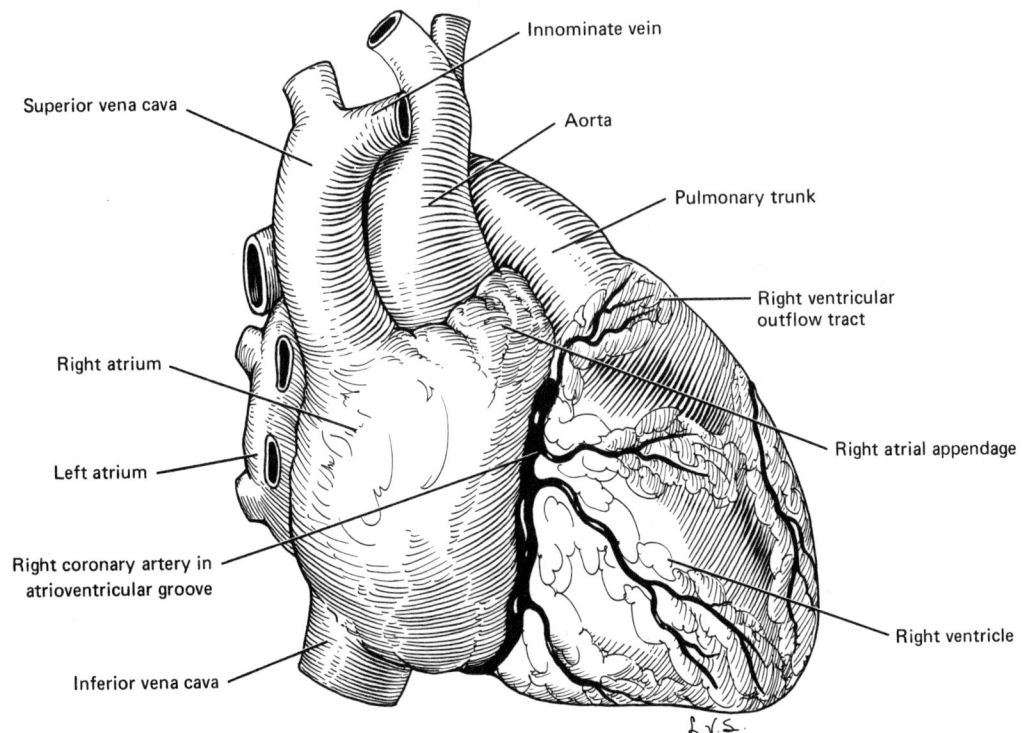

Figure 1-4. The heart viewed from the right side.

while the right branch turns laterally behind the ascending aorta and the superior vena cava to reach the hilum of the right lung. The bifurcation of the pulmonary artery lies on the roof of the left atrium and above the left main bronchus.

The **aorta** arises deep within the heart, and its proximal portion is covered by the right atrial appendage. It runs upward beside the **superior vena cava** before giving off its first and largest (innominate) branch, which shortly divides into the right common carotid and right subclavian branches. The aortic arch passes backward and to the left, giving off its left common carotid and left subclavian branches before crossing the left pulmonary artery. There is a close relationship between the left pulmonary artery and the aorta. The ductus arteriosus, which connected these 2 structures during fetal development, persists as a remnant—the ligamentum arteriosum—in adults. The point at which it joins the aorta is termed the isthmus of the aorta, because there is sometimes a narrowing at this level. The aorta is weakest at this point, and traumatic aortic tears usually occur at this level.

THE CHAMBERS OF THE HEART

The Right Atrium

The right atrium consists of 2 embryologically distinct portions, as shown in Fig 1-5. The more posterior thin-walled portion into which the venae cavae and coronary sinus empty is formed from the sinus venosus and is composed of tissue similar to that of the great veins. The more anterior muscular portion includes the right atrial appendage and the tricuspid valve ring. The fossa ovalis lies in the middle of the thin-walled portion and is the site of the foramen ovale. This interatrial communication, which is present during fetal life, permits the flow of oxygenated placental blood from the inferior vena cava into the left heart. The foramen ovale remains open or potentially open in about 15% of normal subjects, but since it is a flap valve that only allows flow from right to left, it is normally functionally closed.

The Right Ventricle

The right ventricle is triangular in shape and forms a crescentic, shallow structure wrapped over the ventricular septum. It can be divided, as shown in Fig 1-6, into a proximal inflow portion, containing the tricuspid valve and its chordae, and a distal outflow tract, from which the pulmonary trunk arises. The line of demarcation between the 2 portions consists of bands of muscle formed by the crista supraventricularis, the parietal band, the septal band, and the moderator band. The outflow tract of the right ventricle is derived from the embryologically distinct bulbus cordis—in contrast to the inflow portion, which arises from ventricular tissue.

The Left Atrium

The left atrium, like the right, is composed of a veinlike portion, into which the pulmonary veins drain, and a more muscular anterior portion, which includes the left atrial appendage. Its wall is slightly thicker than that of the right atrium, and the thinner area, corresponding to the fossa ovalis, can be seen on its right upper surface (Fig 1-7).

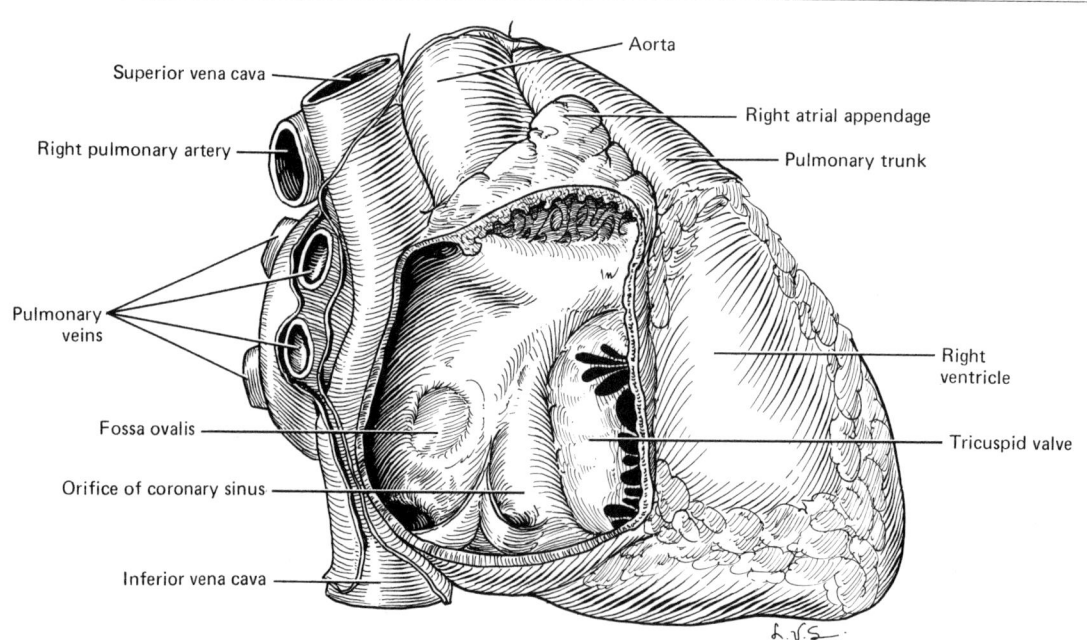

Figure 1-5. View of the right heart with the right wall reflected to show the right atrium.

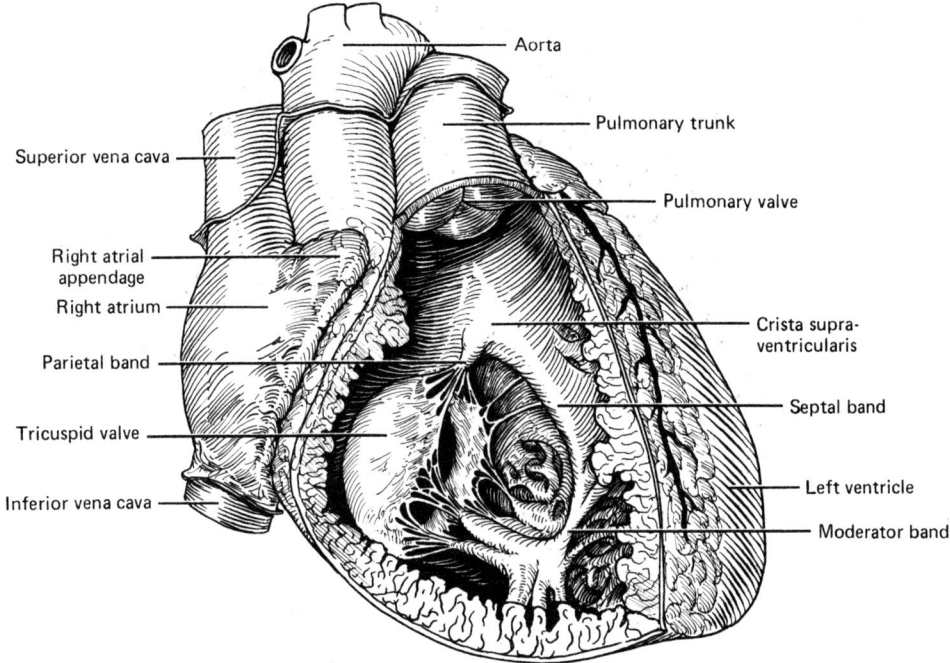

Figure 1-6. Anterior view of the heart with the anterior wall removed to show the right ventricular cavity.

The Left Ventricle

The left ventricular cavity is shaped like an egg. The base of the egg is formed by the mitral valve ring. The wall of the left ventricle is 3–4 times as thick as that of the right ventricle and accounts for about 75% of the mass of the heart. The aortic and mitral valve rings lie close to each other, with the larger anterior mobile cusp of the mitral valve adjacent to the left and posterior cusps of the aortic valve. The posterior immobile cusp of the mitral valve is shorter and, together with the anterior cusp, is tethered to the anterior and posterior papillary muscles in a parachutelike fashion by chordae tendineae, some of which are shared by the 2 cusps as shown in Fig 1–8. The interventricular septum, which forms the anterior aspect of the left ventricle, bulges into the right ventricle, making

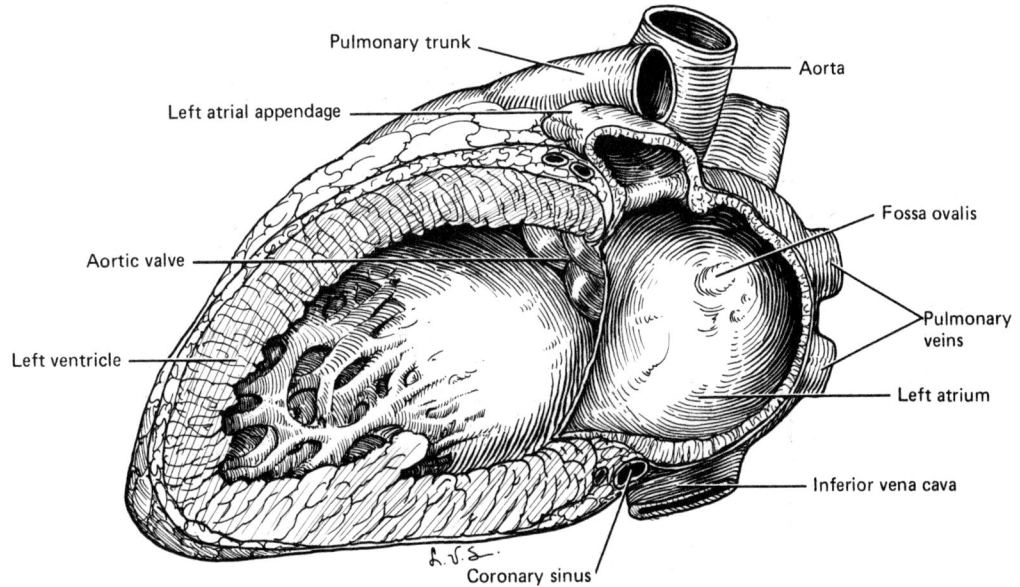

Figure 1-7. View of the left heart from the left side with the left ventricular free wall and mitral valve cut away.

the cross section of the mid portion of the left ventricle circular in shape.

CARDIAC VALVES

The **tricuspid valve** is a thin, filmy tripartite structure with anterior, posterior, and medial cusps. The membranous portion of the interventricular septum lies beside its medial cusp. The **mitral valve,** which is thicker than the tricuspid valve, has 2 cusps and is shaped like a bishop's hat (miter) in which the anterior surface (anterior cusp) is longer and wider than the posterior surface. The **pulmonary valve** is composed of 3 pocketlike cusps. Two of the cusps are situated anteriorly (right and left), and the third is posterior. It is constructed of thinner tissue than the **aortic valve,** which lies farther down in the heart. The aortic valve also has 3 cusps—the anterior (right coronary), the left posterior (left coronary), and the right posterior (noncoronary) cusps—associated with corresponding dilatations of the aorta called the aortic sinuses or sinuses of Valsalva.

CORONARY CIRCULATION

The coronary arteries are more variable in pattern than any other part of the cardiac anatomy. The 2 main coronary arteries—left and right—arise from the right and left aortic sinuses within the pockets of the aortic valve cusps. Either vessel may predominate and supply the posteroinferior portion of the heart. In 30% of persons the **left coronary artery** is the smaller of the 2. The left coronary artery is likely to be dominant in patients with congenital aortic stenosis or bicuspid aortic valve. The left coronary artery runs behind the main pulmonary artery as a short main stem about 1 or 2 cm long before dividing into an **anterior** and a **circumflex branch.** The anterior branch usually has a **descending branch** that follows the interventricular groove. The circumflex branch follows the atrioventricular groove, curving around to the posterior surface of the heart. The area between these 2 vessels, each of which is defined by a course within a groove, is supplied by branches from one artery or the other. Thus, the left coronary artery usually consists of 3 branches, with the mid branch arising from one of the more readily definable arteries. The circumflex branch is larger in persons with a dominant left coronary pattern. In this case, the vessel may run as far as the crux of the heart and even give off the posterior descending branch, which runs in the posterior interventricular groove.

The right coronary artery runs in the atrioventricular groove, downward and to the right, before curving around to the back of the heart to reach the crux, giving off a posterior descending interventricular branch. An anterior right atrial branch usually arises near the origin of the right coronary artery. It usually supplies a branch to the sinoatrial node. The atrioventricular node is also commonly supplied by a branch of the right coronary artery that arises from the posterior descending branch.

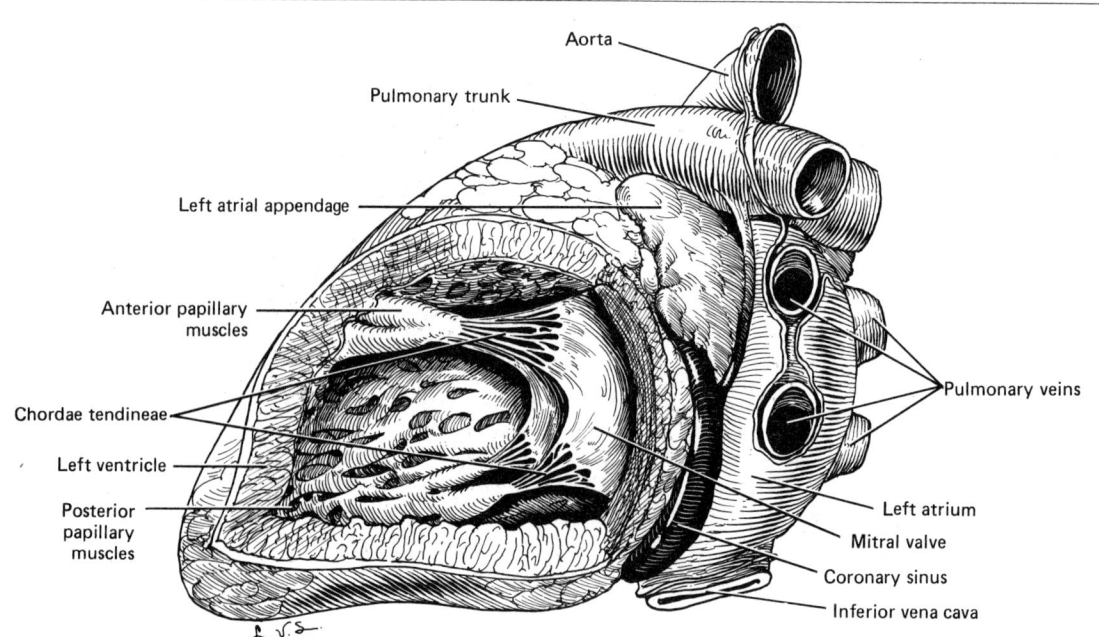

Figure 1-8. View of the left heart with the left ventricular wall turned back to show the mitral valve.

Most of the coronary venous drainage is into the **coronary sinus.** The few veins that drain directly into the cardiac chambers are called thebesian veins. The main venous drainage of the left ventricle is via the great cardiac vein, which runs with the anterior descending branch of the left coronary artery before joining with the posterior cardiac vein to form the coronary sinus.

The anatomy of the coronary vessels is of great importance in the interpretation of coronary arteriograms and in coronary artery surgery. The subject is discussed in more detail in Chapter 8.

CONDUCTION SYSTEM

The **sinoatrial node,** which initiates the normal cardiac impulse, lies at the junction of the superior vena cava and the right atrium. The **atrioventricular node** is located in the right posterior portion of the interatrial septum near the base of the tricuspid valve. The atrioventricular node is continuous with the **bundle of His,** which divides into a left and a right bundle branch at the top of the interventricular septum. The left branch divides again into anterior and posterior branches, and all 3 branches run subendocardially close to the septum before ramifying into the **Purkinje fibers,** which spread to all parts of the ventricular myocardium. The details of abnormal conduction pathways are given in Chapter 14.

LYMPHATICS

The lymphatics of the heart are arranged in 3 plexuses: subendocardial, myocardial, and subepicardial. The drainage is outward to the subepicardial plexus, where the vessels unite to form drainage trunks that follow the coronary arteries. They eventually form a single vessel that leaves the heart on the anterior surface of the pulmonary artery to reach a lymph node between the superior vena cava and the innominate artery. Cardiac transplantation, which inevitably severs the cardiac lymphatics, does not seem to produce any deleterious effect.

CARDIAC NERVES

The heart is innervated both by cholinergic fibers from the vagus nerve and by adrenergic fibers arising from the thoracolumbar sympathetic system and passing through the superior, middle, and inferior cervical ganglia. The efferent cholinergic supply is confined to the atria. Fibers from the right vagus nerve supply the sinoatrial node and serve to control the heart rate and the force of atrial contraction. Fibers from the left vagus nerve supply mainly the atrioventricular node, but there is usually some cross-innervation. The atria also receive sympathetic fibers, but most of the adrenergic nerves pass to the ventricles, where they serve to increase the force of cardiac contraction. The heart also has an autonomic sensory innervation via small, mainly nonmedullated sympathetic fibers. These are thought to respond to nociceptive stimuli and to constitute the pathway through which cardiac pain is mediated.

Vagally innervated receptors are also widely distributed in the atria and ventricles. The atrial receptors discharge into myelinated fibers and send impulses up the vagus nerve that reduce sympathetic output to the kidneys. Their effect is to cause an increase in urinary volume and sodium excretion. The ventricular receptors are served by nonmedullated fibers. The endings are thought to be mechanoreceptors that respond to changes in ventricular pressure and reinforce the effects of the carotid and aortic baroreceptors.

MICROSCOPIC ANATOMY OF THE HEART

The basic heart muscle cell forms part of a syncytium in which the individual cells are joined together in an irregular fashion in bands and spirals without the well-defined tendons and bony attachments characteristic of skeletal muscle. The heart muscle cell differs from the skeletal muscle cell also in that it possesses inherent rhythmicity. This property varies with different types of cardiac muscle; it is most marked in nodal tissue and least notable in peripheral muscle cells. The subcellular arrangement of cardiac muscle cells (Fig 1–9A) is similar to that of skeletal muscle. The cells are about 30×10 μm in size and contain about 20–50 fibrils. Each fibril is about 1 μm in diameter and is composed of a series of sarcomeres, the basic muscle units. The cell contains a nucleus and numerous mitochondria. The limiting membrane is the sarcolemma, from which a sarcoplasmic reticulum invaginates the cell to form a complex tubular (T) system surrounding each fibril. The electrical activity triggering the contraction of each sarcomere passes through this complex membranelike structure.

The Sarcomere

The structural unit of the sarcomere is shown in Fig 1–9B. Its banded appearance results from overlapping of the 2 major muscle proteins—actin and myosin—which accounts for the striated appearance. The wide dark A bands are formed by overlapping of the thicker myosin elements with the thinner, lighter actin filaments. The thinner dark Z lines indicate the end of one sarcomere and the beginning of the next. The lighter I bands represent areas in which only actin filaments are present. The pattern of the sarcomere seen by electron microscopy varies with contraction and relaxation of the sarcomere. With contraction, the I band becomes shorter and the A band more dense. The Z lines come to lie closer together as the muscle contracts. When the muscle fibril is cut in cross section, a specific lattice pattern is seen (Fig 1–9C). In the zone in which the actin and myosin overlap, each thick myosin fiber is surrounded by 6 actin fibers. This

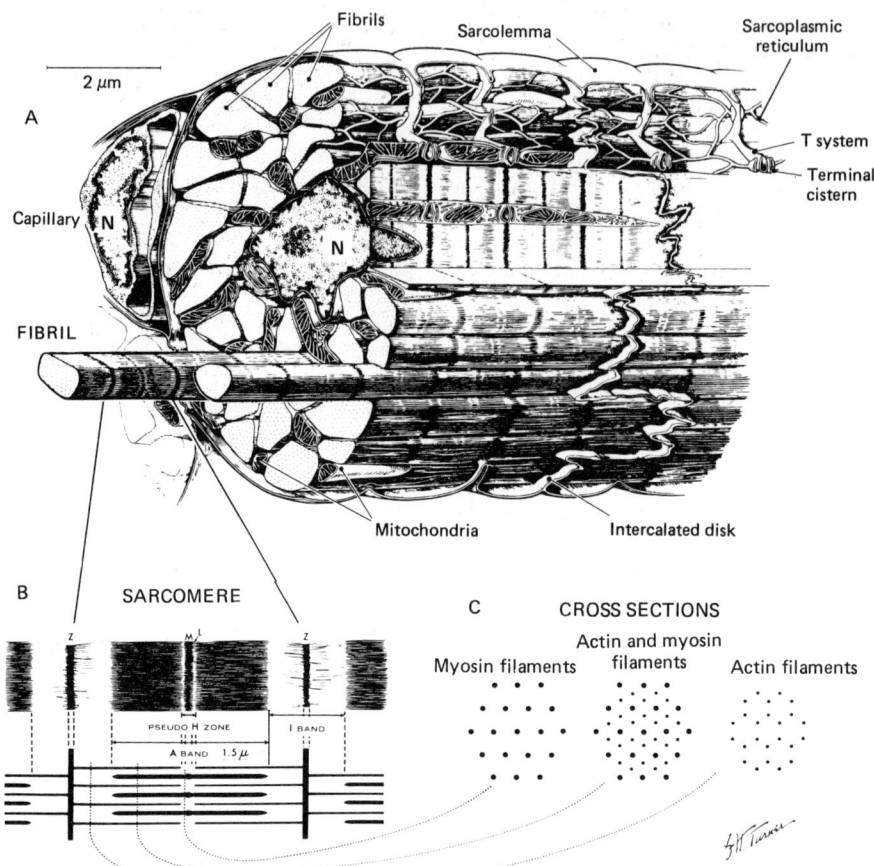

Figure 1–9. Diagram of cardiac muscle as seen under the electron microscope. *A:* A myocardial cell showing the arrangement of the multiple parallel fibrils. N, nucleus. *B:* An individual sarcomere from a myofibril. A representation of the arrangement of myofilaments that make up the sarcomere is shown below. *C:* Cross sections of the sarcomere, showing the specific lattice arrangement of the myofilaments. (Reproduced, with permission, from Braunwald E, Ross J Jr, Sonnenblick EH: Mechanisms of contraction of the normal and failing heart. *N Engl J Med* 1967;**277**:794.)

hexagonal pattern is also seen in the lighter I band region. In the center of the sarcomere, where only myosin is present (M zone), the individual myosin filaments are arranged in a lattice pattern. A similar pattern is seen at the Z lines.

EMBRYOLOGY OF THE HEART

The embryology of the heart is as complex as that of any organ in the body. The heart develops mainly between the second and sixth weeks of gestation; thus, the factors responsible for the development of congenital heart lesions probably operate in most cases before the diagnosis of pregnancy is clinically certain.

Primitive Heart Tube

The heart is formed by the folding of the primitive vascular tube, which appears in the splanchnic mesodermal tissue near the pericardial cavity at about the start of the third week of gestation. At first the primitive heart tube is straight, but differential growth soon forms a cardiac loop, as shown in Fig 1–10. Three more or less distinct portions of the tube can be distinguished, and it is convenient to describe them separately even though their development proceeds in parallel. The 3 portions are (1) the sinus venosus, (2) the cardiac loop, and (3) the aortic and branchial arches.

The Sinus Venosus

The most caudad portion of the primitive heart tube gives rise to the sinus venosus. As shown in Fig 1–11, this is an independent chamber during the early stage of development of the heart. It originally consists of 2 horns, each receiving a duct of Cuvier. The umbilical veins are formed from this structure, which ultimately gives rise to the superior and inferior venae cavae, the pulmonary veins, the coronary sinus, and the posterior portions of the right and left atria.

ANATOMY & PHYSIOLOGY OF THE CIRCULATORY SYSTEM / 9

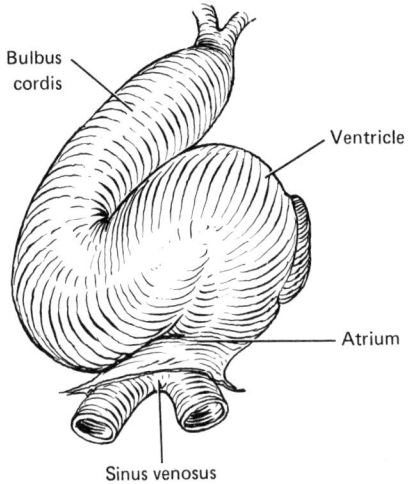

Figure 1–10. Formation of the cardiac loop.

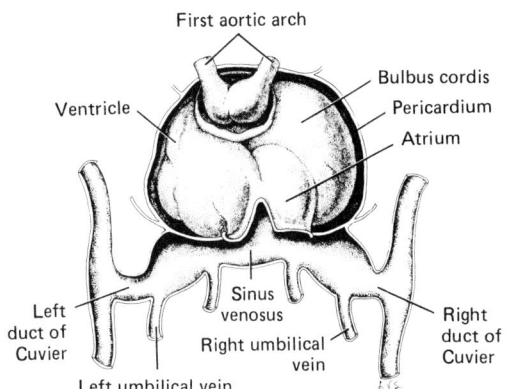

Figure 1–11. The sinus venosus, atrium, and ventricle as seen from the dorsal surface of an embryo at about the fourth week of gestation. (Modified and reproduced, with permission, from Davies J: *Human Developmental Anatomy.* Ronald Press, 1963.)

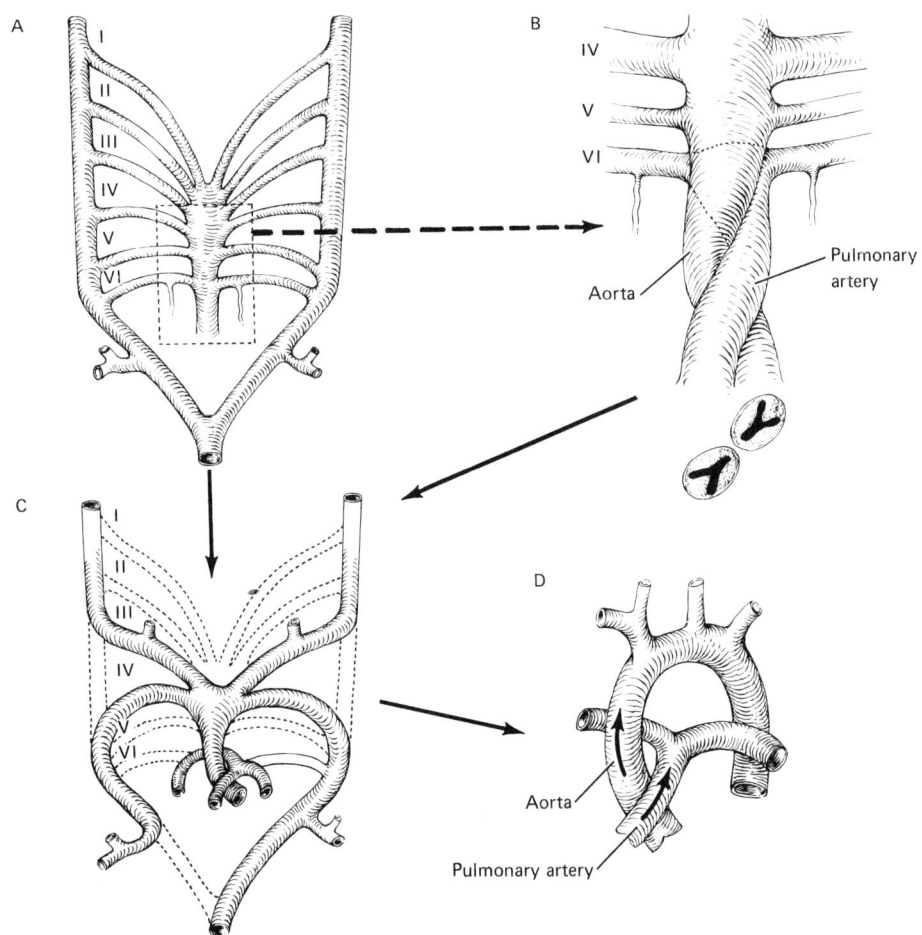

Figure 1–12. *A:* The primitive arches are shown as paired structures. *B:* Rotation and septation of the great vessels. *C:* The third, fourth, and sixth arches persist to form the adult pattern shown in *D.*

The Cardiac Loop

The intermediate portion of the primitive heart tube bends to form the cardiac loop, which twists on itself to form 3 distinct portions: the primitive atrium, the ventricle, and, more distally, the bulbus cordis. In the process of twisting, the primitive heart comes to lie in close apposition to its surrounding pericardial sac, as shown in Fig 1–11. The cardiac chambers are at first single; septation to form separate right- and left-sided atria and ventricles occurs at a later stage.

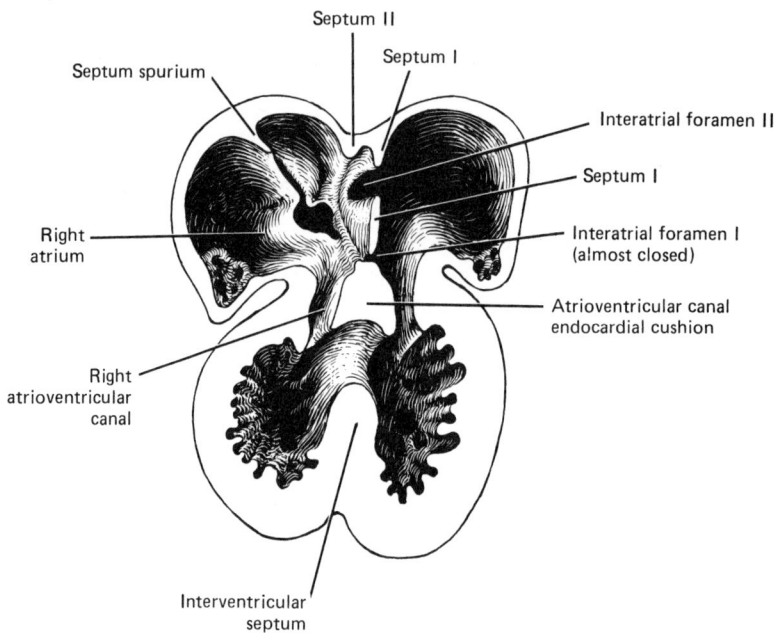

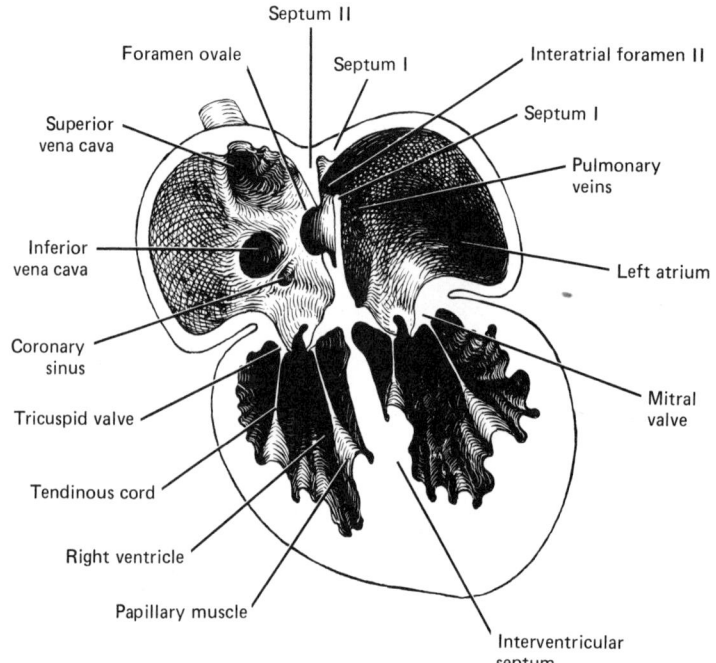

Figure 1–13. Early *(top)* and late *(bottom)* stages of atrial and ventricular septation.

Aortic Arches

The most distal portion of the primitive heart tube forms the aortic sac; distal to this sac, 6 paired aortic arches appear sequentially. Some disappear, but others persist to give rise to the great vessels. The original pattern of arches is shown in Fig 1–12, with the persisting vessels outlined. The third arch persists as the internal carotid artery; the left fourth arch forms the arch of the aorta; and the sixth arch gives rise to the pulmonary arteries and the ductus arteriosus.

Septation

The most complex stage of cardiac embryology is septation of the various parts of the heart. Septation in the atrium is depicted in Fig 1–13. A septum extends downward and forward toward the center of the heart where the endocardial cushions are located and from which the atrioventricular valves subsequently develop. This is the septum primum. A second atrial septum—the septum secundum—grows on the right side of the septum primum. A hole develops in the septum primum in the middle of the atrium, and atrial septation is never complete. The septum secundum does not extend all the way forward and downward to the endocardial cushions, and a persistent interatrial communication between the 2 atrial septa persists as the foramen ovale until birth.

Separation of the primitive ventricle into right and left chambers is accomplished by the development of an interventricular septum, which grows from the anterior wall of the common ventricle. Its free margin is aligned slightly to the right of the midline, toward the region of the endocardial cushions.

The most distal part of the primitive ventricle, the bulbus cordis, dilates to form the truncus arteriosus, which develops between the ventricles and the aortic arches. A spiral septum forms within the bulbus cordis and grows downward toward the center of the heart, where the endocardial cushions are forming the atrioventricular valves and meeting the ventricular septum. The upper (membranous) part of the ventricular septum is formed in this area from endocardial cushion tissue. The spiral bulbar septum separates the truncus arteriosus into right and left portions, forming the root of the aorta and the outflow tract of the right ventricle, respectively, along with their appropriate valves.

Abnormalities of septation account for a large number of congenital heart lesions. In the atrium, defects may occur in the septum primum or septum secundum, and associated abnormalities of the endocardial cushion (atrioventricular canal) area also occur. In the ventricle, the membranous portion of the septum is the site of almost all septal defects; and in the truncus arteriosus, abnormal septation accounts for transposition of the great vessels. The persistence of abnormal aortic arches gives rise to various lesions such as right-sided aortic arch and vascular anomalies of the aortic branches. Persistence of the normal fetal communications (ductus arteriosus and foramen ovale) also gives rise to congenital lesions, while developmental abnormalities of the sinus venosus account for anomalous pulmonary and systemic venous drainage patterns.

PHYSIOLOGIC FUNCTION OF THE CIRCULATION

Normal Metabolic Needs & Their Variations

The cardiovascular system consists of the heart, great vessels, arteries, arterioles, capillaries, and veins, which together function as an integrated circulatory system to supply amounts of blood adequate for the metabolic needs of the body during normal activity, at rest, and during periods of stress. The normal resting metabolic rate, measured as oxygen consumption, is about 250 mL/min. This figure can increase more than 10-fold in normal subjects during strenuous muscular exercise, which is the most stressful physiologic stimulus to which the cardiovascular system can be subjected. Other normal and abnormal stresses—emotional stress, changes in external temperature or gravitational force (posture), sexual activity, pregnancy, changes in body weight, salt deprivation or excess, anemia, and fever—all cause smaller increases in metabolic rate and cardiac output and seldom more than double the resting values. Transport of oxygen (the most conveniently measured overall index of cardiovascular function), elimination of CO_2, transport of nutrients, and control of body temperature are all vital functions of the circulation.

Component Parts of the Circulation

The heart provides all of the power to propel the blood through the body. The force generated in both the right and left ventricles during active depolarization accelerates the blood in a nearly constant manner in both great vessels in early ejection. The pressure in the systemic arterial bed is closely controlled to maintain adequate perfusion of the body so that the needs of different organs are supplied. The arterial bed is an almost lossless transmission system, carrying blood with minimal loss of pressure energy to the arterial bed of each specialized organ system (Fig 1–14). Resistance to the flow of blood is controlled at the level of the arterioles. The velocity of blood flow falls at this point, and the arterioles act as parallel resistance vessels controlling flow to each capillary bed, where gas exchange takes place. The veins act both as return vessels to the heart and as capacitance vessels, whose large volume and marked distensibility play a major part in providing an adequate reservoir of blood for the heart. The reserve capacity of the cardiovascular system is great: the resting output of the heart—about 5 L/min—can increase 5- to 7-fold with exercise. In a person who leads a sedentary life, disease can make significant inroads into cardiac reserve without causing any symptoms.

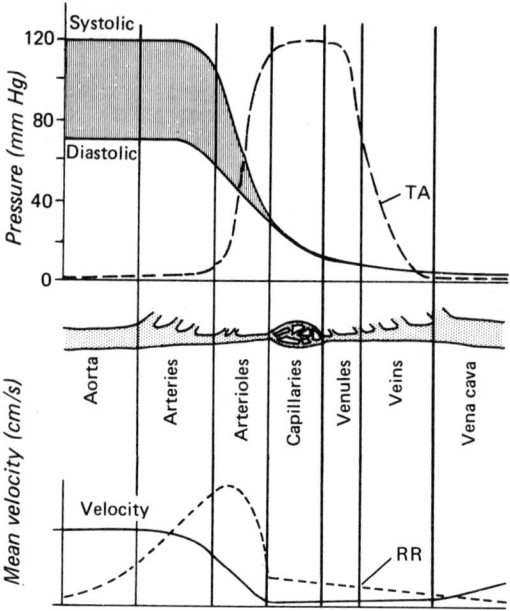

Figure 1–14. Diagram of the changes in pressure and velocity as blood flows through the systemic circulation. TA, total cross-sectional area of the vessels, which increases from 4.5 cm² in the aorta to 4500 cm² in the capillaries. RR, relative resistance, which is highest in the arterioles. (Reproduced, with permission, from Ganong WF: *Review of Medical Physiology,* 12th ed. Lange, 1985.)

Control Mechanisms

The principal force with which the mammalian circulation must contend is that of gravity. Adaptation of the circulation to the varying needs of the body is achieved by the interplay of many complex—often interrelated—regulatory control mechanisms that reinforce one another and have different response times. Neural control mechanisms act rapidly and over a short interval, whereas humoral adjustments come into play more slowly and remain active for longer periods. The control systems support one another so effectively that reasonably satisfactory cardiovascular function can be maintained during exercise even after several important control mechanisms have been rendered inoperative.

PHYSIOLOGY OF THE HEART

The heart consists of a syncytium of striated muscle cells supported by fibrous tissue. The properties of cardiac muscle can be thought of as intermediate between those of skeletal muscle and smooth muscle: Cardiac muscle resembles skeletal muscle in being able to depolarize rapidly to generate the large initial force of cardiac contraction, and it resembles smooth muscle in being able to maintain its contraction for the duration of systole. Specialized muscle cells with a high degree of inherent rhythmicity are present in conduction tissue in the areas concerned with the generation and propagation of excitatory electrical activity.

Although physiologists view the circulatory system as a unit and think of the heart as a relatively simple pump that acts as the power source to maintain the circulation, to the physician, the primary determinant of circulatory function is the heart itself. Since this book deals with diseases of the heart rather than with vascular disorders and their consequences in the tissues, it emphasizes cardiac function and the control systems that regulate cardiac function. The physiology of the heart involves molecular, electrical, mechanical, and functional hemodynamic factors.

1. THE MOLECULAR BASIS OF CARDIAC CONTRACTION

Mechanism of Contraction

The molecular basis of contraction of cardiac muscle is similar to that of other types of muscle throughout the animal kingdom. The muscle cell is composed of a number of muscle fibers that are in turn made up of muscle fibrils. The basic unit of the muscle fibril is the sarcomere, which is described on p 7. The sarcomere consists of 2 main protein components—thick myosin filaments and thin actin filaments—that interdigitate with one another in parallel arrangement. A reaction between these 2 proteins at cross-bridges generates mechanical force by mechanisms similar to those in skeletal muscle. The head of the myosin molecule is composed of heavy meromyosin, which can be split into 2 parts, whereas the tail consists of light meromyosin. Two separate proteins—tropomyosin and troponin—can be distinguished in association with the actin filament.

The sliding filament hypothesis, which is shown diagrammatically in Fig 1–15, is accepted as the most likely explanation of the phenomena associated with muscular contraction. The steps shown depict the influx of calcium as the action potential spreads via the transverse tubules. The actin filaments slide on the myosin filaments, and the Z lines move closer together. Calcium is then pumped back into the sarcoplasmic reticulum, and the muscle relaxes.

The interaction between the myosin head and the actin filament is depicted in Fig 1–16. In the relaxed state (Fig 1–16A), the myosin head is not attached to actin. When the muscle is activated by calcium ions interacting with troponin, ATP is split, and the myosin head is thought to attach to a site on the actin (Fig 1–16B). The "power stroke" (Fig 1–16C) is thought to be associated with generation of force, and the rate of switching between the 2 positions (B and C) is thought to determine the force of contraction. With shortening, the cross-bridges move to the next attachment site. During isometric contraction, they continue to interact with the same site.

ANATOMY & PHYSIOLOGY OF THE CIRCULATORY SYSTEM / 13

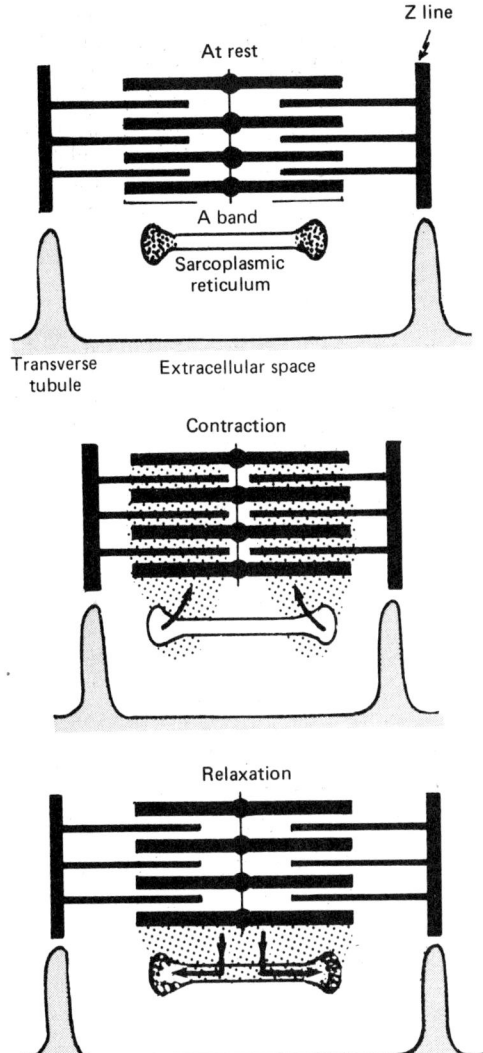

Figure 1–15. Muscle contraction. Calcium ions (represented by black dots) are normally stored in the cisterns of the sarcoplasmic reticulum. The action potential spreads via the transverse tubules and releases Ca^{2+}. The actin filaments (thin lines) slide on the myosin filaments, and the Z lines move closer together. Ca^{2+} is then pumped into the sarcoplasmic reticulum and the muscle relaxes. (Modified and reproduced, with permission, from Layzer RB, Rowland LP: Cramps. *N Engl J Med* 1971;285:31.)

2. ELECTRICAL ACTIVITY OF THE HEART

The Action Potential

The action potential is the electrical charge developed in a cell during activity. Cardiac muscle cells have the capability of generating and propagating electrical activity. At rest, the inside of the cardiac cell has a negative charge compared to the outside, so that the resting membrane potential is about -80 mV. Excitation produces a propagated charge that initiates contraction and causes the sequence of events shown as phases 0–4 in Fig 1–17. Depolarization (phase 0) is initially rapid, lasting a few milliseconds. After an overshoot, there is a short period of repolarization (phase 1), followed by a plateau (phase 2) (corresponding to the ST segment on the ECG). Phase 3 of repolarization (corresponding to the T wave on the ECG) ends with the membrane potential returning to its resting value (phase 4). As in other excitable tissues, changes in K^+ concentration affect the length of the resting potential, while changes in Na^+ affect the intensity of the action potential. The initial rapid depolarization is due to a rapid increase in Na^+ permeability, while the plateau phase is associated with a slower increase in Ca^{2+} permeability of the muscle cell membrane (Fig 1–18). Phase 3 is associated with a slow rise in K^+ permeability. Repolarization time decreases as the heart rate increases, but the rapid depolarization phase remains relatively constant in length.

The Conduction System

Cells with increased rhythmicity that make up the specialized conduction tissue show an unstable membrane potential, with a gradual, slow depolarization toward the end of the cycle (phase 4). The rate of depolarization in phase 4 is more rapid in the sinoatrial node than in any other part of the conduction system (Fig 1–19). Thus, the threshold for firing is first reached at this site, and the electrical impulse that triggers the next impulse normally starts here.

Propagation of the Electrical Impulse

The cardiac cycle can be considered to start with sinoatrial firing, ie, the formation of an impulse in the sinoatrial node in the upper part of the right atrial muscle near the superior vena caval orifice. Electrical events precede mechanical events, and atrial contraction follows the P wave on the ECG and generates the atrial systolic activity (*a* wave). Activation proceeds in an orderly, repetitive fashion as the impulse spreads by several internodal pathways through both atria. When the impulse reaches the atrioventricular node, near the tricuspid valve, the cells of the bundle of His are activated, and the impulse spreads via the Purkinje fibers to activate the ventricles, generating the Q, R, and S waves on the ECG. The impulse passes via the right and left bundle branches, the latter splitting into anterior and posterior divisions. Thus, there is a trifascicular ventricular conduction pathway through which the activating electrical impulse reaches each individual muscle cell at such a time that the result is an orderly sequence of ventricular contractions.

On the ECG, atrial and ventricular depolarization appear as P waves and QRS waves, respectively, and repolarization as ST–T waves. The shape and size of these waves are virtually unrelated to the force of cardiac contraction, in contrast to the uncoordinated,

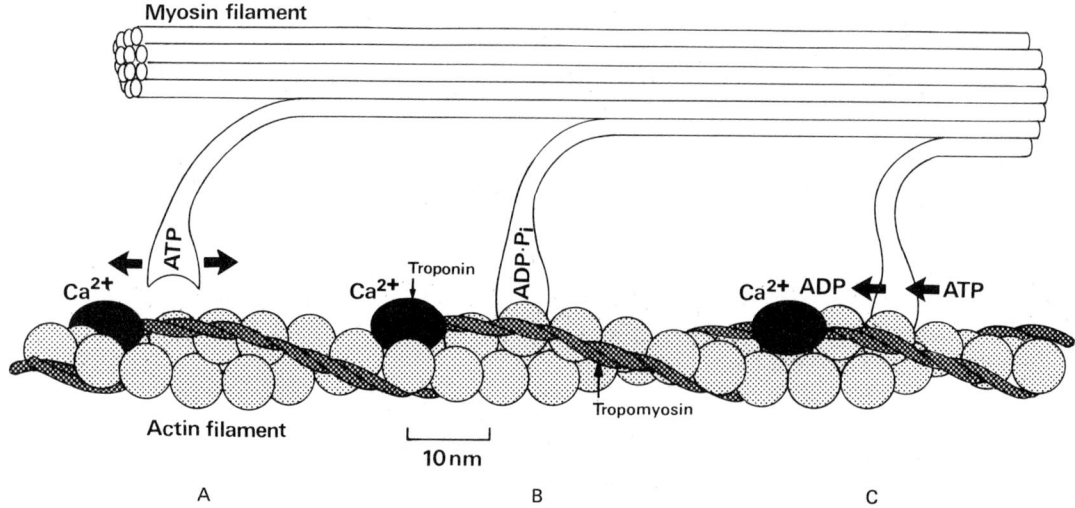

Figure 1–16. Diagram showing mechanism of contraction of striated muscle. For explanation, see text. (Courtesy of R Cooke.)

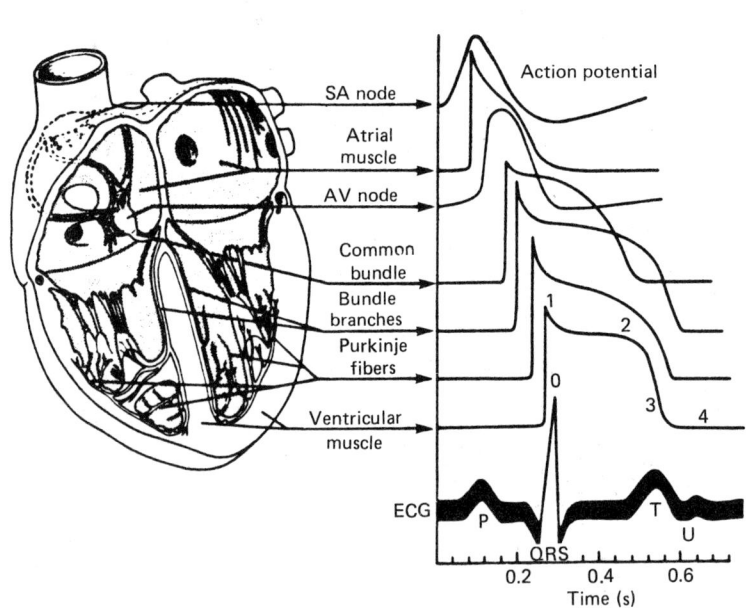

Figure 1–17. Schematic representation of the sequence of excitation in the heart. The relationship to the ECG is shown. (Modified and reproduced, with permission, from Noble MIM: *The Cardiac Cycle*. Blackwell, 1979.)

asynchronous, variable, disorderly electromyographic tracings from contracting skeletal muscle. In skeletal muscle, the number of fibers taking part in a contraction depends on the force required to carry out that task; recruitment of extra fibers causes increased electrical activity when the force of muscular contraction is increased. In contrast, all cardiac muscle cells contract with each heartbeat, and any increase in the force of contraction is achieved by modulating mechanisms that involve each individual muscle cell.

3. MECHANICAL EVENTS OF THE CARDIAC CYCLE

The mechanical events of the cardiac cycle are shown in Fig 1–20. The cardiac cycle can be consid-

ANATOMY & PHYSIOLOGY OF THE CIRCULATORY SYSTEM / 15

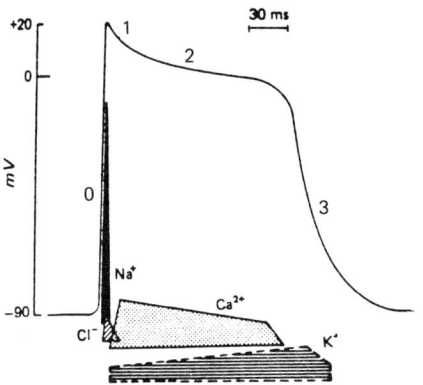

Figure 1–18. Phases of the action potential of a cardiac muscle fiber and the corresponding changes in ionic conductance across the muscle membrane. 0, depolarization; 1, rapid repolarization; 2, plateau phase; 3, late repolarization. (Modified and reproduced, with permission, from Shepherd JT, Vanhoutte PM: *The Human Cardiovascular System: Facts and Concepts.* Raven Press, 1979.)

ered to start with atrial systole (following the P wave on the ECG), which boosts ventricular filling pressure (the *a* wave in the atrial and ventricular pressure pulses).

Ventricular Systole

Contraction of the ventricles is initially isovolumetric (isovolumic), ie, there is increase in tension but no change in volume during contraction. Contraction follows the QRS complex on the ECG. The force of cardiac contraction is determined during development of the action potential (electrical activation) of ventricular muscle. Isovolumetric contraction can be compared to the firing of a charge that expels a bullet from a gun. The velocity of the bullet depends on the force of the explosion, which occurs before the bullet starts to move. In cardiac contraction, the rate of motion of the blood depends on the force of the contraction, which occurs before the blood is ejected. This idea is supported by findings showing that oxygen requirements for a contraction prevented from ejecting blood are the same as requirements for a contraction causing ejection of a normal volume of blood (Monroe, 1961). During isovolumetric contraction, the left ventricle changes shape, becoming more spherical as pressure rises. Ejection results from shortening of the sarcomeres in a mostly radial direction at a rate nearly constant with respect to time. The contraction is isovolumetric, because blood is incompressible, but not truly isometric. Isovolumetric contraction ends when the semilunar valves open.

Left Ventricular Ejection

The following analysis of left ventricular ejection is based on studies of animals by Noble (1968) and of humans by Targett et al (1985), who used pulsed, range-gated Doppler ultrasound to study blood flow velocity in the aorta. This view of hemodynamics differs from conventional descriptions of the cardiac cycle in that ejection is divided into 2 phases: an early active phase and a later more passive phase.

A. Phase 1; Early Active Left Ventricular Ejection: The first phase of ejection is associated with phase 0 of the action potential. It starts when the aortic valve opens and lasts until the velocity of blood flow in the aorta reaches its first peak, after about 50 ms. During this time, pressure in the ventricle exceeds pressure in the aorta (Fig 1–21), and blood in the aorta gains momentum. The rate of increase in blood velocity in early systolic ejection is normally constant (Fig 1–22). A constant rate of increase in velocity entails a constant acceleration. In addition, since the velocity of blood flow depends on the difference in pressure between the left ventricle and the aorta, physical prop-

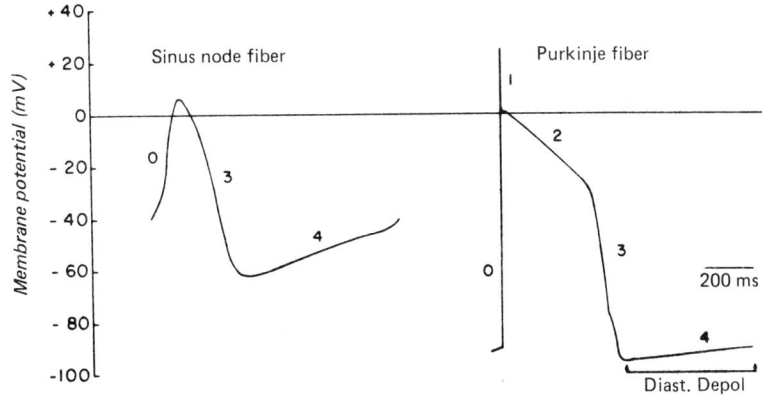

Figure 1–19. Action potential of sinus node and Purkinje fibers. 0, rapid depolarization; 1, rapid repolarization; 2, plateau phase; 3, late repolarization; 4, slow diastolic depolarization. (Modified and reproduced, with permission, from Levy MN, Vassalle M: *Excitation and Neural Control of the Heart.* American Physiological Society, 1982.)

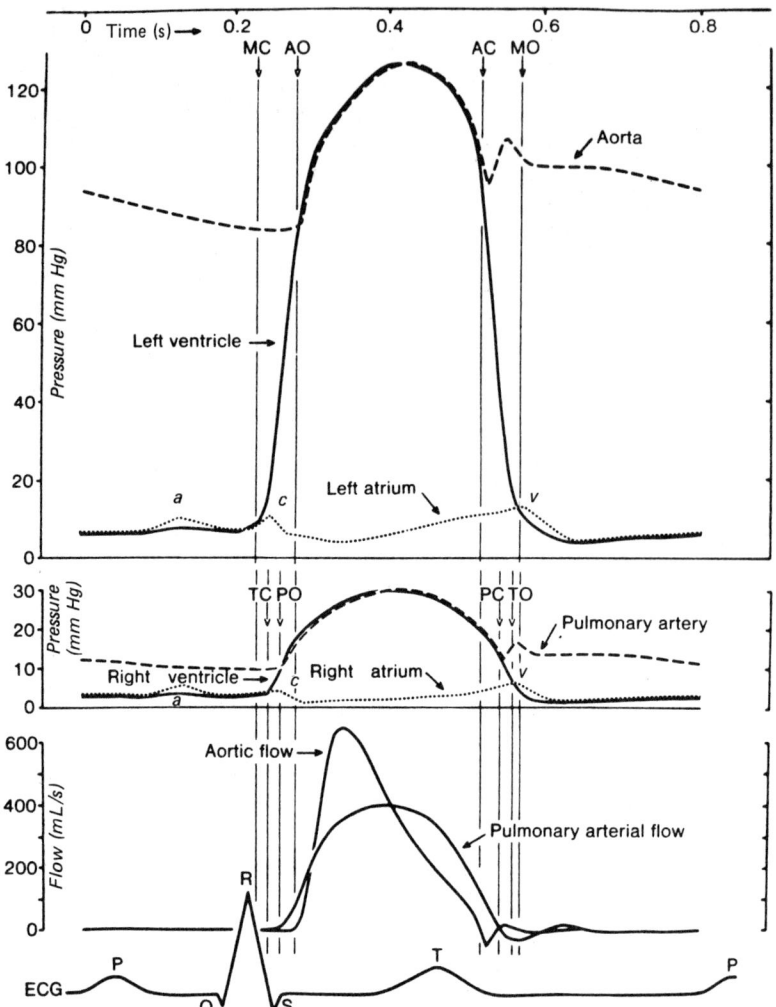

Figure 1–20. Diagram of events in the cardiac cycle. From top downward: pressure (mm Hg) in aorta, left ventricle, left atrium, pulmonary artery, right ventricle, right atrium; blood flow (mL/s) in ascending aorta and pulmonary artery; ECG. Abscissa, time in s. Valvular opening and closing are indicated by AO and AC, respectively, for the aortic valve; MO and MC for the mitral valve; PO and PC for the pulmonary valve; TO and TC for the tricuspid valve. (Modified and reproduced, with permission, from Milnor WR: The circulation. Page 951 in: *Medical Physiology.* 2 vols. Mountcastle VB [editor]. Mosby, 1980.)

---

erties of the aorta must be adjusted to ensure a constant acceleration of blood.

The velocity profile across the aorta in the active phase of ejection is blunt (ie, all blood elements across the aorta move with the same velocity) (Fig 1–23). This pattern of flow results from the convective acceleration of blood passing from the relatively wide-open ventricle into the narrow confines of the aorta. This type of flow is known as "entry flow" and differs from the classic Poiseuille flow, with a parabolic velocity profile, seen in steady flow in rigid pipes.

B. Phase 2; Later, More Passive Left Ventricular Ejection: The second phase of ventricular ejection starts at the point when blood velocity reaches its peak and lasts until the momentum of the blood, which is greatest when velocity is highest, falls to 0. The semilunar valves then close, and blood flow stops and diastole starts. The pressure in the ascending aorta in the second phase of ejection exceeds the left ventricular pressure (Fig 1–21). The ventricular volume decreases in this phase, and the long axis of the ventricle shortens. The ventricle is supporting the aortic pressure at this time, maintaining, rather than actively generating, a force. The blood has enough momentum from the active phase to complete the normal ejection. The ventricular shortening that occurs in this phase represents the mechanical work done during this part of the cardiac cycle, but the oxygen consumption

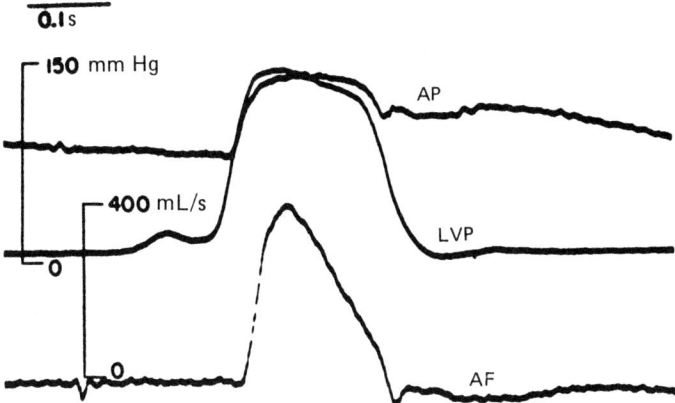

Figure 1–21. Aortic pressure (AP) and left ventricular pressure (LVP) recorded simultaneously, together with aortic flow (AF) via an electromagnetic flowmeter. LVP exceeds AP in the early part of systole. AP exceeds LVP in the latter part of systole. (Modified and reproduced, with permission, from the American Heart Association, Inc., Noble MIM: The contribution of blood momentum to left ventricular ejection in the dog. *Circ Res* 1968;**23**:663.)

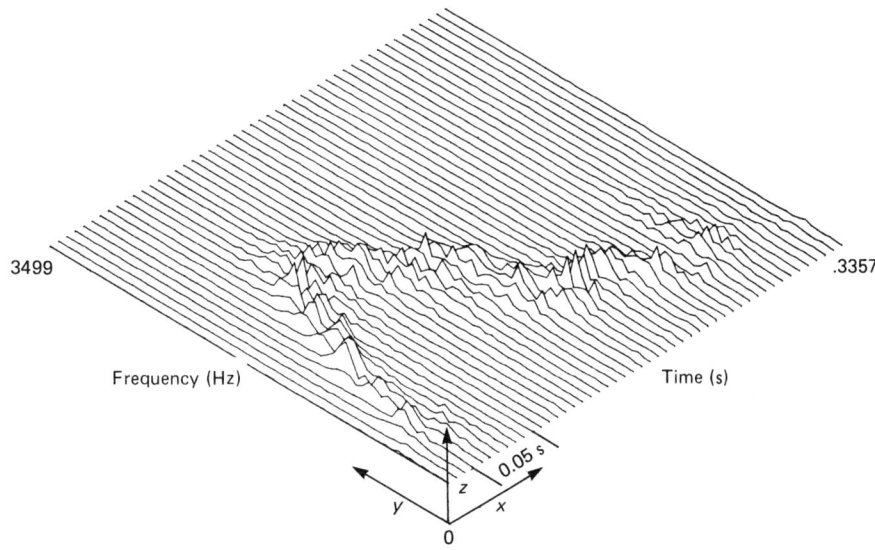

Figure 1–22. Three-dimensional plot of Doppler shift frequency (y axis), time (x axis), and intensity (z axis) during systole in the ascending aorta of a normal subject. The increase in frequency (proportionate to blood velocity) is close to linear in the first 0.05 s of ejection.

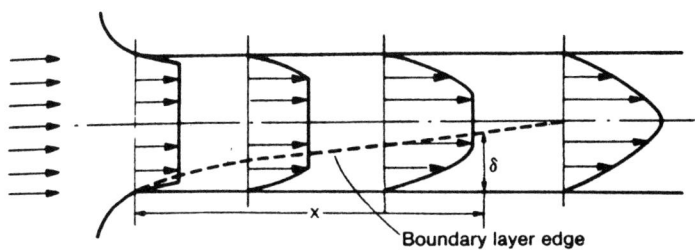

Figure 1–23. Velocity profiles in steady laminar flow at the entrance to a tube, showing the increasing width (δ) of the boundary layer, corresponding to the change from an initially flat profile to a fully developed parabolic profile. (Reproduced, with permission, from Caro CG et al: *The Mechanics of the Circulation.* Oxford Univ Press, 1978.)

involved has been shown to be negligible (Monroe, 1961). The duration of the second phase of ejection varies with the state of the arterial bed. With vasodilatation, systole lasts longer and stroke volume is higher; with vasoconstriction, systole is shorter and stroke volume is lower. Thus, the overall stroke volume consists of a small, relatively constant volume that is actively ejected early in systole and a larger, more variable volume that is passively ejected later in systole.

Ventricular Diastole

When the blood in the aorta loses momentum, the ventricle relaxes and the aortic valve closes. Relaxation does not change ventricular volume until the ventricular pressure falls below the left atrial pressure and filling starts. The rate of isovolumetric relaxation is linked to the rate of isovolumetric contraction. Early diastolic filling should be considered an active process whose rate varies with the rate of isovolumetric relaxation. Filling is most rapid in early diastole and ordinarily ceases before atrial contraction adds the boost that increases the force of the next ventricular contraction.

The diastolic pressure-volume relationship of the ventricle is not linear. The ventricle fills readily at first, with little increase in pressure. In the later phase of filling, pressure increases as the ventricle fills to near capacity. The extent of filling plays an important role in determining the force of the next contraction, because the ventricular muscle responds to increased stretch with an increase in force. The pressure-volume relationship (stiffness) of the left ventricle can be approximated by an exponential curve. The ventricle is stiffer when it is hypertrophied and less stiff when it is dilated.

Right Ventricle

The right ventricle, like the left, generates a constant force and imparts a constant acceleration to the blood ejected in early systole. The duration of the period of constant acceleration in the right ventricle changes with age. In newborn infants, in whom the right and left ventricles are similar in thickness, right ventricular events resemble those in the left ventricle. In adults, in whom the right ventricle is thin-walled and generates about 10-fold lower pressures than the left, the constant acceleration phase lasts longer (100 ms or more). The velocity profile is blunt, and as in the left ventricle, ejection can be separated into an early active phase and a later more passive phase (Fig 1–24).

Timing of Right & Left Ventricular Events

Right atrial systole precedes left atrial systole, and right ventricular contraction starts after left ventricular contraction. However, since pulmonary arterial pressure is lower than aortic pressure, right ventricular ejection starts before left ventricular ejection and lasts longer. Right-sided events are normally influenced by respiration, which alters venous return. During expiration, the aortic and pulmonary valves close at about the same time; but during inspiration, the aortic valve closes before the pulmonary. The later closure of the pulmonary valve is due to prolonged ejection of the increased venous return. When measured over time, the outputs of the 2 ventricles must be equal, but transient differences are seen with respiration.

Myocardial Work & Oxygen Consumption

The work of the heart—the integral of pressure with respect to volume—is not a true measure of the load on the heart. It is the pressure generated during

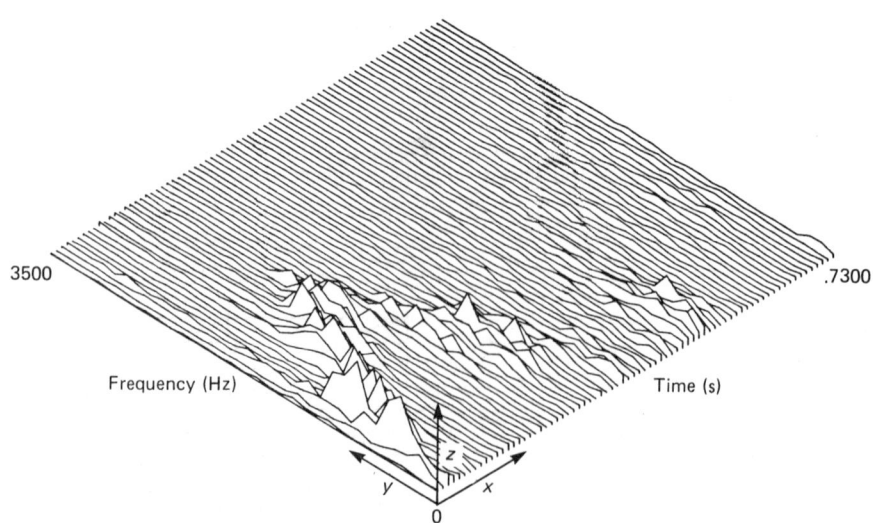

Figure 1–24. Three-dimensional plot of Doppler shift frequency (y axis), time (x axis), and intensity (z axis) in the main pulmonary artery of a normal subject. The increase in frequency (proportionate to blood velocity) is close to linear in the first 0.1 s of ejection.

isovolumetric contraction and early active ejection that is most closely associated with load.

The heart can eject most blood when aortic pressure is normal and cardiac volume is small. High aortic pressure and increased ventricular volume are poorly tolerated. The most important indicator of cardiac load is the metabolic requirement of cardiac activity, which is measured by the oxygen consumption of the myocardium. This is difficult to measure in humans, because it involves knowing both the total myocardial blood flow and the oxygen content difference between the blood in the aorta and that in the coronary venous drainage.

It has been shown in animals that the heart uses more oxygen in performing a given amount of work against increased aortic pressure than in achieving an increase of aortic flow with a normal pressure. This negates the usefulness of measurements of cardiac mechanical work as an indication of cardiac performance. Since work is measured as the product of pressure and stroke volume, any increase in work due to a rise in pressure must be equated with an increase in work due to increased stroke volume. If "pressure work" costs more oxygen than "flow work," stroke work does not accurately reflect the metabolic cost of the increased cardiac activity.

Myocardial oxygen consumption also depends on the mass of the heart muscle. Thus, when the heart hypertrophies in response to an increased mechanical load and the size of the individual muscle cells increases, oxygen consumption increases. Increased coronary blood flow is required; if coronary flow cannot meet the demands of the hypertrophied myocardium, myocardial ischemia may occur.

Myocardial Contractility

Contractility is a poorly defined term often used to denote the force of cardiac contraction as an entity separate from the result of that force (cardiac output)—ie, the force of cardiac contraction independent of filling (preload) or aortic resistance (afterload). The earlier in the cardiac cycle that cardiac contraction is measured, the more likely is the measurement to reflect cardiac, rather than circulatory, forces. Measurement of the maximum rate of change of left ventricular pressure during isovolumetric contraction provides the best indication of contractility. When measurements are made by noninvasive techniques (eg, Doppler ultrasound), the rate of change of aortic velocity (acceleration) in $cm \cdot s^{-2}$ during the early phase of active systolic ejection provides the best index of contractility. Other indices of cardiac function that involve cardiac output (eg, the proportion of ventricular diastolic volume ejected per beat [ejection fraction] or stroke work) reflect afterload and do not provide a true indication of myocardial contractility.

Frank-Starling Law of the Heart

The Frank-Starling law states that *the force of cardiac contraction increases in proportion to the degree of stretching of muscle fibers during diastole*. The law

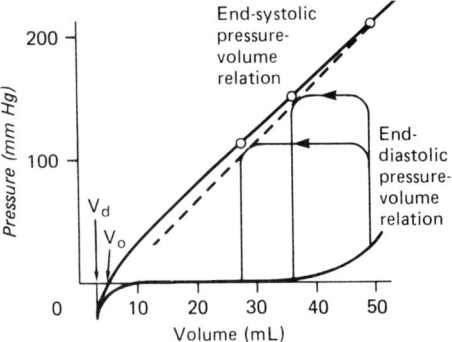

Figure 1–25. Schematic diagram of end-systolic pressure-volume relationship of the left ventricle. The 3 open circles on the solid line represent 3 isovolumetric peak pressures. The broken line represents the end-systolic pressure-volume relation from 2 ejecting beats. (Modified, redrawn, and reproduced, with permission, from the American Heart Association, Inc., Sagawa K: End-systolic pressure-volume relation of the ventricle: Definition, modifications and clinical use. [Editorial.] *Circulation* 1981;**63**:1223.)

thus states a fundamental property of cardiac muscle that can be understood by reference to the sliding filament hypothesis described above. The same property is observed in skeletal muscle and reflects the length-tension relationships of muscle. The law is not absolute, since although increased initial stretch (preload) increases the force of contraction, the actual output per beat (stroke volume) of the contraction depends on pressure during aortic valve opening (afterload). If constant aortic pressure is maintained by artificial means, the heart behaves in a predictable manner, with stroke volume increasing with increased diastolic filling. Starling's analysis provides no information about length-tension relationships, being purely concerned with end-diastolic ventricular volume and volume change (stroke volume). Frank's analysis, on the other hand, which relates end-diastolic volume to aortic pressure, provides no information about cardiac output.

Sagawa has shown that when aortic resistance is fixed, the ratio of end-systolic volume to aortic pressure is constant (Fig 1–25). When aortic resistance is high, stroke volume is small and aortic pressure increases. If aortic resistance is lowered, aortic pressure is reduced and stroke volume is larger.

Differences Between Skeletal Muscle & Cardiac Muscle

The action potentials in skeletal and cardiac muscle are different. There is a sharp initial spike of depolarization in both types of muscle, but repolarization is more rapid in skeletal muscle (being complete in 50 ms or less). In contrast, there is sustained depolarization in cardiac muscle, the duration varying with the heart rate, as shown in Fig 1–26. With rapid heart rates, depolarization lasts less than 250 ms, but with slower heart rates, depolarization may last 350 ms or

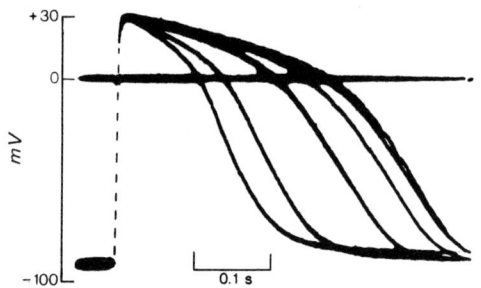

Figure 1–26. Superimposed action potentials from a single fiber in an isolated ventricular trabecula obtained during an operation on a human heart. The record shows shortening of the action potential duration as stimulus frequency is raised in steps from 24/min to 162/min. The initial depolarization (phase 0) is unaffected by changes in rate. (Modified and reproduced, with permission, from the American Heart Association, Inc., Trautwein W et al: Electrophysiologic study of human heart muscle. *Circ Res* 1962;**10**;306.)

more. The time required for initial rapid depolarization (QRS complex on the ECG) is unaffected by heart rate; this indicates that the duration of the initial phase of ventricular contraction is constant and uninfluenced by heart rate. This is in contrast to the QT interval, which shortens as the heart rate increases.

A sustained contraction in skeletal muscle is achieved by repeated firing of different muscle fibers, with relatively short refractory periods. In cardiac muscle, on the other hand, contraction involves the entire heart, and after the initial depolarization phase, tension is maintained for the remainder of systole. Because of these differences, calcium flux lasts much longer in cardiac muscle than in skeletal muscle, causing a longer refractory period.

Calcium channel–blocking drugs, such as verapamil and nifedipine, are therefore more effective in cardiac than in skeletal muscle.

For years, studies of the length-tension relationships of skeletal muscle have been performed with use of supramaximal tetanizing stimuli for production of maximal muscular contraction. More recently, similar studies have been performed with ventricular papillary muscle. Because of its relatively long refractory period, cardiac muscle cannot be tetanized. Thus, although it can be shown that the force of contraction of isolated papillary muscle depends on the degree of stretch, both before (preload) and during the shortening (afterload), the quantitative results, especially the extrapolated values for the maximal speed of contraction during minimal loading, are open to question.

The length-tension relationships of cardiac muscle have been thought to depend on variations in the number of cross-bridges formed between the actin and myosin filaments at any given muscle length. Recent studies indicate that changes in permeability of the sarcoplasmic reticulum and cell membranes to calcium ions play a major part in determining the length-tension relationships in cardiac muscle. It appears that increasing the stretch of the muscle permits release of more calcium and that this, rather than changes in the amount of overlap of actin and myosin filaments, is responsible for the increased force of cardiac contraction (Sugi, 1979).

Length-Tension Relationships & Ventricular Pressure

The length-tension relationships of the individual sarcomeres must be viewed in light of the behavior of the whole heart. Tension must be converted into pressure and length into volume. The relationship between length, tension, and radius for a thin-walled, curved surface as stated by the law of Laplace is shown in Fig 1–27. For a cylinder or a cone, the equation is as follows:

Pressure = 2 × Tension ÷ Radius

If the ventricle increases in size, the wall stress associated with a given pressure increases. These physical principles indicate that there is more mechanical advantage in applying a force to contract a small than a large ventricle. Thus, the larger and more dilated the ventricle, the larger is its radius and the greater the wall stress for a given ventricular pressure.

The second conversion, from a change in length of the individual sarcomere to a change in volume of the whole ventricle, involves assumptions about the shape of the ventricle. It is relatively easy to contrast 2 of the simple shapes that might be envisaged for the left ventricle, a sphere versus a cone. For a sphere in which volume (v) = $4/3\ \pi r^3$, the rate of change of volume (dv/dt) would be $4\pi r^2$ and the acceleration would be $8\pi r$. In contrast, for a cone with radial shortening, volume = $\pi r^2 h$; the rate of change of volume is $\pi r h$; and the acceleration is πh. In a sphere, acceleration should be proportionate to the radius, whereas in a cone, acceleration should be constant—a finding compatible with the pattern of blood flow in the early active phase of ventricular ejection. According to this oversimplified analysis, the left ventricle acts in the

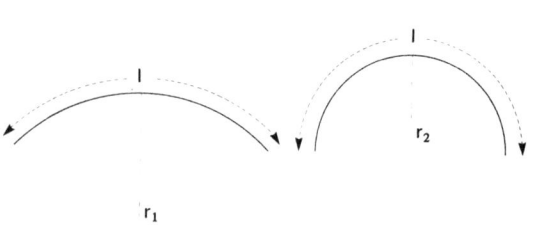

Figure 1–27. Relationship between length and tension underlying the law of Laplace. The tension in the rod of length (*l*) increases as the radius of curvature decreases from r_1 to r_2. For a sphere, pressure is inversely proportionate to the radius for a given tension.

same manner (linear circumferential shortening) as would a conical chamber, so blood is ejected at a constant acceleration during early systole.

Excitation-Contraction Coupling

Changes in the speed of cardiac contraction help modulate the force of cardiac contraction by an electrochemical interaction called excitation-contraction coupling. In contrast to skeletal muscle, in which extra force is provided by recruitment of extra fibers, cardiac muscle relies on a modulating mechanism that involves an increase in the force generated by each individual fiber. It is best thought of as an increase in the rate of cross-bridge attachment and detachment at any given sarcomere length. The 2 cardiac muscle proteins tropomyosin and troponin, which are found in association with the thin actin filament, play a regulatory role in actin-myosin interaction.

The cross-bridges (heads of myosin molecules) are thought to attach and detach from actin sites during their power stroke. The exact nature of the movement of the myosin head associated with sarcomere shortening is not known, but it seems that metabolic activity (ATP splitting) takes place to "cock" the system for its power stroke.

The increased force of cardiac contraction occurring with sympathetic nervous stimulation or use of digitalis therapy is thought to be due to activation of the excitation-contraction coupling mechanism. This mechanism acts via changes in calcium flux in the transverse tubules and sarcoplasmic reticulum in a manner similar to that of the basic Frank-Starling mechanism; the 2 mechanisms are so closely linked that it is difficult to determine the effects of either alone during physiologic experiments.

Digitalis has been shown to have no effect on cardiac output in persons with normal cardiac function, because the normal end-systolic volume is so close to the minimal end-systolic volume described by Sagawa that no increase in stroke volume can occur, although the rate of change of left ventricular pressure increases. In patients with diseased hearts, in whom end-systolic volume is abnormally large, the increased force of cardiac contraction resulting from digitalis therapy can increase stroke volume and improve cardiac output.

Another factor thought by some to increase the force of cardiac contraction is tachycardia. Recent work has shown that oxygen consumption per beat is not increased when the heart rate is increased and that "contractility" is not enhanced.

Thyroid hormone also increases the force of cardiac contraction. The recent work of Morkin suggests that the synthesis of new isoenzymes of myosin with high ATPase activity may be responsible for this effect.

Effect of Control Mechanisms

The circulatory control mechanisms respond to any change in cardiac output by the time approximately 2 heartbeats have occurred and act to modify cardiac performance and change the hemodynamic state. It is thus difficult to determine the cause of changes in cardiac output on a beat-to-beat basis, and clear relationships between cardiac filling and stroke volume, which can be seen in isolated heart preparations in the laboratory, tend to be masked in patients. It is possible, however, to recognize the direction of changes, and if there is an increase in cardiac output with a decrease in filling pressure, this can be considered beneficial, whether it results from the Frank-Starling mechanism, from increased intensity of excitation-contraction coupling, or both.

4. FUNCTIONAL CARDIAC ANATOMY

The basic molecular mechanisms of cardiac muscle contraction must be viewed against the background of the functional anatomy of the heart as it beats within the chest. The change in shape of the heart during each cycle is complex, and using a sphere, cone, or ellipse to approximate the main bulk of the left ventricle is clearly an oversimplification, as is the description of its contraction by a change of one or 2 radii of curvature. Although an adequate description of the complex movements of the contracting left ventricle is not yet possible, a few important points can be made.

Change of Left Ventricular Axis With Contraction

The apex of the left ventricle remains relatively fixed during contraction, as does the ventricular septum. As shown in Fig 1–28, the left and posterior walls of the left ventricle thicken and move anteriorly and to the right during systole. The main axis of the ventricular cavity, which lies in a direct line below the mitral valve during diastolic filling, shifts in an anterior direction during systole, bringing its long axis to a position during ejection in which the ventricular cavity points directly into the ascending aorta.

Descent of the Base of the Heart

The base of the left ventricle, formed by the mitral and aortic valve rings, moves downward toward the apex of the heart during systole, as shown in Fig 1–29. The force of cardiac contraction expelling blood into the aorta produces an equal and opposite recoil that moves the heart in a caudad direction. These changes, which occur with ventricular filling and emptying, are preceded by isovolumetric relaxation and contraction phases, in which changes in ventricular shape occur without any change in volume.

Right Ventricular Shape

The shape of the adult right ventricle is markedly different from that of the left. As shown in Fig 1–30, it has a narrow crescent-shaped cavity that lies on the anterior right-hand surface of the ventricular septum. The thin-walled right ventricle is more compliant and has a lower resting end-diastolic pressure than the left. Right ventricular volume is more likely to change because of changes in intrapericardial and intrathoracic pressure than is left ventricular volume.

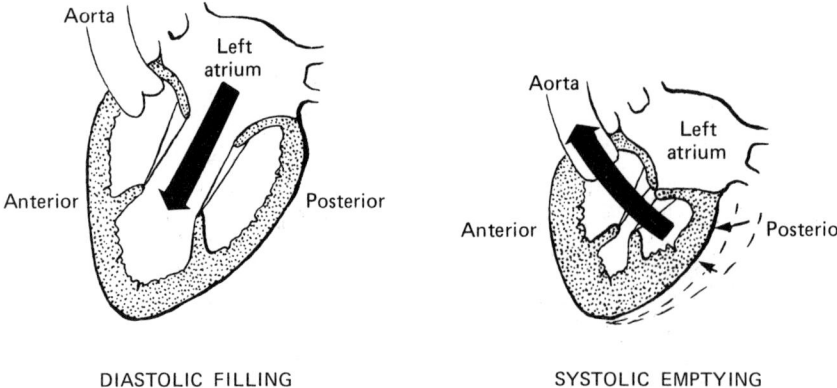

Figure 1-28. Diagram of the heart in the left anterior oblique view showing change in axis of the left ventricle between diastolic filling and systolic emptying.

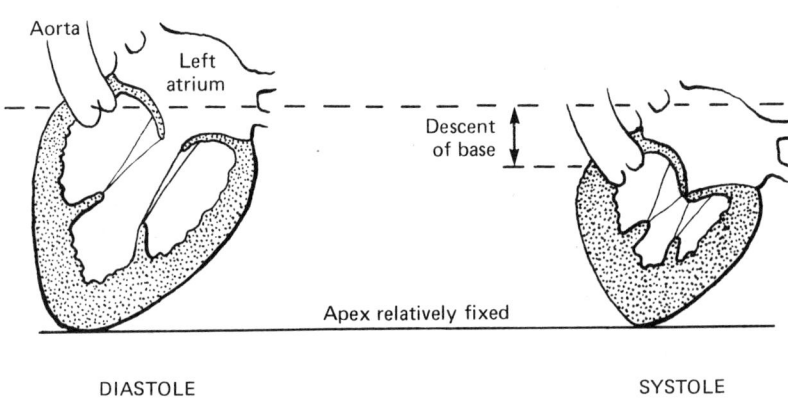

Figure 1-29. Diagram of the heart in the left anterior oblique view showing systolic descent of the base of the heart.

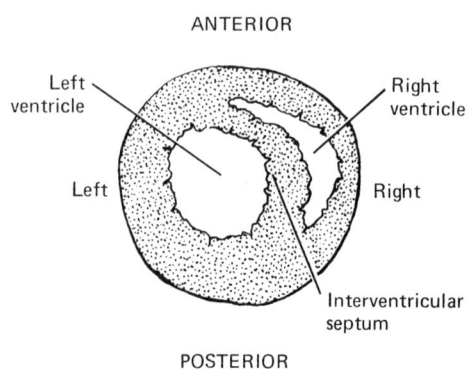

Figure 1-30. Cross section of the heart showing relative positions of the left and right ventricles.

Atrial Anatomy

The atria are composed of even thinner muscle than that of the right ventricle and are thus even more compliant. The atrial musculature is thickest in the atrial appendages, which lie in the most anterior parts of the atria. The more posterior parts of the atria, around the sites of entry of the venae cavae, coronary sinus, and pulmonary veins, contain the least amount of cardiac muscle and resemble veins in structure. Since there are no valves in the great veins on either side of the heart, the venae cavae on the right and the pulmonary veins on the left serve as reservoirs of blood for the ventricles. During ventricular diastole, as the base of the heart moves cephalad, the blood in the atria is transferred to the ventricles by the movement of the heart around it as well as by its own motion.

The atria are smaller than the ventricles. They act not only as reservoirs, filling during ventricular systole, but also as conduits during ventricular diastole, when venous blood flows directly through the atria to fill the ventricles.

Ventricular Enlargement

When either ventricle enlarges, its cavity becomes more spherical. The septum tends to bulge at the expense of the smaller ventricle. Both ventricles eject about the same proportion of their contents with each systole. Approximately two-thirds of the end-diastolic volume of about $100 \text{ mL} \cdot \text{m}^{-2}$ is delivered per beat, but this figure varies with cardiac filling (preload) and aortic resistance (afterload) and is influenced by postural changes in venous return.

Hemodynamics of the Aorta & Arterial Bed

The left ventricle ejects blood into a complex set of branching vessels. The pressure difference between different points in this system determines the pattern of blood flow in the vessels. The resistance encountered by the heart during the cardiac cycle is a complex function of the compliance of the aorta, the inertia of the blood, and the resistance to blood flow. The resistance has generally been viewed as an impedance that varies in a complex manner, both with time during the cardiac cycle and with differing circulatory states. If analysis of the resistance encountered by the left ventricle is confined to the initial, active phase of ejection, the measurement of impedance is greatly simplified. The active phase of ventricular ejection is the most relevant time at which to measure impedance, because it is only then that the heart is actively generating pressure in the arterial bed.

The resistance to active ejection of blood into the aorta generates frictional forces between the blood and the aortic wall that are concentrated in a narrow sleeve of blood close to the wall. It has been shown that this area is occupied by plasma and that red cells are excluded by a process known as "plasma skimming." This serves to reduce the effects of blood viscosity by ensuring that low-viscosity plasma, rather than red cells, interacts with the vessel wall.

Pressure & Flow Wave Transmission

The pulsatile ejection of blood into the aorta generates waves of pressure and blood flow that travel through the arterial bed at speeds greatly in excess of the rate of flow of individual red cells. These waves travel at $5-10 \text{ m} \cdot \text{s}^{-1}$, taking only 100–200 ms to pass from the aorta to the radial artery at the wrist. In contrast, blood flows at an average rate of about $10-20 \text{ cm} \cdot \text{s}^{-1}$ and takes about 5 seconds to travel from the aorta to the hand. The wave speed varies in different blood vessels, being slower in large central arteries and faster in smaller peripheral ones. Wave speed increases with age because the blood vessels become stiffer and transmit the waves more rapidly.

The pressure and flow waves in the aorta and its branches can be simulated by a computer model based on the transient response of a branched electrical transmission line to a linear increase in input voltage lasting about 0.1 s. The impedances and transmission delays in the model depend on the values chosen for inductance and capacitance in the different elements making up the transmission line. The terminal (peripheral) resistance at the arteriolar end of each branch is high, and large reflected waves of pressure and flow travel back up the vessels and cause an increase in pressure and a decrease in flow. The reflected pressure waves maintain a high diastolic pressure in the system.

The initial aortic pressure and flow waves generated by cardiac contraction are not affected by reflected waves during the active phase of ventricular ejection. The pressure and flow waves take a significant time (at least 0.1 s) to travel to the peripheral reflection sites and return to the ascending aorta. Thus, during its "power stroke," the ventricle is uninfluenced by reflections. As a result, the initial waves of pressure and flow travel in a delayed but undistorted form to the periphery. The ventricle is also isolated from the arterial circulation during all but the active phase of its contraction.

In practice, reflected waves returning toward the heart are sometimes reflected a second time at branches in the vessel. They then return to the periphery to cause secondary or even tertiary surges of blood flow of the type seen in Fig 1–31. Reflections from peripheral sites can also cause secondary peaks in aortic flow tracings of the type seen in Fig 1–32.

In disease, especially when there is valvular stenosis, the normal pattern of blood flow (in which turbulence is not seen) is disturbed. Eddies and vortices produced by obstructions to flow result in random motion of the red cells in all directions. The energy losses in turbulent flow are high, and energy dissipation is manifested by sound (murmurs) and increased lateral force causing expansion of the vessel involved (poststenotic dilatation). The pressure required to sustain a given blood flow is larger, and the efficiency of the circulation is impaired. In addition, the red cells are subjected to more trauma and may be damaged.

Ventricular Shape & Pattern of Ventricular Ejection

There is evidence that as a first approximation, ventricular ejection can be thought of as occurring in 2 phases. In the first phase, radial shortening generates the force needed for the initial phase of ejection when aortic pressure builds up rapidly. In the second phase, the long axis of the ventricle shortens, and ejection continues for a length of time influenced by aortic impedance (afterload). Thus, the left ventricle behaves more like a cylinder or a cone than a sphere, and changes in the long axis may be thought of as differing from those in the short (radial) axis.

CORONARY CIRCULATION

Coronary blood flow is an essential determinant of myocardial performance. Flow takes place during both systole and diastole (Fig 1–33) and is precisely adjusted to the needs of myocardial metabolism by the actions of multiple mechanisms. Left coronary artery

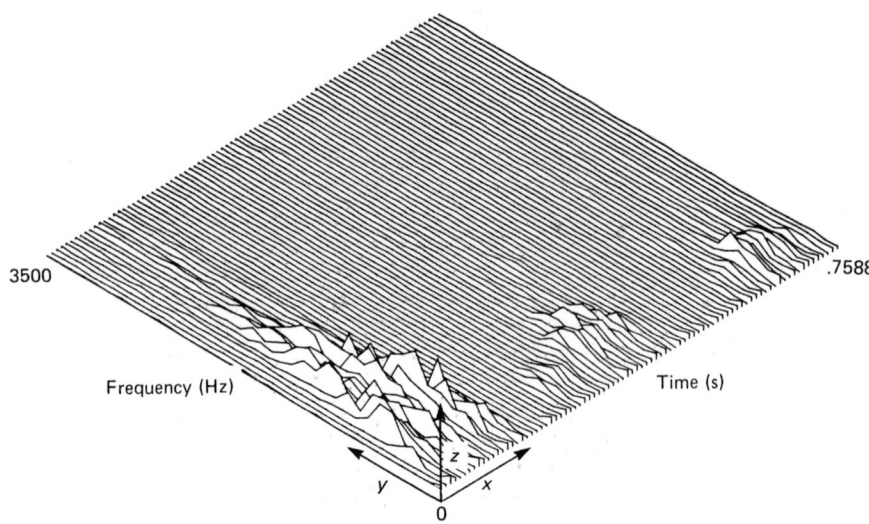

Figure 1–31. Three-dimensional plot of Doppler shift frequency (y axis), time (x axis), and intensity (z axis) during a heartbeat in the radial artery of a normal subject. The increase in frequency (proportionate to blood velocity) at the start of flow is close to linear. The blood flow signal is triphasic.

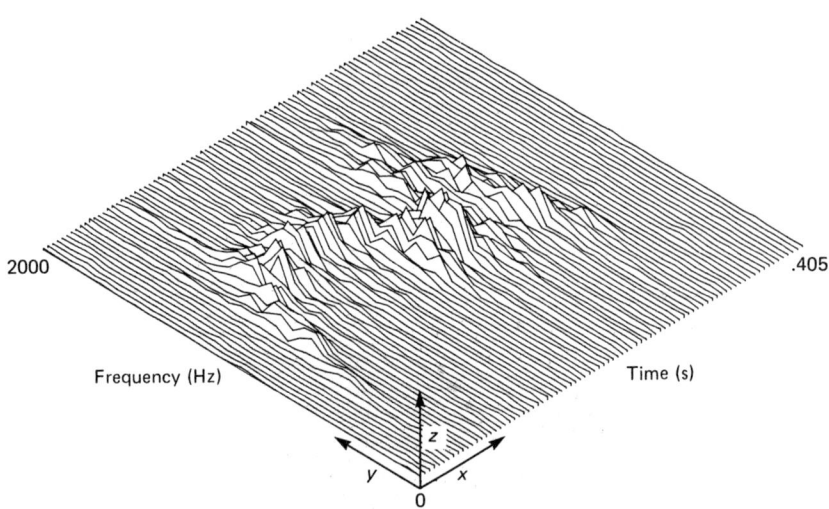

Figure 1–32. Three-dimensional plot of Doppler shift frequency (y axis), time (x axis), and intensity (z axis) during systole in the ascending aorta of a normal subject. Two peaks are seen in the heartbeat. The second peak is attributed to reflection.

flow is mainly diastolic; right coronary flow, which is distributed to the low-pressure right ventricle, is more evenly spread between systole and diastole. The major coronary arteries lie on the surface of the heart, where they are exposed to the relatively low intrapericardial pressure. The branches that penetrate the walls of high-pressure cavities, such as the left ventricle, are exposed to progressively greater systolic pressures as they pass deeper into the wall of the ventricle and come to lie closer to its lumen. It is difficult to see how the innermost subendocardial areas of the left ventricle can be perfused during ventricular systole, and it seems likely that there is a wide range of flows in different parts of the heart at different times during the cardiac cycle.

The tissue pressure in the myocardium is an important factor modifying local blood flow. As shown in Fig 1–34, there is evidence that coronary flow is

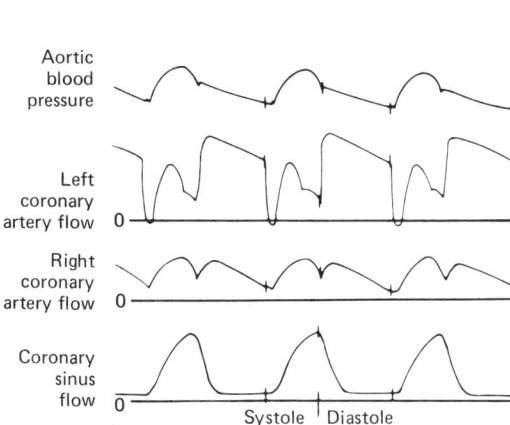

Figure 1–33. Schematic representation of blood flow in the left and right coronary arteries and the coronary sinus of the dog during phases of the cardiac cycle. (After Gregg DE. Reproduced, with permission, from Ruch TC, Patton HD [editors]: *Physiology and Biophysics,* 19th ed. Saunders, 1965.)

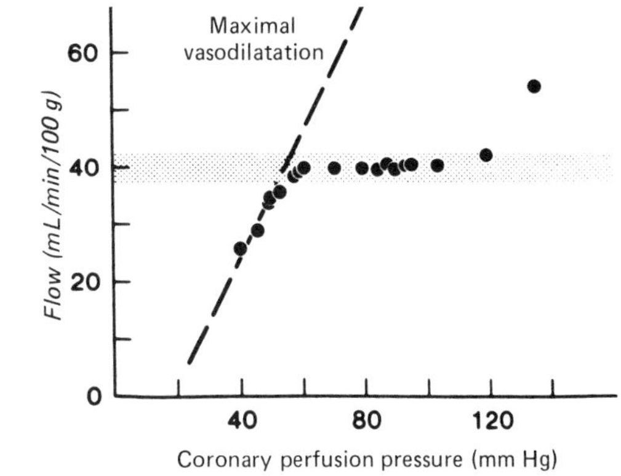

Figure 1–34. Pressure-flow relationships in the coronary circulation during maximal coronary dilatation (broken line) and during normal coronary tone (solid circles). When normal tone is present, coronary flow remains relatively constant over a wide range of perfusion pressures. During maximal coronary dilatation there is a steep relationship between coronary pressure and flow. (Modified and reproduced, with permission, from Marcus ML: *Coronary Circulation in Health and Disease.* McGraw-Hill, 1983.)

not regulated by coronary venous pressure but rather by a higher level of pressure, presumably determined by extravascular tissue forces at the capillary level.

There is thus a gradient of vulnerability between the different layers of the myocardium. The subendocardial regions are more susceptible to ischemia than the superficial ones. Transmural myocardial infarction, manifested by deep Q waves in the ECG, is not usually seen when the coronary circulation is uniformly affected. Thus, in aortic valve disease, severe anemia, rapid arrhythmias, shock, and acute anoxia, evidence of diffuse subendocardial ischemia with widespread ST–T changes is likely to be found.

Effect of Aortic Pressure

Aortic pressure is a major factor in coronary perfusion, and myocardial ischemia may occur in any situation in which blood pressure is acutely lowered, especially in older patients with coronary atherosclerosis.

Autoregulation

Autoregulation is important in maintaining coronary flow, which tends to be kept constant by inherent myocardial mechanisms thought to involve myogenic responses in arteriolar smooth muscle. Autonomic nervous system regulation of coronary blood flow is not thought to be a major factor, but it may induce coronary arterial spasm (also called Prinzmetal's angina; see Chapter 8).

Local Chemical Regulation

Local chemical regulation via vasodilator substances is important, and adenosine, formed by the breakdown of adenosine phosphate compounds, has recently been shown to play an important role. This substance is so rapidly built back into its parent compounds that it persists in the tissues for less than 1 second.

The available evidence indicates that adenosine is by no means the only metabolic product capable of causing coronary vasodilatation. Other vasodilating substances are adenine and guanine nucleotides, hypoxia, increased CO_2, H^+, K^+, lactic acid, and prostaglandins.

Reactive Hyperemia

Reactive hyperemia of the type seen in all metabolizing tissues is readily produced in the heart. Interruptions of coronary blood flow, lasting for as short a time as 1 second, are followed by large increases in flow that more than compensate for the deficiency resulting from the original ischemia. Reactive hyperemia provides a mechanism for maintaining coronary flow in response to local needs and occurs so rapidly that it is difficult to see how neural or humoral factors can be responsible. It seems likely that local myogenic responses mediate this form of control. Thus, any fall in perfusion pressure reduces vascular tone and causes vasodilatation, while a rise in perfusion pressure distends the vessel and evokes a vasoconstrictor response.

Reactive hyperemia closely resembles the increase in coronary blood flow that occurs in response to vasodilator drugs such as amyl nitrite and nitroglycerin. These compounds paralyze smooth muscle in the walls of blood vessels by a direct action that cannot be blocked by any pharmacologic means.

It has been found that radiopaque contrast media injected directly into coronary vessels act as vasodilators and produce significant increases in coronary flow. This action probably depends on interruption of the supply of oxygenated blood to the coronary bed.

Anastomotic Vessels

Coronary vessels drain both directly into the cardiac chambers and also via the coronary sinus. The arteries and arterioles anastomose freely with one another, and small collateral channels appear and grow in number and size when blood vessels are occluded by atherosclerotic changes. There is generally such a well-developed anastomotic network that it is impossible to be certain which major coronary vessel or vessels are involved when a given portion of the myocardium is the site of an infarct. It is also possible for more than one major coronary vessel to be occluded without resulting in an infarct. The rate of development of the lesions seems to be an important variable; if they develop slowly, major lesions may persist for years before symptoms occur.

CONTROL OF THE CIRCULATION

The circulatory system is made up of a systemic circuit (Fig 1–35) composed of multiple (parallel) pathways, each with its own local control mechanisms, plus a pulmonary circulation that is essentially passive in the adult and almost entirely concerned with gas exchange in the lungs. A hierarchy of systemic circuits exists and is based on how long life can be maintained in a given tissue when its circulation is cut off. In descending order of vital importance, these circuits are the cerebral, coronary, renal, visceral, muscular, skin, and reproductive organ circulations.

Dominance of the Cerebral Circulation

The cerebral circulation depends chiefly on the arterial blood pressure, and control of the circulation as a whole can be thought of as aimed primarily at providing the constant arterial pressure needed to maintain cerebral perfusion.

Controlled Variables: Aortic Pressure & Circulating Blood Volume

The 2 main controlled variables in the circulatory system are the central aortic pressure and the circulating blood volume. The servomechanisms that control aortic pressure are reasonably well understood, but the renal salt and water regulation mechanisms by which the blood volume is kept constant are not clear. They involve renin, angiotensin, aldosterone, vasopressin, and osmolality as well as purely physical factors.

Control of Arterial Pressure

A. Baroreceptor Mechanisms: Arterial pressure is kept constant by the baroreceptor servomechanism, which has multiple afferent sensory pathways and several efferent motor pathways. Arterial pressure is sensed via stretch receptors in the carotid sinuses near the bifurcations of the common carotid arteries in the neck (Fig 1–36) and by another set of stretch receptors in the arch of the aorta. Impulses from these receptors pass up the glossopharyngeal nerves to the medulla and provide a frequency-modulated input proportionate to the stretch of the vessel walls. Efferent impulses pass from the medullary centers via the vagus nerves to the sinoatrial (right vagus) and atrioventricular (left vagus) nodes. These impulses influence heart rate and modify the force of atrial contraction by inhibition of sympathetic activity. Other impulses pass via the sympathetic nerves to modify the level of arteriolar smooth muscle contraction in blood vessels in the limbs and in the visceral circulation via the thoracolumbar sympathetic outflow. The net effect of the system is to keep the mean arterial pressure almost constant. A rise in arterial pressure results in bradycardia, reduced force of atrial contraction, and release of peripheral arteriolar constriction. The active phase of the mechanism, which increases the frequency of impulses in the afferent nerves, is a rise in arterial pressure, and the response to a fall in pressure involves the inhibition of the reflex.

B. Speed of Response: The baroreceptor reflex represents a classic example of a short-term neural control mechanism. Heart rate changes take place within 1–2 seconds, whereas changes in vasomotor control take 5 or 6 seconds to act. Baroreceptor mechanisms are most readily brought into operation by changes in posture and also play a part in the increase in cardiac output that occurs in response to the start of exercise. They adapt to slow, prolonged changes in arterial pressure, and in systemic hypertension an abnormal level

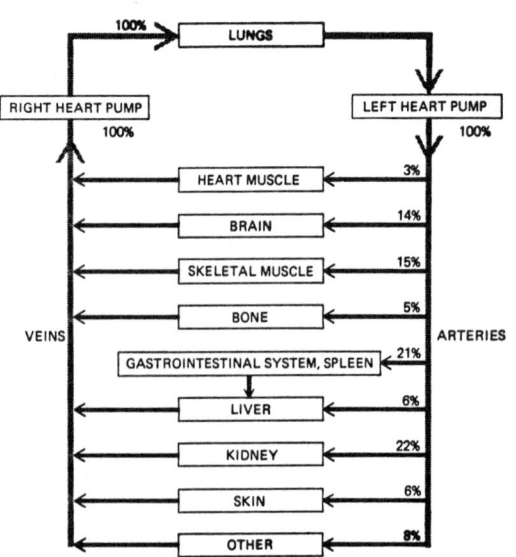

Figure 1–35. Diagram of the circulation showing percentages of cardiac output distributed to different organ systems. (Reproduced, with permission, from Heller LJ, Mohrman DE: *Cardiovascular Physiology.* McGraw-Hill, 1981.)

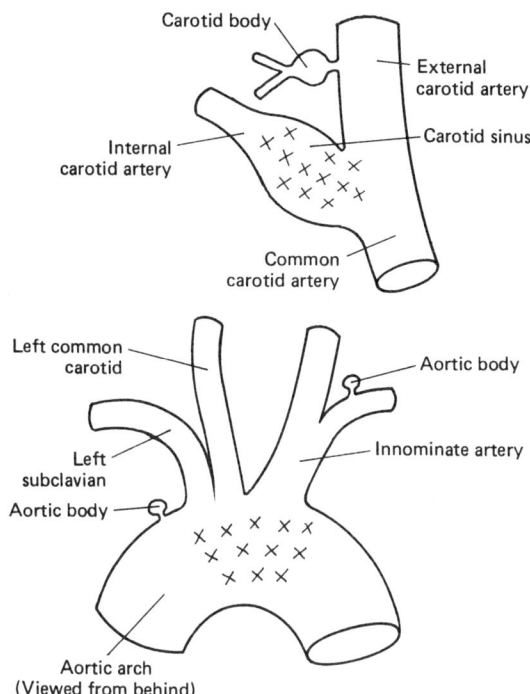

Figure 1-36. Baroreceptor areas in the carotid sinus and aortic arch. (Courtesy of JH Comroe Jr. Reproduced, with permission, from Ganong WF: *Review of Medical Physiology*, 12th ed. Lange, 1985.)

of blood pressure is kept constant on a short-term basis just as effectively as a normal level.

C. Effects of Disease: Normal baroreceptor function is impaired in disease affecting the autonomic nervous system; in conditions in which sensory input to the reflex is reduced, as in prolonged weightlessness; and after the administration of sympatholytic drugs.

D. Baroreceptor Brake–Sympathetic Nervous System Accelerator: The baroreceptor reflex is best thought of as a brake inhibiting the heart through the action of the vagus nerves and protecting the cerebral circulation from excessive increases in perfusion pressure. Conversely, the sympathetic nervous system is thought of as an accelerator that reciprocally comes into play when the baroreceptor brake is removed. The baroreceptor reflex has no direct action on the force of ventricular contraction, and ventricular function plays no direct part in the normal operation of the reflex. If arterial pressure falls because of impaired cardiac function, the reflex will come into play to increase heart rate and constrict the arterial bed even at the expense of further decreasing cardiac function. This type of response is seen after myocardial infarction.

E. Effects of Sympathetic Nervous System on Cardiac Contraction: The force of cardiac contraction is influenced by the sympathetic nerves to the heart. Short-term stimulation of cardiac action occurs reflexly in response to arousal, alarm, excitement, anticipation of exercise, and pain. Any sudden stimulus—usually auditory, visual, or tactile—can cause a sudden increase in cardiac output within a second or less. The subsequent changes in cardiac output depend on whether a true or a false alarm has sounded and are influenced by baroreceptor responses. The circulatory response to isometric exercise is similar to that of arousal. Active muscular contraction causes an increase in heart rate and a disproportionate increase in arterial pressure. Thus, straining, as in lifting heavy objects, causes an increase in blood pressure; and since the response is not directly related to the stimulus, even simple clenching of a fist can cause significant hypertension. The heart also responds to traumatic events such as interference with its blood supply, sudden and intolerable increases in arterial pressure, or obstruction to its output. Such stimuli are thought to affect nonmedullated afferent fibers from endings in the coronary vessels and to result in reflex bradycardia and hypotension mediated through the vagus nerves.

F. Bezold Reflex: The Bezold reflex, discovered in the middle of the last century, involves vagally mediated bradycardia and hypotension after intracoronary administration of veratrum alkaloids. This "chemoreflex" has also been elicited following injection of more physiologically relevant compounds—namely, bradykinin and prostaglandin F_2. The receptors responsible for the Bezold reflex are thought to be stimulated during myocardial ischemia, producing bradycardia and hypotension in the early stages of inferior myocardial infarction. Similar hemodynamic changes often follow injection of contrast material into the right coronary artery. This reflex response is clearly vagally mediated, and atropine blocks the effect.

Control of Blood Volume

One of the most remarkable features of the mammalian circulation (Table 1-1) is the small size of the

Table 1-1. Characteristics of various types of blood vessels in humans.*

	Lumen Diameter	Wall Thickness	All Vessels of Each Type	
			Approximate Total Cross-sectional Area (cm^2)	Percentage of Blood Volume Contained†
Aorta	2.5 cm	2 mm	4.5	2
Artery	0.4 cm	1 mm	20	8
Arteriole	30 μm	20 μm	400	1
Capillary	6 μm	1 μm	4500	5
Venule	20 μm	2 μm	4000	
Vein	0.5 cm	0.5 mm	40	54
Vena cava	3 cm	1.5 mm	18	

*Data from Gregg, in: *The Physiological Basis of Medical Practice*, 8th ed. Best CH, Taylor NB (editors). Williams & Wilkins, 1966.

†In systemic vessels. There is an additional 12% in the heart and 18% in the pulmonary circulation.

circulating blood volume (5 L) and the large proportion contained in the veins. Since the maximum cardiac output during exercise is normally 25 L/min or more, a volume of blood equal to the total contents of the circulation must pass through the aortic valve on an average of once every 12 seconds. Any change in blood volume is likely to have a marked effect on venous return and hence on cardiac output.

A. Difficulty of Measurement: The measurement of blood volume, as either red cell or plasma volume, does not provide a clinically useful indication of the effective blood volume from a cardiovascular functional point of view. This is probably because mixing of the indicators used to measure blood volume with the contents of the circulation tends to be poor in the conditions in which disturbances of blood volume are important, ie, shock and heart failure.

B. Indirect Indications of Effective Blood Volume: Indirect evidence of the degree of filling of the circulation can be obtained by determining the effects of postural changes. When blood volume is large and the capacitance vessels are full, standing up has little or no effect on the heart. The venous return does not decrease, because there is no room for pooling of blood in the lower body and the level of blood in the venous reservoirs does not decrease sufficiently to lower the cardiac output. An adequate systemic arterial pressure can thus be maintained, and no baroreceptor adjustments are necessary. When the effective blood volume is reduced and the capacitance vessels are relatively empty, standing up leads to pooling of blood in the legs. This reduces venous return, which in turn reduces cardiac output, and the arterial pressure falls acutely. Fig 1–37 shows a tracing of arterial pressure in a normal subject in whom venous return is decreased by applying negative pressure to the lower part of the body. Systolic blood pressure falls while diastolic pressure is maintained, and heart rate increases via the baroreceptor system. When the negative pressure is discontinued, blood pressure rises and baroreceptor responses come into play within a couple of beats and restore the arterial pressure level by causing bradycardia and peripheral vasodilatation.

C. Effects of Posture: The simplest means of determining the adequacy of the circulating blood volume is to determine the effects of a simple change in posture on the patient's heart rate and blood pressure. The greater the increase in heart rate on standing, the smaller the effective blood volume. These changes have to be interpreted in light of the patient's build and the soundness of the autonomic control mechanisms. Tall persons are more subject to orthostatic changes, and any person in whom autonomic nervous paralysis is present will almost inevitably show a fall in blood pressure on standing.

D. Mechanisms of Control of Blood Volume: The mechanisms by which blood volume is kept constant are not completely understood. They involve the control of salt and water intake and excretion, transfer of fluid from extravascular to intravascular spaces, control of intracellular water, and hematopoiesis. The role of the kidneys is obviously of great importance, and additional contributions are made by the renin-angiotensin system, aldosterone secretion by the adrenal cortex, and atrial pressure receptors. It has recently been shown that there are important reflex mechanisms linking changes in atrial pressure to renal control mechanisms involving salt and water excretion. It had previously been thought that the atrial receptors only influenced urine flow by means of the effects of antidiuretic hormone from the posterior pituitary. The links between renal and adrenal control mechanisms in the regulation of blood volume and blood pressure will be discussed in Chapter 9.

DEVELOPMENT & AGING

The general physiologic principles set forth in the preceding pages are modified by growth and developmental influences from the fetal and neonatal period through adolescence and adult life up to the stage at which degenerative changes occur with aging. The special aspects of physiology of the fetus, infant, and growing child are outside the scope of this book, but aging is of increasing importance in cardiology in view of the increasing longevity of our population. Age appears to increase the differences between "normal"

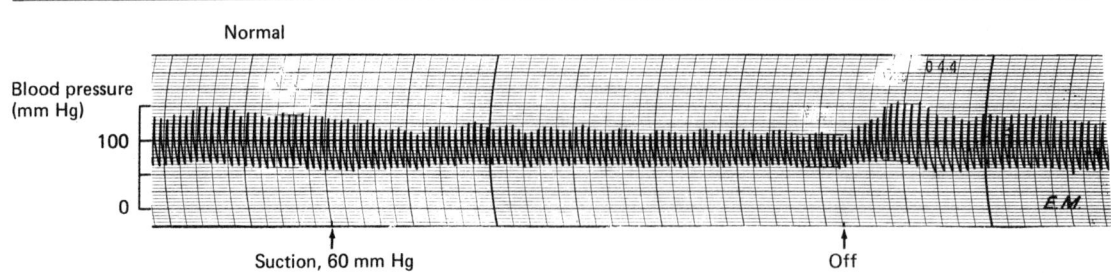

Figure 1–37. Brachial arterial blood pressure tracings in a normal subject. Venous return is reduced by applying suction to the lower half of the body. The baroreceptor reflexes maintain the mean level of arterial pressure, and there is overshoot of pressure when the venous return is restored.

individuals, and the definition of normal and the establishment of ranges of normality become increasingly difficult in older subjects.

Degenerative Changes

Degenerative changes account for most cases of heart disease now seen in the Western world, and the inevitable aging processes seem to occur at widely differing rates in different people. Heart disease due to other causes does not protect patients from degenerative changes, and there is evidence that abnormally stressed tissues degenerate more rapidly than normally stressed ones. Patients with all forms of heart disease are coming to show more and more effects of the aging process as life expectancy increases and treatment to increase longevity becomes more effective.

SPECIAL CIRCULATIONS

Brain

The paramount importance of the cerebral circulation has already been mentioned. The blood supply to the brain, like that to the heart, is provided by an anastomosing system of arteries—the circle of Willis—and obstruction of a main vessel does not necessarily produce cerebral ischemia. As in the heart, it is not possible to be certain which cerebral or extracerebral vessel has been occluded in a patient in whom a particular part of the brain has been infarcted.

The principal factor influencing cerebral blood flow is the arterial CO_2 tension. Hyperventilation, by blowing off CO_2 in the lungs, decreases cerebral blood flow. Conversely, CO_2 administration increases cerebral blood flow. Autonomic reflex control of the cerebral circulation is not well developed, and cerebral perfusion is primarily dependent on the systemic arterial pressure, which is maintained by baroreceptor activity. The cerebral venous system contains no valves, and since the cranial cavity is a closed space with rigid walls, cerebral circulation acts as a siphon to maintain blood flow by physical means. The cerebral circulation is well perfused in relation to its metabolism; thus, the cerebral venous blood is relatively high in oxygen.

Kidney

The renal circulation is under autonomic control, but mechanical and biochemical factors (probably bradykinin and prostaglandins) within the kidney play an important role in distributing flow preferentially to the cortex or medulla. The details of the intrinsic regulation of renal blood flow are not well understood. In normal circumstances, sodium excretion is regulated to maintain a balance between intake and output; however, in conditions of stress, when renal blood flow is compromised, sodium retention occurs. When the cause of inadequate renal perfusion is cardiac failure, the increased water retention that follows sodium retention increases blood volume and contributes to pulmonary and peripheral edema. The renal circulation, being concerned primarily with extraction of metabolites from the blood, has a perfusion rate that is high in relation to its metabolic rate. The renal venous blood is thus high in oxygen, and the kidney extracts relatively little oxygen from its arterial blood supply.

Other Viscera

Visceral blood flow is regulated by reflex hormonal and mechanical factors. The circulatory load imposed by visceral function is small and seldom compromises the general circulation. The viscera, being mainly involved in the transport of nutriments, have (like the kidneys) a low arteriovenous oxygen difference.

Muscle

The circulation to the muscles is potentially the largest in the body, and its regulation to meet the metabolic demands of muscular exercise is complex. The degree of local autonomy is great, and each group of muscles can provide the necessary stimuli to bring about a perfusion adequate to meet its own metabolic needs. The overall cardiac output increases with muscular exercise as a result of sympathetic nervous activity. Any tendency for the blood pressure to fall as a result of the opening of muscle capillaries in response to muscular contraction causes release of the baroreceptor brake on the circulation and increases cardiac output. Increased muscular activity increases venous return to the heart, and this acts via the Frank-Starling mechanism to increase cardiac output. Local effects in the working muscles play an important role in the regulation of blood flow. Vasodilator substances—probably prostaglandins, bradykinin, potassium ions, inorganic phosphate ions, and breakdown products of ATP—are responsible for much of the marked local vasodilation that occurs. The resistance to blood flow in the working muscles falls, and local muscular blood flow increases. It is probable that local neural stimuli from muscle spindles, mediated via nonmedullated fibers, pass to the medulla and help to stimulate increases in cardiac output and ventilation.

The muscular circulation, being concerned with mechanical work, has a high metabolic rate in relation to its blood flow. The blood draining exercising muscles, like that draining the heart, is thus low in oxygen, and the muscles extract more oxygen from their arterial blood supply than do other organs. Muscular contraction raises the tissue tension and interferes with muscular perfusion. The situation is similar to that in the heart in that venous pressure does not regulate muscle blood flow.

Skin

The principal role of the skin circulation is temperature regulation. Since the mechanical efficiency of muscular work is only about 20–25%, large amounts of heat are generated during exercise. The skin acts as a radiator, and the evaporation of water from sweat acts as a means of cooling the blood perfusing the skin. This mechanism also comes into play in response to fever, with marked loss of heat occurring from the skin at times when the fever is subsiding. The converse occurs in response to low external temperatures and in periods when the body temperature is rising in febrile reactions. In this case, shivering and peripheral vasoconstriction act to generate and conserve heat. The demands of the skin circulation can become important in patients with severe heart disease when the cardiac reserves are seriously diminished.

The skin, being concerned primarily with temperature regulation, has the potential for a high perfusion rate in relation to its metabolic rate. The arteriovenous oxygen difference across the skin capillaries is thus small, especially when body temperature is raised and the skin is radiating heat.

Reproductive Organs

The circulation to reproductive organs is most important during pregnancy. The increased load of the placental circulation is sufficient to increase the resting cardiac output and blood volume. The peripheral resistance is lowered, and tachycardia and a wide pulse pressure can be noted as early as the middle of the second month of pregnancy.

Pulmonary Circulation

Whereas appropriate distribution of cardiac output is the most important factor in systemic circulatory dynamics, maximal blood flow with minimal perfusion pressure is what is required in the pulmonary circulation. With increasing right ventricular output, eg, during exercise, there is an increase in the area of the pulmonary capillary bed and little or no increase in pulmonary arterial pressure. Reflex control of the pulmonary bed is minimal when compared to the systemic circulation. For example, occlusion of one pulmonary artery in a normal adult man in the resting supine position causes no detectable change in the circulation, and release of the occlusion does not result in any increase in blood flow to the lung whose circulation was occluded. This lack of reactive hyperemia after pulmonary artery occlusion is in sharp contrast to the finding when systemic flow to any organ is cut off. Reactive hyperemia in the pulmonary circulation probably does occur in human fetal and neonatal life.

The principal factor influencing pulmonary arterial pressure is alveolar hypoxia. A lowered alveolar oxygen tension produces pulmonary arteriolar vasoconstriction. This probably serves as a local mechanism to divert pulmonary blood flow away from areas of the lung in which ventilation is inadequate. Increased CO_2 tension and hydrogen ion concentration are important in enhancing the response to hypoxia.

DISTRIBUTION OF CARDIAC OUTPUT

All of the parallel systemic circulations compete for perfusion, and the total cardiac output reflects the sum of all their demands. The ratio of oxygen consumption to cardiac output represents the average systemic arteriovenous oxygen difference in milliliters of oxygen per liter of blood flow. The resting level of arteriovenous difference reflects the resting "mix" of perfusion of the brain, heart, kidneys, skin, and other viscera. Ordinarily, with normal cardiac function, enough blood flow is available for all circulations both at rest and during mild or moderate exercise. During severe exercise, however, the ability of other circulations to reduce their demands and thus free the maximal amount of blood for muscular perfusion is an important determinant of performance. When the cardiac output is inadequate because of heart disease, blood flow to less essential elements of the circulation (kidneys, viscera, and skin) is reduced, and the average systemic arteriovenous oxygen difference increases. This effect is sometimes interpreted as "an increase in oxygen extraction by the tissues" but in fact represents a redistribution of blood flow rather than a change in the behavior of any of the special circulations.

MUSCULAR EXERCISE

Muscular exercise constitutes the most severe physiologic stress to which the normal circulation is exposed. In mammalian evolution, exercise performance has played an important part in natural selection by influencing either escape from natural enemies or pursuit of other animals in the search for food. All forms of muscular activity are important—from feats of strength and short sprints to long-term endurance running—and the rate of recovery following exertion determines the level of performance that is possible after a short rest.

Isometric (Static) Exercise

Isometric exercise, involving lifting and straining, increases the systemic arterial pressure and heart rate and puts a "pressure load" on the circulation. The rise in blood pressure is partly reflex and partly mechanical. The reflex pathways are poorly understood, and the mechanical element stems from the increase in tissue pressure in the contracting muscles. Increased tissue pressure provides increased resistance, against which the left ventricle must eject blood. An individual's muscular strength bears no necessary relationship to the ability of the heart to increase its output during sustained exercise, and cardiac mechanisms mainly come into play when the muscles relax and perfusion is restored into a vasodilated muscular bed.

Short-Term Exercise

In short bursts of exercise, the muscles rely on fuel stored locally, and cardiopulmonary transport mechanisms are minimally involved. Thus, in a 100-meter dash, an accomplished athlete can take a deep breath before the start of a race and hold his or her breath during the few seconds needed to run the distance. Local substrates plus oxygen stored in the muscles and blood and the breakdown of muscle glycogen are used to provide the high-energy phosphate bonds needed for muscular contractions. These stores must be replenished during recovery.

Long-Term Exercise

In more prolonged intervals of exercise—minutes to hours—the cardiopulmonary transport of oxygen and removal of metabolic products become important considerations. The fuel stored in the muscles is not sufficient to provide the energy requirements, and increasing muscle blood flow leads to an increase in cardiac output and increased delivery of oxygen to the tissues. The sooner the cardiopulmonary transport mechanisms come into operation, the sooner the supply of oxygen can reach the level of the demand and a "steady state" of exercise be achieved. The arteriovenous oxygen difference increases as a larger proportion of the cardiac output is directed to the muscles, and blood flow to the viscera tends to decrease as the level of exercise increases.

In more strenuous and protracted exercise, a steady state becomes progressively more difficult to maintain. Increased heat production by the exercising muscles leads to increased demands for skin perfusion to increase heat elimination, and ultimately, anaerobic metabolism, analogous to the use of energy stored in the muscle at the start of exercise, is superimposed on the steady state picture. The use of glycogen as a source of energy results in lactic acid production and makes available only a small proportion (about 10%) of the high-energy phosphate bonds provided by aerobic metabolism. Metabolic acidosis develops as lactic acid accumulates and escapes from the muscles into the blood. Increased ventilation and disproportionate tachycardia result, and the length of time that exercise can be continued at the same level of work becomes limited. Motivation becomes an important consideration, and all of the factors influencing oxygen transport—pulmonary ventilation, oxygen diffusion, stroke volume, and heart rate—reach their limits at about the same time in normal subjects.

Recovery From Long-Term Exercise

When exercise stops, the metabolic products that accumulated in the underperfused, contracting muscles cause a local vasodilation that imposes an important demand on the circulation. The initial stages of the return of the cardiovascular system toward normal following strenuous exercise are controlled by the baroreceptor reflexes. Muscular perfusion is limited by the need to maintain an adequate arterial pressure for cerebral perfusion. If circulatory function is good and a large cardiac output is available, muscular perfusion is well maintained during recovery, and the heart rate and cardiac output fall rapidly to normal as the load of metabolites that accumulated in the muscles during exercise is transferred to the rest of the circulation. If circulatory function is poor and there is little cardiac output to spare, the rate of recovery is slow, and the heart rate and cardiac output take longer to recover.

In all cases, the rate of return of metabolism and heart rate toward normal follow an exponential pattern in the first few minutes of the recovery stage. In the longer term (first hour), recovery from exercise involves excretion of the metabolic products of exercise from the general circulation. Lactic acid and heat generated by muscular contraction are the most important factors in this phase of recovery, which also follows an exponential pattern but with a longer time constant (15 minutes or more).

Physical Training

Improving a person's physical condition by exercise training involves redistribution of systemic blood flow. In the untrained state, perfusion of visceral and skin circulations continues during exercise, and the cardiac output needed for a given level of submaximal work is increased. By exercise training, which involves habitually increasing the heart rate to moderately high levels (about 150/min) for an hour or so each day, blood flow is more efficiently distributed. Muscular perfusion is increased as blood is diverted from less essential parts of the circulation. The heart rate and cardiac output at submaximal loads are reduced, exercise performance is improved, and the rate of recovery from exercise is speeded up.

LIMITATION OF CARDIAC PERFORMANCE

Performance during sustained activity in normal subjects is always limited by the capacity of the heart to meet the demands of the circulation. Cardiac capacity increases after birth, during the period of growth and development, up to a peak in early adult life. With disease and the degenerative changes associated with aging, the capacity of the heart to perform work decreases and the maximum cardiac output, the maximum oxygen consumption, and the maximal heart rate decrease. Both the maximal values and the rates at which the maximal values are reached decrease with age. When the capacity of the heart to do work falls to a level at which renal or cerebral perfusion is compromised, a chain of events is initiated that leads to a vicious circle resulting finally in a clinical syndrome known as heart failure. This condition is easy to recognize but difficult to define. It is best viewed as a derangement of the normal circulatory control mechanisms mediated through the autonomic nervous system and will be discussed in Chapter 10.

Failure of the heart to maintain its own circulation at an adequate level also leads to a vicious circle that also results in what might just as well be called a form of heart failure but is in fact recognized as myocardial ischemia, discussed in Chapter 8.

The Heart as the Servant of the Circulation

The physiologic bases of these 2 forms of severe impairment of cardiac function—heart failure and myocardial ischemia—involve an understanding of the subservient role of the heart in relation to the overall circulation. The physiologic mechanisms involved in the maintenance of a normal blood pressure and blood volume so dominate the picture that when cardiac function is impaired, the autonomic nervous servomechanisms that ordinarily restore the status quo are activated even though the result is aggravation of the abnormal circulatory state.

Mechanisms of Heart Failure

"Inappropriate" physiologic mechanisms triggered by inadequate cardiac function are thus important in producing the vicious circles that result in the clinical syndromes of heart failure and myocardial ischemia.

To cite specific examples, if the heart cannot maintain an adequate blood pressure, vasoconstriction mediated via the sympathetic nervous system occurs; this increases the work of the heart, causing a vicious circle. If the heart cannot generate a blood pressure adequate to maintain renal perfusion, mechanisms physiologically appropriate for defense against loss of blood volume by dehydration, hemorrhage, or salt deprivation are set in motion. Retention of salt and water with blood volume expansion and restriction of urinary output then result in a vicious circle by overloading the already damaged circulation, causing heart failure.

REFERENCES

General

Amsterdam EA, Wilmore JH, DeMaria AN (editors): *Exercise in Cardiovascular Health and Disease.* Yorke Medical Books, 1977.

Becker AE, Anderson RH: *Cardiac Pathology.* Raven Press, 1983.

Berne RM (editor): The cardiovascular system. Vol 1, Section 2, of: *Handbook of Physiology.* American Physiological Society, 1979.

Berne RM, Levy MN: *Cardiovascular Physiology,* 4th ed. Mosby, 1981.

Campbell EJM, Dickinson CJ, Slater JDH (editors): *Clinical Physiology,* 4th ed. Lippincott, 1974.

Caro CG et al: *The Mechanics of the Circulation.* Oxford Univ Press, 1978.

Dawes GS: *Foetal and Neonatal Physiology.* Year Book, 1968.

Fung YC: *Biodynamics: Circulation.* Springer-Verlag, 1984.

Ganong WF: *Review of Medical Physiology,* 12th ed. Lange, 1985.

Heller LJ, Mohrman DE: *Cardiovascular Physiology.* McGraw-Hill, 1981.

Honig CR: *Cardiovascular Physiology.* Little, Brown, 1981.

Hudson REB: *Cardiovascular Pathology.* 3 vols. Arnold, 1965–1970.

Hwang NHC, Gross DE, Patel DJ (editors): *Quantitative Cardiovascular Studies.* University Park Press, 1978.

Little RC: *Physiology of the Heart and Circulation,* 2nd ed. Year Book, 1981.

McDonald DA: *Blood Flow in Arteries,* 2nd ed. Williams & Wilkins, 1974.

Milnor WR: *Hemodynamics.* Williams & Wilkins, 1982.

Rowell LB: Human cardiovascular adjustments to exercise and thermal stress. *Physiol Rev* 1974;**54**:75.

Shepherd JT, Vanhoutte PM: *The Human Cardiovascular System: Facts and Concepts.* Raven Press, 1979.

Smith JJ, Kampine JP: *Circulatory Physiology: The Essentials.* Williams & Wilkins, 1980.

Wagner NK (editor): *Exercise and the Heart.* Davis, 1978.

Willerson JT, Sanders CA (editors): *Clinical Cardiology.* Grune & Stratton, 1977.

Anatomy of the Heart

Feola M et al: The terminal pathway of the lymphatic system of the human heart. *Ann Thorac Surg* 1977;**24**:531.

Hutchins GM et al: Shape of the human cardiac ventricles. *Am J Cardiol* 1978;**41**:646.

James TN: Anatomy of the coronary arteries in health and disease. *Circulation* 1965;**32**:1020.

Miller AJ: *The Lymphatics of the Heart.* Raven Press, 1982.

Walmsley R, Watson H: *Clinical Anatomy of the Heart.* Churchill Livingstone, 1978.

Yoffey JM, Cortice FC: Pages 272–277 in: *Lymphatics, Lymph and the Lymphomyeloid Complex.* Academic Press, 1970.

Cardiac Contraction

Frank O: Die Grundform des arterielle Pulses. *Z Biol* 1898;**37**:483.

Huxley AF, Simmons RM: Proposed mechanisms for force generation in striated muscle. *Nature* 1971;**233**:533.

Huxley HE: The mechanism of muscular contraction. *Science* 1969;**164**:1356.

Jewell BR: A re-examination of the influence of muscle length on myocardial performance. *Circ Res* 1977;**40**:221.

Langer GA, Brady AJ: *The Mammalian Myocardium.* Wiley, 1974.

Monroe RG, French GN: Left ventricular pressure-volume relationships and myocardial oxygen consumption in the isolated heart. *Circ Res* 1961;**9**:362.

Morkin E, Flink IL, Goldman S: Biochemical and physiologic effects of thyroid hormone on cardiac performance. *Prog Cardiovasc Dis* 1983;**25**:435.

Noble MIM: *The Cardiac Cycle.* Blackwell, 1979.

Noble MIM: The contribution of blood momentum to left ventricular ejection in the dog. *Circ Res* 1968;**23**:663.

Patterson SW, Piper H, Starling EH: The regulation of the heart beat. *J Physiol* 1914;**48**:465.

Sagawa K: The end-systolic pressure-volume relation of the ventricle: Definitions, modifications and clinical use. (Editorial.) *Circulation* 1981;**63**:1223.

Sagawa K: The ventricular pressure-volume diagram revisited. *Circ Res* 1978;**43**:677.

Sugi H, Pollack GH (editors): *Cross-Bridge Mechanisms in Muscle Contraction.* University Park Press, 1979.

Targett RC et al: Simultaneous Doppler blood velocity measurements from aorta and radial artery in normal human subjects. *Cardiovasc Res* 1985;**19**:394.

Trautwein W et al: Electrophysiologic study of human heart muscle. *Circ Res* 1962;**10**:306.

Nerves & Reflexes

Brown E et al: Circulatory responses to simulated gravitational shifts of blood in man induced by exposure of the body below the iliac crests to subatmospheric pressure. *J Physiol (Lond)* 1966;**183:**607.

Coleridge JCG, Coleridge HM: Chemoreflex regulation of the heart. Vol 1, Section 2, p 653, in: *Handbook of Physiology.* American Physiological Society, 1979.

Donald DE, Shepherd JT: Cardiac receptors: Normal and disturbed function. *Am J Cardiol* 1979;**44:**873.

Gauer OH et al: The effect of negative pressure breathing on urine flow. *J Clin Invest* 1954;**33:**287.

Hertzman A: Vasomotor regulation of cutaneous circulation. *Physiol Rev* 1959;**39:**280.

Heymans C, Neil E: *Reflexogenic Areas of the Cardiovascular System.* Churchill, 1958.

Jones RD, Berne RM: Intrinsic regulation of skeletal muscle blood flow. *Circ Res* 1964;**14:**126.

Kirchheim HR: Systemic arterial baroreceptor reflexes. *Physiol Rev* 1976;**56:**100.

Levy MN, Vassalle M: *Excitation and Neural Control of the Heart.* American Physiological Society, 1982.

Linden RJ: Atrial reflexes and renal function. *Am J Cardiol* 1979;**44:**879.

Mark AL: Implications of inhibitory reflexes originating in the heart. *J Am Coll Cardiol* 1983;**1:**90.

Shepherd JT: The lungs as receptor sites for cardiovascular regulation. *Circulation* 1981;**63:**1.

Sleight P: Reflex control of the heart. *Am J Cardiol* 1979;**44:**889.

Special Circulations

Bellamy RF: Diastolic coronary artery pressure-flow relations in the dog. *Circ Res* 1978;**43:**92.

Betz E: Cerebral blood flow: Its measurement and regulation. *Physiol Rev* 1972;**52:**595.

Harris P, Heath D: *The Human Pulmonary Circulation,* 2nd ed. Churchill Livingstone, 1977.

Knox FG (editor): *Textbook of Renal Pathophysiology.* Harper & Row, 1978.

Langitt TW et al (editors): *Cerebral Circulation and Metabolism.* Springer-Verlag, 1975.

Marcus HL: *The Coronary Circulation in Health and Disease.* McGraw-Hill, 1983.

Metcalfe J, Ueland K: Maternal cardiovascular adjustments to pregnancy. *Prog Cardiovasc Dis* 1974;**16:**363.

Rouleau J et al: The role of auto-regulation and tissue diastolic pressures in the transmural distribution of left ventricular blood flow in anesthetized dogs. *Circ Res* 1979;**45:**804.

Zelis R (editor): *The Peripheral Circulations.* Grune & Stratton, 1975.

2 History Taking

A medical history carefully elicited by an understanding and competent clinician is essential to the evaluation of the patient with cardiovascular disease. Because of the great fear of heart disease by most patients, the physician's questioning should be unhurried and nonthreatening but nonetheless thorough. Skillful interrogation, appropriate to the urgency of the situation, must be matched by thoughtful listening. Questions should be as free as possible of the force of suggestion. The patient must be permitted to raise questions at appropriate times. The history is the starting point in the diagnostic process and to a large extent determines the direction and extent (and delays, costs, and inconveniences) of further studies.

Artful history taking brings the patient and physician close together. In many respects, the history, taken properly, is therapeutic in itself. For this reason, it is a critical factor not only in establishing the diagnosis but also in determining the outcome of subsequent therapy.

Subclinical Disease; Asymptomatic Patients

The modern tendency for patients with no symptoms to consult physicians for routine "checkup" examinations has increased the possibility that doctors might cause unnecessary anxiety in their patients even though the intent of such examinations is to discover latent or developing illness. Since symptoms of disease are often exaggerations of normal findings (eg, dyspnea, fatigue), the borderline between normality and disease is often ill-defined. The problem becomes greater as the patient becomes older, because the range of normality widens with advancing years. Some patients deny the existence of symptoms, fearing to be told that they are ill and may die; and some may exaggerate symptoms for secondary gain. Decreasing activity, failing memory, and wishful thinking may lead people to defer seeking advice until disease is far-advanced. Persons with no complaints are technically not "patients," and a distinction should be maintained between conditions discovered during routine examinations and the diseases of patients with true symptoms. Experience in dealing with clinical and laboratory information obtained from checkup examinations is relatively small, and physicians tend to forget that under such circumstances they are dealing with a presymptomatic phase of disease.

DYSPNEA

The problem of interpreting a symptom that may also be a normal physiologic response is perhaps most strikingly demonstrated in the case of the cardinal symptom of heart disease—dyspnea, or shortness of breath. Shortness of breath on exertion is a normal phenomenon. In most cases, exercise performance is limited by shortness of breath rather than by fatigue, chest pain, leg pain, dizziness, or syncope. Dyspnea on progressively less severe exertion is also a normal accompaniment of the common modern combination of a sedentary life, increasing weight, and advancing age. It may therefore be more difficult to determine whether heart disease is present with dyspnea than if there are more obvious symptoms such as hemoptysis or severe chest pain.

Mechanism of Dyspnea

The mechanism of dyspnea in normal and abnormal conditions is not always clear. "The unpleasant sensation of the need for increased ventilation" is the best description of dyspnea. Two main varieties have been distinguished. With the first variety, the patient feels that extra work on the part of the respiratory muscles is required to achieve adequate ventilation. With the second type, the patient is aware of a feeling of smothering and feels an urgent need to take another breath; the smothering sensation is akin to that associated with breath-holding. Dyspnea is a cortical sensation involving consciousness and must be distinguished from hyperpnea (increased ventilation), which may occur without discomfort or distress and which may be seen in unconscious patients.

Dyspnea in Normal Subjects

Dyspnea normally limits exercise performance in almost everyone. A person becomes conditioned to a certain level of discomfort arising from some particular task, such as walking up a familiar hill. The ease with which dyspnea is provoked varies with the amount of ventilation required for that task. This in turn depends on a person's physical condition, weight, age, and life-style. In sedentary persons, the ability of the circulation to distribute maximum blood flow to the exercising muscles while decreasing perfusion of relatively nonessential vascular beds (eg, adipose tissue, skin, and viscera) is impaired.

Dyspnea in Heart Disease

The dyspnea of patients with heart disease most closely resembles the dyspnea of normal exertion and is characteristically directly related to the degree of exertion. The patient complains that some effort that previously did not result in awareness of breathing now causes an unpleasant gasping sensation. The feeling of discomfort is in the chest but is not well localized to any single structure such as the diaphragm or the intercostal muscles.

In contradistinction to cardiac dyspnea, shortness of breath at rest is more common in many lung diseases such as asthmatic attacks, bronchitis, pneumonia, or pneumothorax, but not in emphysema.

A. Dyspnea Associated With Low Cardiac Output: When cardiac output is inadequate to meet the metabolic needs of the body, hyperventilation and subsequent dyspnea occur. Pulmonary congestion need not be present, although the dyspnea is similar to that occurring in pulmonary congestion and is quantitatively related to exertion. Nonmedullated sensory fibers arising from stretch receptors in muscle spindles monitor local metabolic conditions and cause reflex medullary ventilatory stimulation when flow to the exercising muscle is inadequate to meet metabolic needs. These nervous mechanisms involve primitive visceral sensory fibers that are highly resistant to blocking agents. In this form of dyspnea, oxygen inhalation has little effect, because the extra oxygen carried in solution in the plasma is not sufficient to relieve the symptoms.

B. Dyspnea Due to Pulmonary Congestion: Dyspnea on exertion is the cardinal symptom of pulmonary congestion. It results from a rise in left ventricular end-diastolic pressure or a raised left atrial pressure with a normal left ventricle in mitral valve disease. In both cases, increased pulmonary venous and pulmonary capillary pressures increase the stiffness of the lungs and the work of breathing by decreasing the compliance of the lungs, mainly by causing interstitial pulmonary edema. In addition to the mechanical changes, there is also a reflex autonomic visceral sensation, probably mediated through nonmedullated sensory fibers in the lungs and passing up the vagus nerves to the medulla, which contributes to dyspnea by direct autonomic sensory stimulation. In the early stages of heart disease, dyspnea only occurs with severe exertion, but as pulmonary congestion becomes more severe, permanent changes in the lungs occur: Resting lung compliance is reduced, and increased lymphatic drainage, thickening of interstitial tissues, and other compensatory changes occur. Such changes reduce the chances of acute pulmonary edema and enable the body to tolerate high pulmonary capillary pressures because of thickened barriers between the blood in the capillaries and the gas in the alveoli.

C. Dyspnea in Acute Pulmonary Edema: When pulmonary congestion is acute and severe, dyspnea occurs with minimal exertion, and pulmonary edema results as fluid is forced into the alveolar spaces by capillary congestion. This congestion may seriously interfere with gas exchange and cause hypoxia and respiratory acidosis with CO_2 retention. When dyspnea is due to pulmonary edema, gas exchange in the lungs is impaired; inhalation of oxygen can increase the oxygen saturation of blood leaving the lungs, often relieving dyspnea.

D. Dyspnea Associated With Other Forms of Heart Disease: Dyspnea occurs in forms of heart disease other than those involving pulmonary congestion and low cardiac output. In cyanotic congenital heart disease, shunting of venous blood into the systemic circulation lowers arterial oxygen tension and contributes to dyspnea by stimulating the carotid bodies and increasing the ventilation needed for a given work load. In pulmonary embolism and pulmonary infarction, dyspnea may result from reflex stimulation of medullary centers by impulses from vagal nerve endings in the lungs and pulmonary arteries. Dyspnea due to such causes may be in addition to that due to inadequate cardiac output, which has already been described.

Dyspnea Resulting From Chemical Stimuli

Other mechanisms involved in dyspnea include chemical stimuli to ventilation mediated through hypoxia, as seen at high altitude; increase in CO_2 (hypercapnia); and metabolic acidosis. The chemoreceptor cells of the carotid and aortic bodies respond primarily to hypoxia and secondarily to increased CO_2. The central chemosensitive areas in the medulla stimulate respiration primarily in response to acidosis resulting from CO_2 and only secondarily in response to hypoxia. Chemically mediated stimuli to ventilation provide slowly responding and long-lasting control mechanisms and are chiefly involved in controlling depth and rate of breathing rather than causing dyspnea. Hypoxia, as demonstrated by a lowered arterial oxygen tension while the patient is breathing air at rest or during exercise ($P_{O_2} < 70$ mm Hg), is not generally found in dyspneic cardiac patients. Hyperventilation with low P_{CO_2}, low pH, and a normal or raised P_{O_2} is the usual finding. It is caused in cardiac patients by the release of acid metabolites from inadequately perfused tissues rather than by anxiety. Dyspnea also results from acute changes in the permeability of the pulmonary capillaries, as when pulmonary edema develops in heroin overdose, or on exposure to toxic fumes such as chlorine, phosgene, or other noxious gases.

Episodic Dyspnea

Episodic dyspnea and dyspnea at rest that is relieved by sitting up (orthopnea) are important indicators of severe disease. The mechanism of orthopnea involves an increase in pulmonary capillary pressure and a decrease in lung volume when in the supine position. Lung compliance decreases and respiratory resistance increases to cause an acute increase in the work of breathing. Paroxysmal dyspnea classically occurs at night, often after a strenuous day or an evening out dancing or after excessive salt or fluid intake. It characteristically wakes the patient up around 2:00 AM and is so clearly relieved by sitting or standing and made worse by lying flat that a patient who has once experienced this symptom will often never sleep flat in bed again.

When dyspnea is relieved by postural change other than sitting or standing, the possibility of pressure on intrathoracic structures by a tumor or aneurysm should be suspected. In pericardial disease, kneeling face down may relieve pressure on the heart and alleviate distress.

In acute pulmonary congestion in bedridden patients, the least exertion, such as eating, use of a bedpan or commode, washing, or the minor excitement of a visitor, may provoke an episode of dyspnea. The dyspnea of acute pulmonary congestion, if not relieved, will progress to acute pulmonary edema, which can cause circulatory collapse, with restlessness, anxiety, apprehension, sweating, tachycardia, tachypnea, and acute respiratory distress.

Dyspnea Associated With High-Altitude Pulmonary Edema

Dyspnea on exertion is normally seen at high altitude. Dyspnea at rest due to pulmonary edema may occur in persons acutely exposed to hypoxia at altitudes of 2000 m or more. The breathlessness usually comes on in the evening or during the night of the first day at high altitude. The patient often gives a history of unaccustomed exertion during the day. Even previously acclimatized persons returning to high altitude after a stay at sea level may be affected. Dyspnea, cough, frothy pink sputum, and circulatory collapse may develop if treatment is not forthcoming, and mountain climbers have died from the condition. Oxygen inhalation and returning to lower altitude are effective treatment. The causative mechanism is almost certainly increased permeability of the alveolocapillary membrane of the lungs. Left atrial pressure has been shown to be normal in at least one person with the condition, and left heart failure is not the primary cause. The chest x-ray shows dramatic changes (Fig 2–1) that disappear rapidly with treatment.

Diagnostic Value of Dyspnea

Certain features may occasionally help to show that dyspnea is due to specific forms of heart disease. In left ventricular failure, as opposed to pulmonary congestion, dyspnea is often associated with a heavy oppressive substernal discomfort, which tends to merge into angina of effort. Patients with mitral stenosis often complain of anginalike pain, but only when there is severe pulmonary hypertension. The distinction between dyspnea alone and angina plus dyspnea on the one hand, and between angina alone and dyspnea plus angina on the other, is often unclear. Acute left ventricular distention causes both severe discomfort in the chest and dyspnea resulting from acute pulmonary congestion. Similarly, acute imbalance between myocardial oxygen supply and demand often causes an acute rise in left ventricular end-diastolic pressure. In left ventricular failure, dyspnea appears first, and the discomfort never occurs without the dyspnea. The discomfort may radiate like anginal pain and is described as a sensation of heaviness, rather than pain, as in angina. Aortic valve disease, hypertension, and cardiomyopathy are the commonest causes of the discomfort. The basic mechanism is an increase in the work required from the left ventricle, and acute left ventricular distention may be involved.

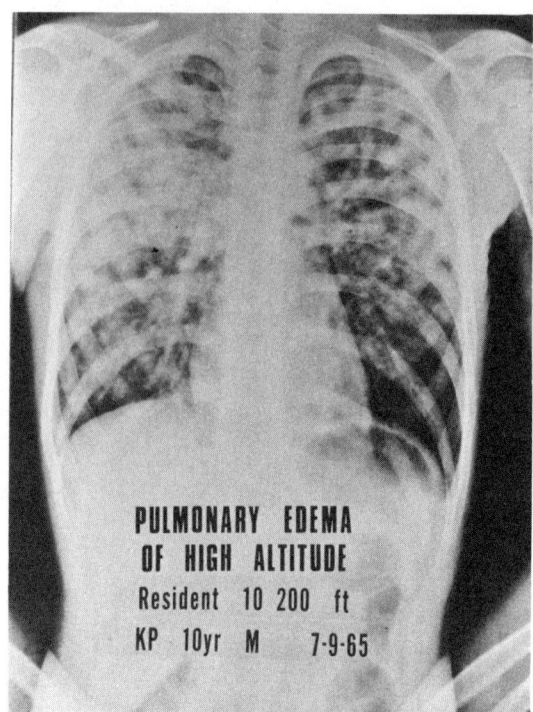

Figure 2–1. Chest x-ray showing high-altitude pulmonary edema in an individual accustomed to living at high altitudes. The edema developed on return from a stay at low altitude. (Courtesy of RF Grover.)

Dyspnea Due to Anxiety

Dyspnea at rest commonly accompanies anxiety. The patient complains that normal breathing is not satisfactory, and it is only by taking deep sighing breaths that relief is obtained. This form of dyspnea is not generally provoked by exertion and is associated with symptoms due to hyperventilation (see Chapter 21).

CHEST PAIN

Chest pain occurs in many varieties of heart disease and also in noncardiac diseases. Its correct interpretation is occasionally almost impossible.

Ischemic Cardiac Pain (Angina Pectoris) (See also p 144.)

Classic ischemic pain (angina pectoris) can be either so obvious that it is easily recognizable or (uncommonly) so atypical that even after complete investigation, significant doubt exists about the nature of the pain. The basic mechanism of ischemic pain is an increase in the demand for both coronary blood flow and oxygen delivery that exceeds the available supply.

The mechanism producing cardiac pain is not clearly understood. Nonmedullated small sympathetic nerve fibers paralleling the coronary vessels are thought to provide the afferent pathway. The pain, like other forms of visceral sensation, is referred to the equivalent spinal segments C8 and T1–5. Relief of angina following nonspecific surgical procedures such as thoracotomy, mammary artery ligation, and pericardial poudrage is well recognized but not consistent. Although it is thought to be a placebo effect, the severing of afferent autonomic nerves may play a role in relieving pain.

A. Angina of Effort:

1. Character and duration–The original subjective description in the late 18th century by William Heberden of his own angina of effort has not been surpassed. He wrote that ". . . they who are afflicted with it, are seized while they are walking (more especially if it be uphill, and soon after eating) with a painful and most disagreeable sensation in the breast, which seems as if it would extinguish life, if it were to increase or to continue; but the moment they stand still, all this uneasiness vanishes. In all other respects, the patients are, at the beginning of this disorder, perfectly well, and in particular have no shortness of breath, from which it is totally different. The pain is sometimes situated in the upper part, sometimes in the middle, sometimes at the bottom of the sternum, and more often inclined to the left than to the right side. It likewise very frequently extends from the breast to the middle of the left arm. Males are most liable to this disease, especially such as have passed their fiftieth year." The pain is described as crushing, squeezing, viselike, and resembling a weight on the chest but not as shooting or jabbing. It is a steady, constant pain that does not wax and wane. Angina pectoris normally subsides rapidly, especially when it is provoked by effort. It usually lasts for minutes rather than seconds and seldom for hours or days. Long-lasting cardiac pain implies myocardial infarction or unstable angina.

2. Site and radiation–Anginal pain is ordinarily substernal or felt slightly to the left of the midline, beside or partly under the sternum. It is not felt solely at the cardiac apex in the inframammary region. It tends to radiate bilaterally across the chest, into the arms (left more than right), and into the neck and lower jaw. It does not radiate into the upper jaw, the lower back, or below the umbilicus and is rarely felt in the abdomen alone. In the arms, the pain passes down the ulnar and volar surface to the wrist and then only into the ulnar fingers, never into the thumb or down the outer (extensor) surface of the arm. Pain may occasionally be felt only in the arm or may start in the arm and radiate to the chest.

3. Provocation and relief–Angina of effort represents the commonest form of cardiac pain. The pain or discomfort is provoked by any effort that raises the metabolic demand for coronary flow above the available supply. The pain is quantitatively related to exertion, and the patient often learns to identify the level of exercise that will bring on pain, and by avoiding that level, may obtain relief of symptoms. Attacks are precipitated by walking uphill or upstairs. Pain is more likely to occur when the patient is outdoors, especially when the temperature is high or low or when the patient is walking against the wind with face unprotected; after the patient has eaten a heavy meal; or when the patient is excited, angry, or tense. Pain sometimes comes on more readily with arm exercise or carrying heavy objects. Hot or cold showers or baths may precipitate pain, as may brisk toweling afterward. The sensory effects of temperature are mediated through the fifth nerve and cause reflex autonomic changes in blood pressure and heart rate. Cold showers raise blood pressure and heart rate; hot showers result in increased cardiac output in response to vasodilation.

Angina of effort is normally relieved by rest, with or without the help of vasodilator drugs such as nitroglycerin. Failure to obtain relief suggests another cause of pain or actual or impending myocardial infarction. In some instances, belching may relieve pain; this does not necessarily indicate a gastrointestinal source of pain. Patients sometimes find that continuing exercise (in some cases at a slower pace) leads to relief of pain ("walk-through angina"). This suggests either relief of vasospasm or an increase in the delivery of substrate to the myocardium.

B. Rest Pain: Anginal pain may be so readily provoked that it occurs at rest (**angina decubitus**). Excitement, mental activity, and physical tension (eg, even simple clenching of a fist) raise arterial pressure and heart rate and increase myocardial oxygen consumption. Rest pain is likely to occur at night and may wake the patient. Increases in blood pressure and cardiac output during dreams may be sufficient to induce ischemia. When the coronary circulation is severely diseased, even minor circulatory changes may provoke pain. Anginal pain comes on more readily in the presence of fever, anemia, or arrhythmia (both bradycardia and tachycardia).

C. Variant (Prinzmetal) Angina: A paradoxic form of angina occurs in some patients as a result of coronary arterial spasm. The pain is like that of classic angina but occurs at rest rather than on effort. In some cases, the pain is relieved, rather than brought on, by exercise. Variant angina is likely to be associated with ST segment elevation rather than depression on the ECG. This form of angina may occur either in patients with normal coronary arteries at angiography or in those with significant coronary atherosclerosis.

D. Coronary Arterial Spasm: While all variant (Prinzmetal) angina is probably due to coronary spasm, not all forms of coronary spasm produce variant angina. Coronary spasm may be provoked by vasoconstrictive drugs, such as ergotamine used for the control of migraine. Coronary spasm is commoner in women and may be associated with increased reactivity in other vascular beds (eg, Raynaud's disease or scleroderma). The pain associated with coronary spasm may be atypical and is not usually accompanied by tachycardia or a rise in arterial pressure. Electrocardiography may show ST segment depression or arrhythmia; it is important to obtain an ECG while the patient is experiencing pain.

E. Unstable Angina: The pain of unstable angina is like that of other forms of myocardial ischemia, but the circumstances in which the pain occurs are different. A diagnosis of unstable angina is suggested when a lower level of exercise is needed to provoke angina, by pain of different duration, by rest pain, or by failure to obtain relief with nitroglycerin. Relatively minor changes in symptoms may indicate impending myocardial infarction. Retrospective analysis of patients with established infarction often reveals one or more premonitory episodes that either the physician or the patient did not consider severe enough to heed. The unpredictability of the clinical course in this, as well as other forms of ischemic heart disease, makes the diagnosis difficult and accurate prognosis impossible.

F. Pain of Myocardial Infarction: The pain of myocardial infarction is similar in character, site, and radiation to that of angina pectoris, but it is more severe and longer-lasting and associated at times with a feeling of impending death (**angor animi**) and also with circulatory collapse and shock. The patient may be short of breath, but pain is usually the dominant symptom. The patient is restless and often seeks, but cannot find, a comfortable position in which the pain is relieved. In myocardial infarction, the pain ordinarily lasts until the patient is given an analgesic such as morphine or meperidine. If such relief is unobtainable, the pain can last for several days.

Pain in Acute Thoracic Disease

Pain similar to that of myocardial infarction also occurs with other acute intrathoracic disorders. **Aortic dissection** can cause severe chest pain. This frequently starts in the back or radiates to it. **Acute pulmonary embolism** also causes acute chest pain and shock that may be indistinguishable from that due to myocardial infarction. The cause is thought to be sudden acute right ventricular distention that stimulates ventricular receptors whose sensory representation resembles that of the left ventricle. Spontaneous pneumothorax and acute pleurisy, especially at the onset of lobar pneumonia, also cause chest pain and must be distinguished from pericardial disease, which causes a pain similar in distribution to other cardiac pains but more related to posture. Like pleural pain, pericardial pain is often worse with respiration, but relief obtained from sitting up and leaning forward or even from crouching on all fours face down is particularly suggestive of pericardial pain. Such maneuvers presumably alter tension on the pericardial sac. Like pleural pain, pericardial pain is often relieved when effusion develops.

Pain Associated With Anxiety States

The most troublesome pain to explain is the noncardiac pain of anxiety states and effort syndrome. The pain is stabbing, felt at the apex of the heart in the left inframammary region, and associated with a feeling of anxiety, breathlessness, and inability to take a satisfying deep breath (Da Costa's syndrome). It seems to be related to the sympathetic nervous system responses of fright. The more knowledge the patient has of heart disease, the more difficult it may be to interpret such pain, because the description may be unconsciously molded to emphasize or minimize a possible illness.

Pain Associated With Herpes Zoster

The pain of herpes zoster classically precedes the rash, and this diagnosis should be borne in mind, especially in older persons. The pain is radicular in nature, gripping, tight, and constricting, and it may be severe. The diagnosis, which may be suspected when hyperesthesia is found in the affected area, becomes obvious when the eruption develops in a few days.

Musculoskeletal Pain

Musculoskeletal pain due to cervical or thoracic spinal bone or joint disease is readily confused with cardiac pain. Dorsal root pain (girdle pain) tends to be gripping and constricting and causes tightness. It is often associated with local tenderness, whereas angina is not. The presence of degenerative changes in spinal radiograms is no positive evidence of a musculoskeletal origin of the pain, any more than ST and T wave changes on the ECG indicate a cardiac origin. Provocation of the pain by movement, jarring, coughing, and sneezing and relief of pain by means of massage, heat, and manipulation are useful in suggesting a musculoskeletal origin. Tenderness of the anterior rib cage suggests costochondritis (Tietze's syndrome).

Abdominal Pain

Abdominal pain sometimes occurs in patients with heart disease, especially in acute, severe right-sided failure. Hepatic distention is usually invoked as the causative mechanism. Abdominal pain also occurs in angina and in myocardial infarction, but the pain is never solely abdominal.

Esophageal spasm and pain associated with hiatal hernia can also be confused with angina. The esophagus and the stomach are innervated by the autonomic nervous system and are capable of causing visceral pain having the same area of radiation as the heart. Any disease of the epigastric viscera can cause chest pain, which can be confused with cardiac pain. The pain of gallbladder disease is also difficult to distinguish from cardiac pain, since gallbladder disease and coronary disease often coexist.

PALPITATIONS

Awareness of the beating of the heart varies with the sensitivity of the patient and the severity of any disturbance of the force or rhythm of the heartbeat. The variation in these factors is great. Awareness of each ectopic beat or even of normal sinus rhythm may be extremely troublesome to some patients. Others may have an extremely forceful heartbeat owing to free aortic incompetence, or they may be subject to episodes of ventricular or supraventricular tachycardia with heart rates of over 180 beats/min without noticing anything. One must therefore differentiate between awareness of forceful heart action and an arrhythmia when the patient complains of palpitations. Most patients notice irregular rhythms more than they do regular tachycardia, but the more rapid the heartbeat, the more likely the patient is to notice an abnormality. In some cases, arrhythmia is only noticed during exercise when the heart rate is rapid.

Associated Symptoms

An important question is whether the palpitations are accompanied by any other symptoms such as dizziness, chest pain, or dyspnea. The functional effect of an arrhythmia may sometimes be a clue to its cause, as for example in mitral stenosis, in which dyspnea is almost always provoked when the arrhythmia occurs.

Examination & Recording of an ECG During an Attack

It is imperative to examine any patient with palpitations and record an ECG during an episode of palpitation. Until this has been done, it is essential to keep an open mind concerning the diagnosis. Palpitations often begin abruptly and cease gradually, and because the sinus tachycardia resulting from anxiety caused by the arrhythmia subsides only gradually, the patient may not be aware that the arrhythmia itself has stopped. The functional consequences of an episode of palpitations depend on the duration, the rapidity of the heart rate, and the state of the heart before the episode started. A paroxysm of tachycardia at a rate of about 140 beats/min may be well tolerated for a day or 2, but any rapid arrhythmia with an acute onset and a duration of more than a week to 10 days is likely to provoke heart failure, even in healthy young persons. In older, sicker patients, especially those with anemia or hypoxia, a shorter time elapses before serious heart failure develops.

DIZZINESS & SYNCOPE

Dizziness and syncope are difficult symptoms to interpret if the patient's consciousness has been impaired and recollection of the events surrounding the attack is hazy. The effects of alcohol or drugs cloud the patient's consciousness and interfere with interpretation of events. Dizziness and syncope both occur more commonly as benign manifestations than as symptoms of serious disease. They are most commonly due to noncardiac causes such as epileptic seizures, transient ischemic attacks due to cerebral or carotid vascular disease, and cerebrovascular accidents and vertigo due to vestibular disease rather than cardiac disease. A description of the episode from witnesses is of great value, but much can be learned from the circumstances surrounding the episode, as related by the patient. Dizziness is a frequent but not a necessary precursor of syncope, and one or both occur in 3 main types of conditions involving the cardiovascular system. The commonest form of cardiac syncope is simple vasovagal fainting resulting from certain autonomic nervous system effects. This is described in the chapter on hypotension (Chapter 21). The next most common is cardiac syncope due to arrhythmia or cardiac standstill, in which the heartbeat does not maintain adequate blood flow to the brain. The least common is syncope on unaccustomed effort, in which the demand for systemic perfusion exceeds the supply during severe stress, and cerebral ischemia ensues. Cardiac syncope is described in the chapter on arrhythmias (Chapter 15), and effort syncope is described under the heading of aortic stenosis (see Chapter 13). Effort syncope can also occur in severe pulmonary stenosis and in primary pulmonary hypertension.

Fainting Attacks in Tetralogy of Fallot

A specific form of syncope occurs in patients with tetralogy of Fallot in whom infundibular obstruction is present. Spasm of the muscle of the outflow tract of the right ventricle results in an acute decrease in pulmonary blood flow. Right-to-left shunting of blood through the ventricular septal defect into the aorta increases as a result, and acute severe arterial hypoxemia occurs, leading to loss of consciousness. The factors precipitating the infundibular spasm are not known.

Carotid Sinus Syncope

Another rare cause of syncope is excessive sensitivity of the carotid sinus baroreceptor mechanism. Extreme bradycardia and peripheral vasodilation may occur in response to minor mechanical stimulation of the neck, as in sharp turning of the head or pressure on the neck from too tight a collar. The condition is generally seen in older atherosclerotic men.

Cough Syncope

Syncope sometimes follows a bout of coughing. In this case, the repeated large (> 100 mm Hg) increases in intrathoracic pressure reduce systemic venous return enough to lower the systemic arterial pressure to levels of 50 mm Hg or less. Syncope results from inadequate cerebral perfusion. Either continuous or intermittent coughing spasms may cause these effects, which are commonest in middle-aged male smokers.

OTHER SYMPTOMS OF HEART DISEASE

Cough & Hemoptysis

Hemoptysis may occasionally be the first symptom of heart disease, and since there can be no hemoptysis without cough, cough is technically the presenting symptom. Mitral valve stenosis is the commonest condition in which hemoptysis is the presenting manifestation, and pulmonary congestion, frank pulmonary hemorrhage due to a ruptured vessel, and pulmonary infarction account for almost all cases. Cough without hemoptysis also occurs in any condition causing pulmonary congestion, and cough on exercise is sometimes seen in patients with mitral stenosis. Dry, unproductive cough is usually the earliest manifestation of impending pulmonary edema and precedes the profuse, watery, frothy pink sputum seen in the fully developed picture of acute pulmonary edema.

Cough may also occur as a manifestation of pressure on the bronchial tree in patients with cardiovascular disease. Left atrial enlargement may compress the left main bronchus in patients with mitral valve disease, and it may irritate the recurrent laryngeal nerve on the left side as it hooks under the aorta. Enlarging aortic aneurysms involving the aortic arch and tumors involving the heart may also cause cough when they compress mediastinal structures. Cough that occurs when the patient lies flat and is relieved when the patient sits up is particularly suggestive of pressure on the bronchial tree.

Fatigue

Fatigue is the most difficult cardiac symptom to evaluate. Whereas other symptoms of heart disease have associated outward manifestations, fatigue is entirely subjective. Although it is sometimes due to heart disease, fatigue is far more frequently due to noncardiac causes. Fatigue as a cardiac symptom is almost never of diagnostic value except as an indication of low cardiac output. It is rarely the first or the only symptom of significant organic heart disease, although it is a prominent symptom of neurocirculatory asthenia (Da Costa's syndrome; see Chapter 21). It commonly accompanies severe long-standing heart disease, especially chronic valvular disease with persistent right heart failure and low cardiac output. It is seen in patients with severe coronary artery disease after myocardial infarction, in mitral stenosis with marked increase in pulmonary vascular resistance, and in primary pulmonary hypertension. Dehydration due to excessive diuretic therapy and potassium depletion are 2 additional contributing factors.

Nocturia & Polyuria

Nocturia is occasionally the earliest symptom of raised left atrial pressure in left ventricular failure or mitral stenosis. The exact mechanism is not known, but transfer of fluid from the legs to the trunk when the patient lies down may play a part. Reflex connections have been demonstrated between left atrial receptors and the central nervous system, and the efferent pathway is known to involve the kidneys. Nocturia implies the passage of an abnormally large amount of urine at night, rather than an increased frequency of micturition at night, as occurs in prostatic disease. In the healthy state, the cardiac output is sufficient to provide adequate renal blood flow during the day, and urine flow at night is therefore conveniently reduced to a minimum. It may be that in early heart failure this mechanism breaks down because of inadequate cardiac output. There is also a connection between cardiac function and urinary output in patients with paroxysmal tachycardia due to any cause. Some patients note an increased urinary volume within 15–30 minutes of the start of tachycardia. The urine is of low specific gravity. The possibility of a reflex mechanism involving left atrial distention remains to be proved.

Squatting

Exertional dyspnea that is relieved by squatting during recovery from exercise strongly suggests the diagnosis of tetralogy of Fallot. The central blood volume and pulmonary blood flow are both increased by squatting. It has been shown that it is the change in the amount of venous return and not the change in posture that is important, because squatting in water has no hemodynamic effect. Thus, in tetralogy of Fallot, squatting increases the arterial pressure and provides more blood flow to the lungs by decreasing the right-to-left shunt across the ventricular defect. A similar result can be obtained by lying down, but children find it easier to squat after exertion. It is the pooling of blood in the legs in the upright position after stopping exercise that is the primary problem; if this does not occur, as in patients with a large pulmonary blood volume, the benefit from squatting is not seen. A tracing showing the time course of the changes in arterial pressure and arterial saturation on standing and squatting in a patient with tetralogy of Fallot is seen in Fig 2–2.

Hoarseness

Hoarseness as a manifestation of heart disease is seldom, if ever, a presenting symptom. It occurs in cardiac patients with gross left atrial enlargement in mitral valve disease, in giant left atrium, and in aortic aneurysm with or without dissection. All of these conditions cause pressure on the left recurrent laryngeal nerve and result in hoarseness. Hoarseness is also seen in patients with myxedema, in whom it may be the first clue to diagnosis.

Edema

Edema due to cardiac disease is a result of right heart failure and is seldom seen early, because right heart failure is a late development in heart disease. A complaint of edema as a primary symptom implies a

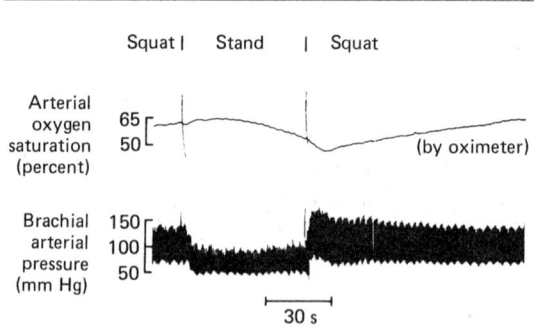

Figure 2–2. Changes in arterial oxygen saturation and blood pressure on standing and squatting in a patient with tetralogy of Fallot.

noncardiac cause such as venous stasis, thrombophlebitis, nephrotic syndrome, lymphedema, or idiopathic edema. Edema is seldom seen in patients with congestive heart failure under good medical control now that effective diuretic therapy is available. Right heart failure can be surprisingly severe, with hepatic enlargement, ascites, and a raised venous pressure, but no significant pitting edema of the ankles.

Cyanosis

Patients occasionally complain of blueness of the extremities, face, and lips. Cyanosis may be **peripheral** and associated with a low cardiac output, peripheral vasoconstriction, and a feeling of coldness. In this case, the blueness is due to a high concentration of reduced hemoglobin in the blood in the veins of the skin, and arterial saturation is normal. In true **central** cyanosis, the arterial oxygen saturation is reduced because of right-to-left shunting or lung disease. In this case, the patient's extremities are often warm, or if they are made warm, the blue color does not disappear.

Loss of Weight (Cardiac Cachexia)

Loss of weight is not a presenting symptom of heart disease, but it does occur in chronically ill cardiac patients, especially when the cardiac output is low. It is probably related to secondary anorexia. The patient characteristically loses weight from the limbs and accumulates fluid in the abdomen. It is difficult to establish the true extent of the cachexia, because the accumulation of fluid tends to maintain total body weight.

FUNCTIONAL & THERAPEUTIC CLASSIFICATION OF HEART DISEASE

The patient's overall disability is conventionally expressed in terms of the New York Heart Association's criteria for functional capacity.

Functional Capacity (Four classes)

Class I: No limitation of physical activity. Ordinary physical activity does not cause undue fatigue, palpitation, dyspnea, or anginal pain.

Class II: Slight limitation of physical activity. Comfortable at rest, but ordinary physical activity results in fatigue, palpitation, dyspnea, or anginal pain.

Class III: Marked limitation of physical activity. Comfortable at rest, but less than ordinary activity causes fatigue, palpitation, dyspnea, or anginal pain.

Class IV: Unable to carry on any physical activity without discomfort. Symptoms of cardiac insufficiency or of the anginal syndrome may be present even at rest. If any physical activity is undertaken, discomfort is increased.

While this classification gives a good overall indication of the patient's status, many physicians prefer to subdivide class II into classes IIa and IIb. In class IIa, the patient can keep up with others walking on the flat but has limitation on more severe exercise such as climbing stairs. In class IIb, the patient has slight limitation on all forms of physical activity.

REFERENCES

Barcroft H et al: Posthaemorrhagic fainting: Study by cardiac output and forearm flow. *Lancet* 1944;**1**:489.

Boucher IAD, Morris JS: *Clinical Skills*. Saunders, 1982.

Frank MJ, Alvarez-Mena SC, Abdulla AM: *Cardiovascular Physical Diagnosis*, 2nd ed. Year Book, 1983.

Grover RF, Hultgren HN, Hartley LH: Pathogenesis of acute pulmonary edema at high altitude. Page 409 in: *Central Hemodynamics and Gas Exchange*. Giutini C (editor). Minerva Medica, 1971.

Heberden W: *Commentaries on the History and Cure of Diseases*. London, 1802.

Herrick JB: Clinical features of sudden obstruction of the coronary arteries. *JAMA* 1912;**59**:2015.

Horwitz LD, Groves BM: *Signs and Symptoms in Cardiology*. Lippincott, 1984.

Hultgren HN et al: Physiologic studies of pulmonary edema at high altitude. *Circulation* 1964;**29**:393.

Johnson AD, Detweiller JH: Coronary spasm, variant angina and recurrent myocardial infarctions. *Circulation* 1977;**55**:947.

Levine H: Difficult problems in the diagnosis of chest pain. *Am Heart J* 1980;**100**:108.

Lewis HP: *The History and the Physical Examination*. Appleton-Century-Crofts, 1979.

McIlroy MB: Breathlessness in cardiovascular disease. Pages 187–202 in: *Manchester Symposium on Breathlessness*. Blackwell, 1966.

Mendel D: *Proper Doctoring*. Springer-Verlag, 1984.

O'Donnell TV, McIlroy MB: The circulatory effects of squatting. *Am Heart J* 1962;**64**:347.

Parry CH: *An Inquiry Into the Symptoms and Causes of the Syncope Anginosa, Commonly Called Angina Pectoris: Illustrated by Dissections*. London, 1799.

Prinzmetal M et al: Angina pectoris. 1. A variant form of angina pectoris. *Am J Med* 1959;**26**:375.

Sandler G: The importance of the history in the medical clinic and the cost of unnecessary tests. *Am Heart J* 1980;**100**:928.

Sharpey-Schafer EP: The mechanism of syncope after coughing. *Br Med J* 1953;**2**:860.

Silverman ME: *Examination of the Heart*. Part 1: *The Clinical History*. American Heart Association, 1975.

Weiss S, Baker JP: The carotid sinus reflex in health and disease: Its role in the causation of fainting and convulsions. *Medicine* 1933;**12**:297.

Wood P: Attacks of deeper cyanosis and loss of consciousness (syncope) in Fallot's tetralogy. *Br Heart J* 1958;**20**:282.

Wood P: *Diseases of the Heart and Circulation*, 3rd ed. Lippincott, 1968.

Wood P: Polyuria in paroxysmal tachycardia and paroxysmal atrial flutter and fibrillation. *Br Heart J* 1963;**25**:273.

3

Physical Examination

This chapter deals with only the more general or introductory aspects of the physical examination of the patient with heart disease. Details of the physical manifestations of cardiac disease appear under the description of each disease.

It is important to emphasize that examination of the cardiac patient is not confined to those parts of the body in which manifestations of cardiac disease are most commonly seen. Physicians should remember that cardiac disease can be associated with any disease from acromegaly to Zollinger-Ellison syndrome and that clues to the existence of noncardiac disorders which simulate, complicate, or merely coexist with heart disease may be apparent on methodic physical examination.

Approach to the Physical Examination

The general appearance and behavior of the patient are noted as the medical history is recorded. Similarly, the history-taking process may continue during the physical examination. The patient may be questioned about any findings and asked about awareness of signs and duration of such manifestations.

Examination of the patient usually starts from the head and proceeds downward. Inspection precedes palpation, percussion, and auscultation. The cardiologist traditionally feels the patient's pulse while carrying out the preliminary inspection, and many physicians start by recording the vital signs—pulse, temperature, and respiration—and blood pressure.

PULSES

The Radial Arterial Pulse

Palpation of the pulse wave that results from transmission of the pressure wave down the artery is usually performed on the patient's right wrist, with the examiner using the first 3 fingers of the right hand. The frequency, regularity, amplitude, rate of upstroke, and volume of the radial pulse require only one finger for their evaluation, but the rate of propagation of the wave (pulse wave velocity) and the thickness of the artery can only be properly examined with 3 fingers. The amplitude of the pulse (small or large) depends mainly on the pulse pressure and gives a rough indication of stroke volume. Thus the "small" pulse of severe mitral stenosis contrasts with the "large," jerky pulse seen in patients with mitral incompetence. In aortic stenosis, the rate of travel of the wave is slow; the "pulsus tardus" in this condition means that the pulse takes longer to pass under the examiner's fingers. The ease with which the pulse can be obliterated is felt by compressing the artery with the proximal finger and palpating with the other 2 in order to ascertain when the wave has disappeared. It is a rough indication of the systolic arterial pressure (Fig 3–1) and is considerably less accurate than the measurement obtained by sphygmomanometry. The thickness of the undistended arterial wall can be felt using the middle finger to palpate while the proximal and distal fingers simultaneously occlude the vessel. It gives an indication of the degree of atherosclerosis.

A. Sinus Arrhythmia: In sinus arrhythmia, the heart rate varies with the phase of respiration. Inspiration increases and expiration decreases the rate via vagally mediated reflexes. Expiration favors left ventricular filling by increasing the return to the left heart of blood that was stored in the lungs during inspiration. If the heart obeys **Starling's law,** increased filling increases stroke volume, and the consequent increase in arterial pressure provokes reflex bradycardia. Sinus arrhythmia is commoner in young, healthy athletes. It is not seen in patients with heart failure or large left-to-right shunts and is less marked in sick sinus syndrome.

B. Atrial Fibrillation: In atrial fibrillation, the heartbeat is irregular in rate and in force. The irregular beats occur in an irregular pattern, and the force of cardiac contraction varies from beat to beat. The irregularity is usually more obvious during exercise.

C. Ectopic Beats: In ectopic beats, the heart rate is irregular but the pattern is often regular. Beats may occur in pairs (**pulsus bigeminus**) or in runs of 3 or more. Ectopic beats in persons with normal cardiovascular function often disappear on exercise.

Other Arterial Pulses
(See also Neck, p 46.)

It is important to feel the pulse bilaterally to check for differences in timing and intensity. Brachial, radial,

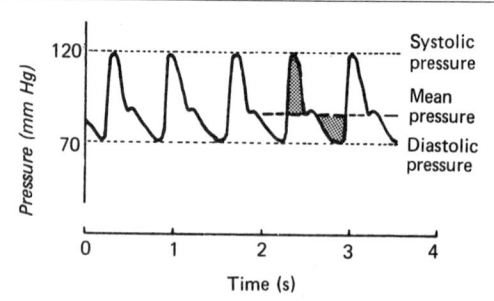

Figure 3–1. Brachial artery pressure curve of normal young person, showing the relation of systolic and diastolic pressure to mean pressure. The shaded area above the mean pressure line is equal to the shaded area below it. (Reproduced, with permission, from Ganong WF: *Review of Medical Physiology,* 12th ed. Lange, 1985.)

carotid, femoral, popliteal, and posterior tibial pulses are usually examined routinely. By this means, the physician may obtain clues about peripheral vascular disease, aortic dissection, and coarctation of the aorta. The closer the vessel lies to the heart, the more reliable the pulse is as an indicator of aortic pressure wave characteristics. Thus, the carotid arterial pulse is best for assessment of aortic valve disease. If there is a prominent pulse in the neck or if coarctation of the aorta is suspected for any other reason, it is important to feel the radial and femoral pulses simultaneously. In normal subjects, the 2 pulses are synchronous, whereas in coarctation of the aorta the femoral pulse is felt up to 0.15 second after the radial.

BLOOD PRESSURE

Measurement of Blood Pressure

A. Measurement in the Arms: Indirect measurement of the systemic arterial pressure is conventionally performed using a sphygmomanometer on the right arm. A 12.5-cm cuff is wrapped around the upper arm and connected to a mercury or aneroid manometer. The arm is placed at heart level and the cuff is inflated to a level above the systolic pressure. The absence of a radial pulse is checked at the wrist. The cuff is slowly deflated (around 2 mm/beat) while the examiner feels the radial pulse. The pressure level at which the pulse is first felt is noted, and the cuff is reinflated. The cuff is then deflated a second time, with the examiner listening over the brachial artery with the stethoscope. The pressure level at which a sound is first heard over the artery is recorded as the systolic pressure. As deflation of the cuff continues, the sound arising from the vessel wall increases in intensity, decreases, becomes muffled, and finally disappears. Differences of opinion exist about the accuracy of considering the muffling or disappearance of sound as an indication of the diastolic pressure. Because the appropriate world cardiologic governing bodies are still undecided about whether it is the muffling of the sounds or their disappearance that is the "correct" level to use, both should be recorded. Correlation between direct arterial pressure measurement and sphygmomanometry has shown reasonable agreement between the 2 methods, especially in normal subjects, but the differences are sometimes marked in individual cases.

Blood pressure should be measured in both the standing and the supine positions in patients who might have hypotension or hypertension, and the pulse rate should always be measured and recorded along with the pressure. Blood pressure should be measured in both arms when the patient is first seen. On subsequent visits, it is taken in the right arm, except when the pulse in that arm is significantly reduced, as, for example, after a Blalock-Taussig operation for tetralogy of Fallot. The site of the measurement and position of the patient should be recorded.

Artifacts in measurement. Artifacts in indirect measurement occur when the arm is large in relation to the cuff (Fig 3–2); when a patient has aortic incompetence, in which the indirectly measured diastolic pressure is usually falsely low; and when the patient is in shock. An erroneously low systolic pressure may be obtained in some hypertensive patients in whom the systolic pressure is not checked by palpation. An

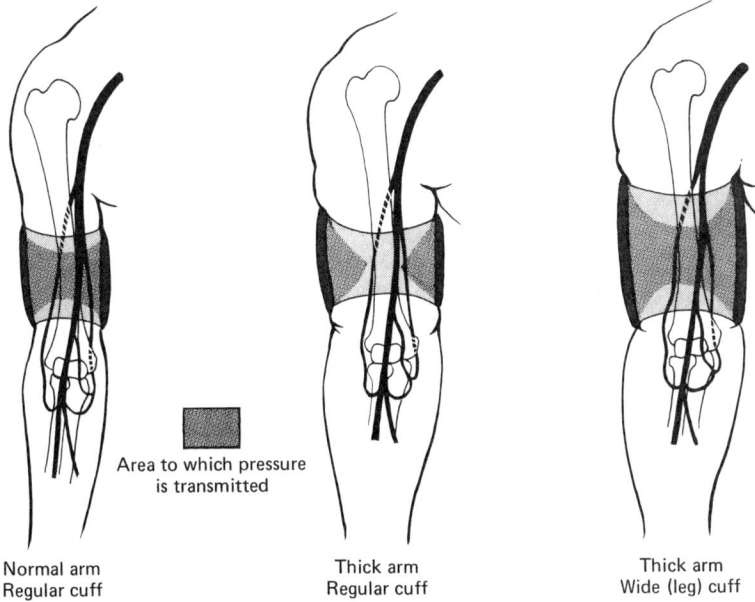

Figure 3–2. Diagram showing that pressure is not transmitted to the brachial artery when a regular cuff is used to measure blood pressure in a thick arm.

"auscultatory gap" may be present in such patients and in those with aortic stenosis and localized arteriosclerosis. The auscultatory gap is a range of pressures over which arterial sounds are absent even though arterial flow is present and the cuff pressure is not above the arterial pressure.

B. Measurement in the Legs: The measurement of arterial pressure in both arms and both legs is advocated by some as a routine measure. If the leg pressure is to be measured, a special wide (20 cm) cuff is used; such a cuff is also needed for patients with thick or fat arms. The diagnosis of coarctation of the aorta is usually made on other grounds. In difficult cases, simultaneous brachial and femoral arterial tracings obtained during exercise may be needed.

Pulsus Alternans & Pulsus Paradoxus

Pulsus alternans and pulsus paradoxus should be sought when the blood pressure is measured. In pulsus alternans, every other heartbeat produces a higher systolic pressure. The alternation of small- and large-amplitude beats with a regular rhythm can be detected by palpation. The mechanism is unknown although many theories have been proposed, and the finding, which is seen in left ventricular failure, carries a poor prognosis, especially if the heart rate is slow. Fig 3-3 shows an example of pulsus alternans in a brachial arterial pressure tracing in a patient with aortic stenosis.

A similar form of alternation in the force of cardiac contraction occurs in the right heart in response to right heart failure. Pulsus alternans sometimes starts after an ectopic beat and lasts for several beats. It may occur when the patient stands or starts to exercise. The more constant the pulsus alternans, the worse the prognosis.

Pulsus paradoxus is principally associated with pericardial disease in which cardiac filling is compromised. The abnormality shown in right and left ventricular pressure tracings in Fig 3-4 consists of an exaggeration of the normal respiratory fluctuation in

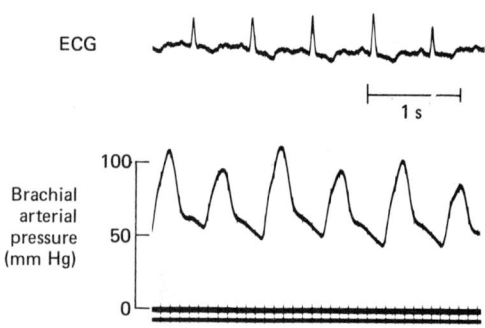

Figure 3-3. ECG and brachial arterial pulse pressure in a patient with pulsus alternans.

systolic pressure (ie, weakening of the pulse during inspiration). The arterial pressure (systolic, diastolic, and mean) normally falls by a few mm Hg when intrathoracic negative pressure increases during inspiration. If the systolic fall amounts to greater than 10 mm Hg (or more than 10% of the systolic pressure), pulsus paradoxus is present. The phenomenon can be due to an increase in the amplitude of intrathoracic pressure fluctuations resulting from changes in the mechanical properties of the lungs, as occurs in large pneumothorax, pleural effusion, or obstructive lung disease. It is more commonly due to pericardial disease, especially cardiac tamponade. As fluid accumulates in the pericardial cavity in the course of pericardial effusion, the intrapericardial pressure rises. If the fluid is formed more rapidly than the pericardium can stretch, the rise in pressure may be sufficient to compress the heart in diastole. If pericardial fluid is formed slowly, as in myxedema, the pericardium has time to stretch, and cardiac tamponade does not occur.

Cardiac tamponade occurs when the pericardial pressure reaches the level of the diastolic pressure in the heart. Since the right-sided pressures are lower than those of the left, the right heart is the first to be

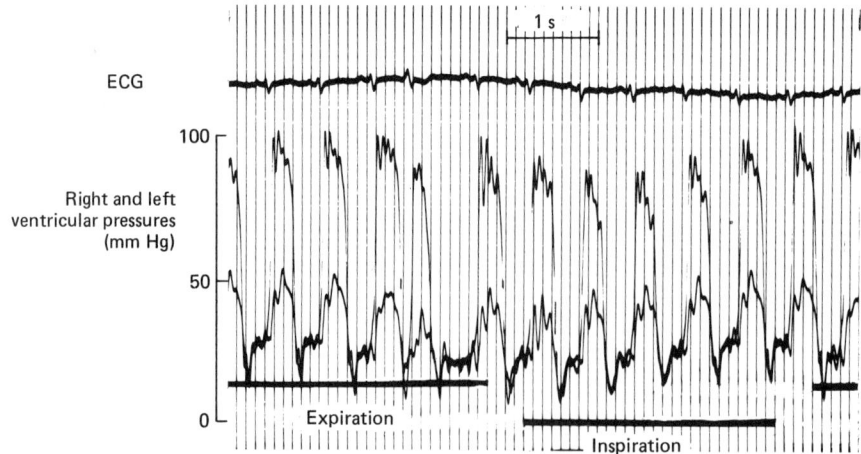

Figure 3-4. Pulsus paradoxus in right and left ventricular pressure tracings in a patient with chronic constrictive pericarditis.

compressed. In tamponade, the maintenance of cardiac volume depends on the level of the venous pressure (right- and left-sided), and the 2 ventricles compete for blood with which to fill in diastole. Respiration has a marked effect on hemodynamics, with inspiration favoring the right ventricle both by increasing its filling, volume, and output and also by pooling blood in the lungs, decreasing left-sided venous return and occasionally displacing the ventricular septum in severe cases. Conversely, on expiration, the extra blood passes from the lungs to the left ventricle as the right ventricle is compressed and left-sided output enhanced. Pulsus paradoxus is the most obvious clinical sign of this process. It does not occur in cardiac tamponade until the pericardial pressure has risen to the level of the right atrial pressure, and it disappears when sufficient fluid is withdrawn to make the pericardial pressure lower than the atrial pressure. The pericardial pressure must rise to equal or exceed that in both the left and the right ventricles before pulsus paradoxus occurs. If the left ventricle is hypertrophied, as in hypertension associated with chronic renal disease, it is less readily compressed by pericardial effusion, and right ventricular tamponade can occur before left ventricular tamponade. Pulsus paradoxus does not occur until filling of both ventricles is impaired, because the reciprocal effect of respiration is an essential part of the mechanism in pericardial tamponade.

EXAMINATION OF ORGANS & REGIONS OTHER THAN THE HEART

Examination of organs of the body other than the heart can provide important clues in the diagnosis of heart disease. Clinical findings and the symptoms and signs that may be noted on examination of various body structures are noted below.

SKIN & MUCOUS MEMBRANES

The state of the peripheral circulation can be determined by inspection and palpation of the skin. If there is vasoconstriction, the skin will be pale, blue, and cold, with diminished flow in the superficial veins. There may be cold, clammy perspiration in low-output states. If there is widespread vasodilatation, as seen in high-output states (Chapter 20) or aortic incompetence, the skin is warm, pink, and moist. The forearm veins are usually distended, and venous flow is high. Pallor of the skin and mucous membranes suggests anemia, and coarse, dry, scaly skin is seen in myxedema. In scleroderma, the skin is tight, smooth, and shiny. These changes are best seen in the fingers and backs of the hands and in the face over the nose.

Cyanosis

The color of the skin and mucous membranes can reflect the oxygen saturation of the blood. Bluish, cyanotic skin may be due to increased concentration of reduced hemoglobin in the arterial blood, indicating arterial anoxemia, or to reduced blood flow in the skin, leading to pooling of blood in the skin (peripheral cyanosis). The detection of cyanosis and the distinction between central (arterial) and peripheral (venous) cyanosis should be based on measurements of arterial oxygen levels.

With reversed (right-to-left) shunting through a patent ductus arteriosus, mixed venous blood is shunted to the legs, while arterial blood reaches the arms through the left side of the heart. There may be cyanosis and perhaps clubbing of the toes but normal color in the hands and no clubbing of the fingers. This characteristic abnormality is more easily recognized if the arms and legs are compared after a hot bath.

Nodes & Other Skin Lesions

A. Rheumatic Nodules: Rheumatic nodules are seen around the joints in both rheumatic fever and rheumatoid arthritis. They are painless, mobile, subcutaneous lesions measuring up to about 1 cm in diameter, occurring around the elbows, knees, and knuckles and also in the occipital region.

B. Osler's Nodes: Osler's nodes are small, tender, red lesions that should be looked for in the pulp of the fingers and toes and on the palms and soles. They are transient embolic lesions characteristic of infective endocarditis (Chapter 16). They last for 4–5 days and gradually darken before fading and becoming painless. Such lesions seldom, if ever, suppurate.

C. Erythema Nodosum: Erythema nodosum causes pinkish-red, raised, tender lesions on the shins or forearms that represent a nonspecific allergic response to antigens, including streptococcal infections associated with rheumatic fever and sarcoidosis.

D. Xanthoma Tuberosum: Xanthoma tuberosum causes pale, yellowish skin lesions that are often superficial extensions of tendinous xanthomas. The lesions are seen on the hands and feet and around the elbows and knees and represent deposits of lipid material in familial hypercholesterolemia.

E. Lesions Associated With Osler's Disease: The lesions of Osler's disease (hereditary hemorrhagic telangiectasia) are also seen on the skin. They are multiple dark-red lesions 1 or 2 mm in diameter that often occur on mucous membranes in the nose and mouth. They may also occur in the viscera and cause hemorrhage. Pulmonary arteriovenous fistulas (Chapter 19) may occur in association with this condition.

F. Petechiae: Petechiae are due to minute hemorrhages into the skin, resulting from increased capillary fragility. They tend to occur in crops and fade over several days, in contrast to telangiectases, which are permanent.

G. Spider Nevi: Spider nevi, seen in liver disease, are also permanent telangiectatic lesions. They are seen on the skin over the upper part of the body. As

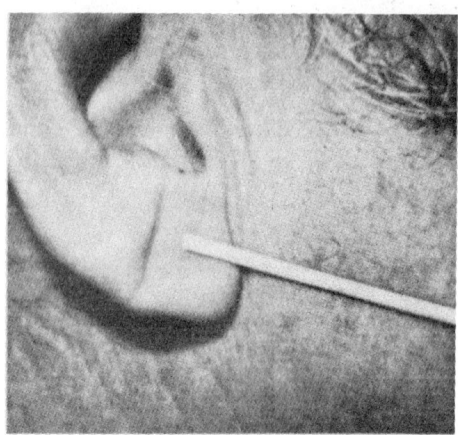

Figure 3–5. The earlobe sign—a deep crease in the lobular portion of the auricle. (Reproduced, with permission, from Frank ST: Aural sign of coronary-artery disease. *N Engl J Med* 1973;289:327.)

their name implies, there is a central body with radiating vascular channels.

EYES

Examination of the conjunctival membranes may detect petechial hemorrhages. An abnormal pupillary reflex in which the reaction to light is lost but the accommodation reaction is retained **(Argyll-Robertson pupil)** is strong evidence for the presence of cardiovascular syphilis. The presence of a hazy gray ring about 2 mm in diameter in the cornea **(arcus senilis)** is, as its name implies, commonly seen in older persons. It is of no clinical significance. Direct visual examination of small arteries and arterioles in the fundus offers an important opportunity to assess the condition of the blood vessels, the retina, and the optic disk. The findings and their classification are discussed in Chapter 9. Hemorrhages and embolic phenomena (Roth spots) can also be seen in the retinas of patients with infective endocarditis.

EARS

Inspection of the earlobe may reveal a deep crease at the site shown in Fig 3–5. Ear creases are associated with age and are present in most people over age 60. However, their occurrence in younger people is associated with a high incidence of premature atherosclerotic changes involving the cerebral, coronary, or aortoiliac vessels.

NECK

The nature of the jugular venous pulse and pressure and the carotid pulse, and the presence of a goiter are sought in the examination of the neck. Thyroid swellings are best detected by the examiner standing behind the seated patient, with both hands around the neck. The upward movement of the gland with swallowing is the most important means of identifying a thyroid origin for a palpable mass. Marked pulsation in the base of the neck on the right side is seen in elderly atherosclerotic people. It is due to kinking of the right carotid artery resulting from dilatation of the aortic arch, which causes the aorta to occupy a higher position in the mediastinum. This benign condition is more common in women.

Jugular Venous Pulse & Pressure

The level of the venous pressure and the nature of the venous pulse are perhaps the most important observations to be made in the examination of the neck. The internal jugular vein should be examined because it lies deep to the sternocleidomastoid muscle and is in free communication with the right atrium. The external jugular vein is often easier to see, but it may be constricted as it passes through the fascial planes of the neck and may give an inaccurate assessment of venous events. The positioning of the patient is most important in examining the veins in the neck. The angle at which the patient is supported in the bed should be adjusted to bring the meniscus of blood in the vein to a level between the clavicles and the angle of the jaw (Fig 3–6). The higher the venous pressure, the more erect the patient should be; patients with severe venous congestion may have to stand up and breathe in deeply in order to bring the level of the meniscus into view. The head should be comfortably supported in order to relax the neck muscles. Any movement of the earlobes should be noted, because this is always due to venous rather than arterial pulsation. Timing of the venous waves against the carotid pulse is carried out by feeling the artery on the opposite side of the neck or by listening to the heart, and *not* by feeling the radial pulse. Interpretation of the pulse wave pattern is sometimes facilitated by observ-

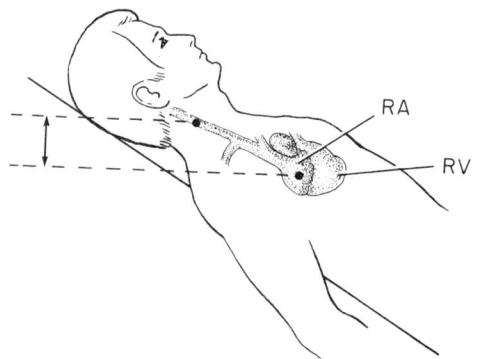

Figure 3–6. Examination of jugular venous pulse and estimation of venous pressure. RA, right atrium; RV, right ventricle.

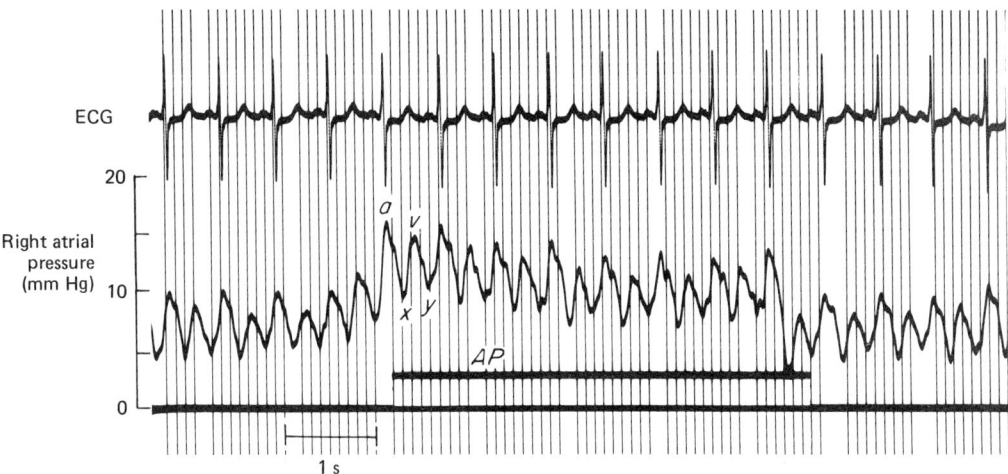

Figure 3–7. ECG and right atrial pressure in a normal subject showing the response to external abdominal compression (AP).

ing when the venous pressure falls. The first venous trough, the x descent, coincides with the carotid arterial pulse. Distinguishing arterial from venous pulses in the neck can be difficult. Venous pulses can be palpable; they are diffusely expansile and influenced by respiration.

Some authorities advocate exerting pressure over the abdomen to distend the neck veins; the results of this technique are shown in Fig 3–7. They maintain that the magnitude of the resulting venous distention (hepatojugular reflux) reflects the level of venous congestion. We believe that although hepatojugular reflux is especially marked in right heart failure, it can also be seen in normal subjects, and that proper positioning of the patient, relaxation with the mouth open, and quiet normal breathing are more important factors in evaluating venous pressure.

Direct bedside assessment of right atrial pressure requires skill and practice, but it can obviate the need for central venous pressure measurement, which requires use of a catheter. The level of the venous pressure is most important in distinguishing cardiac failure with edema and ascites from hepatic or renal disease with similar findings. Unfortunately, it is often in those patients with highest venous pressures that the examiner fails to note the raised pressure.

A. Normal Venous Pulse: The normal waves seen in the venous pulse in the neck are shown in the first and fourth beats in the tracing in Fig 3–8. The positive waves are a, c, and v, and the troughs are x_1, x_2, and y. The a wave is due to atrial contraction. It follows the P wave of the ECG and is absent in atrial fibrillation. The origin of the c wave is more controversial. It was originally noted in tracings of the venous pres-

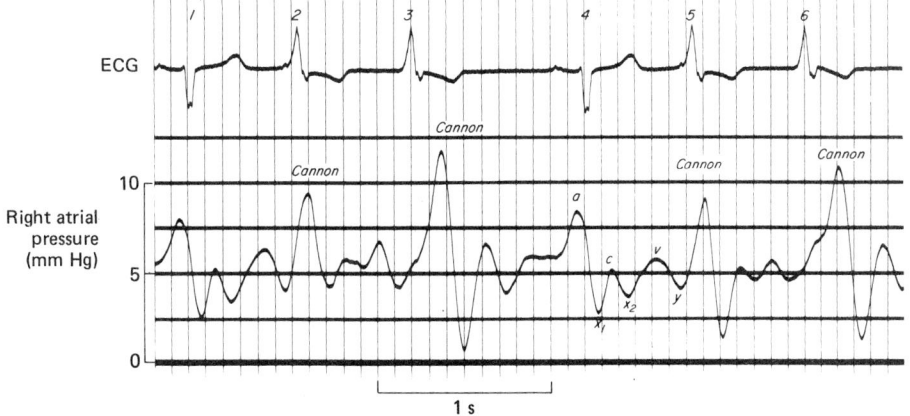

Figure 3–8. Right atrial pressure tracing in a patient with junctional ectopic beats. Beats 1 and 4 are sinus beats and produce normal venous pressure pulses. The other beats are junctional and give rise to cannon waves of varying sizes.

sure in the neck and attributed to the effects of carotid arterial pulsation. When it was also observed in right atrial pressure tracings, however, this explanation became untenable. It is now thought to be due to bulging of the tricuspid valve back into the atrium at the start of ventricular systole. The v wave is associated with atrial filling; pressure in the atrium rises to the v peak and falls as the tricuspid valve opens and the atrium empties into the ventricle. The x_1 and x_2 troughs are attributed to descent of the base of the heart during ventricular systole. The backward bulging of the valve interrupts this process to produce the c wave. The c wave is not always seen. When it is absent, there is a single x descent. The y descent to the y trough is due to atrial emptying, and its rate is influenced by stenosis or insufficiency of the atrioventricular valve.

B. Abnormal or Exaggerated Venous Pulse:

1. Cannon waves–The magnitude of the a wave resulting from atrial contraction varies with the PR interval. In the tracing shown in Fig 3–8, all but beats 1 and 4 are ectopic, with the P wave occurring at the start of the QRS complex. The a waves associated with these beats are larger and are referred to as cannon waves because of their explosive appearance when seen in the neck. The largest cannon waves are seen when atrial contraction occurs at a time when the tricuspid valve is closed, as in beats 3 and 6 in the tracing. Here the P wave is buried in the QRS complex, and large cannon waves can be seen. Irregular cannon waves of this type are also seen in complete atrioventricular block with atrioventricular dissociation. Regular cannon waves are seen in junctional tachycardia and in atrial tachycardia with rapid rates and a long PR interval.

2. Giant a wave–The a wave is increased in force and amplitude in the presence of right ventricular hypertrophy. It is best seen as the "giant a wave" of pulmonary stenosis, shown in Fig 3–9, which is a short, sharp, flicking wave occurring just before ventricular systole. A large a wave is also seen in pulmonary hypertension and in tricuspid valve disease with stenosis.

3. Giant v wave–A large v wave is seen in patients with tricuspid incompetence, especially when atrial fibrillation is present, as in the tracing in Fig 3–10. Tricuspid incompetence is seldom seen in patients with sinus rhythm, but when it occurs, a, x, v, and y peaks and troughs are present. The x descent is usually absent in patients with either tricuspid incompetence or pericardial constriction, and the y descent may be the principal event in the venous pulse.

4. Effect of inspiration–Inspiration may stretch the tricuspid valve and make it incompetent, thus increasing the height of the v wave and the depth of the y trough, as shown in Fig 3–10. When right heart filling is severely impaired, inspiration causes a rise in venous pressure, as shown in Fig 3–11. This rise is known as **Kussmaul's sign,** and it is seen in pericardial constriction and severe right heart failure. The overfilled right heart cannot accommodate the increased venous return associated with the inspiratory fall in intrathoracic pressure. The venous pressure therefore shows a rise with inspiration, instead of the normal fall. In tricuspid incompetence, it is the amplitude of the pulsations that tends to increase (Fig 3–10) rather than the mean pressure, as in pericardial disease (Fig 3–11).

ARMS

Brachial and radial pulses should be compared between the 2 arms, and they should also be compared with the femoral pulses. The fingers, nails, and palms should be examined for evidence of embolism.

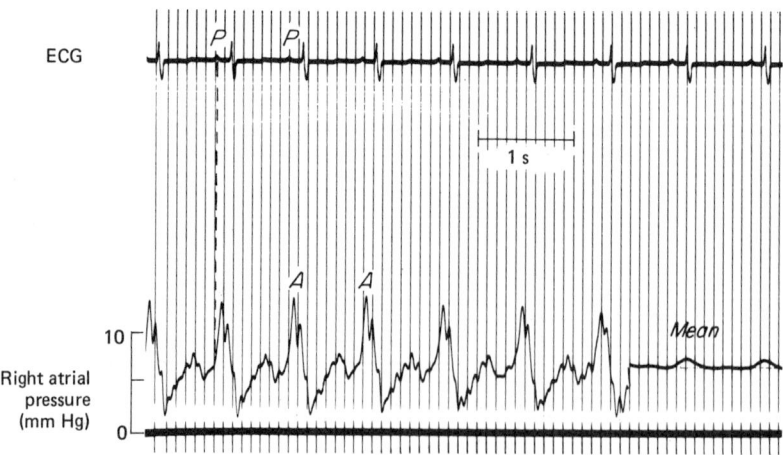

Figure 3–9. Right atrial pressure tracing showing giant a wave (A) in a patient with severe pulmonary stenosis. The a wave follows the P wave of the ECG.

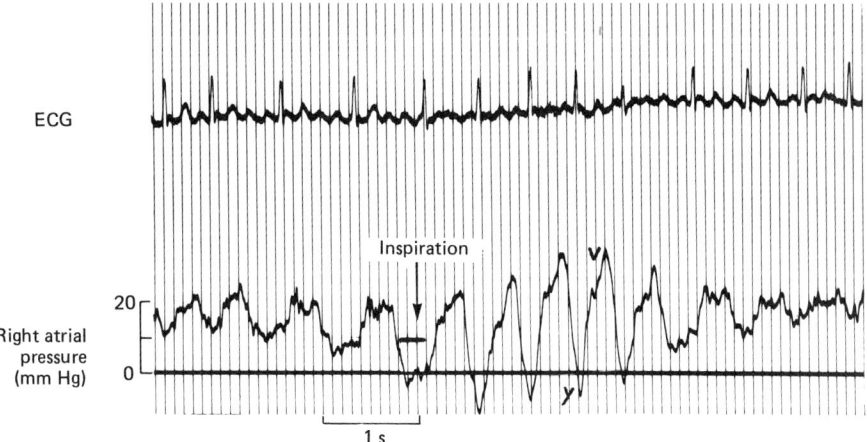

Figure 3-10. Right atrial pressure tracing in a patient with tricuspid incompetence and atrial fibrillation. The v peak and the y trough are exaggerated during inspiration.

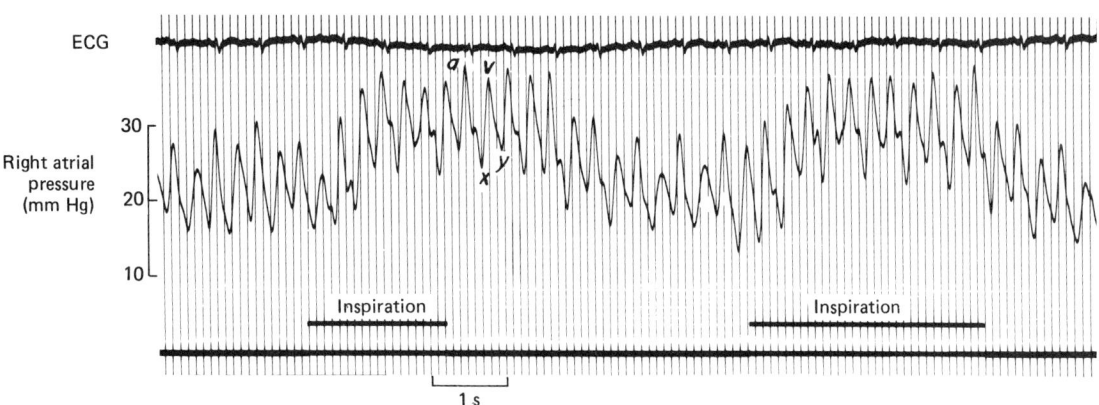

Figure 3-11. ECG and right atrial pressure tracings in a patient with constrictive pericarditis, showing inspiratory increase in pressure (Kussmaul's sign).

FINGERS

Clubbing of the fingers and nail beds (Fig 3-12) is seen in cyanotic congenital heart lesions, infective endocarditis, cor pulmonale, and occasionally in left atrial myxoma. Clubbing of the fingers is also seen in chronic pulmonary infections, cirrhosis of the liver, and bronchial carcinoma. In the latter, severe clubbing with hypertrophic osteoarthropathy may occur; clubbing is sometimes unilateral and may disappear after resection of the tumor.

Splinter hemorrhages in the nail beds should be sought as an indication of endocarditis, although it should be noted that similar findings may sometimes be seen in normal people. Other finger abnormalities associated with congenital heart disease include arachnodactyly, in which the fingers are long and spidery. This is seen in Marfan's syndrome and in some patients with atrial septal defect.

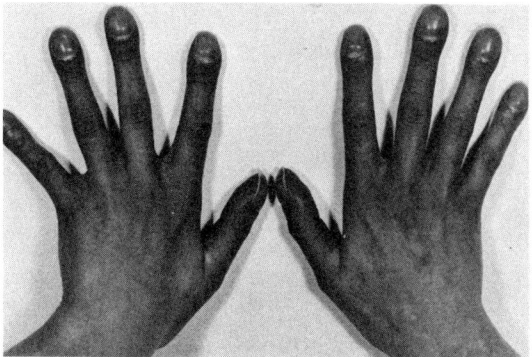

Figure 3-12. Clubbing of the fingers in a patient with congenital heart disease.

LUNGS

Examination of the lungs in patients with heart disease focuses on the detection of pleural fluid and a search for rales and crepitations, especially at the base of the lungs posteriorly. Such findings reflect raised pulmonary venous pressure. Added sounds are noted when there is fluid in the alveoli, but the signs are not specific, and they may be absent in some cases of obvious pulmonary edema. They are often due to other causes. Pleural effusion due to heart failure is usually bilateral; in unilateral cases, it is commoner on the side on which the subject habitually lies. Evidence of collapse of the left lower lobe should be sought in patients with marked left atrial enlargement.

BACK

Some cardiac murmurs are heard well in the back. The best examples are the murmurs of coarctation of the aorta, increased bronchial collateral flow, and peripheral pulmonary artery stenosis; the last is often heard well in the axilla as well. Evidence of systemic collateral vessels in coarctation of the aorta is also well seen and felt in the back. Large, pulsating vessels can be detected near the angles of the scapulas. Edema of the lumbar region and sacrum is also sought while the physician examines the patient's back.

ABDOMEN

In examining the abdomen, enlargement and tenderness of the liver and spleen should be sought as evidence of systemic venous congestion. The spleen may also be the site of a friction rub in infective endocarditis. Ascites and pitting edema of the ankles are evidence of congestive heart failure. Disproportionate ascites with minimal leg edema suggests pericardial constriction or prolonged diuretic therapy.

LOWER EXTREMITIES

In examining the lower extremities, the physician palpates the femoral pulse; if its palpability is in question or if the patient is hypertensive, it is useful to look for delay between the radial and femoral pulse (see p 354). Absence of femoral pulsations and inequality between the 2 sides may suggest embolic disease or aortic dissection. Calf tenderness and pain on dorsiflexion of the foot (**Homans' sign**) are evidence of venous thrombosis. Clubbing of the toes is seen in cyanotic congenital heart disease. In addition to looking for edema of the sacrum, the examiner should check for edema in the flanks and medial aspects of the thighs in bedridden patients.

URINE

Examination of the urine is an important adjunct to the physical examination. Proteinuria should be sought in heart failure, in hypertensive patients, and in primary renal disease. Hematuria suggests renal infarction; if microscopic, infective endocarditis. Specific gravity should be recorded and the urinary sediment examined for casts and other abnormalities.

EXAMINATION OF THE HEART & CHEST

INSPECTION

Examination of the chest starts with inspection of the shape and movements of the thorax and a search for visible pulsations. Chest deformities such as kyphosis and scoliosis may cause heart disease, but in general, it is remarkable how a severe deformity can exist without causing cardiac embarrassment. Depressed sternum with pectus excavatum is obvious on inspection, and although it is often associated with benign heart murmurs, it is seldom of more than cosmetic importance. The left parasternal area sometimes bulges in patients who have had heart disease since early in life. Ventricular septal defect is the commonest lesion causing this sign.

Visible Pulsations

The cardiac impulse can sometimes be seen in normal subjects either in the area of the left nipple or in the epigastrium. Pulsation in the second or third left interspace over the right ventricular outflow tract can be seen in normal thin persons, but it can also suggest pulmonary hypertension or increased pulmonary blood flow. Pulsation to the right of the sternum is always abnormal, and when seen in the second or third interspace, it indicates aneurysmal dilatation of the ascending aorta.

Periodic Breathing

Abnormalities of respiratory rhythm should be noted during inspection of the chest. The commonest abnormality is periodic breathing. This can occur in normal subjects at high altitude and may also be seen after head injuries. When it is due to heart disease, the cycle of hyperventilation followed by hypoventilation and apnea with subsequent gradual increase of ventilation lasts 40–120 seconds. The phenomenon results from oscillation of the feedback control mechanisms regulating respiration. In a patient with severe ventricular failure, there is an abnormal lag between the timing of the neurologic stimulus to breathe and the arrival back at the control center in the brain of the humoral signal resulting from respiratory changes in blood gases following the breath. This lag is thought to play an important part in the mechanism of periodic breathing. Periodic breathing is usually referred to as **Cheyne-Stokes breathing.** In the classic description, apnea was present, but this feature is not necessarily a component. The length of the lung-to-brain circulation time determines the length of the period of one cycle. By following this measurement, the examiner can note the progress of left ventricular failure. Periodic breathing is usually a manifestation of hyper- rather than hypoventilation and is generally abolished by giving oxygen, CO_2, or aminophylline. It tends to occur at night when sensory input is low and to disappear when a mouthpiece and nose clip are used to obtain spirometric tracings.

PALPATION

Palpation of the chest is used to confirm the presence of pulsations that have been noted on inspection. The cardiac impulse is routinely sought and can be elicited by having the patient roll over to the left side. The examiner should note the nature of the impulse and distinguish between the feel of a large left ventricle and a right ventricle. The site where the impulse is felt is of primary importance in distinguishing the 2 impulses; in addition, the right ventricular impulse is more lifting than the left, is perceived as being farther from the hand, and less readily moves the examining fingers. The feel of a ventricle with a large stroke volume should be distinguished from the feel of a hypertrophied ventricle. Hypertrophy imparts a forceful sustained thrust (heave) with relatively little movement of the examiner's hand, whereas increased stroke volume gives a more dynamic movement of greater amplitude. A "tapping" impulse is found in patients with mitral valve disease. This reflects the palpable vibrations of a loud first heart sound felt at the apex.

Apex Beat

The position of the apex beat should always be located by palpation. It is the point farthest downward and outward at which the cardiac impulse can be clearly felt. Before the determination of cardiac size by chest radiography became routine, the position of the apex beat in the absence of lung disease was the most important measure of heart size. Its position should be described in relation to the intercostal space and to the distance from the midline, the nipple, or the midclavicular, anterior axillary, or midaxillary lines. These are imaginary lines drawn vertically through various planes. Palpation of the base of the heart may detect an impulse caused by closure of the aortic or pulmonary valves or arising from an aneurysm. The findings should be interpreted in light of the patient's build.

Thrills

The significance of palpable thrills is similar to that of cardiac murmurs and is discussed below (see Auscultation). Thrills are palpable, sustained high-frequency vibrations associated with the same disturbances of flow that cause heart murmurs. A murmur that is associated with a thrill is likely to have an organic cause.

Palpable Impulses

Palpable impulses over the precordium must be interpreted in light of their associated findings; it is not always possible to be certain of their origin. In a patient with mitral incompetence, a substernal impulse may be due to systolic expansion of the left atrium rather than to right ventricular overactivity. Epigastric pulsations may arise from the abdominal aorta or the right ventricle or be transmitted from the right atrium to an enlarged liver in tricuspid incompetence.

Paradoxic rocking impulses can sometimes be felt after myocardial infarction, especially when a left ventricular aneurysm is present. When the aneurysm involves the free ventricular wall, the outward motion of the aneurysmal sac can sometimes be felt in early systole.

Palpable Gallops

The vibrations produced by loud third and fourth heart sounds can often be felt. If the sounds are of very low pitch, the gallop may be easier to appreciate on palpation than on auscultation. In most cases in which a gallop is palpable, it is also audible.

PERCUSSION

Percussion of the heart has virtually no place in physical examination today because it is open to error and because the size of the heart is better determined by chest radiography.

AUSCULTATION

Auscultation of the heart is performed with a properly fitting stethoscope that uses either an open bell or a closed diaphragm as the means of coupling the examiner's ear to the patient's chest. The diaphragm transmits more sound and is better for listening to high-pitched sounds (such as the second heart sound) and murmurs. The bell is better for low-pitched noises, and variation of the pressure of the bell on the skin can be used to alter the intensity of the sounds and murmurs heard. Auscultation focuses more on the timing of events within the cardiac cycle than on their intensity or the site at which they are heard best. It is important to move the chest piece of the stethoscope to sites where specific sounds can best be heard. Do not restrict examination to the classic "valvular" areas described in older textbooks. Listen selectively (eg, to heart sounds or murmurs, but not both at once).

Heart Sounds

The timing of the different heart sounds is diagrammatically shown in Fig 3–13. First and second heart sounds are normally audible, and an early (dia-

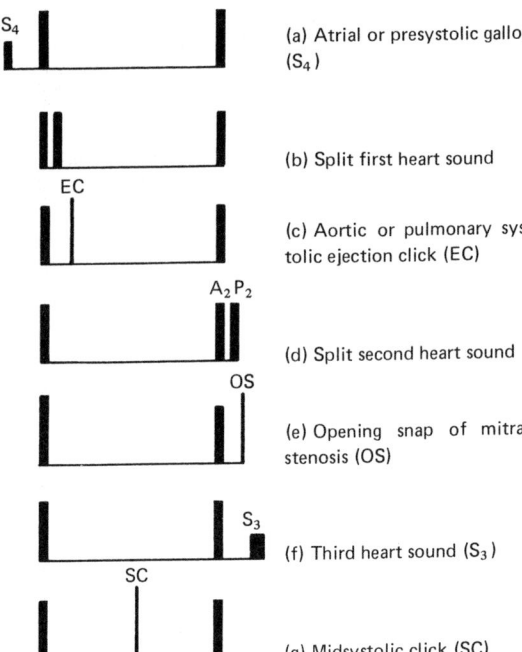

Figure 3–13. Timing of the different heart sounds and added sounds. (Modified and reproduced, with permission, from Wood P: *Diseases of the Heart and Circulation*, 3rd ed. Lippincott, 1968.)

stolic gallop) third sound is often present in children and young adults. In addition, a fourth (atrial) sound can sometimes be recorded by phonocardiography.

A. First Heart Sound: The first heart sound (S_1) is attributed to closure of the mitral and tricuspid valves at the start of ventricular systole. The 2 components can sometimes be clearly distinguished, and although the right atrial contraction precedes the left, the mitral valve closes before the tricuspid, and the first component of the first heart sound is mitral in origin. The position of the valve leaflets at the time of the start of systole influences the loudness of the first sound. In general, the first heart sound is louder, longer, and lower pitched than the second heart sound at the apex. In normal resting subjects, the atrioventricular valve leaflets have drifted into an almost closed position by the time systole starts, because diastolic flow is more or less complete by late diastole. Atrial contraction tends to reopen the valves. Consequently, the length of the PR interval affects the loudness of the first sound. When flow across an atrioventricular valve is increased for any reason or lasts longer than normal, the valve tends to shut from a more open position and produces more noise. The situation is similar to that encountered in closing an open door: the wider the door stands open before it is slammed shut, the louder the resulting noise. Thus, a loud first sound is heard in patients who are exercising, in patients with mitral stenosis in whom flow lasts throughout the whole of diastole, and in patients with left-to-right shunts and increased atrioventricular flow, eg, atrial septal defect. In complete atrioventricular block in which the PR interval varies, the loudness of the first sound varies, being loudest when the PR interval is slightly shortened to about 0.1 second, as shown in Fig 3–14.

B. Second Heart Sound: The second heart sound (S_2) is due to closure of the semilunar valves and normally consists of 2 components (Fig 3–15). The earlier component is normally aortic in origin; the later one arises from the pulmonary valve (P_2). The location at which the second heart sound is best heard varies. It is normally heard well at the base and is almost always louder than the first sound in that area. It is sometimes necessary to listen at the apex or even in the epigastrium. Hearing the pulmonary valve closure sound at the apex suggests the presence of pulmonary hypertension.

1. Splitting of the second heart sound–Right and left ventricular stroke volumes vary reciprocally with quiet respiration when there is adequate venous return. Inspiration favors right ventricular output, and expiration favors left ventricular output. Thus, in normal subjects resting quietly and breathing easily, the time of pulmonary valve closure with inspiration can be shown to move later in the cardiac cycle by 0.02–0.04 second, as seen in Fig 3–16. Increased filling of the right heart is associated with a more negative pressure within the thorax during inspiration, which increases right ventricular output in accordance with the Frank-Starling mechanism. The extra output has a longer ejection time; consequently, the pulmonary valve closure sound is delayed. The opposite occurs with aortic valve closure during expiration, but the magnitude of the changes is less. Thus, although both

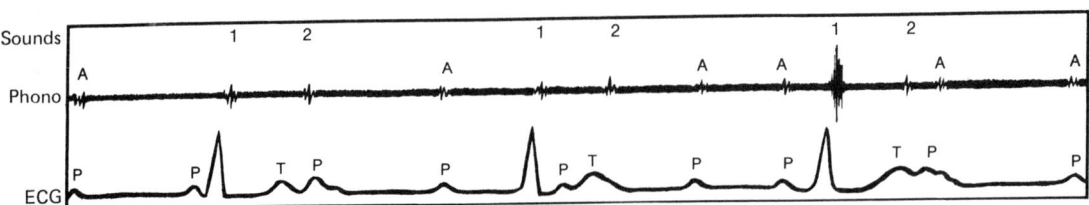

Figure 3–14. Phonocardiogram and ECG showing intensity of first sound varying with position of P wave on the ECG and atrial sound in complete atrioventricular block. (Courtesy of Roche Laboratories Division of Hoffman-La Roche, Inc.)

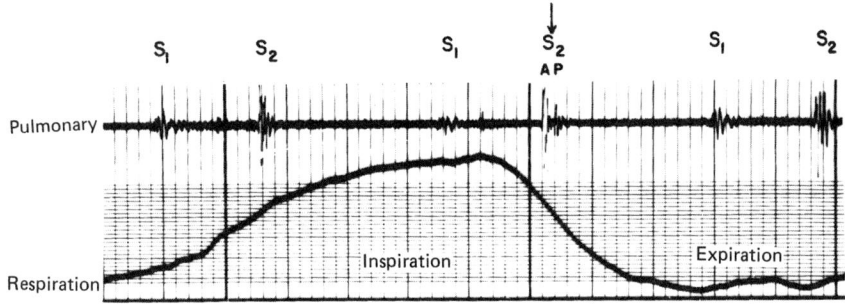

Figure 3-15. Phonocardiogram taken from the pulmonary area in a healthy 28-year-old man. It shows that splitting of the second sound becomes distinct after inspiration. The curve of respiration moves upward during inspiration. (Reproduced, with permission, from Dressler W: *Clinical Aids in Cardiac Diagnosis.* Grune & Stratton, 1970.)

the aortic and pulmonary components of the second heart sound move, the pulmonary component moves more. The net effect is that the interval between the 2 components of the second sound increases with inspiration and then decreases until the interval between the 2 sounds is not appreciable during expiration. The process is conventionally referred to as **physiologic splitting of the second heart sound.** When right ventricular systole is prolonged because of right bundle branch block, pulmonary valve closure is delayed. In this case, both the first and the second heart sounds tend to be split throughout the respiratory cycle, with the split widening further with inspiration (Fig 3–16). When right ventricular stroke volume is increased and venous return is high, as in atrial septal defect with large pulmonary blood flow, respiration has relatively little effect on right ventricular output. In this case, pulmonary valve closure is greatly delayed and the second sound is widely split; respiration has no effect, and the split is "fixed" even during expiration (Fig 3–17). Splitting of the second heart sound is almost always found in atrial septal defect with left-to-right shunt, but the finding of a **fixed split** is indicative of a significant left-to-right shunt. If the venous return is reduced when the patient stands up, the splitting of the second sound will become more normal, becoming either movable with respiration or less widely split.

2. Paradoxic splitting of the second sound– When left ventricular contraction is prolonged (eg, poor contractility, aortic stenosis), aortic valve closure is delayed and occurs after pulmonary closure. Aortic valve closure can be identified by timing it against the dicrotic notch of the carotid artery tracing (Fig 3–18). In paradoxic splitting, aortic and pulmonary valve closure sounds coincide toward the end of inspiration, and splitting is greatest during expiration. This is also referred to as "reversed" splitting of the second sound and is found in patients with left bundle branch block, in aortic stenosis, and in any other condition that greatly overloads the left ventricle. The effect of respiration on the second heart sound in paradoxic splitting is shown in Fig 3–19. Aortic valve closure tends to be delayed and diminished in aortic stenosis and may be absent when the lesion is severe.

3. Intensity–The second heart sound is also important in patients with pulmonary stenosis. Here the timing and intensity of the sound vary with the severity of the stenosis. In mild cases, the second sound is normal. In cases with more severe stenosis,

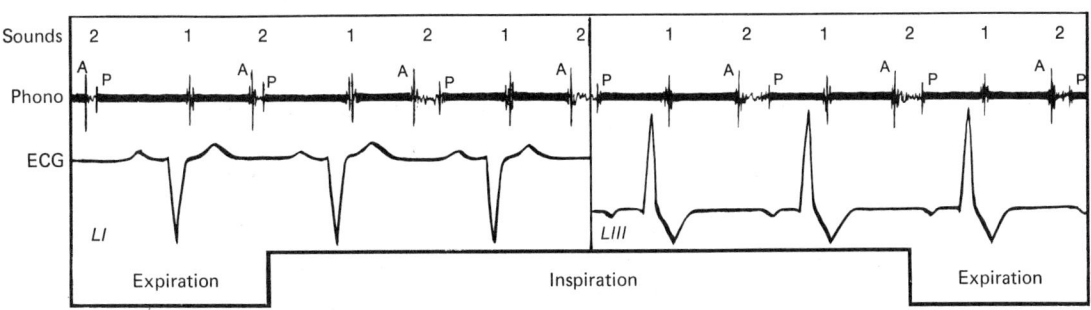

Figure 3-16. Phonocardiogram showing widely split second sound in right bundle branch block with P_2 even later on inspiration. (Courtesy of Roche Laboratories Division of Hoffman-La Roche, Inc.)

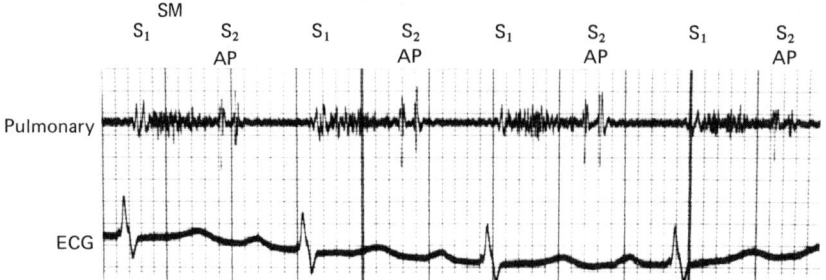

Figure 3–17. Phonocardiogram from the pulmonary area in a patient with ostium secundum atrial septal defect showing wide splitting of the second heart sound that remained constant although normal breathing was not interrupted while the phonocardiogram was obtained. SM, systolic murmur. (Reproduced, with permission, from Dressler W: *Clinical Aids in Cardiac Diagnosis.* Grune & Stratton, 1970.)

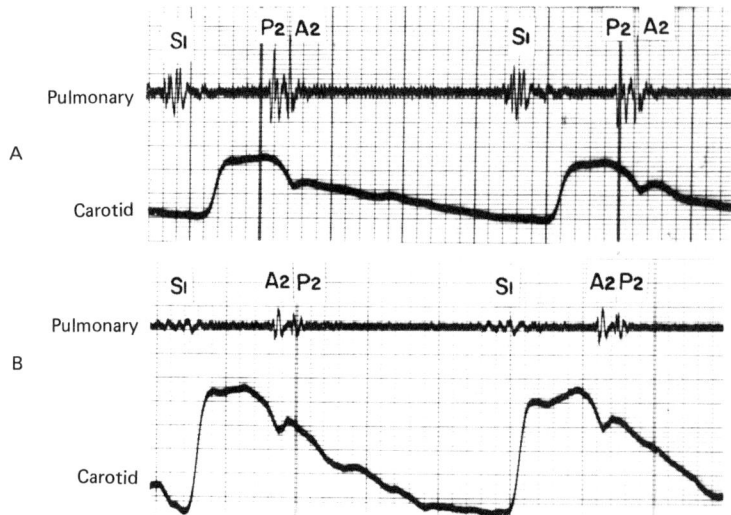

Figure 3–18. Paradoxic splitting of S_2 in a 55-year-old patient with Stokes-Adams syndrome with artificial pacing. *A:* The electrical pacemaker is in the right ventricle. The phonocardiogram shows splitting of the second sound. Comparison with the carotid pulse shows that the aortic element, which occurs 0.03 second prior to the dicrotic notch, follows the pulmonary component. *B:* The electrical pacemaker is in the left ventricle. The aortic element now precedes the pulmonary component of the second sound. (Reproduced, with permission, from Dressler W: *Clinical Aids in Cardiac Diagnosis.* Grune & Stratton, 1970.)

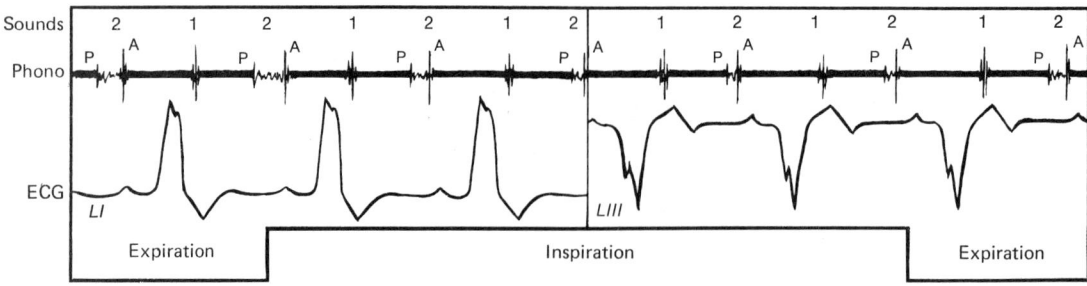

Figure 3–19. Phonocardiogram showing paradoxic splitting (split on expiration, narrower on inspiration) in left bundle branch block. (Courtesy of Roche Laboratories Division of Hoffman-La Roche, Inc.)

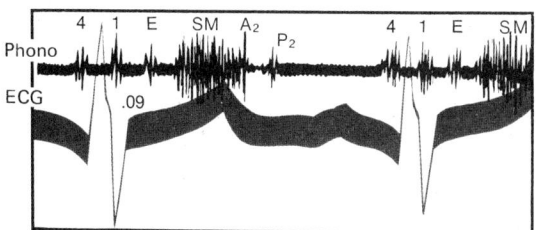

Figure 3-20. Phonocardiogram from a patient with pulmonary stenosis showing the typical presystolic gallop (4), ejection click (E), systolic murmur (SM), and delayed pulmonary valve closure sound (P_2). Recorded at left sternal border. (Courtesy of Roche Laboratories Division of Hoffman-La Roche, Inc.)

the second sound is delayed and diminished because pulmonary blood flow is less (Fig 3–20). Thus, in severe cases the sound of pulmonary valve closure is inaudible. However, it can usually be detected by phonocardiography and is shown to occur up to 0.12 second after aortic valve closure. The loudness of each component of the second sound varies with the pressure in the corresponding vessel. Thus, a loud pulmonary valve closure sound is heard in pulmonary hypertension and a loud aortic second sound in systemic hypertension (Fig 3–21). Loudness of the components of the second sound is not an accurate indicator of pressure, which should be directly measured in doubtful cases. The character of the aortic valve closure sound is altered in patients with aortic disease. In patients with syphilitic aortitis and other diseases that dilate the root of the aorta, aortic valve closure has a high-pitched, drumlike, "tambour" quality. The reason for this is not known. In systemic hypertension, the aortic valve closure sound is not only loud but also clear and ringing.

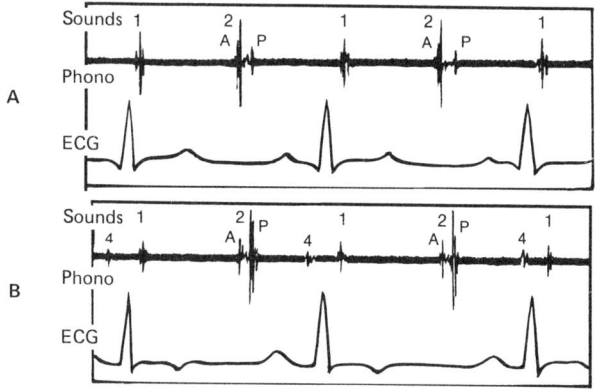

Figure 3-21. *A:* Phonocardiogram demonstrating loud aortic valve closure sound (A_2) in systemic hypertension. *B:* Phonocardiogram demonstrating loud P_2 in pulmonary hypertension. (Courtesy of Roche Laboratories Division of Hoffman-La Roche, Inc.)

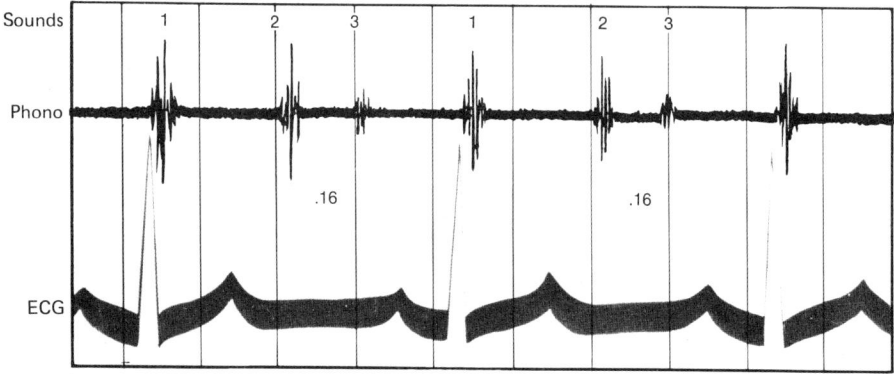

Figure 3-22. Phonocardiogram showing typical third heart sound (S_3). It follows the second sound (S_2) by 0.16 second. (Courtesy of Roche Laboratories Division of Hoffman-La Roche, Inc.)

C. Third Heart Sound: The third heart sound (S_3) shown in Fig 3–22 is associated with ventricular filling. It is not clear why it is normally present in young persons and disappears with age. An audible third heart sound is also found when there is an abnormally large diastolic flow into a normal ventricle or a normal flow into an abnormal ventricle. The former occurs in patients with left-to-right shunt and also occurs in mitral or tricuspid incompetence. The latter is seen in patients with right or, more commonly, left ventricular disease. The third heart sound is a dull, low-pitched, localized sound occurring about 0.12–0.16 second after the second sound. If the sound arises from the right heart, it increases in intensity during inspiration and is heard at the lower sternal edge. Conversely, a left-sided third sound increases on expiration.

D. Fourth Heart Sound: The fourth heart sound (S_4) results from atrial contraction and is thought to be a filling sound arising within the ventricle. Although it can often be recorded by phonocardiography, it is not normally audible. A fourth heart sound is heard shortly before the first heart sound in any condition in which the force of either the right or the left atrial contraction is increased. This means that atrial sounds are heard in conditions in which the ventricle is working against high pressure and the atria are contracting against increased resistance, as shown in Fig 3–23. Thus, pulmonary or aortic stenosis and pulmonary or systemic hypertension are the commonest causes of a fourth heart sound. A fourth heart sound is also often audible during an episode of angina pectoris. Here, too, the ventricular compliance is reduced, and the left atrium contracts against increased resistance. Right and left atrial sounds can often be distinguished on the basis of their response to respiration and the site where they are most clearly heard.

E. Gallop Rhythm: When a third or a fourth heart sound is present, the extra heart sounds give rise to a gallop, or triple, rhythm. When the extra sound is presystolic, it is difficult to distinguish the rhythm from that of a split first sound or even an ejection click following the first sound. The presystolic gallop is said to have the cadence of the word "Tennessee," whereas diastolic gallop has been likened to "Kentucky." In some cases, both third and fourth heart sounds can be heard. If the heart rate is rapid—about 120/min—the third and fourth sounds may be superimposed, giving rise to **summation gallop** (Fig 3–24). In this case, 2 inaudible sounds may combine to give an audible sound. It is possible to slow the heart rate by carotid sinus massage and listen to hear whether the gallop disappears or whether either the third or the fourth sound or both can be distinguished; this causes a quadruple rhythm. A prominent filling sound is also heard in patients with impaired ventricular filling in pericardial constriction. This can be as loud a sound as the second heart sound and is sometimes called a "pericardial knock." It is thought to be caused by the sudden cessation of right ventricular filling.

A loud early diastolic sound is sometimes heard in left atrial myxoma. It is attributed to a pedunculated tumor falling into the mitral orifice as cardiac filling starts. This sound has been called "tumor plop."

F. Opening Snap: The opening snap of the atrioventricular valve heard in patients with rheumatic valvular disease is also considered as a heart sound. It is heard 0.06–0.12 second after the second heart sound and is shown in Fig 3–25. It may be the loudest and most widely heard sound in the cardiac cycle and is heard best in the third or fourth left interspace in most cases.

The interval between the second heart sound and the opening snap can vary with posture, decreasing when the patient stands up and the left atrial pressure falls. It also varies with the severity of mitral stenosis (see p 371).

G. Systolic Clicks: Extra intracardiac sounds are also heard during systole. These, like the opening snap, arise from valves. The commonest is the systolic ejection click, which can arise from either the aortic or

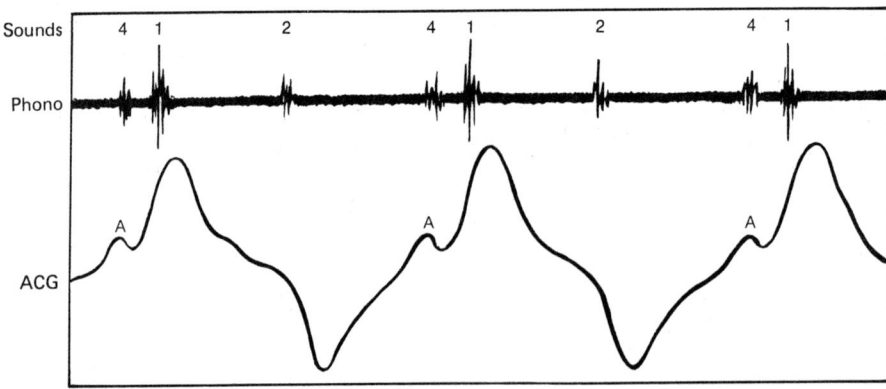

Figure 3–23. Phonocardiogram showing a fourth heart sound (S_4) and its relation to first sound (S_1). Below, an apexcardiogram (ACG) shows the occurrence of the wave of atrial contraction together with the presystolic gallop sound. (Courtesy of Roche Laboratories Division of Hoffman-La Roche, Inc.)

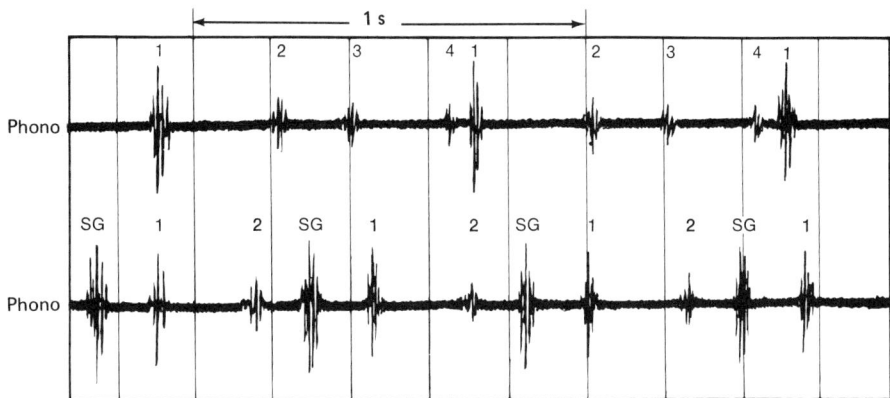

Figure 3-24. The phonocardiographic strip above shows separate presystolic and diastolic gallop; the strip below shows their fusion, which results in a summation gallop (SG). (Courtesy of Roche Laboratories Division of Hoffman-La Roche, Inc.)

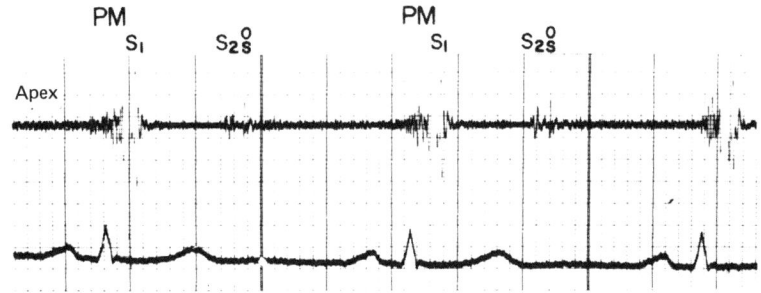

Figure 3-25. From a 24-year-old woman with mitral stenosis and sinus rhythm. The first sound (S_1) shows high-amplitude vibrations that merge with a presystolic murmur (PM). There is also a mitral opening snap (OS). The opening snap occurs about 0.06 second after the onset of S_2. (Reproduced, with permission, from Dressler W: *Clinical Aids in Cardiac Diagnosis.* Grune & Stratton, 1970.)

the pulmonary valve. The click occurs early in systole, about 0.02 second after the first sound. It usually ushers in a systolic ejection murmur, as shown in Fig 3-26. Ejection clicks commonly occur when dilatation of the great vessel (aorta or pulmonary artery) with which they are associated is combined with normal or increased flow through the vessel. A pulmonary ejection click is louder during expiration because tension in the valve structures is less when intrathoracic pressure is less negative. Ejection clicks are sometimes heard in normal subjects but are most common in patients with insignificant or mild stenosis of the valve. A different variety of systolic click is heard in patients with insignificant mitral disease, as shown in Fig 3-27. The clicks, which may be multiple, occur in mid or even late systole and may precede, follow, or accompany the late systolic murmur heard in this lesion **(click-murmur syndrome).** In some cases, the click occurs without any murmur. The basic lesion is prolapse of the mitral valve cusp, and although the sound is thought to originate in the valve, the exact mechanism of its production is not known.

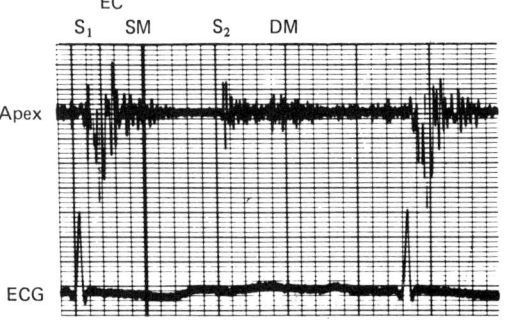

Figure 3-26. From a patient with rheumatic aortic regurgitation. The diastolic murmur is most distinct in the apical area. A phonocardiogram taken from that region shows a first sound of marked intensity. It is closely followed by a systolic murmur (SM) that starts with an ejection click (EC). The systolic murmur occupies the first half of systole. The second sound is immediately followed by a diastolic murmur that extends over the entire diastolic phase. (Reproduced, with permission, from Dressler W: *Clinical Aids in Cardiac Diagnosis.* Grune & Stratton, 1970.)

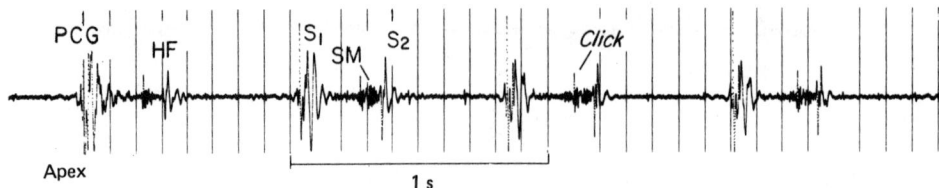

Figure 3-27. Apical high-frequency (HF) phonocardiogram (PCG) showing late systolic click and murmur (SM) in a patient with hemodynamically insignificant mitral incompetence.

(a) Presystolic murmur of mitral stenosis

(b) Pansystolic murmur of mitral or tricuspid incompetence or of ventricular septal defect

(c) Aortic systolic ejection murmur following an ejection click and ending before the second heart sound

(d) Long pulmonary systolic ejection murmur in severe pulmonary stenosis lasting through left ventricular systole and ending before a delayed and diminished pulmonary valve closure

(e) Immediate diastolic murmur of aortic or pulmonary incompetence

(f) Delayed diastolic murmur of mitral stenosis following the opening snap

(g) Short diastolic inflow murmur following a third heart sound

(h) Continuous murmur of patent ductus arteriosus; loudest at the time of the second heart sound

(i) Late systolic murmur of hemodynamically insignificant mitral incompetence

First sound   Second sound

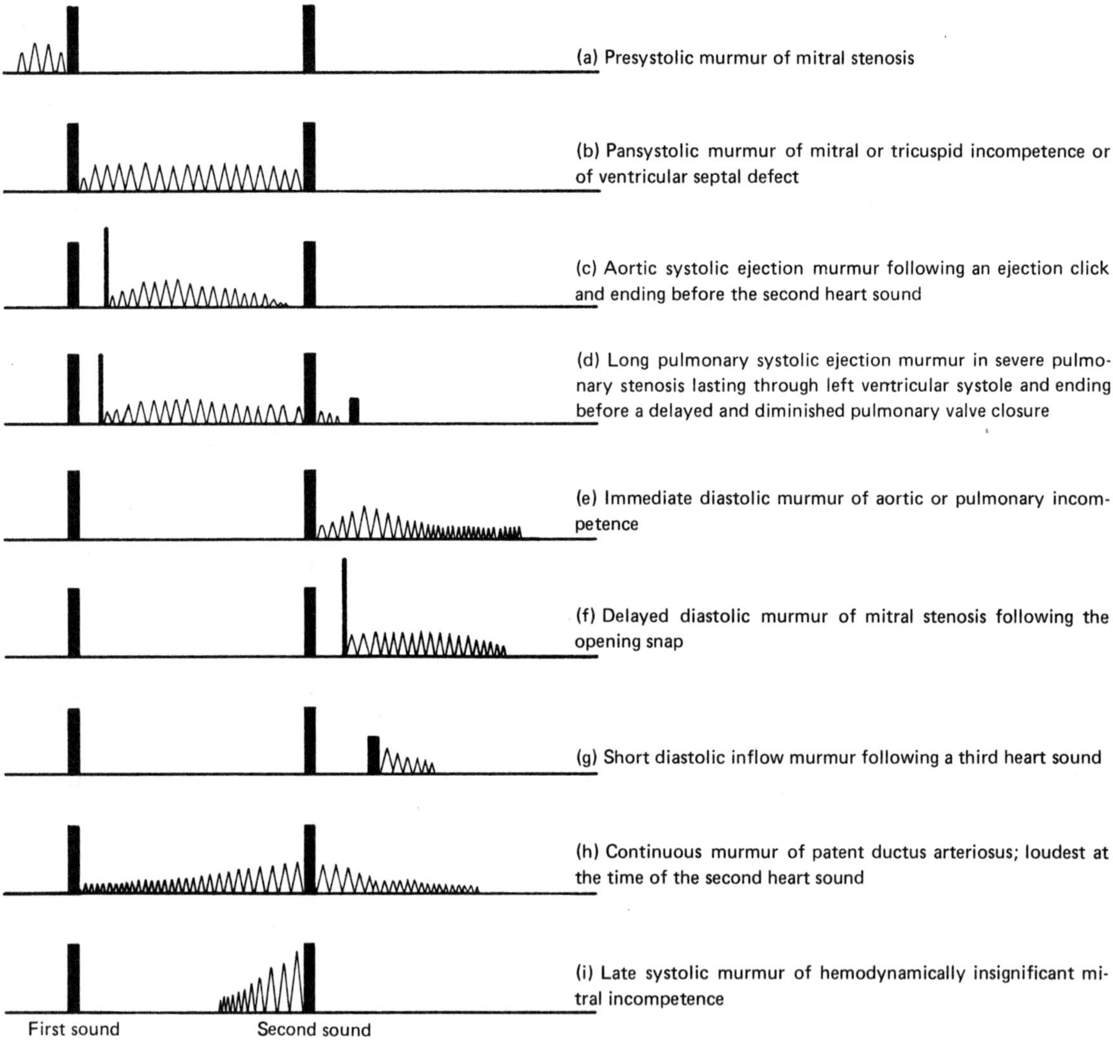

Figure 3-28. The timing of the principal cardiac murmurs. (Modified and reproduced, with permission, from Wood P: *Diseases of the Heart and Circulation,* 3rd ed. Lippincott, 1968.)

Heart Murmurs

The timing of the principal heart murmurs is shown diagrammatically in Fig 3–28. Cardiac murmurs are thought to result from disturbances of normal blood flow patterns in the heart and great vessels. They are classified on the basis of their timing as systolic, diastolic, and continuous murmurs.

A. Systolic Murmurs: Systolic murmurs are generally less significant than diastolic murmurs and may occur in patients in whom no evidence of heart disease can be found.

1. Ejection murmurs–An abnormally large flow through a normal valve may cause a systolic murmur that is ejection in timing. An ejection murmur begins when flow starts in one of the great vessels and finishes before the time of valve closure. It thus starts after the first heart sound and ends before the second heart sound. Murmurs of this type do not necessarily indicate the presence of heart disease and may be "innocent." Trained athletes with slow heart rates may have systolic murmurs, especially when they are examined while supine. The murmur usually disappears when the heart rate increases as the subject stands up or exercises. Care must be taken in interpreting new murmurs in adults as "innocent," because the murmur may signify early aortic stenosis. Systolic ejection murmurs can be heard in high-output states such as anemia, pregnancy, or thyrotoxicosis and also in patients with dilated aortic root due to atherosclerosis, hypertension, syphilis, or other forms of aortitis. They occur when there is a high stroke volume, as in complete atrioventricular block with bradycardia. Increased flow through the pulmonary valve occurs in patients with left-to-right shunts, especially in atrial septal defect, and a systolic ejection murmur is virtually always found in such conditions (Fig 3–29).

The most important causes of systolic ejection murmurs are aortic and pulmonary stenoses at a valvular level. The intensity and duration of such murmurs vary with the severity of the stenosis and with the stroke volume. When the stroke volume is low, the murmur may be of low intensity, and it does not last as long as it does when there is normal flow. Because a systolic ejection murmur can also occur

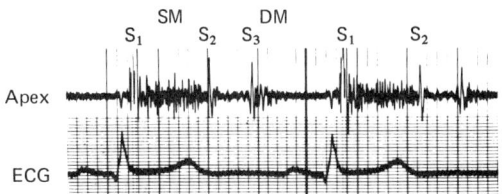

Figure 3–30. From a 25-year-old woman with a rheumatic lesion of the mitral valve. Mitral incompetence is dominant. The phonocardiogram shows a pansystolic murmur (SM) and a third heart sound (S_3) that is followed by a short diastolic murmur (DM). (Reproduced, with permission, from Dressler W: *Clinical Aids in Cardiac Diagnosis.* Grune & Stratton, 1970.)

when the stenosis is mild and the valve is merely thickened, it is unwise to base any assessment of the severity of the stenosis on the intensity of the murmur.

2. Pansystolic murmurs–Pansystolic (holosystolic) murmurs start with the first sound and continue up to the second sound, as shown in Fig 3–30. They are commonly due to incompetence of the mitral or tricuspid valve. The valve leaks throughout systole, and the relatively high pressure difference across the valve accounts for the murmur. The murmur is high-pitched and more musical (of purer tone) than an ejection murmur. A similar murmur is heard when there is flow across a ventricular septal defect with a large pressure difference between the 2 ventricles (Fig 3–31).

3. Late systolic murmurs–Mitral incompetence can also result in a late systolic murmur that increases in intensity up to the second sound, as shown in Fig 3–27. This murmur has a peculiar quality, and inexperienced observers may find it difficult to time. Once recognized, it is never forgotten. This late systolic murmur may become pansystolic when the degree of incompetence increases, eg, when peripheral resistance is increased during the overshoot that occurs following Valsalva's maneuver.

4. Other systolic murmurs–Although in theory it is easy to classify murmurs as ejection or pansystolic, it may be difficult to make this distinction in practice. In some cases, the murmur exhibits features of both varieties, and it varies in timing at different sites. In infundibular stenosis involving the outflow tract of the right ventricle or in hypertrophic obstruc-

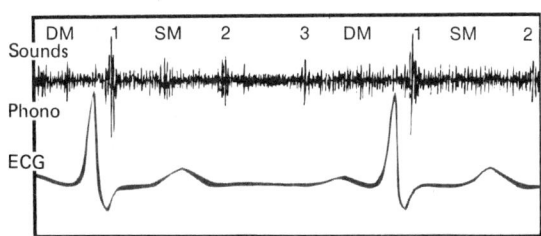

Figure 3–29. Phonocardiogram in atrial septal defect showing a systolic ejection murmur (SM), split second sound, and tricuspid diastolic murmur (DM). (Courtesy of Roche Laboratories Division of Hoffman-La Roche, Inc.)

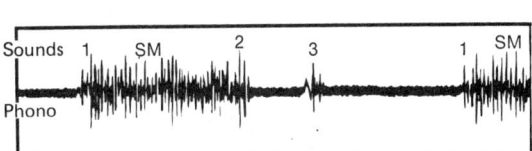

Figure 3–31. Pansystolic murmur (SM) and third heart sound (3) recorded at left sternal border in a patient with ventricular septal defect. (Courtesy of Roche Laboratories Division of Hoffman-La Roche, Inc.)

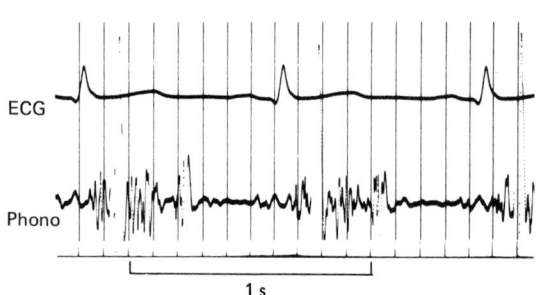

Figure 3-32. Long pansystolic ejection murmur in hypertrophic obstructive cardiomyopathy.

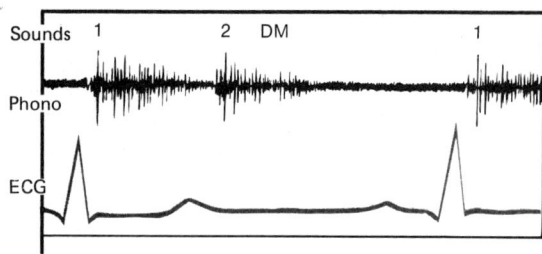

Figure 3-33. Phonocardiogram showing typical diastolic murmur in aortic incompetence and, in this instance, a systolic murmur although no aortic stenosis is present. (Courtesy of Roche Laboratories Division of Hoffman-La Roche, Inc.)

tive cardiomyopathy, which produces a rather similar lesion in the left ventricle, there is usually a harsh murmur that lasts throughout systole but peaks in intensity in the middle of systole, when flow is greatest (Fig 3-32). Similarly, when pulmonary stenosis and ventricular septal defect coexist, the murmur has characteristics of both pansystolic and ejection murmurs.

A special type of systolic murmur may occur in coarctation of the aorta or peripheral pulmonary arterial stenosis. In these conditions, there may be a murmur late in systole owing to the late peaking of flow across the narrowing in the vessel. In coarctation, there may also be a systolic murmur that lasts longer and is due to flow through collateral vessels in the chest wall that have developed in response to the lesion. This murmur is similar to that of bronchial collateral flow, which is heard in patients who have markedly reduced flow to the lungs via the pulmonary artery, as in pulmonary atresia. This systolic murmur also resembles the bruit heard over an arteriovenous fistula or over an extremely active toxic goiter. Systolic bruits are also heard over stenotic lesions in peripheral vessels. Carotid arterial and renal arterial stenotic lesions are the most important examples. These murmurs can be systolic or diastolic in timing and are ejection in character. They tend to occur late in the cardiac cycle.

B. Diastolic Murmurs: Diastolic murmurs are almost always due to significant lesions, although they can rarely occur in severe anemia. They are either **immediate,** caused by incompetence of the aortic or pulmonary valve, or **delayed,** caused by actual or relative mitral or tricuspid stenosis. A special form of diastolic murmur that is commonest in mitral stenosis is the **atrial systolic (presystolic) murmur.**

1. Immediate (early diastolic) murmurs– Immediate, or early, diastolic murmurs start immediately after the time of closure of the valve, as shown in Fig 3-33. They decrease in intensity during diastole and are high-pitched and difficult to hear. They are heard best using the diaphragm of the stethoscope, with the subject sitting up and leaning forward and the breath held in expiration. These murmurs are heard on either side of the sternum in the third, fourth, and fifth interspaces. Their duration is roughly related to the degree of aortic or pulmonary valvular incompetence. Similar murmurs are heard when there is diastolic flow from the aorta into any low-pressure chamber, eg, the right ventricle or an atrium.

2. Delayed (middiastolic) murmurs–The delayed, or middiastolic, murmur does not start until the ventricular pressure has fallen below the level of the atrial pressure. There is thus a sound-free interval between the second heart sound and the start of the murmur, as shown in Fig 3-30. The murmur is low-pitched and rumbling, and its duration is related to the severity of the stenosis and the size of the stroke volume. Mitral stenosis is the commonest cause of such a murmur; patent ductus arteriosus and ventricular septal defect on the left side and atrial septal defect and tricuspid stenosis on the right side are other causes. An example of a tricuspid flow murmur in a patient with atrial defect is shown in Fig 3-29. Pure tricuspid stenosis is extremely rare, but mixed incompetence and stenosis occasionally gives rise to a delayed diastolic murmur. The right-sided murmurs increase with inspiration and are heard near the sternum. The left-sided murmurs are best heard with the patient lying in the left lateral position and the stethoscope applied directly over the point of maximal cardiac impulse.

3. Presystolic murmurs–Presystolic accentuation of a delayed diastolic murmur is characteristic of mitral stenosis. In some cases, the presystolic murmur is all that can be heard with the patient supine and at rest, as in Fig 3-25. The delayed diastolic murmur is often elicited by having the patient exercise and then lie on the left side. Presystolic accentuation of a murmur is also encountered in patients with severe aortic incompetence (**Austin Flint murmur**). The aortic cusp of the mitral valve tends to be caught between 2 streams of blood during diastole. One stream flowing from the aorta through the leaking valve encounters another from the left atrium during diastolic ventricular filling. The valve leaflet tends to vibrate in the 2 streams and

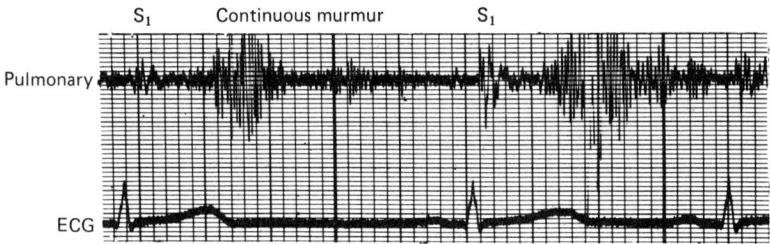

Figure 3-34. Patent ductus arteriosus characterized by a continuous murmur. The phonocardiogram, taken from the pulmonary area, shows a murmur that occupies the entire length of the cardiac cycle. It waxes at the end of systole and during early diastole, reaching at that point its highest frequency and intensity and enveloping the second sound. Only the first sound is distinctly visible. (Reproduced, with permission, from Dressler W: *Clinical Aids in Cardiac Diagnosis.* Grune & Stratton, 1970.)

cause what Austin Flint described as a blubbering murmur. This murmur may appear or become louder at the time of atrial systole and thus be confused with the murmur of mitral stenosis. In practice, the 2 lesions—mitral stenosis and aortic incompetence—are readily distinguished, and it is only when the lesions are thought to coexist that difficulties in diagnosis arise (see Chapter 13).

C. Continuous Murmurs: Continuous murmurs arise when there is a pressure difference between 2 communicating vessels or chambers at all times in the cardiac cycle. The commonest example is that found in patent ductus arteriosus with left-to-right shunt (Fig 3-34). This lesion gives rise to a continuous "machinery" murmur. The characteristic feature of the murmur is that it is loudest at the time of the second heart sound. At this time, right ventricular ejection is coming to an end and pulmonary arterial pressure is falling, while aortic pressure is remaining high. Similar continuous murmurs are heard with aortopulmonary fistulas and after surgical creation of a shunt for the relief of tetralogy of Fallot (Blalock's operation).

D. Differential Diagnosis: Murmurs that come close to being continuous can be readily confused with the "machinery" murmur if their relationship to the second heart sound is not taken into account. In mixed aortic stenosis and incompetence, there is a to-and-fro systolic and diastolic murmur that can appear almost continuous. There is, however, a gap at the time of the second heart sound. Similarly, in patients with ventricular septal defect and aortic incompetence, the murmur may appear continuous. Coronary arteriovenous fistula and anomalous drainage of a coronary vessel into the pulmonary artery also give continuous murmurs, and in cases of rupture of a sinus of Valsalva aneurysm into a chamber with a lower pressure, the murmur is continuous or near continuous. The murmur of a patent ductus may only be heard high in the left chest below the left clavicle. In some patients, it may be confused with a venous hum. This is a sound that may be continuous and results from partial occlusion of a large vein. Such a bruit is abolished by pressure over the root of the neck or by a change in the patient's position. The hum is never loudest at the time of the second heart sound.

E. Transmission of Murmurs: The interpretation of the origin of murmurs can be assisted by determining the direction of transmission of the murmur. The stethoscope is moved over various areas of the precordium to determine where the murmur can still be heard. Murmurs arising from the mitral valve are transmitted toward the axilla. Aortic and pulmonary diastolic murmurs are transmitted down the sides of the sternum. Aortic stenotic murmurs are usually but not always transmitted into the neck. The information obtained from determining the direction of transmission of murmurs is only of secondary value, however.

F. Hemodynamic Factors Influencing Murmurs: Any factor that alters hemodynamics can change the auscultatory findings and may on occasion be useful in diagnosis (Table 3-1).

Table 3-1. Hemodynamic factors influencing auscultatory findings.

	Stroke Volume	Heart Rate	Systemic Vascular Resistance
Physical factors			
Respiration			
Inspiration	−	+	+
Expiration	+	+	−
Posture			
Standing	−	+	+
Squatting	+	−	−
Exercise			
Upright	+	+	+
Supine	+−	+	+
Isometric handgrip	+−	+	+
Carotid sinus massage	−	−	−
Valsalva's maneuver	See Chapter 4.		
Cold pressor test	+−	+	+
Pharmacologic factors			
Vasodilators (nitrites)	+	+	−
Beta blockers	−	−	+−
Beta-agonists	+	+	−
Alpha-agonists	−	+	+

1. Inspiration and expiration–Inspiration increases venous return to the right heart and tends to accentuate right-sided murmurs. This effect is of more significance than any tendency for a left-sided murmur to be louder during expiration. All intrathoracic sounds tend to become less loud with inspiration, simply because the stethoscope moves farther away from the origin of the sound and because lung tissue is likely to be interposed and decreases sound transmission. Thus, exaggeration of a murmur with inspiration is of greater significance than exaggeration with expiration.

2. Posture–Although examination of the heart is ordinarily performed with the subject supine, it is also useful to have the patient assume the left lateral decubitus position, so that mitral murmurs can be heard, especially after the patient has done several sit-ups to increase cardiac output. Having the patient sit up, lean forward, and breathe out can make an aortic diastolic murmur more readily audible. Examining the patient when standing tends to increase the systemic vascular resistance, as pooling of blood in the legs causes a fall in arterial pressure that triggers peripheral vasoconstriction via the baroreceptor reflexes. Standing may thus increase mitral incompetence and convert a late systolic murmur in a patient with click-murmur syndrome to a pansystolic murmur. Squatting, like lying down, increases venous return and shifts blood into the central circulation, increasing the pulmonary and left heart blood volumes. Thus, squatting tends to increase left ventricular volume and reduce or abolish the murmur of hypertrophic obstructive cardiomyopathy.

The effects of postural change on murmurs must be interpreted in the light of associated circulatory changes. If the heart rate does not slow on squatting and quicken on standing, postural effects on murmurs should be discounted. In general, the absence of change in a murmur with posture is not of significance.

3. Isometric handgrip; cold pressor test–An isometric handgrip and the cold pressor test (immersion of a hand in ice water for 1 minute) produce a relatively pure increase in systemic arterial pressure. This increases the intensity of aortic diastolic and mitral systolic murmurs and also tends to reduce the intensity of aortic systolic murmurs.

4. Carotid sinus massage–Carotid sinus massage, which slows the heart rate and may facilitate auscultation, should be used with caution and only in a supine patient, preferably with electrocardiographic control. It should never be performed bilaterally and is contraindicated when there is a carotid bruit. The patient should turn the head to one side, and the area of the carotid sinus, below the angle of the jaw, should be gently massaged (not occluded) for no more than 5 seconds, in order to determine if bradycardia is present. The maneuver can be useful in separating the sounds of summation gallop.

5. Valsalva's maneuver–Listening during the period of strain in Valsalva's maneuver or during the overshoot after the release of strain can help in diagnosis. Right-sided murmurs disappear or diminish early during strain and return early after release of pressure in Valsalva's maneuver. The increase in pressure during the period of overshoot tends to accentuate the murmur of mitral incompetence and decrease the intensity of murmurs in aortic stenosis and hypertrophic obstructive cardiomyopathy.

6. Drugs–Vasodilator drugs such as amyl nitrite by inhalation and sublingual nitroglycerin reduce systemic resistance. This accentuates the murmurs of aortic stenosis and obstructive cardiomyopathy and decreases the murmur of mitral incompetence. The actions of alpha-adrenergic and beta-adrenergic blockade and stimulation can be inferred from their effects on the systemic circulation.

Pericardial Friction Rubs

Pericardial friction rubs are heard over the precordium as harsh, grating sounds related to the cardiac cycle and having a systolic component. When they have several components—most typically they have 3—they may be confused with murmurs. They tend to vary with time, posture, and the phase of respiration. Their intensity tends to vary with the degree of pressure of the bell of the stethoscope on the chest, and they sound superficial, like the noise of hair rubbing against the diaphragm of the stethoscope.

REFERENCES

Abrams J: Precordial motion in health and disease. *Mod Concepts Cardiovasc Dis* 1980;**49**:55.

Basta LL, Bettinger JJ: The cardiac impulse: A new look at an old art. *Am Heart J* 1979;**97**:96.

Brooks N, Leech G, Leatham A: Factors responsible for normal splitting of first heart sound: High-speed echophonocardiographic study of valve movement. *Br Heart J* 1980;**42**:695.

Bruns DL: A general theory of the causes of murmurs in the cardiovascular system. *Am J Med* 1959;**27**:360.

Cochran PT: Bedside aids to auscultation of the heart. *JAMA* 1978;**239**:54.

Constant J: *Bedside Cardiology*, 2nd ed. Little, Brown, 1976.

Dressler W: *Clinical Aids in Cardiac Diagnosis*. Grune & Stratton, 1970.

Flint A: On cardiac murmurs. *Am J Med Sci* 1862;**91**:27.

Fowler NO: *Inspection and Palpation of Venous and Arterial Pulses.* Part 2 of: *Examination of the Heart.* American Heart Association, 1972.

Frank ST: Aural sign of coronary artery disease. *N Engl J Med* 1973;**289**:327.

Goldstein S, Killip T: Comparison of direct and indirect arterial pressures in aortic regurgitation. *N Engl J Med* 1962;**267**:1121.

Grassman E, Blomqvist CG: Absence of respiratory sinus arrhythmia: A manifestation of the sick sinus syndrome. *Clin Cardiol* 1983;**6**:151.

Hada Y, Wolfe C, Craigie E: Pulsus alternans determined by biventricular simultaneous systolic time intervals. *Circulation* 1982;**65**:617.

Horwitz LD, Groves BM: *Signs and Symptoms in Cardiology.* Lippincott, 1984.

Hurst JW, Schlant RC: *Inspection and Palpation of the Anterior Chest.* Part 3 of: *Examination of the Heart.* American Heart Association, 1972.

Kincaid-Smith P, Barlow J: The atrial sound in hypertension and ischemic heart disease. *Br Heart J* 1959;**21**:479.

Kirkendall WM et al: *Recommendations for Human Blood Pressure Determination by Sphygmomanometers.* American Heart Association, 1967.

Kussmaul A: Uber schwielige Mediastino-Pericarditis und den paradoxen Puls. (3 parts.) *Berl Klin Wochenschr* 1873;**10**:433, 445, 461.

Lange RL, Hecht HH: The mechanism of Cheyne-Stokes respiration. *J Clin Invest* 1962;**41**:42.

Leatham A: *Auscultation of the Heart and Phonocardiography,* 2nd ed. Churchill Livingstone, 1975.

Leatham A: *An Introduction to the Examination of the Cardiovascular System,* 2nd ed. Oxford Univ Press, 1979.

Leatham A: Splitting of the first and second heart sounds. *Lancet* 1954;**2**:607.

Leatham A, Vogelpoel L: The early systolic sound in dilatation of the pulmonary artery. *Br Heart J* 1954;**16**:21.

Leatham A, Weitzman D: Auscultatory and phonocardiographic signs of pulmonary stenosis. *Br Heart J* 1957;**19**:303.

Leech G et al: Mechanism of influence of PR interval on loudness of first heart sound. *Br Heart J* 1980;**43**:138.

Leonard JJ, Kroetz FW: *Auscultation.* Part 4 of: *Examination of the Heart.* American Heart Association, 1967.

Mackenzie J: *Disease of the Heart.* Oxford Univ Press, 1908.

McDonald DA: Murmurs in relation to turbulence and eddy formation in the circulation. *Circulation* 1957;**16**:278.

Mendel D, McIlroy MB: The mechanical properties of the lungs in patients with periodic breathing. *Br Heart J* 1957;**19**:399.

Mills PG et al: Echographic and hemodynamic relationships of ejection sounds. *Circulation* 1977;**56**:430.

Mounsey P: The early diastolic sound of constrictive pericarditis. *Br Heart J* 1955;**17**:143.

Perloff JK: The physiologic mechanisms of cardiac and vascular physical signs. *J Am Coll Cardiol* 1983;**1**:184.

Ravin A: *Auscultation of the Heart,* 2nd ed. Year Book, 1967.

Reid JVO: Mid-systolic clicks. *S Afr Med J* 1961;**35**:353.

Settle HP et al: Echocardiographic study of paradoxical arterial pulse in chronic obstructive lung disease. *Circulation* 1980;**62**:1297.

Shearn MA: Nails and systemic disease: A review of fingernail findings in various systemic disorders. *West J Med* 1978;**129**:358.

Stein PD: *A Physical and Physiological Basis for the Interpretation of Cardiac Auscultation.* Futura, 1981.

Tavel ME (editor): *Dynamic Auscultation and Phonocardiography: The Contribution of Vasoactive Drugs to the Diagnosis of Heart Disease.* Charles Press, 1979.

Thompson R: *An Introduction to Physical Signs.* Blackwell, 1980.

Vogelpoel L et al: The use of amyl nitrite in the diagnosis of systolic murmurs. *Lancet* 1959;**2**:810.

Weitzman D: The mechanism and significance of the auricular sound. *Br Heart J* 1955;**17**:70.

4

Clinical Physiology

Knowledge of the pathophysiologic changes that occur in heart disease is essential for understanding and interpreting the results of diagnostic investigations in clinical cardiology and for assessing the results of treatment. An introductory discussion of the function and control of the normal cardiovascular system has been given in Chapter 1.

Clinical physiology is additionally concerned with 2 different but interrelated sets of measurements. The first set of measurements relates to overall circulatory function, more particularly to the transport systems for oxygen and CO_2. The second set comprises purely cardiac measurements such as cardiac output, intracardiac pressures, cardiac volumes, assessment of valvular stenosis and incompetence, intracardiac shunts, coronary blood flow, and assessment of cardiac function. Both applied physiology and normal basic physiology must be understood before the physician can develop a rational approach toward the special investigations undertaken for some patients and toward the interpretation of data obtained at the bedside or in the clinical laboratory. Practical experience in applying the clinical techniques to patients is invaluable.

OXYGEN & CO_2 TRANSPORT

The basic mechanisms involved in cardiopulmonary function are oxygen uptake in the lungs, oxygen-CO_2 exchange in the tissues, and elimination of CO_2 in the lungs.

Gas Tension

A. Partial Pressure: It is the partial pressure, or tension, of each gas that provides the force which determines how the gas will pass across the various membranes involved in gas transfer. The partial pressure of any gas in a mixture of gases is equal to the total pressure (barometric pressure) multiplied by the fraction of that gas in the mixture. Thus, since there is 20.9% oxygen in the atmosphere, the partial pressure of oxygen (P_{O_2}) in the atmosphere at normal barometric pressure (760 mm Hg) is (20.9/100) × 760, or 159 mm Hg. If any liquid such as blood is allowed to equilibrate with a gas, the partial pressure of the gas in the liquid will come to equal that in the gas. The amount of gas entering the liquid will depend on the solubility of the gas in the liquid and on any chemical reaction occurring between the gas and the liquid. If the barometric pressure is reduced, as at high altitude, the same fraction of oxygen in the atmosphere (20.9%) exerts a lower partial pressure because the total pressure is lower. Thus, at 3000 m the barometric pressure is about 525 mm Hg, and the partial pressure of oxygen is reduced to 110 mm Hg. Similarly, a gas mixture of higher oxygen content (50%) exerts a higher P_{O_2} at sea level: (50/100) × 760, or 380 mm Hg.

B. Oxygen Tension, Saturation, and Content: Hemoglobin, the respiratory pigment of blood, has an affinity for oxygen and combines reversibly with it. Hemoglobin exists in 2 forms, a red (oxygenated) form and a blue (reduced) form, depending on the oxygen content of the blood. The proportion of oxygenated blood can vary from 0 to 100%; this is the oxygen saturation of blood. Arterial oxygen saturation is reduced in cyanotic congenital heart disease and hypoxic patients. The complex relationship between oxygen tension and oxygen saturation is illustrated by the dissociation curve of hemoglobin shown in Fig 4-1 and is influenced by the temperature and acidity of the blood. The hemoglobin concentration in blood varies with the degree of anemia or polycythemia, and the oxygen-carrying capacity is directly related to hemoglobin concentration. One gram of hemoglobin when fully saturated can carry 1.34 mL of oxygen. Thus, a normal person with 149 grams of hemoglobin per liter of blood has an oxygen capacity of 149 × 1.34, or

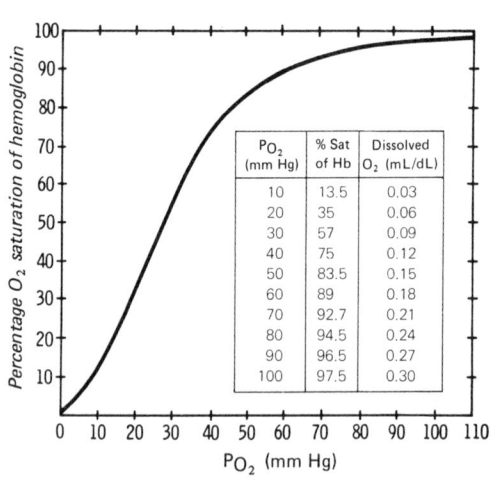

Figure 4-1. Oxygen hemoglobin dissociation curve. pH 7.40, temperature 38 °C. (Redrawn and reproduced, with permission, from Comroe JH et al: *The Lung: Clinical Physiology and Pulmonary Function Tests*, 2nd ed. Year Book, 1962.)

200 mL oxygen per liter of blood. Hemoglobin becomes effectively fully saturated with oxygen at a P_{O_2} of 150–200 mm Hg. At this P_{O_2} there is also a small amount (5–6 mL/L) of oxygen in solution in the plasma.

At a normal arterial P_{O_2} of 70–100 mm Hg, hemoglobin is about 97% saturated. Further increase in P_{O_2} to about 200 mm Hg will almost completely saturate hemoglobin and also result in an increase in the amount of oxygen in solution. Thus, on exposure to 100% oxygen, blood is fully saturated with oxygen and, in addition, contains about 21 mL/L of oxygen in solution, since solution of the gas in blood is directly proportionate to P_{O_2}.

It is important to distinguish between P_{O_2}, oxygen saturation, and oxygen content. P_{O_2} is the force driving oxygen across cellular membranes; oxygen saturation determines the color of the blood; and oxygen content is the volume of oxygen in the blood. The last measurement is most relevant to the cardiopulmonary transport of oxygen.

Oxygen content depends on hemoglobin level and is influenced by oxygen in solution, especially during oxygen breathing. Blood pH, temperature, and hemoglobin level must be known if oxygen content is to be accurately calculated from arterial P_{O_2}. The Severinghaus slide rule provides a convenient means of making this calculation.

CO_2 Transport

CO_2 production, which results from metabolism of substrates in the tissues, is the other aspect of gas exchange that equals oxygen consumption in importance. In addition, the regulation of the level of CO_2 in the blood plays a major role in determining the acid-base balance of the blood and of the body as a whole. It also sets the level of arterial pH (negative logarithm of the H^+ ion concentration). CO_2 is carried in the blood in 3 different ways. Like oxygen it dissolves in blood, but to a much greater degree (25 times greater, or about 27 mL/L at a normal P_{CO_2} of 40 mm Hg in arterial blood). CO_2 is also carried as bicarbonate in the buffering system of the blood and in combination with hemoglobin as a carbamino compound. Arterial CO_2 tension is the most closely controlled variable in the respiratory system. The normal value of 40 mm Hg is equivalent to $(40/760) \times 100$, or 5.25% CO_2 in the alveolar gas, and free equilibration takes place across the pulmonary membrane. Pulmonary ventilation is the most important determinant of arterial P_{CO_2}; hypoventilation raises the P_{CO_2} level. The level of ventilation is normally closely controlled by servomechanisms, and the arterial P_{CO_2} is maintained within a few mm of 40 mm Hg. The level of metabolism and the adequacy of tissue perfusion determine the pH and P_{CO_2} of venous blood returning to the lungs, and the adequacy of ventilation determines the extent to which the products of metabolism are cleared from the blood by the lungs. Abnormalities of the arterial P_{CO_2} result both from abnormalities of ventilation and from disturbances of acid-base balance.

Relationship Between P_{CO_2} & pH

Alterations in the relationship between arterial P_{CO_2} and pH may be grouped into 4 categories, 2 of which are respiratory and 2 of which are metabolic.

Ventilation is the most important means of influencing P_{CO_2} and pH. (1) With hyperventilation, arterial pH rises and P_{CO_2} falls as CO_2 is washed out of the blood (respiratory alkalosis). (2) With hypoventilation, arterial pH falls and P_{CO_2} rises as CO_2 accumulates in the blood (respiratory acidosis).

Metabolism influences P_{CO_2} in the reverse direction. (1) In metabolic acidosis, although blood pH falls, the increased acidity of the blood stimulates ventilation so that arterial P_{CO_2} also falls. A low pH associated with a low P_{CO_2} is common in cardiac failure, because inadequate tissue perfusion results in excessive anaerobic metabolism and lactic acid accumulation. (2) In metabolic alkalosis, the arterial pH and P_{CO_2} are both elevated. This is by far the least common disturbance of the group and may occur as a result of alkali ingestion or following prolonged vomiting with loss of acid gastric contents.

	pH	P_{CO_2}
Respiratory acidosis	↓	↑
Respiratory alkalosis	↑	↓
Metabolic acidosis	↓	↓
Metabolic alkalosis	↑	↑

Assessment of Acid-Base Balance

Unless calculations are performed, it is not always easy to see the accommodation of pH level to changes in P_{CO_2}, both because renal compensatory forces may come into operation and because pH involves a logarithmic scale. The Severinghaus slide rule is particularly helpful in calculating a value for base deficit or base excess from arterial P_{CO_2} and pH, and it takes into account the buffering properties of hemoglobin. Using it enables the clinician to accurately determine the acid-base balance of acutely ill patients and to plan appropriate therapy for acid-base disturbances. The various disturbances of blood gas tensions are commonly followed by measurements of the P_{O_2}, P_{CO_2}, and pH of arterial blood. These measurements are indicated in almost all acutely ill patients with cardiopulmonary disease and also in postoperative care of patients after major surgery, especially after cardiac surgery. These measurements are thus routinely available in most intensive care and coronary care units, where specially trained nurses and technicians can perform the analyses on the spot, without sending the specimen to a laboratory, and the information is available at any time.

Fick Principle

Cardiac output is most commonly measured by the Fick principle, which states that in a steady state the flow of blood through an organ (eg, the lungs) is equal to the amount of a substance (eg, oxygen) absorbed by the blood flowing through the organ, divided by the difference in oxygen concentration between the blood entering and blood leaving the organ. Thus, pulmonary blood flow is the oxygen consumption in milliliters per minute divided by the arteriovenous difference across the lungs (pulmonary venous oxygen content minus pulmonary arterial oxygen content in milliliters per liter). The same principle applies to the systemic capillary beds of the entire systemic circulation. Thus, systemic blood flow is equal to the oxygen consumption of the body (equal in the steady state to the uptake in the lungs) divided by the difference in oxygen content between arterial blood going to the tissues and mixed venous blood (pulmonary arterial blood) returning to the lungs for oxygenation. In normal subjects, blood flow through the lungs is virtually equal to blood flow to the body, and no substantial right-to-left or left-to-right shunt is present.

In a normal subject the oxygen consumption is about 250 mL/min. The arterial oxygen content is about 200 mL/L, and the mixed venous (pulmonary arterial blood) content is about 150 mL/L. Thus, the cardiac output is 250/50 or 5 L/min. This value in liters per minute is often adjusted to the size of the subject by dividing it by the body surface area derived from standard tables and expressed in m^2. The adjusted value is called the cardiac index; the normal value is about 4 L/min/m^2.

Indicator Dilution Method

The Fick principle also forms the basis for the indicator dilution method of measuring cardiac output, which uses green dye (indocyanine green), a radioactive isotope, or cold saline (thermodilution) injected into one place in the circulation and measured in another. A known amount of indicator is injected, usually into the right atrium, and the concentration of the indicator is subsequently measured at a downstream site after the indicator has thoroughly mixed with the blood. If cold saline is used, the temperature of blood in the pulmonary artery is measured continuously with a thermistor at the tip of a catheter (Swan-Ganz catheter). If green dye is used, the concentration is measured in systemic arterial blood by drawing a sample continuously through a photoelectric instrument (cuvette densitometer) that measures the optical density of blood at an appropriate wavelength. If a radioisotope is used, a counter is positioned over the heart or lungs. The cardiac output equals the amount of indicator injected, divided by its average concentration during its passage past the sampling site (Fig 4–2). The indicator must not leave the circulation between the injection and the sampling sites, nor can it cause harmful effects or those that alter hemodynamic status.

In practice, when green dye is used, the logarithm of the concentration of dye is plotted against time as the concentration rises to a peak, falls, and then rises again as recirculation of dye occurs. With thermodilution, recirculation is negligible, and the disappearance follows an exponential pattern (straight line on a semilog plot). With dye, the exponential disappear-

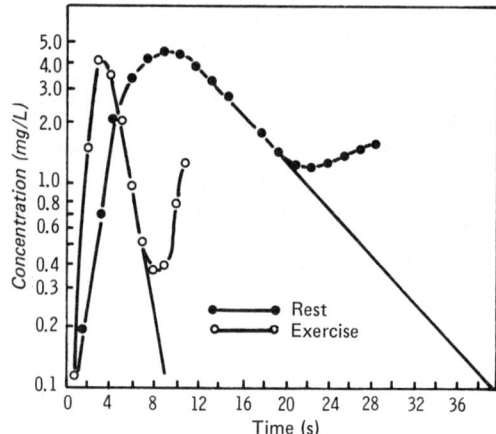

$$F = \frac{E}{\int_0^\infty C \, dt}$$

F = flow
E = amount of indicator injected
C = instantaneous concentration of indicator in arterial blood

In the *rest* example above,

$$\frac{\text{Flow in 39 s}}{\text{(time of first passage)}} = \frac{5\text{-mg injection}}{1.6 \text{ mg/L}}$$
$$\text{(avg concentration)}$$

Flow = 3.1 L in 39 s

Flow (cardiac output)/min = 3.1 × $\frac{60}{39}$ = 4.7 L

For the *exercise* example,

Flow in 9 s = $\frac{5 \text{ mg}}{1.51 \text{ mg/L}}$ = 3.3 L

Flow/min = 3.3 × $\frac{60}{9}$ = 22.0 L

Figure 4–2. Determination of cardiac output by indicator (dye) dilution. (Data and graph from Asmussen E, Nielsen M: The cardiac output in rest and work determined by the acetylene and the dye injection methods. *Acta Physiol Scand* 1952;**27**:217.)

ance is interrupted by recirculation of dye, as shown in Fig 4–2, and the initial linear portion of the curve must be extrapolated to zero concentration to define the time-concentration curve during the first passage of the dye. Cardiac output is then calculated as shown in Fig 4–2. In practice, computers are used to extrapolate the curves and calculate cardiac output.

MEASUREMENT OF CARDIAC SHUNTS

Use of Fick Principle to Estimate Shunts

Methods based on the Fick principle can be used to estimate and investigate intracardiac and intrapulmonary shunts seen in congenital heart disease in which blood passes from one side of the circulation to another without traversing a capillary bed.

Right-to-Left Shunts

The characteristic feature of a right-to-left shunt is a reduction in systemic arterial saturation resulting from mixing of venous blood with oxygenated blood returning from the lungs. The right-to-left shunt can be calculated by applying the Fick equation to both the pulmonary and systemic circuits and subtracting the pulmonary flow from the systemic. As an example, in a patient with Fallot's tetralogy with mild polycythemia (hemoglobin 18.6 g/dL; oxygen capacity 250 mL/L; $\dot{V}_{O_2}$ 200 mL/min), pulmonary arterial (mixed venous) saturation might be 70% (oxygen content [70/100] × 250, or 175 mL/L); systemic arterial saturation 85% (oxygen content 212.5 mL/L); and end-pulmonary capillary saturation 97% (oxygen content 242.5 mL/L). The Fick principle can be used to calculate systemic flow ($\dot{Q}_s$):

$$\text{Systemic flow} = \frac{225}{(194 - 144)} = \frac{225}{50} = 4.5 \text{ L/min}$$

The Fick principle can also be used to calculate pulmonary flow ($\dot{Q}_p$):

$$\text{Pulmonary flow} = \frac{200}{(242.5 - 175)} = \frac{200}{67.5} = 3 \text{ L/min}$$

In this example, the right-to-left shunt is 5.3 − 3.0, or 2.3 L/min.

Left-to-Right Shunts

The characteristic feature of left-to-right shunts is an increase in oxygen content and saturation in the chamber into which the shunt flows. In other words, the oxygen content is higher than in the immediately preceding cardiac chamber. The magnitude of left-to-right shunts can be conveniently calculated by applying the Fick equation to both the pulmonary and systemic circuits as illustrated above for right-to-left shunts.

For example, in a patient with an atrial septal defect, samples from the right heart chambers might show 85% saturation in the pulmonary arterial blood, 86% in the right ventricle, 83% in the right atrium, 67% in the superior vena cava, and 73% in the inferior vena cava. Arterial saturation and pulmonary venous saturation are 97% each. The oxygen capacity is 200 mL/L and the oxygen consumption 225 mL/min. The increase in this example occurs between the venae cavae and the right atrium; the venae cavae samples represent venous blood returning from the tissues, whereas the right atrial blood is of higher saturation because the blood shunted across the atrial defect is mixed with it. Assuming that the inferior vena cava drains two-thirds of the body and the superior vena cava one-third, the mixed venous saturation can therefore be calculated as

$$\frac{67 + (2 \times 73)\%}{3}$$

or 71% (oxygen content 144 mL/L). The Fick equation can be applied to calculate systemic flow ($\dot{Q}_s$):

$$\text{Systemic flow} = \frac{200}{(212.5 - 175)} = \frac{200}{37.5} = 5.3 \text{ L/min}$$

The Fick principle can be similarly used to calculate pulmonary flow ($\dot{Q}_p$):

$$\text{Pulmonary flow} = \frac{225}{(194 - 166)} = \frac{225}{28} = 8 \text{ L/min}$$

In this example, the left-to-right shunt is 8 − 4.5, or 3.5 L/min.

Pulmonary to Systemic Flow Ratio

The size of left-to-right shunts is often expressed in terms of the ratio of pulmonary to systemic flows. In the example above, the ratio is (8/4.5) or 1.8:1. This is a small flow ratio, and values of 3 or 4:1 are not uncommon.

Accuracy of Shunt Estimations

The accuracy of shunt flow calculations based on intracardiac samples is not high. Bloodstreams tend not to mix fully in the right heart chambers, and if there is valvular incompetence, blood from a more distal chamber can contaminate the next most proximal one. As the pulmonary arteriovenous oxygen difference becomes smaller in patients with large left-to-right shunts, the magnitude of the calculated pulmonary blood flow comes to vary widely in response to small differences in pulmonary arterial oxygen content. Blood oxygen content measurements are usually accurate to within ± 2 mL/L, and when the pulmonary arterial oxygen saturation is 90% or more, the pulmonary arteriovenous oxygen difference may be as low as 14 mL/L. Measurement errors then have a marked effect.

Bidirectional Shunts

The calculation of blood flow in bidirectional shunts in congenital heart disease is even more inaccurate than that in left-to-right shunts. The most satisfactory method of calculation is the measurement of "effective" blood flow. The concept of "effectiveness" of flow implies that any blood flow that fails to traverse a capillary bed is "ineffective." Thus, left-to-right shunt constitutes ineffective pulmonary flow and right-to-left shunt ineffective systemic flow. Effective flow ($\dot{Q}_{eff}$) is calculated from the Fick equation as

$$\text{Effective cardiac output} = \frac{\text{Oxygen consumption in mL/min}}{\text{Pulmonary venous} - \text{Mixed venous oxygen content in mL/L}}$$

In a patient with Eisenmenger's syndrome and a bidirectional shunt at ventricular level, samples from the right heart might show a pulmonary arterial saturation of 80%, right ventricle 78%, right atrium 65%, superior vena cava 63%, and inferior vena cava 67%. With oxygen consumption at 250 mL/min, oxygen capacity 210 mL/L, end-pulmonary capillary saturation 97%, and arterial saturation 92%, the systemic flow is calculated from the arterial and mixed venous (right atrial) samples as follows:

$$\text{Systemic flow} = \frac{250}{(193.2 - 136.5)} = \frac{250}{56.7} = 4.4 \text{ L/min}$$

Pulmonary flow is calculated from end-pulmonary capillary and pulmonary arterial blood:

$$\text{Pulmonary flow} = \frac{250}{(203.7 - 168)} = \frac{250}{35.7} = 7 \text{ L/min}$$

Effective flow is calculated from end-pulmonary capillary and mixed venous blood:

$$\text{Effective flow} = \frac{250}{(203.7 - 136.5)} = \frac{250}{67.2} = 3.7 \text{ L/min}$$

The left-to-right shunt equals the difference between the pulmonary and effective flows (7−3.7), or 3.3 L/min, and the right-to-left shunt equals the difference between the systemic and effective flows (4.4−3.7), or 0.7 L/min. It is easy to see that these calculations may be subject to error when the arteriovenous difference becomes small and when mixing may be incomplete. It is important to realize that all shunt calculations must be regarded as semiquantitative measurements only.

End-Pulmonary Capillary Oxygen Saturation

The clinician must realize the importance of the value selected for end-pulmonary capillary saturation in all the calculations noted above. Pulmonary venous samples are seldom available, and arterial samples are not relevant if a right-to-left shunt is present. Therefore, the clinician must arbitrarily select a value for end-capillary saturation, and it is necessary to decide whether the conventional value of 97% is appropriate in any given case. The effect of oxygen breathing on arterial oxygen content provides some indirect evidence about the validity of assuming a normal end-pulmonary capillary saturation. If arterial oxygen is 97% or higher there is no problem, because end-capillary oxygen content must be normal and no significant right-to-left shunt can be present. When arterial saturation is low, however, it is not possible to tell whether arterial hypoxia is due to right-to-left shunt or to abnormal pulmonary function.

Effect of Oxygen Breathing

Breathing 100% oxygen eliminates oxygen exchange problems in the lungs and raises end-pulmonary capillary content to supernormal levels. If arterial hypoxia is due to lung disease, arterial oxygen content rises markedly with oxygen breathing. In patients with arterial hypoxia due to right-to-left shunt, end-pulmonary capillary saturation is normal, and oxygen breathing has only a small and predictable effect on arterial oxygen content.

Breathing 100% oxygen raises end-pulmonary capillary oxygen content by increasing the amount of oxygen carried in solution in the blood. An increase of 18 mL/L in end-pulmonary capillary blood occurs if alveolar P_{O_2} changes from 100 mm Hg to 700 mm Hg. As long as the hemodynamic status of the patient remains unchanged, an equal increase of 18 mL/L in oxygen content will occur in all sites of the body. The rise of 18 mL/L corresponds to an increase in saturation of 9% if the oxygen capacity is 200 mL/L. If the oxygen capacity is higher than 200 mL/L, the percentage change in saturation is lower, and vice versa.

Qualitative Estimation of Shunts by Indicator Dilution Methods

Indicator dilution curves using dye or radioactive isotope provide qualitative information about shunts. In right-to-left shunts, a portion of the injected dose of indicator—which passes from an injection site in the right heart through the shunt—traverses a shorter path through the circulation than does the main bolus, as shown in Fig 4–3. It thus appears earlier as a hump on the build-up phase of dye curve recorded in the arterial tree. In left-to-right shunts, blood containing indicator recirculates abnormally early and produces a hump on the disappearance curve (Fig 4–4).

Detection of Small Shunts

A number of methods are available for the detection of shunts that are too small to be detected from differences in the oxygen content of blood samples. These techniques generally involve sampling blood from the right side of the heart after the patient has

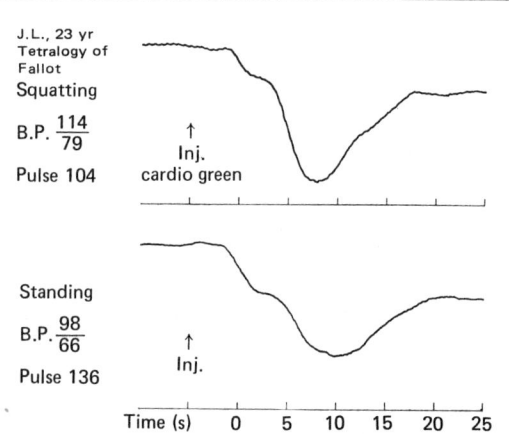

Figure 4–3. Indicator dilution curves showing early appearance of dye injected into the right atrium in a patient with Fallot's tetralogy. The size of the initial hump due to right-to-left shunt is greater in the standing position.

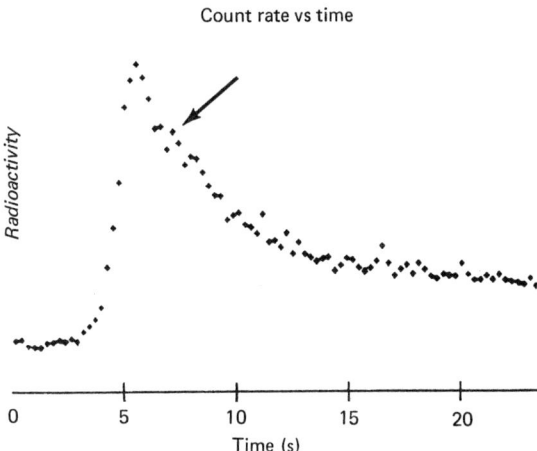

Figure 4-4. Indicator dilution curve in a patient with left-to-right shunt due to atrial septal defect (pulmonary/systemic flow ratio 2:1). Radioactivity is plotted on the ordinate and time on the abscissa. The hump on the disappearance curve results from early recirculation of shunted blood. (Courtesy of E Botvinick.)

inhaled gaseous indicators such as hydrogen, nitrous oxide, or radioactive krypton that enter the pulmonary capillary blood. Hydrogen has the advantage that it can be detected with a platinum electrode at the tip of a catheter, thus eliminating the need for blood sampling. In practice, the detection of small shunts that are not discovered by means of right heart sampling of oxygen content or angiocardiography is of little clinical significance.

Other Methods for Measurement of Blood Flow

A. Clearance Methods: Inert gas methods for the measurement of flow in regional circulations, such as the brain or the heart, are based on the approach introduced by Kety and Schmidt in 1945. The principle involves following the saturation or desaturation of the tissue in question with an inert gas indicator introduced into the circulation via the lungs. The increase or decrease in the arterial and venous concentrations of the indicator is measured over the time of equilibration, and the reciprocal of the time taken for the process to reach completion reflects flow to the tissue in mL/min/100 g of tissue. Nitrous oxide was the first gas to be used for this purpose; subsequently, helium, hydrogen, and argon have proved equally useful. The method is slow, a single measurement taking 5–30 minutes, and a steady state must be assumed to be present over this time.

A more invasive method using the same principle involves injecting radioactive xenon (Xe 133), dissolved in saline, into a tissue or a blood vessel (eg, a coronary artery) and measuring the rate of decay of radioactivity over the tissue (eg, over the precordium). The reciprocal of the clearance time gives a value related to the blood flow in mL/min/100 g of tissue.

B. Local Thermodilution: Another form of indicator dilution has been applied to the invasive measurement of coronary flow (Ganz, 1971). In this method, a special catheter is passed into the coronary sinus and a continuous infusion of cold saline made through a lumen near the tip at a rate of 35–55 mL/min for up to 20 seconds. The temperature of the blood at a site several centimeters back from the tip of the catheter is measured with a thermistor. The method uses the form of the Fick equation dealing with continuous infusion of indicator (I) at a constant rate:

$$\dot{Q} = I \div C$$

where $\dot{Q}$ is blood flow and C the steady concentration of indicator (temperature difference in this case) resulting from the infusion. This method provides absolute measurements in milliliters per minute rather than relative flow per 100 g of tissue. It assumes adequate mixing of the cold saline with blood in the short distance between the injection and sampling sites in the coronary sinus.

C. Flowmeter Techniques: More direct methods for the measurement of the velocity of blood flow include electromagnetic and Doppler blood velocity meters. Catheter-tip electromagnetic flowmeters can be used in the great vessels to measure blood velocity, but calibration and finding a stable position for the catheter away from the wall of the vessel present problems. Ultrasonic Doppler blood velocity meters, either continuous wave or pulsed, have also been used to measure aortic and pulmonary blood flow (see Chapter 5). In addition, both electromagnetic and ultrasonic Doppler flowmeters have been used during surgery to measure the blood velocity in exposed vessels, eg, through aortocoronary grafts and in coronary arteries.

BLOOD VOLUME

The circulating blood volume can be determined either from measurements of red cell volume or from plasma volume plus hematocrit. The values, although statistically valid, are subject to considerable variation, and the range of normal values is wide. The principle in blood volume measurement is the injection of a tracer material that mixes with the total blood volume before it is excreted. The degree of dilution of the tracer is measured in a sample of blood drawn after mixing is complete. Commonly used tracers are radioactive chromium–labeled red cells, which measure red cell volume, or iodine-labeled albumin, which measures plasma volume. The total blood volume is calculated from the hematocrit:

$$\frac{\text{Red cell volume}}{\text{Red cell volume + Plasma volume}}$$

Thus, total blood volume equals

$$\text{Red cell volume} \times \frac{1}{\text{Hematocrit}}$$

or,

$$\text{Plasma volume} \times \frac{1}{1 - \text{Hematocrit}}$$

In practice, mixing of the indicator is not always complete before the indicator begins to be excreted, and incomplete mixing of indicator often gives falsely low values, especially in patients with heart disease in whom the cardiac output is low.

Angiographic Measurements of Cardiac Chamber Volumes

Left ventricular volume is most commonly measured from cineangiograms recorded following the injection of iodine-containing contrast material into the ventricle during left heart catheterization. Ventricular volumes are calculated from the dimensions of opacified areas of individual films or cine frames exposed at the end of systole and the end of diastole.

The angiographic image of the left ventricle may be recorded in a single plane (usually the left anterior oblique) or in 2 planes: posteroanterior (shown in Fig 4–5) and lateral or 2 obliques. The examiner must make some assumption about the shape of the ventricle in the axis of revolution about the plane or planes in which measurements are made. The simplest assumption is to consider the left ventricle as a sphere, but the slightly more complex figure of a prolate ellipse is frequently used. Computer programs are commonly used to calculate left ventricular volume from a small number of specific angiographic measurements.

Errors of Method

The process of defining the edge of the ventricular shadow is often subjective. Blood trapped between the trabeculae carneae cordis, which form muscular projections into the body of the left ventricle, may not show up on end-systolic films as an opacity. The assumption made about a particular geometric shape for the ventricle introduces an unknown error. The end-diastolic volumes are more accurate than the end-systolic values, which are probably too small.

Ventricular volume can also be estimated from 2-dimensional echographic images. Several geometric approaches have been used, and most give smaller volumes than angiography. The reason for this discrepancy is not clear, and errors are possible with both techniques.

Ejection Fraction

The ratio of stroke volume (end-diastolic minus end-systolic volume) to end-diastolic volume (the ejection fraction) has become a widely accepted measure of left ventricular function. It is a nondimensional number that expresses the percentage of blood in the ventricle that is ejected per beat. The normal value obtained from a measurement in 2 planes is 67 ± 9%. This value tends to be falsely high, because the end-systolic volume from which it is calculated is falsely low. The injection of contrast material into the left ventricle is usually made with a catheter in the chamber, although less invasive methods using intravenous radioactive indicators or right-sided injections of contrast media are sometimes used. The injection of contrast media into the left ventricle often provokes ectopic beats, as shown in Fig 4–6. This can be significant in the evaluation of left ventricular function. A false idea of ejection fraction can also be obtained from the abnormally forceful left ventricular contraction that usually follows a run of ectopic beats.

Ejection fraction can also be measured from 2-dimensional echocardiograms. The measurement is greatly facilitated if a "light pen" is used to outline the ventricle and calculations made using computer techniques (Fig 4–7).

Wall Motion Abnormalities

Localized abnormalities of the motion of the heart can be detected from angiograms. These abnormalities almost always involve the left ventricle and are due to coronary artery disease. Changes in the shape of the left ventricle as seen on angiography also give clues to the site of ischemic areas of the left ventricular myocardium. It is difficult to obtain quantitative measurements of regional ventricular function, but a qualitative impression of the site of noncontracting or poorly contracting areas can be readily obtained. Similar information is available from echocardiographic studies, especially those using 2-dimensional sector scan-

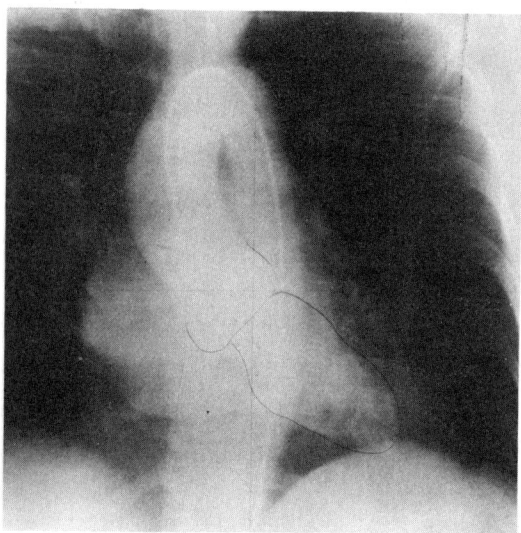

Figure 4–5. Posteroanterior view of the left ventricle following injection of contrast material. The outline of the ventricle from which volume was calculated is drawn on the x-ray.

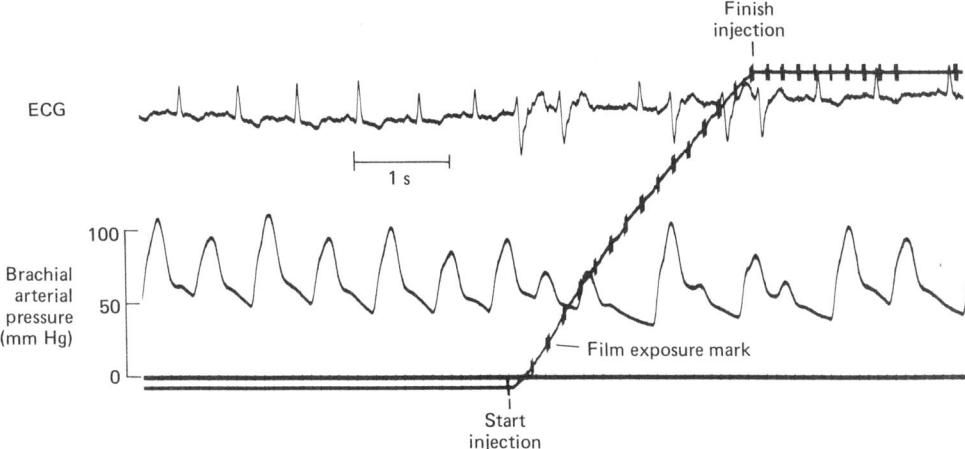

Figure 4-6. ECG and brachial arterial pressure tracing obtained during an injection of contrast material into the left ventricle in a patient with aortic stenosis. The timing of the angiographic film exposures is indicated. Pulsus alternans is present, and ectopic beats are seen during the injection.

ning. Although nuclear medical techniques are also being used for this purpose, the clarity of the image obtained using radiographic methods is the best.

The errors inherent in calculations based on angiography are even more of a problem in echocardiographic and nuclear medical techniques, because their level of resolution is relatively low. Their main advantage lies in their noninvasiveness.

Effects of Contrast Material

The contrast material itself also influences left ventricular function, mainly because of its hyperosmolarity. This factor is thought to be unimportant in the first 7 beats following injection, however, and it generally influences left ventricular end-diastolic pressure rather than ejection fraction. Left ventricular ejection fraction has proved to be a useful functional measurement that is greatly preferred to a visual impression of the force of contraction, which can be misleading. The right ventricle is of a completely different shape from the left and varies more in shape in disease. It is inappropriate to apply methods developed for computing left ventricular volume to the right side of the heart.

Measurement of Valvular Incompetence

Angiographic measurements of stroke volume include all the blood pumped by the ventricle, whereas

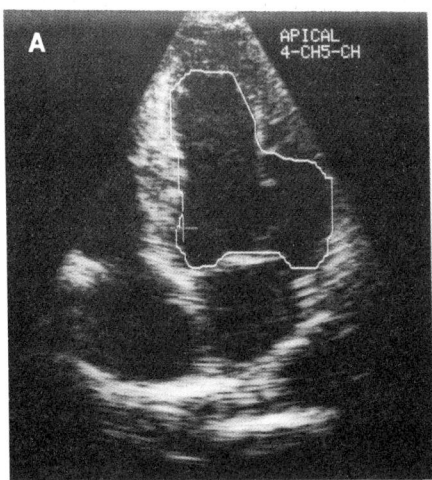
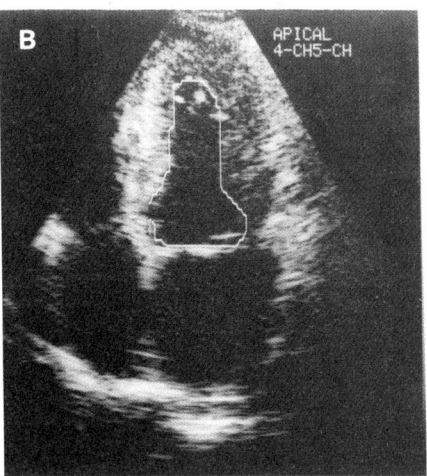

Figure 4-7. End-diastolic *(A)* and end-systolic *(B)* 2-dimensional echographic images of the left ventricle with the cavity outlined with a "light pen." Ejection fraction is calculated from the ratio of the areas at end-systole and end-diastole. (Courtesy of Elscint Inc.)

methods based on the Fick principle measure only the blood that flows forward to the systemic arterial bed. It is thus possible by combining the 2 methods to measure the volume of blood returning to the ventricle or atrium through the incompetent aortic or mitral valve. The angiographic stroke volume minus the forward (Fick) stroke volume gives a measure of the amount of backflow, which is usually expressed as the "regurgitant fraction," the proportion of the angiographic stroke volume flowing back per beat. A value of 50% or more indicates severe valvular incompetence.

MEASUREMENT OF BLOOD PRESSURE

Technique

Measurements of pressures in the heart and great vessels are almost always made through long small-bore catheters connected to electromanometers of the strain-gauge type. Obtaining accurate pressure recordings presents significant problems, especially when the catheter is subject to motion because of the action of the heart. The only satisfactory solution is to use catheter-tip manometers. Unfortunately, these are so expensive that their use outside research laboratories has not yet become practical. Experience and comparison of conventional and catheter-tip manometer tracings have made it possible to recognize high-quality pressure tracings and know when serious artifacts are present. Excessive damping of pressure tracings resulting from leaky stopcocks, bubbles of air in the catheter or manometer, or blockage of the catheter should be easily recognized, as shown in Fig 4–8. Excessive overswing due to catheter fling in hyperdynamic hearts is more difficult to deal with. The problems in this case mainly relate to inertia and depend on the magnitude of the accelerative forces involved; they are thus greatest with rapidly changing pressure signals. Electrical and mechanical damping systems are of some help but are still not entirely satisfactory. Obtaining acceptable readings of intravascular pressure depends more on skill and experience in positioning the catheter than on any objective knowledge of the scientific principles involved in damping. Part of the expertise of cardiac catheterization is recognizing an adequate tracing.

Configuration of Pressure Tracings

The pressures in each cardiac chamber are different. Examples are found in the sections on different diseases.

Systemic Arterial Pressure

Systemic arterial pressure is the most important pressure, because it is the most closely controlled. Control is established mainly by the action of the baroreceptor system. The normal arterial wave form is shown in Fig 4–9. Peak arterial pressure roughly coincides with the T wave of the ECG. There is often a prominent (dicrotic) notch on the downstroke associated with aortic valve closure. The normal values (110–120 mm Hg peak systolic and 70–80 mm Hg minimal diastolic pressure) change in response to physiologic stimuli such as exercise, excitement, mental stress, sleep, external temperature, posture, pregnancy, growth and development, and age. The range of normal values is wide and increases with age. Mean arterial pressure is usually recorded as the average pressure during the cardiac cycle and is obtained by electrically averaging the pressures recorded during the cycle. The pulse pressure (the difference between systolic and diastolic pressure) is usually about 40 mm Hg and mirrors stroke volume. It changes magnitude in the same direction as stroke volume in exercise,

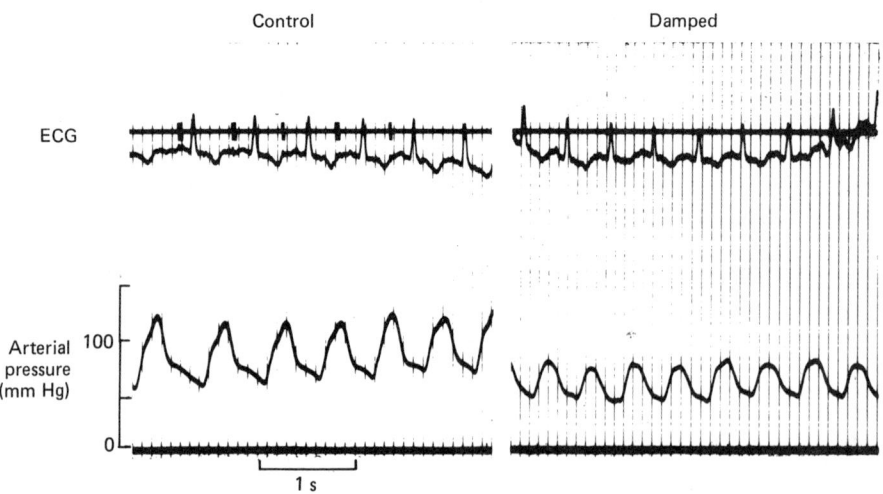

Figure 4–8. Control and damped brachial arterial pressure tracings obtained several minutes apart from a patient with aortic stenosis. Both the amplitude and the mean pressures decreased as the pressure was damped.

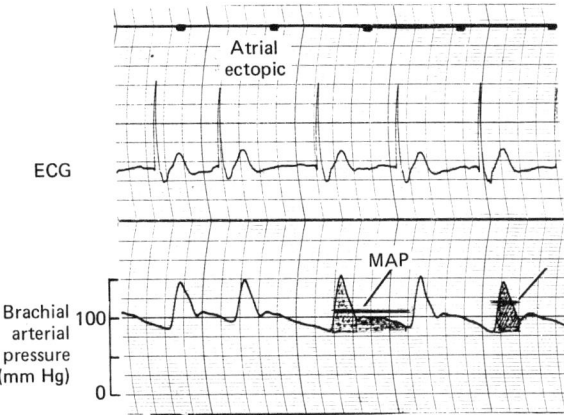

Figure 4-9. ECG and brachial arterial pressure in a normal subject. Mean arterial pressure (MAP) and mean systolic pressure (MSP) are indicated. One atrial ectopic beat is shown.

shock, or heart failure. The mean arterial pressure is roughly equal to the diastolic pressure plus one-third of the pulse pressure.

The mean systolic pressure (the average pressure during ventricular systole) can be measured by planimetry of an arterial pressure tracing, as shown in Fig 4-9. The mean systolic pressure gives an indication of the force against which the left ventricle must eject blood. This is not the same as the mean arterial pressure (also indicated in Fig 4-9), which is lower because it is an average taken over the whole cardiac cycle. The systemic arterial bed senses the mean arterial pressure as the force pressing against the walls of the blood vessels and influencing the rate of wear and tear on vascular tissues. In atrial fibrillation, especially in association with mitral valve disease, the systolic arterial pressure varies with the RR interval, being lower after a short pause and higher after a long pause, as shown in Fig 4-10. This reflects the effect of ventricular filling on the subsequent ventricular systole in accordance with the Frank-Starling mechanism. A similar effect is seen with an ectopic beat, even if it is atrial, as shown in Fig 4-9, in which the level of systolic arterial pressure in the beat after the pause following the ectopic beat is higher. When the ectopic beat is ventricular, the arterial pressure is increased by another mechanism. This is termed postectopic potentiation and involves the excitation-contraction coupling mechanism. It is seen in Fig 4-10, in which the beat following the ventricular ectopic beat shows the highest systolic arterial pressure in the strip. If regular ectopic beats are produced by pacing the heart

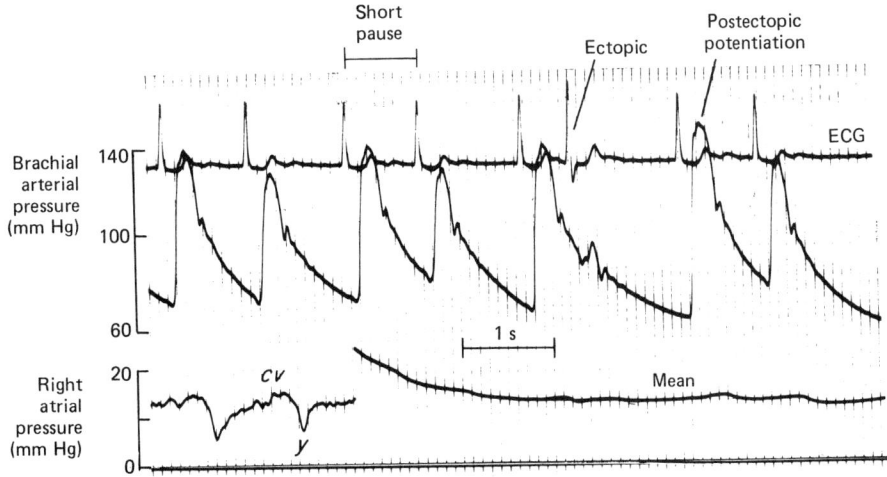

Figure 4-10. Brachial arterial and right atrial pressure tracings in a patient with mitral valve disease in atrial fibrillation. The effect of varying cycle lengths and an ectopic beat on arterial pressure are shown.

after each normal beat (paired pacing), an increase in cardiac output results. This is not achieved without an increase in myocardial oxygen consumption.

Pressure Gradients

The pressure difference between different chambers or across valves constitutes a clinically important measurement. The difference between the peak systolic left ventricular pressure and the aortic systolic pressure is called the gradient across the aortic valve. Similarly, the difference between the diastolic left atrial, or wedge, pressure and the left ventricular diastolic pressure is the gradient across the mitral valve. The gradient is often used as an indication of the severity of stenosis of the affected valve.

A simplified form of the Bernouilli equation has been used for the indirect measurement of pressure gradients across stenotic valves using Doppler ultrasound. The peak velocity in a jet of blood passing through a stenosed valve bears a significant relationship to the pressure difference across the valve. The simplified form of the Bernouilli equation is

$$P = 4 \times V^2$$

where P is the pressure gradient in millimeters of mercury and V the maximal velocity in centimeters per second. An equivalent method has been applied to the pressure difference across the mitral valve. Here the relationship has been expressed as

$$P = 220 \div t$$

where P is the pressure of gradient in millimeters of mercury and t is the time in milliseconds the diastolic mitral valve flow takes to fall to half its maximal value. The pressure gradients measured by these techniques have been compared with directly measured values, and reasonable agreement has been demonstrated (Stamm and Martin, 1983). The methods have the advantage of being noninvasive, but it is important to take into account the blood flow at the time that pressure measurements are being made. The pressure difference across stenotic valves varies with the flow across the valve, and the relationship is nonlinear. Thus, doubling the blood flow does not merely double the pressure difference but produces closer to a 4-fold increase in pressure difference. These considerations are most important in patients with mitral and aortic stenosis, since they affect calculations concerning the severity of the stenosis. The situation in patients with stenosis is further complicated by changes in heart rate that alter the relative lengths of systole and diastole. Whenever possible, cardiac output and the difference in pressure between 2 chambers should be measured simultaneously. In some cases this is not practical, and withdrawal tracings are obtained as the catheter is pulled from one chamber to another. Such tracings have the advantage that errors in calibrating 2 strain gauges are avoided, since only one gauge is used. It is important to record the heart rate at the time that each pressure measurement is made as a rough indication that the hemodynamic status of the patient has not changed significantly.

Measurements of Valve Area

Hydraulic formulas have been adapted for use in estimating valve area based on pressure differences and flows across valves. The formulas are most commonly applied to stenotic lesions of the mitral and aortic valves. They are based on steady turbulent flow under stable conditions in smooth, cylindric pipes and should not be used when there is valvular incompetence unless the extra forward flow resulting from the incompetence can somehow be incorporated in the calculations. Although the assumptions underlying the formulas clearly do not apply to flow across cardiac valves, these valve area calculations represent the best available means of obtaining numerical estimates of valve orifice size and do take into account both pressure and flow.

The formula for mitral valve area (MVA) is

$$\text{MVA in cm}^2 = \frac{\text{Diastolic mitral flow in mL/s}}{31 \times \sqrt{\Delta P \text{ in mm Hg}}}$$

where ΔP is the average pressure difference in mm Hg between the left atrium and the left ventricle during the period of diastolic flow. The value of 31 represents an arbitrary constant required to adjust the units appropriately.

The formula for aortic valve area (AVA) is

$$\text{AVA in cm}^2 = \frac{\text{Systolic flow in mL/s}}{44.5 \times \sqrt{\Delta P \text{ in mm Hg}}}$$

where ΔP is the mean pressure difference across the valve during the time of systolic flow and 44.5 is the arbitrary constant.

CARDIAC MEASUREMENTS & ELECTRICAL ANALOGS

Vascular Resistance

In describing the relationships between pressure and flow in the circulation, it is customary to measure vascular resistance as the ratio of pressure to flow. This is a simplistic application of Ohm's law, and it assumes that the circuits involved are linear and that there is a lack of phase difference between pressure and flow. In spite of these inaccuracies, pulmonary and systemic resistances are useful clinical measurements if their limitations are kept in mind.

Conductance (Calculations of Pulmonary & Systemic Vascular Resistance)

In some situations the reciprocal relationship—conductance—is used and the ratio of flow over pressure is calculated. Pulmonary vascular resistance (PVR) is a useful index of the degree of pulmonary vasoconstriction, especially in patients with pulmonary hypertension. It is calculated as follows:

$$\frac{\text{PVR in mm Hg}}{\text{L/min}} = \frac{\text{Mean pulmonary arterial pressure} - \text{Mean left atrial pressure}}{\text{Pulmonary blood flow}}$$

If pressure is expressed as dynes/cm^2 and flow in cm^3/s, the units can be expressed as dynes-s-cm^{-5}. However, these units do not show how the measurement is derived, and the equivalent units of mm Hg/L/min are preferable. One can convert mm Hg/L/min to dynes-s-cm^{-5} by multiplying by 80. Systemic vascular resistance (SVR) is the analogous measurement in the systemic circulation. It is calculated as

$$\frac{\text{SVR in mm Hg}}{\text{L/min}} = \frac{\text{Mean arterial pressure} - \text{Mean right atrial pressure}}{\text{Systemic blood flow}}$$

Vascular Compliance

Compliance is the term used in clinical physiology to describe the elastic behavior of elements involved in cardiovascular phenomena. It also refers to the storing of energy in a system, as in a spring. Like the term resistance, it is borrowed from the nomenclature of electrical theory, in which its analog is capacitance. Compliance is the ratio of volume change to pressure change and is measured in terms of units of volume change per unit of pressure change. Decreased compliance involves increased stiffness. Compliance when applied to the atria and ventricles refers to a change in pressure proportionate to a given amount of diastolic filling. If a chamber is compliant, it can accept a large volume with little rise in pressure. The word compliance first came into use in pulmonary physiology as a ratio expressing the volume of lung distention resulting from a given inflating transpulmonary pressure change. The term compliance is also used to describe the elastic behavior of the pulmonary and systemic arterial beds. A compliant bed can distend more with a given pressure change. The venous bed is referred to as a high compliance or high capacitance part of the circulation. The use of a single value to express the compliance of a structure implies a linear relationship between volume and pressure. This is seldom seen in the cardiovascular system. The left ventricle is more compliant at low volumes and becomes less compliant as it is distended. Thus, diastolic pressure tends to remain low until greater levels of distention occur, after which pressure rises more steeply. In general, acute heart failure causes higher diastolic ventricular pressures than do chronic lesions; thus, left ventricular compliance is said to increase with time as the ventricle distends in response to stretching. An indirect indication of ventricular compliance is given by the height of the *a* wave. If the ventricle is stiff and noncompliant, atrial contraction results in a larger pressure wave per given force of atrial contraction.

Time Constant

As a further extension of the electrical analogy it is possible to think in terms of the product of resistance and compliance. The units of this product are

$$\text{Time in min} = \frac{\text{mm Hg}}{\text{L/min}} \times \frac{\text{L}}{\text{mm Hg}}$$

The time constant is used in describing the change in left atrial pressure during diastole in a patient with mitral valve disease. In this case, the rate of left atrial pressure fall depends on both the resistance to flow across the mitral valve and the compliance (stiffness) of the left atrium. Either a high resistance to mitral valve flow (stenosis) or a large overdistended compliant atrium can increase the time constant of left atrial emptying. The time constant is the time taken for the pressure to fall to 1/e times (37%) the original value, where *e* is the base of natural logarithms (2.718). The time constants of the systemic and pulmonary circulations can also be determined from the diastolic fall of pressure in the system.

ASSESSMENT OF CARDIAC FUNCTION: "CONTRACTILITY"

One of the most important aspects of clinical cardiac physiology is the assessment of cardiac function. The reserve capacity of the heart is so large that disease must generally be far advanced before resting cardiac function is detectably impaired. Cardiac function normally deteriorates with age and is poor in sedentary people. Therefore, there is usually a mixed load on the heart in patients with cardiac symptoms. In addition to structural and mechanical problems there may be a functional myocardial factor and also an element of poor function owing to disuse. Assessment of cardiac function involves identifying each of these components in any individual patient, and it is most commonly required in patients in whom surgical correction of an anatomic defect is under consideration.

There are many measurements and indices available to assess cardiac dysfunction. None is entirely satisfactory. It is not possible to predict with certainty how a given patient's heart will function when a mechanical load such as valvular stenosis or incompetence is relieved. Thus, the severity of the cardiac lesion is of the greatest importance. There are a number of measurements that give an indication of ventricular function. They involve different levels of invasiveness. Although they are of value in prognosis, their results are almost never a complete contraindication to attempts to correct severe valvular lesions such as aortic stenosis.

Evidence of Impaired Ventricular Function

One of the most readily detectable indicators of poor ventricular function is pulsus alternans. In this condition, every other ventricular beat generates a lower pressure. The slower the heart rate and the bigger the pressure difference between alternate beats, the more significant the finding. The mechanism of mechanical pulsus alternans is unknown, and the finding is significant only if the heartbeat is regular.

An abnormally low cardiac output, usually reflected by an increased arteriovenous oxygen difference, is another finding that suggests myocardial disease, provided that an adequate venous return is present. These findings are not entirely reliable, because healthy, well-trained athletes often exhibit similar results, and resting values bear no necessary relationship to findings during exercise.

Valsalva's Maneuver

One of the most readily performed tests of cardiac function is to determine the patient's response to straining (Valsalva's maneuver), in which the subject blows against a mercury manometer to raise the intrapulmonary pressure to 40 mm Hg for 10 seconds. The height of the pressure and the duration of the period of strain can be varied, but 40 mm Hg and 10 seconds are conventionally used. The subject should not inhale deeply before straining; introducing a small leak into the system forces the subject to use the thoracic and abdominal muscles (rather than the cheeks) to generate the pressure. The sudden strain of the maneuver causes a complex sequence of mechanical and reflex changes in the circulation that depend on 2 factors, the level of cardiac function and effective central blood volume, and the speed and magnitude of the baroreceptor responses to a change in arterial pressure. The maneuver is best performed with a continuous recording of arterial pressure and is shown in Fig 4–11.

A. Normal Response: The first effect is a rise in arterial pressure owing to the transmission of applied pressure to the intrathoracic structures (heart and great vessels). The magnitude and speed of the rise depend on the suddenness and force of the strain. The arterial pressure then starts to fall, the pulse pressure narrows because the venous return is cut off, and the normal heart responds to a decrease in filling with a fall in output. The rate and magnitude of the fall during this period of strain reflect the size of the central blood volume.

B. Square Wave Response: In the extreme case of a large central blood volume, there is sufficient blood in the central circulation to maintain a constant pressure throughout the period of strain. This type of response is termed a square wave response and has in the past been incorrectly termed the heart failure response. It is seen in congestive heart failure but is also found in overhydrated normal subjects and in symptom-free patients with large left-to-right shunts, especially those with atrial septal defects. Fig 4–12 shows an example from a patient with atrial septal defect. The rate at which the heart empties during the period of straining depends on cardiac output. In congestive heart failure, the central circulation is overloaded and the cardiac output is low, so that the heart does not empty; thus, a square wave response is due to a combination of factors.

The reflex changes of Valsalva's maneuver depend on baroreceptor activity. In a normal response to Valsalva's maneuver, the falls in blood pressure and pulse pressure trigger reflex tachycardia within about 5–7 seconds and a rise in peripheral resistance a few seconds later. Thus, the arterial pressure stops falling and starts to rise toward the end of the period of strain. When the strain ends, the blood pressure falls and venous return is restored. The cardiac output increases and the blood pressure rises. The peripheral resistance is still raised in response to the previously low pressure, and the surge of blood into constricted vessels causes an overshoot of pressure. This overshoot in turn causes vagally mediated reflex bradycardia within 3–5 seconds and is followed by vasodilation, which restores the pressure to normal.

The response to Valsalva's maneuver offers a con-

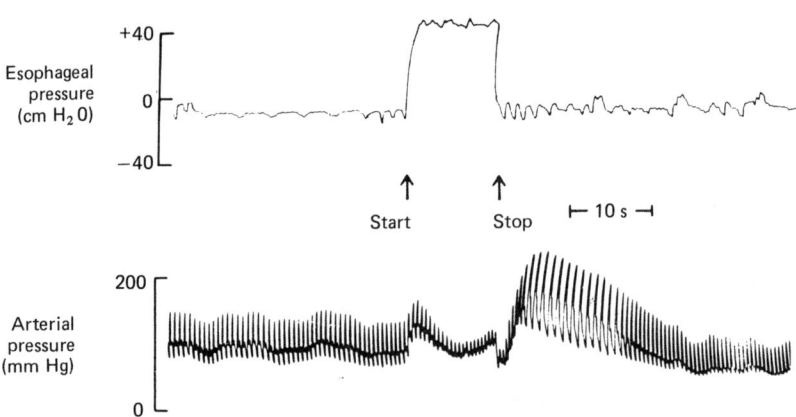

Figure 4–11. Tracing of the normal blood pressure and pulse response to straining (Valsalva's maneuver) in a normal man, recorded with a needle in the brachial artery.

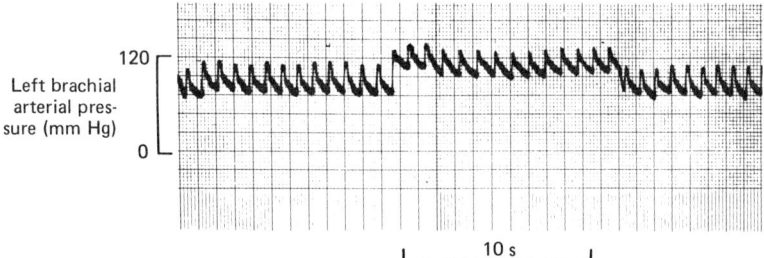

Figure 4–12. Arterial pressure tracing showing the response to Valsalva's maneuver in a patient with atrial septal defect and a large pulmonary blood flow. The pulse pressure is maintained during the period of strain, and there is no overshoot on release of the strain.

venient means of testing the reactivity of the baroreceptor reflex arc. It is primarily used in the investigation of patients with disease of the autonomic nervous system (Chapter 21). The intense vagal stimulation associated with the overshoot after Valsalva's maneuver may be sufficient to stop paroxysmal atrial tachycardia, and the maneuver may be useful therapeutically.

Left Ventricular Function

The difficulty of defining "contractility" and the lack of any satisfactory means of directly measuring the force of cardiac contraction have been mentioned in Chapter 1.

Maximum dp/dt. The maximum rate of change of left ventricular pressure (dp/dt_{max}) during the phase of isovolumetric contraction is probably the purest indicator of ventricular performance (Fig 4–13). The measurement is valid only if a catheter-tip manometer is used.

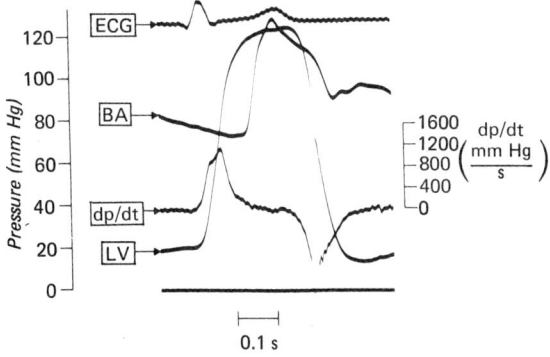

Figure 4–13. Pressure tracings and ECG showing the rate of change of left ventricular pressure. BA, brachial artery pressure; dp/dt, first derivative of left ventricular pressure; LV, high-fidelity left ventricular pressure. (Reproduced, with permission, from the American Heart Association, Inc., Kreulen TH et al: The evaluation of left ventricular function in man: A comparison of methods. *Circulation* 1975;**51**:677.)

Aortic acceleration. The best noninvasive indication of ventricular function is given by the speed of ejection in early systole. This can be measured by Doppler ultrasound as the average rate of increase in aortic or pulmonary blood velocity over the first 45 ms of ventricular ejection (see Chapter 5). This represents the linear acceleration in $cm \cdot s^{-2}$ imparted to the blood in the aorta or pulmonary artery in the early ejection phase of systole. The normal value in resting adults is about 700 $cm \cdot s^{-2}$ for the left and about 300 $cm \cdot s^{-2}$ for the right ventricle. Like all measurements made after the start of ejection, it depends in part on the quality of the match of aortic impedance (afterload) to the force of cardiac contraction. More conventional indicators of ventricular function can be obtained angiographically, by M mode or 2-dimensional echocardiography, or by radionuclear techniques. The size of the left ventricle and its ejection fraction, although well established as indicators of cardiac function, are not strictly measures of "contractility," because both are influenced by afterload. The values obtained by left ventricular angiography are better established than those for echocardiographic or radionuclear methods. The time resolution of these methods is unsatisfactory, because measurements can only be made 30–60 times a second by all but M mode echocardiography, and it gives only a one-dimensional view. The period of constant acceleration of blood flow out of the left ventricle lasts for only about 50 ms, so that only one or 2 frames of a left ventricular angiograph will be exposed during the rapid phase of ejection, and acceleration cannot be accurately assessed from 2 frames. Similar problems arise with 2-dimensional echocardiography and radionuclear measurements, but they have the advantage of being applicable during exercise. It is important to remember that several crucial assumptions are made whenever left ventricular volumes are calculated. For example, the measurement of ventricular volume is likely to involve an assumption about the shape of the ventricle (spherical, conical, or elliptical), and if the measurement uses M mode echocardiography, a single dimension is ordinarily measured and the radius cubed to give a volume measurement. Such measurements as the rate of circumferential shortening involve similar assumptions that must not be forgotten by those interpreting the studies.

It seems clear that no assessment of ventricular function can predict how the heart will behave after a mechanical load is removed. Even retrospective analysis of preoperative studies cannot distinguish between those who will survive and those who will succumb to an operation. There is thus no alternative to accepting patients for surgical treatment even though operative risks may be high. Statistical analysis has shown that left ventricular function measurements are significant indicators of the prognosis, but they should not be used to make absolute predictions or to make the decision in individual cases. The most logical approach—although it is not easy to achieve—is to follow patients as closely as possible, recognize surgically treatable lesions at an early stage, and operate before severe myocardial damage occurs.

NORMAL VALUES

Rest

The normal resting cardiac output of about 6 L/min (cardiac index about 4.05 L/min/m^2) varies from about 3.5 to 7.5 L/min. The values in the Fick equation that give this figure are blood oxygen capacity about 200 mL/L, arterial oxygen saturation 97%, arterial oxygen content 194 mL/L, mixed venous oxygen saturation 72%, mixed venous oxygen content 144 mL/L, arteriovenous oxygen content difference 50 mL/L, and oxygen consumption 300 mL/min.

The normal blood volume of about 5 L is composed of about 2.75 L of plasma and 2.25 L of red cells to give a hematocrit of 2.25 ÷ 5, or 45%. The volume of blood in the heart and lungs (central blood volume) totals about 1.5 L. About 0.9 L is contained in the pulmonary arteries, capillaries, and veins, but only about 75 mL is in the pulmonary capillaries at any instant. The total volume of blood in the heart is about 0.6 L. Left ventricular volume at the end of diastole is about 150 mL; with a stroke volume of 100 mL and an ejection fraction of 67%, the end-systolic volume is 50 mL. The conventional normal values for arterial pressure of 120 mm Hg systolic and 80 mm Hg diastolic should be thought of as normal for young adults. Arterial pressure varies with age. The problem of deciding the upper limit of normal is dealt with in Chapter 9. Mean arterial pressure changes little with posture; systolic pressure may fall when the patient stands up after having been supine. Depending on the effective blood volume, diastolic pressure rises, pulse pressure decreases, and heart rate increases.

The normal mitral valve area is greater than 3 cm^2. Values of about 1.5 cm^2 indicate slight stenosis and 1 cm^2 or less, significant stenosis. Aortic valve area is greater than 2 cm^2. Values of about 1 cm^2 indicate mild stenosis and 0.7 cm^2 or less, significant stenosis. The normal pulmonary vascular resistance is less than 2 mm Hg/L/min, or less than 160 dynes-s-cm^{-5}. The normal systemic resistance is less than 20 mm Hg/L/min, or less than 1600 dynes-s-cm^{-5}.

The maximal rate of change of left ventricular pressure is about 1200 mm Hg/s, and the corresponding figure for the right ventricle is about 250 mm Hg/s.

The normal resting ventilation is about 5 L/min. Normal arterial P_{O_2} is between 70 and 100 mm Hg, P_{CO_2} is 37–42 mm Hg, and pH is 7.36–7.43.

Exercise

During moderate exercise (sufficient to increase heart rate to about 120/min), oxygen consumption increases from about 250–300 mL/min to 1200–1500 mL/min. Arteriovenous oxygen difference increases from 50 mL/L to about 100 mL/L; and cardiac output to about 15 L/min. Blood gas tensions and pH do not change significantly. Ventilation increases to 30–40 L/min. Stroke volume increases to about 125 mL and arterial pulse pressure to about 60 mm Hg, with a systolic pressure of 130 mm Hg and a diastolic pressure of 70 mm Hg. With more severe exercise (oxygen consumption about 2500 mL/min), most untrained normal subjects show evidence of metabolic acidosis, with an increase in arterial lactate, a fall in pH, and a fall in arterial P_{CO_2} to about 35 mm Hg. The maximal heart rate in young adults of about 195/min falls to about 170 at the age of 60 years. Most patients with heart disease do not complain of dyspnea until their maximal oxygen consumption falls to less than 1200–1500 mL/min. By the time they are seriously disabled, their maximal cardiac output is about 10 L/min.

REFERENCES

AHA Committee Report: Recommendations for human blood pressure determination by sphygmomanometers: *Circulation* 1980;**62**:1145A.

Antman EM et al: Blood oxygen measurement in the assessment of intracardiac left to right shunts: A critical appraisal of methodology. *Am J Cardiol* 1980;**46**:265.

Carlsson E: *Measurement of Cardiac Chamber Volumes and Dimensions by Radiographic Methods: A Methodological Study With Some Physiological Applications.* Univ of California Press, 1970.

Chaitman BR et al: Objective and subjective analysis of left ventricular angiograms. *Circulation* 1975;**52**:420.

Cournand A et al: Measurement of the cardiac output in man using technique of catheterization of the right auricle or ventricle. *J Clin Invest* 1945;**24**:106.

Currie PJ et al: Continuous wave Doppler echocardiographic

assessment of severity of calcific aortic stenosis: A simultaneous Doppler-catheter correlative study in 100 adult patients. *Circulation* 1985;**71**:1162.

Dodge HT, Sandler H, Baxley WA: Usefulness and limitations of radiographic methods for determining left ventricular volume. *Am J Cardiol* 1977;**18**:10.

Dodge HT, Sheehan FH: Quantitative contrast angiography for assessment of ventricular performance in heart disease. *J Am Coll Cardiol* 1983;**1**:73.

Fick A: Ueber die Messung des Blutquantums in den Herzventrikeln: Sitzungsberichte der phys-med. *Gesellschaft zu Würzburg* 1870;**16**.

Filley GF: *Acid-Base and Blood Gas Regulation*. Lea & Febiger, 1971.

Fry DL: Physiologic recording by modern instruments with particular reference to pressure recording. *Physiol Rev* 1960;**40**:753.

Gaasch WH et al: Left ventricular compliance: Mechanisms and clinical implications. *Am J Cardiol* 1976;**38**:645.

Ganz W, Swan HJC: Measurement of blood flow by thermodilution. *Am J Cardiol* 1972;**29**:241.

Ganz W et al: Measurement of coronary sinus blood flow by continuous thermodilution in man. *Circulation* 1971;**44**:181.

Gelberg HJ et al: Quantitative left ventricular wall motion analysis: A comparison of area, chord and radial methods. *Circulation* 1979;**59**:991.

Goerke RJ, Carlsson E: Calculation of right and left cardiac ventricular volumes. *Invest Radiol* 1967;**2**:360.

Gorlin R, Gorlin SG: Hydraulic formula for calculation of the area of the stenotic mitral valve, other cardiac valves, and central circulatory shunts. *Am Heart J* 1951;**41**:1.

Greene DG et al: Estimation of left ventricular volume by one-plane cineangiography. *Circulation* 1967;**35**:61.

Hatle L, Angelsen BA, Tromsdol A: Noninvasive assessment of aortic stenosis by Doppler ultrasound. *Br Heart J* 1980;**43**:284.

Hatle L, Angelsen BA, Tromsdol A: Noninvasive assessment of atrioventricular pressure half time by Doppler ultrasound. *Circulation* 1979;**60**:1096.

Holen J et al: Determination of pressure gradient in mitral stenosis with a noninvasive ultrasound Doppler technique. *Acta Med Scand* 1976;**199**:455.

Holmgren A: Circulatory changes during muscular work in man. *Scand J Clin Lab Invest* 1956;**8 (Suppl 24)**:1.

Hossack KF et al: Maximal cardiac output during upright exercise: Approximate normal standards and variations with coronary disease. *Am J Cardiol* 1980;**46**:204.

Jefferson K, Rees S: *Clinical Cardiac Radiology*. Butterworth, 1973.

Klinke WP et al: Use of catheter-tip velocity–pressure transducer to evaluate left ventricular function in man: Effects of intravenous propranolol. *Circulation* 1980;**61**:946.

Klocke FJ: Measurements of coronary blood flow and degree of stenosis: Current clinical implications and continuing uncertainties. *J Am Coll Cardiol* 1983;**1**:31.

Levy B et al: Quantitative ascending aortic Doppler blood velocity in normal human subjects. *Cardiovasc Res* 1985;**19**:383.

Lewis BS, Gotsman MS: Current concepts of left ventricular relaxation and compliance. *Am Heart J* 1980;**99**:101.

Marshall RJ, Shepherd JT: *Cardiac Function in Health and Disease*. Saunders, 1968.

McIlroy MB: Pulmonary shunts. In: *Handbook of Physiology*. Vol 2. Fenn WO, Rahn H (editors). American Physiological Society, 1965.

Murray JF: *The Normal Lung: The Basis for Diagnosis and Treatment of Pulmonary Disease*. Saunders, 1976.

Parker JO, Case RB: Normal left ventricular function. *Circulation* 1979;**60**:4.

Ross JJ: Cardiac function and myocardial contractility: A perspective. *J Am Coll Cardiol* 1983;**1**:52.

Saksena FB: *Hemodynamics in Cardiology*. Praeger, 1983.

Severinghaus JW, Bradley AF: Electrodes for blood P_{O_2} and P_{CO_2} determination. *J Appl Physiol* 1958;**13**:515.

Severinghaus JW: Blood gas calculator. *J Appl Physiol* 1966;**20**:1108.

Sharpey-Schafer EP: Effects of Valsalva's manoeuver on normal and failing circulation. *Br Med J* 1955;**1**:693.

Shepherd JT, Vanhoutte PM: Role of the venous system in circulatory control. *Mayo Clin Proc* 1978;**53**:247.

Stamm RB, Martin RP: Quantification of pressure gradients across stenotic valves by Doppler ultrasound. *J Am Coll Cardiol* 1983;**2**:707.

Stewart GN: Researches on the circulation time and on the influences which affect it. *J Physiol* 1897;**22**:159.

Swan HJC: Indicator-dilution methods in the diagnosis of congenital heart disease. *Prog Cardiovasc Dis* 1959;**2**:143.

Tzivoni D et al: Analysis of regional ischemic left ventricular dysfunction by quantitative cineangiography. *Circulation* 1979;**60**:1278.

West JB: *Pulmonary Pathophysiology*. Williams & Wilkins, 1977.

Woodcock J: *Theory and Practice of Blood Flow Measurement*. Butterworth, 1975.

Wynne J et al: Estimation of left ventricular volumes in man from biplane cineangiograms filmed in oblique projections. *Am J Cardiol* 1978;**41**:726.

5 Special Investigations: Noninvasive

INTRODUCTION

Special cardiologic investigations are dealt with under the headings of noninvasive and invasive studies. This distinction is maintained in the subsequent chapters dealing with individual diseases. The descriptions of special investigations given here and in Chapter 6 deal in general terms with the principles involved in the various studies. They are not intended to provide sufficient technical details to enable a person to carry out the procedures but rather to aid in the understanding and interpretation of the various tests. Direct involvement in performance of any of the tests, learning from an experienced clinician, and application of the techniques to patients who have been personally seen and examined constitute the best means of acquiring proficiency in the technical aspects of special cardiologic investigations.

Routine Cardiologic Investigations

The clinical examination of all cardiac patients is incomplete without the recording of a 12-lead ECG and a chest x-ray. The physician should interpret the ECG and chest x-rays independently before reading the opinions of the radiologist or electrocardiographer who may have provided a written interpretation of the findings. Both investigations form such an important aspect of the clinical evaluation of the patient's condition that a valid opinion about a patient cannot be given until both have been seen by the physician.

Special Investigations

All investigations other than chest x-rays and ECG are considered to be special studies indicated by some clinical finding. Standard laboratory tests of blood, urine, feces, sputum, bone marrow, and cerebrospinal fluid may be required in the diagnostic investigation of the patient with cardiovascular disease. The laboratory findings in each type of cardiac disease are covered in the chapters dealing with that disease.

Special Cardiovascular Studies

Two main types of information are sought by cardiologic studies: anatomic (structural) and physiologic (functional). Although the relationship between structure and function is usually close, it is important to keep clearly in mind what specific information is being sought in any study. In many types of investigations, both structural and functional information is provided (eg, cardiac catheterization). In general, anatomic abnormalities relate to a specific diagnosis, whereas physiologic findings are more pertinent to degrees of functional impairment.

Most forms of cardiac investigation start as research procedures. Whether any new procedure will ultimately be accepted by the medical community is not usually decided for several years. The decisive factors include the clinical usefulness of the procedure, the prevalence of the conditions for which it is indicated, and economic factors such as cost of equipment that are outside the scope of this book. Not surprisingly, the current cardiologic literature is largely preoccupied with new forms of investigation that are still in the uncertain stage between research studies and standard procedures.

In all forms of investigation, it is important for the physician to bear in mind the cost to the patient in danger, discomfort, and expense and to make a clear distinction mentally between clinically indicated studies and ancillary confirmatory procedures. In many cases an accurate diagnosis is required, and in cases in which cardiac surgery is contemplated, an accurate diagnosis is in fact essential in every case. Because being right 85–90% of the time is not enough, studies must sometimes be done for confirmatory purposes even though the diagnosis is clinically almost certain.

Interpretation of Results

The greatly increased use of noninvasive tests to diagnose disease, especially in its early, presymptomatic stages, has led to problems in the interpretation of test results. The importance of the result of a given test is difficult to determine accurately. The significance of a "positive test" is reflected in the sensitivity of the test, which expresses its ability to detect "the disease" in patients in whom it is present. Sensitivity is defined as

$$\frac{\text{Positive}}{\text{Positive} + \text{False-negative}} \text{ Tests \%}$$

The significance of a negative test is reflected in the specificity of the test, which expresses its ability to exclude "the disease." Specificity is defined as

$$\frac{\text{Negative}}{\text{Negative} + \text{False-positive}} \text{ Tests \%}$$

The concept of "false-positive" and "false-negative" tests implies a "gold standard" or accurate means of deciding whether a given disease is present or not. Disease is not an all-or-none phenomenon, especially in its early stages, and "gold standards" of diagnosis are necessarily fallible and subject to change. The prevalence of "the disease" in the population under study is also an important variable that influences the probability of finding a given test positive or negative. (See also Chapter 8.) In practice, especially in patients with coronary artery disease, the finding of agreement (for or against the diagnosis) in several elements in the diagnosis—history, ECG, exercise test, or radionuclide study—is the most important evidence for or against.

The problem of dealing with asymptomatic persons is difficult. Most cardiac diseases cannot be defined in terms of a single specific abnormality but consist of constellations of findings. Firm diagnoses of conditions such as coronary artery disease, mitral valve prolapse (click-murmur syndrome), and hypertrophic cardiomyopathy should not be made on the basis of abnormalities discovered on a single test in an asymptomatic, otherwise normal person. The overenthusiastic use of a particular test to find persons with subclinical disease is of doubtful value unless specific treatment is available.

RECORDING OF THE ECG

Technique

The simplest diagnostic procedure with which every physician must be familiar is the taking of a standard 12-lead electrocardiogram (ECG). Modern electrocardiographs have become simple to use, and problems are most likely to be related to matching wall plugs, connecting the cables to the electrodes properly, and eliminating electrical interference. With any type of electrode, providing adequate localized skin contact with the right amount of electrode paste is important. Correct and consistent precordial electrode placement is important, especially when serial records are needed. Interference from other electrical equipment, especially electric blankets in domiciliary practice, should be suspected when 60-cycle noise is encountered. Increased electronic filtering should not be used to eliminate this, as it will almost certainly decrease the frequency response of the equipment and give a damped and inaccurate ECG.

Each lead of the ECG should be properly calibrated.

Safety

The examiner should remain alert to the possibility of ground loops, which present a risk of electrocution when more than one electrical device is attached to the patient. Patients with temporary artificial pacemakers are particularly vulnerable, because currents as low as 10·microamperes applied directly to the endocardium via the pacemaker catheter can cause ventricular fibrillation.

Electrocardiographic Interpretation

The details of electrocardiographic interpretation per se are not presented in this book. The electrocardiographic findings are discussed in the chapters dealing with individual diseases. For further information on the theory and practice of electrocardiographic interpretation, the reader is referred to Goldman MJ: *Principles of Clinical Electrocardiography*, 12th ed. Lange, 1986.

Reporting Results; Display of Tracings

The tracing should be examined, mounted, and reported and the results returned to the patient's chart as soon as possible (within 24 hours). Care must be taken to correctly identify the ECG with the patient's name and hospital number. The role of the frontal plane axis in determining heart position is important. The interpretation should include the rhythm; rate; axis; duration of the PR, QRS, and QT_c intervals; and description of P, QRS, and ST–T abnormalities in each lead, followed by an estimate of the significance of the findings.

Serial records or comparisons with previous tracings are often necessary for proper interpretation. Records obtained over 1–5 minutes or 4- to 24-hour monitoring or those obtained during or after exercise or interventions such as carotid sinus massage may clarify the relationship between symptoms and electrocardiographic abnormalities. The role of medications and metabolic or electrolyte state must be considered in interpretation. For example, digitalis or quinidine therapy or hypokalemia or hyperkalemia can often be confused with primary myocardial disease (Figs 5–1 to 5–4).

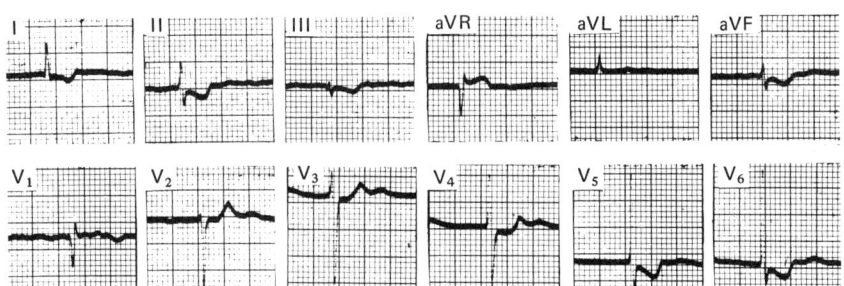

Figure 5–1. Digitalis effect. Note the ST segment depression. This produces an oblique downward configuration of the first portion of the ST in leads I, II, III, aVF, and V_{5-6}. There is a rounded ST segment depression in V_{3-4}. As a result, the T waves are "dragged" downward. There is reciprocal ST elevation in aVR. The above changes are indicative of digitalis effect but do not indicate digitalis toxicity. The rhythm is atrial fibrillation. (Reproduced, with permission, from Goldman MJ: *Principles of Clinical Electrocardiography*, 12th ed. Lange, 1986.)

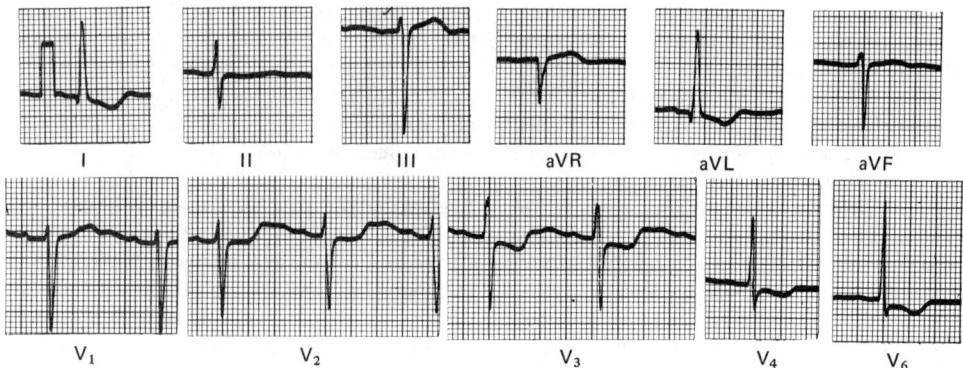

Figure 5–2. Effect of quinidine. The rhythm is regular sinus; PR = 0.2 second. The R in aVL = 14 mm. There is ST depression and T wave inversion in I, aVL, and V_{2-6}. The measured QT interval (see V_{2-3}) = 0.6 second (QT_c = 0.65 second). *Clinical diagnosis:* Aortic stenosis; quinidine therapy for previous ventricular arrhythmias. The R voltage in aVL and some of the ST–T changes are due to left ventricular hypertrophy. The long QT interval is due to quinidine. (Reproduced, with permission, from Goldman MJ: *Principles of Clinical Electrocardiography,* 12th ed. Lange, 1986.)

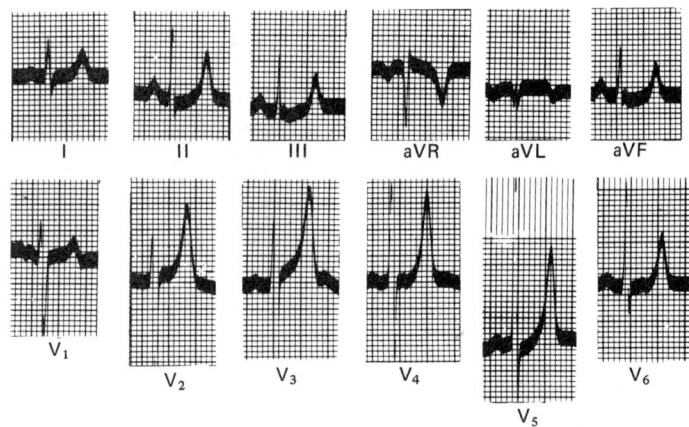

Figure 5–3. Hyperkalemia (chronic glomerulonephritis with uremia). Tall slender T waves are seen in I, II, III, aVF, and V_{2-6}. The rhythm is regular sinus; QRS interval = 0.09 second. Serum potassium = 7.2 meq/L. (Reproduced, with permission, from Goldman MJ: *Principles of Clinical Electrocardiography,* 12th ed. Lange, 1986.)

CHEST X-RAYS

Size of Heart Shadow

The posteroanterior chest x-ray should be taken with the x-ray tube 6 feet* from the x-ray so that distortion of heart size is avoided. This film is used for overall assessment of heart size. As a rough guide, the widest part of the heart should be less than half the diameter of the thorax. The Ungerleider tables, which relate the transverse diameter of the heart to the patient's height and weight, are probably more reliable than the simple measurement.

Lung Fields

Interpretation of the chest x-ray also involves examination of the lung fields for evidence of pulmonary congestion, redistribution of blood flow, pulmonary plethora in left-to-right shunts, and pulmonary oligemia with reduced pulmonary blood flow. Pulmonary edema tends to be central in origin and to spread out from the root of the lung. It is not infrequently asymmetric, perhaps because the patient lies on one side or the other. An example is shown in Fig 5–5.

ULTRASONOGRAPHY, ECHOCARDIOGRAPHY, & DOPPLER ECHOCARDIOGRAPHY

Ultrasonography has developed rapidly as an important form of noninvasive cardiac investigation. Ultrasonic energy within the range of frequencies used in clinical studies has proved to be harmless in more

*This distance varies in countries using the metric system.

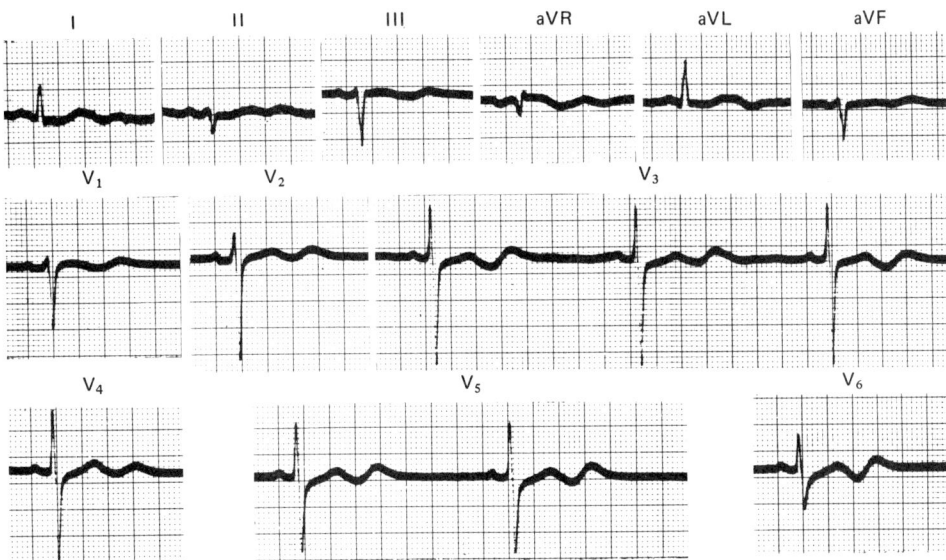

Figure 5–4. Hypokalemia (Cushing's syndrome). Regular sinus rhythm; PR = 0.16 second; QRS = 0.1 second. The frontal plane QRS axis = −40 degrees. There is ST depression in leads I, aVL, and V_{3-6}. Prominent U waves are seen in all precordial leads. The measured QT interval = 0.51 second, but when corrected for a heart rate of 37, the QT_c = 0.39 second. Serum potassium = 2.5 meq/L. (Reproduced, with permission, from Goldman MJ: *Principles of Clinical Electrocardiography*, 12th ed. Lange, 1986.)

than a decade of use. The standard ultrasound transducer consists of a piezoelectric crystal that is excited electronically to transmit sound waves at frequencies between 2 and 13 MHz. The beam of sound waves penetrates soft tissues and is reflected at interfaces, eg, between blood and heart muscle or heart valves. Blood is a poorer reflector than tissue, but as it moves, it causes a shift in the frequency of reflected ultrasound that can be detected and used to measure flow in the circulation using the Doppler principle (see Chapter 4). The ultrasound reflected from cardiac tissues is received at the transducer and electronically processed to provide images of the heart. The penetration of tissues by ultrasound depends on the frequency of the ultrasound. High frequencies (10 MHz) penetrate poorly and can only be used for tissues within a few millimeters of the surface. Low frequencies (2 MHz) penetrate more deeply (up to 20 cm) and can reach all intracardiac structures. Ultrasound does not penetrate bone or air-containing lung tissue, because it is strongly reflected at interfaces where there is a large acoustic impedance mismatch. Thus, access to the heart in adults is limited to areas where the heart abuts against the intercostal spaces and to suprasternal and subcostal approaches. An aqueous gel is used to couple the transducer to the skin, and the transducers are usually focused at a depth of 5–10 cm. The several modes available for the display of the ultrasonic signals are illustrated in Fig 5–6.

The time required for the reflected sound signals to return to the transducer varies with the distance traveled and provides a form of echo ranging. The transducer is switched to receive when it is not transmitting and puts out an electronic signal proportionate to the intensity of the echoes.

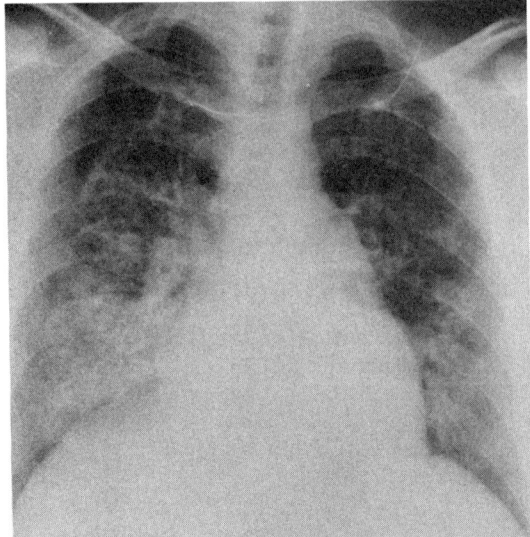

Figure 5–5. Chest x-ray of a patient with pulmonary edema showing perihilar ("bat's wing") distribution, especially on the right side. The lung periphery is relatively free of infiltrate.

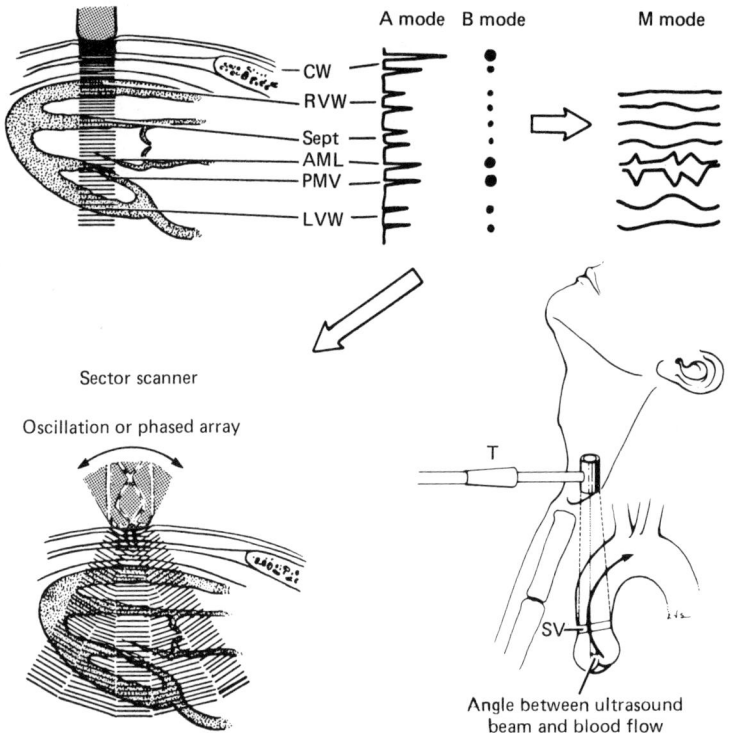

Figure 5–6. Diagram showing different modes of display of ultrasonic information. The structures displayed in A mode, B mode, M mode, and sector scanning, from front to back, are the chest wall (CW), the right ventricular wall (RVW), the interventricular septum (Sept), the anterior mitral valve leaflet (AML), the posterior mitral valve leaflet (PMV), and the posterior wall of the left ventricle (LVW). The Doppler transducer (T) is depicted in the suprasternal notch with its sample volume (SV) in the ascending aorta. (Courtesy of NH Silverman and NB Schiller.)

A Mode

In an A mode echo system, the intensity of the returning echoes is displayed on one axis of an oscilloscope (x axis in Fig 5–6), and the time required for the transmitted wave to travel from the transducer to the target and back is displayed on the other axis (y axis in Fig 5–6). The highly reflective structures in the ultrasound beam are thus shown, one above the other, with the nearest at the top and the farthest at the bottom of the oscilloscope screen. Since the heart is moving, these echoes dance up and down during the cardiac cycle. The most rapidly moving structures are the mitral valve leaflets, and in the view depicted in Fig 5–6, the anterior leaflet of the mitral valve is the most prominent structure. It abuts against the posterior leaflet during systole and moves anteriorly during diastole. A mode was the first form of echographic display to be developed and is seldom used today.

B Mode

In B mode echocardiography, the intensity of the echo signal is displayed on the z (brightness) axis of the oscilloscope screen, and the distance from the transducer appears on the y axis. Pure B mode echoes are seldom used but form the basis of M mode echocardiography.

M Mode

In M mode (motion) echocardiography, a B mode echo signal is recorded on the y axis, with time on the x axis, either by sweeping the oscilloscope screen or by photographing the oscilloscope face on moving paper. Thus, the conventional M mode display shows time on the x axis, distance on the y axis, and intensity of the echo on the z axis. An ECG is recorded for timing, and the movement of the structures within the beam is displayed during the cardiac cycle. As shown in Fig 5–6, the movement of the mitral valve is readily seen, giving a pattern that is repeated with each heartbeat. In M mode echocardiography, the transducer is excited at 2–7 MHz with 1000 pulses per second (repetition rate 1 kHz). The image is thus updated every 1 ms, giving a signal with an excellent frequency response.

Two-Dimensional (2-D) Echocardiography

A more complicated and expensive scanning technique is now widely used. In 2-dimensional studies, a B mode echographic tracing is rapidly and sequentially scanned across a sector field at a rate sufficient to provide a continuous image to the unaided eye (frequency 20–30 Hz). The scanning process, depicted in Fig 5–6, can be either mechanical, with rapid oscillation of the transducer; or electronic, with an array of crystals being sequentially and repeatedly excited to provide a similar form of scan (phased array). The sector scanner provides a pie-shaped image within which the reflective cardiac structures move in 2 dimensions. By placing the transducer appropriately, transverse, sagittal, or coronal sections can be displayed and the scope of the ultrasonic examination greatly increased. The frequency response of sector scanners is inferior to that of M mode echocardiography and is comparable to that of x-ray angiography. However, the advantages of seeing the motion of the heart in 2 dimensions in real time far outweigh any loss of resolution resulting from the use of 2-dimensional instruments. It is not possible to do justice to the technique with single-frame pictures, and it is not surprising that 2-dimensional echocardiography has become the primary form of ultrasonic investigation, with M mode being relegated to an ancillary role.

Doppler Ultrasound

In Doppler studies, the velocity of blood flow is detected via the frequency shift of reflected ultrasound. The process is governed by the Doppler equation:

$$\Delta f = \frac{2 \times f \times v \times \cos \theta}{c}$$

where Δf is the shift in frequency, f the transmitted frequency, v the velocity of the target, θ the angle between the ultrasound beam and the target, and c the speed of sound in the tissues.

Two forms of Doppler ultrasonic instrument are used: continuous wave Doppler and pulsed, range-gated Doppler. In the simpler, continuous wave instruments, separate transmitting and receiving crystals are continuously active, and reflected signals are obtained from all structures within the ultrasound beam. In pulsed, range-gated instruments, a single crystal is used to transmit pulses at a rate of 7–10 kHz. Between transmitted bursts, the transducer is switched to receive signals from moving targets. The longer the time between the burst (pulse) of ultrasound and the time of reception of reflected signals, the farther the target is from the transducer. By opening the "gate" at specific times and receiving reflected signals at varying intervals after transmission, it is possible to restrict the received signals to structures at specific distances from the surface of the chest. Pulsed, range-gated Doppler instruments can thus detect blood flow in specific blood vessels (aorta or pulmonary artery) and cardiac chambers.

When Doppler techniques are combined with echocardiography (2-dimensional or M mode), it is possible to obtain a combination of anatomic and physiologic information and correlate structure with function. Doppler techniques have been used in the assessment of valvular lesions. The pattern of blood flow is altered when valve lesions are present; and disturbed flow associated with both stenosis and incompetence and also with shunt lesions—such as ventricular septal defect and patent ductus arteriosus—can be recognized using this technique.

The optimal angle for echographic investigations is not generally compatible with that for Doppler studies. The best definition of echographic signals is obtained when the ultrasound beam intersects its target at right angles. The shift in frequency is, in theory, zero with this aim, since the value for Cos θ in the Doppler equation should be zero. Doppler signals are best recorded from blood vessels with near axially aimed transducers. These considerations make quantitative measurements with simultaneous echo and Doppler recordings difficult. Intracardiac recordings present less of a problem, and using an apical 4-chamber view of the heart, it is possible to aim the transducer in the axis of flow through either the mitral or the aortic valve and obtain satisfactory echographic signals with the same transducer position. Pulsed, range-gated Doppler instruments are limited in the range of frequencies (velocities) they can record, because of factors related to the repetition rate. High velocities cause ambiguity in the reflected signals, because the Doppler-shifted signals become confused with the results of the next transmission burst.

Cardiac Output Measured by Doppler Ultrasound

Doppler measurements of cardiac output from signals in the aorta and pulmonary artery are now possible. It is necessary to know the cross-sectional area of the vessel involved, and this can be measured from an A mode or M mode recording from the left parasternal (aorta) or second or third left intercostal space (pulmonary artery). The angle between the ultrasound beam, directed either from the suprasternal notch (aorta) or second or third left intercostal space (pulmonary artery), can be close enough to axial to reduce the error in the calculation of Cos θ to less than 5%. The mean velocity of blood flow and evidence about the flow profile can be obtained from spectral analysis of the Doppler signals. This analytic technique usually employs Fourier analysis to convert the audio Doppler signal into its frequency components at discrete intervals during the cardiac cycle. An example of a microcomputer-based plot of a Fourier-analyzed aortic blood velocity signal is shown in Fig 5–7. The frequency (proportionate to velocity) is shown on the y axis, time on the x axis, and intensity of the Doppler-shifted signal on the z axis. Two beats are shown, and the flow can be seen to be systolic. The velocity of blood flow can be seen to increase in a linear manner in the early, rapid ejection phase of left ventricular systole. Doppler-based measurements of cardiac output, made in the ascending aorta, have been compared with simultaneously measured thermodilution outputs. The agreement has been good (correlation coefficient about

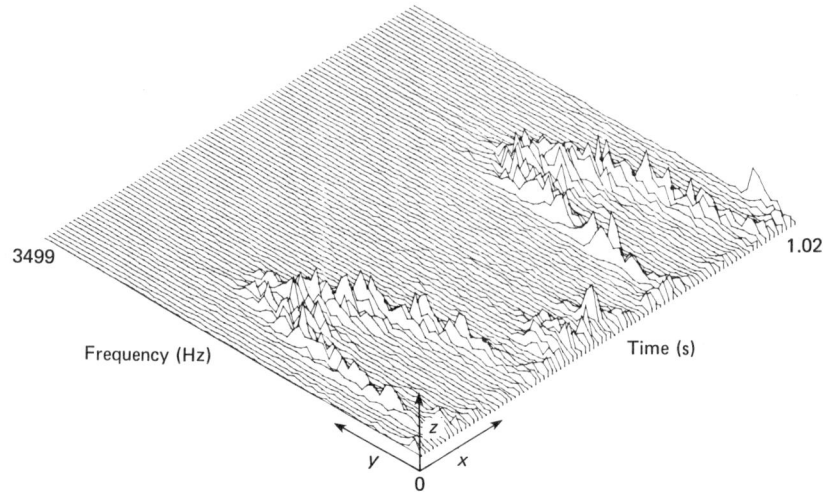

Figure 5–7. Doppler signal recorded from the ascending aorta via the suprasternal notch in a normal subject. The 3-dimensional plot shows frequency on the y axis, time on the x axis, and intensity on the z axis. The Doppler frequency shift (proportionate to blood flow velocity) increases in near-linear manner in early ejection.

0.93) in studies in patients in intensive care units. Some disagreement exists about the validity of similar measurements made using continuous wave instruments.

Measurement of Pressure Gradients

The use of measurements of the peak velocity of blood flow in a jet of blood passing through a stenosed valve to calculate the pressure gradient across the valve has already been described (Chapter 4). The method, which uses a continuous wave instrument, has been validated in patients with aortic stenosis and mitral stenosis.

Normal M Mode Findings

The structures that can be observed in what has come to be the basic echocardiographic scanning maneuver are shown in Fig 5–8.

A. Mitral Valve: With the transducer (T) in constant contact with the patient's skin through a layer of coupling jelly, the beam is aimed posteriorly through the fourth intercostal space to the left of the sternum. In position 1, indicated in Fig 5–8, the mitral valve leaflet echo is readily picked up. The beam intersects the right ventricular cavity, the interventricular septum, and the left ventricular cavity before passing through the mitral valve to reach the posterior wall of the left ventricle. In the example shown in Fig 5–8, there is an echo-free space anterior to the right ventricle and behind the left ventricle owing to pericardial effusion. Clearer pictures can usually be obtained when the heart is surrounded by fluid, which appears to act like aqueous coupling jelly to improve the quality of the signals. A more detailed picture of the mitral valve and its motions is shown in Fig 5–9. During systole, the anterior leaflet lies close to the posterior leaflet. Diastole starts from a point designated "D," and the anterior leaflet moves forward toward the septum, reaching the "E" point. As flow falls off in mid diastole, the anterior leaflet moves backward to a minimum point (F) before moving forward again as a result of atrial contraction to an "A" point. Throughout the whole of diastole, the posterior leaflet remains close to the posterior wall of the left ventricle.

B. Left Ventricle: By tilting the transducer in the direction of the feet, a picture of the left ventricular cavity is obtained. This is shown in detail in Fig 5–10. The posterior motion of the ventricular septum during systole, combined with the anterior motion of the posterior wall of the left ventricle, reduces the anteroposterior diameter of the ventricular cavity. The mitral valve is seen in this view, and in the patient in Fig 5–10 the range of motion of the heart wall and the valve is increased because of a high-output state. The dominant left ventricle pulls the right ventricle posteriorly during systole, and the narrowing due to posterior systolic movement of the anterior wall of the right ventricle is not well shown.

C. Aortic Valve: Tilting the transducer upward and slightly medially through position 2 to position 3 in Fig 5–8 brings the aortic valve into view. The details seen in this view are illustrated in Fig 5–11. The right ventricular outflow tract comes to lie at the front of the display, and the left atrium, rather than the left ventricle, comes to lie behind the aorta as the mitral valve falls out of the picture. Its position in the center of the display is taken by the aorta, whose dense walls move forward during systole. The aortic valve leaflets can be seen during systole. They are less reflective than the mitral valve leaflets in normal

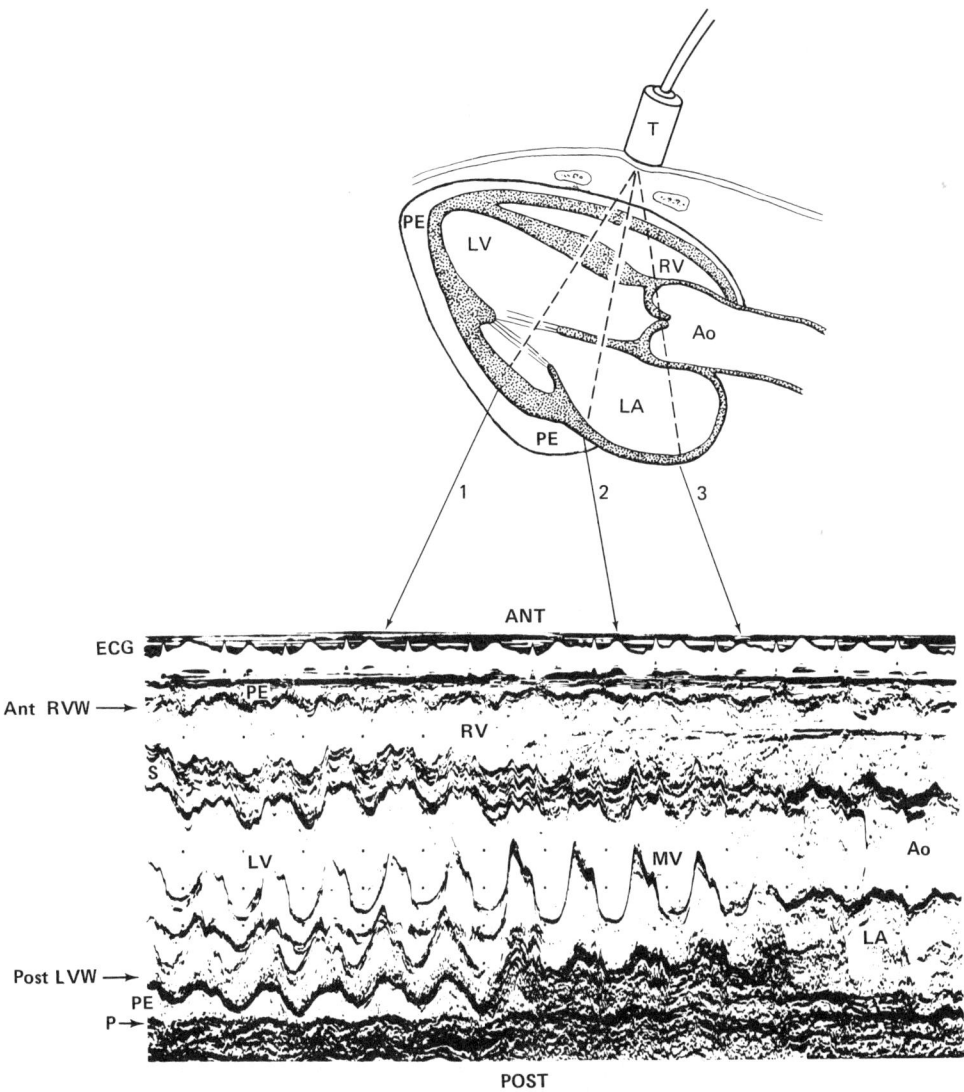

Figure 5–8. M mode echocardiogram showing normal intracardiac structures in a patient with pericardial effusion. The transducer (T) was moved from position 1 to position 3 during the recording. ANT, anterior; RV, right ventricular cavity; LV, left ventricular cavity; S, septum; MV, mitral valve; Ao, aorta; LA, left atrium; PE, pericardial effusion; POST, posterior; Ant RVW, anterior right ventricular wall; Post LVW, posterior left ventricular wall; P, pericardium. (Courtesy of NB Schiller.)

subjects. The diastolic diameter of the aorta in Fig 5–11 is greater than normal because the patient had Marfan's syndrome. The left atrial diameter in this view is smaller than the aortic diameter. Normally, the left atrial dimension is greater than the aortic.

Normal 2-Dimensional Findings

The 3 standard orthogonal imaging planes used in 2-dimensional echocardiography are illustrated in Fig 5–12. In the long-axis view, the transducer is placed in the third or fourth left intercostal space, beside the sternum. The scanner sweeps in a sagittal plane, intersecting the aortic and mitral valves, both ventricles, and the left atrium. The apex of the pie-shaped display is closest to the outflow tract of the right ventricle. The actions of the aortic and mitral valves are well seen in this view.

The short-axis view is obtained from the same position on the chest but with the axis of the scanner turned through 90 degrees, as shown in Fig 5–12. In this view, the body of the left ventricle occupies most of the field, with the right ventricle in front and to the left side of the image. Two-dimensional images in the coronal plane are conventionally displayed as if they were seen from the feet of the subject, with the left ventricle on the right and vice versa.

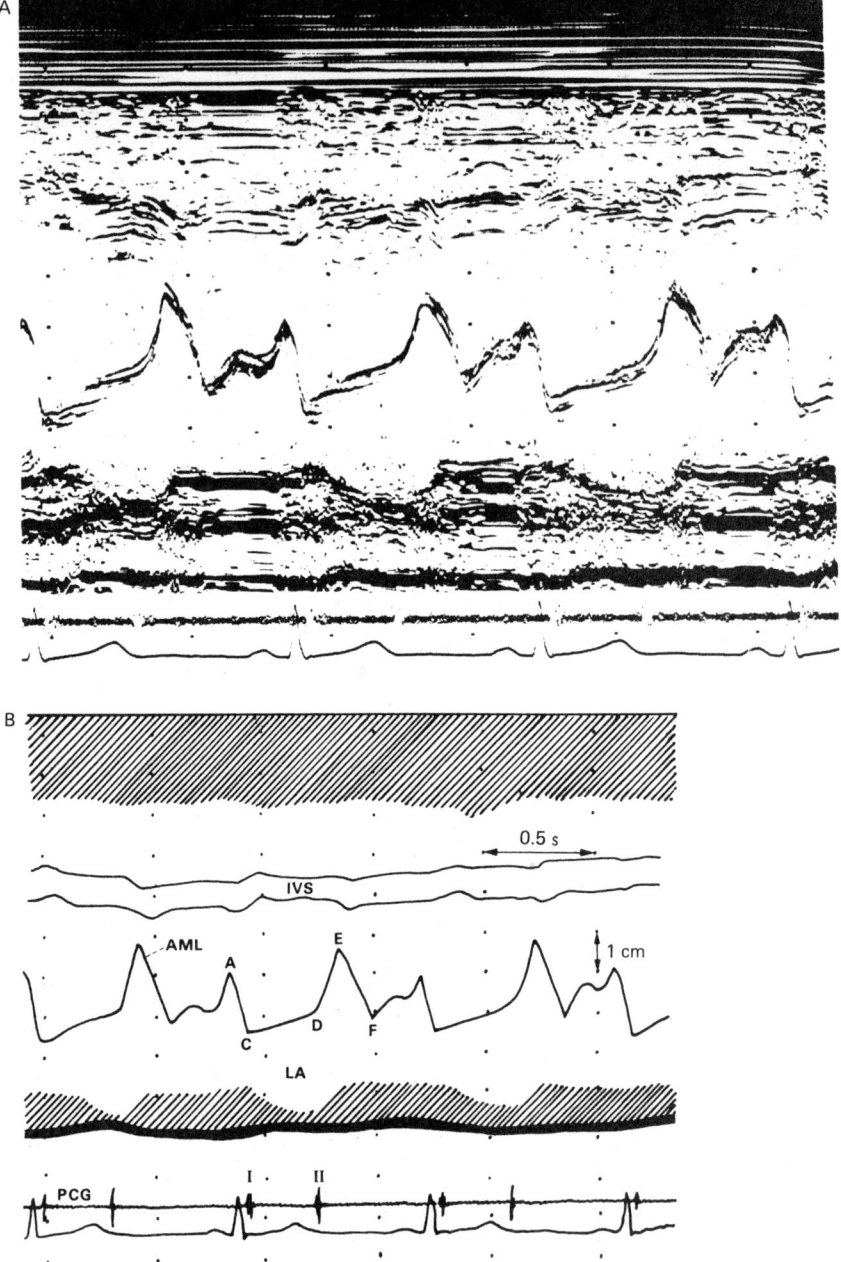

Figure 5-9. *A:* M mode echocardiogram showing details of the motion of a normal mitral valve. *B:* Diagrammatic representation of *A*. IVS, interventricular septum; AML, anterior mitral leaflet; PCG, phonocardiogram; I and II, first and second heart sounds. Points A, C, D, E, and F are peaks and troughs of mitral valve motion. (Modified and reproduced, with permission, from Omoto R, Kobayashi M: *Atlas of Essential Ultrasound Imaging.* Igaku-Shoin, 1981.)

The 4-chamber view is obtained from the apex of the heart, with the scanner being aimed in a plane that is close to frontal. The left ventricle and atrium are on the right in this view, which intersects both the tricuspid and the mitral valves. Additional views, illustrated in Fig 5–13, can be obtained by using the subcostal and suprasternal transducer positions.

Clinical Uses of Echocardiography

A. M Mode: The clinical value of M mode echocardiography is now clearly established. The findings in individual diseases are described in the appropriate chapters. The main use of echocardiography is as a preliminary screening test: It has not yet displaced cardiac catheterization and angiography as a definitive preoperative diagnostic study. M mode studies are of

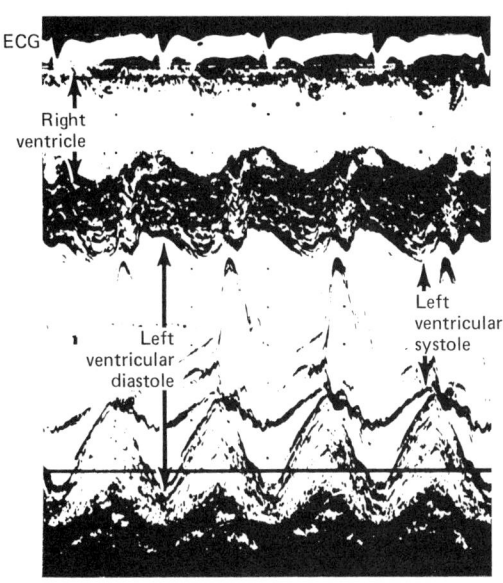

Figure 5–10. M mode echocardiogram showing the right and left ventricles in a patient with a high cardiac output. The arrows indicate the relative dimensions of the left ventricular systole and diastole. (Courtesy of NB Schiller.)

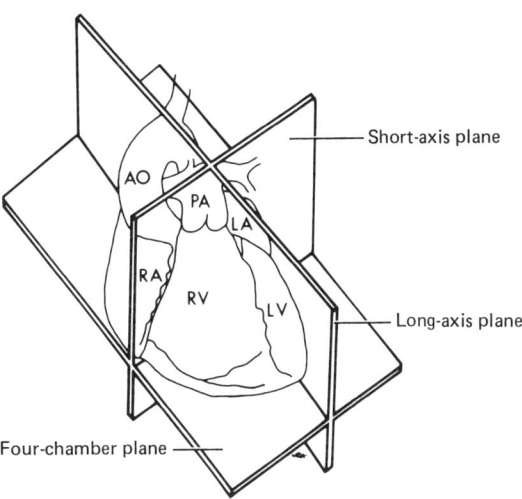

Figure 5–12. Diagram of the 3 orthogonal imaging planes used to visualize the heart with 2-dimensional echocardiography. Ao, aorta; LA, left atrium; LV, left ventricle; PA, pulmonary artery; RA, right atrium; and RV, right ventricle. (Reproduced, with permission, from the American Heart Association, Inc., Henry WL et al [editors]: Report of the American Society of Echocardiography Committee on Nomenclature and Standards in 2-Dimensional Echocardiography. *Circulation* 1980;**62**:212.)

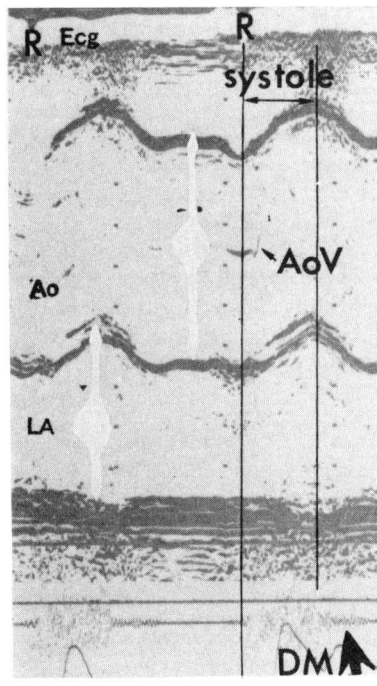

Figure 5–11. M mode echocardiogram showing the aortic valve (AoV) and the aorta (Ao) in a patient with Marfan's syndrome. The left atrium (LA) is seen to lie posteriorly. DM refers to an aortic diastolic murmur seen in the phonocardiogram. R, R wave of ECG. (Courtesy of NB Schiller.)

value in evaluating nearly all the manifestations of heart disease (pericardial, valvular, congenital, hypertensive, coronary, and primary myocardial disease) and are of particular value in pericardial effusion (Fig 5–8) and in mitral valve disease—either incompetence or stenosis—especially in detecting prolapse of the valve leaflets during systole. An example is shown in Fig 5–14 from the same patient (with Marfan's syndrome) as in Fig 5–11. During systole, a portion of the valve can be seen to be displaced posteriorly, giving the appearance of separation of the leaflets.

Another condition in which M mode echocardiography is particularly valuable is hypertrophic obstructive cardiomyopathy. In this condition, as illustrated in Fig 5–15, there is systolic anterior motion of the mitral valve. The tip of the anterior leaflet and the chordae tendineae abut against the hypertrophied interventricular septum during systole, and the motion coincides with the development of a systolic murmur.

B. Two-Dimensional Echocardiography: Two-dimensional echocardiographic scanning can be used to display all the features that can be seen with M mode techniques. The extra dimension adds greatly to the flexibility of the study, and it is difficult with still photographs to give an adequate idea of the advantages of this technique. It has now superseded M mode echocardiography in the routine investigation of almost all forms of heart disease. Examples of images from normal hearts showing the 6 conventional views (1, long-axis; 2, short-axis; 3, apical 4-chamber; 4, apical 2-chamber; 5, subcostal [inferior

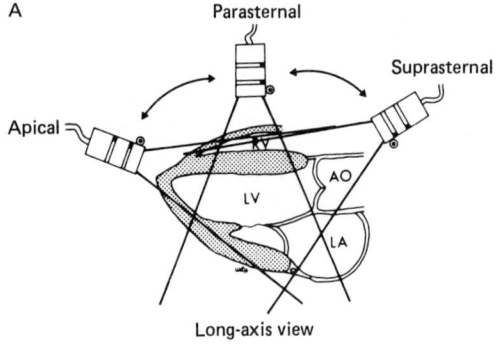
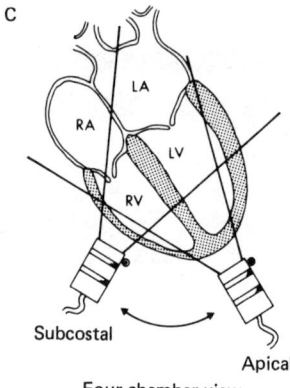
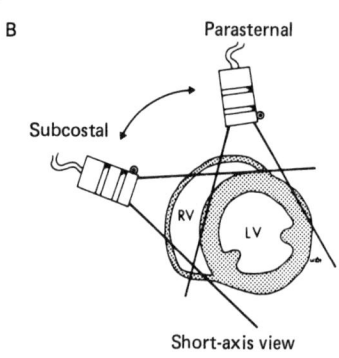

Figure 5–13. Diagram of the transducer orientations used to obtain long-axis views *(A)*, short-axis views *(B)*, and 4-chamber views *(C)* of the heart. Note that the transducer index mark is always pointed either in the direction of the patient's head or the patient's left side. Abbreviations are as in Fig 5–12. (Reproduced, with permission, from the American Heart Association, Inc., Henry WL et al [editors]: Report of the American Society of Echocardiography Committee on Nomenclature and Standards in 2-Dimensional Echocardiography. *Circulation* 1980;**62**:212.)

vena cava]; and 6, suprasternal) are shown in Figs 5–16, 5–17, 5–18, 5–19, 5–20, and 5–21.

C. Left Ventricular Function: Both M mode and 2-dimensional echocardiography have been used to investigate left ventricular function.

1. Ventricular volume and ejection fraction–M mode echocardiography provides only a single measurement from which to calculate ventricular volume. The errors inherent in this approach preclude its use for this purpose.

Two-dimensional signals provide much superior images of the ventricle in long-axis and short-axis views. Their use for the calculation of left ventricular volume and ejection fraction is described in Chapter 4, and examples of end-systolic and end-diastolic views with the ventricular cavity outlined are shown in Fig 4–7.

2. Left ventricular mass–The thickness of the septal and posterolateral walls of the left ventricle can be readily estimated by echocardiography. Using assumptions about ventricular shape, it is possible to calculate a value for left ventricular mass that has been shown to correlate well with measurements made at autopsy. When left ventricular hypertrophy is developing, the increase in mass precedes electrocardiographic changes and is a more reliable indicator of the hypertrophic process.

3. Velocity and extent of shortening–Attempts have been made to assess ventricular "contractility" from measurement of the rate of change of position of echographic images. Such measurements should probably not be made using 2-dimensional techniques, because the rate of imaging (20–30 Hz) is too slow for adequate temporal resolution. M mode signals have a better frequency response (1000 Hz), but the assumptions involved make the calculation of shortening rates only marginally acceptable.

4. Wall motion–The movement of the left ventricular wall can be readily investigated using 2-dimensional scanners. An accurate visual impression of the extent and timing of the motion of different areas can be obtained that is clinically valuable, but translating this into numerical terms presents significant difficulties.

Limitations of Echocardiography

The principal limitation of ultrasonic examinations, as compared to conventional radiography, is that sound waves travel more slowly through tissue (about 1.5 km/s) than do x-rays (2.99×10^5 km/s). The longer wave length of the more slowly moving sound waves limits the resolution of ultrasonic examinations. Ultrasound is, however, much less damaging to tissues than x-rays, and there is as yet no clinical evidence of ill effects despite extensive use of the technique over more than a decade.

Skill, experience, and judgment are involved in the interpretation of echocardiographic studies. The variability and the effects of observer error on the interpretation of echocardiography are now becoming

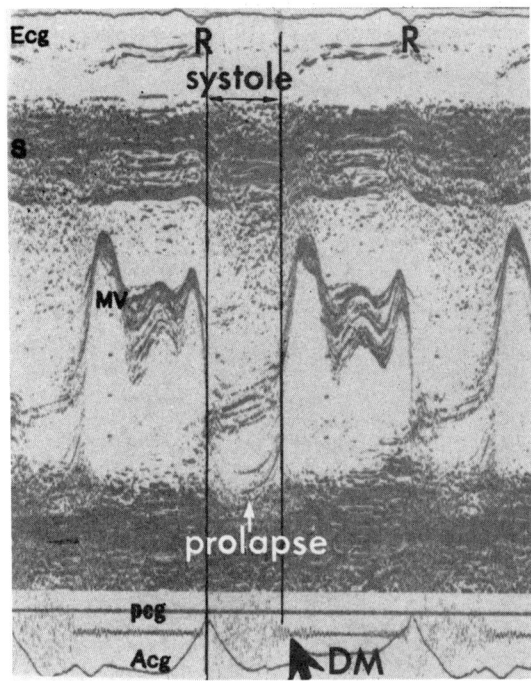

Figure 5–14. M mode echocardiogram of the mitral valve (MV) showing systolic prolapse in the same patient with Marfan's syndrome shown in Fig 5–11. A phonocardiogram (pcg) and apexcardiogram (Acg) are included, and the same diastolic murmur (DM) is shown. R, R wave of ECG; S, ventricular septum. (Courtesy of NB Schiller.)

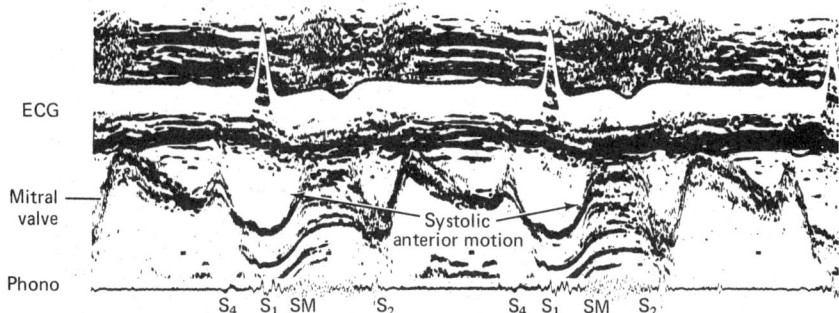

Figure 5–15. Echocardiogram, ECG, and phonocardiogram showing systolic anterior motion of mitral valve in a patient with hypertrophic obstructive cardiomyopathy. SM, systolic murmur. (Courtesy of NB Schiller.)

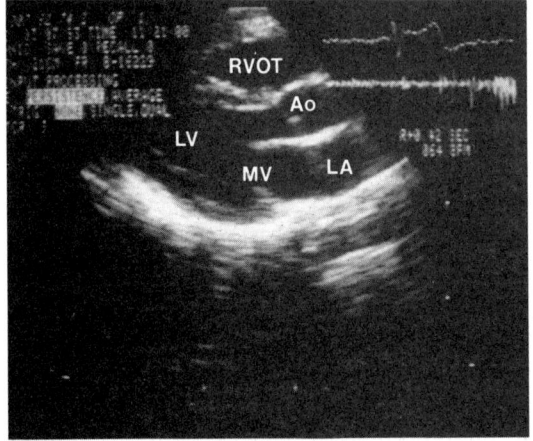

Figure 5–16. Normal 2-dimensional echocardiogram, long-axis view. LV, left ventricle; MV, mitral valve; LA, left atrium; RVOT, right ventricular outflow tract; Ao, aorta. (Courtesy of NB Schiller.)

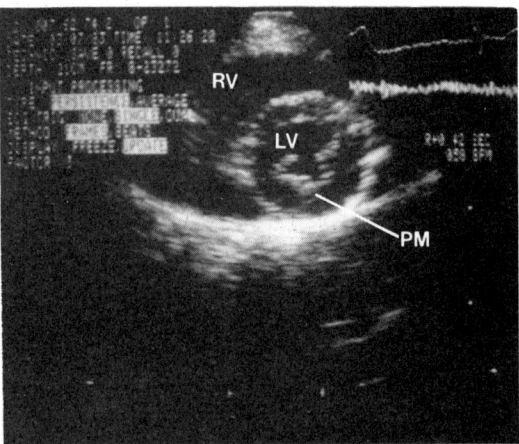

Figure 5–17. Normal 2-dimensional echocardiogram, short-axis view at ventricular level. LV, left ventricle; RV, right ventricle; PM, papillary muscles. (Courtesy of NB Schiller.)

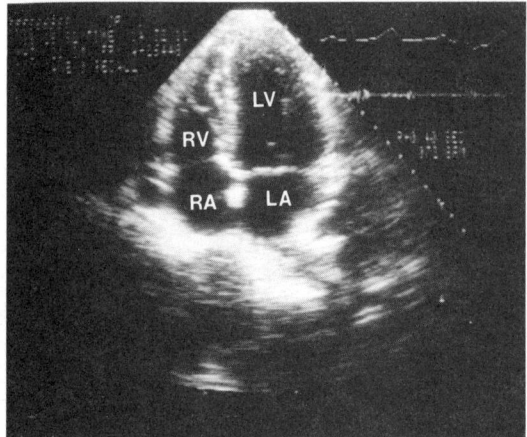

Figure 5-18. Normal 2-dimensional echocardiogram, apical 4-chamber view. LV, left ventricle; RV, right ventricle; LA, left atrium; RA, right atrium. (Courtesy of NB Schiller.)

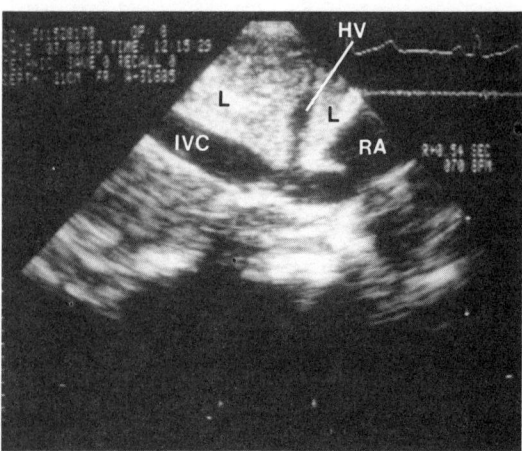

Figure 5-20. Normal 2-dimensional echocardiogram, subcostal view. L, liver; IVC, inferior vena cava; HV, hepatic vein; RA, right atrium. (Courtesy of NB Schiller.)

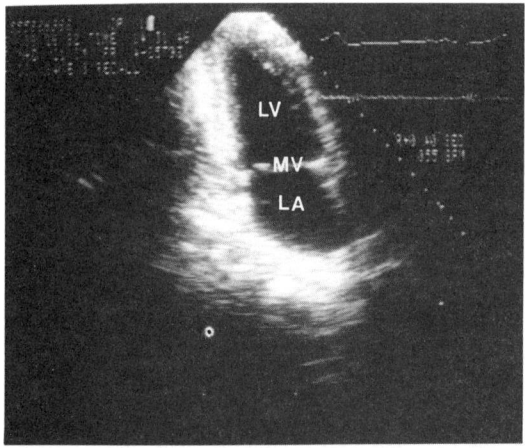

Figure 5-19. Normal 2-dimensional echocardiogram, apical 2-chamber view. LV, left ventricle; LA, left atrium; MV, mitral valve. (Courtesy of NB Schiller.)

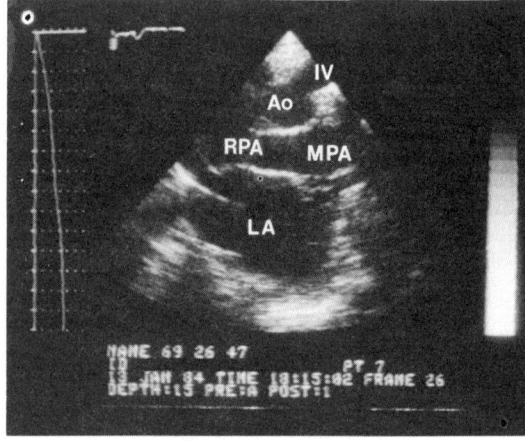

Figure 5-21. Normal 2-dimensional echocardiogram, suprasternal view. Ao, aorta; MPA, main pulmonary artery; RPA, right pulmonary artery; IV, innominate vein; LA, left atrium. (Courtesy of NB Schiller.)

apparent. The measurements made are valid in that they are made in millimeters. There is, however, a certain element of subjectivity in setting the controls that determine the intensity, and it is possible to have structures drop out or to introduce artifacts. The technique, in spite of these minor disadvantages, has proved extremely useful in clinical cardiology, and the full potential of ultrasonic examination has yet to be realized.

Detection of Bubbles

Ultrasound is particularly sensitive to the presence of microscopic bubbles in the circulation. The interface between the air in the bubble and the blood reflects ultrasound strongly. Any freshly made solution or forceful injection of liquid contains or generates sufficient intravascular bubbles to be detectable in either echocardiographic or Doppler recordings from the heart. These effects have been used to carry out the equivalent of indicator dilution curves, to identify intracardiac shunts by means of ultrasound, and to establish connections between different areas of the heart and great vessels. The techniques are qualitative rather than quantitative and are harmless.

PHONOCARDIOGRAPHY

Phonocardiography is a standard (but not routine) study that is perhaps the most difficult and subjective of all noninvasive investigations. The apparatus is not expensive and is available in most large hospitals. Although modern bedside auscultation owes an enormous debt to phonocardiography, a recording of heart sounds is seldom of critical clinical importance. Phonocardiography is most valuable as a means of timing the events of the cardiac cycle and demonstrating their relationship to indirectly recorded pressure tracings such as the apexcardiogram, indirect carotid pulse tracings, external phlebograms, and stethographic recordings of respiration. It is of little value in analyzing the sound content of murmurs and heart sounds because the harmonic content of the recordings obtained is so dependent on the electrical filters used, the placing of the microphones, and the position of the patient. In consequence, phonocardiography is of most practical value in teaching auscultation and in settling differences of opinion. Its value in confirming the auscultatory findings is well established. Most people find it easier to appreciate sensory information when it is received simultaneously by 2 senses. Thus, listening to a patient's heart with a stethoscope and watching an oscilloscopic recording of the sounds at the same time is most valuable in teaching. After the student has become experienced in auscultation, the phonocardiograph is less often needed. In practice, the principal reason for recording a phonocardiogram is to obtain a permanent tracing of the auscultatory findings. The tracing is thus an adjunct to and not a substitute for careful auscultation by a trained clinical observer. A possible exception to this generalization is in patients with artificial heart valves. Prosthetic valves give relatively clear sounds in which changes can indicate the development of thrombotic material on the valve, changes in ball size in a ball and cage device, or the early stages of valve dehiscence. Serial phonocardiography can be useful in following the postoperative course of patients with artificial valves on a long-term basis.

SPECIAL ELECTROCARDIOGRAPHIC INVESTIGATIONS

1. VECTORCARDIOGRAPHY

Vectorcardiography is a well-established electrocardiographic technique that has never achieved great popularity. The apparatus required is not expensive but differs from that needed for routine scalar electrocardiography. The electrical potentials generated by the heart during the cardiac cycle are displayed in a form that emphasizes their spatial orientation as vectors in the 3 conventional planes of the body: horizontal, sagittal, and frontal. Various lead systems are available, but the Frank lead system is the most popular. The electrocardiographic signals are displayed on the x and y axes of an oscilloscope, and the dimension of time is indicated by interrupting the ECG signal every 2 milliseconds. The ECG signal traces out loops on the screen during the P, QRS, and T phases of the cardiac cycle. The standard 12-lead ECG was so well established by the time vectorcardiography became available that the dominant position of the ECG as an empiric pattern-recognition system has never been seriously challenged.

2. CONTINUOUS ELECTROCARDIOGRAPHIC MONITORING

Continuous electrocardiographic monitoring outside a laboratory has become a standard means of identifying arrhythmias and conduction defects; this technique should be considered in any patient in whom an exact diagnosis of an arrhythmia or conduction defect has not yet been established. The apparatus required, which is moderately expensive, is available in most large hospitals. It is also routinely used in coronary care units to obtain the earliest possible indication of the onset of arrhythmia or conduction defect or to monitor the frequency of premature beats. Monitoring for up to 12 hours can readily be carried out in patients going about their normal business. One lead of an ECG is usually recorded on a tape recorder that is strapped around the patient's waist. The tape recording of the ECG is played back at speeds of 10–100 times the recording speed and scanned for abnormalities, either visually or using a special computer program. These areas of interest are then recorded at standard speed for analysis. Both arrhythmias and ST–T wave changes of ischemia can be detected in this way and the time of their occurrence correlated with events in the patient's life. In continuous monitoring in a coronary care unit, the ECG is usually continuously displayed on an oscilloscope and can be recorded on chart paper by simply pressing a button. Alarms are often arranged to provide a signal when the patient's heart rate falls outside a prescribed range. These are not always desirable, because displacement of electrocardiographic electrodes and disconnection of leads tend to trigger the alarm systems inappropriately. It is especially valuable to use a system that includes a memory loop. In this case, the immediate past portion (say the last 20 seconds) of the patient's electrocardiographic signal is continuously stored in a memory, which is continuously erased after 20 seconds. When some untoward event occurs, it is then possible to stop erasing the memory and examine the ECG during the period immediately preceding the untoward event.

3. EXERCISE ELECTROCARDIOGRAPHY (See also Chapter 8.)

Exercise electrocardiography is a standard procedure for investigation of patients in whom a diagnosis of angina pectoris is being considered. The apparatus required is not expensive, and the test is available in many doctors' offices. The aim of an exercise test is to induce the symptoms of which the patient is complaining in the laboratory, in the presence of a physician, and with an ECG running continuously.

Safety Precautions

There is a small but significant (1:10,000) risk in exercising patients with angina until they develop pain. The risk mainly stems from the possibility that the patient may have developed a myocardial infarction since last seen, but ventricular arrhythmias, myocardial infarction, collapse, and sudden death may occur during the test. Care must be taken to make sure that the patient's symptoms have not changed, and a 12-lead ECG is taken at rest in the supine and upright positions and compared with the most recent previous ECG. An exercise test should never be done without a doctor present and resuscitation equipment available. The physician in charge must strike a balance between failing to stress the patient enough to bring out symptoms and encouraging excessive and dangerous overexertion. It is, however, safer for patients with angina to bring on their pain in a laboratory than in the course of their daily activities.

Technique

The exercise stress consists of walking on a motor-driven treadmill or pedaling a cycle ergometer. Several patterns of graded exercise are in common use. The commonest is the Bruce protocol, in which the test is divided into 4 stages, each lasting 3 minutes. In stage I, the patient walks at 1.7 mph at a 10% grade; in stage II, the speed is increased to 2.5 mph at a 12% grade; in stage III, the speed is 3.4 mph and the grade 14%; and in stage IV, the speed is 4.2 mph and the grade 16%. Comparable protocols are used for cycle ergometer exercise.

Blood pressure is often measured by sphygmomanometry during the test, but the values obtained tend to be unreliable because of the motion of the patient and the noise of the treadmill.

The patient is instructed to stop exercise when he or she would ordinarily stop in daily life. The physician stops the test if arrhythmia develops or the patient shows obvious signs of distress. Marked (> 3 mm) ST depression or a falling blood pressure is also an indication to stop.

The heart rate is monitored and the ECG continuously observed during the test. A significant increase in heart rate is sought. Since the maximal heart rate that can be achieved during exercise by normal subjects decreases with age, the expected heart rate for a given patient is obtained from tables, and about 80% of this value used as a target. A rough guide to the maximal heart rate is 220 beats/min minus the patient's age in years. In practice, most patients with angina of effort develop chest pain at heart rates below 130/min. The ECG is recorded during the first 3 minutes of recovery, since ST–T wave changes sometimes do not develop until after exercise.

The technical aspects of recording an ECG during exercise have largely been overcome, so that with improved electrodes it is now possible to obtain stable tracings even during severe exercise on a cycle ergometer or treadmill. Although various lead systems have been used, a single unipolar lead or a bipolar lead from the right subclavicular region to the apex beat, with an indifferent electrode on the head or left shoulder, will detect ischemic changes in the ECG during exercise almost as effectively as more complicated lead systems.

Results

The changes of myocardial ischemia occur during exercise and are virtually always visible in the left ventricular leads (V_5 is probably the best). They consist of ST–T wave depression with T wave inversion. Junctional depression and upsloping ST segments are not significant, although ST depression of 2 mm and a duration of 0.08 second are considered definite positive findings indicating ischemia. ST depression of 1–2 mm is deemed equivocal.

There is some relationship between the ease with which electrocardiographic changes can be provoked, their magnitude, and the severity and prognosis of the coronary lesions. Patients with significant left main coronary artery lesions often show marked ST depression with minimal exercise.

Interpretation

The significance of electrocardiographic changes during exercise is greatest in patients with a normal resting tracing who develop "their pain" during the test. Digitalis therapy and the presence in the body of beta-adrenergic blocking agents make interpretation difficult. Digitalis produces ST–T wave changes that may mimic ischemia, and propranolol reduces the heart rate and makes pain less likely to be the limiting factor during exercise. The accuracy of the results of an exercise test as a means of establishing a diagnosis of ischemic heart disease is not easily determined. Results are generally interpreted as "false-positive" if changes occur in the ECG in patients whose coronary arteries are found to be normal at angiography. Conversely, "false-negative" results are assumed if coronary disease is seen on angiography in patients in whom no changes occurred in the ECG during exercise.

False-positive results may be due to misinterpretation of the coronary angiograms. Typical angina with a normal coronary angiogram does, however, undoubtedly occur, especially in young women. The results of exercise tests are less reliable in patients with abnormal resting ECGs and in those in whom pain does not develop. The magnitude of the ST depression is also related to the significance of the test. "False-negative" results are common, especially in patients who do not develop pain or a high enough heart rate or in asymptomatic persons. If the coronary arteriograms are taken as the "gold standard" for diagnosis, this result is not surprising. There is no necessary or inevitable relationship between the presence of obstructive lesions in the coronary circulation and the presence of ischemic pain or changes on an ECG, but significant lesions are usually present when angina and electrocardiographic changes are found on exercise. Coronary artery disease is undoubtedly present in a presymptomatic (latent) form in many "normal" persons past middle age.

Exercise tests are also used to assess the fitness of normal persons in particular occupations, eg, airline pilots. The interpretation of changes in the ECG induced by exercise in such cases is less reliable than in patients with chest pain.

In recent years, exercise tests have been commonly used as a means of assessing patients with recent myocardial infarction. If the patient develops chest pain or changes in the ECG during the test, convalescence should be prolonged and the prognosis is worse. The time after an infarction at which it is safe to do an exercise test is open to question. The present vogue for earlier testing seems unwarranted, and we believe that 2 or 3 months should elapse before an exercise test is performed.

4. MYOCARDIAL ST SEGMENT MAPPING

This procedure, still in the research phase, is another form of investigation designed to follow the progress and assess the size of myocardial infarctions. It is moderately expensive and involves multiple ECGs recorded from different sites of the precordium. In patients with anterior infarcts, the extent of the area over which ST elevation can be detected bears a relationship to the size of the infarcted area. By summing the total extent of ST elevation in 30 or so electrocardiographic leads placed in standard positions on the surface of the left chest, it is possible to obtain a numerical assessment that bears a relationship to infarct size. Unfortunately, changes in position of the heart and thickness of the chest wall vary greatly from patient to patient, and this detracts from the general usefulness of the technique.

MYOCARDIAL ENZYME DETERMINATIONS

A number of enzymes (eg, glutamic-oxaloacetic transaminase [GOT], lactate dehydrogenase [LDH], creatine phosphokinase [CPK]) are released into the blood following myocardial infarction. Necrosis of tissue with rupture of cell membranes and release of intracellular components must occur before the increased levels of enzyme are found. More specific enzymes and enzymatic fractions have now been identified, and the relatively specific myocardial MB ("myocardial band") fraction of creatine phosphokinase isoenzyme has become the standard test used to confirm that myocardial infarction has occurred. The level of this enzyme gives more specific information about myocardial necrosis than any other available at the moment. Attempts have been made to relate serial measurements of enzyme levels to the size of the infarction and the patient's clinical progress, with the examiner seeking evidence of healing on the one hand or extension with increasing enzyme levels on the other. Since the enzyme mixes with a large and potentially variable blood volume at an undetermined rate, such measurements tend to be relatively insensitive.

SPECIAL RADIOLOGIC INVESTIGATIONS

1. CINEFLUOROSCOPY

Cinefluoroscopy is of greatest value in establishing the presence of calcification in the heart valves, the myocardium, the coronary arteries, or the pericardium or in recognizing paradoxic motion of a left ventricular aneurysm. It is also valuable in patients with prosthetic heart valves in whom the question of valve dehiscence is raised. A permanent postoperative record of artificial valve movement should therefore be obtained in all patients subjected to valve replacement for comparison with later studies if trouble arises.

2. COMPUTER-ENHANCED DIGITAL ANGIOGRAPHY

Recent advances in computer technology have led to the development of this new radiologic technique. An analog-to-digital converting system is used to transform the information in a fluoroscopic x-ray image or a television (video) image into a set of numbers (commonly 512×512 picture elements; "pixels"). Once entered into the computer, the information in the stored images can be manipulated in a number of ways, being amplified linearly or logarithmically or subtracted. One technique (temporal subtraction angiography) subtracts a "blank" or "mask" image, recorded without contrast injection and stored in the computer, from a second image recorded while intravenously injected contrast material is passing through the circulation. The patient must be in exactly the same position for the 2 images and must have a similar level of lung inflation. A more complex type of imaging employs "energy subtraction." In this case, the energy of the x-ray generator is changed rapidly to provide 2 different types of image, one favoring the "blank" or "mask" image and the other the image with contrast material in the heart and vessels. In this form of imaging, the time between the recording of the 2 images is shorter, and movement of the patient is less of a problem.

The spatial resolution of the images recorded with digital angiography is not yet up to the standard of conventional angiography, but satisfactory images of major blood vessels and cardiac chambers can be

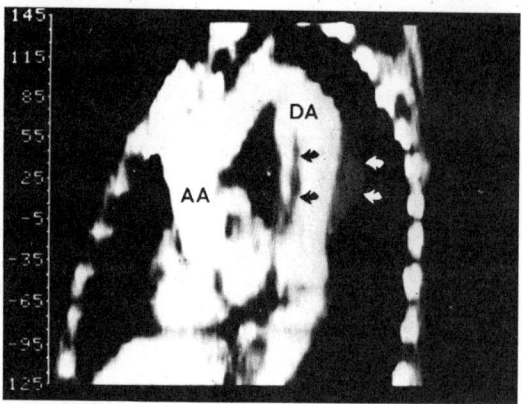
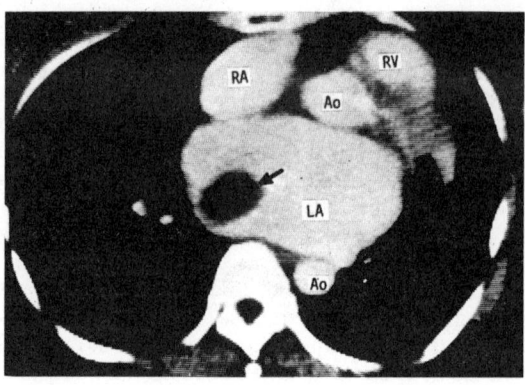

Figure 5–22. Oblique reconstruction of a series of transverse computer-based x-ray tomographic scans obtained during contrast drip infusion demonstrating aortic dissection. The intimal flap (black arrows) and an associated hematoma (white arrows) are shown. AA, ascending aorta; DA, descending aorta. (Reproduced, with permission, from Brundage BH, Lipton MJ: The emergence of computed tomography as a cardiovascular diagnostic technique. *Am Heart J* 1982;**103**:313.)

Figure 5–23. Computer-based x-ray tomographic scan of the thorax showing thrombus in the left atrium (black arrow) of a patient with mitral valve disease. RA, right atrium; LA, left atrium; Ao, aorta; RV, right ventricle. (Reproduced, with permission, from Tomoda H et al: Evaluation of left atrial thrombus with computed tomography. *Am Heart J* 1980;**100**:306.)

obtained with peripheral venous injections of relatively small amounts of contrast material. The technique has proved valuable for demonstrating the patency of coronary bypass grafts and for ventricular ejection fraction measurements. Selective injections through arterial catheters can be avoided and studies performed on outpatients. The technique has not yet been developed to a stage at which it can compete successfully with conventional selective coronary angiography.

3. COMPUTER-BASED X-RAY TOMOGRAPHY

Computer-based x-ray tomography is coming to be more widely used in specialized centers for cardiologic investigation. The equipment used is extremely expensive; significant amounts of ionizing radiation are employed; and the imaging of moving structures such as the heart and blood vessels presents serious problems. The technique relies on variations in tissue density to distinguish between different structures in the line of an x-ray beam sequentially aimed in a radial direction through cross sections of the body. The reconstruction of an image from the basic density data depends on complicated computer methods. With present-day instruments, the "scan time" for a single cross-sectional image is about 2–3 seconds, and the patient is expected to keep still and not breathe during scanning. Intravenous injections of radiopaque contrast material are generally used to enhance the density differences between circulating blood and cardiac tissue. A bolus injection of contrast can be followed through the circulation, or a continuous infusion can be used with multiple recordings of different cross-sectional images. These can then be "stacked" to give a reconstructed image resembling a conventional radiograph. The technique can accurately determine the patency of aortocoronary artery bypass grafts. It can detect many anterior (not posterior) myocardial infarctions and outline aortic dissections, as shown in Fig 5–22. It is well suited to the detection of calcification in coronary arteries or in the pericardium and can also delineate intracardiac tumor or thrombus, as shown in Fig 5–23. The resolution with this technique is inevitably inferior to that with conventional angiography, both in space and in time; but new instruments with shorter scan times (about 0.06 second) are under development.

NUCLEAR MEDICAL INVESTIGATIONS

The various techniques used in radionuclear investigations fall into the general domain of radiology. They involve the injection of specially prepared radioactive materials that can be detected either in the bloodstream or in the tissues. Radioactivity is detected with a nuclear (gamma) camera. Radioactivity is converted into light energy in the crystals of the camera. This is in turn converted to electrical signals by photomultiplier tubes. The x,y coordinates of the energy from each part of the crystal are stored in an x,y matrix of a computer and converted into a "time activity" curve for the areas covered by the camera. The apparatus required for recording the patterns of radioactivity is expensive, and the procedures have not as yet become standardized.

Lung Scanning

A gamma camera can be used to determine the distribution of radioactivity in the lungs following intravenous injection of 99m technetium (^{99m}Tc)–labeled albumin particles. This technique has proved valuable in localizing pulmonary arterial emboli and is most specific in patients with a normal chest x-ray (see Chapter 19). The technique is available in many large hospitals and is useful in pulmonary as well as cardiac disease.

Myocardial Imaging

A. Perfused Areas: Scanning of the precordium after the intravenous injection of thallium 201 (^{201}Tl) outlines perfused areas of the heart. Imaging can start 5–10 minutes after injection of the isotope through a short intravenous catheter. The advantage of this technique is that the injection can be made within a few seconds of the end of a maximal exercise test, and the scanning can be carried out with the subject at rest after recovery. Images are produced by a gamma camera in anteroposterior, left anterior oblique, and left lateral views. If the study is technically satisfactory and no defect is seen in the image, ischemia can be excluded with about 90% accuracy. If an area of abnormality (''cold spot'') is seen, a further image is obtained 3–24 hours later to distinguish between reversible ischemia that disappears after redistribution of the isotope and permanent impairment of blood supply to the region, such as scarring from a previous infarct, or some other cause of myocardial fibrosis. No further injection is needed for the second scan. Alternatively, a resting image can be obtained, but this requires a second injection of radionuclide after a delay to allow the isotope to clear from the heart. An example of this type of study is shown in Fig 5–24.

This form of scanning is useful for the detection of ischemia in groups of patients with a low prevalence of coronary disease, eg, patients with atypical pain or airline pilots with equivocal electrocardiographic changes and no symptoms. A normal test can exclude significant ischemia with a high degree of confidence and make coronary angiography unnecessary. The test can also be used to assess the significance of minor abnormalities found on coronary angiography or electrocardiographic studies, either at rest or during exercise, by determining whether the myocardium in the territory supplied by a given artery does or does not become ischemic on exercise. The effect of surgical treatment can also be assessed by establishing whether an ischemic area, present before operation, is adequately perfused postoperatively. Tomographic images of the heart obtained with this technique increase the chance of detecting a lesion. An example of this type of study is shown in Fig 5–25. Imaging with thallium (^{201}Tl) detects ischemia, not obstruction of coronary arteries. The test thus detects the effects of coronary disease on myocardial perfusion and not coronary lesions per se. Radionuclear studies are also useful in patients with equivocal

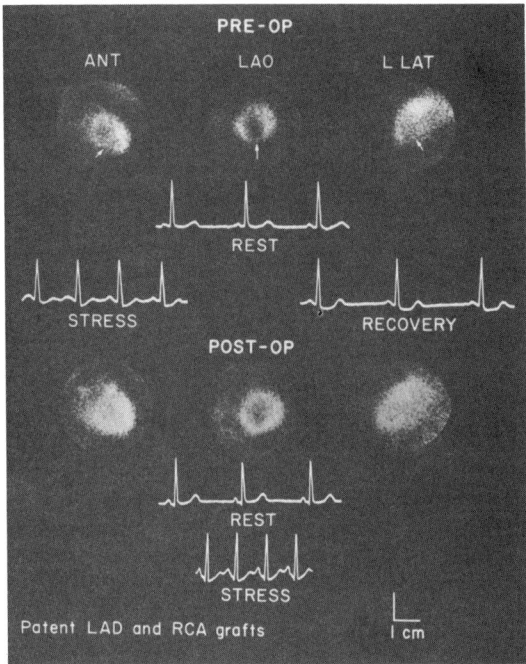

Figure 5–24. Pre- and postoperative thallium 201 stress scintigrams and ECGs obtained before and after placement of right coronary (RCA) and left anterior descending (LAD) grafts for treatment of angina pectoris. The preoperative study revealed an inferior wall perfusion abnormality (arrows). Perfusion is normal in the postoperative stress scintigram, and the patient was symptom-free. ANT, anterior; LAO, left anterior oblique; LLAT, left lateral. (Reproduced, with permission, from Greenberg BH et al: Thallium-201 myocardial perfusion scintigraphy to evaluate patients after coronary bypass surgery. *Am J Cardiol* 1978;**42**:167.)

findings, eg, if the ECG shows bundle branch block or permanent abnormalities due to previous myocardial infarction.

B. Infarcted Areas: The injection of radionuclear materials that are concentrated in necrotic tissue can be used to detect myocardial infarctions. In this type of study, technetium (^{99m}Tc)–labeled pyrophosphate is injected intravenously, and imaging is done with a gamma camera about 2 hours later. The isotope is concentrated about 11-fold in infarcted heart muscle, and the image becomes visible 10–12 hours after the infarction occurs. The intensity of the image is greatest at about 72 hours, and, while it usually fades in about a week, it may persist for months. Anterior myocardial infarcts produce better images than posterior infarcts, and if the first image is negative, a later scan after another 24–48 hours may be positive. More than 95% of patients with transmural infarcts imaged within 6 days of the onset of infarction give positive scans. The technique gives a valuable indication of the extent of myocardial infarction. The detection of subendocardial infarcts is less reliable. False-positive results occur in 1–2% of cases due to

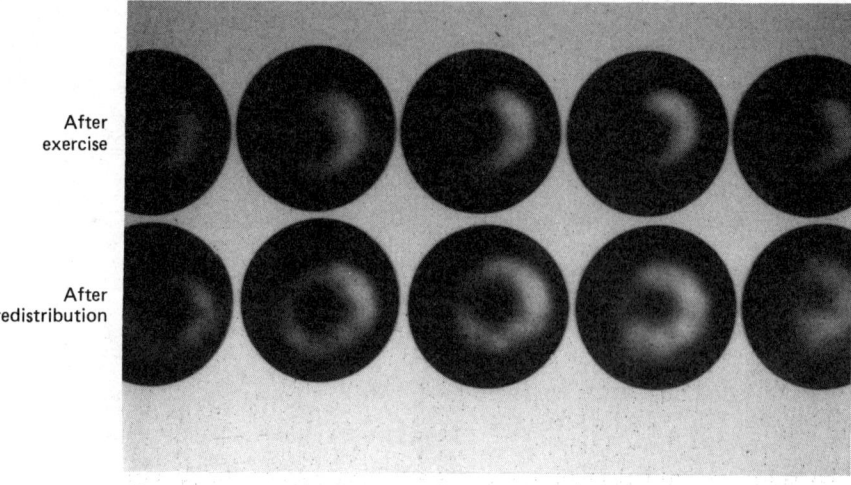

Figure 5–25. Tomographic thallium (^{201}Tl) scintigraphic images in the left anterior oblique position after exercise (above) and redistribution (below). The tomographic slices are from base (left) to apex (right). The septal area is ischemic during exercise and well perfused after recovery. (Courtesy of EH Botvinick.)

rib fractures related to resuscitative measures or breast or chest wall lesions.

This form of imaging is useful in patients who are not seen until a week or so after the onset of symptoms. The electrocardiographic and enzyme changes may have cleared, and radionuclear examination may establish the diagnosis of infarction. Perioperative infarcts can be detected when nonspecific electrocardiographic changes and trauma-related enzyme elevation cause confusion. Traumatic myocardial contusion produces a positive test, usually without specific electrocardiographic changes. An example of a positive scan is shown in Fig 5–26. The radioisotope is concentrated in the sternum and ribs, in addition to the infarcted area in the heart.

C. Radionuclide Angiography: Radionuclide angiography has developed to a stage at which it can provide significant structural and functional infor-

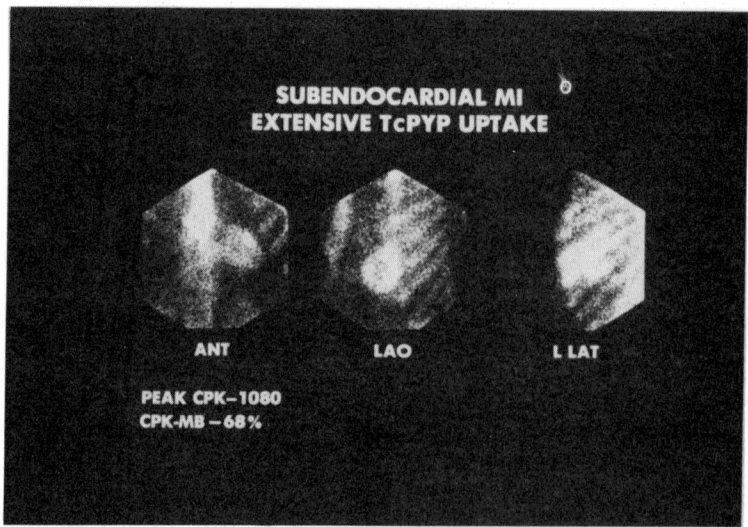

Figure 5–26. Anterior (ANT), left anterior oblique (LAO), and left lateral (LLAT) views of the left chest showing technetium ^{99m}Tc–labeled pyrophosphate taken up by infarcted cardiac tissue in a patient with extensive subendocardial infarction. (Courtesy of EH Botvinick.)

mation. It is best thought of as a noninvasive equivalent of cineangiography in which resolution is comparatively low. It relies heavily on expensive equipment and computer-based analyses, but it has a major advantage in that it can be applied during exercise. Two types of study are used: first-pass and gated equilibrium techniques.

1. First-pass technique—A bolus of sodium pertechnetate (^{99m}Tc) is injected intravenously and followed through the right and left heart chambers. The examination is carried out in the 30-degree right anterior oblique position in order to separate the atrial and ventricular images. The right and left sides of the heart overlap in this view, but radioactivity has normally cleared from the right heart by the time the left heart is imaged. The technique provides a quick, relatively simple means of outlining the cardiac chambers. Appropriate positioning of the patient is important, and serial studies require repeated injections. Two injections ordinarily constitute a full dose of radioactivity. This method provides the best estimate of right ventricular ejection fraction, especially when the ECG is recorded and used to identify end-systolic and end-diastolic images. The ratio of the number of counts in the area of interest at end-systole and end-diastole provides a measure of ejection fraction that depends not on the assumption of a specific geometric shape for the ventricle but rather on delineating the borders of the ventricular image. Computer assistance with this task is often sought.

2. Gated equilibrium technique—In this method, the radionuclide (usually ^{99m}Tc–labeled red cells) is injected intravenously and allowed to equilibrate with the blood volume for 5–10 minutes before imaging starts. Imaging can continue for up to 6 hours, and the patient's position or circulatory state can be altered between images. This technique is particularly applicable to exercise studies. The images are "gated" to the ECG, so that imaging is restricted to certain times during the cardiac cycle. Gating to end-systole and end-diastole, shown in Fig 5–27, is used in ejection fraction measurements, and data from several hundred beats are stored in a computer to obtain signals of adequate intensity. The start of imaging is linked to the R wave, and the subsequent images are recorded at regular intervals during the cardiac cycle. Both this technique and the first-pass method have the potential for identifying wall motion abnormalities in the left ventricle. Images are usually obtained in the left anterior oblique position to minimize overlap between the right and left ventricles. Computer-assisted "region of interest" delineation is commonly used to outline the edges of the left ventricular image in ejection fraction measurements. The values for ejection fraction by this method correlate well (correlation coefficient about 0.9) with angiocardiographic measurements. The radionuclear studies can be done during exercise on a cycle ergometer, but loss of resolution due to patient movement is inevitable. With all radionuclear techniques, the visual impact of the images is not outstanding, and spatial and temporal resolution

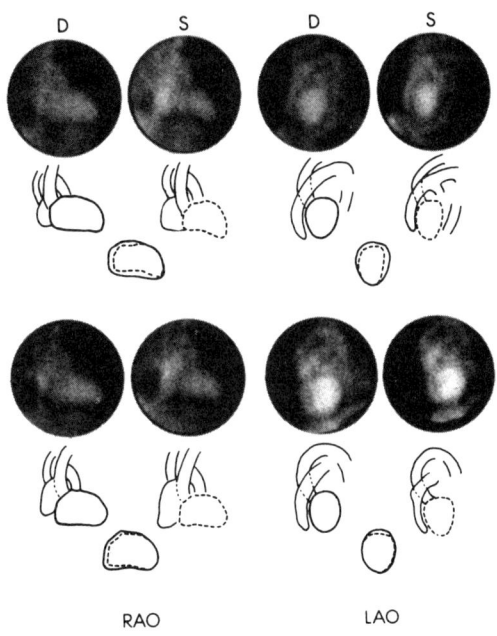

Figure 5–27. Diastolic (D) and systolic (S) frames from an equilibrium multiple-gated blood pool scintigram in the right anterior oblique (RAO) and left anterior oblique (LAO) positions. The upper images were obtained on the second day after the patient suffered a myocardial infarction. Left ventricular function was better on this occasion than in the study illustrated below, obtained 3 weeks later when left ventricular failure had developed. (Reproduced, with permission, from Botvinick EH, Shames DM: *Nuclear Cardiology: Clinical Applications*. Williams & Wilkins, 1979.)

are poor compared to radiologic and ultrasonic techniques. Computer assistance with data analysis is almost essential, and color coding helps in the display of data. The possibility for distortion of results based on the operator's bias exists. "Computer enhancement" of images and edge detection are subjective activities, and care must be taken to obtain an unbiased measurement.

D. Phase Image Analysis: The pattern of ventricular activation can be determined by phase image analysis. In this technique, the time that radioactivity is detected in different areas of the heart is coded in terms of a gray scale. By this means, the sequence of contraction of different areas (eg, left versus right ventricle) can be demonstrated. The technique may be valuable in the analysis of complex arrhythmias.

POSITRON EMISSION TOMOGRAPHY

Positron emission tomography represents a new radionuclide-based imaging technique that has potential for the quantitative analysis of metabolic processes. It uses physiologically relevant radioisotopes of common elements (^{15}O, ^{13}N, ^{11}C, or ^{18}F) with such short half-lives (2 minutes–2 hours) that a cyclotron or its equivalent must ordinarily be located in the building in which the studies are performed.

The radioisotopes are incorporated into biochemically relevant compounds—eg, ^{11}C palmitate or FDG (^{18}F-2-fluoro-2-deoxy glucose)—and their radioactivity followed in cardiac tissue. The tomographic technique depends on the emission of positrons ("antielectrons") that combine with electrons in the tissue, emitting 2 photons that travel in opposite directions (180 degrees apart). These photons readily pass through the tissues and are simultaneously detected by counters placed on opposite sides of the body. The process is called "annihilation coincidence detection" and has a better signal-to-noise ratio than conventional gamma counting.

This type of imaging is particularly well suited to tomography. Computer-based reconstruction techniques analagous to those used in x-ray tomography are used to generate images of the tissues under study. The spatial resolution of the images (about 18 mm) is similar to that of conventional radionuclear techniques and inferior to those of x-ray tomography imaging or magnetic resonance imaging. The absorption of radioactivity by the tissues is not as great as—and more constant than—that with gamma-emitting compounds, and the potential for accurate metabolic studies is clear. The technique has been used to distinguish between old and new myocardial infarctions and to study ^{11}C palmitate metabolism in the heart. The wide range of substrates that the heart can metabolize is a complicating factor, and large differences between fed and fasted subjects have been seen. Imaging following the injection of 2 isotopes (^{13}N ammonia for blood labeling and FDG for heart muscle) has been reported (Marshall RC et al, 1983). The time between the 2 injections must be at least 45 minutes, and several minutes are needed for the acquisition of each image.

MAGNETIC RESONANCE IMAGING

Magnetic resonance detection is a complicated analytical technique that has been used to perform spectroscopy of biologic materials in biochemistry laboratories for more than a decade. The new application that has great potential for clinical use requires computer-based reconstruction of images derived from measurements involving proton density in the tissues. While the nuclei of many compounds exhibit the phenomenon of magnetic resonance, the proton (^{1}H) is the only element that can now be used effectively for imaging. The next most suitable element, phosphorus (^{31}P), is 5 orders of magnitude less effective.

The apparatus used is large and expensive, principally because of the size and power of the permanent magnets needed for imaging the heart. The principle of magnetic resonance imaging depends on the ability of external radio-frequency fields of appropriate frequency to induce resonance in protons lined up in a powerful magnetic field. The protons behave as tiny bar magnets that spin like tops. When an external pulse of appropriate radio frequency is applied at 90 degrees to the alignment of the protons by means of an external coil, the protons rotate from the longitudinal to the transverse plane. When the pulse is turned off, the magnetized protons swing back in an exponential manner to their original position. A receiver coil, surrounding the patient, detects an electrical signal during the "magnetic relaxation time," and this forms the basis of the imaging technique.

Four factors determine the intensity of the signal detected by the receiver coil: (1) the proton density in the tissue; (2) and (3) the magnetic relaxation time constants—τ_1 for the return of the proton in its long axis to its rest position (spin-lattice relaxation) and τ_2 for the return of the proton in its transverse axis (spin-spin relaxation); and (4) blood flow, based on the entry of blood, containing undisturbed protons, into the field. The values for τ_1 and τ_2 vary from tissue to tissue, so that by varying the sequence and duration of the distorting radio-frequency pulse in the coil and the time of data collection, it is possible to alter the intensity of the signals obtained from different tissues. Signal collection takes about 10–30 ms, using a 512 × 512 matrix, and serial images are obtained at about 1-second intervals. The patient must lie still in the scanner for several minutes. Gating of the signals to the ECG has been achieved by using fiberoptic techniques to conduct the electrocardiographic signals through the strong electromagnetic fields surrounding the patient. The technique cannot be applied to patients with magnetizable material in their bodies, eg, pacemakers, artificial valves, prosthetic joints, or metal clips. Care must be taken to keep metal objects and magnetized materials (watches, keys, floppy disks, etc) away from the powerful magnets needed for this form of investigation. The technique is just beginning to be applied clinically. An example of a magnetic resonance image of the heart is shown in Fig 5–28.

CARDIOPULMONARY FUNCTION TESTING

Pulmonary function testing of varying degrees of complexity is available in most hospitals of moderate size. It is used mainly for the study of patients with lung disease, but since pulmonary function is likely to be impaired in patients with heart disease, tests of pulmonary function are often needed in the assessment of cardiac patients. The 3 main elements of pulmonary function—ventilation, diffusion, and pulmonary blood flow—and the relationships between

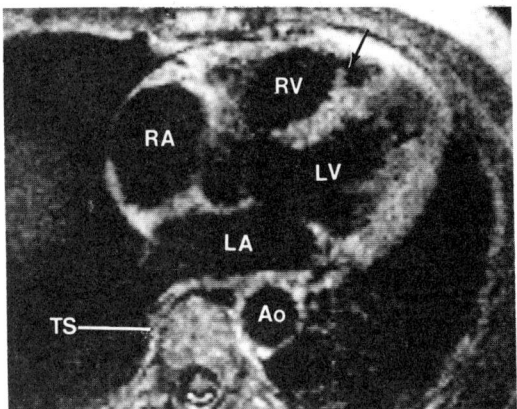

Figure 5-28. Magnetic resonance image of a normal heart. LV, left ventricle; RV, right ventricle; LA, left atrium; RA, right atrium; Ao, aorta; TS, thoracic spine. The black arrow points to the moderator band in the right ventricle. (Reproduced, with permission, from Herfkens RJ et al: Nuclear magnetic resonance imaging of the cardiovascular system: Normal and pathologic findings. *Radiology* 1983;**147**:749.)

them need to be tested, both at rest and during exercise. The conventional measurements of vital capacity and maximum expiratory flow rate give an indication of the maximal ventilation the patient can achieve voluntarily. Maximal exercise ventilation may be a more relevant measurement, since it tests the response to natural stimuli rather than the ability to perform a respiratory maneuver. Diffusion of oxygen across the alveolar membrane is assessed by measuring the transfer of carbon monoxide into the blood. This process may be impaired in severe pulmonary congestion with edema. Measurement of the concentrations of physiologically relevant gases (oxygen and CO_2) or inert gases (usually helium) in the respired air at the mouth gives information about the adequacy of ventilation, its distribution, and its relationship to perfusion. Specific gas analyzers and flowmeters are now available with which to make appropriate measurements of cardiopulmonary function in patients at rest and during exercise. The mechanical properties of the lungs can be tested by measuring the force applied to the lungs (intrathoracic pressure) from esophageal pressure records using an air-filled balloon connected to a pressure transducer by a plastic tube. The compliance (stiffness) of the lungs and the resistance to air flow in the bronchial tree can be calculated. Arterial oxygen saturation can be measured noninvasively with an ear oximeter. The absorption of light transmitted through the illuminated ear is recorded at different wavelengths, and the concentration ratio of oxygenated and reduced hemoglobin is calculated. Arterial desaturation is more commonly found in lung disease but occurs in pulmonary edema and in patients with cyanotic congenital heart disease. Arterial oxygen and CO_2 tensions can also be measured via the heated skin by using electrodes.

EXERCISE TESTING

Exercise testing, in which physiologic measurements are made, in addition to recording of an ECG, is not in routine use in the USA. The apparatus involved varies in complexity and in cost. The information obtained by exercise testing is almost entirely functional. Muscular exercise is the most significant, repeatable, and physiologically relevant stress to which a patient can be subjected. It can be conveniently performed either on a cycle ergometer or on a motor-driven treadmill. *An ECG must always be recorded, and resuscitation equipment must be available.* Standardized exercise tests are routinely done in cardiac patients in the Scandinavian countries. They provide objective evidence of the patient's work capacity and record work load, heart rate, changes in the ECG, and blood pressure. They are most helpful in following individual patients and assessing the effects of therapy and the progress of disease. Additional measurements such as ventilation, oxygen consumption, respiratory exchange ratio, cardiac output, and lung-to-ear circulation time by oximetry can be added to give additional physiologic information using noninvasive methods. Patients with heart disease show excessive exercise ventilation, a high respiratory exchange ratio owing to disproportionate metabolic acidosis, a low maximal cardiac output, and a prolonged lung-to-ear circulation time.

OTHER GRAPHIC METHODS

1. BALLISTOCARDIOGRAPHY

Ballistocardiography, one of the oldest of these methods, purports to measure the accelerative forces imparted to the body by cardiac contraction. The procedure is not in common use, and it has been the difficulty encountered in standardization and calibration of the records obtained that has probably limited its usefulness. In principle, since the force of cardiac contraction is determined during the period of isovolumetric contraction, the accelerative forces during this period of constant ventricular volume are potentially of great functional significance. The technical problems involved in measuring the accelerative forces imparted to the body by the beating heart have not yet been mastered, and clinical ballistocardiography tends to be overly influenced by the effects of the damping properties of the body tissues.

2. APEXCARDIOGRAPHY

Apexcardiography attempts to record the same type of accelerative forces as ballistocardiography but concentrates on the displacement of the apex beat during the cardiac cycle. Apexcardiography is claimed by its advocates to help in understanding the hemodynamic events associated with cardiac filling and emptying, in distinguishing between an opening snap and a third heart sound, and in investigating patients with cardiomyopathy. The apparatus is not expensive, but the technique is not in routine use.

3. SYSTOLIC TIME INTERVALS

These noninvasive measurements do not require expensive apparatus but are not widely used. In systolic time interval measurements, the ECG, phonocardiogram, and an externally recorded carotid pulse tracing are used to provide a tracing from which specific time intervals are measured. The important intervals are the QA_2 interval, ie, the interval between the Q wave of the ECG and the aortic component of the second heart sound on the phonocardiogram, and the left ventricular ejection time (LVET), measured from the start of the upstroke of the carotid pulse tracing to the dicrotic notch on the downstroke. The difference between these 2 time intervals—the preejection period (PEP)—is the time from the Q wave to the start of the upstroke of the carotid arterial tracing. The PEP/LVET ratio is considered to reflect left ventricular function, the normal ratio of about 0.35 increasing to about 0.6 in patients with heart failure. The fidelity of the external recordings of carotid arterial pulsations is not high, and similar information can be obtained from echocardiographic recordings of aortic valve opening and closing. Systolic time intervals are most useful for following the progress of individual patients with left ventricular disease. As with other indirect methods, a definitive diagnosis or a serious decision, such as whether or not to submit a patient to cardiac surgery, would never be based solely on this measurement.

REFERENCES

Electrocardiography

Chaitman BR et al: The importance of clinical subsets in interpreting maximal treadmill exercise test results: The role of multiple-lead ECG systems. *Circulation* 1979; **59**:560.

Chou T, Helm RA: *Clinical Vectorcardiography*, 2nd ed. Grune & Stratton, 1974.

Dunn RF et al: Exercise-induced ST-segment elevation: Correlation of thallium-201 myocardial perfusion scanning and coronary arteriography. *Circulation* 1980;**61**:989.

Frank E: An accurate, clinically practical system for spatial vectorcardiography. *Circulation* 1956;**13**:737.

Goldman MJ: *Principles of Clinical Electrocardiography*, 12th ed. Lange, 1986.

Hardarson T et al: Variability, reproducibility and applications of precordial ST-segment mapping following myocardial infarction. *Circulation* 1978;**57**:1096.

Holter NJ: New method for heart studies: Continuous electrocardiography of active subjects over long periods is now practical. *Science* 1961;**134**:1214.

Lipman BS, Massie E, Kleiger RE: *Clinical Scalar Electrocardiography*, 6th ed. Year Book, 1972.

Littmann D: *Examination of the Heart*. Part 5 of: *The Electrocardiogram*. American Heart Association, 1973.

Marriott HJL, Fogg E: Constant monitoring for cardiac dysrhythmias and blocks. *Mod Concepts Cardiovasc Dis* 1970;**39**:103.

Meijler FL, DeMedina EOR, Helder JC: Future of computerised electrocardiography. *Br Heart J* 1980;**44**:1.

Muller JE, Maroko PR, Braunwald E: Evaluation of precordial electrocardiographic mapping as a means of assessing changes in myocardial ischemic injury. *Circulation* 1975;**52**:16.

Muller JE, Maroko PR, Braunwald E: Precordial electrocardiographic mapping: A technique to assess the efficacy of interventions designed to limit infarct size. *Circulation* 1978;**57**:1.

X-Ray Investigations

Booth DC, Nissen S, DeMaria AN: Assessment of the severity of valvular regurgitation by digital subtraction angiography compared to cineangiography. *Am Heart J* 1985;**110**:409.

Brundage BH, Lipton MJ: The emergence of computed tomography as a cardiovascular diagnostic technic. *Am Heart J* 1982;**103**:313.

Brundage BH et al: Detection of patent coronary bypass grafts by computed tomography: A preliminary report. *Circulation* 1980;**61**:826.

Cooley RN, Schreiber MH: *Radiology of the Heart and Great Vessels*, 3rd ed. Williams & Wilkins, 1978.

Detrano R et al: Videodensitometric ejection fraction from digital subtraction right ventriculograms: Correlation with first pass radionuclide ejection fraction. *J Am Coll Cardiol* 1985;**5**:1377.

Foster CJ et al: Computed tomographic assessment of coronary artery bypass grafts. *Br Heart J* 1984;**52**:24.

Goldberg HL et al: Digital subtraction intravenous left ventricular angiography: Comparison with conventional intraventricular angiography. *J Am Coll Cardiol* 1983;**1**:858.

Jefferson K, Rees S: *Clinical Cardiac Radiology*. Butterworth, 1973.

Mehlman DJ, Resnekov L: A guide to the radiographic identification of prosthetic heart valves. *Circulation* 1978;**57**:613.

Ovitt TW: Intravenous angiography utilizing digital video subtraction techniques. *Am J Cardiol* 1982;**49**:1365.

Ritman EL et al: Quantitative imaging of the structure and function of the heart, lungs and circulation. *Mayo Clin Proc* 1978;**53**:3.

Skiöldebrand CG et al: Assessment of ventricular wall thickness in vivo by computed transmission tomography. *Circulation* 1980;**61**:960.

Tomoda H et al: Evaluation of left atrial thrombus with computed tomography. *Am Heart J* 1980;**100**:306.

Ungerleider HE, Clark CP: A study of the transverse diameter of the heart silhouette with prediction table based on the teleoroentgenogram. *Am Heart J* 1939;**17**:92.

Ultrasonography

Abdulla AM et al: Limitations of echocardiography in the assessment of left ventricular size and function in aortic regurgitation. *Circulation* 1980;**61**:148.

Baker DW, Rubenstein SA, Lorch GS: Pulsed Doppler echocardiography: Principles and applications. *Am J Med* 1977;**63**:69.

Bansal RC et al: Feasibility of detailed two-dimensional echocardiographic examination in adults: Prospective study of 200 patients. *Mayo Clin Proc* 1980;**55**:291.

Crawford MH et al: Accuracy and reproducibility of new M-mode echocardiographic recommendations for measuring left ventricular dimensions. *Circulation* 1980;**61**:137.

Feigenbaum H: Assessment of echocardiography in clinical practice. *Prog Cardiovasc Dis* 1978;**20**:329.

Feigenbaum H: *Echocardiography*, 2nd ed. Lea & Febiger, 1976.

Felner JM et al: Sources of variability in echocardiographic measurements. *Am J Cardiol* 1980;**45**:995.

Fraker TD Jr et al: Detection and exclusion of interatrial shunts by two-dimensional echocardiography and peripheral venous injection. *Circulation* 1979;**59**:379.

Goldberg SJ et al: Evaluation of pulmonary and systemic blood flow by 2-dimensional Doppler echocardiography using fast Fourier transform spectral analysis. *Am J Cardiol* 1982;**50**:1394.

Hagan AD et al: *Two-Dimensional Echocardiography*. Little, Brown, 1983.

Hatle L, Angelsen B: *Doppler Ultrasound in Cardiology*. Lea & Febiger, 1982.

Henry WL et al: Report of the American Society of Echocardiography Committee on Nomenclature and Standards in 2-Dimensional Echocardiography. *Circulation* 1980;**62**:212.

Hirschfeld DS, Schiller N: Localization of aortic valve vegetations by echocardiography. *Circulation* 1976;**53**:280.

Huntsman LL et al: Noninvasive Doppler determination of cardiac output in man: Clinical validation. *Circulation* 1983;**67**:593.

Kleid JJ, Schiller NB: *Echocardiography Case Studies*. Medical Examination Publishing Co., 1974.

Kotler MN et al: Clinical uses of two-dimensional echocardiography. *Am J Cardiol* 1980;**45**:1061.

Lew W, Karliner JS: Assessment of pulmonary valve echogram in normal subjects and in patients with pulmonary arterial hypertension. *Br Heart J* 1979;**42**:147.

McDonald IG, Feigenbaum H, Chang S: Analysis of left ventricular wall motion by reflected ultrasound: Application to assessment of myocardial function. *Circulation* 1972;**46**:14.

Mills P, Craige E: Echophonocardiography. *Prog Cardiovasc Dis* 1978;**20**:337.

Mills PG et al: Echocardiographic and hemodynamic relationships of ejection sounds. *Circulation* 1977;**56**:430.

Morganroth J, Pohost GM (editors): Symposium: Two dimensional echocardiography versus cardiac nuclear imaging techniques. *Am J Cardiol* 1980;**46**:1093.

Omoto R, Kobayashi M: *Atlas of Essential Ultrasound Imaging*. Igaku-Shoin, 1983.

Popp RL: Echocardiographic assessment of cardiac disease. *Circulation* 1976;**54**:538.

Popp RL et al: Optimal resources for ultrasonic examination of the heart: Echocardiography study group. *Circulation* 1982;**65**:423A.

Ports TA et al: Echocardiography of left ventricular masses. *Circulation* 1978;**58**:528.

Reneman RS: *Cardiovascular Applications of Ultrasound*. American Elsevier, 1974.

Schiller NB, Snider AR: Key references: Echocardiography in congenital heart disease. *Circulation* 1981;**63**:461.

Schiller NB et al: Left ventricular volume from paired biplane two-dimensional echocardiography. *Circulation* 1979; **60**:547.

Serruys PW et al: Intracardiac right-to-left shunts demonstrated by two-dimensional echocardiography after peripheral vein injection. *Br Heart J* 1979;**42**:429.

Silverman NH, Schiller NB: Apex echocardiography: A two-dimensional technique for evaluating congenital heart disease. *Circulation* 1978;**57**:503.

Tajik AJ et al: Two-dimensional real-time ultrasonic imaging of the heart and great vessels. *Mayo Clin Proc* 1978; **53**:271.

Talano JV, Gardin JM: *Textbook of Two-Dimensional Echocardiography*. Grune & Stratton, 1983.

Valdes-Cruz LM, Sahn DJ: Two dimensional echo Doppler for non-invasive quantitation of cardiac flow: A status report. *Mod Concepts Cardiovasc Dis* 1982;**51**:123.

Valdez RS et al: Evaluation of the echocardiogram as an epidemiologic tool in an asymptomatic population. *Circulation* 1979;**60**:921.

Radionuclide Investigations

Bailey IK et al: Detection of coronary artery disease and myocardial ischemia by electrocardiography and myocardial perfusion scanning with thallium 201. (Abstract.) *Am J Cardiol* 1976;**37**:118.

Bodenheimer MM, Banka VS, Helfant RH: Nuclear cardiology. 1. Radionuclide angiographic assessment of left ventricular contraction: Uses, limitations and future directions. *Am J Cardiol* 1980;**45**:661.

Bodenheimer MM et al: Detection of coronary heart disease using radionuclide determined regional ejection fraction at rest and during handgrip exercise: Correlation with coronary angiography. *Circulation* 1978;**58**:640.

Botvinick EH, Shames DM: *Nuclear Cardiology: Clinical Applications*. Williams & Wilkins, 1979.

Botvinick EH et al: An accurate means of detecting and characterizing abnormal patterns of ventricular activation by phase image analysis. *Am J Cardiol* 1982;**50**:289.

Botvinick EH et al: Myocardial stress perfusion scintigraphy with rubidium-81 versus stress electrocardiography. *Am J Cardiol* 1977;**39**:364.

Botvinick EH et al: Phase image evaluation of patients with ventricular pre-excitation syndromes. *J Am Coll Cardiol* 1984;**3**:799.

Burrow RD et al: Analysis of left ventricular function from multiple gated acquisition (MUGA) cardiac blood pool imaging: Comparison to contrast angiography. *Circulation* 1977;**56**:1024.

Federman J et al: Multiple-gated acquisition cardiac blood-pool imaging: Evaluation of left ventricular function correlated with contrast angiography. *Mayo Clin Proc* 1978;**53**:625.

Geltman EM et al: Characterization of nontransmural myocardial infarction by positron-emission tomography. *Circulation* 1982;**65**:747.

Greenberg BH et al: Thallium-201 myocardial perfusion scintigraphy to evaluate patients after coronary bypass surgery. *Am J Cardiol* 1978;**42**:167.

Marshall RC et al: Identification and differentiation of resting myocardial ischemia and infarction in man with positron computed tomography, F-labeled fluorodeoxyglucose and N-13 ammonia. *Circulation* 1983;**67**:766.

Phelps ME, Schelbert HR, Mazziota JC: Positron computed tomography for studies of myocardial and cerebral function. *Ann Intern Med* 1983;**98**:339.

Reduto LA et al: Sequential radionuclide assessment of right and left ventricular performance after acute transmural myocardial infarction. *Ann Intern Med* 1978;**89:**447.

Sprengelmeyer J, Weisberger CL: *Practical Nuclear Cardiology.* Harper & Row, 1979.

Strauss HW, Pitt B: *Cardiovascular Nuclear Medicine,* 2nd ed. Mosby, 1979.

Strauss HW et al: Thallium 201 for myocardial imaging: Relation of thallium 201 to regional myocardial perfusion. *Circulation* 1975;**51:**641.

Wackers FJ et al: Multiple gated cardiac blood pool imaging for left ventricular ejection fraction: Validation of the technique and assessment of variability. *Am J Cardiol* 1979;**43:**1159.

Wagner HN: Radioisotope scanning in pulmonary embolic disease. In: *Pulmonary Embolic Diseases.* Sasahara AA, Stein M (editors). Grune & Stratton, 1965.

Walton S et al: Phase analysis of the first pass radionuclide angiogram. *Br Heart J* 1982;**48:**441.

Magnetic Resonance Imaging

Brownell GL et al: Positron tomography and nuclear magnetic resonance imaging. *Science* 1982;**215:**619.

Friedman BJ et al: Comparison of magnetic resonance imaging and echocardiography in determination of cardiac dimensions in normal subjects. *J Am Coll Cardiol* 1985;**5:**1369.

Herkens RJ et al: Nuclear magnetic resonance imaging of the cardiovascular system: Normal and pathologic findings. *Radiology* 1983;**147:**749.

Higgins CB, Kaufman L, Crooks LE: Magnetic resonance imaging of the cardiovascular system. *Am Heart J* 1985;**109:**136.

Kaufman L et al: The potential impact of nuclear magnetic resonance imaging on cardiovascular diagnosis. *Circulation* 1983;**67:**251.

Levy GC, Craik DJ: Recent developments in nuclear magnetic resonance spectroscopy. *Science* 1981;**214:**291.

McNamara MT et al: Detection and characterization of acute myocardial infarction in man with the use of gated magnetic resonance imaging. *Circulation* 1985;**71:**717.

Radda GK: Potential and limitations of nuclear magnetic resonance for the cardiologist. *Br Heart J* 1983;**50:**197.

Steiner RE et al: Nuclear magnetic resonance imaging of the heart: Current status and future prospects. *Br Heart J* 1983;**50:**202.

Young SW: *Nuclear Magnetic Resonance Imaging: Basic Principles.* Raven, 1983.

Other Types of Noninvasive Investigations

Ayotte B et al: Assessment of left heart function by noninvasive exercise test in normal subjects. *J Appl Physiol* 1973;**34:**644.

Bates DV, Christie RV, Macklem PT: *Respiratory Function in Disease.* Saunders, 1971.

Bruce RA: Exercise testing of patients with coronary heart disease: Principles and normal standards for evaluation. *Ann Clin Res* 1971;**3:**323.

Bruce RA et al: Noninvasive predictors of sudden cardiac death in men with coronary heart disease. *Am J Cardiol* 1977;**39:**833.

Chung EK (editor): *Non-Invasive Cardiac Diagnosis.* Lea & Febiger, 1976.

Comroe JH et al: *The Lung: Clinical Physiology and Pulmonary Function Tests,* 2nd ed. Year Book, 1962.

Ellestad MH, Blomqvist CG, Naughton JP: AHA Committee report: Standards for adult exercise testing laboratories. *Circulation* 1979;**59:**421A.

Epstein SE: Implications of probability analysis on the strategy used for noninvasive detection of coronary artery disease. *Am J Cardiol* 1980;**46:**491.

Gibson TC et al: The A wave of the apexcardiogram and left ventricular diastolic stiffness. *Circulation* 1974;**49:**441.

Irving JB, Bruce RA: Exertional hypotension and postexertional ventricular fibrillation in stress testing. *Am J Cardiol* 1977;**39:**849.

Jones NL, Campbell EJM: *Clinical Exercise Testing.* Saunders, 1982.

Leatham A: *Auscultation of the Heart and Phonocardiography,* 2nd ed. Churchill Livingstone, 1975.

Lewis RP et al: A critical review of the systolic time intervals. *Circulation* 1977;**56:**146.

McIlroy MB: The clinical uses of oximetry. *Br Heart J* 1959;**21:**293.

Morganroth J, Parisi AF, Pohost GM: *Noninvasive Cardiac Imaging.* Year Book, 1983.

Murray JF: *The Normal Lung: The Basis for Diagnosis and Treatment of Pulmonary Disease.* Saunders, 1976.

Oliver MF: *Modern Trends in Cardiology–3.* Butterworth, 1975.

Parisi AF, Tow DE: *Noninvasive Approaches to Cardiovascular Diagnosis.* Appleton-Century-Crofts, 1979.

Rapaport E: The fractional disappearance rate of the separate isoenzymes of creatine phosphokinase in the dog. *Cardiovasc Res* 1975;**9:**473.

Sheffield LT, Roitman D: Stress testing methodology. *Prog Cardiovasc Dis* 1976;**19:**33.

Sobel BE, Shell WE: Serum enzyme determinations in the diagnosis and assessment of myocardial infarction. *Circulation* 1972;**45:**471.

Starmer CF, McIntosh HD, Whalen RE: Electrical hazards and cardiac function. *N Engl J Med* 1974;**284:**181.

Starr I, Noordegraaf A: *Ballistocardiography in Cardiovascular Research.* Lippincott, 1967.

Tavel ME: *Clinical Phonocardiography and External Pulse Recording,* 3rd ed. Year Book, 1978.

Wagner GS et al: The importance of identification of the myocardial specific isoenzyme of creatine phosphokinase (MB form) in the diagnosis of acute myocardial infarction. *Circulation* 1973;**47:**263.

Weissler AM: Current concepts in cardiology: Systolic-time intervals. *N Engl J Med* 1977;**296:**321.

Weissler AM (editor): *Non-Invasive Cardiology.* Grune & Stratton, 1974.

Whalen RE, Starmer CF: Electric shock hazards in clinical cardiology. *Mod Concepts Cardiovasc Dis* 1967;**36:**7.

Special Investigations: Invasive 6

The descriptions of invasive investigations in this chapter are of a general nature, principally of the techniques involved and not of the findings in different diseases. The latter are included in the chapters dealing with specific cardiac disorders. The varieties of investigation available, their indications and techniques, precautions in their use, their complications, and some broad generalities about interpretation are offered in this chapter. An attempt has been made to show that a range of choices of approach is available, and it will be noted that the personal preference of the investigator, based upon a familiarity with a particular technique, plays a logical part in determining which procedure will be used.

It should be apparent from the term invasive that such investigations are carried out in hospitalized patients for valid indications and only after adequate preliminary appraisal. In many instances, however, invasive diagnostic methods provide important information that cannot be obtained by simpler methods of cardiac diagnosis. The patient should be advised about the nature, risks, and benefits of such procedures. It is necessary to obtain the patient's written informed consent before all studies.

BEDSIDE VERSUS LABORATORY PROCEDURES

Invasive investigations fall into 2 main categories: those carried out at the bedside in severely ill patients and those performed in a cardiac catheterization laboratory. There is some overlap between the two, but, in general, arterial and venous pressure monitoring and pulmonary arterial and wedge pressure recording with a Swan-Ganz catheter are done at the bedside. Formal diagnostic catheterization studies and angiography are performed in specially equipped laboratories.

BEDSIDE CATHETERIZATION

Whereas arterial blood sampling has become a routine procedure in most hospitals, arterial catheterization, together with central venous or pulmonary arterial pressure monitoring, is mainly confined to intensive care areas where specially trained personnel are constantly available to keep the catheters patent and make certain that they are appropriately positioned. This form of monitoring of the patient's hemodynamic status is indicated only in severe, life-threatening illnesses such as myocardial infarction with shock or heart failure and in acute pulmonary edema or in the postoperative period after cardiac surgery. The disturbance, loss of sleep, and psychologic effect on the patient must be weighed against the therapeutic benefit, ie, early recognition of complications and assessment of the effects of therapy.

ARTERIAL CATHETERIZATION

Arterial puncture is a standard and routine procedure used to obtain samples for blood gas analysis and for direct recording of arterial pressure. Arterial blood can be obtained from a number of different sites, and the principles involved are generally similar. Arterial puncture is more painful than venipuncture, and local anesthesia is advocated in all cases. The risks of hemorrhage and hematoma formation are much greater than with venipuncture, especially in patients receiving anticoagulant therapy, but infection of the puncture site and the development of blood-borne infections are much less apt to occur. Local thrombosis with consequent interruption of blood supply to the distal tissues is perhaps the greatest danger.

Repeated blood sampling and arterial pressure recording are greatly facilitated by the use of an indwelling arterial catheter. This is usually a short (25 cm) plastic tube whose proximal end holds a female adapter plus stopcock. After cannulation of the artery, a plastic or plastic-coated guide wire is inserted, and after removal of the arterial needle, the catheter is passed over the guide wire into the artery. The system is flushed with heparinized saline, or a slow (0.1 mL/min) infusion of heparinized saline (1000 units in 200 mL) is maintained.

PERCUTANEOUS VENOUS & RIGHT HEART CATHETERIZATION

Venous puncture and venous catheterization present few problems in patients with large veins that have not previously been the site of multiple punctures. More peripheral, smaller veins should be used for infusions and for taking single blood samples. The larger veins in the antecubital fossa should be preserved for the introduction of catheters into the central circulation. Most difficulty is encountered in dealing with the veins of persons who habitually use intravenous drugs, especially heroin; in such patients it is sometimes necessary to make a cutdown to expose the venae comitantes of the brachial artery. Superficial veins can be made to relax by flicking the skin with a finger, by warming the arm, and, if necessary, by exercising the limb. The vein should be palpated rather than inspected to find a good puncture site, and the skin and the vein should be punctured sequentially. If a catheter is to be inserted, either a plastic fishing line or a catheter can be introduced through the needle. Successively larger catheters can be used to dilate the puncture site until a catheter with a large enough bore is introduced. For central venous pressure measurements, a plastic catheter equivalent to No. 5 French is sufficient, and a percutaneous approach is often successful.

Swan-Ganz Catheter

If a balloon-tipped catheter is to be placed in the pulmonary artery (Swan-Ganz catheter), a percutaneous technique with insertion in the arm is only feasible if the patient has large veins, and a cutdown over the vein is usually needed. Catheter insertion in the subclavian (p 129) or internal jugular vein provides a short, direct route to the heart and makes it easier to immobilize the catheter, but complications such as hemorrhage, air embolism, and pneumothorax are more frequent. The standard balloon-tipped catheter used to monitor pulmonary and indirect left atrial (wedge) pressure can be introduced without fluoroscopic control in most cases. The length of catheter that has been introduced should be carefully measured. When it is felt that the tip is in the right atrium, the balloon is partially inflated with carbon dioxide and the catheter allowed to float forward through the right ventricle with the bloodstream. *Electrocardiographic monitoring is mandatory,* and if fluoroscopic control is not available, a record of pressure at the tip is essential in order to check the position of the catheter.

Inflation of the balloon to measure indirect left atrial (wedge) pressure should be kept to a minimum to avoid pulmonary infarction. The catheter tends to move forward with blood flow, and care must be taken to ensure that it does not become accidentally wedged. Catheters must be kept filled with heparinized saline, as leaks in the pressure recording system that permit blood to enter the catheter readily cause blockage of the lumen.

Pressure Recording

Arterial and venous pressures are usually recorded at the bedside with strain-gauge pressure transducers. The operator should be familiar with the steps required to balance the gauge and set the operating pressure range appropriately. Provision must be made for calibrating the manometer against a column of water or mercury, setting the zero level at the middle of the thorax, and providing a drip of heparinized normal saline to flush the catheter. The physician should be familiar with the characteristics of the pressure tracings in each of the right heart chambers. The recording of indirect left atrial (wedge) pressure is checked by observing the appropriate change in the tracing when the balloon is inflated. If there is any doubt, a blood sample can be obtained. It should show a high P_{O_2} (about 100 mm Hg) and a low P_{CO_2} (< 30 mm Hg).

Thermodilution Catheters

Special catheters are available for the recording of cardiac output by thermodilution. Cold saline is injected through a proximal lumen that lies in the right atrium. The resulting temperature change is recorded at the tip of the catheter in the pulmonary artery by means of a thermistor bead embedded in the wall of the catheter.

Indications for Bedside Catheterization

Catheterization is most clearly indicated in patients with myocardial infarction in whom heart failure with hypotension, pulmonary edema, or shock develops. Complications such as rupture of the ventricular septum, right ventricular infarction, or papillary muscle dysfunction are best managed when hemodynamic information about cardiac output and left atrial pressure is available. Vasodilator therapy can be more closely controlled, and the course of postoperative recovery in cardiac surgical patients can be monitored efficiently. Patients with virtually any condition warranting admission to a general medical or surgical intensive care unit are also candidates for invasive monitoring (eg, patients with extensive trauma, burns, massive pulmonary embolism, cardiac tamponade, respiratory failure, or drug overdose).

Complications of Bedside Catheterization

The complications of bedside arterial and venous catheterization increase with the length of time the catheter is left in place. It is difficult to maintain sterility, especially when an incision is made in the skin. Infection is much more readily introduced through a venous than an arterial catheter, and infection of arterial puncture sites virtually never occurs. Thrombophlebitis, pulmonary embolism, and endocarditis can all occur following venous catheterization, and if phlebitis occurs, removal of the catheter and reinsertion in another site should be undertaken without delay. The catheter itself may be accidentally severed and may enter the right heart if care is not taken to secure it properly. Air embolism is a possible hazard, especially when the jugular vein is the site used and when the slow drip of heparinized saline used to maintain patency is exhausted and the bottle is empty.

Complications following use of a Swan-Ganz catheter include arrhythmias, pulmonary artery perforation, pneumothorax, damage to heart valves, and intravascular knot formation. Deaths have been reported, but severe complications are few considering the widespread use of such catheters.

ELECTIVE DIAGNOSTIC CARDIAC CATHETERIZATION

Cardiac catheterization has become a standard procedure for the diagnosis and assessment of severity of cardiovascular disease. It is now almost always combined with some sort of angiographic procedure. The range of possible investigations is wide, and the morbidity and mortality rates of the different procedures vary widely with the age of the patient, the severity of the disease, and the skill and experience of the operator. *Cardiac catheterization should only be undertaken by a physician who has personally seen and evaluated the patient's problem clinically before the study.* The techniques require constant practice, and the procedure should not be done occasionally in laboratories that are only used once or twice a week. The study combines anatomic diagnosis with functional assessment, and especially in congenital heart disease, it cannot be known what information should be obtained until the procedure is actually under way. Thus, it is not always a routine procedure in which a previously decided list of data must be obtained, but rather an investigation in which the operator should be continuously aware of what has been established and what remains to be done. The study optimally requires the cooperation of a cardiologist, a radiologist, a nurse, and a technician.

Indications for Diagnostic Cardiac Catheterization

Cardiac catheterization is indicated in preparation for all cardiac surgical procedures in order to make the diagnosis as certain as possible and thereby to provide maximum help to the surgeon. What procedure is chosen depends to some extent on the facilities available as well as on the preference of the investigator. In general, combined right and left heart catheterization with angiography has gradually come to be the most widely used approach. In some centers, thoroughness of the investigation, using all types of studies that could possibly throw light on the problem, is the preferred approach, but in the authors' opinion excessively prolonged procedures expose the patient to unnecessary risks. For example, we do not believe that coronary arteriography is routinely indicated in all patients on the chance that surgically important lesions will be identified. Cardiac catheterization should rather be looked on as an investigation with about the same importance as the history, physical examination, ECG, and chest x-ray.

It is possible to obtain misleading information from cardiac catheterization, and the possibility that an error has been made in a laboratory investigation should not be discounted when collateral facts support that inference.

It has recently been suggested (St. John Sutton, 1981) that routine cardiac catheterization need not be performed preoperatively in selected patients when clinical and noninvasive findings indicate that valvular disease is severe enough to warrant surgical treatment. This position has not won widespread acceptance, and routine preoperative catheterization and angiography are still recommended. The morbidity and mortality rates of invasive studies are now acceptably low, and it is a great advantage if the diagnosis and level of severity of functional impairment can be clearly defined before cardiac surgery is undertaken.

Selection of Studies

It is often more difficult to decide what studies should be undertaken in a given patient than to decide which patient should be studied. The operator must consider how much the patient can tolerate, especially the time involved in any given procedure. High-risk patients—eg, those with severe mitral stenosis, pulmonary hypertension, recent myocardial infarction, or severe aortic stenosis—are much more likely to suffer complications from prolonged procedures. It is often better to postpone part of the study to a later date than to add a procedure such as coronary arteriography to the end of a 3-hour session. The operator must always bear in mind the primary aim of the study, which may be to establish a diagnosis in a patient with congenital heart disease, measure the pressure difference and flow across an aortic valve, or measure the pulmonary vascular resistance in a patient with pulmonary hypertension.

RIGHT HEART CATHETERIZATION

Technique

The conventional approach is via the right medial basilic vein at the bend of the elbow, but almost any vein in the arm or leg can be used. The cephalic vein often makes an awkward bend at the shoulder, and it is impossible to enter the thorax by this route in about one-third of patients.

Wedging the Catheter in a Branch of the Pulmonary Artery

When the catheter enters the pulmonary artery, a wedge pressure is obtained by advancing the catheter firmly until its tip becomes wedged in the tapering vessel. A tracing is obtained, and a and v waves are sought if the patient is in sinus rhythm or a v wave if the patient is in atrial fibrillation. The right lower lobe of the lung is the usual site for wedging the catheter. The tracing obtained is called a pulmonary capillary (PC), or wedge, pressure tracing.

Validity of Wedge (PC) Pressure

In the 40 years since wedge pressure was first introduced, it has been repeatedly shown to give an accurate measure of left atrial pressure, delayed by about 0.1 second. An example of simultaneous left atrial and pulmonary capillary tracings is shown in Fig 6–1. Experience and judgment are needed to determine whether a satisfactory measurement of wedge pressure has been obtained, especially in patients with pulmonary hypertension, mitral stenosis, or acute mitral incompetence. The best way to determine that the catheter is wedged is by recording the pressure change as it is withdrawn. It "pops out" of the wedge position, and pressure rises at that instant, with the tracing changing from a wedge to a pulmonary arterial con-

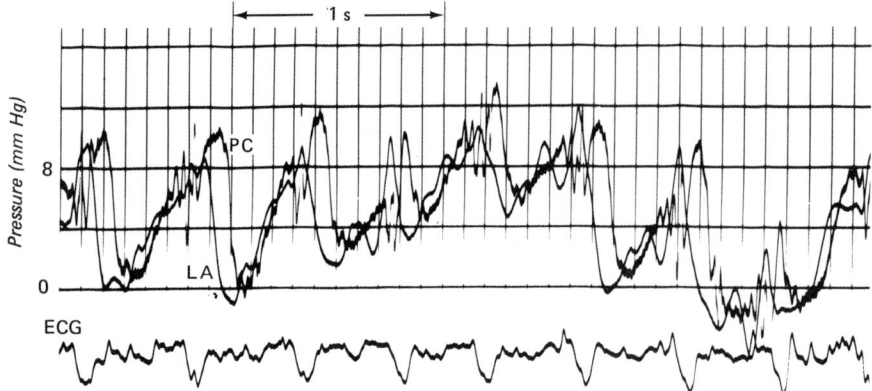

Figure 6–1. Simultaneous left atrial (LA) and wedge (PC) pressure tracings in a patient with aortic stenosis obtained during simultaneous transseptal and right heart catheterization. The patient is in atrial fibrillation, and the PC pressure can be seen to lag about 0.1 second behind the LA pressure. The waveforms are similar.

figuration, as shown in Fig 6–2. A catheter in the wedge position can be flushed easily, but withdrawal of blood samples may be difficult. In any case, the sample obtained is physiologically irrelevant, since the blood obtained equilibrates with an overventilated and underperfused area of lung on the way to the sampling catheter. However, the characteristic high P_{O_2}, low P_{CO_2}, and high pH found in wedge samples are a good means of confirming that the catheter has been properly placed to obtain a satisfactory wedge pressure tracing. It is also possible in a patient with an atrial septal defect to pass a catheter through the defect and to wedge the catheter in the reverse direction by pushing the catheter far out from the left atrium into a pulmonary vein. The pressure obtained resembles that of the pulmonary artery, but the measurement is liable to be incorrect in the presence of pulmonary hypertension.

PRESSURE RECORDINGS

Pulmonary Artery

Phasic and mean pulmonary arterial tracings should always be recorded in the main pulmonary artery. The right pulmonary artery is more readily entered than the left, and the lower lobes of the lungs are more easily catheterized than the upper lobes.

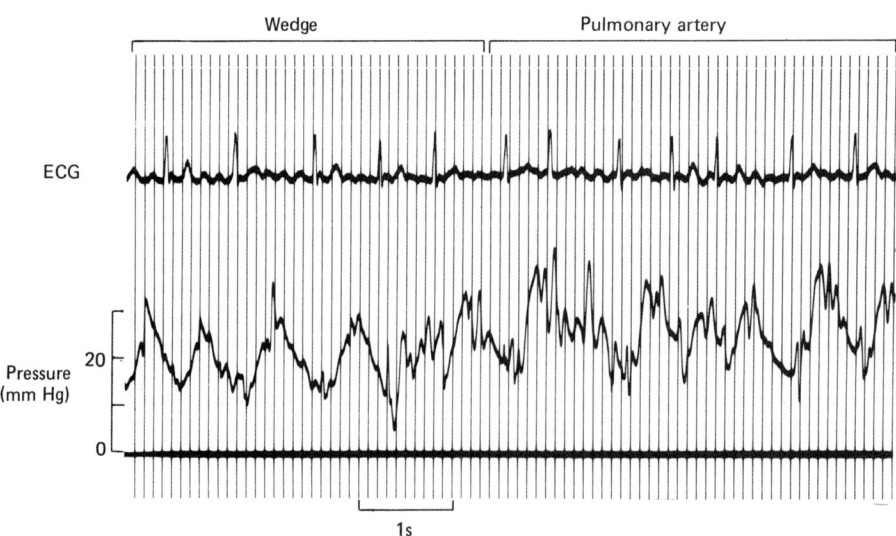

Figure 6–2. Pressure tracing and ECG showing withdrawal of a catheter from the wedge to the pulmonary artery in a patient with mitral valve disease in atrial fibrillation.

Right Ventricle

Right ventricular pressure tracings are conventionally recorded on withdrawal of the catheter from the pulmonary artery. Mean ventricular pressures are not obtained. Right ventricular tracings are particularly liable to be interrupted by ectopic beats, and it is difficult to place a catheter in the right ventricle in a stable position.

Blood Sampling

At the time that withdrawal tracings from the pulmonary artery are obtained, blood samples are taken from each chamber, especially if there is any question of a left-to-right shunt. A sample from the superior vena cava should be followed by a high caval or innominate vein sample if an atrial defect is suspected, because anomalous venous return into the superior vena cava must be excluded. Opinions differ about the importance of obtaining a sample from the inferior vena cava. We believe that a sample should be taken after positioning the catheter approximately 2.5 cm below the diaphragm and pointing to the left, away from the hepatic vein. This may be difficult, and streams of blood from the renal vein tend to give falsely high saturations if the catheter is placed too low.

Measurement of Cardiac Output

Cardiac output is ordinarily measured during right heart catheterization when the right heart catheter is in the main pulmonary artery (mixed venous blood) and an arterial sample is available from a systemic artery. A 3-minute expired gas collection is made, and simultaneous pulmonary arterial and systemic arterial samples are drawn during the gas collection and analyzed for oxygen content and capacity. An ECG is obtained during the gas collection to record the heart rate and to make sure that the patient is in a steady state. Alternatively, the cardiac output may be measured by the indicator dilution method, using Cardio-Green dye or thermodilution.

LEFT HEART CATHETERIZATION

Left heart catheterization is usually carried out in combination with right heart studies. The right heart data are generally obtained first.

Indications for Left Heart Catheterization

Left heart catheterization has come to be widely used in all forms of heart disease affecting the left heart, eg, mitral and aortic valve disease, coronary artery disease, and cardiomyopathy. It is not necessarily indicated in most forms of congenital heart disease, especially when the catheter can be passed from the right heart through a defect into the left heart. In some centers, an attempt is routinely made to enter all cardiac chambers in all patients. We feel that the operator should exercise judgment in choosing procedures and should tailor the study to the needs of each patient.

Different Approaches to Left Heart Catheterization

There is no general agreement about the correct way to approach the left side of the heart. Four methods are in common use in adults: (1) retrograde percutaneous femoral artery catheterization, (2) retrograde brachial arterial catheterization via arterial cutdown, (3) transseptal left heart catheterization via the femoral vein, and (4) direct percutaneous left ventricular puncture.

Almost all laboratories use more than one approach to the left heart, since no one approach is always appropriate, feasible, or successful. The choice depends partly on personal preference and partly on the method used for coronary angiography in that particular laboratory, which in turn depends on the equipment used.

Selection of Method

The nature of the patient's disease plays an important part in the choice of method. Most problems are encountered in patients with aortic stenosis in whom it is difficult to pass a catheter in a retrograde fashion across the aortic valve. If at all possible, the entire left heart study is performed by a single route in an attempt to minimize complications. Thus, the fact that a brachial arteriotomy will be needed to perform coronary arteriography by the Sones technique leads to the selection of the retrograde brachial arterial approach, whereas the need for a study by the Judkins technique for coronary angiography would lead to the selection of a retrograde femoral approach. Transseptal catheterization requires more skill and constant practice than any other form of left heart catheterization and is consequently becoming less popular.

Retrograde Percutaneous Femoral Artery Catheterization Technique

The method used to introduce the catheter is similar to that used in coronary arteriography by the Judkins technique. The femoral artery is punctured with a Cournand needle about 2.5 cm below the inguinal ligament in the groin. A guide wire is threaded via the needle to the abdominal aorta, and the needle is removed. A short (25 cm) dilator is advanced over the wire into the artery and pushed in and pulled out of the artery 2 or 3 times. The dilator is removed and replaced by an end-hole catheter. The catheter and the wire are advanced under fluoroscopic control to the ascending aorta. Several varieties of catheter are available for entering the left ventricle. If the aortic valve is normal, a pigtail catheter can usually be advanced into the left ventricle without a guide wire. Any end-hole catheter should always be used with a soft guide wire projecting 3–10 cm from its tip, because the unoccluded tip may damage the aortic valve when pushed firmly against it. The guide wire rather than the catheter is manipulated to enter the ventricle, the catheter is then advanced over the wire, and the wire is withdrawn. Because it has a curve near the tip, a right coronary artery Judkins catheter is a useful alternative to the standard Gensini Teflon catheter for entering the left ventricle.

This approach is not advocated when the patient has iliofemoral atherosclerosis or has had peripheral vascular surgery, with or without prosthetic replacement. When aortic stenosis is present, retrograde femoral catheterization is unsuccessful in a significant number of patients (15–20%), and in many laboratories another approach is used from the start of the procedure.

Retrograde Arterial Catheterization via a Brachial Arterial Cutdown Technique

Cutting down on the brachial artery and exposing it for 1.5–2.5 cm is the method of choice from the arm, since the vessel is usually too small for percutaneous catheterization. Generous use of local anesthesia, complete familiarity with the anatomy, and an ability to distinguish between the brachial artery and the median nerve are important factors in the success of this approach, which is also used for coronary arteriography by the Sones technique. Adequate exposure through a 5-cm incision, checking for position of the vessel by palpating its pulse, and identification of the tendinous bicipital aponeurosis and its retraction laterally are helpful in the dissection, which usually takes 15–20 minutes. Two plastic tapes are placed around the vessel for control of hemorrhage, and the catheter is inserted either through an arteriotomy or via a puncture site that has been dilated with a tapering plastic cannula. It is helpful to put a loose pursestring suture around the site of entry into the vessel before opening it, using 5-0 silk. The hole in the vessel can then be quickly closed by tightening this suture at the end of the procedure.

A straight, closed-tip catheter with multiple side holes—either a Lehman catheter with a tapered tip, a Sones catheter, or an NIH catheter—is usually used from the arm. Negotiating the bend in the subclavicular area is sometimes a problem in elderly atherosclerotic patients, but the degree of control of the catheter is much greater than with the femoral approach. Crossing the aortic valve is more readily accomplished using the brachial artery than the femoral route. Patients with aortic stenosis present the main problem.

Transseptal Catheterization

Transseptal left heart catheterization provides an alternative approach that is preferred in many centers. A long (>35 cm) needle with a curved tip is introduced into a catheter in the right femoral vein and passed into the right atrium. The catheter, which also has a curved tip and is shaped to fit snugly over the needle, has been placed in the vein either through a cutdown over the saphenous vein or percutaneously. The catheter is advanced until it impinges on the fossa ovalis in the middle of the atrial septum, and the needle is then advanced to puncture the atrial septum. The procedure is carried out under fluoroscopic vision and with a continuously visible pressure record. Once the tip has entered the left atrium, the catheter is advanced over the needle to lie in the left atrium. The catheter itself, or a smaller one passed through it, is then advanced into the left ventricle in the position shown in Fig 6–3. The principal indication for the use of transseptal catheterization is in patients with aortic stenosis in whom a retrograde aortic catheter fails to enter the left ventricle.

The procedure is likely to cause problems in patients with kyphoscoliosis, left atrial thrombus, left atrial myxoma, or giant left atrium. The success rate in entering the left ventricle from the atrium is not 100%, and the fact that aortography and coronary arteriography are now so commonly performed has tended to reduce the number of transseptal studies being done.

Left Ventricular Puncture

Percutaneous transthoracic left ventricular puncture is indicated when a catheter cannot be passed into the left ventricle, as in a patient with calcific aortic stenosis or after valve replacement. This procedure is easier to perform and less dangerous than might be expected and is described in Chapter 13.

Measurements During Left Heart Catheterization

Left ventricular and aortic pressures constitute the principal measurements to be obtained during left heart catheterization. In investigating patients with mitral disease, the left ventricular pressure is measured

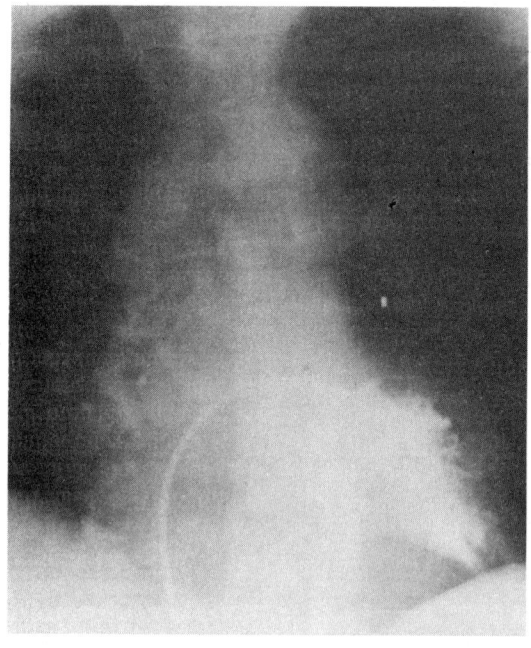

Figure 6–3. Single frame from left ventricular angiography carried out via a catheter passed transseptally into the left atrium and left ventricle.

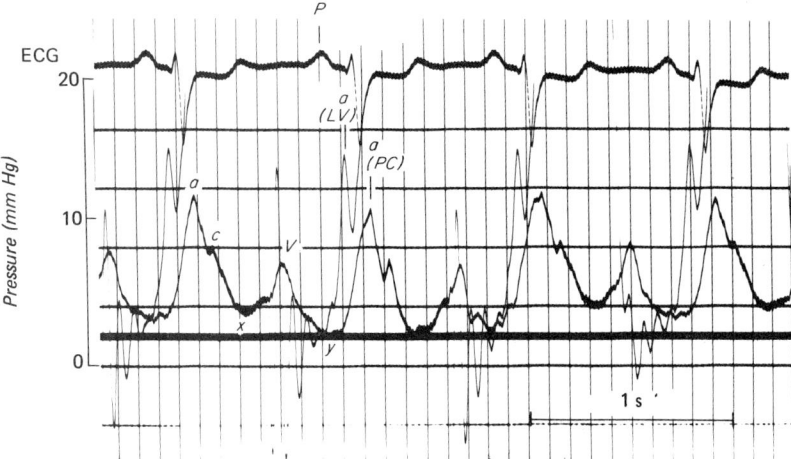

Figure 6-4. Simultaneous wedge (PC) pressure measured by the right heart route and left ventricular (LV) pressure measured by retrograde left heart catheterization. The delay in the PC tracing can be seen at the time of the *a* wave. The systolic LV pressure is "off scale," and the tracings show the diastolic events only.

together with the wedge pressure (via right heart catheterization) in order to assess the pressure difference across the mitral valve. The wedge pressure is inevitably delayed by about 0.1 second and so lags behind the left ventricular pressure. This fact, illustrated in Fig 6-4, must be taken into account in analyzing the tracings and calculating valve area. During transseptal catheterization, the gradient across the mitral valve is recorded on pulling the catheter back across the valve.

Simultaneous arterial or aortic and left ventricular pressures are recorded during transseptal catheterization to assess aortic valve hemodynamics. In retrograde catheterization, the pressures are recorded on pullback. Pressure differences within the ventricle are best sought in retrograde studies on withdrawal of the catheter from the body of the ventricle to the outflow tract. In transseptal catheterization, the operator should be careful to avoid confusing valvular and subvalvular obstructions, which tend to give superficially similar tracings.

ANGIOCARDIOGRAPHY

Angiocardiography has come to play a major role in the clinical assessment of cardiac lesions in the last 20 years. The advent of image intensifiers and cineangiography has greatly improved the quality of the pictures obtained. Left ventricular angiography has come to be an important means of assessing left ventricular function. The performance of the left ventricle can be assessed either by observing the speed and extent of contraction or by measuring the ventricular ejection fraction (see p 70).

Technique

Pressurized injectors are conventionally used, and the dosage of contrast material and the rate of injection vary with the size of the catheter used and the size of the patient. Angiography (other than coronary angiography) requires the use of a multiple-hole catheter, preferably with a closed tip (Lehman or NIH). A small preliminary injection is always given to ensure that the catheter is appropriately positioned. This prevents the injection of large amounts of contrast material into the myocardial tissue. This complication can be serious if it occurs in either the right or the left ventricle when the catheter tip is embedded in trabeculae.

Effects of Contrast Material

Multiple injections of up to 2 mL/kg can be given without fear of complications. The contrast material always affects ventricular function, so that an increase in ventricular diastolic pressure is often seen after an injection. This finding is particularly likely to occur in patients in whom ventricular function is impaired. It may last for half an hour or more and occasionally interferes with assessment of the severity of a lesion.

Quality of Angiograms

Angiocardiography provides the best pictures when the dose of contrast material is large and the dye remains highly concentrated in the heart. Thus, sequential pictures of the chambers of the right and left heart are best taken when cardiac function is good. Conversely, if the contrast material is injected directly into a chamber whose function is poor (eg, the left ventricle in cardiomyopathy), the chamber tends to be well outlined because the dye stays so long in the ventricle.

CORONARY ANGIOGRAPHY

Coronary angiography has come to be an extremely important investigation that is indicated in all patients with coronary artery disease in whom surgical treatment is contemplated. It is also indicated in older patients with other lesions in whom the presence of associated coronary disease is suspected. *Coronary arteriography is not useful in the diagnosis of angina pectoris, which is based principally on the history and the electrocardiographic changes that occur with the onset of the pain.* Abnormalities in the coronary arteriogram can be present without symptoms, and the presence of lesions in an arteriogram cannot be used to show that a given patient's pain is due to ischemia.

Techniques

Two methods are in common use for coronary angiography. The Sones method involves a brachial arterial cutdown using a catheter with a tapered tip. This catheter is manipulated into the aortic root by techniques that require considerable skill in order to enter the right and left coronary arteries. Small (5–10 mL) injections of contrast material are made by hand, and cineangiographic films are taken of the coronary circulation. Multiple views are obtained, and the procedure is made easier if the patient lies strapped in a cradle that can be turned at different angles to the x-ray apparatus. Biplane angiograms are seldom obtained by this method because access to the arm is needed to manipulate the catheter.

The other technique, introduced by Judkins, uses a percutaneous femoral arterial approach. Specially shaped catheters are used for the right and left coronary arteries. The left coronary catheter enters the left coronary ostium quite readily, and little skill is needed for its placement. The right coronary catheter is slightly more difficult to place, but less skill is needed than for the Sones method. Injections of contrast material are again made by hand, and since the arms are free to be placed above the head, biplane angiography can be readily performed. The number of injections of contrast medium, the duration of the procedure, and the severity of the coronary disease determine the morbidity and mortality rates of the Judkins technique. A coronary arteriogram obtained by means of the Judkins technique and showing a normal left coronary pattern is seen in Fig 6–5.

Left ventricular angiography should always be performed as an adjunct to coronary arteriography. Left ventricular volume and ejection fraction are measured, and localized areas of abnormal ventricular motion are sought.

No specific coronary angiographic technique is appropriate for use in every case. In some elderly atherosclerotic patients, access to the aorta via tortuous neck vessels may be impossible, or a previous arteriotomy may have obliterated the brachial artery, making the standard Sones technique impossible. Similarly, previous surgery for peripheral vascular disease may have obliterated the femoral vessels, or iliofemoral grafts may have been inserted at surgery, contraindicating the Judkins technique. In such cases, the axillary arteries may provide an alternative approach.

The possibility of cardiac standstill or complete atrioventricular block developing during coronary angiography has led some physicians to insert a pacing catheter into the right heart as a routine precautionary measure.

Videotape Recorders

It is important to make certain that adequate coronary arteriographic films have been obtained and that it will not be necessary to repeat the studies. Videotape recorders are used to view the results immediately and decide whether the pictures are adequate. The underlying anatomy and the distribution of atherosclerotic disease are so variable that it is difficult to be sure all aspects of the lesion have been demonstrated if only a single pass of the study on a television screen is seen.

Interpretation of Coronary Angiograms

The interpretation of coronary angiograms is of necessity subjective. While complete occlusion of a major vessel can be unequivocally recognized, the percentage of reduction in the size of the lumen may

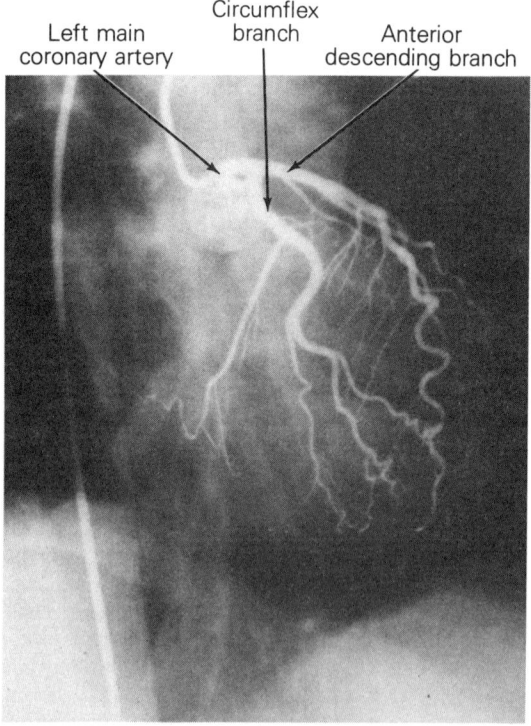

Figure 6–5. Normal left coronary arteriogram using Judkins technique. Right anterior oblique view. (Reproduced, with permission, from Philips Medical Systems, Inc.)

be more difficult to estimate. Multiple views outlining the vessel from different angles help in assessing the degree of obstruction. The arbitrary assignment of numerical ratings (eg, 50% or 70% obstruction) may be misleading. It is customary to assume that the narrowing is concentric, but in fact eccentric lesions are commonly seen at autopsy. Existing arteriographic techniques cannot distinguish between eccentric and concentric lesions, which may cause different types of obstruction to blood flow. In addition, the effects of long segments of narrowing and multiple obstructions in series cannot be adequately assessed.

OTHER DIAGNOSTIC STUDIES

Exercise During Cardiac Catheterization

Exercise is sometimes used during cardiac catheterization to evaluate the effect of stress on the hemodynamic state. However, it is difficult to do physiologic studies in supine patients lying under a fluoroscopic screen with catheters in several vessels. The use of a femoral approach generally restricts the studies to a single leg raising, which does not provide much stress. If the brachial approach is used, the patient can pedal a cycle ergometer attached to the foot of the table, but even this form of exercise is less satisfactory than upright exercise on a cycle ergometer or treadmill. Exercise is most commonly used in patients with mitral valve disease and usually consists of a short, non–steady state period of leg raising.

Coronary Sinus Catheterization & Atrial Pacing

Functional information about the adequacy of coronary perfusion can be obtained by coronary sinus catheterization and by right atrial pacing. It is difficult to use exercise to induce angina in the cardiac catheterization laboratory, and the less "physiologic" stress of progressive levels of tachycardia produced by atrial pacing is more frequently employed. Unfortunately, the electrocardiographic tracing and the level of left ventricular pressure provide unreliable indications of the effects of myocardial ischemia during pacing. The onset of pain and the level of lactate in the coronary sinus blood are the most valuable indicators of ischemia. Selective catheterization of different cardiac venous segments via the coronary sinus and its branches provides some degree of localization of the area of ischemia.

Electrophysiologic Studies

Intracardiac electrocardiography is used in the elucidation of difficult cardiac arrhythmias, eg, in distinguishing supraventricular and ventricular arrhythmias. Intracardiac electrograms are obtained from the conduction system as it runs in the interventricular septum near the tricuspid valve. A special catheter with 4 separate electrodes at different distances from the tip is positioned in the right heart after introduction through a right femoral vein approach. A second catheter is often inserted from the arm to pace the heart by right atrial stimulation. The timing of the electrical signals from the different electrodes against a conventional ECG is used to identify the recording site, and recordings can be obtained from the bundle of His and the right bundle. (See Chapters 14 and 15.)

Programmed stimulation of the right atrium or right ventricle is being used with increasing frequency to induce arrhythmias in the laboratory. The induced forms of arrhythmia have been shown to resemble those that occur spontaneously. The increasing use of surgical ablation of parts of the conduction system has called forth these electrophysiologic studies to define the nature and likely site of origin of the arrhythmia. The effects of different drugs in the prevention and termination of different arrhythmias can also be tested. It is considered safer to find out the most effective form of medication by having the patient experience an episode of arrhythmia in controlled circumstances in the laboratory than to give conventional treatment using trial and error to determine the best regimen for suppressing the arrhythmia.

Provocation & Relief of Coronary Spasm

Now that coronary spasm has come to be recognized as an important cause of cardiac pain, many cardiologists are using drugs to provoke and relieve vessel spasm. Some feel it is important to try to eliminate spasm as a factor in routine studies and give nitroglycerin or a calcium-blocking drug as premedication. Others reserve medication for relief of spasm when it occurs, either spontaneously during catheterization or in response to ergonovine injection. The use of ergonovine maleate to provoke coronary spasm is effective but is contrary to the principle of avoiding procedures that aggravate disease. The drug can be injected either intravenously or into the aorta in an initial dose of 0.0125 mg, which is increased every 5–10 minutes until chest pain occurs or ST–T wave changes appear on the ECG. The maximum total dose used is approximately 0.5 mg. It is generally considered dangerous to try to provoke coronary spasm outside the cardiac catheterization laboratory. The test should be confined to patients with normal coronary vessels or single-vessel disease and should be used only when the cause of chest pain is seriously in doubt. In patients who are repeatedly admitted to the hospital because of pain and in whom spasm cannot be ruled out, coronary angiography shows minimal disease, and ancillary studies are negative, an ergonovine test may help in management. Previous myocardial infarction and significant hypertension are considered contraindications to the test. Hemodynamic and electrocardiographic changes should be sought after each dose of ergonovine; increases in systolic and diastolic left heart pressures are an indication to stop the test. Nitroglycerin and calcium-blocking drugs should be immediately available to reverse spasm.

In spite of all precautions, serious complications of arrhythmia, heart block, and myocardial infarction and death have been reported. The effects of ergonovine are not confined to the coronary circulation. It causes generalized vasoconstriction, and its effect in increasing peripheral resistance may sometimes cause cardiac pain. Ergonovine testing is thus a "nonstandard" procedure that should not be undertaken for the first time unless a physician experienced in using the technique is present.

Endomyocardial Biopsy

Biopsy of myocardial tissue can be carried out through a cardiac catheter. The usual site is the right ventricle in the region of the interventricular septum. A special catheter is used, and a piece of cardiac muscle is sucked into a hole near the end of the catheter and cut off by means of a knife activated from the hub of the catheter. The yield of diagnostic information using this method has not been great, and the principal use of the technique has been to follow the histologic changes that occur in rejection after cardiac transplantation and to adjust the dosage of immunosuppressive drugs according to what is revealed by the biopsy findings. The technique can also be used to establish the benefit of therapeutic regimens (eg, in acute myocarditis) (see Chapter 17). The procedure is painless, and complications are rare.

THERAPEUTIC PROCEDURES INVOLVING CATHETERIZATION

Percutaneous Transluminal Coronary Angioplasty (See also Chapter 8.)

The use of special balloon catheters to dilate narrowed vessels anywhere in the arterial bed, but especially in the coronary circulation, is now an accepted procedure for the palliative treatment of atherosclerosis. The design of the catheters has improved since the technique was introduced by Gruentzig (Grüntzig) in the late 1970s. Sudden inflation of the balloon in the area of stenosis pushes soft atheromatous material back into the vessel wall and relieves the obstruction. Improvement is not necessarily only immediate. According to the Bernouilli principle, localized narrowings in blood vessels tend to become progressively more severe because the pressure in the narrowed part of the vessel tends to fall, further narrowing the vessel. Conversely, acute localized dilatation tends to expand the vessel in the long run because the pressure in the previously narrowed area is increased. According to evidence on angiography, this principle appears to operate in vivo also.

The technique demands skill and judgment, and the results are related to the experience of the operator. It must only be performed in hospitals in which open heart surgery is immediately available to deal with untoward events requiring coronary bypass surgery.

A. Indications and Contraindications: Angioplasty is most clearly indicated in patients with single-vessel disease with a recent onset of angina pectoris. Short, proximal, noncalcified single lesions in the left anterior descending artery are the most satisfactory. The technique is less clearly indicated in lesions of the coronary ostia, but calcification in the neighborhood of the lesion is no longer a contraindication. Age is no bar, and more patients with multivessel disease are now being treated by this method. Patients with unstable angina can also benefit, but restenosis at the site of dilation is always a possibility. A second dilation can produce a satisfactory result.

B. Technique: Preliminary medication with aspirin is started before the procedure. After the lesion has been identified by coronary angiography, spasm is excluded by medication with a calcium-blocking drug and intracoronary nitroglycerin. The special catheters needed for the procedure are inserted via the femoral artery. Full anticoagulation is established with heparin, and a guiding catheter is passed to the orifice of the coronary artery in question. The balloon catheter, inserted through the guiding catheter, is passed across the obstruction while proximal and distal pressures are being monitored. When the position is optimal, as judged by fluoroscopy and contrast injection, the balloon is distended with weak contrast material, initially to a pressure of 3–6 atm for 15–30 seconds. Several inflations at progressively higher pressures up to 10 atm are sometimes needed, and further angiography is performed to assess the results. An example of 2 successful dilations is shown in Fig 6–6. The obstruction in the circumflex branch was dilated first, followed by the lesion in the anterior descending coronary artery. The balloon catheter is shown positioned within each artery in Fig 6–7.

C. Results: At present, 10–20% of patients are suitable candidates for dilation. Dilation is feasible in about 80% of such suitable candidates, and 70–80% show objective evidence of benefit as measured by exercise testing, including electrocardiographic or radionuclear investigations. The rate of restenosis is about 20%, and in about 30–40% of cases a second dilatation produces benefit. Lesions of coronary grafts are also amenable to dilatation, but lesions involving branches are less suitable.

D. Complications: Cardiac pain or arrhythmia may develop when the catheter passes through the obstruction or the balloon is inflated. Spasm, dissection, or occlusion of the vessel by a displaced plaque may occur when the balloon is inflated. In addition, the multiple manipulations of catheters in the iliofemoral vessels of fully heparinized patients can cause vascular complications. About 5% of patients require immediate coronary bypass surgery for complications, and the overall mortality rate is about 1%.

Intracoronary Thrombolytic Therapy for Myocardial Infarction

Recent documentation, by coronary arteriography, that complete or near-complete obstruction of coronary vessels is common (> 80%) early in the

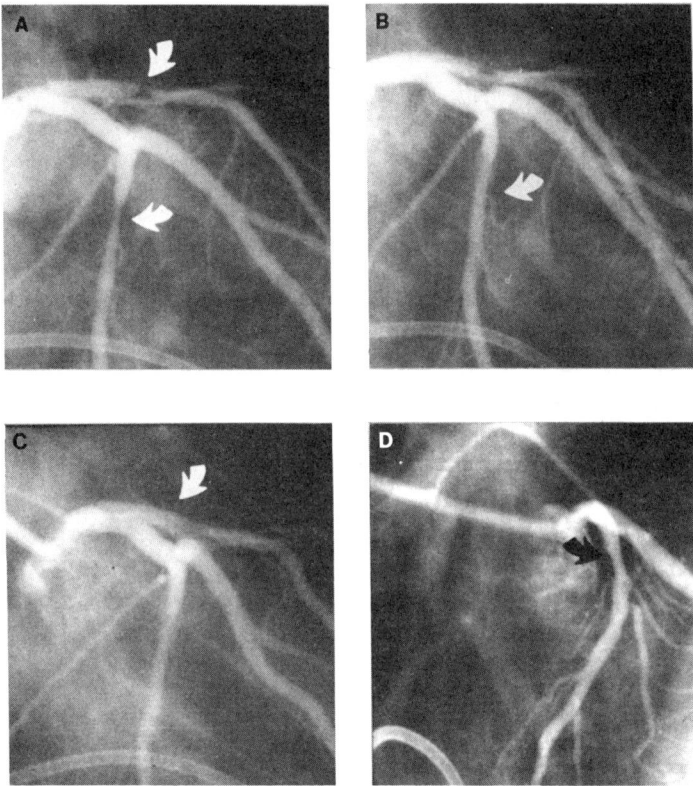

Figure 6-6. Coronary arteriograms showing effects of percutaneous transluminal coronary angioplasty in a patient with obstructions in the circumflex and anterior descending branches of the left coronary artery. In *A*, both lesions are seen. In *B*, the circumflex lesion has been dilated and the anterior descending lesion is still present. In *C*, the anterior descending lesion has been dilated. A different view is shown in *D*. (Courtesy of TA Ports.)

course of myocardial infarction has led to the development of new methods of treatment.

Catheter recanalization. Using special catheters or guide wires, attempts have been made to displace recently formed thrombus in obstructed coronary vessels and reestablish patency. Not surprisingly, the technique is associated with significant complications and has largely been superseded by the use of fibrinolytic methods.

Thrombolysis with streptokinase. The infusion of streptokinase, a fibrinolytic enzyme, into an obstructed coronary artery results in recanalization within 20–30 minutes in about 80% of cases of acute myocardial infarction. The ultimate effects of reperfusion are not completely established. Relief of pain, short-term improvement in left ventricular function, reversal of electrocardiographic changes, and early peaking of myocardial enzyme levels indicate that thrombolysis has beneficial effects. An increased incidence of arrhythmia is associated with reperfusion, but this can be controlled with lidocaine injections. Hemorrhage into the ischemic area following reperfusion has not proved to be a problem.

A. Indications and Contraindications: Streptokinase infusion is more effective if given early (<3 hours) after the onset of symptoms, and it is contraindicated after 18 hours. It should not be used in patients in shock or within 10 days of any surgical operation. Allergic subjects and those with peptic ulcers, cerebrovascular accidents, recent bleeding, or bleeding diatheses are unsuited for this form of treatment, because it tends to cause hemorrhage. The results are better in younger patients (under 50 years).

B. Technique: Intracoronary streptokinase therapy requires angiographic identification of the obstructed artery. After the injection of nitroglycerin to eliminate spasm, a loading dose of 10,000 units of streptokinase is given into the obstructed artery, followed by a constant infusion of 2000 units/min for up to 60 minutes. The effects of the medication are followed via the effects on the patient's pain, electrocardiographic changes, and the results of repeated angiography. In some centers, attempts are made to place the catheter within the obstructed branch of the left coronary artery (circumflex or left anterior descending). In others, such placement is only used if the initial infusion does not result in recanalization. Vigorous anticoagulation with intracoronary heparin is used after recanalization and appears to be important in preventing reocclusion.

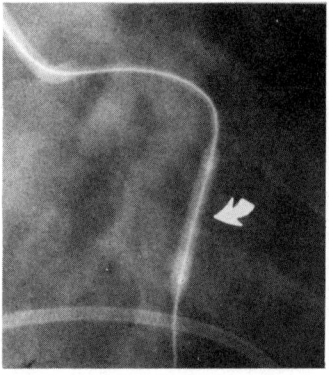 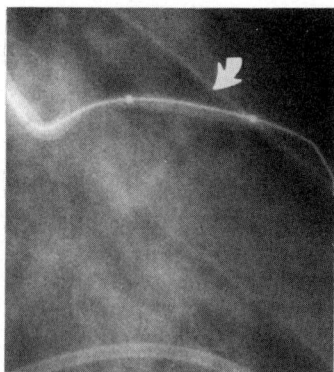

Figure 6–7. Radiographs showing a balloon catheter positioned within each of the coronary arterial lesions shown in Fig 6–6. At left, the balloon is in the circumflex lesion. At right, the balloon is in the left anterior descending lesion. (Courtesy of TA Ports.)

C. Results: An example of the effect of an intracoronary infusion of streptokinase followed by transluminal angioplasty is shown in Fig 6–8. The obstruction in the left anterior descending coronary artery was partially relieved by the infusion. Subsequent angioplasty restored full patency of the vessel.

The long-term results of intracoronary streptokinase infusion are not yet clear. The therapy is expensive in terms of the participation of physicians and technical staff; keeping a laboratory available on a few hours' notice, with cardiac surgical backup, presents logistic problems. Treatment with intravenous streptokinase (see p 179) is clearly easier and more widely applicable. A randomized trial comparing the results of intracoronary streptokinase with those in a control group, in whom left ventricular angiography and coronary arteriography were also carried out, has shown significant reduction in the mortality rate in the treated group (Kennedy, 1983). A tissue-type plasminogen activator (rt-PA) has been found to be more effective than streptokinase in recent studies. If the vessel fails to reopen, the prognosis is worse. It seems clear that obstructed vessels can usually (75%) be shown to recanalize, but the incidence and effects of reocclusion are not clearly established.

D. Complications: Reperfusion arrhythmias present only minor problems. More importantly, streptokinase therapy creates a bleeding tendency which, combined with the anticoagulation needed to maintain patency of the reopened vessel, can lead to hemorrhagic complications.

COMPLICATIONS OF CARDIAC CATHETERIZATION

COMPLICATIONS COMMON TO ALL FORMS OF CATHETERIZATION

Vessel Spasm

Spasm of the vessel into which a catheter is inserted—either an artery or a vein—almost invariably results from excessive trauma, often due to the use of too large a catheter for the size of the vessel. It is more common in young, nervous persons, and prior sedation, which is not needed routinely, may help to minimize it.

Vasovagal Attacks

Vasovagal attacks with bradycardia, hypotension, and ultimately loss of consciousness can occur in any study but are sufficiently common in coronary arteriography (especially when the catheter is near the orifice of the right coronary artery) so that atropine, 0.4–0.8 mg intravenously, is recommended as a routine form of premedication. In other studies, it is sufficient to watch for the early signs—bradycardia, often associated with yawning—and to raise the patient's legs and give atropine via the catheter.

Pulmonary Edema

Cardiac catheterization involves keeping the patient lying flat for several hours. If the patient has pulmonary congestion, this may provoke pulmonary edema. The first hint of development of edema is often restlessness, with a dry cough.

Arrhythmia

Atrial or ventricular arrhythmias are commonly provoked during cardiac catheterization. Fortunately, they usually subside upon removal of the catheter,

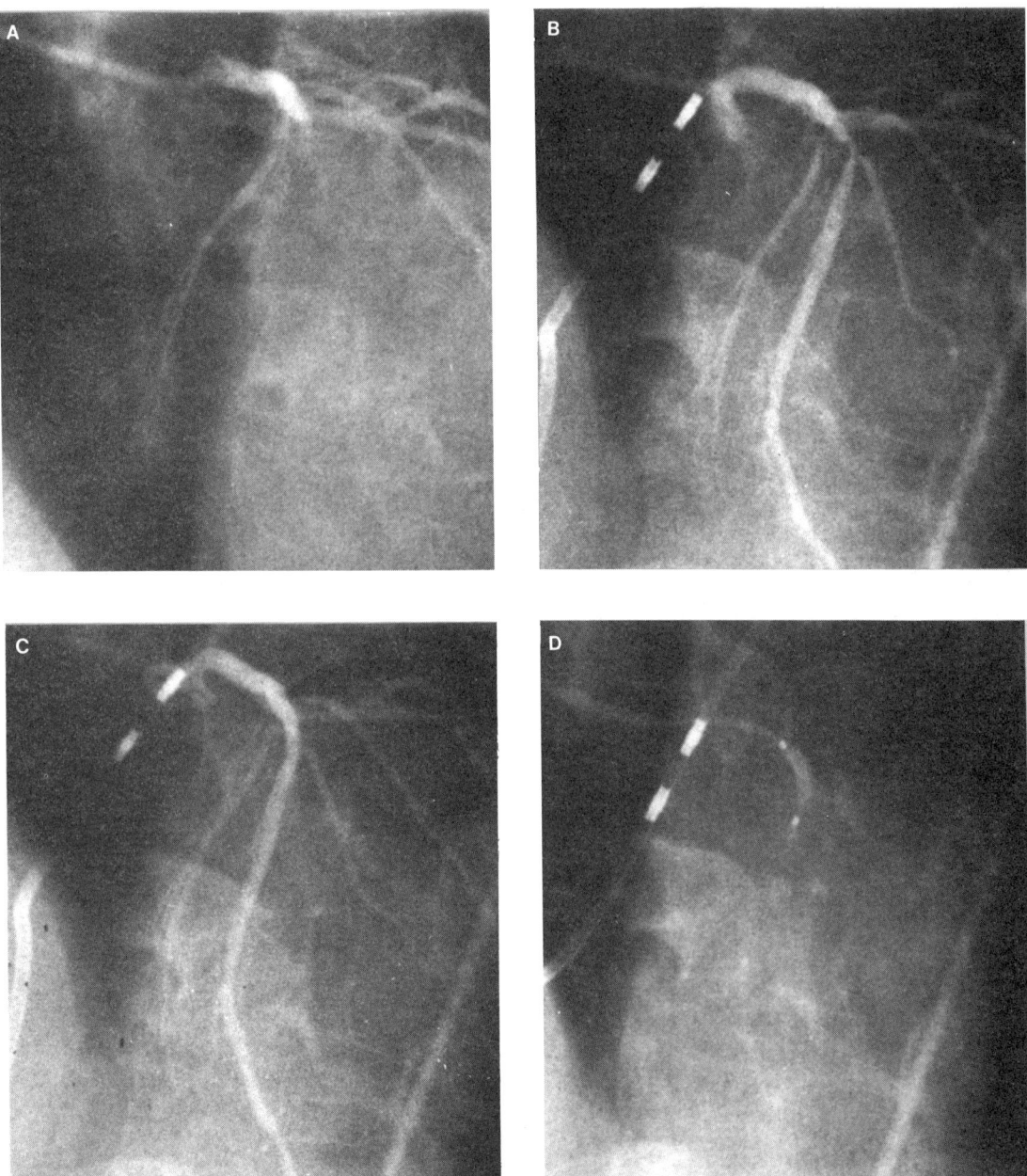

Figure 6–8. Coronary angiograms of a patient with thrombosis of the left anterior descending coronary artery. *A:* Before streptokinase infusion. *B:* After streptokinase infusion. *C:* After transluminal angioplasty. *D:* Angioplasty balloon in position. (Courtesy of TA Ports.)

which is thought to be responsible for their provocation by direct mechanical stimulation. Atrial arrhythmias are common when the catheter is in the right atrium in patients with atrial septal defect or mitral valve disease. Runs of ventricular ectopic beats are particularly frequent when the catheter is in the right ventricle. If the patient has left bundle branch block and electrical activation of the heart depends solely on the right bundle branch, cardiac standstill often takes the place of the run of ectopic beats. A pacemaker should always be available in the laboratory but is seldom needed. Ventricular tachycardia and ventricular fibrillation are rarely seen in right heart catheterization. They are most likely to occur during coronary arteriography (incidence about 1%). A sharp blow on the chest—or, if that is not successful, DC countershock—should restore sinus rhythm. A defibrillator should be available in the room where cardiac catheterization is being done for use in an emergency situation.

Arteriovenous Fistula

Since cardiac catheterization involves the puncture or dissection of arteries and veins as they lie in close proximity in the groin or at the elbow, the possibility of creating an arteriovenous fistula always exists.

Dissection

Dissection of an artery by a guide wire passed up between the media and the intima is a potentially dangerous complication. The actual process of dissection is painful, and advancing guide wires while a patient is experiencing pain is ill advised. It is possible for a dissection begun in the femoral or external iliac artery to spread up into the abdominal aorta, thereby compromising blood flow to the viscera.

Broken Catheters

There is always a risk of breaking a catheter or forming a knot that cannot be extracted by manipulation. When the catheter fragment is radiopaque, it is possible to insert a long looped guide wire in the form of a snare and to extract the fragment as it is carried through the circulation. In other cases, thoracotomy may be necessary, with or without cardiotomy.

Prevention of Complications

In general, the sooner the onset of a complication is recognized, the easier it is to restore the patient's status to normal and complete the study. Most complications are due to the study, and stopping the procedure is usually an effective but unsatisfactory method of treatment.

SPECIAL COMPLICATIONS OF PARTICULAR PROCEDURES

Right Heart Catheterization

Right heart catheterization should result in minimal morbidity and a zero mortality rate in adults. Adequate data should be obtainable in 99% of cases. Venous spasm is probably the most common problem, and anatomic variations in venous anatomy may interfere with the passage of the catheter to the right atrium.

It has recently been reported that asymptomatic pulmonary arterial occlusion, presumably embolic in origin, not uncommonly occurs after right heart catheterization. New pulmonary perfusion defects are found after the studies, and the implication is that venous stasis associated with the procedure has encouraged thrombosis in the venous system. We have not encountered this problem, and in our experience pulmonary infarction has never followed cardiac catheterization.

Left Heart Catheterization

Percutaneous femoral catheterization is the procedure most likely to lead to arterial occlusion. Thrombus forms on the outside of the catheter, and as the catheter is withdrawn from the vessel, a sheath of thrombus is pulled off that coils up and blocks the artery. This complication is likely to occur when the catheter is left for a long time in the arterial tree. A low cardiac output and a small femoral artery, as seen in thin female patients with mitral stenosis and raised pulmonary vascular resistance, favor the occurrence of the complication.

Following brachial arterial arteriotomy, control of hemorrhage is sometimes a problem. Hemorrhage usually stops with prolonged pressure over the vessel. On removal of the catheter at the end of the study, a jet of blood should spurt from both the proximal and distal ends of the artery. When this does not happen, the presence of a blood clot should be suspected. Gently probing the vessel with a soft plastic catheter often dislodges soft thrombus. Passage of a Fogarty balloon catheter is the next step, and a vascular surgeon should be summoned when these measures do not meet with success. Since the brachial artery can usually be tied off without compromising the circulation to the hand and arm, the complications of the brachial approach are seldom serious, but the median nerve may be damaged.

In transseptal catheterization, it is possible to puncture the free wall of the right atrium, the aortic wall, or the tricuspid valve inadvertently, and complications can be serious. Hemorrhage and tamponade are the most common causes of death from the procedure.

In direct left ventricular puncture, the principal complication is pneumothorax. If the procedure is done only in patients with severe left ventricular hypertrophy due to aortic stenosis, the danger of intrapericardial hemorrhage and tamponade is minimized.

The dangers associated with all forms of left heart catheterization are about 10 times greater than those of right heart studies. Systemic embolism from thrombus forming on catheters in the left heart is much more dangerous than in the lesser circulation. It is important to flush catheters in the left side of the circulation frequently and forcefully. The catheters used almost always have multiple openings, and a slow drip of heparinized saline, which is used to keep single-hole catheters patent, should not be used with multiple-hole catheters. It is possible for the drip to pass through one of the holes, leaving the others to become clogged with thrombus. The correct procedure is to flush multiple-hole catheters forcefully every 2 minutes or so.

Coronary Angiography

Ventricular fibrillation or ventricular tachycardia occurs during coronary angiography in about 1% of patients with coronary disease. A sharp blow on the chest, a cough, or DC countershock should restore sinus rhythm, and in many laboratories coronary angiography is continued after this treatment has been successful. Coronary angiography is now the commonest precipitating cause of death in the cardiac catheterization laboratory in adults. The procedure is most dangerous in patients with severe 3-vessel or left main coronary disease, those with previous myocardial infarction and heart failure, and those with a low systolic and high diastolic left ventricular pressure. Progressive hypotension during and after the procedure—rather than arrhythmia—is the usual problem. Precipitation of myocardial infarction is another complication of the procedure. This may be due to embolism, trauma to the coronary ostium, or impaction of the catheter, which occludes the ostium completely.

It is important to monitor the pressure at the catheter tip at all times when the catheter is in a coronary vessel. This obviously is not possible during injection, but arrangements should be made to switch off the pressure tracings for the minimal time. Progressive damping of the pressure tracing is an important indication of the need to reposition the catheter. Spasm of the proximal part of a coronary artery can occur during coronary angiography and is usually attributed to mechanical effects of the catheter. Sublingual nitroglycerin is used for prevention and treatment. In some laboratories, it is routinely given before the study; in others, it is withheld until some indication of spasm is recognized.

The contrast material used in angiography tends to act as an osmotic load and increase the blood volume. This can lead to complications, especially in patients on the verge of pulmonary edema. It is unwise to inject large amounts of contrast material into the pulmonary arteries of patients with mitral stenosis, especially if the pulmonary vascular resistance is raised.

Hypersensitivity responses to the iodine in the contrast material are rare. It seems that injections into the left side of the heart, bypassing the lungs, cause less trouble than intravenous injections, as in intravenous urography.

MORBIDITY & MORTALITY RATES

Patients in whom trouble is to be expected include those with severe mitral stenosis with or without pulmonary hypertension, patients with pulmonary hypertension due to any cause, pulmonary or aortic stenosis of severe degree, Ebstein's malformation, left bundle branch block, and severe ischemic heart disease with heart failure. The mortality and morbidity statistics are highly dependent on the types of patients studied and the experience of the operator. A rate of serious complications (eg, embolism, arrhythmia, and hemorrhage) of more than 3% and a mortality rate of more than 0.3% call for review of the operations and standard procedures in selecting and studying patients by means of these techniques.

REFERENCES

Bedside Catheterization

Bernéus B et al: Percutaneous catheterization of peripheral arteries as method for blood sampling. *Scand J Clin Lab Invest* 1954;**6**:217.

Connors AF et al: Evaluation of right-heart catheterization in the critically ill patient without acute myocardial infarction. *N Engl J Med* 1983;**308**:263.

O'Toole JD et al: Pulmonary valve injury and insufficiency during pulmonary artery catheterization. *N Engl J Med* 1979;**301**:1167.

Pace NL: A critique of flow-directed pulmonary arterial catheterization. *Anesthesiology* 1977;**47**:455.

Rapaport E, Scheinman M: Rationale and limitations of hemodynamic measurements in patients with acute myocardial infarction. *Mod Concepts Cardiovasc Dis* 1969;**38**:55.

Russell RO, Rackley CE: *Hemodynamic Monitoring in a Coronary Intensive Care Unit,* 2nd ed. Futura, 1981.

Silver GM et al: Arterial complications of attempted Swan-Ganz insertion. *Am J Cardiol* 1984;**53**:340.

Spodick DH: Physiologic and prognostic implications of invasive monitoring: Undetermined risk/benefit ratios in patients with heart disease. *Am J Cardiol* 1980;**46**:173.

Swan HJC et al: Catheterization of the heart in man with use of a flow-directed balloon-tipped catheter. *N Engl J Med* 1970;**283**:447.

Cardiac Catheterization

Bloomfield DA: The nonsurgical retrieval of intracardiac foreign bodies: An international survey. *Cathet Cardiovasc Diagn* 1978;**4**:1.

Braunwald E, Swan HJC (editors): Cooperative study on cardiac catheterization. *Circulation* 1968;**37**(**Suppl 3**): III-1. [Entire issue.]

Brewster H, McIlroy MB: Blood gas tensions and pH of pulmonary "wedge" samples in patients with heart disease. *J Appl Physiol* 1973;**34**:413.

Brock RC et al: Percutaneous left ventricular puncture in the assessment of aortic stenosis. *Thorax* 1956;**2**:163.

Fisher R, Ferreyo R: Evaluation of current techniques for nonsurgical removal of intravascular iatrogenic foreign bodies. *AJR* 1978;**130**:541.

Fogarty TJ et al: A method for extraction of arterial emboli and thrombi. *Surg Gynecol Obstet* 1963;**116**:241.

Forssmann W: Die sondierung des rechten Herzens. *Klin Wochenschr* 1929;**8**:2085.

Grossman W (editor): *Cardiac Catheterization and Angiography.* Lea & Febiger, 1974.

Hellems HK et al: Pulmonary capillary pressure in man. *J Clin Invest* 1948;**27**:540.

Kennedy JW et al: Complications associated with cardiac catheterization and angiography. *Cath Cardiovasc Diagn* 1982;**8**:5.

Kory RC, Tsagaris TJ, Bustamente R: *A Primer of Cardiac Catheterization.* Thomas, 1965.

Mendel D: *A Practice of Cardiac Catheterisation,* 2nd ed. Blackwell, 1974.

Morton MJ et al: Risks and benefits of postoperative cardiac catheterization in patients with ball valve prostheses. *Am J Cardiol* 1977;**40**:870.

Primm RK et al: Incidence of new pulmonary perfusion defects after routine cardiac catheterization. *Am J Cardiol* 1979;**43**:529.

Ross J et al: Transseptal left heart catheterization: A new diagnostic method. *Prog Cardiovasc Dis* 1959;**2**:315.

St. John Sutton MG et al: Valve replacement without preoperative cardiac catheterization. *N Engl J Med* 1981;**305**:1233.

Selzer A: *Principles of Clinical Cardiology*. Saunders, 1975.

Verel D, Grainger RG: *Cardiac Catheterization and Angiography*, 3rd ed. Churchill Livingstone, 1978.

Welton DE et al: Value and safety of cardiac catheterization during active infective endocarditis. *Am J Cardiol* 1979;**44**:1306.

Yang SS et al: *From Cardiac Catheterization Data to Hemodynamic Parameters*, 2nd ed. Davis, 1978.

Zimmerman HA: *Intravascular Catheterization*. Thomas, 1966.

Angiography

Abrams HL (editor): *Angiography*, 2nd ed. (2 vols.) Little, Brown, 1971.

Adams DF, Fraser DB, Abrams HL: The complications of coronary arteriography. *Circulation* 1973;**48**:609.

Brown R et al: The effect of angiocardiographic contrast medium on circulatory dynamics in man. *Circulation* 1965;**31**:234.

Cipriano PR et al: The effects of ergonovine maleate on coronary arterial size. *Circulation* 1979;**59**:82.

Dodek A, Hooper RO: Coronary spasm provoked by ergonovine. *Am Heart J* 1984;**107**:781.

Friesinger GG et al: Hemodynamic consequences of the injection of radiopaque material. *Circulation* 1965;**31**:730.

Gensini GG: *Coronary Arteriography*. Futura, 1975.

Hastey CE, Erwin SW, Ramanathan KB: Ergonovine-induced coronary spasm refractory to intracoronary nitroglycerin but responsive to nitroprusside. *Am Heart J* 1984;**107**:778.

Heupler FA: Provocative testing for coronary arterial spasm: Risk, method and rationale. *Am J Cardiol* 1980;**48**:335.

Judkins MP: Selective coronary arteriography. 1. A percutaneous transfemoral technic. *Radiology* 1967;**89**:815.

Klocke FJ: Measurement of coronary blood flow and degree of stenosis: Current clinical implications and continuing uncertainties. *J Am Coll Cardiol* 1983;**1**:31.

Sones FM, Shirey EK: Cine coronary arteriography. *Mod Concepts Cardiovasc Dis* 1962;**31**:735.

Therapeutic Interventions

Bentvoglio LG et al: Percutaneous transluminal coronary angioplasty (PCTA) in patients with relative contraindications: Results of the National Heart, Lung, and Blood Institute PCTA registry. *Am J Cardiol* 1984;**53**:82C.

Block PC et al: Percutaneous angioplasty of stenoses of bypass grafts or of bypass graft anastomotic sites. *Am J Cardiol* 1984;**53**:666.

Dorros G et al: Percutaneous transluminal coronary angioplasty in patients with prior coronary artery bypass grafting. *J Thorac Cardiovasc Surg* 1984;**87**:17.

Feldman RL et al: Intracoronary streptokinase in evolving acute myocardial infarction. *Am Heart J* 1984;**107**:823.

Gruentzig AR: Percutaneous transluminal coronary angioplasty: Six years' experience. *Am Heart J* 1984;**107**:818.

Gruentzig AR, Meier B: Current status of dilatation catheters and guiding systems. *Am J Cardiol* 1984;**53**:92C.

Grüntzig A, Kumpe DA: Technique of percutaneous transluminal angioplasty with the Grüntzig balloon catheter. *AJR* 1979;**132**:547.

Grüntzig AR, Senning Å, Siegenthaler WE: Nonoperative dilatation of coronary-artery stenosis: Percutaneous transluminal coronary angioplasty. *N Engl J Med* 1979;**301**:61.

Kennedy JW et al: Western Washington randomized trial of intracoronary streptokinase in acute myocardial infarction. *N Engl J Med* 1983;**309**:1477.

Kent KM et al: Percutaneous transluminal coronary angioplasty: Report from the registry of the National Heart, Lung, and Blood Institute. *Am J Cardiol* 1982;**49**:2011.

Khaja F et al: Intracoronary fibrinolytic therapy in acute myocardial infarction: Report of a prospective randomized trial. *N Engl J Med* 1983;**308**:1305.

Leiboff RH et al: A randomized angiographically controlled trial of intracoronary streptokinase in acute myocardial infarction. *Am J Cardiol* 1984;**53**:404.

Mock MB et al: Percutaneous transluminal coronary angioplasty (PCTA) in the elderly patient: Experience in the National Heart, Lung, and Blood Institute PCTA registry. *Am J Cardiol* 1984;**53**:89C.

Schwarz F et al: Thrombolysis in acute myocardial infarction: Effect of intravenous followed by intracoronary streptokinase application on estimates of infarct size. *Am J Cardiol* 1984;**53**:1505.

Williams DO et al: Evaluation of the role of coronary angioplasty in patients with unstable angina pectoris. *Am Heart J* 1981;**102**:1.

Zeitler E, Grüntzig A, Schoop W (editors): *Percutaneous Vascular Recanalization: Technique–Application–Clinical Results*. Springer-Verlag, 1978.

Electrophysiology

Bahler RC, MacLeod CA: Atrial pacing and exercise in the evaluation of patients with angina pectoris. *Circulation* 1971;**43**:407.

Damato AN, Gallagher JJ, Lau SH: Application of His bundle recordings in diagnosing conduction disorders. *Prog Cardiovasc Dis* 1972;**14**:601.

Damato AN et al: Study of atrioventricular conduction in man using electrode catheter recordings of His bundle activity. *Circulation* 1969;**39**:287.

Hariman RJ et al: Method for recording electrical activity of the sinoatrial node and automatic atrial foci during cardiac catheterization in human subjects. *Am J Cardiol* 1980;**45**:775.

Mason JW, Winkle RA: Electrode-catheter arrhythmia induction in the selection and assessment of antiarrhythmic drug therapy for recurrent ventricular tachycardia. *Circulation* 1978;**58**:971.

Sung RJ et al: Initiation of two distinct forms of atrioventricular nodal reentrant tachycardia during programmed ventricular stimulation in man. *Am J Cardiol* 1978;**42**:404.

Vandepol CJ et al: Incidence and clinical significance of induced ventricular tachycardia. *Am J Cardiol* 1980;**45**:725.

Watson RM, Josephson ME: Atrial flutter. 1. Electrophysiologic substrates and modes of initiation and termination. *Am J Cardiol* 1980;**45**:733.

Therapeutic Procedures 7

This chapter deals with the techniques of therapeutic procedures used in the management of cardiac disorders. Whenever possible, the patient's status should be monitored by the methods described in Chapters 5 and 6 to observe the response to therapy. However, since therapeutic procedures are often needed in emergency situations, the techniques described must on occasion be used in circumstances that are less than ideal.

CARDIOPULMONARY RESUSCITATION

All physicians should be familiar with the emergency procedures involved in cardiopulmonary resuscitation. These vary with the nature of the emergency and the circumstances surrounding the episode. Resuscitation in a highly equipped area such as an intensive care or coronary care unit differs significantly from that carried out in some public place.

The principles involved are similar in all circumstances, and speed in applying the appropriate treatment is of paramount importance. Establishment of the nature and, if possible, the cause is essential.

The situations encountered in practice in public are (1) sudden collapse without warning, (2) choking on food in the airway (in restaurants), and (3) epileptic seizures.

Resuscitation in a Public Place

When a patient falls to the ground or is found incapacitated, the presence of a pulse should be sought at the carotid artery in the neck and the presence of a heartbeat determined by direct palpation or auscultation. At the same time, the state of consciousness should be established by determining whether the patient can respond to simple commands. The cortical state of consciousness and cerebration should be checked by observing the size of the pupils and testing their response to light. The circumstances surrounding the collapse should be determined, if possible, by questioning witnesses, but nothing should delay the start of resuscitative measures if breathing has stopped and cardiac function is ineffective. It is important in this preliminary assessment to establish whether the patient is breathing and whether the airway is patent, for this determines the priorities of treatment, especially when no help is available.

A. Pulseless, Breathing Patient: If the patient is pulseless and breathing, closed chest cardiac resuscitation should be started. A sharp blow on the lower sternum sometimes stops ventricular arrhythmia or restarts the heart after sudden cardiac arrest (it is equivalent to an electric shock of about 1 J). The patient must be placed on a firm support, usually on the floor, and rhythmic pressure applied to the lower sternum sufficient to move the rib cage one-fifth of the anteroposterior diameter of the chest with every stroke (Fig 7–1). The rate of compression should be about 80–100/min. The patient's head should be as low as possible to encourage cerebral perfusion, and a carotid or femoral pulse should be sought during the procedure if possible. The patient's breathing should be observed to make certain it is being maintained.

B. Pulseless Patient Not Breathing: If neither pulse nor respiration is present, the mouth and pharynx must be cleared of obstructions such as blood, vomitus, mucus, or a bolus of food to open the airway so that mouth-to-mouth resuscitation can be started. The nostrils are pinched closed, the airway kept clear by backward and upward pressure on the chin, and the lungs inflated by forced expiration, as shown in Fig 7–2. After a few inflations, chest compression is begun. Combined cardiac and pulmonary resuscitation is given in alternating fashion, 15 strokes of cardiac compression to every 2 or 3 lung inflations. When help arrives, someone else should take over one of the resuscitative tasks. When qualified and specially equipped persons come on the scene, a plastic airway and a bag with a one-way valve may be substituted for mouth-to-mouth resuscitation and arrangements

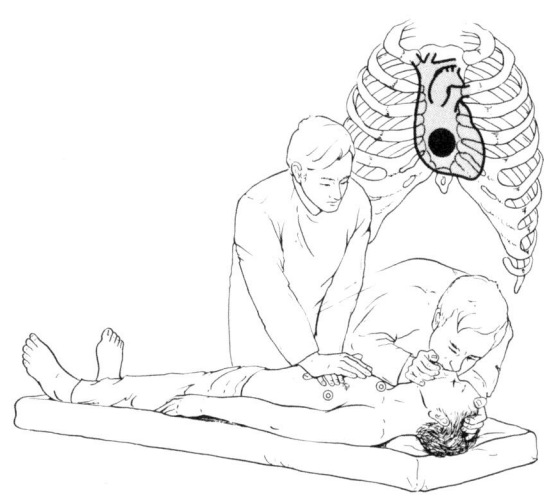

Figure 7–1. Technique of external chest compression. Heavy circle in heart drawing shows area of application of force. Circles on supine figure show points of application of electrodes for defibrillation. (Reproduced, with permission, from Krupp MA, Chatton MJ, Tierney LM Jr [editors]: *Current Medical Diagnosis & Treatment 1986.* Lange, 1986.)

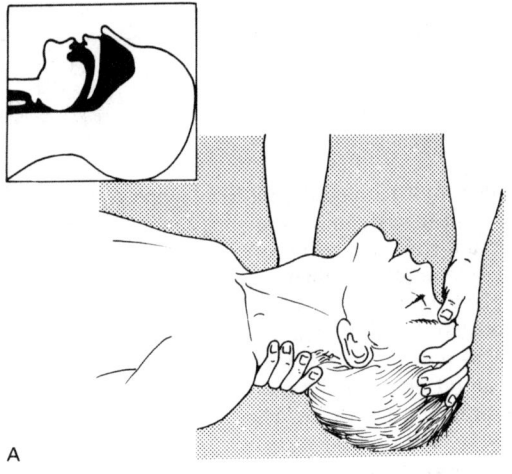

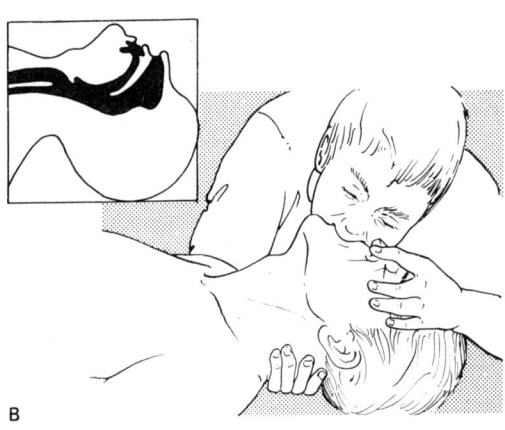

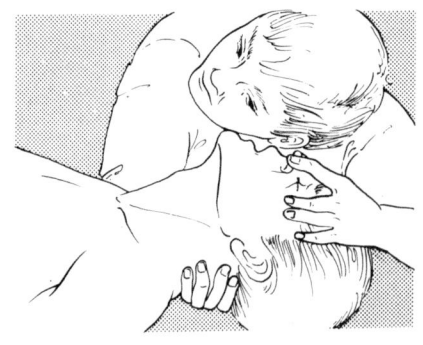

Figure 7–2. Proper performance of mouth-to-mouth resuscitation. *A:* Open airway by positioning neck anteriorly in extension. Inserts show airway obstructed when the neck is in resting flexed position and opening when neck is extended. *B:* Rescuer should close victim's nose with fingers, seal mouth around victim's mouth, and deliver breath by vigorous expiration. *C:* Victim is allowed to exhale passively by unsealing mouth and nose. Rescuer should listen and feel for expiratory air flow. (Reproduced, with permission, from Krupp MA, Chatton MJ, Tierney LM Jr [editors]: *Current Medical Diagnosis & Treatment 1986.* Lange, 1986.)

can be made to move the patient to an appropriate place for further care as needed.

C. Patient With Pulse But Not Breathing: If the patient is not breathing but has a pulse, the procedures described above to open the airway should be followed, and mouth-to-mouth resuscitation should be performed. The circulation must also be checked at intervals to determine that adequate cardiac function is being maintained.

Mechanism of Action of External Chest Compression

Until recently, it was assumed that the mechanism of "closed chest cardiac massage" was to squeeze the heart between the sternum and spine and thus to expel blood from the thorax. Studies have now indicated that it is the rise in intrathoracic pressure associated with chest compression that expels blood from the thorax into the extrathoracic arteries. The effect is not transmitted to the great veins, since they collapse in response to raised intrathoracic pressure. Corollaries to these findings are that "cardiac massage" should be more effective if the chest is compressed at high rather than low lung volumes and that compression during inflation is more effective than compression during deflation. The effectiveness of raising intrathoracic pressure is limited, because ultimately the intrathoracic arteries are compressed and blood flow out of the thorax is impaired. Although these findings have changed the explanation for the mechanism involved, they have not changed the recommended practical procedures for closed chest cardiopulmonary resuscitation. The term "cardiac massage" should no longer be used.

Choking on Food

Choking on food is commonly seen in restaurants in persons who have overindulged in alcohol. It is also a risk in nursing homes among elderly, debilitated, edentulous patients who may be oversedated. Acute respiratory distress associated with airway obstruction resulting from blockage by food is often apparent because the patient jumps up, coughs and splutters, and shows clear signs of respiratory distress. If airway obstruction is only partial, as evidenced by wheezing, forceful coughing, and adequate airway exchange, *do not* interfere with the patient's attempt to expel the foreign body. *If the patient is able to speak, even in a whisper, do not go on to the following steps in treatment.* If the patient cannot speak, the rescuer should take up a position behind the victim, who should stand still in the upright position. The rescuer's arms are then placed around the victim's waist, the hands formed into fists against the victim's epigastrium, and pulled in forcibly on the victim's abdomen several times (Heimlich maneuver). The forced expiratory air flow will usually dislodge the obstruction, at least partially, and it may then be possible to grasp it with the fingers down the throat and remove it if the patient cannot spit it out. If the victim is lying on the floor, the rescuer should kneel beside or astride the victim's body and attempt to expel the obstruction by blows with the fist to the epigastrium. If these maneuvers fail, emergency tracheostomy may have to be performed using the sharpest knife available.

Epileptic Seizure

Make certain that the pulse and respiration are present and that the airway is patent. Lay the patient on a flat surface and support the chin to maintain a free airway. Place the best available padded object between the teeth to prevent tongue biting. Try to establish a diagnosis and summon assistance.

Resuscitation in a Hospital Setting

All hospitals should have an emergency resuscitation team available at all times capable of responding to a telephone call for assistance anywhere in the hospital. The emergency is usually announced over a public address system, and the appropriate persons—usually a cardiologist, an anesthetist, and a surgeon—should go as quickly as possible to the scene. The emergency procedures are instituted by persons already at the scene as described above for resuscitation in a public place. In a hospital setting, it is usually easier to make a rapid diagnosis because the reasons for the patient's hospitalization will be known. The same principles apply in deciding whether chest compression or mouth-to-mouth resuscitation (or both) is required, and since more than one person is usually present, one must take charge and direct operations, maintaining resuscitative measures until further assistance arrives. Note should be made of the time the resuscitation team arrives on the scene, since this will be important in deciding when to abandon resuscitation efforts if they are unsuccessful.

Three basic questions must be considered when the full team is assembled: (1) What is the nature of the problem? (Arrhythmia? Asystole? Respiratory failure?) (2) What is the underlying cause of the problem and is it correctable? (Myocardial infarction? Pulmonary embolism? Hemorrhage? Trauma?) (3) What further measures are needed?

During this period, someone should be attaching electrocardiograph leads, starting an intravenous drip if one is not already set up, preparing the DC defibrillator, preparing drug doses in appropriate syringes for immediate use, and taking an arterial blood sample for analysis of P_{O_2}, P_{CO_2}, and pH. An endotracheal tube is usually inserted to facilitate lung inflation.

Emergency Defibrillation

If ventricular fibrillation or tachycardia is the cause of the emergency, defibrillation should be carried out with a minimum of delay. In emergency situations, a DC shock of 400 J is routinely given and repeated as necessary. The paddles, which should already have been smeared liberally with ECG electrode paste, are applied, one over the cardiac apex and the other over the base of the heart, in the positions shown in Fig 7–1. Everyone except the holder of the paddles breaks physical contact with the patient, and the shock is administered by pressing the button to complete the circuit and discharge the electric impulse through the patient. Since the patient is already unconscious, no anesthetic is required. The instant of the shock is clearly visible as the patient's body jerks because of electrical stimulation of the thoracic muscles. When the response to the shock has been determined, a decision is made whether to restart chest compression and ventilation, whether to try to improve the state of perfusion and oxygenation by some other means, or whether to try another shock.

Defibrillation by Paramedical Personnel

Early treatment of patients with myocardial infarction by specially trained ambulance and fire department personnel is becoming more widespread. Administration of drugs (atropine or lidocaine) and especially electrical defibrillation are the principal forms of treatment available. Advances in the design and portability of equipment, use of the tongue-abdominal pathway for electrocardiographic recording, pacing, and defibrillation, and the introduction of special "foolproof" logic-based instruments may lead to improved results.

Further Measures

If defibrillation is unsuccessful, one should consider the possibility of giving lidocaine, 50 mg, as an intravenous bolus, and repeating the DC shock. The drug can be repeated up to a total dose of 500 mg. If asystole is present and a pacemaker is not immediately available, intravenous or intracardiac epinephrine (0.5 mg, or 5 mL of a 1:10,000 aqueous solution) should be tried. The drug may start cardiac contractions and produce ventricular fibrillation that can then be treated by DC countershock. Acidosis develops rapidly with cardiac arrest and inhibits cardiac contractility. Since chest compression provides only 15–20% of a normal output, acidosis must be treated in all cases that do not respond within 3–5 minutes. Sodium bicarbonate solution, 3.75 g (44.6 meq), should be given intravenously and the dose repeated every 5 minutes until the circulation is restored. A slow infusion of 5% sodium bicarbonate at 100–150 drops/min is often more convenient. The effect of the infusion should be monitored by arterial blood gas measurements whenever possible.

If asystole is present, calcium chloride, 10 mL of a 10% solution, should be tried as a cardiac stimulant. If this fails, the question of cardiac pacing arises. External cardiac pacemakers require high voltage (up to 100 volts) to stimulate cardiac contraction using electrodes at the cardiac apex and right second interspace. External pacing is sometimes effective in primary asystole, but it is traumatic and not tolerable in a conscious patient. It is sometimes possible to stimulate the heart to contract by tapping the precordium rhythmically about 60 times per minute with the ulnar edge of the hand, using a modified "karate chop"; if this is successful, it is much preferred to external pacing. External pacing is only used as an emergency procedure to bridge the gap until a temporary transvenous pacemaker can be inserted. If bradycardia is present after DC countershock, atropine (0.4–0.8 mg intravenously) should be tried.

Isoproterenol is often used as a general supportive measure when the heart rate is slow. It is given as an intravenous drip with 1 mg of the drug in 500 mL of 5% dextrose in water at a rate of 0.03 mg per 5 minutes. A patient who recovers should be carefully examined, transferred to an intensive care area, and observed for the development of shock and for complications arising from the precipitating cause of the original circulatory collapse.

Follow-Up Measures

After the patient has responded to resuscitative measures, evaluation of central nervous system function deserves careful consideration. Each case must be treated on its merits, and it must be decided whether the physician is prolonging life or simply prolonging dying in patients with serious brain damage. Apparently complete central nervous system recovery has been reported in a few patients who have remained unconscious for as long as a week after resuscitation.

Hypothermia at 30 °C for 2–3 days may lessen the degree of brain damage. It is also important to look for complications associated with resuscitation, such as broken ribs, ruptured abdominal viscera, or pneumothorax.

OXYGEN THERAPY

Oxygen therapy should be considered in all patients in whom hypoxia is present and in those who are dyspneic at rest. The objective is to maintain an arterial P_{O_2} greater than 60 mm Hg. Oxygen is ordinarily available as the pure 100% gas either from a cylinder or via a wall outlet in intensive care areas. The ease with which the patient tolerates oxygen therapy depends on the benefit derived from its use. When dyspnea and hypoxia are severe at rest, as in acute pulmonary edema or in lung disease, and the oxygen both raises the arterial P_{O_2} and relieves the dyspnea, the patient tolerates the therapy well. If the dyspnea is not relieved by oxygen, as in right-to-left shunts, severe low cardiac output states, and shock, the patient often tolerates the mask or catheter poorly.

It is difficult to achieve an alveolar oxygen level of more than 40% by the use of masks or nasal catheters, especially in dyspneic patients, and thus it is mainly in those patients in whom a small increase in alveolar P_{O_2} produces a large increase in arterial P_{O_2} that oxygen therapy is effective.

It is possible to achieve higher alveolar oxygen levels by careful administration of oxygen with a trained person in constant attendance and constant monitoring available; 100% oxygen increases the oxygen content of blood leaving the lungs in patients with normal lung function by increasing the amount of oxygen carried in solution in the blood. This effect is small in patients with normal levels of hemoglobin, amounting to 17 mL/L, or equivalent to an increase in saturation of about 8.5% in a person with an oxygen capacity of 200 mL/L. This extra oxygen does not generally produce a significant clinical effect in patients in heart failure with a low cardiac output and normal lungs. In anemic patients, however, the effects are greater, amounting to the equivalent of an increase in oxygen saturation of 34% in a patient with an oxygen capacity of 50 mL/L (hemoglobin level 3.7 g/dL).

Effective oxygen therapy is not without its dangers, since alveolar collapse (atelectasis) is likely to occur if nitrogen is eliminated from the lungs. Since it is so difficult to achieve alveolar oxygen levels of 90% or more in clinical practice, atelectasis is seldom a problem except when increased barometric pressures are used. It is the danger of lung damage that contraindicates the use of hyperbaric chambers for the delivery of increased amounts of oxygen in the treatment of heart disease.

Oxygen Therapy in Specific Conditions

Oxygen therapy is indicated in the treatment of high-altitude pulmonary edema, especially when the patient cannot return to a lower altitude. It should be tried in all patients with myocardial infarction in whom severe myocardial damage has occurred. Ventilation-perfusion mismatching may be present, and hypoxia is not infrequently seen.

If oxygen therapy is well tolerated, it can increase the oxygenation of marginally perfused tissues. If the patient is disturbed by the mask or catheter used for its administration, the resulting increase in cardiac output may offset the benefits obtained. Oxygen is indicated in any patient with pulmonary edema irrespective of the underlying cause. Oxygenation of the blood leaving the lungs is incomplete in pulmonary edema, and oxygen is usually effective and well tolerated in all but the most restless patients.

It is in patients with lung disease, especially those with cor pulmonale, that oxygen is most clearly indicated. Oxygen often reduces the pulmonary artery pressure by reversing hypoxic pulmonary arterial vasoconstriction. This may break the vicious circle responsible for right heart failure and thus play a major part in the patient's recovery.

Respiratory depression due to oxygen therapy can occur in patients who have lost their respiratory sensitivity to CO_2 (eg, in emphysema and chronic bronchitis). In such patients, oxygen therapy can result in respiratory depression and CO_2 retention, with loss of consciousness due to "CO_2 narcosis." The cerebral blood flow increases, the blood pressure rises, and the cerebrospinal fluid pressure may also increase, leading to papilledema and convulsions. However, the chance of this sequence of events occurring has been exaggerated, and it rarely occurs even in patients with chronic pulmonary disease. Artificial or assisted ventilation can be used if hypoventilation develops.

Positive Airway Pressure

Maintenance of a continuous positive airway pressure and the use of positive pressure to inflate the lungs have a place in the treatment of pulmonary edema. Positive end-expiratory pressure (PEEP) can be achieved by having the patient breathe from a mask fitted with a demand valve, breathing out into a tube the end of which is submerged in water to a level of several centimeters. The extra end-expiratory pressure serves to increase the lung volume and, by increasing the intra-alveolar pressure, prevents the transudation of fluid into the alveoli. A similar effect can be obtained by the use of patient-cycled respirators. The aim of their use in pulmonary edema is not to assist in lung inflation but to provide a constant positive pressure airway throughout the respiratory cycle and maintain a normal alveolar volume. They can be used with either air or oxygen, and a considerable amount of cooperation is required from the patient. This form of therapy is preferable to continuous positive pressure breathing, in which active lung inflation is produced by an artificial respirator. The patient is much more likely to struggle and fight the respirator when it is used to inflate the lungs.

Ventilatory assistance is seldom needed in patients who have heart disease alone, but it may become necessary if respiratory failure develops in a patient who already has heart disease. Artificial ventilation via a cuffed endotracheal tube with pressure-cycled or volume-controlled respirators tends to reduce venous return and decrease cardiac output. The possibility of compromising cardiac function must be borne in mind when ventilatory assistance is used, especially in the case of older patients with coronary artery disease.

VENESECTION

Venesection is a traditional means of treating cardiac failure that is seldom used today. Venous blood is ordinarily removed from an antecubital vein with the patient semirecumbent. Blood should not be removed rapidly, and a total of 500 mL is removed in about 15 minutes through a large (16-gauge) needle. If the patient shows any evidence of distress, the foot of the bed can be raised and venous return improved. The great increase in the effectiveness of diuretic drugs has markedly reduced the need for this procedure. It is now almost confined to the treatment of hemochromatosis and of polycythemia in adult patients with cyanotic congenital heart lesions in whom cardiac surgery is not indicated (eg, Eisenmenger's syndrome).

Bloodless Venesection

The use of tourniquets applied to the limbs in rotation to reduce venous return has been advocated in the treatment of acute pulmonary edema. Blood pressure cuffs are inflated on 3 limbs to a level of about 40 mm Hg (between venous and arterial pressure) in order to trap blood in the periphery. The cuff is removed and reapplied on another limb in rotation every 15 minutes. Up to 700 mL of blood can be trapped in the limbs by this means.

BLOOD TRANSFUSION IN CARDIAC PATIENTS

Blood transfusion is seldom indicated in the treatment of heart disease but is not infrequently needed when anemia occurs for other reasons. The patient should always receive the transfusion in the supine position so that the earliest manifestations of pulmonary congestion can be readily recognized. The patient can then sit up to relieve pulmonary congestion while the transfusion is slowed or stopped. Packed cells should be routinely used, and transfusion should be given as slowly as possible after taking into account the underlying reason for the transfusion. The use of sodium citrate as the anticoagulant imposes a severe load on the circulation, and the use of heparinized blood is preferable.

AFTERLOAD REDUCTION
(See also Chapter 8.)

The use of vasodilator drugs to combat the peripheral vasoconstriction seen in acute forms of heart failure provides a useful emergency means of relieving the load on the left ventricle. This technique is particularly helpful in patients with acute aortic or mitral incompetence, which often causes acute pulmonary edema. The treatment also has a place in some cases of acute myocardial infarction with heart failure. The dose of the vasodilator drug must be carefully titrated against its effects on the systemic arterial pressure, heart rate, and cardiac output, and direct monitoring of hemodynamic events is mandatory. The benefits of reducing the load against which the left ventricle must eject blood must be weighed against any increase in cardiac oxygen consumption that may result from increase in heart rate. When valvular incompetence is present, the additional benefit resulting from the decrease in backflow across the incompetent valves provides an important indication for the use of afterload reduction as an emergency measure to tide the patient over until surgery can be performed. The use of the treatment in chronic left heart failure is advocated by some, but the results are less dramatic.

There is no entirely satisfactory drug with which to produce systemic vasodilatation. Phentolamine, which acts as an alpha-adrenergic blocking agent, can be used either intravenously or orally. Sodium nitroprusside is relatively short-acting and is given intravenously, and hydralazine can be given by mouth. The optimal dosage of all of these drugs must be determined by trial and error in each individual patient. The most satisfactory regimen is to start with a small dose (5 mg of phentolamine, 15 μg/min of nitroprusside, or 25 mg of hydralazine) while monitoring the hemodynamic status closely and to gradually increase the medication until a full hemodynamic response is obtained. The dose is then reduced by 15–20% to a maintenance level.

Several other drugs have been tried in an attempt to obtain longer-lasting effects. Sublingual, intravenous, or topical nitroglycerin and sublingual or oral isosorbide dinitrate have been shown to be effective, but their effects on capacitative vessels (veins) are greater, and a fall in output may occur. Their therapeutic effects are less predictable than those of intravenous drugs. Newer drugs that are given orally, such as minoxidil, prazosin, and captopril, are coming into more general use. Their actions are more long-lasting, but as a result their dosage for afterload reduction may be more difficult to titrate in acute cases. Long-term therapy, however, is easier with these drugs than with the above-mentioned ones.

PERICARDIOCENTESIS
(See also Chapter 18.)

This procedure is more commonly required in chronic than in acute pericardial effusion. It is best carried out in a cardiac catheterization laboratory under fluoroscopic control. In traumatic cases and after thoracic surgical procedures when tamponade is suspected, it is best combined with surgical exploration, which is needed to check for bleeding points. The puncture site of choice is in the subxiphoid region, with the subject semirecumbent, but any precordial site can be used. The needle used should not be too small (18-gauge or larger), especially if purulent effusion is suspected, and should have a short bevel. The procedure is more safely carried out if the exploring (chest) electrode of an electrocardiograph is connected to the needle by means of a sterile wire with alligator clips at each end. By this means, any contact between the needle tip and the myocardium can be detected as a sudden elevation of the ST segment, and inadvertent cardiac puncture can be avoided. Examples of electrocardiographic recordings obtained with the needle tip in different sites are shown in Fig 7–3. The procedure is done under local anesthesia similar to that used in thoracocentesis, and precautions should be taken to avoid the intercostal blood vessels that run behind the lower edges of the ribs. It is advantageous to have a central venous pressure recording available at the time of removal of pericardial fluid. A significant fall in central venous pressure indicates that relief of tamponade has occurred, and the final pressure gives an indication of the state of right ventricular function and the level of blood volume. All pericardial taps should be regarded as diagnostic as well as therapeutic procedures, and fluid should always be sent for appropriate laboratory examination, including culture. If a large volume of fluid is to be removed, it is helpful to insert a soft plastic catheter through the needle to avoid myocardial and coronary artery injury. In some cases, fluid may be replaced by air in an attempt to prevent adhesion with possible later constriction. A plastic catheter may be left in situ if effusion is deemed likely to recur rapidly.

ELECTIVE CARDIOVERSION

Restoration of sinus rhythm by DC countershock applied to the chest, when carried out electively, is always performed with the patient under anesthesia. The procedure is painful, and analgesia with morphine or meperidine is not sufficient. The indications for the use of this treatment are similar to those for restoration of sinus rhythm by means of drugs and are

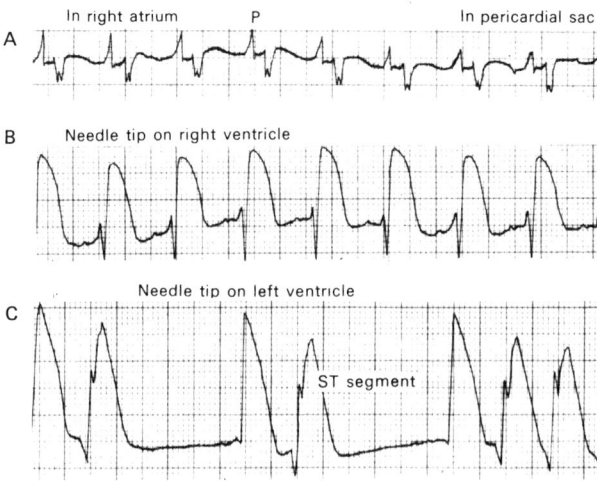

Figure 7–3. Electrocardiograms obtained from the needle tip during pericardiocentesis. In *A*, the amplitude of the P wave decreases when the needle is removed from the right atrium. In *B* and *C*, large-amplitude deflections are seen when the needle touches a ventricle, and in *C*, ectopic beats occur. (Courtesy of A Hollman.)

dealt with elsewhere (see p 487). An antiarrhythmic agent, either quinidine by mouth (0.2 g 4 times daily) for 2 days before, or intravenous procainamide (0.2 g) immediately, is given before the procedure. This premedication is intended to reduce the tendency for the rhythm to revert to the precardioversion state. The premedication may on occasion restore sinus rhythm and make countershock unnecessary. An adequate 12-lead ECG should be taken at the start of the procedure. The rhythm should be identified and a lead chosen in which the characteristics of the arrhythmia are clearly seen. Lead V_1 or V_2 is usually best for patients with atrial fibrillation. The patient's recent medication must be accurately known, especially the level of digitalis dosage and, if possible, the digitalis blood level. If there is any possibility of an element of digitalis toxicity, elective cardioversion should be postponed until digitalis toxicity is resolved, or the first shock after the patient has been anesthetized should be small (about 5 J). At least 3 persons should be in attendance: a nurse, an anesthesiologist, and a cardiologist. The anesthesiologist chooses the method of anesthesia; the nurse runs the electrocardiographic recording, which should also be displayed on a monitor oscilloscope if possible; and the cardiologist applies the paddles to the chest and administers the shock. The large current passing through the body must not be allowed to feed back through the electrocardiographic leads and damage the electrocardiograph. Everyone except the holder of the paddles breaks physical contact with the patient in order to avoid an electric shock. The paddles are insulated. The minimum shock necessary to restore sinus rhythm varies. In most cases, an initial dose of 80 J is used in atrial fibrillation except when digitalis has been given. In that case, a trial dose of 5 J is given and the shock is gradually increased. Atrial flutter usually responds to lower doses. Electrical countershock almost always restores sinus rhythm for at least a few beats, but in many instances the abnormal rhythm recurs. If the first shock is ineffective, a second shock with a larger dose should be given. If multiple shocks (6 or more) are not effective, the physician should consider leaving the patient in the abnormal rhythm, especially if it is atrial fibrillation. The dosage of antiarrhythmic drug, usually quinidine, is continued after the procedure if sinus rhythm is restored.

PACEMAKERS

Significant advances in pacemaker technology have occurred in the past decade. Simple, fixed-rate devices, used for demand pacing of the ventricle, have been superseded by externally programmable instruments that can be used to pace both atrium and ventricle and also to trigger pacing from the intracardiac electrogram. Advances in the design of integrated circuits and microcomputer technology have played an important role. In addition, the design of pacing wires and electrodes has been improved, and the methods for their introduction and stabilization are now more reliable.

The 4 components of any pacemaking system are (1) the battery, (2) the hermetically sealed housing, (3) the lead system, and (4) the signal generator. Failure of any of these components will lead to failure of the whole system, and it was not until advances had been made in the first 3 that sophisticated developments in the signal generator began to be applied. The modern pacemaker is a complex instrument whose function can be changed by setting multiple switches. The pacemaker's program, which is set at the time it is implanted, can be changed noninvasively by means of a magnet or a radio-frequency signal from a coil placed over the implanted unit. A receiver coil in the pacemaker changes the switches appropriately. The implanted unit weighs 50–100 g and is powered by a lithium battery that can last 5–15 years. The variables that can be programmed include the mode of operation (unipolar or bipolar), rate, output (in terms of voltage and duration), sensitivity, atrioventricular delay, and refractory period.

The mode of operation of the modern pacemaker is now conventionally described by a 3-letter code (Fig 7–4): The first letter identifies the chamber paced (A for atrium, V for ventricle, and D for double chamber); the second letter denotes the chamber whose electrical activity is sensed by the pacemaker (A, V, D for double, or O for no sensing function); and the third letter designates the mode of response (I for inhibited, T for triggered, D for both functions, and O for "none" or fixed rate). The simplest, oldest form of ventricular pacemaker is thus designated "VOO," indicating that it paces the ventricle with no sensing of the patient's heartbeat. The commonest form of demand pacemaker is designated "VVI," indicating that it paces the ventricle, sensing the ventricular electrogram and inhibiting the pacing function for a time after sensing an appropriate R wave in the patient's electrogram.

If the standard VVI, R wave–inhibited pacemaker is inserted for sinoatrial disease, the "pacemaker syndrome" (Erbel, 1979) may develop. In such a case, when ventricular pacing starts in response to sinus bradycardia, the lack of atrioventricular coordination causes the cardiac output and blood pressure to drop to levels that cause symptoms. This should not happen with sequential—"physiologic"—pacing. Sequential pacing is, however, never indicated if atrial flutter or fibrillation is suspected.

The 3-letter code describing pacemaker functions has recently been expanded to include 2 more pacemaker capabilities, ie, "programmable functions" and "special antitachyarrhythmic functions" in the fourth and fifth positions, respectively. If these extra functions are not applicable, the 3-letter code is used. A "P" in the fourth position indicates a simple programmable function such as rate or output modification, and "M" indicates a multiprogrammable device; "C" stands for communicating (telemetry) functions, and "O" stands for "none." The available letters in

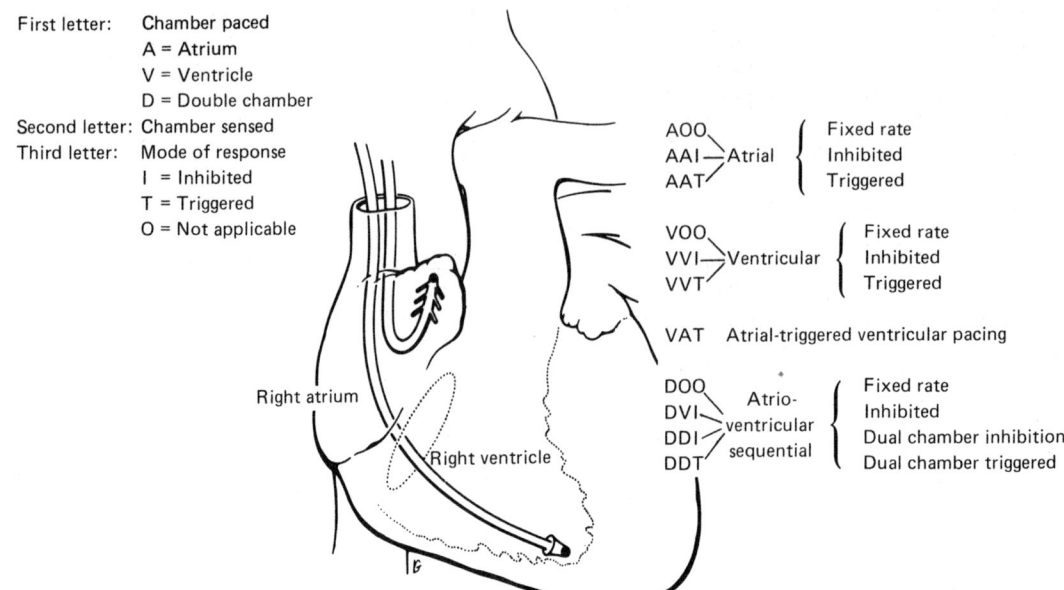

Figure 7-4. International code of modes of pacing. A dual-lead system is illustrated to emphasize that either one or both may be employed clinically. (Modified and reproduced, with permission, from Harthorne JW: Indications for pacemaker insertion: Types and modes of pacing. *Prog Cardiovasc Dis* 1981;**23**:393.)

the fifth position are "B," indicating bursts of impulses; "N," for normal rate competition; "S," for a scanning function; and "E," for external control via a magnet or radio-frequency coil.

With this new code, the standard demand pacemaker is redesignated as VVIPE, indicating that with this form of pacemaker (cost about $2500), the rate and output of the pacemaker can be changed noninvasively. More complex dual units with outputs to atrial and ventricular electrodes are capable of operating in several different modes and of transmitting information back to the external programming coil. This may be an intracardiac electrogram or information about the state of the switches in the unit. The ultimate level of sophistication in this system of classification of pacemakers is "DDDME," which denotes a pacemaker that can be programmed in all the possible modes.

These capabilities are not achieved without raising problems. More complex pacemakers are more expensive (about $5000) and require technical expertise in programming. It is possible for a pacemaker to initiate arrhythmias or to be oversensitive and triggered either by the T wave of the ECG or by muscle action potentials from the diaphragm or chest wall muscles. If the sensitivity is set too low, the pacemaker may not fire. The program of each pacemaker must be readily available at follow-up visits and be capable of transmission over the telephone in case of emergency. Different manufacturers use different techniques and detailed information, and records must be available on a 24-hour basis. The design details of the various commercially available pacemakers are beyond the scope and intention of this book.

Pacemakers are also used to treat arrhythmias. Thus, automatic antitachycardia pacemakers can be used to initiate atrial pacing for the interruption of supraventricular tachycardia (AATON). Higher levels of energy are needed to treat ventricular tachycardia or fibrillation with an automatic internal defibrillator. These more complex varieties of pacemaker should generally not be used unless an electrophysiologic study has been done.

The ability to vary the modes of operation of pacemakers has made it possible to minimize the expenditure of electrical energy and thus prolong the life of the battery. In addition, it has improved the efficiency of troubleshooting and reduced the number of pacemakers that need to be replaced. The increased complexity of pacemakers makes it likely that management of patients with pacemakers will require even more expertise in the future, and skill in the programming of microcomputers will be required of physicians involved in this activity. Thus, the control of pacemakers is coming to be more and more concentrated in specialized units.

Electrodes & Leads

Improvements in the design of electrodes and leads have come close to eliminating lead failure as a problem. Maintenance of a stable position for atrial electrodes has been made easier by use of J-shaped and "screw-in" electrodes. The new polyurethane lead casings are sufficiently slippery to permit simultaneous manipulation of 2 leads in the same vein, and reduction in the stimulation thresholds of new atrial electrodes has increased the life of the whole system.

Method of Introduction: Temporary

The transvenous approach is used unless a pacemaker is inserted at open heart surgery. The site of choice is the subclavian vein (Fig 7–5), with the external or internal jugular, femoral, or antecubital veins as alternatives. Pneumothorax, air embolism, hemorrhage, thrombosis, and phlebitis are the principal complications of the procedure. The pacemaker is almost always inserted under fluoroscopic control. The position of the leads is checked by fluoroscopy at the time of insertion, and the leads are sutured to the skin at the entry site. Use of the subclavian route of entry leaves the patient's arms free during temporary pacing. In emergency situations, the electrode catheter may be inserted without fluoroscopy, with its position guided by recordings of the intracardiac electrogram and tests of the ability to achieve adequate capture of the ventricular impulse. In extreme emergencies, percutaneous transthoracic insertion may be required.

Permanent Pacemaker

Permanent pacemakers are now frequently placed by cardiologists rather than by surgeons. Since thoracotomy is no longer used, the creation of a subclavicular pocket to hold the pulse generator is a relatively simple procedure, compared to the positioning of the intracardiac leads. A cephalic branch of the axillary vein is often used, with the subclavian or external jugular vein as an alternative. A temporary pacemaker is usually left in situ until the permanent device is functioning properly. A temporary pacemaker may sometimes be introduced to provide adequate maintenance of heart rate during insertion of the permanent device. The permanent pacemaker wires may be introduced into the vein after the skin incision has been made. When the wires have been passed into the right atrium, they are positioned under fluoroscopic control. Stylets are now available whose shape can be altered to provide appropriate curves. Placing ventricular leads is generally easier than placing atrial leads.

Checking Operation of the Pacemaker

The threshold of operation of the pacemaker must be checked by determining the minimal voltage needed to capture the rhythm. The voltage is then turned up to determine whether the diaphragm or chest wall muscles contract with each stimulus. Unipolar devices are more likely to respond to external potentials, and changing to a bipolar mode of operation may be helpful. The operation of other aspects of the pacemaker's function (eg, sensing the intracardiac electrogram) is tested and optimized. The patient's ECG is continuously monitored for the first 2 postoperative days, and a follow-up schedule, which must be strictly adhered to, is started. An overpenetrated posteroanterior and lateral chest x-ray should always be taken before discharge. Comparison with subsequent x-rays will be important in determining whether the position of the electrodes has changed. The threshold for pacing often rises in the first few weeks after operation, and the output may well have to be adjusted at this time. A temporary pacemaker is removed when the permanent unit is working satisfactorily. Removal is always done under fluoroscopic control.

Indications for Pacemaker Insertion

Details of the indications for the use of pacemakers are given in the chapters (8, 14, and 15) dealing with different diseases. Complete heart block with episodes of syncope is the longest-established indication, but many pacemakers are now inserted for control of bradycardia and prevention or control of arrhythmia. The principal advantage of the newer pacemakers is their ability to provide sequential atrioventricular ("physiologic") pacing. The hemodynamic effects of this form of pacing have been shown to be significant, but the clinical benefits and the effect on prognosis are not clear. It has been suggested that some physicians may have been overenthusiastic in their use of pacemakers in recent years. There is still some difference of opinion about the indications for pacemaker insertion, and assessment of the benefit is mainly clinical. The huge increase in the last 5 years in the use of this expensive form of therapy, which is usually employed in older pa-

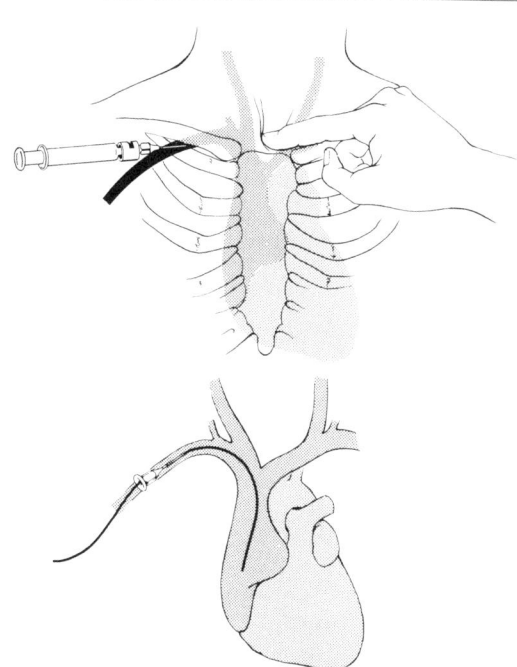

Figure 7–5. Percutaneous subclavian catheterization. (Reproduced, with permission, from Dunphy JE, Way LW [editors]: *Current Surgical Diagnosis & Treatment*, 5th ed. Lange, 1981.)

tients, has raised problems related to the cost of health care.

Complications of Pacemakers

Migration of the pacing electrodes, with erratic pacing or sensing, is a common problem. The electrode may work its way through the myocardium into the pericardial space. This may cause chest pain, pericardial effusion, or stimulation of the diaphragm. Displacement or fibrosis around the electrode tip may necessitate an increase in the stimulating voltage or may decrease the voltage of the electrogram to a level that interferes with proper sensing. Temporary pacemakers are more likely to be affected by external radio-frequency emissions—eg, electric shavers, electrocautery, or magnetic resonance scanners—and some of the more modern devices are sensitive to levels of ionizing radiation used in treatment.

Surgical complications such as hemorrhage, venous thrombosis, and sepsis may occur after permanent pacemaker insertion. Problems with the wires attaching the signal generator to the leads can occur, and displacement of the intracardiac electrodes is commonest in the first 2 months after operation. Battery depletion and ultimately failure are inevitable complications that require operation for their correction.

Regular follow-up with clinic visits is often supplemented by checks on pacemaker function over telephone lines. It is important to try to prevent or alleviate the patient's natural worry over dependence on an electronic instrument.

INTRA-AORTIC BALLOON PUMPING (COUNTERPULSATION)

This specialized circulatory support technique is used only in intensive care areas. The principle is to reduce the load on the heart and increase coronary perfusion by lowering the systolic and raising the diastolic pressure. A plastic balloon is placed in the thoracic aorta and alternately inflated and deflated in time with the heartbeat. Inflation takes place in diastole and deflation during systole. Improvements in design have made it possible to introduce a catheter, around which the deflated balloon is furled, percutaneously via a No. 12 F sheath in the femoral artery. This technique is preferable to insertion through an arteriotomy.

This procedure is effective as a short-term measure but is not widely used except in specialized centers. It may have a place in the postoperative management of cardiac surgical patients. Its medical use has been almost entirely confined to patients with cardiogenic shock following myocardial infarction.

It has been used in conjunction with cardiac surgery, both for the temporary support of patients with cardiogenic shock in the immediate preoperative period and for patients in the postoperative period who cannot be weaned from cardiopulmonary bypass equipment following open heart surgery. The length of time for which intra-aortic balloon pumping can be safely maintained is measured in hours rather than days. Complications include dissection of the aortoiliac arteries, ischemic changes in the legs, and migration of the balloon up the aorta. Timing of the counterpulsation may cause problems in patients with atrial fibrillation or frequent premature beats.

The most satisfactory results are reported in patients with surgically treatable conditions (rupture of the papillary muscles and ventricular septal perforation are the commonest) in whom balloon pumping can be used to tide the patient over a short period of circulatory collapse. Indications for this form of treatment remain controversial, however, as it is highly invasive and therefore not to be undertaken lightly. In spite of the widespread use of this technique in shock following severe myocardial infarction, the mortality rate—especially over the first year—remains high.

EXTERNAL COUNTERPULSATION

There has been a revival of interest in this noninvasive form of circulatory support that was introduced several years ago. In external counterpulsation, the legs are encased in rigid containers with balloons that can be inflated to provide external compression and raise peripheral resistance. The device is triggered from the R wave of the ECG to provide diastolic compression and raise aortic pressure in order to improve coronary perfusion. There is no reciprocal systolic sucking phase. Opinions differ regarding the effectiveness of the procedure, which clearly causes fewer complications but, conversely, is less effective than intra-aortic pumping.

REFERENCES

Amsterdam EA et al: Clinical assessment of external pressure circulatory assistance in acute myocardial infarction. *Am J Cardiol* 1980;**45:**349.

Angello DA: Principles of electrical testing for analysis of ventricular endocardial pacing leads. *Prog Cardiovasc Dis* 1984;**27:**57.

Barold SS, Mugica J: *The Third Decade of Cardiac Pacing.* Futura, 1982.

Bregman D et al: Percutaneous intraaortic balloon insertion. *Am J Cardiol* 1980;**48:**261.

Brundage BH et al: The role of balloon pumping in postinfarction angina: A different perspective. *Circulation* 1980;**62(Suppl 2):**119.

Chardack WM: Heart block treated with implantable pacemaker. *Prog Cardiovasc Dis* 1964;**6:**507.

Chatterjee K, Parmley WW: The role of vasodilator therapy in heart failure. *Prog Cardiovasc Dis* 1977;**19:**301.

Erbel R: Pacemaker syndrome. *Am J Cardiol* 1979;**44:**771.

Frye RL et al: Guidelines for permanent pacemaker implantation. *Circulation* 1984;**70:**331A.

Gordon AS (chairman): Standards for cardiopulmonary resuscitation (CPR) and emergency cardiac care (ECC). *JAMA* 1974;**227(Suppl):**837.

Hancock EW: Symposium on cardiac emergencies: Cardiac tamponade. *Med Clin North Am* 1979;**63:**223.

Harthorne JW: Indications for pacemaker insertion: Types and modes of pacing. *Prog Cardiovasc Dis* 1981;**23:**393.

Heimlich HJ: A life-saving maneuver to prevent food-choking. *JAMA* 1975;**234:**398.

Hess DS et al: Permanent pacemaker implantation in the cardiac catheterization laboratory: The subclavian vein approach. *Cathet Cardiovasc Diagn* 1982;**8:**453.

Hines GL et al: Intra-aortic balloon pumping: Two-year experience. *J Thorac Cardiovasc Surg* 1979;**78:**140.

Isner JM et al: Complications of the intraaortic balloon counterpulsation device: Clinical and morphologic observations in 45 necropsy patients. *Am J Cardiol* 1980;**45:**260.

Jaggarao NS et al: Use of an automated external defibrillator-pacemaker by ambulance staff. *Lancet* 1982;**2:**73.

Kleiger R, Lown B: Cardioversion and digitalis. *Circulation* 1966;**33:**878.

Krikorian JG, Hancock EW: Pericardiocentesis. *Am J Med* 1978;**65:**808.

Kuhn LA: External pressure circulatory assistance: No light on the shadow. *Am J Cardiol* 1980;**46:**1069.

Labovitz AJ et al: Noninvasive assessment of pacemaker hemodynamics by Doppler echocardiography: Importance of left atrial size. *J Am Coll Cardiol* 1985;**6:**196.

Langou RA et al: Surgical approach for patients with unstable angina pectoris: Role of the response to initial medical therapy and intraaortic balloon pumping in perioperative complications after aortocoronary bypass grafting. *Am J Cardiol* 1978;**42:**629.

Levine FH et al: Management of acute myocardial ischemia with intraaortic balloon pumping and coronary bypass surgery. *Circulation* 1978;**58:**I-69.

Lown B: Electrical reversion of cardiac arrhythmias. *Br Heart J* 1967;**29:**469.

Lown B et al: New method for terminating cardiac arrhythmias. *JAMA* 1962;**182:**548.

McEnany MT et al: Clinical experience with intraaortic balloon pump support in 728 patients. *Circulation* 1978;**58(3–Part 2):**I-124.

Mirowski M et al: Implanted automatic defibrillator to convert malignant arrhythmias. *N Engl J Med* 1980;**303:**322.

Obel IWP: *Physiological Pacing.* Pitman Medical, 1981.

Parsonnet V: The proliferation of cardiac pacing: Medical, technical, and socioeconomic dilemmas. *Circulation* 1982;**65:**841.

Parsonnet V, Rodgers T: The present state of programmable pacemakers. *Prog Cardiovasc Dis* 1981;**23:**401.

Parsonnet V et al: Optimal resources for implantable cardiac pacemakers. *Circulation* 1983;**68:**227A.

Rudikoff MT et al: Mechanisms of blood flow during cardiopulmonary resuscitation. *Circulation* 1980;**61:**345.

Scherf D, Bornemann C: Thumping of the precordium in ventricular standstill. *Am J Cardiol* 1960;**5:**30.

Sowton E: Hemodynamic studies in patients with artificial pacemakers. *Br Heart J* 1964;**26:**737.

Unger F (editor): *Assisted Circulation.* Springer-Verlag, 1979.

Walker PR: Pacemakers: Techniques, indications, results and complications. In: *Scientific Foundations of Cardiology.* Sleight P, Vann Jones J (editors). Heinemann, 1983.

8 Coronary Disease

OVERVIEW OF CORONARY HEART DISEASE

Coronary heart disease is one of the most common fatal diseases in the industrialized countries. In the USA, it is the cause of one-third to one-half of all deaths and 50–75% of all cardiac deaths; approximately 500,000 people a year die from the disease. The disease affects men in the prime of life; the average age at the time of the first myocardial infarction is the mid fifties. Women are spared for about 10 years relative to men.

The importance of coronary heart disease extends beyond the high morbidity and mortality rates. Clinical manifestations are unpredictable or absent; the course is variable; and in one-third to one-half of patients, death is sudden and unexpected ("sword of Damocles"). The recognition of coronary heart disease in any of its clinical forms raises the possibility of sudden death, and even minimal symptoms may portend more serious disease.

In about 99% of cases, coronary artery disease is due to atherosclerotic changes. Other causes include syphilis, various forms of arteritis, coronary embolism, and connective tissue disorders (eg, systemic lupus erythematosus). In some instances, coronary spasm alone may be the cause of myocardial ischemia, although more frequently coronary spasm complicates coronary atherosclerosis. The discussion here will be limited to atherosclerotic coronary heart disease.

GENERAL CLASSIFICATION OF CORONARY HEART DISEASE

The classification of coronary heart disease by type and degree is arbitrary and unsatisfactory, because the clinical manifestations merge into one another and represent a diverse spectrum of progressive ischemia, necrosis, spasm, fibrosis, and left ventricular dysfunction. Any of the manifestations may be the first one to appear, and the patient may present with one, develop another, and then stabilize at any manifestation. Fig 8–1 illustrates the presenting clinical manifestations in the Framingham Study. Furthermore, the disease can have acute and chronic phases, and the patient may be critically ill during one phase and capable of full activity a few months later with or without another manifestation. The correlation between symptoms, clinical manifestations, and pathologic findings is so imprecise that one cannot be predicted

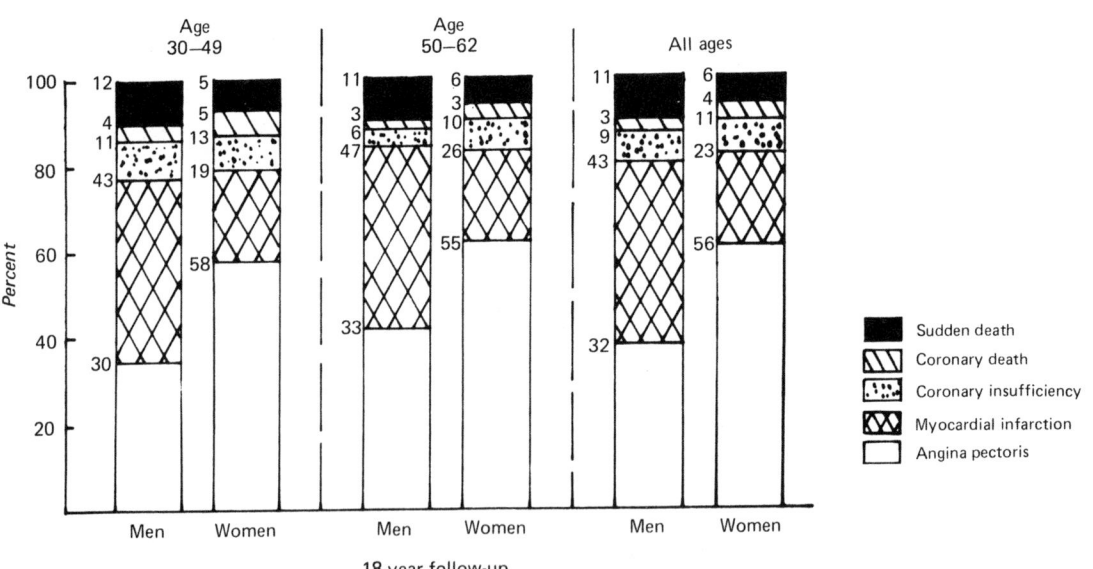

Figure 8–1. Presenting clinical manifestations of coronary heart disease: Framingham Study, men and women age 30–62 years at entry. (Reproduced, with permission, from Kannel WB: Some lessons in cardiovascular epidemiology from Framingham. *Am J Cardiol* 1976;**37**:269.)

on the basis of the other. The clinical expression of the various phases of coronary heart disease is not self-limited or specific. In coronary heart disease, therefore, the patient may present with—or may develop—any of the following:

(1) Asymptomatic coronary disease, manifested by induced myocardial ischemia.
(2) Sudden death.
(3) Angina pectoris of effort; variant (Prinzmetal's) angina; coronary spasm.
(4) Unstable angina pectoris (acute coronary insufficiency).
(5) Acute myocardial infarction.
(6) Cardiac failure.
(7) Cardiac arrhythmias or atrioventricular conduction defects.

PATHOGENESIS OF ATHEROSCLEROTIC CORONARY HEART DISEASE

The clinical entity of coronary heart disease (ischemic heart disease) must be differentiated from its underlying pathologic process, coronary atherosclerosis. Robbins (1976) defines atherosclerosis as follows: "Basically, the disorder comprises the development of focal fibrofatty elevated plaques or thickenings, called atheromas, within the intima and inner portion of the media. As the disorder advances, the atheromas undergo a variety of complications—calcification, internal hemorrhages, ulceration, and sometimes superimposed thrombosis."

The clinical manifestations have become more common and now occur at an earlier age, but the pathologic process has not changed (Fig 8–1). Atherosclerosis is an age-related degenerative process, occurring with increasing frequency with advancing age. Yet its occurrence is not inevitable, because some octogenarians have minimal or no evidence of coronary atherosclerosis on postmortem examination.

Atherosclerosis may begin early in life. During the Korean War, evidence of atherosclerosis was found in about three-fourths of young soldiers killed in battle, and about one-fourth had stenosis of at least 50% of one coronary artery. The extent of coronary atherosclerosis is greater in those who have more severe clinical manifestations of coronary heart disease, but the correlation is far from perfect. With the exception of the left main coronary artery, isolated stenosis of one coronary artery is rarely the cause of sudden death in coronary heart disease. Extensive disease of 2 or 3 arteries is usually found at autopsy.

Lesion of Atherosclerosis

Atherosclerosis occurs in the muscular arteries, including the aorta and the coronary, femoral, iliac, internal carotid, and cerebral arteries. The typical lesion is the fibrous plaque, which grossly is dull white and slightly elevated and impinges on the arterial lumen but, when uncomplicated, rarely occludes it. Histologically, it is characterized by a protrusion of smooth

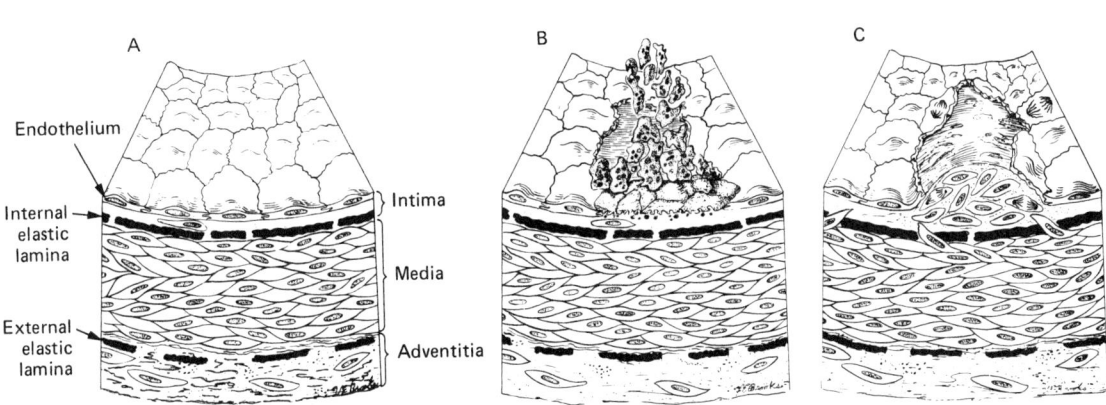

Figure 8–2. Mechanisms of production of atheroma. **A:** Structure of normal muscular artery. The adventitia, or outermost layer of the artery, consists principally of recognizable fibroblasts intermixed with smooth muscle cells loosely arranged between bundles of collagen and surrounded by proteoglycans. It is usually separated from the media by a discontinuous sheet of elastic tissue, the external elastic lamina. **B:** Platelet aggregates, or microthrombi, which may form as a result of adherence of the platelets to the exposed subendothelial connective tissue. Platelets that adhere to the connective tissue release granules whose constituents may gain entry into the artery wall. Platelet factors thus interact with plasma constituents in the artery wall and may stimulate events shown in the next illustration. **C:** Smooth muscle cells migrating from the media into the intima through fenestrae in the internal elastic lamina and actively multiplying within the intima. Endothelial cells regenerate in an attempt to re-cover the exposed intima, which thickens rapidly owing to smooth muscle proliferation and formation of new connective tissue. (Reproduced, with permission, from Ross R, Glomset JA: The pathogenesis of atherosclerosis. [Part 1.] *N Engl J Med* 1976;**295**:369.)

muscle cells containing lipids surrounded by a matrix of connective tissue cells, collagen, elastic fibers, and mucopolysaccharides. As the fibrous plaque enlarges, it may become calcified, may undergo necrosis, may bleed internally, and may develop a superimposed mural thrombus—and in these ways may ultimately partially or completely occlude the artery. Hemorrhage into old atherosclerotic plaques in the coronary arteries may occur. The lesions are focal, tend to occur at points where the arteries branch, and do not impair flow through the artery until stenosis exceeds 70% of the lumen of the artery.

The structure of a normal muscular artery is illustrated in Fig 8–2A. The effect of endothelial injury and the subsequent deposition of platelet aggregates (microthrombi) and infiltration of smooth muscle cells into the damaged intima from the media are illustrated in Fig 8–2B and C. The lipid particles that accumulate in the fibrous plaque arise from the plasma lipid flowing through the artery, as shown by the similarity of the lipid composition of the plasma and of the atherosclerotic plaque.

Pathogenesis of Atherosclerosis

There are 2 major schools of thought about the pathogenesis of atherosclerosis: (1) that coronary artery thrombosis is the initiating event and that the atheroma is the result of the healing process combined with infiltration of lipids; and (2) that intimal injury caused by elevated pressure, deposition of lipid, and infiltration of hypertrophied smooth muscle cells from the media leads to obstruction of the coronary artery, fibrosis, lipid deposition, and atheroma formation (Ross, 1976). Pathologic features of atherosclerosis are shown in Fig 8–3.

A. Coronary Artery Embolism: This is the cause of 10% of myocardial infarctions. (See also p 604.) Mural thrombi occur in the left atrium or left ventricle in patients with valvular (usually mitral) heart disease, previous myocardial infarction, cardiomyopathy, and chronic atrial fibrillation due to any cause. Bits of the thrombi break off and occlude any of the branches of the left coronary artery, usually the more distal ones.

B. Endothelial Damage Theory: Evidence has been offered that atherosclerosis is a response of the intima to endothelial injury, resulting in platelet aggregation on the damaged endothelial surface and proliferation and extension of smooth muscle cells from the media into the intima. This produces the fibrous plaque, which may then undergo calcification, hemorrhage, and thrombosis (Ross, 1976). Endothelial injury may also result from a number of physical and biochemical factors.

Arterial endothelial cells have been cultured in the laboratory, allowing direct study of the role of injury, risk factors, and LDL receptor defects in endothelial damage.

Diagnosis of Stenosis by Coronary Arteriography

Coronary arteriography (see p 151), which is used to delineate the anatomy of the coronary arteries, often underestimates the extent of coronary stenosis shown at autopsy. There is usually good agreement between the radiologic interpretation of the coronary arteriogram and the findings of the pathologist if the stenosis exceeds 85%; if the stenosis is less than this, or if the lesions are peripheral, there is great variation in opinion about the degree of stenosis. Furthermore, the lesions may be obscured in one radiologic plane, and multiple views with different projections are required to avoid missing or underestimating the lesions. Proximal lesions are more prevalent than distal ones—a fact of considerable operative significance. Not only do proximal lesions more adversely affect blood flow to the myocardium, but the beneficial effect of bypassing a proximal stenosis is correspondingly greater. Collateral vessels between a relatively normal coronary artery and a companion coronary artery distal to a stenosis are found in practically all cases of severe stenoses—compensating, in part, for the decreased flow through the stenotic channel.

Risk Factors in the Development of Atherosclerosis

Hyperlipidemia, hypertension, diabetes, a family history of atherosclerosis, cigarette smoking, age, prostaglandin deficiency, male sex, and use of oral contraceptives increase the prevalence and incidence of atherosclerosis. Physical inactivity and personality or sociocultural factors are less important. Combinations of risk factors greatly enhance the probability of a cardiovascular event.

The mechanisms by which these risk factors operate to enhance the likelihood of atherosclerosis are not precisely known. A comprehensive analysis of risk factors and the response to interventions has been published by Stamler (1984).

A. Hyperlipidemia: Hyperlipidemia is thought to foster atherogenesis by increasing the deposition of lipid in the intima because of its increased concentration in plasma. The importance of lipid disorders

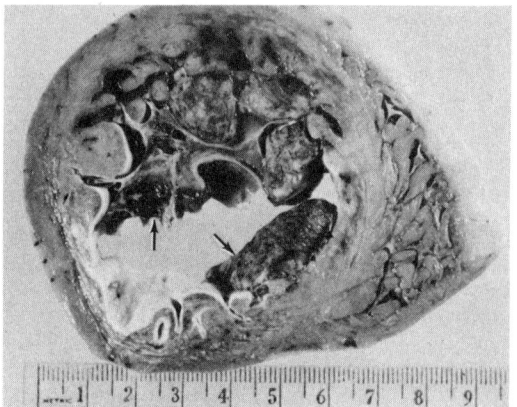

Figure 8–3. Mural thrombosis of the heart superimposed on underlying atherosclerosis. The arrows outline the thrombus. (Courtesy of O Rambo.)

is strikingly emphasized by the course of coronary disease in hypercholesterolemia. Myocardial infarction has been shown to occur in 85% of subjects by age 60—in contrast to 20% of the population at large (Slack, 1969).

The NHLBI Type II Coronary Intervention Study (Brensike, 1984) studied 3086 men with type II hypercholesterolemia who were placed on a low-fat, low-cholesterol diet and given cholestyramine ester, 24 g/d in divided doses. Over a 7.4-year period, total plasma cholesterol levels were reduced by an average of 13.4% and there was a 19% decrease in the incidence of coronary heart disease, nonfatal myocardial infarction, and deaths. Men with a 25% decrease in total cholesterol had about half the incidence of coronary disease of those with no decrease in total cholesterol. No data were presented regarding women or regarding men with lesser elevations of cholesterol (Lipid Research Clinics Program, 1984). In another NHLBI study (Levy, 1984), 115 men and 28 women with type II hypercholesterolemia were studied over a 5-year period. Use of diet and cholestyramine to produce lower total and LDL cholesterol levels and increased HDL cholesterol levels was associated with lower rates of progression of coronary disease. Patients had average pretreatment total cholesterol levels of 253 mg/dL, greater than the levels reported in 95% of the population. Again, no data were available for lesser elevations of cholesterol. These data strongly support the use of diet and cholesterol-lowering drugs in the treatment of hypercholesterolemia. Furthermore, there are several subgroups of HDL, not all of which are equally important in pathogenesis. Data on the fasting plasma triglyceride and total cholesterol levels in both men and women in a large series of subjects are presented in Fig 8–4.

The estimated sex- and age-adjusted plasma cholesterol and triglyceride levels in control subjects were found by Goldstein (1973) to be, respectively, 270 and 147 mg/dL at the 90th percentile; 285 and 165 mg/dL at the 95th percentile; and 314 and 200 mg/dL at the 99th percentile. Cholesterol and triglyceride values in survivors of myocardial infarction are often in the top 20% of the levels found in control subjects.

A decrease in high-density lipoprotein (HDL) may be more important than an increase in low-density lipoprotein (LDL) or total cholesterol in the pathogenesis of atherosclerosis (Fig 8–5). The ratio of HDL cholesterol to total cholesterol (<0.15 mg/dL) may be a better predictor of coronary disease than either level alone, or levels of apoprotein A, B, or E (Schmidt, 1985). HDL increases the absorption of cholesterol from peripheral tissues, including the arterial wall ("scavenger" effect), and transports it to the liver, where metabolic breakdown and excretion occur. The cholesterol in atheroma is derived from that in the plasma, whereas that in the arterial wall is normally synthesized in situ. Decreased HDL may impair the clearance of cholesterol from the arterial wall, leading

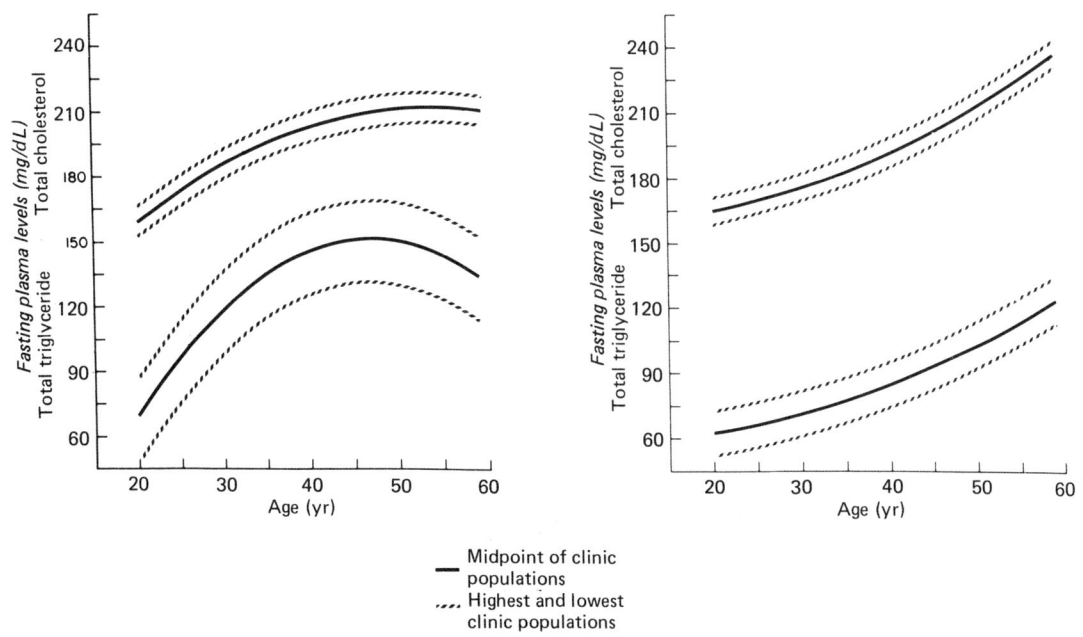

Figure 8–4. Regression estimates of mean plasma lipid values by age and clinic. *Left:* White males, ages 20–59 years. *Right:* White females not taking sex hormones, ages 20–59 years. (Reproduced, with permission, from the American Heart Association, Inc., Heiss G et al: Lipoprotein-cholesterol distributions in selected North American populations: The Lipid Research Clinics Program Prevalence Study. *Circulation* 1980;**61**:302.)

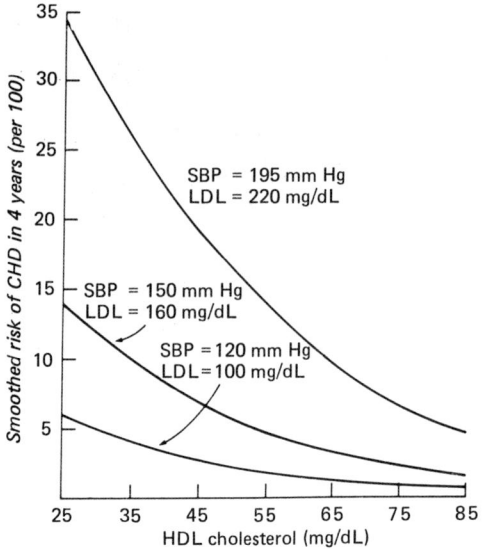

Figure 8–5. Risk of coronary heart disease according to levels of high-density lipoprotein cholesterol in 55-year-old men. Framingham Study 24-year follow-up. CHD, coronary heart disease; SBP, systolic blood pressure; LDL, low-density lipoprotein; HDL, high-density lipoprotein. (Reproduced, with permission, from Kannel WB, Castelli WP, Gordon T: Cholesterol in the prediction of atherosclerotic disease. *Ann Intern Med* 1979;**90**:85.)

to an imbalance between filtration of cholesterol from plasma and its clearance, thereby causing increased deposition of cholesterol.

The mechanism of familial hypercholesterolemia is thought to be a primary genetic defect in the cell membrane surface receptors that bind LDL, the major cholesterol-containing lipoprotein in plasma. In the homozygous form, functional LDL receptors are much decreased or completely absent in cultured fibroblasts, amniotic fluid cells, smooth muscle cells, or lymphocytes; in the heterozygous form, more LDL receptors are present but there are fewer than normal. When this occurs, lipoprotein cannot bind to receptors and enter cells to be used for intracellular metabolism and membrane synthesis. Premature atherosclerosis may occur (most markedly in the homozygous form), and there may be other signs such as tendon and plantar xanthomatosis. The system that regulates the rate of cellular uptake of LDL is complex because of the number of alternative pathways for dealing with excessive serum cholesterol when there are few or no LDL receptors.

Several studies have supported this hypothesis. In one report, cultured amniotic fluid cells were studied from a 20-week-old fetus whose brother had died at age 8 years of homozygous hypercholesterolemia. The cells showed an almost complete absence of LDL cell surface receptors. The serum cholesterol of the aborted fetus was 9 times the average of control fetuses of the same age (Brown, 1978). More recently, studies of Watanabe-heritable hyperlipidemic rabbits have also supported this theory (Goldstein, 1983). This strain of rabbits has a genetic defect and disease similar to those found in humans. Striking hypercholesterolemia and atherosclerosis develop even when the rabbits are fed a cholesterol-free diet. This animal model has aroused considerable interest, and investigations are under way to determine the mechanisms and treatment of the defect.

B. Hypertension: Hypertension increases the filtration of lipid from plasma to the intimal cells by virtue of increased arterial pressure, especially in the presence of elevated plasma lipids. Hypertension as well as hyperlipidemia may injure the intima, leading to platelet aggregation and proliferation of smooth muscle cells in the media. Increased susceptibility to injury from shear forces, torsion, and lateral wall pressure changes may also be important. Hypertension is now the most common and most important risk factor in the pathogenesis of atherosclerosis; atherosclerotic complications constitute the most common causes of death in hypertensive patients.

The average degree of coronary artery sclerosis in a large group of routine autopsies was grade 9 (on a scale of 1–10) in hypertensives in the 40- to 49-year age group, whereas this degree of coronary sclerosis was not reached in nonhypertensives until age 60–70 years (Lober, 1953). Purely hypertensive complications (cardiac failure, accelerated or malignant hypertension, hemorrhagic stroke, and renal failure) have been sharply reduced by present-day antihypertensive treatment. The evidence for reduction of atherosclerotic complications (myocardial infarction or cerebral infarction) is less convincing. In the Hypertension Detection and Follow-Up Program Study, patients who received stepped-care treatment had significantly decreased mortality rates following acute myocardial infarction as compared to patients who received referred care. In other clinical trials, patients with diastolic pressures of 90–104 mm Hg and no major target organ damage or electrocardiographic abnormalities at baseline did not have a significantly decreased incidence of coronary disease following antihypertensive treatment. However, in these cases, mortality rates associated with coronary heart disease were 40% lower in the group receiving stepped care (Stamler, 1984).

C. Diabetes: The asymptomatic hyperglycemia of adults with diabetes mellitus may be a risk factor independent of and additive to the effect of blood pressure and serum lipids. Diabetes affects the capillary basement membrane (microangiopathy) of all tissues. It produces abnormalities in the myocardium, in small coronary vessels, and in the major arteries. Pathologically, atherosclerosis occurs more frequently and at an earlier age in diabetic patients (Waller, 1980). The adverse effect of diabetes on cardiovascular disease cannot be explained by known risk factors. The roles of serum glucose and serum insulin are unknown and the conclusions conflicting. Even when coronary disease is excluded, rates of cardiac failure in diabetes are increased; this may be due to diabetic cardiomyopathy unrelated to small-vessel disease. It is not rare to see angina and myocardial infarction in young people with type I (insulin-dependent) diabetes mellitus. In subjects with impaired glucose tolerance, the mortality rate from coronary heart disease was approximately doubled as compared to that in patients with normal glucose tolerance after a 7½-year period of observation (Fuller, 1980). Control of hyperglycemia in type II (non–insulin-dependent) diabetes mellitus has not been shown to influence subsequent coronary disease. Rigid control of type I diabetes has been claimed by some to be preventive, although this opinion has been challenged.

D. Family History: A positive family history may reflect (1) genetic predisposition to the development of hypertension, hyperlipidemia, or diabetes or (2) environmental influences such as diet, stress, and lifestyle. After all known risk factors for coronary disease are eliminated, there is still a 2-fold risk of myocardial infarction among first-degree relatives of survivors of myocardial infarction as compared to first-degree relatives of those who have not had myocardial infarction (ten Kate, 1982). Sons of fathers with coronary disease were found both to develop the disease and to die at an earlier age than their fathers (Hamby, 1981).

For men under age 55, a coronary death in a first-degree male relative under age 55 increases the risk of coronary death to 3 times that of the general population. For women under age 65, a coronary death in a first-degree male relative under age 55 increases the risk of coronary death to 5 times that of the general population (Slack, 1968). The risk of coronary death in these cases is greater than it is in middle-aged men with elevated serum cholesterol or blood pressure. Men with risk of dominantly inherited familial hypercholesterolemia have a 15-fold increase in risk, and 50% die of coronary heart disease before age 60 (Slack, 1969).

E. Cigarette Smoking: The principal importance of cigarette smoking is that it precipitates arrhythmias and is a factor in sudden death in patients with coronary artery disease. In addition, *smoking is a definite risk factor in promoting atherosclerosis.* Cigarette smoking is strongly associated with reduced serum HDL cholesterol, and this may be one of the mechanisms for its adverse effect. Cigarette smoking is the most prominent risk factor for myocardial infarction in women under age 50 years. The incidence of sudden death is significantly greater in smokers (Fig 8–6). The risk of cigarette smoking is independent of other major risk factors but aggravates them. The risk is reduced when smoking is stopped. The mechanism of atherogenesis due to cigarette smoking is not clear.

The frequency of cigarette smoking is high in patients with atherosclerosis; at the outset of the Framingham Study, in 1949, 60% of the men and 40% of the women were smokers. Cigar and pipe smoking are considerably less important as risk factors.

F. Prostaglandins: The pathway of prostaglandin synthesis from arachidonic acid is illustrated in Fig 8–7. Blood platelets synthesize thromboxane (TXA_2), which both aggregates platelets and constricts arteries. Endothelial cells synthesize prostacyclin (PGI_2), which inhibits platelet aggregation and dilates arteries. Both TXA_2 and PGI_2 are local hormones, which by their balance affect coronary blood flow. It has been speculated that imbalance, especially if TXA_2 is predominant, may foster atherosclerosis (Vane, 1983), and a number of researchers are testing this hypothesis.

G. Estrogens and the Menopause: Women taking estrogens have an average HDL cholesterol approximately 20% higher than those not taking the compounds.

The mechanisms by which the menopause influences coronary disease have not been established. Coronary disease in young menstruating women is rare—much rarer than in men of the same age—and it usually occurs in association with one of the other major risk factors noted above. However, there is an unexplained substantial increase in cardiovascular disease with menopause—especially surgically induced menopause—most evident in the age group 40–44 years.

Premenopausal women with severe hypertension (diastolic pressure >120 mm Hg) are not protected from coronary disease.

H. Oral Contraceptives: There is increasing evidence that women taking oral contraceptives, especially agents with high estrogen content, have increased risk of myocardial infarction, particularly if they are cigarette smokers, are older, and have been taking the drugs for longer than 5 years. The mechanism is unclear. The rate of infarction is increased 3- to 4-fold in women under age 50, as compared with women who have never used the agents (Slone, 1981). It remains to be determined whether the agents with

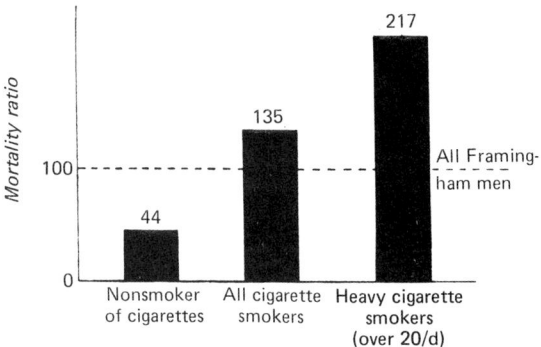

Figure 8–6. Framingham Study 12-year follow-up mortality ratios for sudden death in nonsmokers, all smokers, and heavy smokers among men originally aged 30–62. (Modified and reproduced, with permission, from Kannel WB: *Habits and Coronary Heart Disease: The Framingham Heart Study.* Public Health Service Publication No. 1515, National Heart Institute, 1966.)

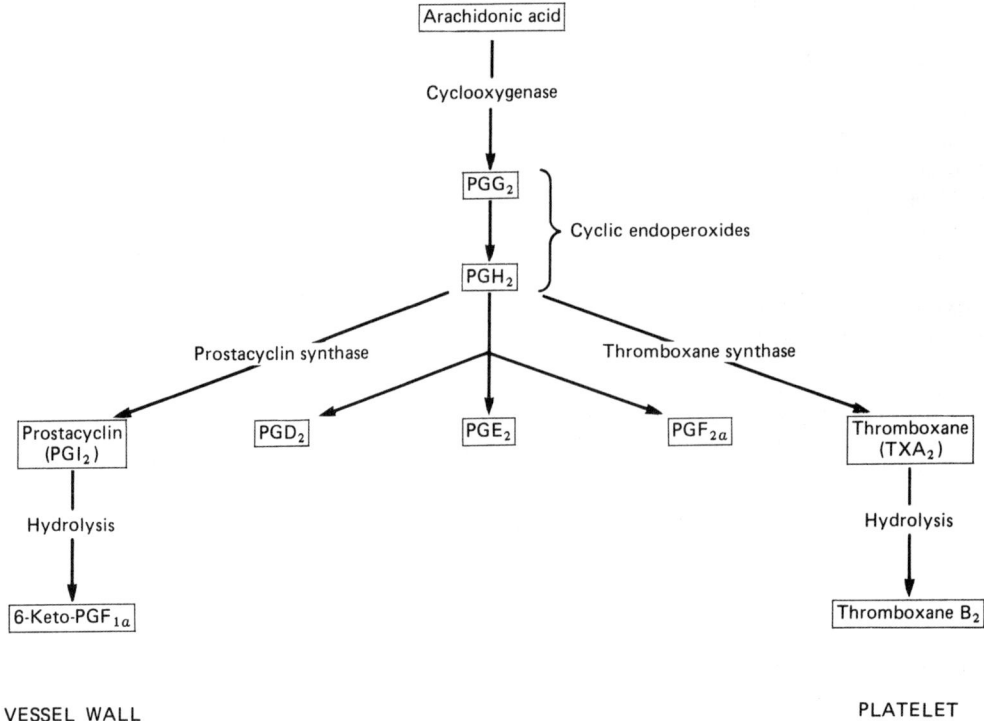

Figure 8–7. Pathway of prostaglandin biosynthesis. (Redrawn, modified, and reproduced, with permission, from Kuo PT: Lipoproteins, platelets, and prostaglandins in atherosclerosis. *Am Heart J* 1981;102:949.)

lower estrogen content will lessen or nullify the increased risk.

I. Physical Inactivity: A sedentary habit of life may produce its effects through associated obesity, which may predispose to diabetes and possibly hypertension. Obesity per se is a marginal risk factor. Preliminary data suggest that because inactive people have fewer collateral coronary vessels, physical inactivity may merely decrease the chance for survival when myocardial infarction occurs; it does not influence the atherosclerotic process itself. The high incidence of myocardial infarction in vigorous northeastern Finns who consume a diet high in saturated fats and cholesterol suggests that exercise affords only minimal protection against coronary disease. Although exercise improves morale, fitness, and evidences of left ventricular function and provides a sense of well-being, cardiovascular morbidity and mortality rates are not convincingly decreased (as independent risk factors) by exercise programs. The National Exercise and Heart Disease Project (Shaw, 1981) found that mortality rates did not differ significantly between men who engaged in high-intensity exercise for approximately 3 years after a myocardial infarction and those who did not. The Ontario Exercise Heart Collaborative Study (Rechnitzer, 1983) found that the recurrence rate of myocardial infarction over a 4-year period did not differ significantly in men who participated in a program of high-intensity exercise compared with those who participated in light exercise. The number of fatal and nonfatal reinfarctions did not differ between the 2 groups.

The various opinions about the benefits of physical exercise in preventing coronary disease or its complications are contradictory. Confounding factors such as family history, the association of other risk factors, preselection of individuals, the large number of dropouts, and the difficulty in quantifying the amount of exercise make interpretation of the studies difficult. The independent preventive benefits of vigorous exercise programs appear to be slight and not as clear-cut as the primary risk factors of high serum cholesterol, hypertension, positive family history, smoking, or diabetes.

J. Personality and Sociocultural Factors: Rosenman (1976) has postulated that personality and behavior characteristics such as pressure of time and work, competitiveness, and aggressiveness (type A) are variables independent of other risk factors. They found that the incidence of coronary disease was lower in type B (more relaxed) individuals.

However, multicenter trials found no relation between type A behavior and subsequent coronary disease in subjects previously free of it (MRFIT Study, 1982) or in late cardiac morbidity or mortality rates in survivors of acute myocardial infarction (Case, 1985).

These studies throw doubt on the independent specificity of type A characteristics but not necessarily of other personality traits that may be risk factors.

Each risk factor discussed above is not only significant in itself but is also additive and perhaps synergistic when combined with one or more other risk factors. Hypertension and atherosclerosis, for example, are independent disease processes, yet hypertension accelerates atherosclerosis.

Pathogenesis of Coronary Heart Disease

The Framingham Study was designed to determine the factors influencing the development of coronary heart disease in 2282 men and 2845 women aged 30–62 who were found to be clinically free of coronary heart disease when first entering the study. Through clinical examinations at 2-year intervals and other methods of follow-up over more than 20 years, the study has traced the natural history of the various manifestations of coronary disease, as well as stroke and peripheral artery disease, and has meticulously related their development to host and environmental factors. The study has provided an elaborate epidemiologic survey of coronary disease and has explored risk factors that increase the likelihood of developing coronary disease. The established risk factors are hyperlipidemia, hypertension, diabetes, a family history of atherosclerosis, cigarette smoking, age, prostaglandin deficiency, male sex, and use of oral contraceptives. Physical inactivity and personality or sociocultural factors are thought to be less important.

The relationship between mural thrombosis of the coronary arteries and myocardial infarction has been the subject of considerable debate. For many years it was thought that the 2 were synonymous, but either one may occur without the other. Thrombosis usually superimposed on a stenotic atherosclerotic lesion is the most frequent cause of myocardial infarction. Such lesions were found in more than 80% of patients with acute infarction studied by coronary arteriography in the first few hours (DeWood, 1980). Ruptured plaques with intimal hemorrhage and occlusive thrombosis were identified in 82% of patients with fatal ischemic disease (Falk, 1983).

The exact reasons for the apparently haphazard onset of angina, myocardial infarction, ventricular arrhythmias, or sudden death are often unknown.

A. Pathophysiology of Coronary Blood Flow: Myocardial oxygen extraction is almost complete even when coronary blood flow is normal. There is thus little reserve capacity to increase oxygen delivery. When delivery is insufficient, anaerobic metabolism is initiated with the production of lactate from glycogen. The presence of increased lactate production can be determined by comparing the lactate content in the coronary sinus with that in arterial blood.

Coronary blood flow is increased further by vasoactive substances that, as a result of hypoxia, increase flow by causing coronary vasodilation. Vasoactive substances include potassium, lactate, adenosine, and prostaglandins.

Another important factor is autoregulation, which relates intra-arterial pressure to vascular tone. For example, in hypertension, blood vessels may stretch, causing contraction of arteriolar muscle. In myocardial ischemia, local vascular pressure levels may fall, causing vasodilation. Brief coronary occlusion results in a fall in intracoronary pressure and induces vasodilatation.

Pathologic studies have shown that the subendocardium is more vulnerable to myocardial ischemia or transmural infarction than the subepicardium. During systole, the subendocardial coronary flow is opposed by pressure in the left ventricular cavity, whereas subepicardial flow is not. The extravascular forces acting on the intramural coronary arteries therefore reduce flow to the subendocardium, especially during exercise (Bache, 1981).

The functional importance of stenosis of a coronary artery is related to the degree of stenosis and the magnitude of flow through it. Resistance increases in a nonlinear fashion and may become 3 or more times as great as stenosis worsens. When coronary blood flow increases, the pressure drop across the stenosis becomes more pronounced when stenosis is severe. With stenosis of 30–50%, the pressure gradient is only slightly more pronounced when coronary flow is increased, but with stenosis of 70%, the gradient is markedly more pronounced (Klocke, 1983) (Fig 8–8).

Myocardial ischemia, which results when coronary blood flow is inadequate to meet the demands of the muscle at any moment, may be due to decreased oxygen supply (vasoconstriction, spasm, or obstruction) or increased demand. The latter occurs when factors such as heart rate, left ventricular wall stress, inotropic state of the myocardium, or preload cause increased myocardial oxygen consumption. Myocardial ischemia is regional, not global, and results from decreased perfusion in the area of a particular stenosed coronary artery. Myocardial ischemia can be documented by regional myocardial perfusion defects, decreased regional wall motion abnormalities, and ST elevation or depression on the ECG. Coronary spasm due to alpha-adrenergic receptor-mediated coronary constriction has been shown to be responsible (1) for variant (Prinzmetal's) angina; (2) for worsening of some cases of stable angina of effort; and (3) infrequently, for induction of myocardial infarction, presumably because of platelet aggregation resulting from endothelial injury consequent to the spasm (Maseri, 1980).

B. Pathologic Lesions and Serum Lipoprotein Studies: Patients with abnormal serum lipoprotein values who died of coronary heart disease showed at autopsy 75% stenosis of at least one, and often of 3, coronary arteries. A similar degree of stenosis is sometimes found in persons who had normal serum lipoproteins. Thus, lipoprotein abnormalities are not essential to the development of atherosclerosis.

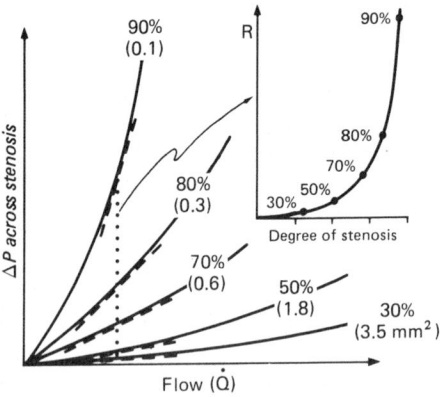

Figure 8–8. Relation between pressure reduction across a stenosis (ΔP) and flow through the stenosis (Q̇). Relations are shown for concentric stenoses of 30, 50, 70, 80, and 90% internal diameter. The numbers in parentheses below each percent diameter stenosis represent residual luminal cross-sectional area, calculated on the basis of a normal internal diameter of 3 mm and cross-sectional area of 7.1 mm^2. A potentially important advantage of the absolute area measurements is that they avoid underestimates of percent stenosis related to the inadvertent use of a narrowed segment adjacent to an arteriographic lesion when defining the severity of the lesion in relation to normal vessel diameter. In the formulation shown here, blood density and viscosity and stenosis length and divergence angle are assumed to be constant. The level of flow corresponding to basal metabolic needs is represented by the vertical dotted line; stenosis resistances for this level of flow are shown as the dashed tangent lines to the individual pressure-flow relations. In the inset on the right, stenosis resistance (R) is plotted as a function of degree of stenosis. (Redrawn, modified, and reproduced, with permission, from the American Heart Association, Inc., Klocke FJ: Measurements of coronary blood flow and degree of stenosis: Current clinical implications and continuing uncertainties. *Newsletter of the Council on Clinical Cardiology of the American Heart Association* [July] 1982;**7**[No.3].)

Arteriograms of patients studied within 1 year of onset of ischemic symptoms reveal stenosis of 1–3 coronary arteries. These changes may be seen very soon after onset of symptoms; this suggests that extensive atherosclerosis and even complete occlusion can precede the onset of symptoms.

C. Onset of Myocardial Infarction: Three mechanisms have been postulated to explain the onset of myocardial infarction: coronary thrombosis, subintimal hemorrhage, and coronary artery spasm (see p 139). Maseri believes that coronary spasm leads to platelet aggregation, which in turn leads to a sequence of events ending in thrombosis that may cause myocardial infarction (Maseri, 1983). (See also Angina Pectoris, pp 144 and 161.)

D. Ventricular Arrhythmias: Fibrosis and chronic ischemia of subendocardial fibers ("blighted zone") containing Purkinje cells induce variable excitability, automaticity, velocity of conduction, refractory periods, and repolarization in neighboring fibers, leading to electrical instability with ventricular fibrillation and sudden death. Ventricular fibrillation is the chief mechanism of cardiac arrest in apparently healthy individuals and in those with known coronary disease who have been resuscitated after apparent death in cardiac arrest. Sudden death is rarely due to conduction defects or Stokes-Adams attacks in the absence of acute anterior myocardial infarction. Emotional factors, with intense sympathetic discharge from the central nervous system, have been incriminated in some patients who have developed ventricular tachycardia or fibrillation or acute myocardial infarction. Vagal stimulation may decrease the heart rate and lead to an increased incidence of arrhythmia, aggravated by sympathetic stimulation.

E. Unusual Demands and Myocardial Ischemia: Unusual demands (unaccustomed severe exertion, rapid ventricular rates, intense emotion, acute hypoxemia, severe anemia, or blood loss) on a myocardium already compromised by decreased flow from coronary artery stenoses may precipitate local chemical and pathophysiologic events in patients with coronary atherosclerosis and may explain unexpected myocardial infarction.

F. Mural Obstruction of Left Anterior Descending Coronary Artery: Muscular bridges may obstruct the left anterior coronary artery in its intramyocardial portion and may lead to myocardial ischemia and sudden death in the absence of coronary atherosclerosis (Morales, 1980).

GENERAL CONSIDERATIONS IN CORONARY HEART DISEASE

Coronary heart disease has a wide variety of clinical manifestations ranging from asymptomatic to angina pectoris of effort, unstable angina, acute myocardial infarction, coronary spasm, or sudden death. The basic disease is almost always coronary atherosclerosis. Its course is variable, and symptoms and signs may occur singly or in combination, often with asymptomatic intervals.

The basis for clinical diagnosis is a history of angina pectoris, myocardial infarction, cardiac failure, or arrhythmias. Risk factors must be noted and evaluated. Various exercise and noninvasive tests can be used to evaluate possible abnormalities in coronary circulation and degrees of myocardial ischemia and dysfunction (see p 168). Ultimately, however, coronary angiograms must be used to define coronary arteries and ventricular angiography to determine impaired contractility or aneurysmal dilatation in localized areas. The evaluation of patients with coronary disease may be complex and best performed by cooperating specialists in related disciplines.

LATENT CORONARY HEART DISEASE

Initial Symptoms in Latent Coronary Heart Disease

Sudden death may be the first and only clinical manifestation of coronary heart disease; this means that asymptomatic coronary heart disease must have existed in the time immediately preceding this event.

Middle-aged individuals may present not with angina but with ventricular arrhythmias or atrioventricular or bundle branch conduction defects that may be the first manifestation of coronary heart disease. Asymptomatic atrial fibrillation is rarely such a manifestation, because it is uncommon even in patients with stable angina pectoris. Stokes-Adams attacks in patients with complete atrioventricular block usually occur during the initial phase of acute myocardial infarction or in the months following an acute anterior myocardial infarction, but Stokes-Adams attacks occur infrequently as an isolated manifestation of coronary disease in asymptomatic patients. Short bouts of ventricular premature beats of tachycardia are a more important manifestation and may be the precursors of ventricular fibrillation and sudden death. Ventricular premature beats, however, are so common and variable in the older population at large that it is difficult to classify them as manifestations of asymptomatic coronary disease. Furthermore, various studies have shown that premature beats in the absence of clinical coronary disease do not presage sudden death.

Noninvasive Investigation of Possible Myocardial Ischemia in Asymptomatic Individuals

Increasingly, efforts are being made by use of noninvasive tests to recognize the presence of ischemic coronary disease in asymptomatic individuals who want to be reassured about the absence of coronary disease. These include persons whose occupations have public safety implications (airline pilots, bus drivers, railroad engineers); executives being considered for promotion or transfer to a new position; persons at high risk of coronary disease by virtue of a history of early coronary disease in first-degree relatives; persons who have multiple risk factors for coronary disease (familial hypercholesterolemia, hypertension, diabetes); or middle-aged persons who simply want the evaluation. Controversy exists over the desirability of performing such noninvasive procedures as electrocardiography or radionuclide studies at rest or after exercise, because of the likelihood of both false-positive and false-negative tests. The sensitivity, specificity, and predictive value of such tests (see below and Fig 8–12) depend upon the selection of subjects, the criteria for a positive test, the degree of stenosis of the coronary artery, the presence of noncoronary cardiac disease, and the skill of the cardiologist. The procedure to be followed in the event of a positive test is also controversial. Should one proceed to coronary arteriography if the exercise ECG shows significant ST depression in an asymptomatic middle-aged man? For further discussion, see Noninvasive Tests, p 148.

SUDDEN DEATH

Sudden death is the first and only clinical manifestation of coronary heart disease in about one-fourth of patients. Most sudden deaths are not totally unexplained or unexpected; often, the patient has had coronary or hypertensive heart disease or has recently sought medical care for symptoms that were disregarded or misinterpreted. One study showed that about a third of the patients had seen a physician within 2 weeks before death complaining of various prodromal symptoms (Table 8–1). The recurrence rate of ventricular fibrillation—the mechanism of "sudden death syndrome"—is high: about 30% in the first year and 50% by 3 years (Cobb, 1975, 1980).

Survivors of out-of-hospital ventricular fibrillation subsequently studied by cardiac catheterization and coronary arteriography demonstrated a high prevalence of advanced coronary atherosclerosis (in one or more major coronary arteries), and three-fourths had abnormalities of left ventricular wall motion, indicating the likelihood of previous myocardial infarction. Of the patients who were resuscitated but died in subsequent months, at least two-thirds had "recurrent sudden death," indicating that the final event was similar to the initial event, usually ventricular fibrillation. Clinical findings in patients who were initially resuscitated but who subsequently died in the hospital are shown in Table 8–2.

Electrophysiologic studies in survivors of cardiac arrest have revealed sustained or unsustained ventricular tachycardia in about three-fourths of patients. Treatment of these patients with conventional drugs or newer drugs such as amiodarone decreases the likelihood of recurrence of cardiac arrest. Patients with recurrent ventricular arrhythmias associated with car-

Table 8–1. Distribution of prodromal symptoms in the 2 weeks before death among 208 arteriosclerotic heart disease sudden deaths and data on whether the symptom was increasing in frequency.*

Symptom	Total		Increasing in Frequency	
	Number	Percent	Number	Percent
Chest pain	77	37	28	13
Shortness of breath	88	42	38	18
Coughing	64	31	25	12
Fainting	10	5	4	2
Dizziness	29	14	19	9
Palpitations	22	11	9	4
Undue fatigue	116	56	78	38
Difficulty sleeping	59	28	28	13

*Reproduced, with permission, from Kuller L, Cooper M, Perper J: Epidemiology of sudden death. Arch Intern Med 1972; 129:714.

Table 8-2. Common clinical findings on admission among 92 deaths in hospital.*†

On Admission	Number	Percent
Clinical shock	32	35
Pulmonary edema	30	33
Coma	13	14
Ventricular fibrillation	6	7
Ventricular tachycardia	1	1
Complete heart block	4	4
Left bundle branch system block	6	7
At least one of the above	56	61

*Reproduced, with permission, from Kuller L, Cooper M, Perper J: Epidemiology of sudden death. Arch Intern Med 1972; 129:714.
†Excludes 2 incomplete cases.

diac arrest should undergo two-dimensional echocardiography or left ventricular angiography to identify ventricular aneurysm, which occurs in a substantial percentage of these patients. If an aneurysm is found, aneurysmectomy and endocardial resection should be considered (see p 176; see p 142 for Prevention of Sudden Death).

One-fourth of deaths due to coronary disease in the USA and UK are investigated by a coroner. Autopsy usually discloses severe atherosclerosis involving 2 or 3 coronary arteries even though the patient had had no prior symptoms. Of patients who died within an hour of the onset of the acute episode, more than 90% had coronary artery disease. Recent coronary thrombosis, intramural or subintimal hemorrhage, and recent myocardial infarction are also found, suggesting that sudden death is due to arrhythmia, probably ventricular fibrillation. This hypothesis is reinforced by the ECGs obtained by mobile coronary ambulance crews, which demonstrated ventricular fibrillation in most patients who have collapsed and were apparently "dead." If and when these patients are resuscitated and subsequently studied, myocardial infarction can be demonstrated in half of them, but a history of cardiovascular disease can be elicited in about three-fourths of patients. Interviews with relatives of people who died indicate that the most significant relationship between sudden death and other identifiable factors was that with acute psychologic stress (Myers, 1975). The age-adjusted incidence of sudden death increased with increasing blood pressure, serum cholesterol, relative weight, and cigarettes smoked per day at the time of the initial examination in the Framingham Study (Kannel, 1982).

Differential Diagnosis

In deaths investigated by the coroner's office, sudden unexpected, unexplained deaths that occur within 1 hour after onset of symptoms are almost always due to coronary heart disease. When death is delayed more than 2 hours, coronary disease is less commonly the cause but is still the cause in at least half of cases. Other causes are overwhelming sepsis; other cardiac disorders such as myocarditis, cardiomyopathy, aortic stenosis or aortic dissection; cerebral hemorrhage; shock due to any cause; or bowel obstruction (Table 8-3). The so-called café coronary, which is due to tracheal obstruction by food while eating, may be confused with sudden death from coronary disease. (See also p 155.)

Prevention of Sudden Death

Sudden death can be prevented both by management of cardiac arrest or acute myocardial ischemia and by longer-term approaches designed to prevent cardiac arrest (see pp 178-192). Since most deaths due to coronary heart disease occur suddenly, usually owing to ventricular fibrillation, successful resuscitation depends upon how quickly trained persons can

Table 8-3. Principal conditions other than coronary artery disease associated with or causing sudden death in adults.*

Cardiovascular
  Rheumatic heart disease
  Bacterial endocarditis
  Myocarditis
  Cardiomyopathies (primary myocardial disease)
  Ruptured aortic aneurysm
  Aortic dissection
  Coronary embolism
  Coronary microembolism
  Mitral valve prolapse
  Long QT interval syndrome
  Conduction defects associated with diseases of the myocardium (eg, sarcoidosis, scleroderma, Chagas' disease)
  Cardiac failure

Respiratory
  Pulmonary thromboembolism
  Pneumonias
  Asthma
  Bilateral midline fixation of cricoarytenoid joint

Central nervous system
  Intracerebral hemorrhage
  Subarachnoid hemorrhage
  Meningitis
  Encephalomyelitis

Gastrointestinal
  Gastrointestinal hemorrhage
  Peritonitis associated with perforated peptic ulcer
  Alcoholism and nutritional fatty liver or cirrhosis

Other
  Trauma
  Poisoning and drug reactions
  Fulminating infections, including meningococcemia
  Amniotic embolism
  Air embolism
  Fat embolism
  Myxedema
  Amyloidosis
  Hemochromatosis
  Endocrine dysfunction
  Leukemia

*Modified and reproduced, with permission, from Schwartz CJ, Walsh WJ: The pathologic basis of sudden death. Prog Cardiovasc Dis 1971;13:465.

institute appropriate measures to sustain the patient until defibrillation can be accomplished. There is no doubt that lives have been saved in communities where specially equipped, trained paramedics are available and can reach the patient within 2–3 minutes, recognize arrhythmias, administer atropine or lidocaine, and accomplish defibrillation.

The data summarized in Tables 8–1 and 8–2 show that about two-thirds of patients who are resuscitated subsequently testify to having had premonitory symptoms in the preceding 1–2 weeks, and one-fourth of them saw a physician in the preceding 1–2 days, not necessarily for a recognizable cardiac complaint. However, because so many sudden deaths are unwitnessed or occur so soon after the development of acute symptoms that the mobile coronary care team cannot arrive in time, it can be fairly stated that most patients with ventricular fibrillation do not survive—even those resuscitated during the acute phase. In one study, only about 30% of 1106 patients found to be in ventricular fibrillation by the mobile team were eventually discharged from the hospital, although over 40% had been initially resuscitated (Cobb, 1980).

A. Coronary Care Unit: Prompt diagnosis of acute myocardial ischemia, preferably in coronary care units, and immediate recognition and treatment of ventricular arrhythmias, ventricular fibrillation, cardiac failure, and cardiogenic shock may prevent secondary ventricular fibrillation. The early recognition and treatment of the sequelae of acute myocardial ischemia or infarction (eg, conduction defects, arrhythmias, extension of infarction, ventricular septal defect, papillary muscle dysfunction, subacute rupture with pseudoaneurysm, left ventricular aneurysm, and other conditions) are discussed in the treatment of acute myocardial infarction on pp 172–189.

B. Automatic Implantable Defibrillator: This device, now undergoing trial, monitors cardiac rhythm continuously and is designed to detect ventricular fibrillation or ventricular tachycardia and deliver automatically a discharge of 25 J within 20 seconds. This promising device has been tested in experimental animals and in the laboratory and has now been used successfully in patients who have had a number of cardiac arrests and have not responded to multiple antiarrhythmic drugs. Details of insertion and modification of the equipment can be found in Mirowski (1982).

C. Cigarette Smoking: The relationship between cigarette smoking and sudden death has been extensively documented. In cases studied by the coroner's office, for example, sudden deaths from coronary heart disease are 2–3 times as common in smokers as in nonsmokers, which suggests that cigarette smoking may predispose to ventricular fibrillation in susceptible individuals. Although sudden death occurs at an older age in women than in men, it occurs in younger women who are heavy smokers. The electrophysiologic mechanism by which smoking causes ventricular fibrillation in patients with coronary artery disease is not fully understood. Coronary disease is progressive, and there may come a point at which obstruction is critically balanced with respect to supply and demand, so that smoking may result in less successful perfusion of myocardial cells and in this way produce the electrical instability that results in ventricular fibrillation.

D. Drug Therapy: Preventive measures may include long-term use of beta-adrenergic blocking agents, possible long-term use of calcium entry–blocking agents, use of antiplatelet drugs, and vigorous use of antiarrhythmic agents in high-risk patients, especially those with previous episodes of ventricular fibrillation or with known coronary disease and complex ventricular arrhythmias.

E. Physical Activity: The high incidence of both coronary disease and coronary deaths in the lumberjacks of northeastern Finland indicates that strenuous physical activity does not effectively protect against coronary disease. Increased physical activity may lead to increased food intake, and there is some evidence that serum cholesterol is slightly higher in eastern than in western Finland, where the coronary mortality rate in men is half that of eastern Finland.

F. Surgical Measures: Coronary bypass surgery has been shown to decrease the incidence of sudden death in patients with left main coronary stenosis exceeding 70%, and probably in patients with 3-vessel coronary disease associated with easily induced ischemia and only moderately impaired left ventricular function. For further details, see pp 192–194.

Emergency Measures

A. Resuscitation: (See also Chapter 7.) The value of resuscitation efforts on behalf of patients with ventricular fibrillation has been demonstrated in a number of community studies in which the 1-year survival rate of those who were resuscitated was about 70%. Resuscitated patients with primary ventricular fibrillation are often able to return to work with adequate left ventricular function. There is an increased likelihood of recurrence of ventricular fibrillation within the next year, and the long-term prognosis is guarded unless antiarrhythmic agents are given and attention is paid to social, psychologic, and environmental factors in order to reduce adrenergic impulses operating "through the mind" that may produce coronary vasoconstriction.

B. Patient Education: The high mortality rate of ventricular fibrillation in acute myocardial infarction and the high incidence of sudden death within 1–3 hours after the acute ischemic episode have highlighted the need for shortening the interval between onset of symptoms and admission to a coronary care unit. There should be no delay in getting the patient to the hospital, and this means within 1 hour at most after onset of symptoms. The best advice is to get to the hospital and *then* call the personal physician.

In spite of public education efforts, even patients with previous coronary heart disease and those who have been told to seek immediate care should new symptoms or a change of symptoms appear sometimes delay seeking medical care, perhaps because patients fail to realize the significance of the symptoms or try to combat the fear of death with the psychologic mechanism of denial.

Although excessive physical activity or intense emotion may be responsible in some instances, especially when death is instantaneous (within seconds), most sudden deaths occur during the patient's usual activities and not as a result of some determinable unusual event.

Delays in treatment in the emergency room must be minimized. Emergency rooms should be equipped for immediate monitoring and resuscitation. Patients who are not accustomed to strenuous physical exertion should be warned of its risks, especially in a setting of emotional stress or on unusually cold, windy, or unusually hot, humid days. Shoveling snow after dinner and pushing stalled automobiles in the winter or in cold weather are particularly dangerous activities. Hot, humid weather increases the blood flow to the skin and increases the work of the heart.

C. Reversibility of Sudden Death: There is no doubt that sudden death due to primary ventricular fibrillation is reversible in many cases. Many survivors have had no episodes of acute myocardial infarction after resuscitation, as shown by serial enzyme and electrocardiographic examination. Most have the same left ventricular function 1 year later as they had before the episode of fibrillation. Furthermore, when cardiac arrest occurs during electrocardiographic monitoring of these patients, the arrhythmia is ventricular fibrillation rather than ventricular standstill. Therefore, a major public health effort should be directed toward identifying groups of people most likely to have primary ventricular fibrillation and devising methods of preventing the attacks. The most important of these preventive measures is treatment of ventricular arrhythmias in patients with known coronary heart disease. Unfortunately, the currently available antiarrhythmic agents (quinidine, procainamide, phenytoin, and propranolol) are of limited effectiveness and often produce side effects that make continued therapy difficult (Jelinek, 1974). The value of beta blockers has been established (see p 157). Newer investigational drugs such as lorcainide, encainide, flecainide, mexiletine, and others are being extensively studied and will probably prove more effective, despite side effects.

D. Defibrillation: When ventricular fibrillation occurs in coronary care units, it often is preceded by ventricular tachycardia or multifocal ventricular premature beats. A small electric shock during this period may depolarize the reentry circuit, terminating the ventricular tachycardia. A sharp thump on the chest is not quite as effective but may do the same. Electrophysiologic studies have demonstrated that myocardium which has been damaged by fibrosis or by ischemic episodes has a variable recovery of excitability and duration of refractoriness in neighboring cells; this can lead to multiple reentry circuits, which in turn may initiate ventricular fibrillation. Prompt treatment of ventricular tachycardia in susceptible patients may prevent ventricular fibrillation. Use of the automatic implanted pacemaker shows considerable promise (Mirowski, 1982).

E. Café Coronary: See p 121.

SPECIFIC TYPES OF CORONARY HEART DISEASE

ANGINA PECTORIS OF EFFORT; VARIANT (PRINZMETAL'S) ANGINA (CORONARY SPASM)

Angina pectoris is usually due to atherosclerotic heart disease, but rare cases occur in the absence of significant coronary disease as a result of severe aortic stenosis or insufficiency; syphilitic aortitis; increased metabolic demands (eg, in hyperthyroidism or after thyroid therapy); marked anemia; paroxysmal tachycardias with rapid ventricular rates; emboli, arteritis, or as has recently been reemphasized, coronary spasm. The underlying mechanism is a discrepancy between myocardial demands for oxygen and substrate and the amount delivered through the coronary arteries. Four groups of variables determine the production of relative or absolute myocardial ischemia:

(1) Limitation of oxygen delivered by the coronary arteries: (a) Vessel factors: atherosclerotic narrowing; inadequate collateral circulation; reflex narrowing in response to emotion, cold, upper gastrointestinal disease, or smoking. (b) Blood factors: anemia, hypoxemia, polycythemia (increased viscosity). (c) Circulatory factors: fall in blood pressure due to arrhythmias, bleeding, and Valsalva's maneuver; decreased filling pressure of or decreased flow to the coronary arteries due to aortic stenosis or insufficiency.

(2) Increased cardiac output: (a) Physiologic factors: exertion, excitement, digestive and metabolic processes following a heavy meal. (b) Pathologic factors (high output states): anemia, thyrotoxicosis, arteriovenous fistula, pheochromocytoma.

(3) Increased myocardial demands for oxygen: Increased work of the heart, as in aortic stenosis, aortic insufficiency, diastolic hypertension; increased oxygen consumption due to thyrotoxicosis or to any state characterized by increased catecholamine excretion (pheochromocytoma, strong emotion, hypoglycemia).

Patients who develop exercise-induced angina during cardiac catheterization show a rise in arterial pressure and left ventricular end-diastolic pressure just before the appearance of angina and the ischemic changes in the ECG. Myocardial oxygen consumption increases similarly. The changes indicate that left ventricular failure or decreased compliance often coincides with the appearance of angina.

(4) Decreased myocardial supply secondary to coronary spasm: (See also p 146.) Coronary artery spasm contributes to manifestations of ischemic cardiac disease (Fig 8–9). "Variant" angina has been attributed to spasm of the large coronary arteries, because coronary arteriograms are frequently negative and because ECG may show elevation and not depression of the ST segment during pain.

Decreased coronary blood flow may result from coronary spasm in the absence of increased myocardial demands. Furthermore, it has been shown that angina pectoris and even myocardial infarction may occur in the absence of visible obstructive coronary artery disease (normal coronary arteriogram). It has therefore been postulated that coronary artery spasm alone in the absence of arteriosclerotic coronary artery disease may be sufficient to produce myocardial ischemia and infarction, although most instances of coronary spasm occur in the presence of coronary stenoses.

Increased coronary vascular resistance due to coronary artery vasoconstriction has been demonstrated experimentally and the mechanism clarified by the use of agents that activate and inhibit alpha-adrenergic receptors (norepinephrine and phentolamine, respectively). Transient localized spasm relieved by nitrates has been noted in about 5% of cases during coronary angiography. Spasm may be confined to an area near the tip of the catheter and therefore is presumably due to mechanical irritation, or it may occur some distance away from the catheter, in which case it is thought to indicate neural or neurohumoral activation. It is therefore necessary to exclude spasm before diagnosing organic stenosis of a coronary artery during coronary arteriography, and it is routine to obtain the arteriogram in multiple views and to give sublingual nitroglycerin or isosorbide dinitrate in an attempt to reverse possible spasm.

Clinical Findings

The term angina denotes a specific type of chest discomfort associated with myocardial ischemia and is now used only in that sense. Pain in the chest is one of the most common complaints the physician is called upon to assess.

A. Symptoms:

1. Characteristics of anginal pain–(See also Chapter 2.) The discomfort is described by most patients as a sensation of tightness or pressure that starts in the center of the chest and subsequently radiates to the lower jaw, to the inner surface of the left arm, and to the volar surface of the fourth and fifth fingers.

a. Precipitating factors–The pain is induced by anything that increases the oxygen requirements of the myocardium; examples are exercise, sexual activity, emotional stress, cold weather, wind, a large meal, anemia, an increase in blood pressure, tachycardia, high altitude, or decreased oxygen content of the inspired air. The essential features of the history include the circumstances that precipitate or relieve the discomfort and the characteristics of the discomfort itself, including its location, radiation, and duration. The essential feature is that the discomfort is precipitated in circumstances that increase the oxygen demands of the myocardium; the most common occasion is

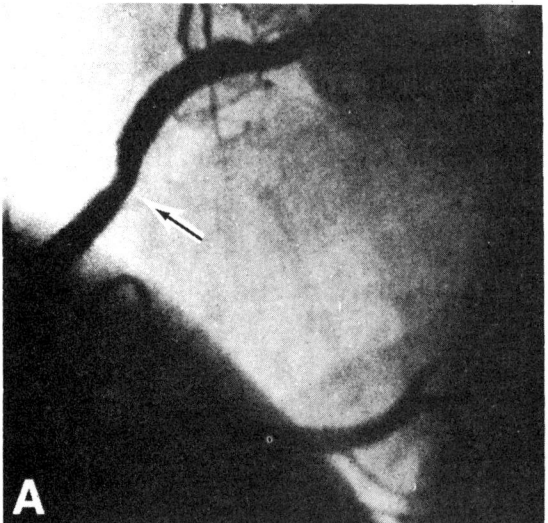 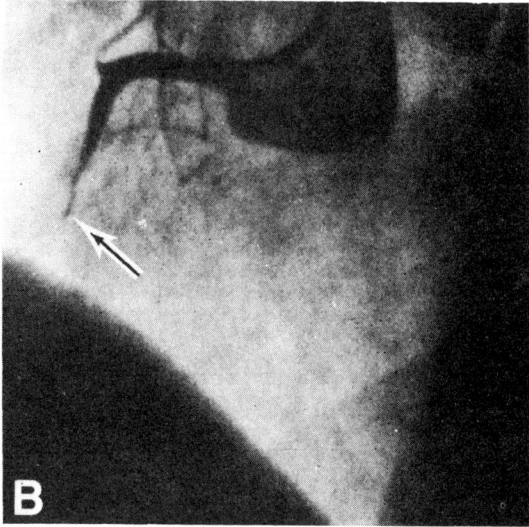

Figure 8–9. Arteriograms of the right coronary artery in left anterior oblique projection demonstrate localized 40% narrowing in the proximal right coronary artery (arrow) after nitroglycerin *(A)* and total obstruction in the same area (arrow) after ergonovine maleate *(B)*. Angina and ST segment elevation in the inferior electrocardiographic leads developed during spasm. (Reproduced, with permission, from Heupler FA Jr, Proudfit WL: Nifedipine therapy for refractory coronary arterial spasm. *Am J Cardiol* 1979;**44**:798.)

during walking, especially when the patient is hurrying or walking up an incline or a flight of stairs.

Prinzmetal (1959) described one type of angina occurring at rest and sometimes relieved with exercise as "variant angina"; it is thought to be due to coronary vasoconstriction. Variant angina occasionally occurs in patients with minimal coronary stenosis or spasms, but usually with substantial coronary artery lesions.

Usually, however, the discomfort of angina occurs during exertion and subsides promptly if the patient stands or sits quietly. If other factors upset the balance between myocardial oxygen supply and demand, less activity is required to produce angina, especially after meals, during times of emotional excitement, or on exposure to a cold wind. Heavy meals and strong emotion can provoke an attack even with trivial exertion.

The discomfort of angina of effort lasts but a short time if the effort is discontinued—almost always less than 10–15 minutes and usually much less. The discomfort develops and subsides fairly quickly but not abruptly. If the effort is continued unabated, the discomfort increases until the patient must stop. Occasionally, a patient learns to decrease activity until discomfort subsides and thus "walks through" the angina.

b. Quality of anginal pain–Patients describe anginal pain as pressing, squeezing, a tightness, a weight on the chest—rarely as though the chest is in a vise. They may describe it as burning and may have difficulty finding the right word but will convey the type of discomfort by pressing on the chest with both hands. Many patients use the term discomfort or distress rather than pain and will answer "No" to the question, "Do you have or have you had chest pain?" The pain is rarely stabbing, lancinating, pointed, or piercing.

c. Location of anginal pain–The pain usually covers a fairly broad area in the central chest and has diffuse, ill-defined edges. Although it may be dominantly left precordial, it almost always involves the central chest and is rarely solely left precordial, lateral, or epigastric. Anginal pain may involve the lower area of the sternum and extend into the epigastrium. Rarely is there localized tenderness during or between attacks—in contrast to patients with musculoskeletal or radicular disease, in whom this is common.

d. Radiation of anginal pain–The pain radiates to the lower jaw (never to the upper jaw), upper neck, left shoulder, and inner surface of the arm to the ulnar surface of the hand in the fourth and fifth fingers. It may be felt only as a sensation of pressure across the volar surface of the wrist. Rarely, a patient with angina may go to the dentist with a "toothache" or to an orthopedist complaining of upper back pain. Chest discomfort is often the only symptom, but there may be associated dyspnea if there is some element of left ventricular failure during episodes of pain. Angina and left ventricular chest pain are often difficult to distinguish.

The pain or discomfort of angina pectoris is a visceral pain from the heart referred from C8–T4 segmental dermatomes. Small pain fibers run with the autonomic nerves and enter the spinal cord in the C8–T4 segments. As with all visceral pain, it is poorly localized. The diaphragm is innervated by T4, and neck pain may be related to the cutaneous pattern of this segment. The thumb is innervated by C5 and C6 and is rarely involved in anginal pain.

e. Ease of production of pain–The ease of production of the pain during effort varies on different days, often depending upon how the patient feels emotionally, whether the patient is out of doors or not, how cold and windy it is, and how much time has elapsed since eating. All of these factors increase the work of the heart. When patients with "stable" or chronic angina are exercised in a comfortable laboratory on an empty stomach in a relaxed state of mind, the amount of exercise required to induce pain is fairly constant (within 10%).

f. Patient response to pain–Patients learn to avoid pain by recognizing the earliest manifestations of pressure or tightness in the chest when they are walking or start to get excited. Most patients must slow down or stop walking and stand still, since otherwise the pain worsens until they are forced to stop. A patient may have discomfort hurrying to the bus in the morning but may find that a similar amount of effort later in the morning or in the afternoon causes no discomfort. Similarly, an individual may have discomfort during the first one or 2 holes of golf and then play the rest of the game in comfort. This uncommon "second wind" phenomenon is presumably explained by local vasodilatation caused by metabolites accumulated during the ischemic pain period.

g. Coronary spasm (Prinzmetal's variant angina)–(See also p 139.) Prinzmetal's variant angina differs from ordinary angina of effort in that it is more apt to occur at rest than with effort, may occasionally be relieved with exercise, may occur at odd times during the day or night (even awakening patients from sleep), and is more likely to be associated with various types of arrhythmias or conduction defects; the ST segment is more commonly elevated rather than depressed, as occurs during angina of effort. There are hemodynamic differences as well (Fig 8–10). Both variant angina and angina of effort respond rapidly to sublingual nitrates as well as to nifedipine. Patients with variant angina usually have no history of previous myocardial infarction, whereas those with the usual angina of effort often have such a history. Variant angina is more common in women under age 50, whereas angina of effort is uncommon in women of this age in the absence of severe hypercholesterolemia, hypertension, or diabetes mellitus.

The observation of coronary spasm during coronary arteriography; the demonstration of perfusion defects by radioisotope studies during induced spasm; and the recognition of angina pectoris at rest, of myocardial infarction, and of ventricular arrhythmias in the absence of stenoses of the coronary arteries have

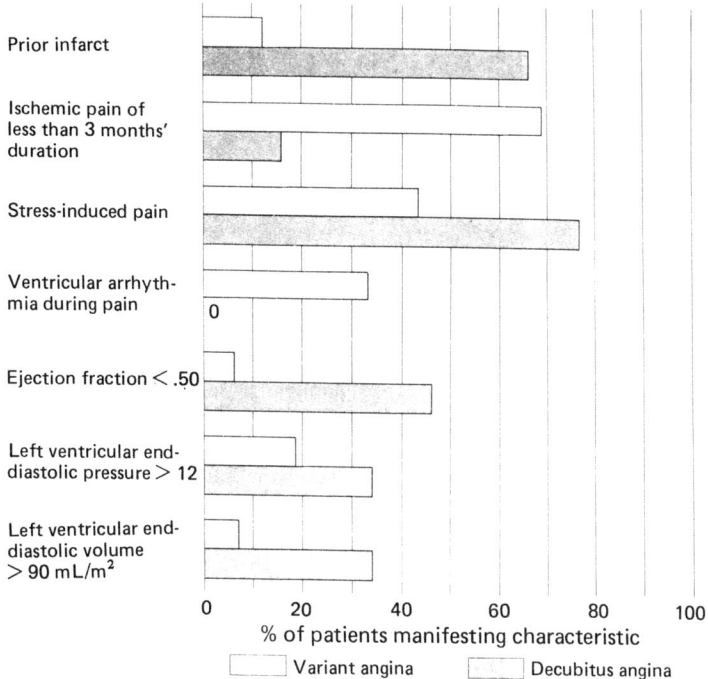

Figure 8–10. Comparison of clinical and hemodynamic findings in 42 variant and 50 decubitus angina patients (mean age 52 and 54 years, respectively) supports the view that the 2 syndromes are distinct entities. With one exception, left ventricular end-diastolic pressure, differences in all parameters analyzed were statistically significant. (Reproduced, with permission, from Johnson AD: Management of variant angina and coronary spasm. Hosp Pract [March] 1978;4:57.)

widened the entire concept of the role of coronary spasm in clinical disease.

Angina has been provoked by ergotamine used for the treatment of migraine and has been specifically induced by ergonovine for diagnosis during coronary arteriography. Because the resulting spasm may be intense and may induce angina, arrhythmias, or myocardial infarction, the drug should be used with considerable caution, in small doses, under close clinical observation, and with resuscitation equipment at hand.

If patients with angina due to coronary spasm do not respond rapidly to nitrates, coronary vasodilators such as verapamil, diltiazem, or nifedipine may be given not only in Prinzmetal's variant angina but also in the usual angina of effort in which spasm may be superimposed. Coronary artery spasm due to neurohumoral influences may occur in patients with or without coronary artery stenoses and may play a role in the frequent association of emotional events and angina pectoris.

2. Interpretation of pain of angina pectoris–The interpretation of the symptom must be based on the history alone, because about one-fourth of patients have no objective clinical findings of coronary atherosclerosis to support the history. The diagnosis may be simple or extremely difficult. The diagnosis of angina is more probable if there is electrocardiographic evidence of myocardial ischemia or a history of myocardial infarction. The likelihood that an uncertain history represents angina is increased by the presence of resting or induced myocardial ischemia or of other atherosclerotic manifestations such as intermittent claudication, cerebral ischemic attacks, or bruits over the major arteries.

3. Induction of pain as support for the diagnosis of angina–The diagnosis is strongly supported (1) if the patient's chest discomfort is induced by procedures (such as exercise, rapid atrial pacing, or isoproterenol infusion) that increase myocardial oxygen demand and if production of chest discomfort is associated with electrocardiographic evidence of myocardial ischemia; (2) if wall motion contraction abnormalities can be demonstrated by radioangiography; (3) if thallium perfusion defects are seen during exercise, with redistribution at rest; or (4) if transiently raised left ventricular end-diastolic pressure occurs with evidence of left ventricular dysfunction. Continuous electrocardiographic tape recordings (Holter) for 12–24 hours can be used to look for the presence of ischemic ST segments during episodes of pain or in the absence of pain (Fig 8–11).

Coronary arteriography is rarely justified for diagnosis alone except in unusual circumstances (see p 151).

B. Signs: Examination is often completely negative in patients with angina pectoris who have not

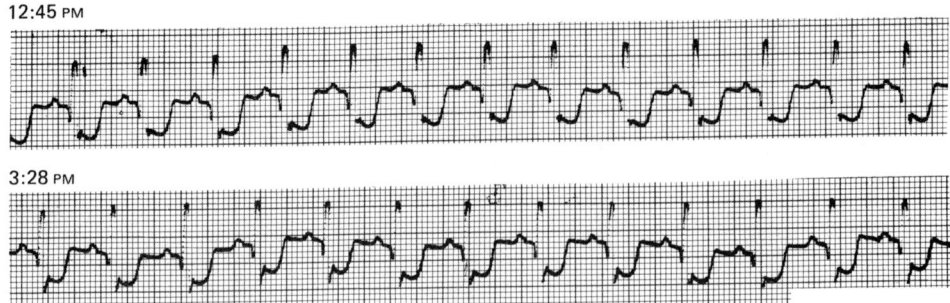

Figure 8-11. Holter monitor ECG of a 65-year-old man showing marked ST depression of myocardial ischemia when the patient carried out his ordinary work routine as a salesperson. There were no symptoms during the time of the ischemic changes on the ECGs, but angina pectoris of effort occurred at other times. (Courtesy of Dr William Atchley.)

had a previous myocardial infarction and who show no evidence of hypertensive or aortic valve disease. During an attack, the systolic and diastolic blood pressures are usually significantly elevated, and there may be a third or fourth heart sound, pulsus alternans, or transient pulmonary rales.

C. Hemodynamic Observations: The clinical signs mentioned in ¶B, above, have been shown in some patients during cardiac catheterization. The pulse rate may be increased, and carotid sinus massage to slow the ventricular rate may abruptly reverse the process. This maneuver (carotid sinus massage) can be used as a diagnostic test.

D. Laboratory Findings: Routine laboratory findings in stable angina pectoris are usually normal. Anemia, hypercholesterolemia, hypertriglyceridemia, diabetes mellitus, hypoglycemia, hyperthyroidism, and upper gastrointestinal tract diseases should be investigated as possible contributing factors. A chest x-ray is valuable to exclude pulmonary or skeletal abnormalities that might be the cause of pain. The resting ECG is normal in about one-fourth of patients with stable angina. In the remainder, abnormalities include patterns of left ventricular hypertrophy, old myocardial infarction, nonspecific ST–T abnormalities, and atrioventricular or conduction defects.

E. Special Investigations: Fig 8-12 indicates the specificity and sensitivity of noninvasive tests in the diagnosis of angina pectoris and defines the terms used. Noninvasive tests are described in the next section, followed by a section on invasive special procedures.

Noninvasive Tests

Noninvasive tests may be important because a clear history of angina pectoris is sometimes difficult to obtain.

A. Routine ECG: An electrocardiographic abnormality on routine examination may reveal unexpected characteristic features of previous myocardial infarction such as typical abnormal Q waves or unequivocal ST–T abnormalities. Acute myocardial infarction may occur without symptoms, or the symptoms may be so atypical that the diagnosis of old infarction can only be made on the basis of electrocardiographic abnormalities.

B. Stress Electrocardiographic Tests: (See also Chapter 5.) Induction of chest discomfort by exercise has for many years been the commonest noninvasive technique used to provide objective evidence of myocardial ischemia. The current method uses a cycle ergometer or treadmill and the Bruce protocol, with progressive, graded exercise (stages 1–6). The physician may terminate the exercise at any stage (see Precautions, below).

1. Criteria for a positive electrocardiographic stress test–Table 8–4 gives the criteria for the diagnosis of coronary disease.

The original criteria for a positive test were the same for all studies, consisting of a horizontal downsloping ST segment depression of a degree that varied from 1 mm to 1.5 or 2 mm. Refinements of the electrocardiographic stress tests attempt to measure the degree of positivity and not merely to classify results as positive or negative. Factors considered in these refinements include the contour, depth, and area of the ST segment change (depression or elevation); the time of appearance (which stage of the Bruce protocol); the duration of the ST segment changes; the pulse rate achieved in relation to the maximum predicted for the age and sex of the patient; the coexistent development of anginal pain; and the appearance of hypotension or complex ventricular beats during exercise. These have led to attempts at quantitative grad-

Table 8–4. Criteria for diagnosis of coronary disease with exercise stress test (assuming normal baseline ECG and no digitalis).

Horizontal downsloping ST depression ≥ 2 mm.
Duration of ST depression > 3 min.
Angina pectoris during or immediately after the test.
Exercise associated with hypotension or blood pressure ≤ 130 mm Hg.

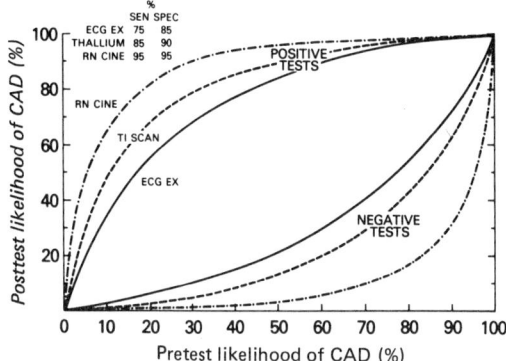

Figure 8–12. Probability of coronary artery disease (CAD). Comparison of electrocardiographic exercise testing (ECG EX), thallium perfusion scanning (Tl SCAN), and radionuclide cineangiography (RN CINE). (Sensitivity [SEN] and specificity [SPEC] values are approximations derived from published series.) (Reproduced, with permission, from Epstein SE: Implications of probability analysis on the strategy used for noninvasive detection of coronary artery disease: Role of single or combined use of exercise electrocardiographic testing, radionuclide cineangiography and myocardial perfusion imaging. *Am J Cardiol* 1980;40:491.)

Definitions

Predictive value of a positive test
= the probability that a patient has disease, given a positive test outcome

$$= \frac{\text{number of patients with disease}}{\text{total number of patients with a positive test}}$$

Predictive value of a negative test
= the probability that a patient does not have disease, given a negative test outcome

$$= \frac{\text{number of subjects without disease}}{\text{total number of subjects with a negative test}}$$

Sensitivity
= the probability a patient with disease will have a given test result

$$= \frac{\text{number of patients with disease with a given test result}}{\text{total number of tested patients with disease}}$$

Specificity
= the probability a patient without disease will not have the given test result

$$= \frac{\text{number of disease-free subjects not showing the test result}}{\text{total number of disease-free subjects tested}}$$

Pretest likelihood (= prior probability)
= the probability of disease in a subject to be tested

$$= \frac{\text{number of patients with disease in the test population}}{\text{total number of patients in the test population}}$$

Posttest likelihood (= posterior probability)
= the probability of disease in a subject showing a given test result

$$= \frac{\text{number of patients with disease showing a given test result}}{\text{total number of subjects showing the test result}}$$

ing of symptoms, in order to permit gradations of positivity by combining the ECG and clinical responses. A strongly positive test consists of marked ST changes (> 2 mm) that appear early and at a heart rate less than 85% of predicted maximum, and are associated with angina, hypotension, or complex arrhythmias. Additional refinements include having the patient perform the exercise test following use of beta-adrenergic blocking agents or with a hand placed in ice water, so that the effects of a cold pressor and an exercise electrocardiographic test are combined. It is difficult to interpret many of the published reports, because different criteria are used by different authors. It seems clear, however, that the greater the abnormality, the more marked the positivity and the more likely the presence of multivessel disease, including left main coronary disease. Care must be taken not to interpret a J junction depression as a positive test, because this occurs often in normal individuals, is of short duration, and immediately precedes the ST segment. Upsloping ST depression likewise is less significant than downsloping depression, and it may occur when a deep J junction ascends to the T wave. Elevated ST segment changes may also occur, possibly because of the association of coronary spasm with the effort (see p 146).

2. Precautions during exercise stress test– Exercise should not be performed if a recent myocardial infarction or unstable angina is suspected or if the patient is in a condition in which exercise would be unwise. Acute myocardial infarction may be precipitated if exercise testing is done in patients with acute or subacute myocardial ischemia and with pain of recent origin. The test must be done under the supervision of a physician, who should observe and examine the patient during the exercise and be able to perform resuscitative measures in the event of ventricular fibrillation. A continuous electrocardiographic recording should be obtained during exercise so the test can be stopped if necessary.

3. Prognostic significance of a positive exercise stress test–Ellestadt (1975) and Bruce (1977) both have shown that patients who have had positive exercise studies have increased rates of subsequent clinical coronary disease or death due to coronary disease (Figs 8–13 and 8–14).

4. General significance of a positive exercise stress electrocardiographic test–There is controversy about the desirability of performing exercise tests in asymptomatic middle-aged persons. Some of the same considerations pertain to patients with probable or definite angina pectoris. The specificity and predictive accuracy of an abnormal exercise ECG test is high in symptomatic individuals but generally less than 50% in asymptomatic individuals. The prevalence of the disease in the population being studied influences the reliability of any test. Even marked ST depression may represent a false-positive test, and a negative test is unreliable in excluding coronary disease. All clinical data must be taken into account in the interpretation of a positive test.

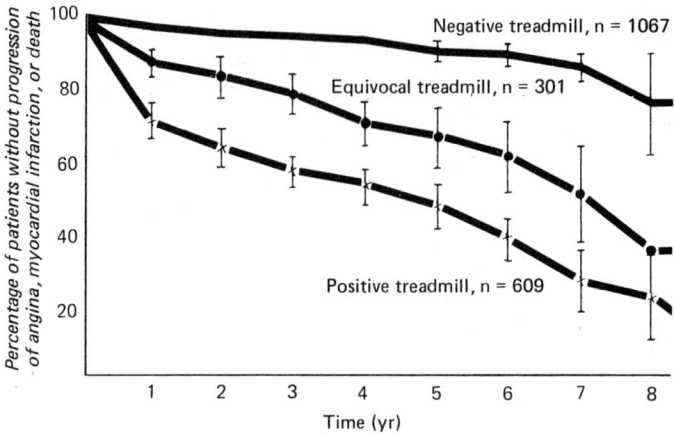

Figure 8–13. Life table display of an 8-year experience of absence of complications in approximately 2000 ambulatory individuals who had a negative, equivocal, or positive (ST depression of 1.5 mm or more) treadmill response (n, number of patients). (Reproduced, with permission, from the American Heart Association, Inc., Ellestad MH, Wan KC: Predictive implications of stress testing: Follow-up of 2700 subjects after maximum treadmill stress testing. *Circulation* 1975;**51**:363.)

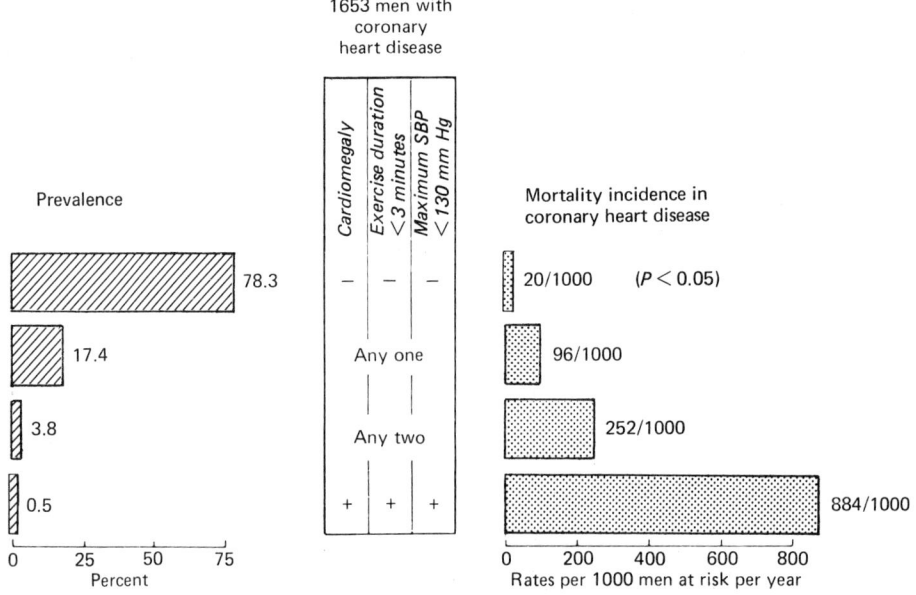

Figure 8–14. Mortality incidence in men with coronary heart disease, according to the presence or absence of 3 predictors: cardiomegaly, peak systolic pressure less than 130 mm Hg, and exercise duration not exceeding 3 min. P for the first row applies in combination with the second, third, and fourth rows and is based on Poisson confidence intervals. SBP, systolic blood pressure. (Reproduced, with permission, from Bruce RA: Exercise for evaluation of ventricular function. *N Engl J Med* 1977;**296**:671.)

Patients with known coronary disease can be divided into low- and high-risk subgroups on the basis of ease of production of pain and duration of exercise or electrocardiographic changes. Fig 8–15 shows a greatly increased survival rate in the low-risk group. Exercise testing is also useful in the assessment of left ventricular function, especially if the symptoms seem out of proportion to other clinical findings. Comparison of the functional capacity of the ventricles during exercise and at rest may reveal the onset of angina, dyspnea, or hypotension on slight effort of short duration and is therefore an important index of cardiac function. Noting changes on the ECG in association with maximal oxygen uptake during exercise also gives useful information about cardiovascular function.

C. Radioisotope Studies: If patients with atyp-

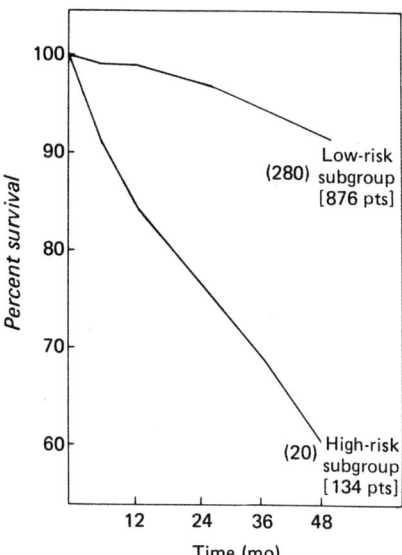

Figure 8–15. Cumulative life table survival rates in low- and high-risk subgroups. Numbers in parentheses represent the number of patients followed for 48 months. Numbers in brackets represent the number of patients in each subgroup. The low-risk subgroup includes those patients with a negative test or exercise duration ≥ stage IV or a maximum heart rate ≥ 160. The high-risk subgroup includes those patients with a positive test and exercise duration < stage III. (Reproduced, with permission, from the American Heart Association, Inc., McNeer JF et al: The role of the exercise test in the evaluation of patients for ischemic heart disease. *Circulation* 1978;57:64.)

ical chest pain thought possibly to be anginal have negative or equivocal exercise stress studies or if the presence of abnormalities at rest (such as conduction defects, ST–T changes, or changes due to medication) makes interpretation of stress ECG unreliable, radioisotope evaluation with thallium 201 during exercise and after redistribution should be obtained. Hypoperfusion (myocardial ischemia) with a discrete defect or "cold spot" that disappears after redistribution of the isotope a few hours later is a more reliable indication of ischemia than electrocardiographic exercise studies. False-negative results occur in a small percentage of patients.

Radionuclide angiography is the recommended radioisotope study when such studies are indicated in angina pectoris, because it may be more sensitive though less specific than thallium 201. Either the first-pass or the equilibrium-gated blood pool technique (see p 168) can be used. Whereas the appearance and disappearance of hypoperfusion defects with thallium indicate the presence of myocardial ischemia, radionuclide angiography assesses overall and regional left ventricular function by determining ejection fraction and the location and degree of wall motion (contraction) abnormalities. Ejection fraction can be determined from the difference between the systolic and diastolic isotope images of left ventricular volume. Outlines of these images in both phases of the cardiac cycle allow various segments of the left ventricle to be analyzed for localized areas of hypokinesia, akinesia, or dyskinesia. These areas correlate positively with myocardial fibrosis found at autopsy.

If a thallium defect is present at rest but does not increase and then resolve during and after exercise, one cannot infer the induction of myocardial ischemia or even the presence of an old myocardial infarct. The defect at rest may represent scar from any cause or chronic myocardial ischemia. The appearance and disappearance of a thallium defect is necessary to document that myocardial ischemia has been induced.

D. Two-Dimensional (2-D) Echocardiography: Two-dimensional echocardiography is valuable for qualitative but not quantitative evaluation of left ventricular function in patients with angina pectoris. It is difficult to perform and evaluate during exercise. It is valuable in identifying left ventricular aneurysm and associated pericardial effusion and for estimating ejection fraction (see p 186).

Left ventricular angiography and coronary angiography are the reference standards against which the noninvasive radioisotope studies must be judged.

E. Comparison of Exercise Electrocardiographic Testing, Radionuclide Studies at Rest and Exercise, and Coronary Arteriography: (See also pp 148 and 150 and Fig 8–12.) There is significant correspondence of results in these 3 methods of evaluation. Generally, hypoperfusion (transient or permanent) with thallium 201 and wall motion abnormalities with gated blood pool cardiac imaging are considered more specific than stress electrocardiographic tests.

The greatest sensitivity (the proportion of patients with established coronary disease who have a positive test) and specificity (the proportion of negative tests in patients proved not to have coronary disease) will be obtained when all 3 tests (ECG, thallium perfusion, and radionuclide angiography) are combined. The ultimate diagnostic procedure to establish coronary stenoses is invasive coronary arteriography combined with contrast ventriculography.

F. Newer Investigational Noninvasive Procedures: In an effort to avoid invasive procedures such as angiography, new diagnostic techniques utilizing computer processing are being developed. These include digital subtraction angiography used in association with CT scan, positron emission tomography (for the determination of abnormal myocardial metabolism), and magnetic resonance imaging (MRI) used alone or in combination with other methods (see Chapter 5).

Invasive Special Procedures

A. Coronary Arteriography: Coronary arteriography, because of its risk potential, should not be used solely for diagnosis and prognosis until the indications for coronary bypass surgery are more definitely established. Experienced workers find that the

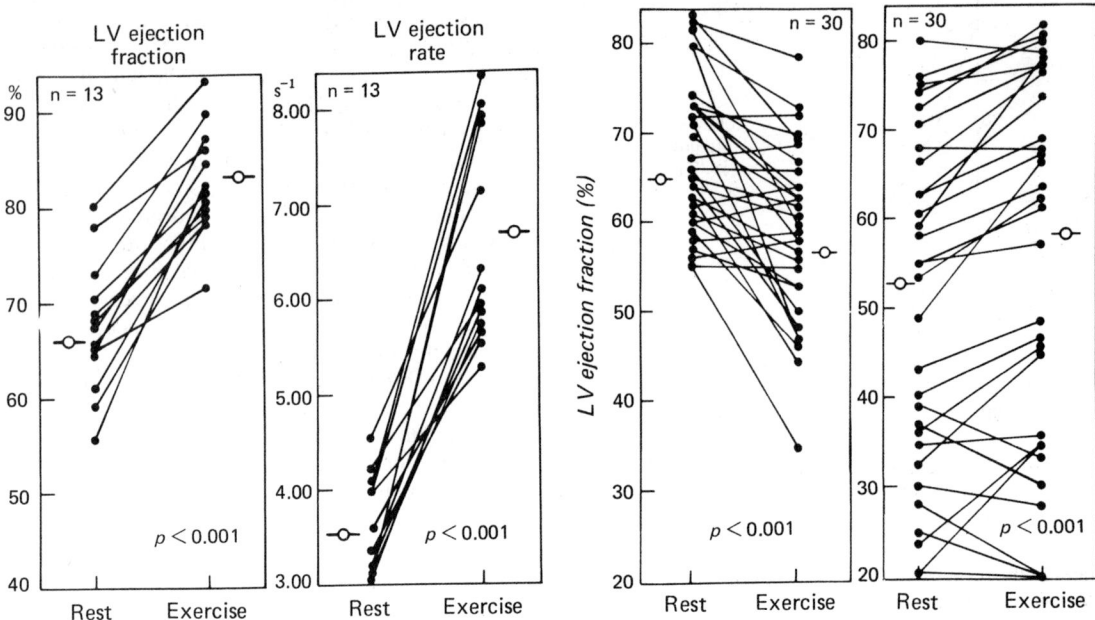

Figure 8-16. Left ventricular (LV) ejection fraction and ejection rate at rest and during exercise in 13 normal control subjects; LV ejection fraction in 60 patients with coronary artery disease. Individual patients are represented by closed circles connected by solid lines. The open circles at the sides of each panel are the means. (Reproduced, with permission, from Berger JH et al: Global and regional left ventricular response to bicycle exercise in coronary heart disease: Assessment by quantitative radionuclide angiocardiography. *Am J Med* 1979;**66**:13.)

procedure involves only a slight risk in their hands. The anatomy of the coronary arteries cannot be predicted from the history of angina and the patient's responses to exercise testing. Patients with stable angina may have one-, 2-, or 3-vessel disease. Even in mild angina there may be major stenoses of 2 or 3 coronary arteries; thus, coronary angiograms are required if the physician wishes to know the anatomy of the coronary arteries in any particular case.

The anatomy and distribution of the coronary arteries and the topography of infarction are illustrated in Fig 8-17. Multiple views and projections are usually necessary to evaluate the coronary angiogram. Fig 8-18 shows examples of branches of the right and left coronary arteries seen in the usual coronary angiograms.

1. Complications–Nationwide surveys have shown that the morbidity and mortality rates associated with coronary arteriography are directly related to the experience of the operator and the frequency with which the procedure is done in the particular hospital. Ventricular fibrillation, acute myocardial infarction, hemorrhage, and thrombosis of the artery are the major problems encountered. Embolism is the least common complication. The mortality rate in various series is about 0.1–0.5%. The risk rises with the degree of severity of left main coronary artery disease.

The interpretation of coronary angiograms is hampered by the difficulty of quantitating partial stenosis, of determining the significance of collaterals, and of deciding whether arterial spasm or some technical artifacts are present.

2. Indications for coronary arteriography–A number of studies have shown that survival in patients with angina pectoris depends upon (1) the dominance (whether posterior descending coronary arteries come from right or left systems) of the stenotic artery; (2) the location, severity, and number of coronary stenoses (whether there is a single severe proximal stenosis or more moderate multiple distal stenoses); (3) the proximity of the stenosis to the first perforator (left anterior descending); (4) left ventricular function as estimated by the ejection fraction, left ventricular volumes, and the presence and degree of wall motion abnormalities; and (5) the presence and adequacy of collateral circulation.

Coronary arteriography is indicated for the following classes of patients:

(1) Patients being considered for coronary bypass surgery because of disabling stable angina and failure to improve on an adequate medical regimen.

(2) Patients being considered for coronary bypass surgery because of myocardial infarctions in rapid succession or because of repeated unstable angina causing hospital admissions.

(3) Patients with aortic valve disease who have angina pectoris, especially if the aortic valve gradient is only modest, to determine whether the angina is

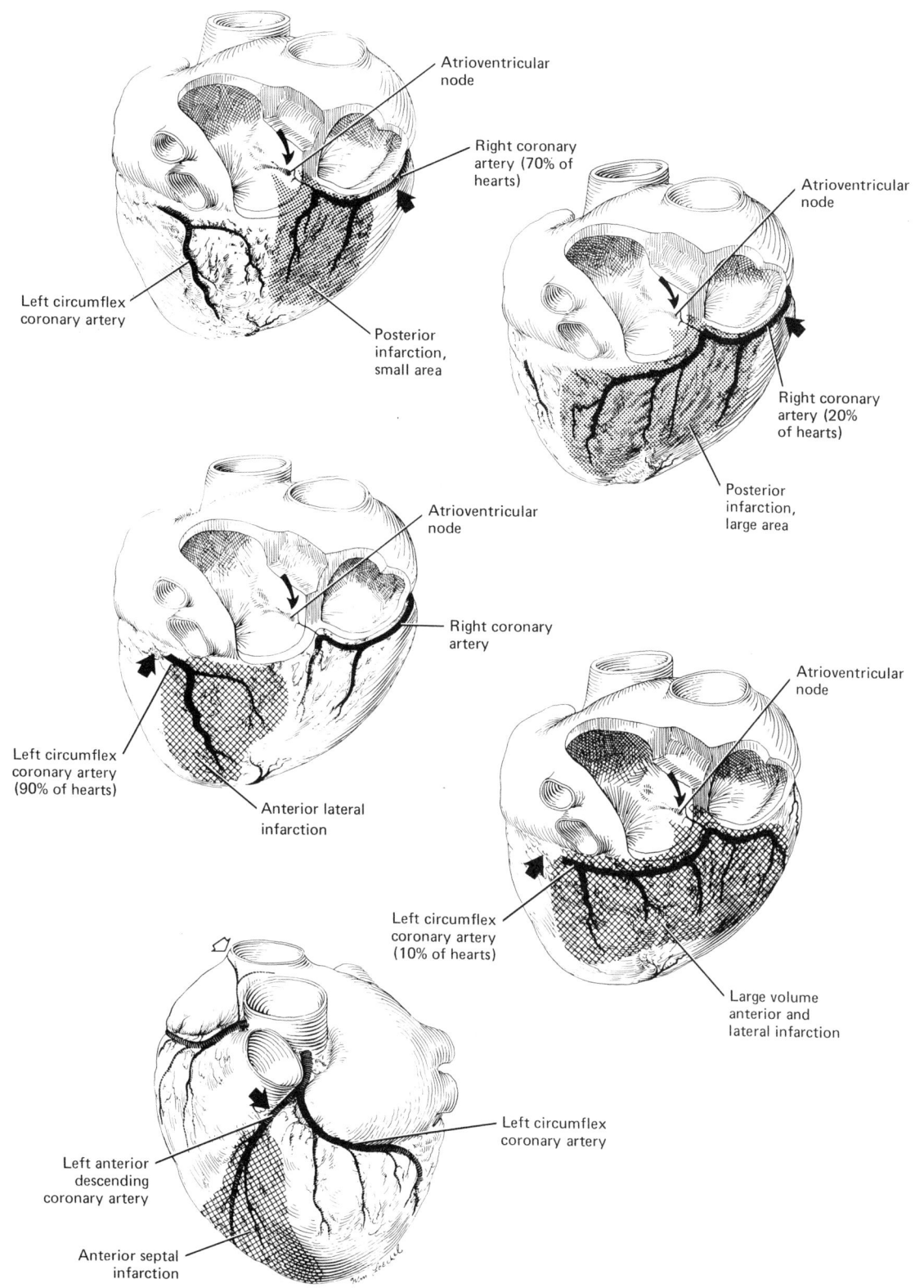

Figure 8–17. Anatomy and distribution of the coronary arteries and the topography of infarction. (Reproduced, with permission, from James TN: Arrhythmias and conduction disturbances in acute myocardial infarction. *Am Heart J* 1962;**64**:416.)

154 / CHAPTER 8

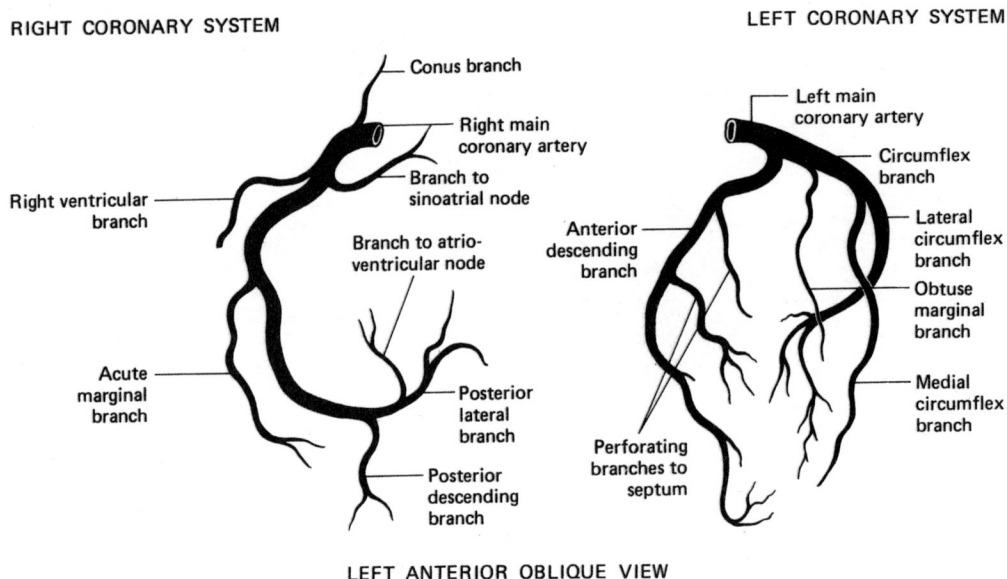

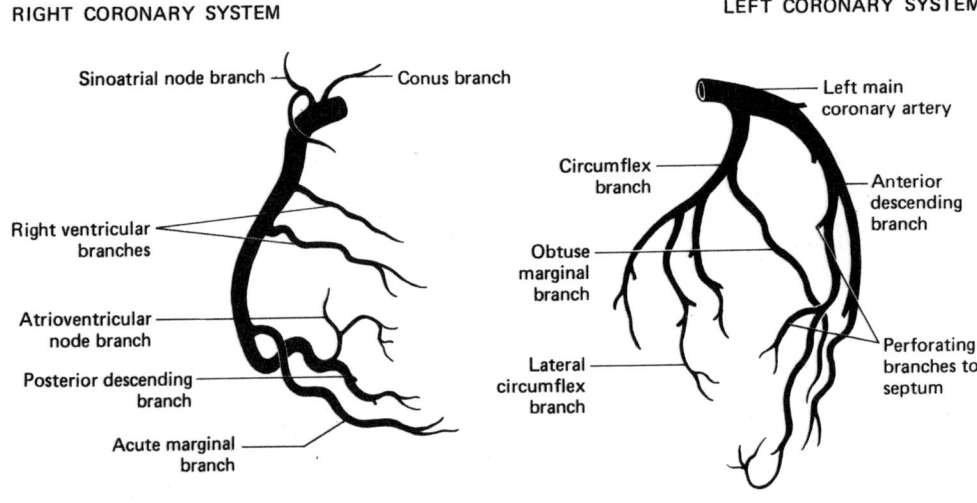

Figure 8-18. Example of branches of the left and right coronary arteries as seen in the usual coronary angiograms, left and right oblique views. (Modified and reproduced, with permission, from Cosby RS et al: Clinicoarteriographic correlations in angina pectoris with and without myocardial infarction. *Am J Cardiol* 1972;**30**:472.)

due to coronary disease or aortic stenosis. Severe angina in the presence of aortic stenosis is not invariably associated with coronary artery stenosis.

(4) Patients who have had coronary bypass surgery with initial improvement and subsequent relapse of symptoms, to determine whether or not the bypass graft is patent or occluded.

(5) Patients with coronary disease, ischemic cardiomyopathy, and cardiac failure in whom a left ventricular aneurysm is suspected.

(6) For diagnostic purposes in patients who have chest pain of uncertain cause believed not to be anginal, if the patient will be benefited in knowing for certain that the pain is not due to coronary disease.

B. Contrast Left Ventricular Angiography: (See also Chapter 6.) Left ventricular cineangiograms should be performed in conjunction with coronary arteriograms because of the information the former give on left ventricular function; size of the heart during systole and diastole; wall motion abnormalities; the presence of ventricular aneurysm; and the absence of other conditions such as valvular disease, hypertrophic cardiomyopathy, mitral valve prolapse, and other unsuspected abnormalities. It is unwise to perform coronary arteriography alone without contrast left ventricular angiography.

Differential Diagnosis

The differential diagnosis of chest pain requires great skill in history taking. The physician can usually decide that the pain is or is not angina, but in some cases even the most careful and thoughtful inquiry may leave the issue in doubt. Chest pain in someone with coronary disease is not necessarily angina.

A. Psychophysiologic Reactions: Psychophysiologic cardiovascular reactions are a loosely defined group of disorders having in common dull aching chest pains often described as "heart pain," lasting hours or days, often aggravated by exertion but not promptly relieved by rest. Darting, knifelike pains of momentary duration at the apex or over the precordium are often present also. Emotional tension and fatigue make the pain worse. Hyperventilation, palpitations, fatigue, and headache are also usually present. Constant exhaustion is a frequent complaint.

B. Anterior Chest Wall Syndrome: This disorder is characterized by sharply localized tenderness of intercostal muscles, and pressure at these sites reproduces the chest pain. Sprain or inflammation of the chondrocostal junctions, which may be warm, swollen, and red (so-called Tietze's syndrome), may result in diffuse chest pain that is also reproduced by local pressure. Intercostal neuritis (herpes zoster, diabetes mellitus) may confuse the diagnosis.

Xiphoid tenderness and lower sternal pain may arise from and be reproduced by pressure on the xiphoid process.

Any of the above may also occur in a patient with angina.

C. Degenerative Thoracic or Cervical Spine Disease: Cervical or thoracic spine disease (degenerative disk disease, postural strain, "arthritis") involving the dorsal roots produces sudden sharp, severe chest pain similar to angina in location and "radiation" but related to specific movements of the neck or spine, recumbency, straining, or lifting, and there are usually sensory changes in the skin. Pain due to cervical thoracic disk disease involves the outer or dorsal aspect of the arm, thumb, and index fingers rather than the ring and little fingers, as in angina pectoris.

D. Gastrointestinal Disorders: Peptic ulcer, chronic cholecystitis, cardiospasm, and functional gastrointestinal disease are often suspected because some patients indisputably obtain relief from angina by belching. In these disorders, symptoms are related to food or alcohol intake rather than physical exertion. X-ray and fluoroscopic study are helpful in diagnosis. The pain is relieved by appropriate diet and drug therapy.

Hiatal hernia with esophagitis is characterized by lower chest and upper abdominal pain after heavy meals, occurs in recumbency or upon bending over, and is made worse with the acid or alcohol test. The pain is relieved by bland diet, antacids, the Fowler position, and walking.

E. Shoulder Origin of Pain: Degenerative and inflammatory lesions of the left shoulder or cervical rib and the scalenus anticus syndrome differ from angina in that the pain is precipitated by movement of the arm and shoulder, paresthesias are present in the left arm, and postural exercises and pillow support to the shoulders in bed give relief.

F. Pain of Pulmonary Hypertension: "Tight" mitral stenosis or pulmonary hypertension resulting from chronic pulmonary disease can on occasion produce chest pain which is indistinguishable from that of angina pectoris, including ST segment depression. The clinical findings of mitral stenosis or of lung disease are evident, and the ECG invariably discloses right axis deviation or right ventricular hypertrophy. Pulmonary embolism must also be considered.

G. Spontaneous Pneumothorax: Spontaneous pneumothorax may cause chest pain as well as dyspnea and create confusion with angina pectoris as well as myocardial infarction.

H. Pericarditis: See Chapter 18.

Complications

The major complications of stable angina are unstable angina, myocardial infarction, arrhythmias, and sudden death.

Treatment

Treatment will be discussed in 3 main categories: (1) overall considerations, (2) treatment of the acute attack of angina pectoris, and (3) management of chronic angina pectoris. See pp 144 and 161 in considering whether the individual case is chronic or acute. In addition, exclude acute myocardial infarction; evaluate the presence of an old infarction or segmental wall motion abnormalities; and evaluate left ventricular function.

A. Overall Considerations:

1. Approach to atherosclerosis in general–One must distinguish between efforts to prevent or relieve anginal pain; efforts to prevent myocardial infarction or arrhythmias; and efforts to avert the fundamental process of atherosclerosis by lowering the blood pressure, reducing fat and carbohydrate intake, losing weight, and giving up cigarettes.

Recent data demonstrate that a low-calorie, low-fat diet combined with use of cholestyramine resin decreases serum cholesterol and the incidence of initial coronary events. In patients with known coronary disease, this regimen decreases the progression of coronary disease (see p 135). The Hypertension Detection Study and the Oslo Study have shown a decreased incidence of clinical coronary disease following antihypertensive therapy, but other trials were less convincing (Stamler, 1984) (see also p 135). Weight reduction with diets that decrease carbohydrate and alcohol intake may produce striking decreases in serum triglyceride and smaller decreases in serum choles-

Table 8–5. Nondietary treatment of primary hyperlipidemias.*

Disorder	Drugs	Other Treatment
Monogenic or oligogenic hyperlipidemias		
Familial hypercholesterolemia		
Heterozygous	Resin plus nicotinic acid;† resin plus neomycin	Distal ileal bypass
Homozygous	Resin plus nicotinic acid	Plasmapheresis†
Familial multiple type hyperlipoproteinemia		
Elevated LDL	Resin, nicotinic acid, or combination	
Elevated VLDL	Nicotinic acid or clofibrate	
Elevated VLDL and LDL	Resin, nicotinic acid, or combination	
Familial hypertriglyceridemia		
Mild	Clofibrate or nicotinic acid	
Severe (with chylomicronemia)	Nicotinic acid†	Eliminate aggravating factors
Familial dysbetalipoproteinemia	Clofibrate (small doses);† nicotinic acid	
Familial lipoprotein lipase of apolipoprotein C-II deficiency	None	
Other primary hyperlipidemias		
Polygenic or unclassified hypercholesterolemia	Resin;† nicotinic acid or clofibrate	
Exogenous hypercholesterolemia	Beta-sitosterol	
Sporadic or unclassified hypertriglyceridemia	Clofibrate or nicotinic acid	

*Modified and reproduced, with permission, from Havel RJ, Kane JP: Therapy of hyperlipidemic states. *Annu Rev Med* 1982;**33**:417.
†Indicates drug or other treatment of choice.

terol. Exogenous type IV hyperlipidemia may therefore appear or disappear depending upon the amount of carbohydrate in the diet and the weight of the patient. A combination of colestipol (20 g/d in 3 doses) and nicotinic acid (as well as cholestyramine ester in combination with a low-calorie, low–saturated fat diet) will result in lowered levels of LDL and increased levels of HDL (Samuel, 1980; Levy, 1983). There are at least 5 subgroups of HDL, with variable response to these drugs.

Prevention of coronary disease should be started in childhood or adolescence, because hypertension and genetic disorders of lipid and carbohydrate metabolism are manifest early in life.

2. Prevention of myocardial infarction– Prevention of myocardial infarction is one of the aims of treatment of angina. While most infarctions come "out of the blue" and cannot be predicted by patient or physician, an effort should be made to avoid factors that sometimes precipitate the event. The list includes physical stresses (eg, bursts of unaccustomed strenuous activity, shoveling snow in the cold after a heavy meal, running with heavy luggage to a departure gate) and emotional stresses associated with a rise in blood pressure or coronary vasoconstriction (eg, arguments at home or on the job). The physician should help patients to develop insight into the effects of stress and to learn healthy ways of responding to it. In spite of such efforts, however, acute myocardial infarction may develop without apparent reason at any time.

3. Risk factors– It is desirable to eliminate or control known risk factors (hypertension, hyperlipidemia, diabetes, cigarette smoking, emotional stress, obesity) that aggravate atherosclerosis. Cigarette smoking, which may precipitate ventricular arrhythmias and sudden death in patients with coronary disease, should be stopped permanently. There is no statistically convincing evidence that physical fitness achieved by exercise programs prolongs life. Weight reduction decreases the work of the heart, and a reducing diet low in calories and animal fats is desirable. Sedatives or tranquilizers may reduce the frequency of attacks but are of only marginal benefit except in hyperactive or emotionally stressed individuals.

B. Use of Nitrates and Amyl Nitrite in Angina Pectoris: (Table 8–6.) Nitrates and amyl nitrite are the drugs of choice to terminate an acute anginal attack. The choice of drug and dosage depends on the patient's experience. Nitroglycerin must be fresh (replenish supplies every 6 months), kept in a tightly closed glass container, and stored in a refrigerator. A 0.3-mg tablet dissolved sublingually is usually sufficient, but the dose may be increased to 0.4–0.6 mg if needed. A burning sensation on the tongue, flushing, or a headache are to be expected if the drug is active.

Crushing an amyl nitrite ampule and inhaling the vapor gives relief in 10–45 seconds. Some patients dislike the odor and the attention drawn to them by the procedure. Isosorbide dinitrate, 2.5–10 mg dissolved sublingually, acts somewhat more slowly. (The chewable preparation is irregularly absorbed.) Pentaerythritol tetranitrate has not been much used recently. If these preparations are ineffective even in larger doses or are poorly tolerated, nifedipine, 10 mg sublingually, may be of benefit.

All preparations mentioned (except for nifedipine) have a half-life of less than 10 minutes and all cause

Table 8–6. General principles of medical treatment of stable angina pectoris of effort.

1. Use sublingual nitroglycerin or nifedipine for acute relief when discomfort starts or sublingual or oral isosorbide dinitrate for prevention of attacks or more prolonged effect.
2. Use transdermal nitroglycerin for long-term effect, including nocturnal discomfort.
3. Use beta blockers to prevent attacks, lower blood pressure, and prevent or treat ventricular arrhythmia; if coronary spasm is present, use calcium entry–blocking agents.
4. Avoid physical and emotional factors that precipitate the pain.
5. Avoid exercise in the presence of other precipitating factors that increase work of the heart (cold weather, heavy meals, emotional upset).
6. Exercise caution in the face of unusual and unaccustomed effort.
7. Reduce work activity (speed of effort, regulation of time, intermittent rest periods).
8. Treat hypertension if present.
9. Treat arrhythmias if present.
10. Treat cardiac failure if present.
11. Stop cigarette smoking.
12. Reduce weight if overweight.
13. Manage adverse emotional responses.
14. Institute supervised physical fitness program (perhaps beneficial).

relaxation of vascular smooth muscle. This results in peripheral pooling of blood and decreased venous return, thereby lowering ventricular volume, intraventricular pressure, and cardiac output, causing reduced oxygen demand of the myocardium. Cineangiography can demonstrate decreasing venous return, with relaxation of large veins, decreased cardiac volume, and left ventricular filling pressure and increasing ejection fraction of the left ventricle. Total coronary blood flow does not appear to be increased, but there may be some redistribution of blood flow, eg, vasodilation of epicardial coronary arteries.

The major untoward effects accompanying relief of angina are the result of vasodilatation (flushing, dizziness, throbbing headache, tachycardia, faintness [orthostatic hypotension]), and the patient should therefore sit or lie down when using nitrates or amyl nitrite. Obviously, the patient should cease whatever activity brought on the acute attack until the pain is gone. In a few patients, carotid sinus massage or Valsalva's maneuver may provide relief.

C. Management of Chronic Angina Pectoris:

1. Avoidance of precipitating factors–Patient and physician should review carefully the situations causing physical or emotional stress that result in anginal attacks and should make specific plans to avoid or diminish these situations. If this proves unfeasible, drug prophylaxis should be considered.

2. Drug prophylaxis–Less obvious precipitating factors are paroxysmal arrhythmias, hypotension, hyperthyroidism, left ventricular outflow obstruction, left ventricular failure, anemia, and obesity. Left ventricular failure may be obvious or incipient, and treatment with digitalis or diuretics (or both) may be helpful.

a. Nitrates–When undertaking an activity that usually causes acute angina, the patient can prevent angina by use of sublingual nitroglycerin in a dosage known to be effective; prevention, however, is brief. For longer-lasting prevention, nitroglycerin ointment, ½–2 inches of 2% ointment placed on a hairless area of skin, can be effective for 3–6 hours. Topical slow-release preparations (5–30 mg), which provide prophylaxis for 6–12 hours and are particularly suitable for nighttime use, are used in the form of transdermal patches of ointment placed on a hairless area of skin and covered by plastic. When this form of medication is discontinued, the dosage must be tapered over a 2-week period. These preparations can increase exercise tolerance and can prevent coronary spasm of variant angina. Side effects include headache and hypotension.

Another longer-lasting nitrate medication is isosorbide dinitrate, 10–30 mg orally every 4–6 hours. When taken at bedtime, this agent tends to prevent nocturnal pain.

b. Beta-adrenergic blocking agents–Propranolol, timolol, atenolol, nadolol, metoprolol, alprenolol, and other similar agents are beneficial because of their hemodynamic effects (decreased heart rate, blood pressure, and contractility), all of which decrease myocardial oxygen requirements. They also may prevent cardiac arrhythmias and decrease the likelihood of myocardial infarction or sudden death. Propranolol (Inderal), 10–40 mg 3–4 times daily, has long been used for prophylaxis. It should not be given to patients with a history of ventricular failure, bronchospasm, or atrioventricular conduction defects. Undesirable effects of beta-blocking agents include slowing of the heart rate, with an increase in end-diastolic volume and an increase in ejection time. These deleterious effects are commonly mediated by the concomitant use of nitrates.

Among the growing number of beta blockers, cardioselective drugs may be of wider use because they are less likely to cause bronchospasm. Beta blockers must not be withdrawn abruptly, because myocardial ischemia or infarction may be precipitated.

c. Calcium entry–blocking agents–Agents of this class (eg, nifedipine, verapamil, diltiazem) inhibit calcium influx and decrease the myocardial contractile force, which in turn reduces myocardial oxygen requirements. These agents also decrease arteriolar tone and systemic vascular resistance, resulting in decreased arterial and intraventricular pressure—again reducing myocardial oxygen requirements. They tend to relieve and prevent focal coronary artery spasm; this is important in variant angina, for which they are effective treatment. Calcium blockers are effective in the long-term management of chronic stable angina, with an increase in exercise duration and a significant delay in the onset of effort angina. They are likewise helpful in unstable angina, cardiac arrhythmias, hypertrophic cardiomyopathy, and hypertension. In

Table 8–7. Oral calcium entry–blocking drugs.

	Inhibition of Atrioventricular Conduction	Coronary Vasodilatation	Decreased Inotropic Action	Hypotension, Edema	Dose (Initial; Daily)*
Verapamil	+++	++	++	++	40–80 mg; 240–360 mg
Diltiazem	+ to ++	++	+	+	30–60 mg; 180–240 mg
Nifedipine	0 to +	+++	0	+++	20 mg; 40–120 mg

*Give in divided doses.

unstable angina with coronary spasm, patients who fail to respond favorably to rest, sedation, nitrates, and beta blockers may respond to nifedipine (10–20 mg 2–3 times daily), verapamil (80–120 mg 2–3 times daily), or diltiazem (30–90 mg 2–3 times daily). This may permit deferral of invasive diagnostic studies and coronary surgery until conditions have stabilized. However, the 3 drugs have different hemodynamic and electrophysiologic actions: nifedipine has the greatest vasodilator effect; verapamil has the greatest inhibiting effect on the atrioventricular node; and diltiazem has effects intermediate between these 2 agents. In the presence of cardiac failure, beta blockers and calcium–entry blockers in combination must be used with caution, because both have negative inotropic effects.

d. Aminophylline–In some patients with incipient left ventricular failure and bronchospasm, aminophylline, 250–500 mg in rectal suppositories, may provide relief of angina and dyspnea.

3. Control of ventricular premature beats and ventricular arrhythmias–Ventricular arrhythmias are common in patients with coronary heart disease. Arrhythmias may precipitate myocardial ischemia, angina pectoris, and sudden death by decreasing cardiac output and coronary perfusion and inducing ventricular fibrillation. Both ventricular premature beats and the more complex ventricular arrhythmias are more apt to be noted by 24-hour ambulatory electrocardiographic monitoring than by graded exercise. One-third to one-half of patients with no premature ventricular beats (or only one) on a routine ECG show a variety of ventricular premature beats that are frequent, multiform, early, or occur in runs when monitoring is employed. The degree of angiographically demonstrated coronary stenosis is greater in patients with more complex premature ventricular beats. Prophylactic treatment with digitalis, quinidine, procainamide, or beta-blocking agents may prevent attacks of angina (including nocturnal angina) precipitated by complex premature beats.

Although it is difficult to prove, since most cases of sudden death syndrome are due to ventricular fibrillation often preceded by ventricular premature beats, control of the premature beats may prevent ventricular fibrillation and sudden death. Antiarrhythmic drugs may decrease ventricular premature beats, but with the exception of beta blockers (see above), it has not been established that they prevent sudden death.

Tables 8–8 and 8–9 set forth some of the data that have been accumulated about ventricular arrhythmias in patients with coronary heart disease. One-third to one-half of patients with no premature ventricular beats (or only one) on a routine ECG show a variety of ventricular premature beats that are frequent, multiform, early, or in runs when monitoring is employed. It is important to determine the grade of ventricular premature beats (simple or complex) because the degree of angiographically demonstrated coronary stenosis is greater in patients with more complex premature ventricular beats.

4. Treatment of hypertension–Episodes of angina are often preceded by rises in blood pressure, and treatment of hypertension may be valuable in these patients (see Chapter 9). Beta-adrenergic blockers may be particularly effective, because they may relieve the symptoms of angina pectoris, lower the blood pressure, and prevent ventricular arrhythmias. They may also be combined with hydralazine in the treatment of hypertension in patients with angina pectoris, in order to prevent the reflex tachycardia that results from the vasodilator.

5. Treatment of cardiac failure if present–(See Chapter 10.)

6. Social and psychologic factors–Knowing that one has "a bad heart" is a heavy psychologic burden, and some patients respond by denial, anger, depression, or regression. Sympathetic listening and discussion are an essential part of good management.

Table 8–8. Distribution of ventricular premature beats during a 24-hour monitoring session in 184 patients with coronary heart disease. (Each patient is presented once on the basis of maximal grade reached during monitoring.)*

Grade	Description	Percent of Patients
0	No ventricular ectopic beats	12
1	Occasional, isolated ventricular premature beats	17
2	Frequent ventricular premature beats (> 1/min or 30/h)	6
3	Multiform ventricular premature beats	25
4	Repetitive ventricular premature beats	
4A	Couplets	27
4B	Salvos	14

*Reproduced, with permission, from the American Heart Association, Inc., Lown B et al: Monitoring for serious arrhythmias and high risk of sudden death. *Circulation* 1975;52(Suppl 3):189.

Table 8–9. Comparison of the nature of complex ventricular premature complexes (VPCs) during 1 hour of baseline monitoring in coronary heart disease patients with and without prior myocardial infarction (MI).*

	Angina Only		Prior MI	
	(n)	(%)	(n)	(%)
Men with any complex form in hour	65	100.0	462	100.0
Qualitative features				
Early VPC (R on T)	12	18.5	83	18.0
Runs of 2 or more VPCs	19	29.2	172	37.2
Early and/or runs	27	41.5	202	43.7
Bigeminy	26	40.0	208	45.0
Multiform VPCs	53	81.5	362	78.4
Multiformity is sole complex feature	28	43.1	158	34.2
Total number of VPCs in hour				
1–9	12	18.5	109	23.6
10 or more	53	81.5	353	76.4

*Reproduced, with permission, from the American Heart Association, Inc., Ruberman W et al: Ventricular premature complexes in prognosis of angina. *Circulation* 1980:**61**:1172.

The high percentage of patients (50–60%) who report decreased frequency of attacks and decreased need for nitroglycerin when given a placebo attests to the role of emotional factors in increasing the frequency of anginal attacks. An attempt should be made to improve the patient's general emotional health and state of mind. Factors that cause unhappiness, resentment, or hostility should be eliminated if possible. Everyone associated with the patient must be considered as a possible source of emotional stress, including the employer, colleagues at work, spouse, and children. The physician who has a good personal relationship with the patient is in the best position to suggest creative solutions to problems of this sort.

Patients with driving personalities who lead hectic lives must learn to moderate their activities, quit smoking, use alcohol only in moderation, take rest periods in the afternoon and frequent short holidays, and avoid all activities shown by experience to bring on attacks. Rest and relaxation in a totally different environment often produce dramatic results when drugs do not.

7. Anticoagulant therapy–Anticoagulants have been tried, both in patients with angina of effort and in patients who have survived an acute infarction, in order to prevent subsequent infarction and death, but the results have shown only minimal benefit if any. The same can be said about chronic aspirin usage, now being studied experimentally. Routine anticoagulant therapy is used today only when thromboembolic complications are present or believed to be a substantial risk.

8. Increased physical activity–A planned program of daily exercise may not prevent myocardial infarction and death, but it can have beneficial physiologic and psychologic effects. The same degree of exercise that is well within the bounds of tolerance in the laboratory or on a pleasant day may not be tolerated under less favorable circumstances.

9. Referral for coronary angiography and possible coronary bypass surgery–See section on coronary heart surgery for indications for coronary surgery in patients who have unacceptable angina pectoris.

10. Preparation for survival–

a. Education of family–When an attack occurs, the patient should be taken promptly to a nearby hospital with good coronary care facilities unless mobile ambulance crews trained in resuscitation are readily available.

b. Education of lay people and ambulance crews–Various communities provide physician and lay educational programs in order to minimize the time between onset of symptoms of a coronary event and hospitalization. Emergency paramedics and medical technicians in specially equipped ambulances and fire department personnel with rescue vehicles have been taught to recognize arrhythmias, to accomplish defibrillation, and to inject drugs such as atropine and lidocaine. Good prehospital care of this kind in patients with angina can be lifesaving.

Prognosis

A. Overall Mortality Rate: The overall mortality rate of patients with stable angina varies from 0.3 to 8% (Frank, 1973). The influence of congestive heart failure and hypertension is shown in Fig 8–19. Factors adversely influencing survival include complex

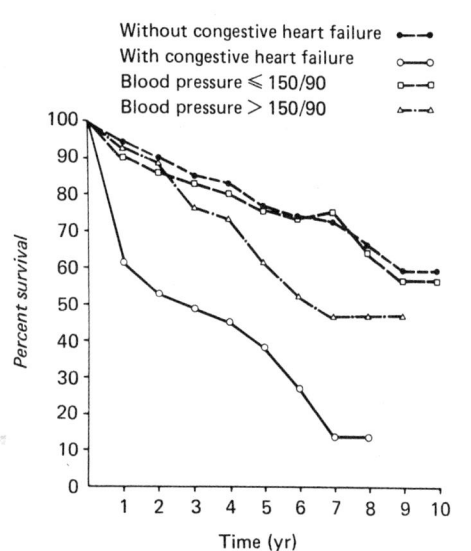

Figure 8–19. Survival with coronary artery disease related to heart failure and blood pressure. (Reproduced, with permission, from the American Heart Association, Inc., Burgraf GW, Parker JO: Prognosis in coronary artery disease: Angiographic, hemodynamic, and clinical factors. *Circulation* 1975;**51**:146.)

Table 8–10. Causes of death in patients with stable angina of effort.*

Cause	Number	Percent of Deaths
Noncardiac	8	11
Sudden (outside hospital)	24	34
Chronic congestive heart failure	10	14
Acute myocardial infarction		
Arrhythmia	16	23
Pump failure	13	18
Total	71	100

*Reproduced, with permission, from the American Heart Association, Inc., Burggraf GW, Parker JO: Prognosis in coronary artery disease: Angiographic, hemodynamic, and clinical factors. *Circulation* 1975;**51**:146.

arrhythmias, easily induced myocardial ischemia, large perfusion or contraction abnormalities, low ejection fraction, and left main coronary artery disease.

The causes of death are listed in Table 8–10.

B. Role of Coronary Artery Anatomy: Angina is often the initial manifestation of coronary disease, and the prognosis depends chiefly on the anatomy of the coronary arteries (Fig 8–20) and the left ventricular function. The mortality rate is higher when left ventricular function is impaired. Three-vessel disease with diffuse left ventricular functional abnormalities with a low ejection fraction was found by Sheldon (1975) to have an almost 100% 5-year mortality rate, whereas 3-vessel disease with normal left ventricular function had a 35% 5-year mortality rate. Most deaths occur in the year following the onset of angina pectoris or myocardial infarction.

Another means of estimating the severity of coronary disease involves recognition of the extent of coronary calcification in one, 2, or 3 vessels (Fig 8–21).

C. Importance of Previous Myocardial Infarction: Patients presenting with angina pectoris may have had a previous myocardial infarction that either was silent or coincided with the onset of angina. The mortality rate of such patients is higher than that of patients who have not had a previous myocardial infarction. Patients who have had a previous myocardial infarction with diffuse fibrosis from healed ischemic areas often have evidence of left ventricular failure; in these patients, the 2-year mortality rate is 40–50% regardless of the number of vessels involved. Patients with orthopnea and paroxysmal nocturnal dyspnea have enlarged hearts and an unfavorable prognosis.

The anatomic changes revealed by coronary arteriography show that the most hazardous lesion is stenosis of the left main coronary artery and then (in decreasing order of risk) the left anterior descending, the left circumflex, and the right coronary artery. Patients with stenosis of the left main coronary artery have at least twice the mortality rate over a period of 1–3 years of those with equivalent stenoses in the other 2 vessels.

D. Need for Better Definition of Stenosis: Better methods are needed to define precisely the location and degree of stenosis and the amount of blood flow across stenotic coronary vessels. More objective, less opinionated measurements are needed to permit eval-

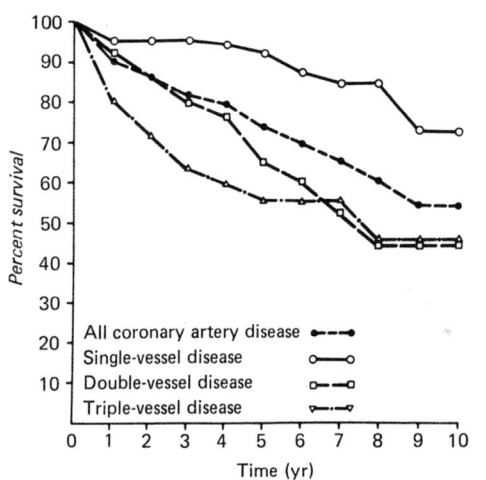

Figure 8–20. Survival related to extent of coronary artery involvement. (Reproduced, with permission, from the American Heart Association, Inc., Burggraf GW, Parker JO: Prognosis in coronary artery disease: Angiographic, hemodynamic, and clinical factors. *Circulation* 1975;**51**:146.)

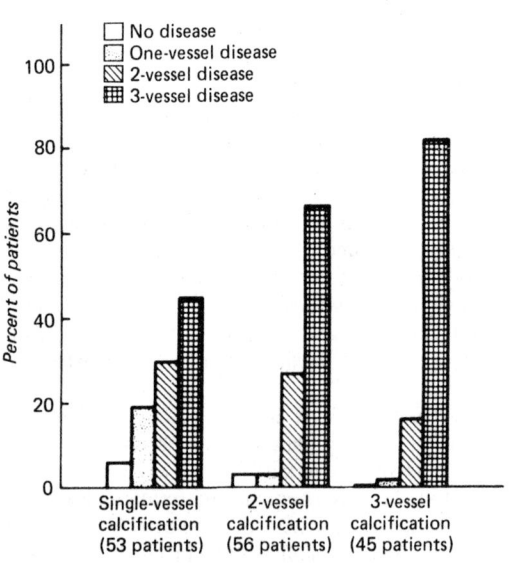

Figure 8–21. The severity of coronary disease increased progressively with the extent of coronary calcification. No "false-positives" were found in patients with 3-vessel calcification. (Reproduced, with permission, from the American Heart Association, Inc., Bartel AG et al: The significance of coronary calcification detected by fluoroscopy: A report of 360 patients. *Circulation* 1974;**49**:1247.)

uation of interacting factors to yield a better basis for decision making and determination of prognosis.

E. Assumption of Coronary Disease With Normal Angiograms: Possible explanations of normal coronary arteriograms in the presence of what is considered to be definite angina pectoris or a clear history of myocardial infarction include improper technique, errors of interpretation, small-vessel coronary disease, recanalization of a previously thrombosed single coronary artery, previous prolonged coronary spasm, or lysis of a previous embolus or thrombus (Michaelson, 1977; Selzer, 1980).

About 5–10% of patients with recurrent myocardial infarction are believed to have had angina pectoris in spite of normal coronary angiograms. One must always exclude vasculitis and arteritis as the cause of angina in patients with normal coronary angiograms. Rheumatic disease, connective tissue disorders, and syphilis involving coronary arteries must be excluded as causes of vasculitis.

UNSTABLE ANGINA PECTORIS

The foregoing discussion pertained to angina of effort, which is relatively stable. In stable angina, patients can relate frequency of angina to effort expended, emotional state, weather, and meals, and the occurrence of attacks is relatively predictable within a broad range of activities. Intermediate between this stable angina and acute myocardial infarction is a clinical state variously referred to as unstable angina, acute coronary insufficiency, and preinfarction angina.

Definition of Unstable Angina

Patients with unstable angina are not a homogeneous group but can be divided into several subgroups. This may explain the widely differing estimates of prognosis in these patients.

The usual condition is **crescendo angina,** in which a patient known to have had stable angina of effort (1) develops angina on less exertion, (2) develops angina at rest or during sleep, (3) has pain with a somewhat different duration or radiation, (4) has pain that is not relieved as promptly with nitroglycerin as before, or (5) has angina that gradually worsens over a period of days and in many instances develops into acute myocardial infarction. However, infarction often does not follow. Some patients with unstable angina have already had a small myocardial infarction. Its divergent features in patient subgroups may explain the different mortality rates in unstable angina. Angina that occurs for the first time in a patient is also considered unstable because it may result in acute myocardial infarction. However, such first-time angina, unless it occurs at rest and requires hospitalization, has a better prognosis than does angina that progresses to pain at rest or is of the crescendo type and recurs at increasingly shorter intervals or lesser degree of effort or lasts longer.

Pathophysiology of Unstable Angina

The pathophysiology of unstable angina is uncertain when aggravating factors such as arrhythmias, cardiac failure, and anemia are excluded. Coronary occlusion or near occlusion due to subintimal hemorrhage or rupture of an atherosclerotic plaque, clumping of platelets or fibrin, or coronary spasm may be involved. Reduced regional coronary blood flow is the mechanism for rest angina; this could be due to increased metabolic demands or to decreased flow caused by coronary obstruction or spasm.

Most patients with unstable angina and chest pain at rest have coronary obstruction, but about one-third have decreased coronary blood flow due to coronary vasoconstriction. Many episodes of such pain are associated with ST elevation and decreased left ventricular wall motion. In these episodes, Chierchia (1983) found no changes in pulse or blood pressure prior to the pain and the heart rate–blood pressure product was not altered, indicating that myocardial oxygen demand was not increased. The National Cooperative Study Group to Compare Surgical and Medical Therapy (1980) in unstable angina found that two-thirds of patients with unstable angina had ST depression during chest pain and about one-third had ST elevation.

Classification & Symptoms of Unstable Angina

It is logical to subdivide unstable angina as follows: (1) initial angina that promptly subsides with bed rest; (2) initial angina that continues despite bed rest and medical treatment; (3) crescendo angina in patients with previous stable angina; (4) angina at rest or during sleep; and (5) angina that changes in character and duration.

A. Puzzling Diagnosis of Unstable Angina: When unstable angina is the first manifestation of coronary disease, the diagnosis can be very puzzling because there is no history of angina of effort. Often the patient states that effort does not induce pain but that pain occurs at unpredictable times during periods of rest. But the quality of the discomfort is typical of ischemic pain.

B. Possible Presence of Unproved Myocardial Infarction: Radioisotope imaging may help identify areas of myocardial necrosis in this group of patients. Discrete hypoperfusion defects with thallium 201 indicate a myocardial infarction (see p 168). Diffuse hypoperfusion occurs with unstable angina and should not be used to diagnose infarction. The presence of acute myocardial infarction in a patient considered to have unstable angina is associated with a higher rate of complications during emergency coronary angiography, angioplasty, or bypass surgery.

C. Hazards of Unstable Angina: The possibility of development of an acute myocardial infarction within the next few hours, days, or weeks after the development of unstable angina makes it a hazardous manifestation of ischemic heart disease. The mortality rate of acute myocardial infarction is greatest in the first few hours (see the section on acute myocardial infarction); therefore, it is prudent to monitor all patients with unstable angina in a coronary care unit for at least 2–4 days both because they might be developing a myocardial infarction that can become obvious at any time and because unstable angina may be associated with serious ventricular arrhythmias requiring immediate care (Fig 8–22). Restriction of all activity and appropriate medication (see below) may turn the tide, and infarction may be prevented.

Treatment

A. Medical Therapy: With unstable angina, the goals of therapy are to control the major determinants of oxygen demand and coronary spasm. If the coronary arteries are severely stenotic, an ordinary stimulus causing a small degree of vasoconstriction or minor changes in cardiac work can cause intermittent ischemia. If transdermal or sublingual nitrates do not relieve pain, give nitroglycerin intravenously in an initial dose of 5 μg/min, increased by 5-μg increments at 2- to 5-minute intervals until pain is relieved or systolic pressure decreases by 20 mm Hg. The average maximal rate of infusion is about 50 μg/min.

Vigorous medical therapy with bed rest, nitrates, beta-adrenergic and calcium entry–blocking agents as well as other vasodilator therapy should be used, because in many patients with unstable angina but without infarction the acute process subsides. When beta blockers are used, begin with 20 mg of propranolol or its equivalent and increase the total daily dose to 300 mg/d in divided doses every 4 hours until bradycardia (<50 beats/min) or hypotension <90–100 mm Hg systolic) occurs. Calcium entry–blocking agents are superior to beta blockers in angina at rest; nifedipine can be given, 10 mg 3 times a day. Beta blockers do not cause dilation of the large coronary arteries, whereas calcium blockers do. Calcium blockers prevent ergonovine-induced spasm, but beta blockers do not. Beta blockers reduce myocardial oxygen consumption and metabolic demands, whereas calcium blockers cause dilation of the large arteries (Maseri, 1983). Verapamil should be used with caution if the ejection fraction is less than 30%. Side effects of calcium blockers are headache, hypotension, and dizziness. The goals of treatment are to increase blood flow to the myocardium, relieve pain, prevent myocardial infarction, and enhance survival.

Activity should be restricted. Recurrent pain at rest lasting 10–15 minutes and requiring opiates occurs in about 20% of patients despite full medical treatment.

In a recent Veterans Administration Cooperative Study (Lewis, 1983), aspirin was reported to decrease the incidence of acute myocardial infarction and the mortality rate in a 12-week trial in patients with unstable angina. The difficulties of precise diagnosis and the high percentage (81.7%) of patients meeting the original diagnostic criteria who were excluded from the study weaken the argument that aspirin is protective in unstable angina.

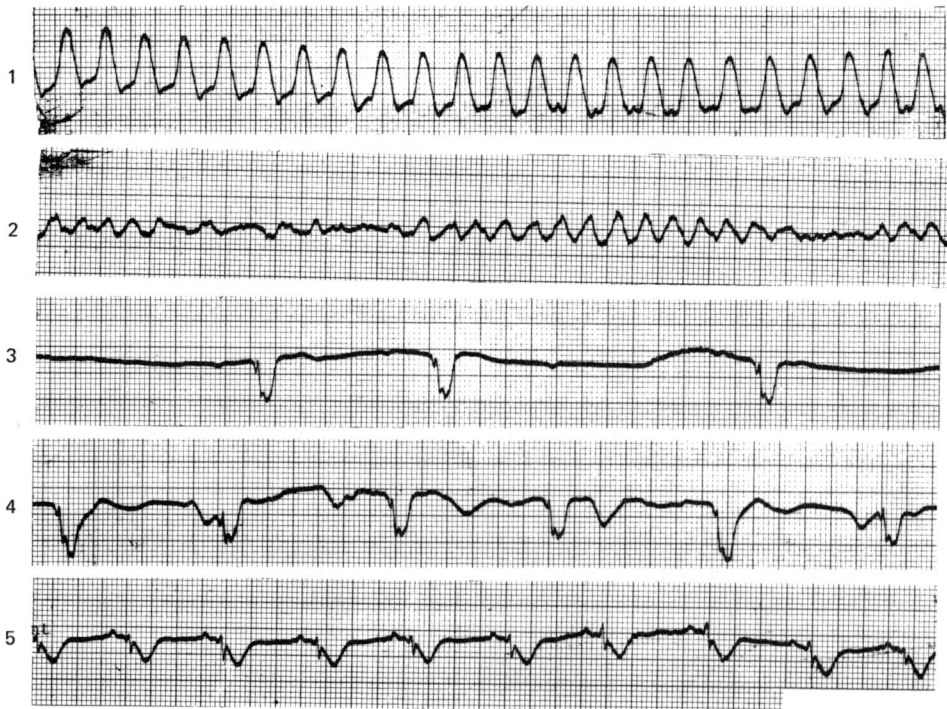

Figure 8–22. Sequential changes after cardiac arrest in a 55-year-old woman with unstable angina: Strip 1 shows ventricular tachycardia. Strip 2 shows ventricular fibrillation. Strip 3 shows idioventricular rhythm after defibrillation. Strip 4 shows ventricular premature beats. Strip 5 shows sinus rhythm. (Courtesy of K Gershengorn.)

A large prospective, randomized national cooperative study compared intensive medical therapy with coronary bypass surgery for the acute management of patients with unstable angina who had ST elevation during pain. There was no difference in the rate of hospital deaths (3–5%) or myocardial infarction (5–6%) in the 2 groups, but over a period of 4 years about half of the medically treated patients underwent coronary bypass surgery for unacceptable angina. Thus, most patients with unstable angina can be stabilized with good medical therapy without an increased risk of early myocardial infarction or death. Elective surgery can be considered later (National Cooperative Study Group, 1980).

B. More Aggressive Therapy: If it becomes clear that medical treatment is ineffective, an aggressive approach can be initiated. Intra-aortic balloon pumping controlled by hemodynamic monitoring may decrease myocardial ischemia and relieve angina (see p 184). When stabilization occurs, one can proceed to coronary arteriography, and if the stenotic lesions are anatomically suitable, coronary bypass surgery or percutaneous transluminal angioplasty can be performed. Early surgical treatment is confined to the 10–20% of cases that fail to respond to maximum medical treatment; nifedipine or other calcium entry–blocking agents relieve rest angina in 75% of those patients who fail to get relief with nitrates and beta blockers.

Because of the frequency with which angina recurs in patients with crescendo or unstable angina (excluding initial-onset angina after discharge from the hospital), exercise electrocardiography and radionuclide studies are usually performed 1–2 months after discharge. If early, markedly positive ischemic ST changes or complex ventricular arrhythmias are found, coronary arteriograms are recommended with a view to performing surgery.

The National Cooperative Study Group (1978, 1981) found mortality rates in unstable angina to be 4.1% for patients treated medically in the hospital and 5% for patients treated surgically. After 2 years, mortality rates for this group of patients were 5% for those treated medically and 5.2% for those treated surgically. The rate of late infarction was 13% in both groups. Three times as many medically as surgically treated patients had class III or class IV angina after 2 years.

Coronary angioplasty has been tried in unstable angina. In several small series of patients, most had relief of angina, increase in functional capacity, and objective improvement in previously ischemic myocardium, as seen with exercise electrocardiographic testing and thallium 201 images.

Prognosis

The prognosis of unstable angina is controversial because of the difficulties of definition, as stated previously. The outcome is influenced by (1) the extent and nature of the anatomic disease in the coronary arteries, (2) the presence or absence of a previous myocardial infarction or multiple areas of wall motion abnormalities, including fibrosis; (3) the existence of acute myocardial infarction, which may be suggested by ST segment abnormalities, new Q waves, or an increase in serum enzymes by serial determination; and (4) other factors such as cardiac failure, ventricular arrhythmias, and hypertension or hypotension.

The imbalance between supply and demand of oxygen, even at rest, is precarious, and myocardial ischemia and myocardial necrosis can be imminent if demands are even slightly raised, as after meals or during bathing or defecating.

Most patients with unstable angina have severely stenosed coronary arteries, and the prognosis is considered intermediate between stable angina pectoris and unequivocal acute myocardial infarction.

A. Differentiation of Unstable Angina and Myocardial Infarction: It may be very difficult to differentiate unstable angina from myocardial infarction that is already present. The absence of ischemic changes in the ST–T segment, the absence of serum enzyme elevations, and the absence of discrete increased uptake on radioisotopic imaging with technetium ^{99m}Tc pyrophosphate are needed to rule out infarction in a patient with prolonged or rest pain. Serum enzyme measurements and myocardial imaging may demonstrate that infarction has already occurred in some patients in whom the ECG failed to show infarction.

B. Prospective Studies to Establish Prognosis: There is a need to establish the prognosis for sharply defined subgroups. At present, the mixing of different subgroups in reported series results in widely differing estimates. Accurate prognosis is particularly important, because it influences the choice of therapy.

C. Effect of Treatment on Prognosis: The prognosis of unstable angina is influenced by the treatment given. It is not reasonable to compare the outcome in patients who are ambulatory and at work with others who are at strict bed rest.

The evidence is not convincing that survival rates are improved by treating unstable angina as an acute surgical emergency. In most cases, symptoms are relieved by medical treatment. Surgery performed after the patient has been stabilized should be considered.

ACUTE MYOCARDIAL INFARCTION

In myocardial infarction there is ischemic necrosis of a variable amount of myocardial tissue as a result of an abrupt acute decrease in coronary flow or an equivalent abrupt increase in myocardial demand for oxygen that cannot be supplied by an obstructed coronary artery. Coronary flow may be impaired by a thrombus in one of the coronary arteries, by hemorrhage within or beneath an atherosclerotic plaque, or by coronary vasoconstriction or spasm. Decreased flow may be due to shock, dehydration, or hemorrhage, leading to poor perfusion of all tissues, including the myocardium. Rapid ventricular rates due to ventricular tachycardia or uncontrolled atrial fibrillation may also contribute to myocardial ischemia because of the decreased diastolic filling time. Transient temporary ischemia is reversible, but persistent ischemia (approximately 1 hour) results in a central area of complete necrosis surrounded by viable cells that are ischemic. The histologic pattern is illustrated in Fig 8–23.

The site and extent of necrosis depend upon the degree of occlusion of the coronary artery, the disproportion between flow and demand resulting from the anatomic distribution of stenoses within the coronary vessels, the adequacy of the collateral circulation between neighboring coronary arteries, and the presence and extent of previous infarctions. The infarct may involve the full thickness of the myocardium from endocardium to epicardium (transmural infarction) or may be confined to the subendocardium (nontransmural, or subendocardial, infarction). An infarct is usually caused by a thrombus in the coronary artery overlying an eroded atherosclerotic plaque in the distribution of acute myocardial infarction (Horie, 1978; DeWood, 1980). Others believe that coronary thrombosis infrequently precipitates acute myocardial infarction and that thrombosis is a consequence rather than the cause of the coronary occlusion. Acute myocardial infarction may occur from other causes such as acute hypotension or coronary spasm; secondary thromboses are rare in these events. Coronary occlusion and acute myocardial infarction are independent entities. A thrombus may occlude a branch of the coronary artery without producing myocardial infarction. Conversely, infarction may occur in the absence of coronary thrombosis. One must keep in mind the 3 distinct entities: (1) coronary atherosclerosis (a pathologic finding that may or may not be associated with coronary heart *disease*), (2) coronary thrombosis, and (3) myocardial infarction.

Although infarction of the left ventricle is usually assumed when one refers to myocardial infarction, right ventricular infarction is not rare and is usually associated with the inferior myocardial infarction resulting from occlusion of the right coronary artery. (See also p 166.)

The left anterior descending artery is most commonly occluded; this results in infarction of the anteroseptal portion of the left ventricle. Less commonly, occlusion of the right coronary artery leads to infarction of the inferior and posterior left ventricle. Least common is occlusion of the left circumflex artery, producing anterolateral myocardial infarction. When occlusion of the left main coronary artery occurs (rarely without severe disease of its branches), massive infarction of the left ventricle often results, but may not. Decrease in coronary flow in occlusive disease of the coronary artery usually implies occlusion of at least 80% of the artery. A lesser degree of coronary stenosis may increase coronary resistance when coronary flow increases during exercise (Klocke, 1983) (see p 139).

Premonitory Manifestations

Reports of premonitory symptoms such as weakness, shortness of breath, and vague chest discomfort days or weeks before the event in 50–75% of patients with acute myocardial infarction indicate the presence of progressive myocardial ischemia, suggesting that the onset is not as "unexpected" as was once thought. Prodromal symptoms are listed in Table 8–11.

Clinical Findings
A. Symptoms:
1. Pain–Pain is the classic dominant feature of acute myocardial infarction that compels the patient to seek help. It is similar in quality to angina pectoris (pp 145–147) and may be described as a heaviness or tightness or a great weight sitting on the chest. The pain is similar to angina of effort in location and radiation, but it may radiate more widely. Not only may it radiate more widely to the lower jaw and teeth, neck, left shoulder, upper back, or down the left arm to the 2 fingers innervated by the ulnar nerve (as with angina of effort), but it may also involve the upper posterior thoracic area, and the patient may think there is an orthopedic problem. The pain is more severe than that of angina of effort, does not subside with rest, builds up rapidly, may wax and wane, and may reach maximum severity in a few minutes. Nitroglycerin has little or no effect. The pain may last for hours if unrelieved by narcotics and may be unbearable. The

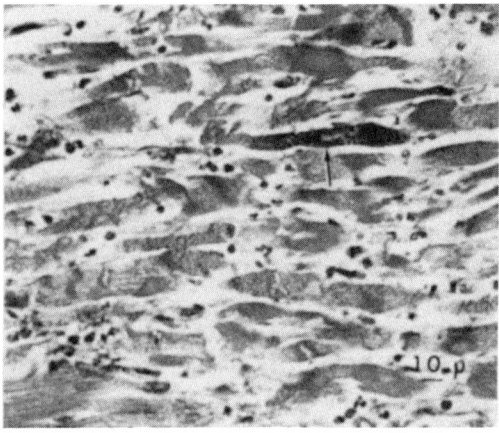

Figure 8–23. Photomicrograph of myocardium in peripheral region 96 hours after coronary artery occlusion. Note extensive myofibril degeneration and necrosis with many contraction bands, fragmented fibers, and loss of myofibrils, with edema and polymorphonuclear neutrophil infiltration. Occasional cells contain mineral deposits (arrow). Hematoxylin and eosin stain. (Reproduced, with permission, from the American heart Association, Inc., Bishop SP, White FC, Bloor CM: Regional myocardial blood flow during acute myocardial infarction in the conscious dog. *Circ Res* 1976;**38**:249.)

Table 8–11. Prevalence of prodromal symptoms in 160 patients hospitalized with acute myocardial infarction and in 138 who died prior to hospitalization.*

Symptoms	Prevalence	
	Hospitalized (112 out of 160) (percent)	Died Out of Hospital (88 out of 138) (percent)
Chest pain	67	35
	$\longleftarrow P < 0.001 \longrightarrow$	
Dyspnea	36	39
Arm and other pain	14	10
Fatigue and weakness	38	42
Dizziness and syncope	10	8
Anorexia and nausea	14	17
Emotional changes	14	20
Ankle edema and ascites	1	7
General malaise	16	17
Miscellaneous	9	16

*Modified and reproduced, with permission, from the American Heart Association, Inc., Alonzo AA, Simon AB, Feinleib M: Prodromata of myocardial infarction and sudden death. *Circulation* 1975;52:1056.

severity of chest pain is not related to the severity or size of the infarct, and the physician must not be misled into considering the event a minor one because the symptoms are not devastating.

2. Systemic manifestations–An indirect measure of the amount of necrotic tissue is the magnitude of the systemic response to acute infarction as evidenced by fever, tachycardia, leukocytosis, and increase in the sedimentation rate. These systemic signs of tissue necrosis usually appear 24–48 hours after the onset of the initial pain and are related to the amount of tissue that has undergone necrosis. They therefore serve as an estimate of the extent of infarction. The delayed systemic response is also helpful in differentiating acute myocardial infarction from such conditions as pneumonia or acute pericarditis, in which systemic abnormalities are present at the onset of illness.

Because necrosis appears 24–48 hours after the initial onset of pain, the temperature course follows this time interval. Substantial fever that is present at onset of pain or occurs after the fifth or sixth day should raise the question of some independent cause of fever. Patients with pulmonary infarction, for example, may have fever on the day of onset of chest pain, whereas in acute myocardial infarction the fever is delayed.

3. Sweating, weakness, and apprehension– The patient often breaks out into a cold sweat, feels weak and apprehensive, and moves about, seeking a position of comfort—in contrast to the discomfort of angina of effort, in which the patient's instinct is to stand still or to sit or lie down.

4. Light-headedness, dyspnea, and hypotension–In association with the pain and sweating, the patient may feel weak, faint, and light-headed. Syncope may occur if there is a rapid onset of ventricular tachycardia or fibrillation or an atrioventricular conduction defect with a Stokes-Adams attack. Syncope and manifestations of cerebral infarction are presumably the effects of decreased cardiac output on a compromised carotid or cerebral arterial supply to the brain.

The presence or absence of pain is important in evaluating the significance of hypotension, especially at the onset of acute myocardial infarction. The vasomotor response to acute pain is hypertension in some individuals but abrupt decrease in cardiac output and vasodilatation in muscles and skin in others, resulting in hypotension with poor tissue perfusion manifested by cold, clammy skin; a gray appearance; sighing respirations; tachycardia; and low blood pressure. These signs must not be taken as evidence of cardiogenic shock until pain is relieved by appropriate medication (see below).

Ventricular arrhythmias in the first few hours after an acute infarction may cause hypotension aggravated by the pain and fear engendered by the infarct. The myocardium often responds to acute ischemia with variable electrophysiologic changes of excitability and refractoriness, increased vulnerability to ventricular ectopia, and ventricular fibrillation.

5. Nausea, vomiting, and "indigestion"– Nausea and vomiting are not rare. The discomfort may extend into the epigastrium and be associated with sensations of indigestion and bloating, so that the patient takes antacids for supposed acute indigestion, but without benefit.

6. Pulmonary edema and left ventricular failure–In 10–20% of cases, the pain is minor and may be misinterpreted or overshadowed by the presence of acute pulmonary edema, rapidly developing left ventricular failure, profound weakness, shock, dyspnea, or cough or wheezing of acute left ventricular failure.

7. Retrospective diagnosis–In perhaps 10% of cases, the initial symptoms are mild enough so that the diagnosis is only recognized in retrospect, when an ECG is taken months later. This is particularly true in patients with autonomic nervous system dysfunction due to diabetes mellitus. The patient may fail to realize that myocardial infarction has occurred, because the pain lasts only 30 minutes and is unrelated to effort, with onset at rest or even during sleep. A patient with previous angina of effort will recognize the unusual features, particularly the severity, radiation, and duration of the discomfort and its failure to respond to nitroglycerin; however, a patient who has not had angina of effort may interpret the discomfort as indigestion or musculoskeletal disease or may merely complain of feeling unwell.

B. Signs: The signs of acute myocardial infarction may be trivial, or the patient may be at the point of death when first seen. The clinical picture is related to the size and extent of the infarction, the presence of previous infarction with left ventricular dysfunction, and the adequacy of the collateral circulation.

1. Initial signs—The initial signs may be more severe than those found 1–2 hours later, especially if the patient has had a ventricular arrhythmia, marked bradycardia with poor output, or abrupt left ventricular failure that subsided as compensatory reflex mechanisms came into play.

2. Signs in mild cases—In mild cases the patient may appear well, with dry skin, normal pulse and blood pressure, and complaining only of prolonged substernal discomfort.

3. Signs in more severe cases—In more severe cases the patient appears acutely ill and may have marked hypotension with low cardiac output; tachycardia; cold, clammy, sweaty skin; and a gray (ashen) appearance due to peripheral cyanosis. If cerebral perfusion is impaired, the patient may be mentally dull and confused and may have either tachycardia or bradycardia. At the onset of acute myocardial infarction, the temperature is usually normal. Fever is delayed for 24–72 hours and is due to myocardial necrosis, which takes time to develop.

4. Combination of shock and cardiac failure—A patient with clinically apparent shock with a systolic pressure less than 80 mm Hg and a urine output less than 20 mL/h may show signs of left ventricular failure with a diastolic gallop rhythm, pulsus alternans, and bilateral rales. The gallop and rales may rapidly progress to acute pulmonary edema or right-sided congestive heart failure or may remain the same. The chest x-ray confirms left ventricular failure by haziness in the central lung fields if there is transudation into the alveoli or redistribution of flow to the upper lobe if there is interstitial edema. Kerley's B lines may also occur after some days but may be out of phase with the clinical signs, and there may be hemodynamic evidence of raised pulmonary artery diastolic pressure. Although the radiologic signs lag behind the hemodynamic ones, x-ray offers valuable evidence of cardiac failure, especially when raised wedge pressure is present.

The venous pressure may be raised, and when hemodynamic studies are done, the right atrial pressure is elevated. If the signs of shock are delayed, venous constriction out of proportion to arteriolar constriction may lead to transudation of fluid out of the capillaries, and the patient may be hypovolemic, in which instance the right atrial pressure is low and volume repletion is indicated.

Right ventricular infarction must be considered in patients with inferior myocardial infarction who have right ventricular failure with raised venous pressure, low cardiac output and hypotension, but little evidence of left ventricular failure. The right atrial pressure is often higher than the wedge pressure. Hypokinesis localized to the right ventricle (on gated blood pool angiography) and abnormal radionuclide uptake localized to the right ventricle aid in the diagnosis. Recognition is important because diuretic therapy is inadvisable and prognosis is better than when right ventricular failure complicates left ventricular failure from anterior infarction.

C. Laboratory Findings:

1. White count and erythrocyte sedimentation rate—The white blood count and sedimentation rate are normal at onset and rise with the fever as myocardial necrosis occurs. As the necrotic area of myocardium extends toward the epicardium, pericarditis may be recognized by pericardial friction rub, but this is often delayed until at least the second day and is transient, usually lasting not more than 2–4 days, and may be intermittent. High fever and leukocytosis indicate extensive infarction in the absence of pneumonia or other diseases. The sedimentation rate often remains elevated for 2–3 weeks after the white blood count and temperature have returned to normal.

2. Myocardial enzymes—With necrosis of cells, myocardial enzymes appear in the serum. The myocardial band (MB) isoenzymes of creatine phosphokinase (CPK) are found within 4 hours. These isoenzymes are derived exclusively from myocardial cells, as compared with the total CPK, which may enter the serum from muscle, brain, or liver (Fig 8–24). Serum glutamic-oxaloacetic transaminase (AST) may not rise for 6–12 hours and returns to normal in 5–7 days; CPK is usually normal in 4–6 days. Serum lactate dehydrogenase may remain elevated for 7–9 days; for this reason, measurement of LDH, especially the

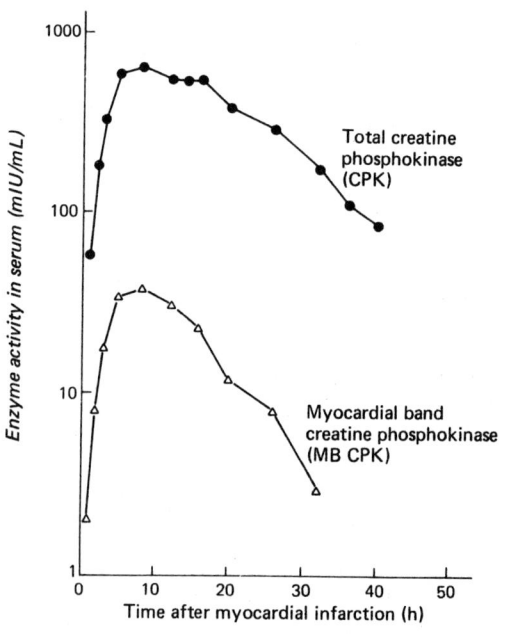

Figure 8–24. Serial changes in total serum CPK activity and serum MB CPK activity in a patient with hemodynamically uncomplicated acute myocardial infarction. The disappearance rate of MB CPK activity exceeded the corresponding rate for total CPK. MB denotes myocardial band of CPK. (Reproduced, with permission, from Sobel BE, Roberts R, Larson KB: Estimation of infarct size from serum MB creatine phosphokinase activity: Application and limitations. *Am J Cardiol* 1976;**37**:474.)

isoenzyme of LDH, may be valuable when the patient is not seen until a few days have elapsed after an acute episode of pain, because these enzymes may remain positive after the MB CPK isoenzymes have returned to normal. Serial determinations of enzymes every 2 hours make it possible to determine the area under the time curve of the increase and decrease in the enzyme and thus permit an estimate of the magnitude of the infarction.

D. Electrocardiographic Findings: A myocardial infarction of significant size, especially if transmural and anterior, produces characteristic electrocardiographic changes in about 95% of patients. Five examples of the electrocardiographic changes in myocardial infarction are seen in Figs 8–25 to 8–29.

1. Early unchanged ECG–At the onset of infarction, the ECG may be within normal limits. A normal ECG at this stage should not rule out the diagnosis.

2. Early electrocardiographic changes–The characteristic pattern may be delayed for hours or days, and the initial slightly convex ST elevation seen over septal leads V_{2-4} in anteroseptal myocardial infarction, over lateral leads V_{5-6} anterolateral infarction, and in inferior leads II, III, and aVF in inferior infarction may be subtle and difficult to distinguish from the normal variant of early repolarization. Over a period of hours or days, however, the characteristic evolution occurs, with subsequent symmetric inversion of T waves in the leads that initially showed convex elevated ST segments.

3. Evolving ECG–If characteristic broad Q waves are present in leads with convex elevated ST segments that subsequently evolve to symmetrically inverted T waves, an unequivocal diagnosis can be made. Q waves are more significant than QS complexes, particularly in the right precordial (V_{1-3}) or septal leads (V_{2-4}) or in the inferior leads (II, III, aVF) in horizontal heart position with left axis deviation. If there is a broad (≥ 0.4 second) slurred, wide Q wave with an amplitude exceeding 30% of that of the succeeding R wave, which is slightly slurred in its upstroke—and especially if a previous ECG did not show the Q waves—the diagnosis is strongly supported.

4. Serial changes–The diagnosis is less certain if there are no diagnostic Q waves, as is the case with nontransmural infarctions. In these instances, serial changes with waxing and then waning of the ST–T abnormalities are more reliable than static changes. If the patient is seen after the infarction has been present for some days and there is no previous ECG for comparison, the initial ST–T changes may appear nonspecific, and further serial records over days to weeks may be necessary before one can interpret the electrocardiographic changes as diagnostic.

5. ECG in presence of old infarct–If the patient has had previous myocardial infarction, if there is left

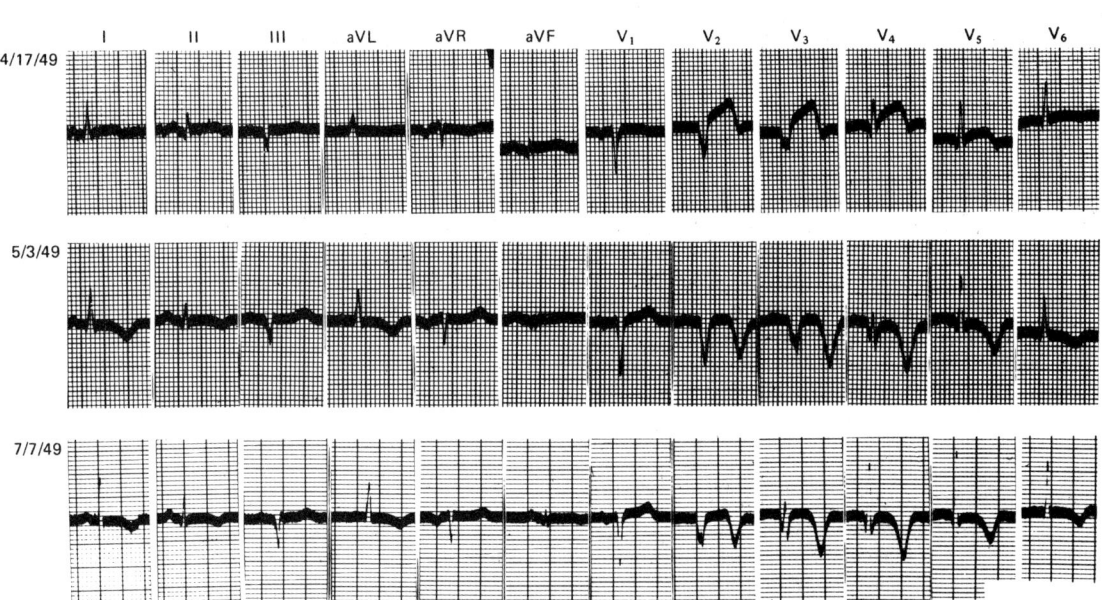

Figure 8–25. ECG of a 65-year-old man with anteroseptal myocardial infarction. Electrocardiographic findings of acute anteroseptal infarction with serial changes were noted on 4/17/49—1 month after the patient developed pain in the posterior aspect of the upper chest that awakened him from sleep and required injection of an analgesic. The pain had recurred the next day, spread to the anterior chest, and was recurrent at rest for the month prior to 4/17/49. The ECG shows a QS complex with elevated ST and late inversion of the T wave, which progressively developed in the 3 months indicated by the dates. Sequential changes resulted in a significant Q wave in V_3 followed by deep inversion of the T wave in V_{2-6}.

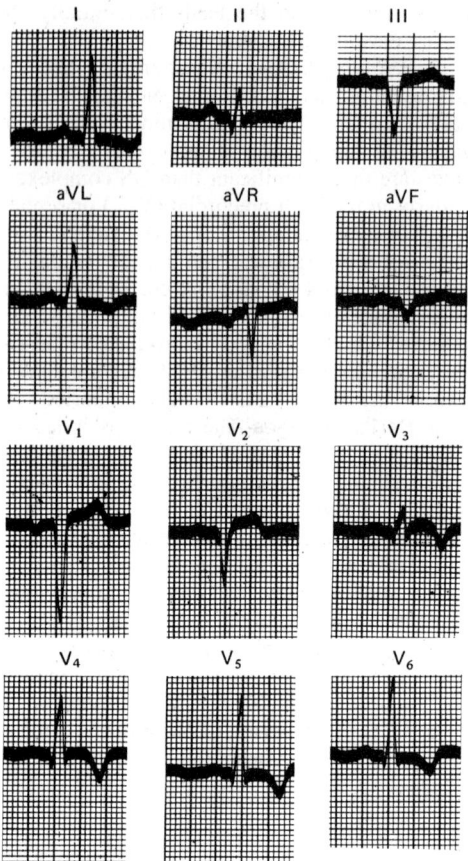

Figure 8–26. ECG of a 59-year-old man showing old inferior myocardial infarction (slurred QS in aVF and slurred Q in lead II) and more recent anteroseptal myocardial infarction with associated left ventricular conduction defects (inverted T waves in V_{3-6}, I, and aVL with a slurred Q in V_3 and a slurred QRS complex in V_4).

---

bundle branch block or significant conduction defects in the peripheral Purkinje system, or if there is underlying left ventricular hypertrophy or digitalis effect, the interpretation is more difficult and the presence of diagnostic Q waves or characteristic serial evolution of the ST–T abnormalities is required to establish the electrocardiographic diagnosis of myocardial infarction. Radioisotopic methods may be especially useful in these situations.

6. Return to normal ECG–The usual evolution of the ST–T changes takes several weeks, but in minor infarction this may occur within 10 days. When the acute infarction is characterized only by ST–T changes, the ECG may return completely to normal in about 20–30% of patients; a normal ECG therefore does not exclude a previous infarction.

7. Abnormal Q waves–Q waves, defined as initial negative deflections followed by positive deflections—in contrast to QS complexes, which are negative deflections not followed by positive ones—have greater diagnostic value when abnormal than ST–T abnormalities. A Q wave of 0.04 second, especially if slightly slurred and followed by a slurred upstroke of the R wave, is considered diagnostic of anterior infarction when it occurs in the precordial leads and of inferior infarction when it occurs in lead aVF. One-half to two-thirds of patients with Q waves have localized segmental wall motion abnormalities demonstrable by left ventricular angiography in the area of the Q wave representing infarction. It is now believed that the immediate subendocardial area does not contribute to the Q waves but that they are the result of necrosis of the mid- and subepicardial areas. The Q waves may be transient and due to functional impairment resulting from hypoxia or ischemia or the development of collateral blood flow and may disappear as the infarct heals. The presence of a Q wave, therefore, does not mean myocardial scar, death of cells, or permanent damage, because during left ventricular angiography the Q waves may disappear, and segmental areas of hypokinesia or asynergy may contract more normally when the load on the myocardium is decreased following administration of nitroglycerin or hydralazine.

Conduction defects that alter pathways of activation may influence the appearance and course of Q waves. The Q waves may disappear when left bundle branch block develops, only to reappear when the conduction delay disappears in intermittent block, as sometimes occurs during the course of an acute infarction.

Persistent Q waves are not a reliable sign of ventricular aneurysm. Many patients with Q waves do not have aneurysms, although they may have segmental localized contraction abnormalities.

In aVF, a Q wave 0.04 second wide with a depth of at least 30% that of the succeeding R wave, and an associated significant Q wave in lead II are the most reliable signs of inferior infarction. Small Q waves may appear in aVF in a vertically placed heart in normal individuals. A Q wave in aVF is more significant if the patient has a horizontally placed heart (left ventricular potentials transmitted to the left arm) than if the heart is vertically placed (left ventricular potentials transmitted to the left leg). When typical evolutionary serial electrocardiographic changes occur in the presence of progressive increases in serum enzymes (particularly the MB isoenzymes of CPK) and a compatible clinical history, the diagnosis is considered to be firmly established.

E. Radioisotope Studies of Myocardial Infarction: (See Figs 8–30 to 8–33.) Coronary perfusion studies using thallium 201 in patients with previous myocardial infarction have shown that the myocardium supplied by the artery may have normal coronary blood flow at rest but hypoperfusion or altered distribution of flow under the stress of exercise. Quantitative thallium 201 scans have been used to determine the location, extent, and persistence of myocardial ischemia at the time of the acute infarction and later before hospital discharge; transient ischemia can be

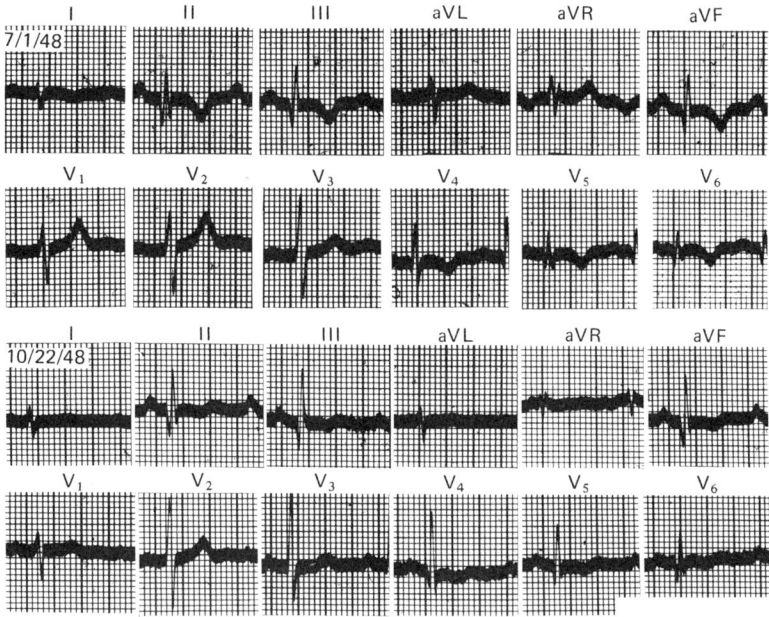

Figure 8–27. ECG of a 59-year-old man with inferolateral myocardial infarction who had dyspnea on exertion for 6 months as well as angina of effort and anginal pain on awakening that lasted about 2 weeks (up until 2 months before the time of the first tracing). Blood pressure was 140/90 mm Hg. Note the prominent Q and inverted T waves in leads II, III, aVF, and V_{4-6} in the record of 7/1/48. The abnormalities have improved in the record of 10/22/48.

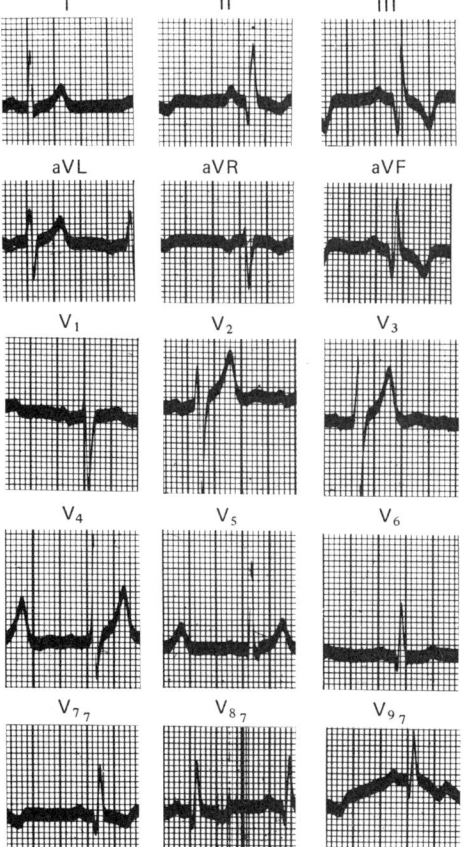

observed by comparison of rest and exercise abnormalities. Perfusion defects in areas distant from that of the acute infarction indicate additional areas of ischemia. Multiple thallium 201 defects usually predict multivessel and more extensive disease with a greater likelihood of left ventricular dysfunction (Gibson, 1983).

Right ventricular infarction can be diagnosed by radioisotope studies as well as clinical findings. Abnormal radionuclide uptake can be localized to the right ventricle, or localized hypokinesis of the right ventricle may be evident on gated blood pool angiography. Infarction of the right ventricle may explain predominant right ventricular failure in patients with acute inferior myocardial infarction. (See also p 166.)

Thallium isotopic perfusion scans do not show small perfusion defects, and reproducibility is variable unless maximum exercise is performed. Resolution of isotopic scans is imperfect, but the reliability of scanning is improved by the use of computer techniques.

In contrast to thallium 201, which reveals defects in perfusion ("cold spots"), intravenous technetium ^{99m}Tc pyrophosphate has the advantage of being actively

Figure 8–28. An example of inferior myocardial infarction with typical findings of prominent Q in leads II, III, and aVF, with inverted T waves in these leads and in the posterolateral leads (V_{7-9}) in the seventh interspace but no diagnostic findings in the routine lateral leads (V_{4-6}).

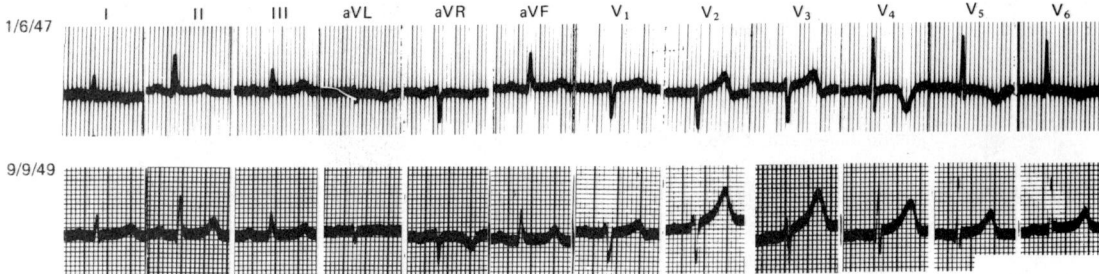

Figure 8–29. ECG of a 63-year-old man with myocardial infarction. The electrocardiographic abnormalities characteristic of myocardial infarction on the first tracing have completely disappeared in the second tracing obtained 2 years later. (Inverted T waves in V_{4-6}.)

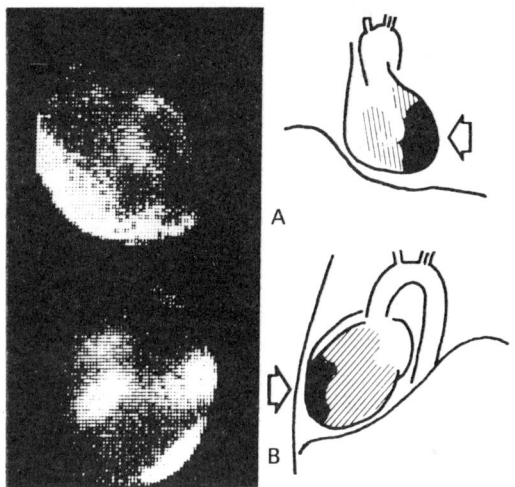

Figure 8–30. Anterolateral infarction. The frontal *(A)* and left lateral *(B)* scintiscans show an area of diminished activity (arrows) at the site of infarction. (Reproduced, with permission, from Wackers FJT et al: Noninvasive visualization of acute myocardial infarction in man with thallium-201. *Br Heart J* 1975;**37**:741.)

taken up by acutely infarcted myocardial cells (but not old scar), producing discrete, well-localized "hot spots" in transmural acute infarction. Technetium pyrophosphate has limitations in nontransmural subendocardial infarction, because diffuse uptake can be seen. Such uptake may also occur in the absence of infarction, and it will cause false-positive interpretations. On the other hand, a definitive, discrete uptake of pyrophosphate demonstrates recent myocardial infarction more effectively than the failure of uptake of thallium by scarred or ischemic cells following induced ischemia.

As imaging techniques improve, especially with 3-dimensional computer processing, it is becoming possible to more accurately determine the size of an infarct, especially if it is anterior. The quantitative estimate of the size of the infarct by radionuclide

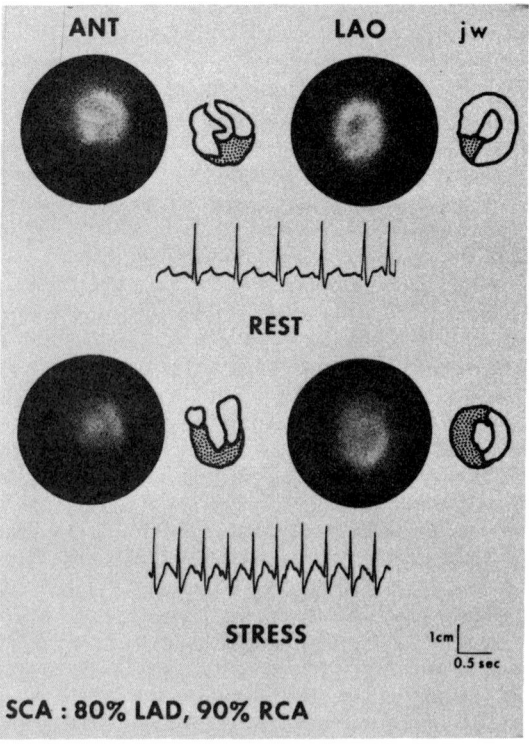

Figure 8–31. Isotopes in myocardial infarction. Man, age 58, with a negative treadmill test but showing, at rest, a residual old infarct abnormality, worse with exercise after administration of thallium. Selective angiogram shows left anterior oblique artery 80% stenotic and right coronary artery 90% stenotic. ANT, anterior; LAO, left anterior oblique; SCA, selective coronary angiogram; LAD, left anterior descending artery; RCA, right coronary artery. (Reproduced, with permission, from Botvinick EH et al: Myocardial stress perfusion scintigraphy with rubidium 81 versus stress electrocardiography. *Am J Cardiol* 1977;**39**:364.)

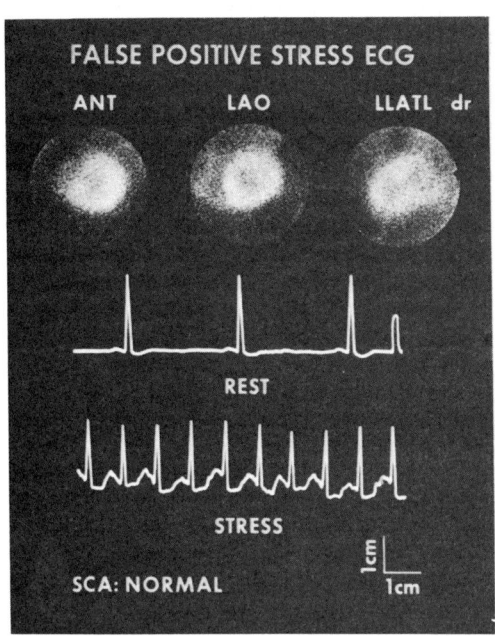

Figure 8–32. Isotopes in myocardial infarction. Positive stress test (?false-positive) with normal image and normal coronary angiogram—not on digitalis. ANT, anterior; LAO, left anterior oblique; LLATL, left lateral; SCA, selective coronary angiogram. (Modified and reproduced, with permission, from Botvinick EH et al: Thallium 201 myocardial perfusion scintigraphy for the clinical clarification of normal, abnormal, and equivocal electrocardiographic stress test. *Am J Cardiol* 1978;**41**:43.)

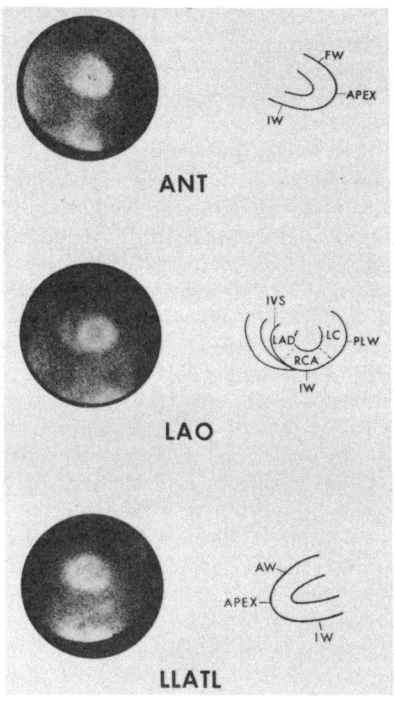

Figure 8–33. Isotopes in myocardial infarction. Normal thallium 201 perfusion image. ANT, anterior; LAO, left anterior oblique; LLATL, left lateral; FW, free wall; IW, inferior wall; IVS, interventricular septum; LAD, left anterior descending artery; RCA, right coronary artery; LC, left circumflex artery; PLW, posterior lateral wall; AW, anterior wall. (Modified and reproduced, with permission, from Botvinick EH et al: Thallium 201 myocardial perfusion scintigraphy for the clinical clarification of normal, abnormal, and equivocal electrocardiographic stress tests. *Am J Cardiol* 1978;**41**:43.)

technique correlates significantly with serial serum enzyme determinations and hemodynamic measurements. The methods are complementary, and both should be used. In patients with old myocardial infarction or myocardial scars, image perfusion defects may be diagnostic of an old infarction or scar at a time when only nonspecific ST segment abnormalities without Q waves are present in the resting ECG. If image defects following exercise do not change, it confirms that the defect seen at rest is due to an old scar.

A promising new technique being tested is the use of radioiodinated fragments of antimyosin antibody, which allows discrete myocardial uptake. Infarcted myocardial cells have increased membrane permeability and permit the intracellular concentration of the specific antibody to myosin. When the radioiodinated fragments were injected intravenously into dogs with an infarct, discrete uptake required approximately 72 hours, but when the isotope was injected into the coronary artery, clear images were demonstrated as early as 7 hours after occlusion (Khaw, 1979).

F. Size of Myocardial Infarct: As a result of the factors mentioned earlier that influence myocardial ischemia, the artery occluded in an extensive myocardial infarction cannot always be predicted accurately. Although we describe myocardial infarction as a disease entity, it is more useful to consider it as a continuum of increasing necrosis from a few cells to massive infarction. The former results in a mild illness mainly with cardiac pain (see below), without disturbance in left ventricular function, and with minimal serum enzyme elevations, although the pattern on the ECG may be diagnostic. When necrosis involves many cells and a large area, especially if there has been previous infarction with segmental scars, the clinical picture is complicated by the presence of ventricular arrhythmias, cardiogenic shock, left ventricular dysfunction with cardiac failure, conduction defects, cardiac arrest, and death. The physician therefore must attempt to estimate the extent of the infarction in terms of its impact on the circulation as well as its site and size. The former is a function of the extent of the previous as well as the current myocardial infarction, which limits left ventricular function. If the amount of previous myocardial scarring is extensive, even a small additional myocardial infarction may produce severe clinical manifestations of cardiogenic shock and failure.

Methods for measuring the size of the myocardial infarction include the following: (1) determination of the extent of abnormalities on the ECG and location of the Q, ST, and T wave changes, whether they occur in just a few leads over the lateral chest or extend across the entire anterior precordium and perhaps the inferior wall as well; (2) ST mapping, in which the magnitude and persistence of ST segment elevation using multiple precordial leads are added up and averaged over a period of days; (3) serial determinations of MB isoenzymes of CPK released into the serum by necrosing myocardial cells; (4) pyrophosphate and thallium radioisotope uptake studies; (5) hemodynamic studies; and (6) cineangiography.

The greater the isoenzyme rise or increased uptake of pyrophosphate (or factors of uptake of thallium), the greater the number of necrosed myocardial cells. Using computer-assisted methods, a thallium defect score can be determined that correlates with infarct size and subsequent mortality rate (Silverman, 1980). Positive scans are usually negative within the first few hours but become positive, showing perfusion defects, in about 12 hours after intravenous injection of the radioisotope. Serial studies can then be done to follow the course, which may demonstrate an increase or decrease in the size of the infarct or allow a small infarction to become visible.

G. Determination of Wall Motion Abnormalities and Left Ventricular Function by Radioisotope and 2-Dimensional Echocardiographic Studies:

Left ventricular function and the presence of complications such as ventricular aneurysm, pseudoaneurysm, ventricular septal defect of papillary muscle dysfunction, or ventricular thrombi can be determined by 2-dimensional echocardiograms. Localized and global ejection fraction and regional wall motion by 2-dimensional echocardiograms may be the earliest finding in acute coronary occlusion (Reeder, 1982; Gibson, 1983). The presence of extensive wall motion abnormalities outside the immediate acute infarcted area is associated with more severe disease and a worse prognosis for survival (Gibson, 1983).

There are also at least 2 noninvasive radioisotope techniques by which wall motion abnormalities and left ventricular function can be estimated. The first is by the recording of images during both systole and diastole after a bolus injection of technetium-labeled albumin, "gated" (synchronized) to the ECG. Disturbances in wall motion can be recognized, and localized areas of hypokinesia or dyskinesia can be noted. Ejection fraction can be determined from the difference between the systolic and diastolic isotope image. The second method is by the so-called single-pass nucleotide angiogram, in which technetium ^{99m}Tc pertechnetate is given intravenously and a computerized, summated series of cardiac cycles is obtained. These cycles resemble a dye-dilution curve. Localized abnormalities of wall motion and ejection fraction can be noted. Both methods correlate reasonably well. Radioisotope special techniques such as radionuclide angiography to determine wall motion abnormalities are still research procedures involving expensive equipment and highly technically trained physicians and are not essential in most patients with acute myocardial infarction.

H. Minor Myocardial Infarction:

The diagnosis of minor myocardial infarction is often obvious only in retrospect when one reviews the entire sequence of events of the illness. Slight increases in serum enzymes, relatively minor ST–T abnormalities, slight fever, the presence of transient gallop rhythm, and serial radioisotopic scans may permit diagnosis. However, myocardial infarction may extend and hemodynamic manifestations may worsen, and a patient who originally presented with what appeared to be minor myocardial infarction may develop a more severe variety. Furthermore, even a small area of myocardial necrosis may induce ventricular arrhythmias or conduction defects.

In general, mild and nontransmural infarction has a lower mortality rate than transmural infarction. Patients with transmural infarction may have a greater prevalence of previous myocardial infarction and therefore a greater area of total myocardial infarction, new and old, than those with nontransmural infarction.

Course & Complications

Table 8–12 compares the complications in patients with acute myocardial infarction with those in patients with acute coronary insufficiency (unstable angina). The late mortality rate is 4–15% per year depending on the number of vessels involved and the degree of left ventricular dysfunction.

In mild cases, after chest pain is relieved by morphine or one of its analogs, the course is uneventful, with no evidences of arrhythmia, cardiac failure, or cardiogenic shock. In more severe infarction, and even in some milder cases, the most common finding is the development of arrhythmias. The most lethal development is cardiogenic shock. Extension of the infarcted area to the epicardium causes pericarditis in about 10% of cases, usually pericardial pain combined with a transient pericardial friction rub.

A. Arrhythmias:

1. Tachyarrhythmias–(See also Chapter 15.) Within hours after an episode of acute myocardial infarction, ventricular arrhythmias develop (usually ventricular premature beats) in 10–15%, and ventricular fibrillation in 5–10% (Table 8–13). The ventricular premature beats may be single or may occur in salvos; may occur frequently or only occasionally; or may be repetitive and lead to ventricular tachycardia or fibrillation. The ischemic cells are usually the sites of onset of abnormal activation leading to arrhythmia. These surviving Purkinje fibers have abnormal electrophysiologic changes that foster arrhythmias. Severe ventricular arrhythmias are 10–20 times more com-

Table 8–12. Comparison of complications and hospital course in patients with acute coronary insufficiency (unstable angina) and a group of 359 concurrently admitted patients with definite acute myocardial infarction.*

	Definite Myocardial Infarction (359 Patients)	Acute Coronary Insufficiency (Unstable Angina) (100 Patients)
Average age (years)	62	62
Men:women	2.5:1	1.8:1
Complications		
Hypotension (<90 mm Hg systolic)†	34%	4%
Bradycardia	16%	12%
Atrial premature beats	15%	15%
Ventricular premature beats†	61%	35%
Ventricular tachycardia†	25%	6%
Atrioventricular block		
First- to second-degree†	13%	5%
Third-degree†	7%	1%
Bundle branch block	11%	7%
Congestive heart failure†		
Mild to moderate	39%	20%
Severe	16%	6%
Acute mortality		
Coronary care unit†	16%	0
Hospital outside coronary care unit†	5%	1%
Average length of stay		
Coronary care unit	6.6 days	4.6 days
Hospital	21 days	14 days

*Reproduced, with permission, from Krauss KR, Hutter AM, DeSanctis RW: Acute coronary insufficiency (unstable angina): Course and follow-up. *Arch Intern Med* 1972;**129**:808.
†$P < 0.05$

mon in the first 4 hours than they are on the second day; for this reason, patients are ideally admitted as soon as possible to a coronary unit with specially trained personnel and equipment permitting continuous electrocardiographic monitoring. The great frequency of early ventricular arrhythmias explains the high mortality rate before the patient receives treatment. The severity of early arrhythmias is related to the size of the infarct and the presence of ventricular asynergy or aneurysm. The abrupt development of ventricular tachycardia or ventricular fibrillation may result in cardiac arrest.

a. Ventricular fibrillation–When ventricular fibrillation or cardiac arrest follows the development of shock or heart failure, it is considered secondary to the poor left ventricular function and not to primary electrical instability of the ischemic myocardium. Prompt recognition and treatment of ventricular arrhythmias in the coronary care unit (see Treatment, below) has been a major factor in reducing the mortality rate of acute infarction in the hospital and in mobile ambulance units. Continuous monitoring of the patient, with a monitor both at the bedside and at the nursing station, permits immediate recognition of the abnormal rhythm, which must be treated promptly (within 30 seconds) in order to prevent irreversible cardiac or cerebral damage. Sudden cardiac death in acute ischemia is usually due to ventricular fibrillation, and at autopsy most patients have severe coronary disease with 2- or 3-vessel involvement; occasionally, only a single vessel is diseased. Although most episodes of ventricular fibrillation occur very early in the course of acute myocardial infarction, a small percentage develop late in the hospital course, especially in those patients with anteroseptal myocardial infarction complicated by right or left bundle branch block. These patients should be monitored by electrocardiography for at least a month (Lie, 1975).

b. Other tachyarrhythmias–(See also Chapter 15.) Accelerated idioventricular rhythm occurs in about 15–25% of patients. It is usually due to enhanced automaticity but may be an "escape" rhythm. Idioventricular rhythms are "benign," because the heart rate is usually relatively slow (60–100/min) and because they infrequently lead to ventricular tachycardia with more rapid rates (150–180/min) or ventricular fibrillation. This is not always true, however; close observation is required, and the possibility of ventricular tachycardia must be considered when ventricular rates exceeding 100–110/min occur. The idioventricular rhythm is often heralded by ventricular premature beats with varying coupling intervals combined with sinus bradycardia.

Atrial arrhythmias, including paroxysmal atrial fibrillation or tachycardia, are less common, are usually short-lived, and do not require rigorous treatment (such as cardioversion) unless symptoms appear or

Table 8–13. Incidence of dysrhythmias among 284 patients seen within the first hour, 1966–1969.*

Dysrhythmia	Number of Patients				Total Number of Patients
	Within 1 Hour	Within 2 Hours	Within 3–4 Hours	After 4 Hours	
Bradyarrhythmia	88 (31%)	10 (3.5%)	6 (2%)	21 (7%)	125 (44%)
Ventricular ectopic beats	70 (25%)	36 (13%)	16 (6%)	41 (14%)	163 (57%)
Ventricular fibrillation	28 (10%)	12 (4%)	2 (0.7%)	12 (4%)	54 (19%)
Ventricular tachycardia	10 (3.5%)	16 (6%)	6 (2%)	55 (19%)	87 (31%)
Atrial fibrillation/flutter	11 (4%)	0	0	15 (5%)	26 (9%)
Supraventricular tachycardia	1 (0.4%)	0	0	10 (3.5%)	11 (4%)

*Reproduced, with permission, from Adgey AA et al: Acute phase of myocardial infarction. *Lancet* 1971;**2**:501.

Table 8–14. Frequency of supraventricular arrhythmias in acute myocardial infarction (222 instances in 154 patients).*

Type of Arrhythmia	Alone	Combined	Total	Incidence	Mortality
	(Number)			(Percent)	
Supraventricular premature contractions	70	58	128	36	24
Supraventricular tachycardia	20	35	55	16	25
Atrial flutter or fibrillation	5	34	39	11	41

*Reproduced, with permission, from Cristal N, Szwarcberg J, Gueron M: Supraventricular arrhythmias in acute myocardial infarction: Prognostic importance of clinical setting; mechanism of production. *Ann Intern Med* 1975;82:35.

hemodynamic deterioration occurs. Their frequency is illustrated in Table 8–14.

When the ventricular rate is rapid—exceeding 140–150 beats/min in atrial fibrillation or atrial tachycardia—coronary perfusion may be decreased and cardiac output may fall. If the patient has incipient left ventricular failure it may worsen, and the adverse hemodynamic effects may increase the area of infarction. In these situations, cardioversion should be used promptly. If the ventricular rate is slower and the patient is tolerating it well, without symptoms or hemodynamic change, one may use conventional antiarrhythmic agents such as digitalis — or edrophonium or rapid atrial stimulation if digitalis toxicity is a possibility. Atrial stimulation must not be used in fibrillation. New compounds are used for the treatment of paroxysmal tachycardia; one of the most effective is verapamil, a drug that selectively increases conduction delay in the atrioventricular node and may terminate reentry rhythm.

2. Bradyarrhythmias–(See Table 8–15 and Chapter 15.) At the onset of acute infarction, sinus bradycardia or sinus standstill may occur in 10–20% of cases, causing junctional escape or idioventricular rhythm. Bradycardia is due to the Jarisch–von Bezold vagal reflex, a chemoreflex which is triggered by chemical stimuli (possibly histamine) from the left ventricular wall or coronary artery and which causes bradycardia or hypotension. Involvement of the sinoatrial nodal artery in right coronary artery occlusion with inferior or posterior myocardial infarction may also cause bradycardia. Most of the slow heart rates noted in the early stages following an acute infarction are due to sinus bradycardia. Sinoatrial block and atrioventricular block are infrequent. Most patients with cardiac arrest have ventricular fibrillation and not sinoatrial or atrioventricular block when first seen under these circumstances.

Slow heart rates allow for a greater degree of nonhomogeneity of excitability and refractoriness in neighboring fibers, and arrhythmias are thus more common in these patients. If evidence of poor cardiac output is present with slow heart rates at the onset of acute myocardial infarction, atropine, 0.3–0.6 mg intravenously, is often beneficial but may produce sinus tachycardia and ventricular arrhythmias if high or repetitive doses are used.

B. Atrioventricular Conduction Defects: Atrioventricular conduction defects are common in acute myocardial infarction, occurring in about 10% of patients, and are associated with a mortality rate of about 50% in third-degree or Mobitz type II block. (For further details, see Chapter 14.)

1. Conduction defects in anterior infarction–Atrioventricular and intraventricular conduction defects are more hazardous in the presence of anterior myocardial infarction because they represent widespread necrosis in the ventricular septum, often involving the bundle of His and its branches and frequently resulting in impaired left ventricular function and hypokinesia. The conduction defect may be recognized early during electrocardiographic monitoring in the coronary care unit. The patient may develop a left anterior fascicular block with left axis deviation of -45 to -60 degrees; this indicates damage to the left anterior superior fascicle of the left bundle with or without right bundle branch block.

2. Stokes-Adams attacks–The patient may also develop partial atrioventricular block with prolongation of the PR interval (>0.21 second) or may have second-degree atrioventricular block with dropped beats (Mobitz type II). The change from a first-degree atrioventricular block or a left anterior fascicular block to second-degree and then complete atrioventricular block with Stokes-Adams attacks may occur within hours, and immediate prophylactic placement of a temporary artificial pacemaker is essential. When complete atrioventricular block occurs in anterior infarction, the ventricular escape pacemaker is usually below the area of destruction in the septum, in one of the branches of the left or right bundle, or even in the ventricular myocardium; as a result, the QRS complex is usually wide (>0.12 second) and the rate of discharge of the ectopic pacemaker in one of the fascicles is usually slow and unreliable.

3. Conduction defects in inferior infarction–The situation is more favorable when atrioventricular conduction defect occurs late in inferior myocardial infarction, because the damage is usually to the atrioventricular node and is more ischemic than destructive. In such instances, although there are exceptions, the patient may have a partial atrioventricular block with a prolonged PR interval or may have second-degree atrioventricular block—so-called Wenckebach phenomenon or Mobitz type I—rather than 2:1 atrioventricular block with dropped beats, Mobitz type II (see Chapter 14). Conduction defects occur 2–4 times more frequently in acute inferior myocardial infarction than in anterior infarction (Table 8–15). Although about one-sixth of patients with acute inferior infarction have a high degree of atrioventricular block, death is due chiefly to a power failure and not to Stokes-Adams attack. The insertion of a right ventricular pacemaker has not been found to

Table 8–15. Incidence of bradyarrhythmias among 284 patients related to time after onset of symptoms and site of infarction, 1966–1969.*

Site of Infarction	Number of Patients				Total Number of Patients
	Within 1 Hour	Within 2 Hours	Within 3–4 Hours	After 4 Hours	
Sinus or nodal bradycardia	75 (26%)	9 (3%)	5 (2%)	19 (7%)	108 (38%)
Anterior infarct	24 (18%)	5 (4%)	1 (0.7%)	2 (1.5%)	32 (24%)
Posterior infarct	48 (36%)	4 (3%)	3 (2%)	16 (12%)	71 (53%)
Atrioventricular block, second degree or complete	17 (6%)	2 (0.7%)	1 (0.4%)	8 (3%)	28 (10%)
Anterior infarct	1 (0.7%)	0	1 (0.7%)	1 (0.7%)	3 (2%)
Posterior infarct	15 (11%)	2 (1.5%)	0	7 (5%)	24 (18%)

*Reproduced, with permission, from Adgey AA et al: Acute phase of myocardial infarction. *Lancet* 1971;2:501.

reduce the mortality rate. High-degree block is present in half of cases when the patient is first seen in the hospital; it rarely occurs less frequently after the first few days. The mortality rate is higher when the block occurs early.

4. Infrequency of Stokes-Adams attacks in inferior infarcts–When complete atrioventricular block occurs in the presence of inferior myocardial infarction, the pacemaker is just below the atrioventricular node, the QRS is usually narrow (>0.11 second), and the heart rate is faster (about 60/min) because the cardiac pacemaker is high in the conduction system. Because of the rarity of Stokes-Adams attacks in this setting, a conservative approach is usually recommended with continued monitoring rather than insertion of a temporary right ventricular pacemaker, unless the block occurs very early and is associated with hemodynamic deterioration. This decision must be individualized and must be considered tentative at present.

5. Complete infranodal block–Complete infranodal block is uncommon in patients with *preexisting* bundle branch block, but in about one-fourth of patients, right bundle branch block or left anterior hemiblock *develops* during acute myocardial infarction. Prophylactic pacing is advised in these latter instances because of the suddenness with which complete block may occur. The abrupt appearance of bundle branch block is an unfavorable sign and is associated with an increased frequency of both atrioventricular block and cardiac failure, with a higher mortality rate than in patients who do not develop bundle branch block.

6. Bilateral bundle branch block–Bilateral bundle branch block is diagnosed when block of either the right or the left bundle is associated with any degree of atrioventricular (bifascicular) block or when there are conduction defects in both branches. The mortality rate is high in these patients. The usual causes of death are ventricular arrhythmias and cardiac failure, rather than complete atrioventricular block. The use of temporary prophylactic pacemakers may be warranted but remains controversial.

The indications for *permanent* ventricular pacing in patients who have developed complete atrioventricular block during acute myocardial infarction are controversial. Some authors have asserted that patients with bifascicular block who develop complete atrioventricular block during the acute infarction are at high risk of recurrent complete atrioventricular block with sudden death if permanent pacing is not performed. Others disagree. Further prospective studies are required to determine whether death can be prevented by insertion of a permanent pacemaker in this specific subset of patients.

C. Cardiac Failure:

1. Acute left ventricular failure–Acute left ventricular dysfunction resulting from acute myocardial infarction may lead to unremitting pump failure or may be transient and associated with acute pulmonary edema, subsiding with relief of pain and the opening of collateral channels. Cardiac failure is the cause of death in two-thirds of hospital deaths except for those deaths occurring in the first 4 hours.

2. Milder cases of left ventricular failure–In less severe cases, the existence of left ventricular failure can be inferred on the basis of dyspnea, pulmonary rales, gallop rhythm, pulsus alternans, raised venous pressure, radiologic evidence of pulmonary venous congestion or redistribution of fluid to the upper lobes. If there is alveolar edema, bat's wing infiltrates near the hilar areas of the lungs may be seen. Increased heart size, sinus tachycardia, and gallop rhythm may be the only signs.

Serial chest films parallel the hemodynamic changes (see below), and the greater the degree of pulmonary venous congestion on admission, the higher the mortality rate. The absence of pulmonary venous congestion in association with normal heart size is an excellent prognostic sign.

3. Bedside hemodynamic monitoring–Monitoring of right atrial and pulmonary artery wedge pressure during the course of acute infarction can be performed with the balloon-tipped Swan-Ganz catheter, which allows repeated measurements of pressure and oxygen saturation in the right side of the heart in the coronary care unit with little disturbance to the patient. Serial determinations of cardiac output utilizing thermodilution (see Chapters 4 and 6) and computerized techniques also make it possible for patients with left ventricular dysfunction to be monitored intermittently for the purpose of determining right atrial pressure, pulmonary arterial pressure, pulmonary arterial wedge pressure, and cardiac output. Treatment can be individualized on the basis of abnormalities disclosed by these studies. Serial determinations of indices of left ventricular performance such as cardiac output, stroke output, or stroke work index can be compared with left ventricular filling pressure by inflating the balloon at the tip of the catheter wedged into the pulmonary artery. One can then determine whether left ventricular function is improving or deteriorating.

With more severe manifestations on presentation, the mean pulmonary artery wedge or diastolic pressure (the left ventricular filling pressure) increases, the left ventricular end-diastolic volume increases, the ejection fraction falls, and the cardiac output decreases. Subsets of acute myocardial infarction in cardiac failure have been defined by relating the left ventricular filling pressure to stroke work or cardiac index, which describes left ventricular performance. When the end-diastolic pressure is high and the stroke work index or cardiac index is low, the prognosis is worse (Table 8–16).

Right ventricular failure secondary to right ventricular infarction can be treated with volume expansion (not diuretics) to increase right ventricular output. Hypotension should be treated with dopamine. If the blood pressure is maintained but right ventricular failure persists, vasodilator therapy can be added.

4. Bedside echocardiography–Echocardiography at the bedside can complement hemodynamic studies and allow estimation of left ventricular dimensions and wall motion, septal and posterior myocardial wall contraction, size of the left atrium, and ejection fraction. Echocardiography can support the diagnosis of severe left ventricular failure in acute myocardial infarction by showing greatly increased left ventricular dimensions and a wide E point separation between the maximum excursion of the anterior mitral valve leaflet and the ventricular septum (see Fig 10–5).

5. Factors precipitating cardiac failure–Although cardiac failure may develop insidiously, it may appear abruptly following an arrhythmia or pulmonary infarction or following complications such as perforation of the ventricular septum or dysfunction of the papillary muscle with the development of acute mitral regurgitation. When either of the latter 2 complications develops, a loud, harsh systolic murmur and thrill suddenly appear over the lower left parasternal area in the case of septal perforation or at the apex in the case of mitral regurgitation. In both instances, severe cardiac failure may develop rapidly. Acute mitral incompetence gives rise to the abrupt development of very large v waves on the wedge tracing and septal rupture to a high oxygen content in the right ventricle, which can be demonstrated by using the Swan-Ganz catheter. Minor degrees of papillary muscle dysfunction are commonly found (about 50% of cases) if careful auscultation is done daily to search for the pansystolic or late systolic murmur of slight mitral insufficiency that accompanies the lesion.

6. Evaluating left ventricular function–The ejection fraction, which can be estimated serially by radioisotope study or by echocardiography, can be used to estimate the size of the infarct and the effectiveness of left ventricular function and helps to determine prognosis.

D. Cardiogenic Shock: Cardiogenic shock with hypotension and poor tissue perfusion with oliguria and cerebral obtundation may be present at the onset of a massive infarction or may develop insidiously and progressively over the next few days. It is more apt to occur when there has been previous infarction or when the current infarction is so massive that at least 50% of the myocardium is destroyed. Three-vessel coronary artery disease, severe proximal left anterior descending artery stenosis, or left main coronary artery stenosis is frequently present in patients with cardiogenic shock. Cardiogenic shock is more common than congestive failure in patients dying from "pump failure" after acute myocardial infarction. It is the most frequent cause of death in the hospital following acute infarction. The large area of damaged myocardium frustrates successful medical treatment.

Hemodynamic studies in patients with cardiogenic shock demonstrate a high left ventricular filling pressure, low cardiac output, low stroke work index, severe hypotension, and no evidence of hypovolemia. Severe cardiogenic shock is a dread event, and patients usually die within a few days. The prognosis is poor even in somewhat milder cases, and aggressive therapy is warranted. Following stabilization by temporary circulatory assist mechanisms such as aortic balloon counterpulsation, vasodilator therapy, and inotropic agents, coronary arteriography and left ventricular cineangiography are performed with a view to possible emergency operation. Cineangiography may also demonstrate the presence of perforation of the ventricular septum or gross mitral regurgitation as well as evidence of hypokinesia or akinesia or left ventricular aneurysm that may require surgical treatment. Even when salvage during the acute episode is possible by heroic effort, 1- or 2-year survivals are infrequent because of the severity of myocardial disease. Left ventricular asynergy with dyskinesia is more common than true aneurysm and occurs in most patients

Table 8–16. Mortality rates in clinical and hemodynamic subsets in acute myocardial infarction.*

Subset	Pulmonary Congestion (PCP > 18 mm Hg)†	Peripheral Hypoperfusion (CI < 2.2 L/min/m²)†	Percent Mortality	
			Clinical	Hemodynamic
I	–	–	1	3
II	+	–	11	9
III	–	+	18	23
IV	+	+	60	51

*Reproduced, with permission, from Forrester JS, Waters DD: Hospital treatment of congestive heart failure: Management according to hemodynamic profile. *Am J Med* 1978;**65**:173.
†PCP, pulmonary capillary pressure; CI, cardiac index.

after transmural infarction. In patients who have recovered from cardiogenic shock or cardiac failure after an acute infarction and are doing well, the Swan-Ganz catheter can be removed and a search for akinetic segments or ventricular aneurysm performed by noninvasive techniques with radioisotopes (Fig 8-34) or 2-dimensional echocardiography. If the patient has persistent or recurrent symptoms of cardiac failure or recurrent ventricular arrhythmias after successful initial management, left ventricular angiography is usually required. (See section on ventricular aneurysm, p 185.) Mitral regurgitation from papillary and free wall muscle dysfunction and ventricular septal defect from perforation of the septum should always be considered with a view to possible surgical treatment in patients who have had cardiogenic shock or cardiac failure.

E. Arterial Embolism: An uncommon occurrence during the course of acute infarction, which may be delayed for days, weeks, or months, is systemic embolism to various arteries (cerebral, coronary, visceral, or peripheral) resulting from dislodgment of a portion of mural thrombus that has developed over the infarct or within a ventricular aneurysm; it can be diagnosed by 2-dimensional echocardiography. This complication is seen less frequently today than formerly, though anticoagulants are now used less commonly.

F. Phlebothrombosis and Pulmonary Embolism: These complications are also less common now than when prolonged bed rest was recommended for acute infarction. Phlebothrombosis with or without pulmonary embolism occurs in approximately 10% of patients with acute myocardial infarction. Fatalities are rare.

G. Cerebral Infarction: The fall of arterial pressure associated with acute infarction in a patient with a compromised cerebral arterial blood supply may produce cerebral infarction. One should suspect acute myocardial infarction in all patients who develop cerebral infarction and should obtain an ECG. Cerebral embolism secondary to a mural thrombus in the left ventricle may also cause cerebral infarction, but the event is usually later in the course of acute myocardial infarction and is of sudden onset.

H. Rupture of the Heart: This an uncommon event (5%) and may cause sudden death owing to acute hemopericardium and tamponade (Fig 8-35). Rupture may be "subacute," with slight penetration of the epicardium to the pericardium, escape of blood, and worsening of the clinical picture. Penetration of a weakened epicardial wall with hemopericardium may be recognized by a change in symptoms and by echocardiography, and immediate surgery has been successful in some patients. Cardiac rupture is more common during the first week, but it can occur later.

I. Acute Renal Failure: Following prolonged hypotension and shock, patients may develop acute tubular necrosis with oliguria, anuria, and acute renal failure. Renal failure may also develop if vasodilator therapy with sodium nitroprusside is unusually vigorous, producing prolonged hypotension.

J. Pericarditis: Extension of the transmural infarct to the epicardial surface may result in inflammatory changes in the pericardium, possibly with hemopericardium, especially if anticoagulants have been used. The pain of pericarditis differs in that it is affected by movement in bed and by swallowing and is often relieved by leaning forward. Definitive diagnosis depends upon recognition of a pericardial friction rub (in about 15% of patients), which may be triphasic if the heart rate is slow but may appear to be uniphasic if the rate is rapid. The rub is usually heard along the left sternal border, is harsh and grating in quality, may be intermittent, and may last only a few days.

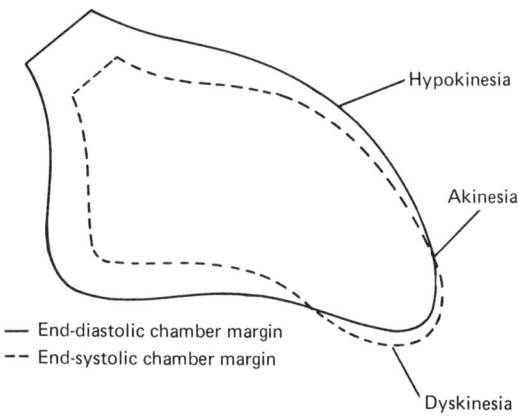

Figure 8-34. Segmental wall motion is analyzed by superimposing end-systolic chamber outline on end-diastolic chamber outline from left ventricular angiograms. Inward excursion is qualitatively estimated as mild, moderate, or severe hypokinesia, akinesia (no systolic motion), and dyskinesia (paradoxic outward systolic motion). (Reproduced, with permission, from Alderman EL: Angiographic indicators of left ventricular function. *JAMA* 1976;**236**:1055. Copyright © 1976, American Medical Association.)

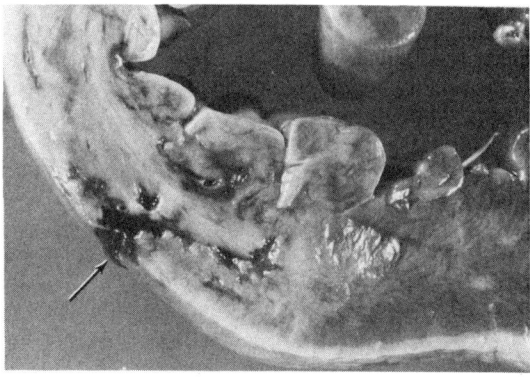

Figure 8-35. Myocardial infarction with early rupture of the left ventricular wall. (Courtesy of O Rambo.)

K. Cardiac Hypertrophy: Cardiac hypertrophy is uncommon in uncomplicated coronary heart disease but develops if myocardial infarction with cardiac failure ensues or if hypertension has been present. The average heart weight in fatal cases of acute myocardial infarction is just over 400 g, slightly heavier than normal.

Prevention

Preventive treatment of primary acute myocardial infarction and reinfarction is similar to that of hypertension. Serum lipids should be reduced with a low-calorie, low-saturated fat diet and use of resins such as cholestyramine and colestipol (see p 135). Primary prevention of coronary artery atherosclerosis by attention to other risk factors and the use of agents that prevent platelet aggregation are undergoing therapeutic trial, and the results are suggestive but not definitive. Beta-blocking drugs have prevented reinfarction and death in a number of studies (Frishman, 1984). Unusual physical or psychologic stress has been thought to precede the acute occurrence of myocardial infarction in some cases, but retrospective studies do not as a rule disclose any activities that might explain the cardiac event.

Treatment

Patients are ideally treated at the onset of myocardial infarction in a coronary care unit equipped for continuous monitoring of the ECG, with alarm signals, arterial and venous pressure recording, pacemaker insertion and resuscitation equipment, and specially trained nurses and physicians in attendance. Facilities for introduction of bedside Swan-Ganz balloon catheters for determination of intracardiac pressures and oxygen content in the right heart, pressure transducers for determination of direct intra-arterial pressure, and equipment to determine the cardiac output by the thermodilution method are valuable in the individualized management of severe manifestations occurring during the course of acute myocardial infarction. Equipment for taking bedside chest films, an echocardiograph, and perhaps equipment to determine the wall motion and perfusion status of the myocardium utilizing radioisotopes are also desirable, either in the unit or nearby.

In the following discussion it is assumed that coronary care unit facilities, equipment, and personnel are available. Of course, there are hospitals where all of these resources may not be available. Nevertheless, every effort to recognize arrhythmias early and to recognize and treat complications of acute myocardial infarction that would otherwise be diagnosed by direct hemodynamic monitoring must be made. Personnel can be taught to recognize changes in a patient's appearance or symptoms or changes on an oscilloscopic monitor and to call for help immediately should an arrhythmia or other changes appear. All such medical facilities should have available at least one nurse and one physician who could then begin appropriate therapy. If no defibrillation equipment is available, one must rely on cardiac massage and intravenous drugs such as lidocaine in hope of reversing the ventricular fibrillation. The minimum requirements are constant surveillance and a trained person who can respond immediately if arrhythmias or other complications occur.

In smaller hospitals, criteria for admission to the coronary care unit must be established to select patients who will benefit most from the services available. The major benefit of the coronary care unit is that it makes possible early recognition of severe ventricular arrhythmias, which may be the prelude to ventricular fibrillation and sudden death. Patients with mild initial episodes of myocardial infarction are at less risk, though arrhythmia may develop and ventricular fibrillations can occur early. Priorities for selection of patients for admission to a limited coronary care unit are not universally agreed upon and may vary with time and place.

A. Home Care of Acute Myocardial Infarction: Some writers believe that relatively mild myocardial infarction should be treated in the home as was routinely done years ago (Hill, 1978). They reason that the psychologic impact of admission to the coronary care unit may induce adrenergic stimuli that increase the likelihood of ventricular arrhythmias, particularly ventricular fibrillation. Where coronary care units are not available, home care for patients with initially mild acute myocardial infarction is acceptable if the minimum requirement for constant surveillance and ready availability of effective treatment of arrhythmias can be met.

B. Hospital Care of Acute Myocardial Infarction: The goals of hospital therapy are (1) to relieve pain and anxiety; (2) to prevent and treat serious ventricular arrhythmias; (3) to recognize ventricular fibrillation immediately and give treatment to prevent sudden cardiac death; (4) to recognize the presence of cardiac failure and treat it vigorously so as to prevent extension of the myocardial infarction; (5) to attempt to decrease the extent of the infarcted and ischemic myocardium; and (6) to protect the damaged myocardium by increased rest and judicious ambulation.

1. Immediate measures—(See Emergency Measures in section on sudden death, p 143.) The risk of ventricular fibrillation and sudden death is greatest in the first 4 hours. Patients with acute myocardial infarction should enter the coronary care unit as soon as possible so that defibrillation can be performed if needed. The extension of coronary care capability to specially equipped ambulances and fire department vehicles manned by personnel trained in defibrillation and resuscitation (so-called pre–coronary care) may reduce the number of deaths in the first hour after the attack.

Arrival at emergency room. Upon arrival at the emergency room, the ECG should be monitored and the patient sent immediately to the coronary care unit with monitoring continued during transfer. Upon arrival in the unit, monitoring is continued during the evaluation procedure. A slow intravenous drip of glucose and water is begun so that an open intravenous line will be in place if needed.

2. Relief of pain—Relief of pain is the first requirement if cardiac rhythm is satisfactory. Pain may cause nausea and vomiting, hypertension or hypotension, sinus tachycardia, sweating, and restlessness due to acute anxiety.

If the pain is severe or if the patient is in shock, give morphine sulfate, 2–5 mg slowly intravenously, repeated every 15 minutes until pain is relieved, or, less desirably, meperidine (pethidine; Demerol), 25–50 mg intravenously, repeated in 15 minutes if necessary. If the pain is not severe but bad enough to be disturbing, give morphine, 10–15 mg intramuscularly, repeated in 1 hour if necessary; or meperidine, 50–100 mg intramuscularly. Morphine or meperidine should not be repeated, however, if respirations are less than 12/min. The patient should be kept supine following injection of morphine to avoid hypotension and fainting. Monitoring of respirations is necessary.

If the pain is not relieved by opiates or oxygen (see below), aminophylline, 0.5 g slowly intravenously at a rate of 1–2 mL/min, can be given. Pentazocine is not recommended as an alternative analgesic for pain of myocardial infarction, because it increases left ventricular filling pressure and cardiac work. Nitroglycerin sublingually or isosorbide dinitrate orally may relieve pain, but the drug must be stopped if tachycardia or hypotension develops. Beta-blocking drugs may relieve persistent pain but should be used cautiously because of their negative inotropic action.

3. Rest—

a. Sedation—Patients with acute myocardial infarction are apprehensive and anxious and often have a feeling of impending doom. Opiates, in addition to relieving pain, produce physical and mental rest by allaying anxiety; if they are ineffective, drugs such as diazepam (Valium), 2.5–5 mg orally every 4–6 hours, may be helpful. If pain is not a problem and patients are restless and unable to sleep, sedatives should be used as necessary, because adequate sleep is vital for physical and mental rest.

b. Bedside care—During the first day or two, patients with myocardial infarction should not be allowed to feed or care for themselves unless the attack is mild. Diet should be mild, low-calorie, and low-residue, with multiple small feedings. Most patients find that a bedside commode, with help getting on and off, requires less effort than use of a bedpan. After the first few days, patients can feed themselves, but modified bed rest is advisable for at least the first week. In mild, uncomplicated cases, sitting should begin after 3 days with 30 minutes in a chair, the time being progressively increased depending upon the individual responses (Table 8–19).

4. Oxygen—The decreased cardiac output and pulmonary venous congestion associated with acute myocardial infarction often result in decreased arterial P_{O_2}; levels as low as 50 mm Hg during breathing of room air are not uncommon. Hypoxemia of this degree may contribute to the development of ventricular arrhythmias, hypotension, unrelieved chest pain, and left ventricular failure. Oxygen by face mask at flow rates of 6–10 L/min is preferable to an oxygen tent or intranasal oxygen. Positive pressure breathing is often resisted by the patient, decreases venous return and cardiac output, and may aggravate myocardial ischemia. Other procedures for the management of left ventricular failure with dyspnea are preferable (see below).

5. Anticoagulant therapy—Anticoagulant therapy during the acute phase is controversial. Anticoagulants are not used routinely in patients with mild attacks. In older patients with cardiac failure in whom prolonged bed rest is anticipated, anticoagulation is often given to prevent venous thrombosis and possible pulmonary emboli unless there are contraindications such as a history of bleeding, peptic ulcer, or hepatic insufficiency. Anticoagulants can be stopped when patients are fully ambulatory. Randomized studies favor continuous rather than intermittent heparin therapy, because major bleeding episodes appear to be more common when boluses of heparin are given intravenously at 4-hour intervals than when heparin is given as a continuous intravenous drip of 1000 units/h. A loading dose of 5000 units is often given in order to keep the activated partial thromboplastin time between 40 and 60 seconds. The value of anticoagulant therapy is at best only marginal in the light of the low incidence of thromboembolic complications currently observed in patients with acute myocardial infarction.

6. Beta-adrenergic blocking agents—The use of these agents at the onset of myocardial infarction is controversial.

7. Thrombolytic agents, including streptokinase—Angiography in the early hours after acute myocardial infarction has demonstrated complete occlusion with thrombosis in 87% of patients (DeWood, 1980). Efforts to recanalize the occluded artery and reestablish coronary arterial flow by thrombolysis have been employed to permit survival of myocardium in patients in whom irreversible necrosis had not occurred and limit the area of infarction.

Intracoronary infusions of streptokinase given within 3–4 hours of the onset of symptoms have been shown to restore the patency of the thrombosed artery in about 60% of cases; a highly skilled team is necessary. Myocardial perfusion and ejection fraction have improved in these cases. In some patients, immediate relief of angina is achieved, reversal of elevated ST segments occurs, and abnormal ECGs change toward normal. Cardiogenic shock may be reversed in some cases.

Intravenous thrombolytic therapy can be given immediately after the onset of acute myocardial infarction, especially in community hospitals with limited or no catheterization facilities. The results with intravenous streptokinase are not as good as with intracoronary infusion; recanalization occurs in about 35–45% of cases. In a preliminary multicenter NHLBI trial (TIMI), intravenous tissue-type plasminogen activator (rt-PA) was compared with intravenous streptokinase. Recanalization occurred with the former in about 60% of cases within 90 minutes without significant adverse effects (Braunwald, 1985). In a European cooperative trial, rt-PA was also found to be more effective than intravenous streptokinase (Verstraete, 1985). Further and more detailed experience is awaited. The convenience, lesser risk, and earlier availability of the intravenous as compared to the intracoronary approach make the former more attractive and useful. Percutaneous transluminal coronary angioplasty is being performed following thrombolytic therapy because of the frequency of significant stenosis underlying the thrombus.

8. General clinical observation–After the patient has been relieved of pain, reassured, sedated, given oxygen, and made comfortable in bed with monitoring devices in place, further therapy depends on the presence or absence of complications.

The physician must be prepared to deal with the patient's regression, denial, anger, and hostility as well as anxiety, because emotional stress adversely affects the course of the disease and its management. The physician's manner is most important in minimizing emotional responses to the illness. Neither excessive gravity nor excessive optimism is warranted; realistic optimism is always both justified and therapeutic.

Clinical observation by the physician at hourly intervals during the first day is required to make certain that pain does not return and that hypotension, cardiogenic shock, ventricular arrhythmias, and cardiac failure do not occur. The function of constant observation by special coronary care nurses is to alert the physician to any new symptoms such as dyspnea, embolism, palpitations, mental confusion, oliguria, syncope or near-syncope from heart block, or arrhythmias.

Activity Following Uncomplicated Infarction

Increasingly, patients are being encouraged to increase their activity in bed after the first 2 days, to sit up on the third or fourth day, and to walk about the room on the fifth to seventh days, provided the course has been mild and uncomplicated and the patient tolerates the increased activity without incident. Cautious controlled ambulation allows the patient with mild myocardial infarction and a good home situation to leave the hospital between the tenth and fourteenth days. Early hospital discharge is unwise if, during the acute phase of infarction, the patient has had multiple ventricular premature beats, ventricular tachycardia or fibrillation, second- or third-degree atrioventricular block, cardiac failure with pulmonary edema or cardiogenic shock, sinus tachycardia, systemic hypotension, atrial arrhythmias, or any evidence of extension of the infarction. These complications eliminate from early ambulation at least half of patients with infarction.

During ambulation and before discharge, the response of the patient should be monitored, so that the pulse rate and blood pressure can be observed and the presence of symptoms determined. If recovery is not smooth, the process of rehabilitation can be slowed until a stable state occurs. The object is for the patient to be partially self-sufficient before discharge.

Exercise Testing Before Hospital Discharge

Many centers recommend submaximal exercise testing approximately 3 weeks after an uncomplicated acute myocardial infarction, just before hospital discharge, in order to estimate long-term prognosis. Low-level exercise testing (with close monitoring of the patient, the ECG, and blood pressure and with resuscitation equipment immediately available) can be limited either by heart rate (up to 120–130/min) or by symptoms. Patients are exercised to the approximate metabolic equivalent of activity that they would be expected to engage in at home (about 4 mets). Patients who have a positive electrocardiographic stress test with ST depression of greater or less than 1 mm or who show complex ventricular arrhythmias have a greater likelihood of reinfarction, sudden death, and cardiac death in the following 1–2 years (Moss, 1983). These patients usually have impairment of left ventricular function, which is an independent prognostic factor. Patients who do not develop angina, ST depression of greater than 1 mm, or complex ventricular arrhythmias and who can exercise beyond stage 3 of the Bruce or Naughton protocol have a distinctly better prognosis than those who show one or more abnormalities.

Results of low-level exercise testing are helpful in planning activities following discharge from the hospital and in adjusting treatment. Opinions differ as to whether ST depression or complex ventricular arrhythmias are more significant; the duration of exercise that can be performed and evidence of left ventricular dysfunction are thought by some to be more important than either of the other 2 findings. An important secondary result of the predischarge exercise test is reassurance of the patient and the family when exercise can be performed without significant symptoms or abnormal findings. If there is any question about the patient's ability to perform even low-level exercise, it should be postponed for 6 weeks.

An exercise program begun early after myocardial infarction and continued for several months was found to have neither adverse nor beneficial physiologic effects. Most patients had marked spontaneous recovery after 3 months with or without the exercise program; after 3 months, no further spontaneous improvement was the rule (Sivarajan, 1982).

Treatment of Complications
A. Arrhythmias:
1. Ventricular arrhythmias–(See also Chapter 15.) The most common adverse event (approximately 90% of acute myocardial infarctions seen within the first 4 hours) (Table 8–13) is the development of an

arrhythmia. Ventricular premature beats are common and must be recognized and treated promptly; they indicate either increased irritability from enhanced spontaneous depolarization of the damaged myocardial cells or reentry phenomena from currents of injury set up by impaired conduction and delayed repolarization in neighborhood fibers. Ventricular premature beats or ventricular tachycardia should be treated with lidocaine, 50–100 mg intravenously, followed by an infusion at a rate of 1–2 mg/min. In some centers, lidocaine is begun as a prophylactic measure immediately upon admission to the coronary care unit. If lidocaine produces central nervous system symptoms of confusion or excitement (usually when the drug is given at a higher rate of infusion), alternative drugs may be used. If lidocaine is ineffective, alternative drugs are procainamide, 50 mg/min intravenously up to a total dose of 1 g, or quinidine gluconate, 0.8 g diluted in 100–200 mL of glucose and water and given at a rate of 1 mL/min. It can be repeated if necessary and controlled by monitoring blood levels. Do not exceed 6 μg/mL in the steady state infusion. If the patient has been receiving digitalis or has hypokalemia resulting from diuretic therapy, potassium salts may be given orally or intravenously depending upon the urgency of need. Prompt treatment of ventricular arrhythmias is indicated to prevent ventricular fibrillation and cardiac arrest.

2. Ventricular tachycardia and fibrillation– Ventricular tachycardia is an emergency and, if not rapidly converted with intravenous lidocaine, should be terminated by electrical cardioversion. Ventricular fibrillation should be instantly recognized by the alarm system at the nursing station, and defibrillation should be accomplished within 30 seconds. Defibrillation should be performed by specially trained personnel, because delay compromises not only cardiac function but also cerebral function. After defibrillation, lidocaine is given by constant intravenous infusion in a dosage of 1–2 mg/min in order to prevent recurrence. This may be discontinued in 24–48 hours if there is no recurrence.

3. Other ventricular or junctional arrhythmias– Nonparoxysmal ventricular tachycardia (accelerated idioventricular rhythm) with junctional tachycardia and aberrant conduction may occur early in the course of acute myocardial infarction and may be confused with either ventricular tachycardia or complete atrioventricular block. Because the prognosis with these arrhythmias is better than that of ventricular tachycardia in general, supportive care is usually sufficient and defibrillation is rarely needed if the differential diagnosis can be made.

4. Atrial arrhythmias– Atrial arrhythmias occur less frequently (about 15% of cases) than ventricular ones. The most common atrial arrhythmia is fibrillation. It is usually transient, lasting hours or 1–2 days, unless the ventricular rate is rapid and hemodynamic deterioration occurs. Treatment consists of digitalization or, if urgent, cardioversion. Conservative therapy is usually more desirable. If frequent atrial premature beats occur—especially if they produce hemodynamic deterioration with resultant symptoms—they should be treated with quinidine sulfate, 0.3 g orally every 4–6 hours. Frequent premature beats often presage atrial fibrillation and may result in a fall in arterial pressure that decreases coronary perfusion and may increase the size of the infarct.

5. Late ventricular fibrillation– The frequency of ventricular fibrillation (10–20% overall) decreases with time and with healing of the infarction. Electrocardiographic monitoring should be continued for several days after the last episode of ventricular arrhythmia. This is of concern in patients who are transferred to general medical wards without monitoring equipment. Ideally, patients should be transferred to an intermediate unit where they can be monitored for another week until it is clear that ventricular arrhythmias are not recurring.

B. Cardiac Failure and Cardiogenic Shock: Left ventricular performance is impaired to some degree in all patients with acute myocardial infarction. A first myocardial infarction of minor extent in a patient with no underlying cardiac disease usually produces little or no impairment of left ventricular performance as judged by symptoms and signs and by hemodynamic monitoring of cardiac output, left ventricular filling pressure, and arterial pressure, but it may cause hypokinesia on radioisotope wall motion studies. If the infarction is large and occurs in an area of previous infarctions with large areas of scar and borderline compensation, the patient may rapidly develop severe cardiac failure. Possibilities thus range from no clinical evidence of impaired cardiac function to cardiogenic shock with a very high (80%) mortality rate. It is thus appropriate to discuss the subject as a continuum with treatment individualized according to the degree of severity (Table 8–17).

Table 8–17. Acute myocardial infarction: Suggested therapeutic measures in relation to hemodynamic indices.*

Left Ventricular Stroke Work Index	Left Ventricular Filling Pressure	Therapy
Normal	Normal	Observation
Normal	Raised	Diuretics
Decreased	Decreased or normal	Volume expansion
Moderately decreased	Raised	Afterload reducing agents with or without diuretics
Markedly decreased (cardiogenic shock)	Raised	Intra-aortic balloon counterpulsation and afterload reducing agents. Use of inotropic agents if other measures do not increase cardiac output, eg, dopamine or dobutamine.

*Modified and reproduced, with permission, from Chatterjee K, Swan HJC: Hemodynamic profile of acute myocardial infarction. Chapter 6 in: *Myocardial Infarction.* Corday E, Swan HJC (editors). Williams & Wilkins, 1973.

1. Mild and moderate cardiac failure–Some degree of cardiac failure, usually left ventricular failure, can be detected in 20–50% of patients with acute myocardial infarction unless the attack is mild. The patient may have dyspnea, pulmonary rales, diastolic gallop rhythm, and accentuated hilar congestion on chest x-ray. The typical central congestion with bat's wing densities does not occur unless the patient develops acute pulmonary edema. The radiologic findings may be out of phase with the clinical findings because they take longer to develop and to regress. In patients who are being monitored by means of a bedside Swan-Ganz catheter (Fig 8–36), elevated pulmonary venous wedge pressure may be noted before the radiologic changes occur.

If left ventricular failure is minimal or subclinical, treatment can be conservative, with oral diuretics (eg, hydrochlorothiazide, 50–100 mg orally), oxygen, and avoidance of sodium-containing fluids and food. Hemodynamic intracardiac monitoring is *not necessary*, because the left ventricular filling pressure is usually normal (< 12 mm Hg) and the cardiac index is also normal (> 2.5 L/min/m^2). The prognosis is good (mortality rate ± 6%).

2. More severe cardiac failure–Left ventricular failure not promptly relieved by cautious sublingual nitroglycerin beginning with 0.4 mg or by diuretic therapy requires more aggressive management (see below). Begin with hemodynamic monitoring of the arterial pressure, pulmonary venous wedge pressure (left ventricular filling pressure), and cardiac output utilizing the Swan-Ganz catheter (Fig 8–36). (See also p 106.) The stroke work index can be computed from these measurements, and rational therapy can be directed at the specific hemodynamic abnormality.

Right ventricular infarction rarely occurs without left ventricular inferior infarction. Right ventricular infarction often is not recognized and may be responsible for right ventricular failure (see p 166). The clinical diagnosis is usually suspected from the presence of high jugular and right atrial pressures, which are often higher than the left ventricular filling pressure; 2-dimensional echocardiography and gated blood pool scans may establish the diagnosis. It is important to recognize right ventricular failure in right ventricular infarction, because the high jugular venous pressure helps generate right ventricular flow; venodilators and diuretics should be avoided. Fluid replacement fosters right ventricular output. Arterial vasodilators (see below) may be used to reduce the afterload.

a. Volume replacement–When monitoring reveals that left ventricular filling pressure is low (< 12 mm Hg) and cardiac output is normal despite the low arterial pressure, hypovolemia is the most probable cause. Treatment consists of volume replacement by the intravenous route in 100-mL increments with dextrose in water or half-normal saline every 5–10 minutes until the left ventricular filling pressure rises to 18 mm Hg. If cardiac output does not increase as the

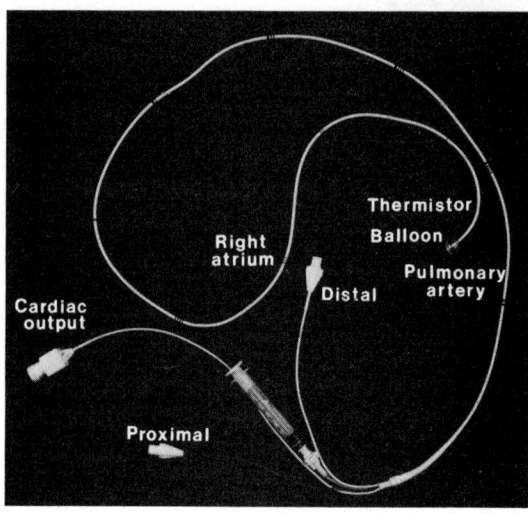

Figure 8–36. Triple-lumen Swan-Ganz thermodilution catheter for monitoring in the coronary care unit. (Courtesy of K Chatterjee.)

Table 8–18. Vasodilators useful in cardiac failure in acute myocardial infarction.*

Vasodilator	Advantages	Disadvantages	Dose Range
Nitroprusside	High potency; immediate effect; half-life extremely short.	Requires hemodynamic monitoring.	15–400 µg/min intravenously.
Phentolamine	High potency; rapid action.	Requires hemodynamic monitoring.	0.25–1 mg/min intravenously.
Isosorbide dinitrate	Sublingual or oral administration.	Less potent than nitroprusside and phentolamine.	2.5–5 mg sublingually; 10–30 mg orally (ingested).
Nitroglycerin ointment	Prolonged duration of action (up to 6 hours); removable.	Topical use may not be well accepted by patients.	1.5–4 inches (cutaneous).
Nitroglycerin, transdermal	Continuous well-controlled absorption for 12–24 hours; removable.	May cause headache or hypotension.	2.5–30 mg/24 h.
Nifedipine	Coronary spasm.		10–20 mg 3 times daily orally.
Verapamil	Coronary spasm; paroxysmal atrial tachycardia.		80–120 mg 2–3 times daily orally.

*Modified and reproduced, with permission, from Forrester JS, Waters DD: Hospital treatment of congestive heart failure: Management according to hemodynamic profile. *Am J Med* 1978;**65**:173.

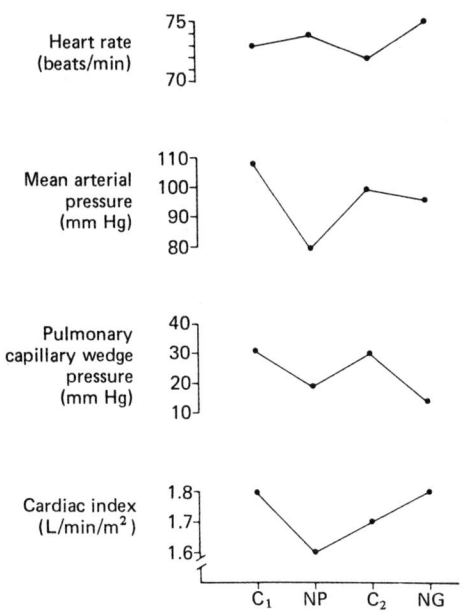

Figure 8-37. Hemodynamic changes following administration of nitroprusside (NP) and nitroglycerin (NG) in a patient with acute myocardial infarction. C_1 and C_2 refer to control periods. (Adapted and reproduced, with permission, from the American Heart Association, Inc., Armstrong PW et al: Vasodilator therapy in acute myocardial infarction: A comparison of sodium nitroprusside and nitroglycerin. *Circulation* 1975;**52**:1118.)

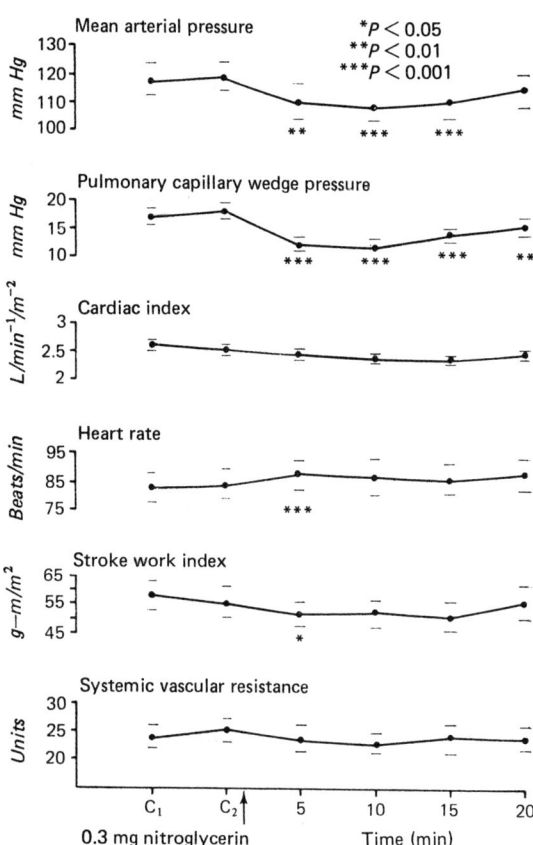

Figure 8-38. Hemodynamic effects of 0.3 mg sublingual nitroglycerin in 14 patients with acute myocardial infarction. The mean values and standard errors are shown during 2 control observations, C_1 and C_2, separated by 20 minutes, and after nitroglycerin. (Reproduced, with permission, from Delgado CE et al: Role of sublingual nitroglycerin in patients with acute myocardial infarction. *Br Heart J* 1975;**37**:392.)

left ventricular filling pressure rises to 15–20 mm Hg, volume replacement should be stopped to prevent pulmonary edema.

b. Diuresis–If the only hemodynamic abnormality is a raised left ventricular filling pressure but blood pressure and cardiac output are normal, more vigorous diuresis can be obtained with large doses (80–160–320 mg) of furosemide. Excessive diuresis must be avoided because the patient may become dehydrated.

c. Vasopressors–Some patients with acute myocardial infarction have hypotension with impaired tissue perfusion primarily due to failure of compensatory peripheral vasoconstriction without a substantial change in filling pressure or cardiac output; these patients often respond with a rise in arterial pressure to the inotropic action of sympathetic amines (norepinephrine, dopamine, or dobutamine) that stimulate the beta-adrenergic receptors of the heart. These drugs are a temporary measure to allow the use of vasodilators or intra-aortic balloon assist (see below). They should be infused at a slow rate to avoid tachycardia, marked increases in blood pressure, and ventricular arrhythmias.

d. Vasodilator therapy–(See Table 8–18.) When cardiac dysfunction is more severe, with reduced cardiac output, increased left ventricular filling pressure (above 20 mm Hg), and arterial blood pressure at or above 90 mm Hg, vasodilator therapy can be cautiously started while the hemodynamic result is monitored. Drugs such as nitroglycerin, sodium nitroprusside, trimethaphan, and phentolamine, given by intravenous drip, decrease the impedance to left ventricular ejection; reduce left ventricular volume and filling pressure; decrease myocardial oxygen consumption; improve perfusion to the brain (Fig 8–37), kidneys, and heart; and may improve the left ventricular stroke work index. Temporary improvement may tide the patient over a critical period (Chatterjee, 1979). Dopamine or dobutamine should be tried in low output states with hypotension. The combination of vasodilator therapy and inotropic therapy may be helpful if the blood pressure is low, with hypoperfusion combined with a high filling pressure documented by hemodynamic monitoring.

Nitroglycerin given sublingually in the acute phase of acute myocardial infarction may decrease the wedge pressure but may also produce arterial hypotension with or without bradycardia (Fig 8–38). The same effect may occur with intravenous sodium nitroprusside or nitroglycerin, but the dose must be titrated to avoid hypotension. In less severe cases, transdermal nitroglycerin (see p 157 under Angina Pectoris) can be used with appropriate safeguards in acute myocardial infarction; this may reduce the left ventricular filling pressure with only a slight fall in arterial pressure.

Efforts should be made to raise arterial pressure to about 100 mm Hg with vasopressors before vasodilator therapy unless vasodilators are required to relieve symptoms of pulmonary venous congestion when cardiac failure is severe. If the patient has cardiogenic shock and a low urine output, dopamine can be tried to increase the urine output and cardiac output and raise the blood pressure. The average dose of dopamine is 15–20 µg/kg/min. Dopamine may increase the myocardial oxygen consumption. The physician must be cautious in treating severe left ventricular failure with dopamine because of the danger of worsening of myocardial function.

e. Aortic balloon counterpulsation–If it is not possible to raise blood pressure with vasopressors, aortic balloon counterpulsation may, in some patients, be a dramatically effective temporary method of raising arterial pressure so that vasodilator therapy can be started; this technique is associated with morbidity and should be used only by skilled personnel. Counterpulsation decreases aortic pressure during systole and increases it in diastole. Decreasing systolic pressure decreases impedance to left ventricular ejection and reduces afterload and the work of the left ventricle. Raising the pressure during diastole increases coronary perfusion and improves left ventricular function. In refractory heart failure without shock, arterial counterpulsation decreases ischemic pain, improves cardiac failure, and increases survival (Sammel, 1979).

f. Combination of aortic balloon counterpulsation and vasodilator therapy–Counterpulsation followed by vasodilator therapy with sodium nitroprusside or nitroglycerin may significantly improve left ventricular "pump" function in cardiogenic shock and thus reduce the mortality rate. Treatment with hydralazine, nitroprusside, and dopamine may make counterpulsation unnecessary in some patients. The long-term prognosis in patients who have needed balloon assist for cardiogenic shock is still poor (approximately 10% survival after 1 year), because of the extensive underlying disease implied by the presence of cardiogenic shock.

g. Counterpulsation as prelude to cardiac surgery–Invasive balloon counterpulsation can be used as a temporary measure to tide the patient over acute "pump failure" and make it possible to perform coronary angiograms as well as to explore the feasibility of coronary bypass surgery. The surgical mortality rate in patients recovering from cardiogenic shock is high. The feasibility and desirability of operative intervention remain uncertain.

h. Hemodynamic parameters guiding treatment–The poor response to medical as well as surgical therapy in patients with cardiogenic shock can be appreciated when one considers that at least half of the left ventricle is often damaged in such patients. Left ventricular stroke work is usually less than 20 g-m/m^2 and often less than 15 g-m/m^2, and hypoxemia with P_{O_2} of less than 40–50 mm Hg is frequently found. The high wedge pressure induces dyspnea; impaired peripheral perfusion from the decreased cardiac output results in cold, clammy skin, cerebral obtundation, and poor urine output.

i. Value of hemodynamic monitoring in prognosis–Monitoring of the hemodynamic parameters is valuable in prognosis. Patients with left ventricular filling pressures under 15 mm Hg and stroke work indices of more than 35–40 g-m/m^2 have a mortality rate of 6%, whereas if the filling pressure exceeds 20 mm Hg and the stroke work index is less than 15–20 g-m/m^2, the mortality rate is 80% (Chatterjee, 1973). In patients with a poor prognosis, aggressive therapy is warranted before severe deterioration occurs. The response of the patient determines the drugs used and their dosages, and these are varied as treatment proceeds. If the blood pressure falls, the physician cannot continue administration of the sodium nitroprusside or nitroglycerin and must use pressor agents to raise the blood pressure.

j. Digitalis–Digitalis is infrequently used today in the treatment of cardiac failure due to acute myocardial infarction, because of its tendency to cause ventricular arrhythmias and its relatively low effectiveness against severe left ventricular pump failure. Digitalis should be tried, however, unless the failure is mild. If ventricular arrhythmias develop, it is difficult to decide whether they are due to digitalis or myocardial ischemia. Digitalis should be used if the patient has atrial fibrillation with a rapid ventricular rate.

C. Conduction Defects:
1. Stokes-Adams attack with heart block (complete atrioventricular conduction defect)–(See Chapter 14.) *This is an emergency!* Complete heart block complicates acute myocardial infarction in 6–10% of cases; it has a high mortality rate (about 60% untreated), usually lasts less than a week, and often can be treated by a ventricular pacemaker. Pacing at a rate of 70–80/min may greatly improve cardiac output and tissue perfusion and prevent Stokes-Adams attacks. Death during a Stokes-Adams attack with syncope is rare in the presence of inferior myocardial infarction. Progression of the electrocardiographic changes of heart block may be rapid and lead to complete atrioventricular block and Stokes-Adams attacks. Temporary pacemakers are usually left in place for a week after the atrioventricular conduction becomes normal. A permanent pacemaker may be considered in anterior infarction associated with Stokes-Adams attacks. The mortality rate is said to be reduced if a permanent pacemaker is used in patients with acute anterior myocardial infarction who have developed complete atrioventricular block in association with bifascicular block during the acute attack; the data supporting this opinion are still incomplete and contradictory.

2. Second-degree heart block, Mobitz I and II–(See Chapter 14.) Second-degree atrioventricular block with Wenckebach pauses (see below) (Mobitz I) and *narrow* QRS complexes is not routinely paced if the patient has inferior infarction. Stokes-Adams attacks are uncommon in inferior infarction with narrow QRS complexes, even if complete block develops. They are common in anterior infarction with wide QRS complexes. The block is usually within the bundle of His or in the bundle branches, with *wide* QRS complexes (Mobitz II); Stokes-Adams attacks with fatalities occur if the patient is not protected by a pacemaker.

3. Prophylactic demand pacemakers in Mobitz II block–(See Chapter 14.) Because asystole may occur unpredictably, electrode catheters should be placed prophylactically in patients with anterior infarctions who have bifascicular block, complete atrioventricular block, or type II Mobitz atrioventricular block or in those who have inferior infarctions with early complete atrioventricular block. Infusions of lidocaine should be given to prevent ventricular fibrillation if atrioventricular block subsides and competition occurs with the patient's own pacemaker.

4. Sinus bradycardia–Sinus bradycardia, especially in inferior infarction, may precede atrioventricular block and provide a setting in which ventricular arrhythmias can occur. Furthermore, when hypotension and decreased cardiac output occur with bradycardia in acute myocardial infarction, perfusion of the vital organs may be inadequate. Atropine, 0.4–0.8 mg intravenously, is desirable in such situations, with close observation to determine its effectiveness and side effects, since ventricular arrhythmias may result. If atropine is ineffective or if the bradycardia is marked or associated with sinoatrial or atrioventricular block, a temporary prophylactic transvenous demand pacemaker should be inserted into the right ventricle.

D. Other Complications:

1. Thromboembolic phenomena–These are usually manifested by phlebothrombosis resulting from enforced bed rest. Pulmonary embolism and arterial emboli from mural thrombi in the left ventricle occur infrequently. Anticoagulants should be administered promptly.

2. Renal failure–Early oliguria and anuria are due to cardiogenic shock; late renal failure may be due to prolonged hypotension caused by vasodilator therapy. Early vigorous treatment of cardiogenic shock and caution in the use of vasodilator agents should decrease the incidence of renal failure. If renal failure with acute tubular necrosis develops after the patient has been stabilized with respect to cardiogenic shock and left ventricular failure, hemodialysis or peritoneal dialysis is indicated.

3. Perforation of the interventricular septum and mitral insufficiency due to papillary muscle and left ventricular wall dysfunction or rupture–These complications may occur together but are usually separate untoward events. Either may result in abrupt worsening of left ventricular failure. Hemodynamic studies are usually required to establish the nature of these lesions. Two-dimensional echocardiograms are effective in diagnosing septal rupture because they provide direct visualization of the septal defect and show air bubbles entering the left ventricle via the septal rupture following intravenous saline contrast injection. Whenever possible, surgical repair of the ventricular septal defect or replacement of the mitral valve should be delayed for several weeks after the lesion has been stabilized by vigorous treatment of cardiac failure (see Chapter 10). Patients having acute mitral insufficiency with acute left ventricular failure requiring surgery have marked pulmonary venous congestion, a very high v wave, raised mean pulmonary capillary wedge pressure, and a reduced cardiac index (< 2.5 L/min/m^2). In both ventricular septal defects and mitral insufficiency, vasodilator therapy may improve or correct cardiac failure, so that surgical repair can be performed with an acceptable mortality rate. Results of surgical repair of both of these lesions are gratifying and allow restoration of normal activity.

4. Left ventricular aneurysm–

a. Spectrum of left ventricular contraction abnormalities–Acute necrosis of a portion of the left ventricle, with resulting healing by fibrosis and scar, may lead to a spectrum of disorders of contraction of the left ventricle, varying from hypokinesia or akinesia of a segment that is fully scarred to a definite left ventricular aneurysm with well-demarcated paradoxic outpocketing during systole. This can be established on cineangiography. Aneurysms, however, may not be disclosed on physical examination or chest x-ray; 2-dimensional echocardiography may be diagnostic and differentiate pseudoaneurysm from true aneurysm—the former has a narrow neck in communication with the left ventricular cavity; the latter has a wide neck (Figs 8–39 to 8–41).

b. Consequences of ventricular aneurysms–The force of left ventricular contraction is wasted

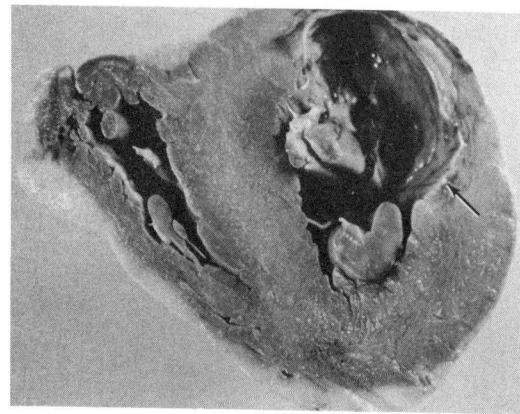

Figure 8–39. Cardiac aneurysm of the posterior wall of the left ventricle following acute myocardial infarction. (Courtesy of O Rambo.)

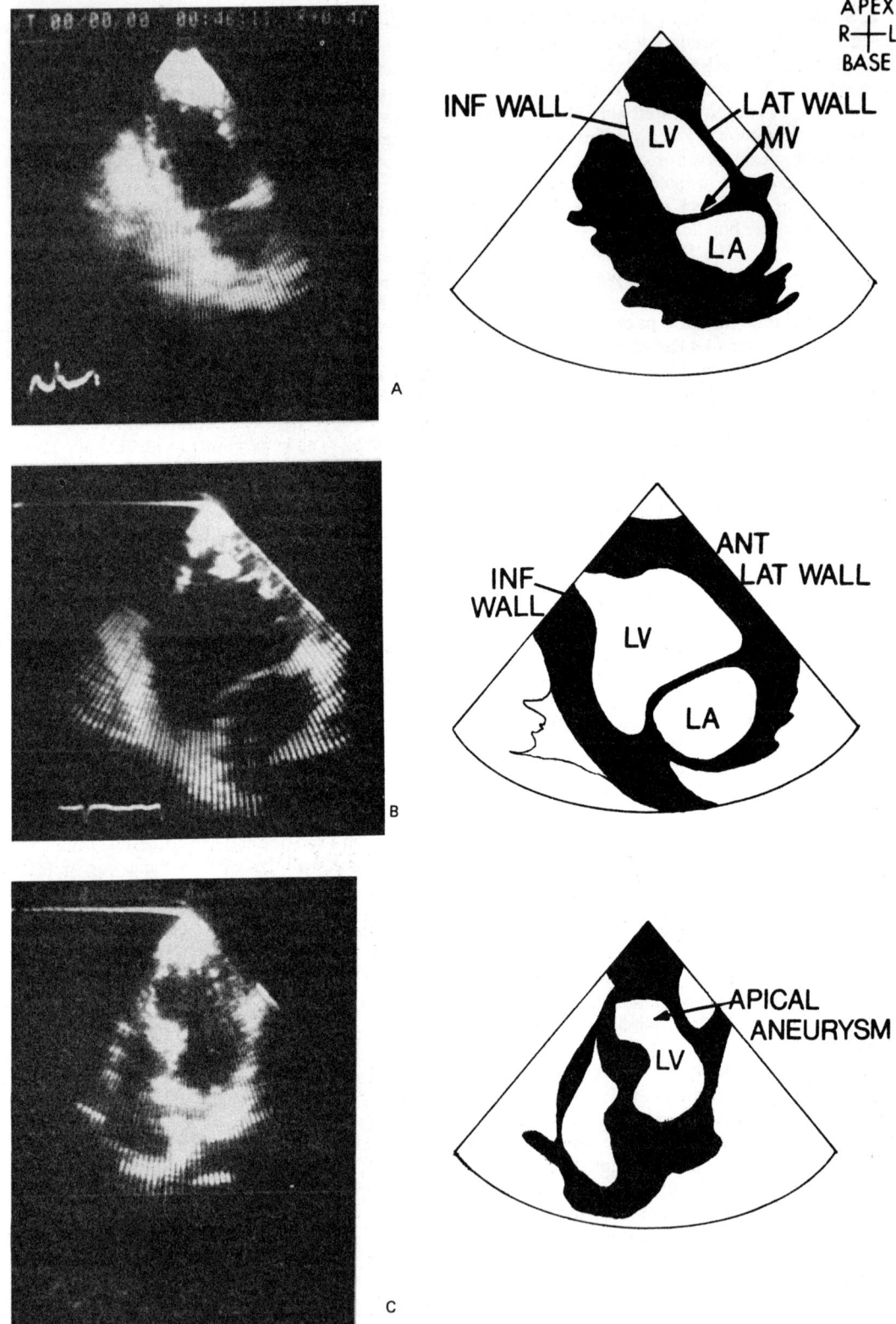

Figure 8–40. Two-dimensional echocardiograms of normal left ventricle and of left ventricular aneurysms. *A:* Normal left ventricle and mitral valve in a modified right anterior oblique position representing a hemiaxial equivalent taken through the apex. *B:* Considerably dilated left ventricle with an aneurysm on the inferior wall. *C:* Apical aneurysm with slightly enlarged left ventricular cavity. (Courtesy of NB Schiller.)

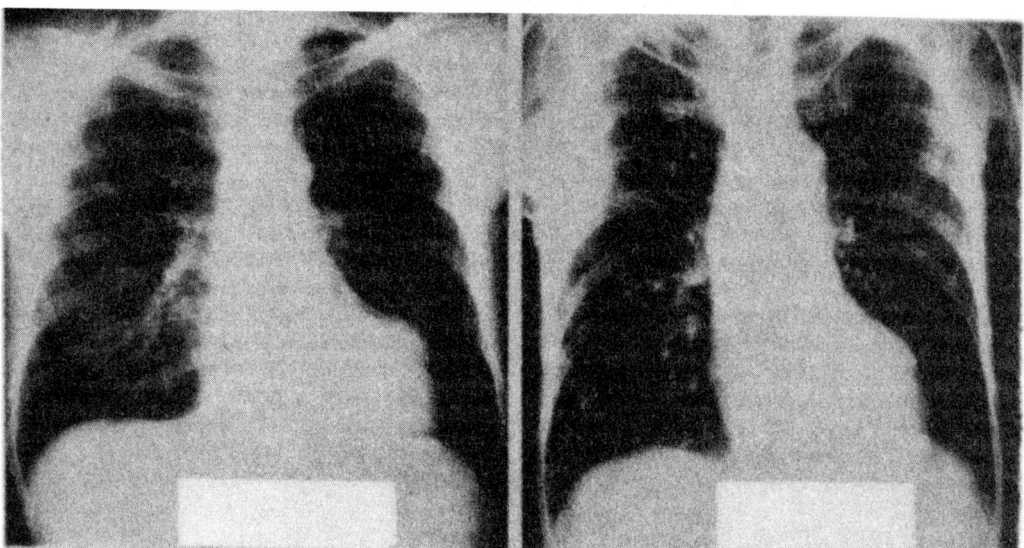

Figure 8–41. Ventricular aneurysm in 2 patients. *Left:* Classic x-ray findings of a discrete left ventricular aneurysm. *Right:* Film from a patient who at autopsy was found to have diffuse thinning and aneurysmal dilatation of the entire apical region of the left ventricle. (Reproduced, with permission, from Davis RW, Ebert PA: Ventricular aneurysm: A clinical-pathologic correlation. *Am J Cardiol* 1972;**29:**1.)

by distention of the aneurysm, increasing the work of the left ventricle. This may lead to persistent cardiac failure or ventricular arrhythmias, or both. When persistent left ventricular failure follows the healing of an acute myocardial infarction, the possibility of left ventricular aneurysm should be excluded by 2-dimensional echocardiograms or cineangiograms, and if an aneurysm is found it should be resected surgically if the remaining portion of the left ventricle has adequate function (see below). Areas of myocardium receiving minimal perfusion, with consequent ischemia on effort, may surround the area of the left ventricular aneurysm and result in frequent ventricular arrhythmias that often are disabling.

c. Surgical resection of aneurysms–Surgical resection can abolish the ventricular arrhythmias as well as cardiac failure in many patients. In patients who have ventricular tachycardia resistant to conventional medical therapy, endocardial electrophysiologic mapping should be performed prior to resection of the aneurysm to determine the site of origin of the ectopic activity. Surgical resection of the endocardial area that originates the ectopic activity can then be combined with resection of the aneurysm. Search for left ventricular aneurysm can be very gratifying; although the mortality rate is about 5%, the results may be dramatic. Surgery should be deferred if possible for 4–10 weeks until cardiac failure has stabilized. Resection of left ventricular aneurysm is often effective in relieving cardiac failure. Resection is unwise unless the remaining regional myocardial contraction is satisfactory (40–50%). Surgical treatment is not indicated in patients with hypokinesia with severe cardiac failure. A minor left ventricular aneurysm in the absence of cardiac failure or severe ventricular arrhythmias is likewise not an indication for surgical resection, because it does not influence prognosis.

5. Cardiac rupture and false aneurysm–The rupture may be subacute with a slight perforation into the pericardium and can be diagnosed on the basis of pericardial pain or effusion or by the recognition of a false aneurysm on 2-dimensional echocardiogram. Progressive enlargement of a "false" or pseudoaneurysm of the left ventricle may result from a slight cardiac rupture, with only the parietal pericardium preventing the expanding false aneurysm from rupturing. With time it may rupture, usually into the lung. The false aneurysm is readily identified by 2-dimensional echocardiography, by radionuclide angiography, and by contrast angiography.

6. Pericarditis–Although pericarditis occurs in about 15% of patients with acute myocardial infarction, pericardial tamponade is rare. Involvement of the pericardium contraindicates anticoagulant therapy, because extensive bleeding in the pericardium may result in tamponade. The differential diagnosis between acute pericarditis and acute myocardial infarction may be difficult, especially if the patient is not seen until the second or third day. Electrocardiographic abnormalities due to involvement of the epicardium and pericardium may complicate the interpretation of electrocardiographic patterns, especially if the patient has a nontransmural infarct.

7. Rare post–myocardial infarction syndromes–
a. Dressler's syndrome–Pericarditis, pericardial friction rub, and fever, with or without pneumonitis,

may occur weeks or months after acute myocardial infarction in a small number of patients. It has been considered to be a hypersensitivity reaction similar to postcardiotomy syndrome (see Chapter 18). It must be differentiated from a new myocardial infarction, pulmonary infarction, pneumonia, or cardiac failure. It subsides spontaneously in a few days or weeks, but improvement is more rapid if corticosteroids or indomethacin is given. Anticoagulants should not be used because of the hazards of hemorrhagic pericardial effusion.

b. Shoulder-hand syndrome—A syndrome consisting of stiffness, limitation of motion, and pain in the shoulder and arm (especially the left) following myocardial infarction is now rare. The condition probably was due to disuse of the arms and shoulders when strict limitation of activity for weeks was recommended for acute myocardial infarction. It may last for days or weeks and is benefited by symptomatic treatment, including physical therapy.

E. Convalescent Activity and Rehabilitation:

1. Initial period of rest—

a. Rest in bed—The period of rest in bed depends on the severity and size of the infarction and the presence or absence of complications.

b. Ambulation—(See pp 180 and 192.) If the infarction is mild and if the family can provide all required services, the patient who can perform 3 mets (metabolic energy equivalents) without symptoms (one met is the energy expenditure per kilogram per minute at rest—about 3.5–4 mL of oxygen per minute) may go home early in the second week. Walking at 2.5 mph, dressing, or taking a shower requires 3 mets.

c. Resuming full activity—As a guide, 2 or 3 weeks of rest, mostly in bed or in a chair, are followed by slow ambulation as noted above; 2 or 3 weeks of slowly increasing activity, including walking and slow stair climbing; and then several weeks of progressive activity before return to part-time work. Even in uncomplicated cases, the patient who has previously been normally active requires 2–3 months of convalescence before returning to full preinfarction activity. Improvement in exercise tolerance progressively continues up to 3–6 months.

d. Usual practice of ambulation—(See p 180.) When the patient first begins to walk slowly, the physician should be present to note any deleterious effects that might occur. The patient should not leave the hospital until the activity status has progressed to the stage of relative self-sufficiency. Early ambulation and self-sufficiency improve morale, prevent cardiac invalidism, and restore the patient's confidence in his or her ability to resume a normal life. Progressive increases in ambulatory effort should be possible without chest pain, dyspnea, or undue tachycardia or fatigue. Severe physical exertion should be avoided for at least 2 months, in order to prevent left ventricular dilatation and subsequent hypertrophy. A balance must be achieved between excessive exertion too early and prolonged inactivity and invalidism. A useful mobilization program is presented in Table 8–19.

Table 8–19. Mobilization program following myocardial infarction. (An adaption of the program used in the Emory University [Atlanta] practice of Wenger.)*

Step	Exercise
I	Active mobilization of ankles and wrists; respiratory exercises
II	Active mobilization of limbs; partial wash-up care in bed; dangle legs on side of bed (5 minutes)
III	Active mobilization in bed; use of a bedside commode; sitting 15 minutes in armchair twice a day
IV	Active mobilization against resistance; complete care in bed; sitting 30 minutes in armchair twice a day
V	Active mobilization in bed; sitting 1 hour in armchair twice a day; 2 short walks in room
VI–VIII	Active mobilization in bed; light gymnastic exercises; sitting in armchair at will; washing at the washstand; walks in corridor
IX–X	As above plus exercises with footstool
XI	As above plus walking down 1 flight of stairs twice a day
XII–XIV	As above plus walking up 1–3 flights of stairs twice a day

*Reproduced, with permission, from Bloch A et al: Early mobilization after myocardial infarction: A controlled study. Am J Cardiol 1974;34:152.

2. Later rehabilitation—Rehabilitation programs utilize the services of physical therapists with the object of encouraging the patient to return to normal activity without neurocirculatory asthenia or cardiac neurosis.

a. Electrocardiographic monitoring during activity—Twelve-hour electrocardiographic monitoring (eg, with a Holter monitor) when the patient first resumes activity (usually about 3 weeks in uncomplicated cases; see steps XI–XIV in Table 8–19) may alert the physician to the presence of residual myocardial ischemia or left ventricular arrhythmias and may require a reduction in activity or the use of antiarrhythmic drugs.

b. Use of graded exercise and Holter electrocardiographic monitoring in early postinfarction period—Graded, limited exercise with cycle ergometers or treadmills up to a ventricular rate of about 130/min is often performed 3–6 weeks after uncomplicated acute myocardial infarction; the presence and degree of ST segment abnormalities or ventricular premature beats provide an estimate of recovery and also have prognostic significance. Patients with ischemic ST depression or complex ventricular premature beats during early postinfarction exercise have a significantly higher incidence of new infarctions or ventricular fibrillation with sudden death syndrome in the succeeding 1–2 years (DeBusk, 1980). Before performing this early exercise test, patients should be free of complications such as cardiac failure, arrhythmia, and conduction defects, and the test should be stopped if the patient develops undue fatigue, angina, frequent or complex premature beats, or marked ST depression. The physician must be aware of drugs that the patient may be taking. Ability to perform the exercise tests is usually a source of great encouragement to the patient. At 3 months the patient has regained about 70% of preinfarction exercise tolerance, and recovery is usually complete by 12 months. Sexual activity in both sexes may be resumed after 1–2 months when the patient has shown the ability to tolerate a heart rate of 130/min. Properly supervised rehabilitation exercise programs have been shown to be safe and helpful in that they foster a sense of well-being, decrease anxiety, and induce a healthier emotional response to the life-threatening event; they have not been shown to prolong life or decrease the frequency of recurrence of myocardial infarction.

Special Precautions in Patients at Increased Risk

The high-risk patient likely to have recurrent acute myocardial infarction or sudden death is one who has survived a previous episode of "sudden death syndrome" or acute myocardial infarction and who has frequent or complex ventricular premature beats. Monitoring such patients electrocardiographically will indicate whether the premature beats are simple or complex. They have been graded by Lown as shown in Table 8–8 (p 158). In addition to ambulatory electrocardiographic monitoring, high-risk patients should have radioisotope or echocardiographic evaluation of wall motion and ejection fraction weeks or months after recovery from the acute episode. Multiple areas of hypokinesis or dyskinesis indicating myocardial fibrosis correlate with frequent ventricular premature beats, and the combination of complex ventricular premature beats and poor left ventricular function considerably increases the likelihood of sudden death and is an indication for coronary angiography with a view to possible coronary surgery. If neither is present, the death rate is low.

Special care in a patient with known coronary disease involves education of the patient and the patient's family about the disease, instruction of the family regarding resuscitation, vigorous treatment of complex ventricular arrhythmias, and the use of drugs to improve left ventricular function. Beta-adrenergic blocking drugs should be considered (see p 191) (unless the patient has a contraindication to their use), because a number of therapeutic trials have shown that several of these agents (timolol, metoprolol, propranolol, and alprenolol) decreased the likelihood of sudden death and nonfatal myocardial infarction and were associated with lower total mortality rates. It is wise to urge the patient and family to have emergency telephone numbers readily available, and they should be instructed to bring the patient (if possible) to a coronary care unit at the first sign suggesting acute myocardial infarction. The patient should be urged to decrease the time interval between the first symptom and the call for medical assistance.

New approved antiarrhythmic drugs are currently available, but it not yet clear what their ultimate role in preventing "sudden death syndrome" or myocardial infarction will be. For antiarrhythmic drugs, some of which are not yet approved by the FDA but are being used in Europe and elsewhere, see Table 15–7 and p 191.

Prognosis

Patients who had a previous myocardial infarction and findings during the second infarction of severe cardiac failure, shock, high left ventricular filling pressure, sinus tachycardia, low ejection fraction, decreased cardiac index, and decreased left ventricular stroke work all had significant left ventricular impairment and a correspondingly worse outcome (Taylor, 1980; Moss, 1983).

A. Overall Mortality Rate: The overall mortality rate during the first month after acute myocardial infarction is about 30%, with most of the deaths occurring in the first 12 hours and one-fourth of them, due to ventricular fibrillation, in the first 1–2 hours. With mild attacks and no complications, the hospital mortality rate is less than 5%. The hospital mortality rate is 50% higher in recurrent as compared to initial infarctions, but cardiac rupture occurs more frequently with the first infarction. Early recurrence or extension of acute myocardial infarction takes place in approximately 15% of patients and can be diagnosed by the appearance of MB isoenzymes of plasma CPK on an average of 10 days after the initial infarct. These patients are at increased risk (Marmor, 1981). Overall figures are misleading in estimating prognosis. Since the average delay between onset of symptoms and arrival at the hospital is 5–6 hours, arrival of the patient alive at the hospital is itself a favorable prognostic sign with respect to electrical instability but not necessarily to pump failure.

B. Factors Influencing Survival: Over a 5-year period, 3-vessel disease with poor left ventricular function has at least 10 times the mortality rate of single-vessel disease with good left ventricular function (Table 8–20). At present, the prognosis is influenced favorably by surgical treatment for (1) repair of perforated ventricular septum; (2) replacement of

Table 8–20. Mortality rates following coronary arteriography by number of vessels diseased and by symptoms of congestive heart failure (CHF). (Mean duration of follow-up = 21 months.)*

Number of Vessels Diseased	No Symptoms of CHF			Symptoms of CHF		
	Dead (No.)	Alive (No.)	Mortality (Percent)	Dead (No.)	Alive (No.)	Mortality (Percent)
0	2	87	2.2	1	8	11.1
1	1	39	2.5	1	5	16.7
2	4	32	11.1	9	5	64.3
3	8	28	22.2	7	9	43.8
Total	15	186	8.1	18	27	40.0

*Modified from Oberman (1972). Reproduced, with permission, from the American Heart Association, Inc., Kouchoukos NT, Kirklin JW, Oberman A: An appraisal of coronary bypass grafting. *Circulation* 1974;50:11.

the mitral valve when there is gross mitral regurgitation resulting from papillary muscle dysfunction; (3) resection of left ventricular aneurysm associated with left ventricular failure; and (4) coronary bypass or angioplasty when the artery involved is the left main coronary artery or in proximal 3-vessel disease with only moderately impaired left ventricular function (see p 192). Thrombolytic agents (see below) may improve prognosis, but long-term data are not available.

C. Life Adjustment After Myocardial Infarction: Patients who were actively employed before an acute infarction are more likely to seek work than those who were not employed before the attack. Only one-third of patients surviving an infarction actually return to their jobs. The prognosis for return to work is less good if the patient is depressed or denies the illness.

D. Variable Postinfarction Health: A long period of good health often follows an initial episode of angina or myocardial infarction. It is difficult to reconcile such a benign course with the downhill course of patients who, following acute myocardial infarction, have progressively worsening symptoms and recurrent myocardial infarctions. The coronary anatomy may differ in patients with such discrepant courses.

CHRONIC (ESTABLISHED) CORONARY HEART DISEASE

Patients with coronary heart disease may continue to have angina pectoris of effort as the sole manifestation of chronic coronary disease. Stable angina may change to unstable angina (see p 161); the patient may have an episode of acute myocardial infarction followed by chronic coronary disease with stable angina, chronic left ventricular failure, recurrent arrhythmias, or "sudden death syndrome"—or following coronary bypass surgery, recurrent angina, or a new myocardial infarction. Specific treatment regimens for recurrent angina, cardiac failure, ventricular arrhythmias, or conduction defects occurring in patients with chronic coronary disease following myocardial infarction are discussed in other chapters. These events may occur alone or in combination in chronic (established) coronary disease, and treatment must be specifically directed at the individual clinical state.

Evaluation of Post-Myocardial Infarction Patients

The mortality rate in the first year following uncomplicated acute myocardial infarction varies from 7 to 10%. Patients with a complicated course (cardiac failure, cardiogenic shock, low ejection fraction, complex ventricular arrhythmias, conduction defects) have a significantly higher mortality rate that may approach 30–50% in the first year (Epstein, 1982; Taylor, 1980).

Because of variability in the clinical course following acute myocardial infarction, it seems prudent to evaluate patients recovering from infarction to identify high-risk subgroups for possible further diagnostic or therapeutic intervention. It is important to note evidences of continuing ischemia, left ventricular dysfunction, complex ventricular arrhythmias, unrecognized ventricular aneurysm, ventricular septal defect, or papillary muscle dysfunction with mitral regurgitation.

Low-level electrocardiographic exercise stress testing and 24-hour Holter electrocardiographic monitoring (see pp 180 and 188) performed just before hospital discharge will demonstrate any evidence of residual ischemia or complex ventricular arrhythmias. If continuing ischemia is demonstrated by a markedly positive ECG (see p 188) and there is also associated recurrent postinfarction angina, coronary and left ventricular angiography is usually advisable 3–6 weeks after discharge because the likelihood of new coronary events (including death) or the presence of significant left main coronary disease is greater in this high-risk subgroup.

Unless the situation is critical, the patient is usually discharged from the hospital on medical therapy with nitrates and beta-adrenergic or calcium entry–blocking agents; is given advice about restricted activities; and is advised to return in 4–6 weeks for clinical evaluation and noninvasive studies.

If clinical and noninvasive studies reveal no angina, a good ejection fraction ($> 50\%$), and no complex arrhythmias, no further investigation is required, and the patient is given medical treatment as for stable angina. If at 6 weeks there is persistent ischemia, complex ventricular arrhythmias, or significant left ventricular dysfunction with an ejection fraction of 30–40% or less, coronary and left ventricular angiograms are advised to assess the coronary anatomy, to estimate the amount of myocardium at risk, and to consider coronary surgery. Both the number of vessels involved and the degree of left ventricular dysfunction are important in prognosis (see Table 8–20). The importance of complex ventricular arrhythmias can be seen in Fig 8–42.

If the patient with postinfarction angina has a strongly positive electrocardiographic stress test and multiple wall motion abnormalities, significant stenosis of the left main coronary artery or multivessel disease with a substantial area of the myocardium at jeopardy is possible. If these are documented by angiography and left ventricular function is only moderately impaired, coronary bypass surgery is advisable. If, however, severe proximal stenosis of the left anterior descending coronary artery is found, angioplasty may be substituted. If considerable left ventricular failure due to coronary cardiomyopathy is found (ejection fraction ≤ 20–30%), medical and not surgical treatment is advised.

If investigation reveals a localized, well-demarcated ventricular aneurysm and if the patient has chronic cardiac failure, surgical resection is indicated.

Late Prognosis Following Myocardial Infarction

The prognosis after infarction is worse (1) the

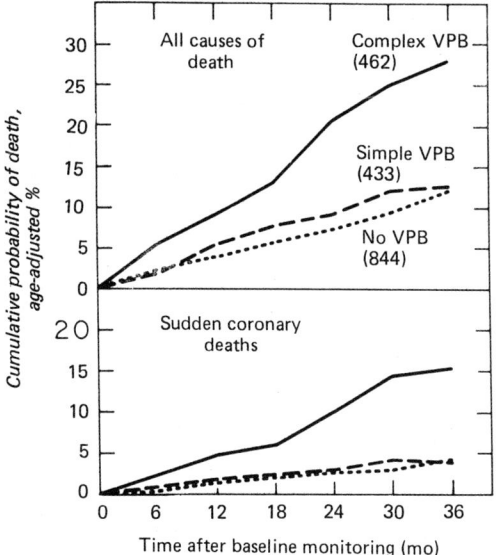

Figure 8–42. Mortality rates over 3 years after baseline monitoring in relation to ventricular premature beats (VPB) in the monitoring hour. (Reproduced, with permission, from Ruberman W et al: Ventricular premature beats and mortality after myocardial infarction. *N Engl J Med* 1977; 297:750.)

greater the area of infarction during the acute episode; (2) the more severe the evidence of left ventricular dysfunction after myocardial infarction; (3) the greater the magnitude and number of areas of wall motion hypokinesis, akinesis, or dyskinesis; (4) the more marked the ST segment depression on exercise (especially if the ST change occurs early at a relatively low heart rate below the predicted maximum); (5) the greater the fall in ejection fraction with exercise; (6) the more prominent or persistent the complex ventricular arrhythmias during exercise or during long-term ambulatory electrocardiographic monitoring; (7) the greater the number of stenosed coronary arteries, especially if the stenoses are proximal and involve the left main vessel; or (8) if the infarction is recurrent, especially with nontransmural infarction.

A large, poorly contracting left ventricle without a well-demarcated aneurysm is usually associated with left ventricular failure and has a poor prognosis.

The mortality rate of patients who survive an acute infarction is higher during the first 3–12 months than later. Patients with anterior infarction who have had transient complete atrioventricular block are at substantial risk of sudden death within the year, and permanent pacemakers are considered more often. Patients who have had severe cardiac failure have a higher mortality rate in the 1–2 years following infarction.

Secondary Prevention of Myocardial Infarction & Sudden Death

A. Lowering of Serum Lipids With Drugs and Diet: See p 135 for detailed discussion.

B. Antiarrhythmic Agents: About 60% of patients with coronary heart disease are victims of sudden death. Those with complex ventricular arrhythmias following acute myocardial infarction are more likely to die suddenly or have early cardiac death, and patients have been given conventional and investigative antiarrhythmic drugs in various trials. Although the prevalence of simple and complex ventricular premature beats was reduced in most studies, there was no convincing evidence that sudden death was prevented.

Among the newer drugs, the most effective appears to be amiodarone, which may prevent recurrent ventricular fibrillation. Aprindine, mexiletine, encainide, tocainide, flecainide, lorcainide, and others have been used in various trials with conflicting results. (See section on treatment of ventricular arrhythmias in Chapter 15.)

C. Beta-Adrenergic Blocking Agents: These drugs decrease myocardial oxygen consumption and cardiac work; are antihypertensive and antiarrhythmic; and inhibit sympathetic impulses to the heart. There have now been a substantial number of placebo-controlled, double-blind intervention trials with both cardioselective and noncardioselective beta-adrenergic blocking drugs. The incidence of sudden death and new myocardial infarction has been reduced by about 30% in each of the trials (Furberg, 1983). The most recent and largest trials are the Norwegian Multicenter Study Group (1981), using timolol, and the Beta Blocker Heart Attack Study Group (1981) in the USA, using propranolol. Taken as a whole, the results are impressive in showing that life is prolonged by these drugs. There is no agreement on when the drugs should be started after the infarction and for how long they should be continued. Unless there are contraindications, disturbing side effects, or the patient is in a very low risk group, serious consideration should be given to the use of such drugs about 10 days after patients have started recovering from a myocardial infarction.

D. Anti–Platelet-Aggregating Agents: Platelet aggregation is thought to be a factor in the development of atherosclerosis and acute coronary thrombosis; drugs that inhibit platelet aggregation have been used in various trials.

1. Sulfinpyrazone—Sulfinpyrazone (Anturane) was given in a dosage of 200 mg 4 times daily for 16 months beginning about 1 month after an acute myocardial infarction; a sharp reduction in the rate of sudden deaths occurred in the treated group up to the seventh month after infarction. It is not clear why the benefits of therapy are so short-lived, and further experience is required.

2. Aspirin—The Aspirin Myocardial Infarction Study Research Group (1980) found that although aspirin interferes with platelet aggregation, it does not reduce the total mortality rate in patients with a history of myocardial infarction. One-fourth of patients receiving aspirin developed symptoms of gastritis or gastric erosion. Aspirin is not recommended for routine use in survivors of acute myocardial infarction, although it is used extensively, often in combination with dipyridamole, but their beneficial effects have not been established. However, because of the trend in favor of aspirin, while not statistically significant, a new large-scale trial of aspirin for primary prevention is now under way in the USA, utilizing physicians as subjects (see p 162). The combination of aspirin and dipyridamole (Persantine) has been used in the so-called Paris trial, but the results were similar to those with the use of aspirin alone. Details of secondary prevention of coronary disease are summarized by May (1983).

E. Rehabilitation Programs: Physician-supervised exercise programs increase the physical work capacity of patients and improve morale. There is no convincing evidence that exercise decreases the likelihood of recurrence of myocardial infarction or the mortality rate. Despite the subjective and objective improvement seen in some patients following exercise rehabilitation, the claims for increased survival are premature (Shaw, 1981; Council on Scientific Affairs, 1981; Rechnitzer, 1983).

F. Anticoagulants: Long-term use of anticoagulants to prevent thromboembolic complications has been recommended by some for at least 20 years, and the risks and benefits have been argued. The treatment is difficult, and benefits seem marginal. Deaths due to thromboembolic complications are infrequent in patients with acute myocardial infarction or chronic coronary disease, possibly because of early ambulation and rehabilitation programs. Patients at particular risk of thromboembolism due to prolonged cardiac failure or a history of venous thromboses should be considered for long-term anticoagulant treatment. Bleeding from various sites in the body is the most important complication of the treatment and may require hospitalization or may even be fatal. The ease with which a stable prothrombin time can be achieved with oral anticoagulants is an important factor in the decision to use the treatment.

G. Coronary Heart Surgery: See below.

Recent Decline in Deaths Due to Heart Disease (Fig 8–43)

The age-adjusted overall ischemic heart disease mortality rate declined by 20% in the USA between 1968 and 1976 (Stamler, 1984). Improved survival was reported in both sexes, in all age groups, and in all major ethnic groups. The cause of the decline may be due to vigorous attempts to manage risk factors. These include (1) identification and treatment of hypertension; (2) efforts to reduce cigarette smoking; (3) extensive availability and use of coronary care units; (4) efforts to encourage a prudent diet to decrease serum lipids and weight; (5) supervised exercise training; and (6) extensive use of coronary bypass surgery.

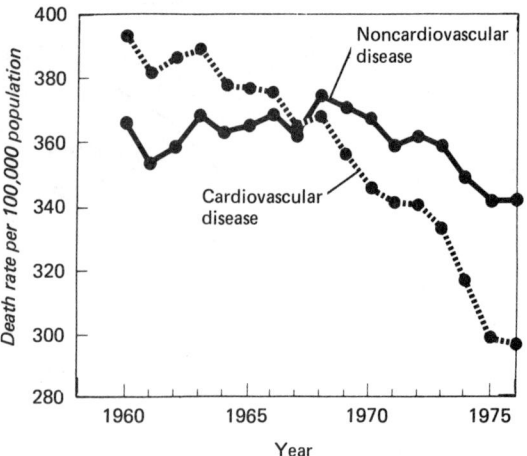

Figure 8–43. Cardiovascular and noncardiovascular mortality rates, 1960–1976. (Reproduced, with permission, from the American Heart Association, Inc., Levy RI: Progress toward prevention of cardiovascular disease: A 30-year retrospective. *Circulation* 1979;**60**:1555.)

CORONARY HEART SURGERY

Over the past 20 years there has been an increasing trend toward use of surgical procedures for revascularization of the heart. The coronary bypass procedure—in which the obstructed coronary artery is bypassed by inserting the saphenous vein into the aorta proximal to the coronary arteries and beyond the obstruction distally or, alternatively, by anastomosing the internal mammary artery to a point distal to the obstructed artery has now been used in more than a half million people.

Results of Coronary Bypass Surgery

A. Relief of Angina Pectoris: Bypass surgery is now performed extensively for single-, double-, and triple-vessel disease. Relief of angina of effort occurs in about 85% of patients. The surgical mortality rate of bypass surgery in stable angina is now 1–3%. The mortality rate is higher if patients have unstable angina or require resection of a ventricular aneurysm, replacement of the mitral valve, or closure of an acquired ventricular septal defect.

B. Prevention of Myocardial Infarction and Death: The benefits of bypass surgery in preventing myocardial infarction and prolonging life are controversial.

The decreased operative risk in the past 5 years has been due to improved anesthetic and surgical techniques, myocardial protection during surgery, and better pre- and postoperative care.

Objective improvement occurs in about half of these patients. Electrocardiography shows less evidence of ischemia induced by graded exercise. There is increased left ventricular contractility with improved ejection fraction and improved left ventricular wall motion in patients who preoperatively had impaired segmental left ventricular walls—especially if the graft to the myocardial segment remains patent following surgery. Most patients have sufficient subjective improvement so that they can return to work. Relapse may occur as a result of occlusion of the previously patent graft when a patient appears to be improving. The long-term effectiveness of bypass surgery in patients who have had a good technical result and a patent graft is now being reported. In a consecutive group of 500 patients (of whom 70% had good left ventricular function) followed for at least 10 years after bypass surgery, 50% were asymptomatic and 41% were improved. Half the patients were on medication and, if younger than age 65 years, were employed full-time. Reoperation was required in 9% of patients. The 10-year survival rate for 3-vessel disease was 48%. The long-term results in this series were notable; the 10-year survival rates for patients with good left ventricular function were 83% for single-vessel disease, 73% for 2-vessel disease, 53% for 3-vessel disease, and 73% for left main disease. These data indicate that the yearly mortality rate for surgically treated 3-vessel disease, for example, was about 5% per year (Lawrie, 1982).

Surgical treatment is indicated when there is severe stenosis of the left main coronary artery; 2- to 3-year survival rates are higher for surgically treated than for medically treated groups (85–90% vs 65–69%) (Chaitman, Am J Cardiol 1981; CASS, 1983). Surgical treatment is most beneficial for patients in whom left main stenosis exceeds 75% and in whom left ventricular function is abnormal. In the CASS study reported by Zimmern (1982), long-term survival is possible despite total occlusion of the left main coronary artery, although in groups of patients, bypass surgery improved survival rates. There were significant lesions of the other major coronary arteries in about 60% of patients in both groups.

Of particular interest are patients rejected for coronary revascularization who by current indications would now be considered operable. Those considered operable in retrospect had a 3-year survival rate of 98%. The major factor influencing survival was left ventricular function; survival was approximately 90% if the ejection fraction exceeded 34% but only 59% if the ejection fraction was less than this figure (Gross, 1978).

The most important recent paper comparing surgical and medical treatment of mild to moderate stable angina pectoris in a large series of cases is CASS (1983). This randomized study found that the surgical mortality rate was only 1.4% and the annual mortality rate in the medically treated group only 1.6%—considerably less than in any of the medically treated control groups in previous trials. This low mortality rate was a function of modern medical therapy. Only some of the patients received beta-adrenergic blocking agents, and none received calcium entry–blocking drugs. Angina was relieved in 80–90% of patients. The results show that there is no difference in survival rates or rates of prevention of myocardial infarction in patients in whom angina can be controlled by medical treatment, even though they had multivessel disease or previous myocardial infarction. However, the study did not include patients with significant left main artery stenosis or those at high risk with grade III or grade IV angina, unstable angina, or post–myocardial infarction angina. It is clear that angina pectoris refractory to medical therapy is a prime indication for surgery, but indications for surgery in high-risk patients with diseases other than left main coronary stenosis were not provided by the CASS report.

C. Factors Influencing Operative Results: (Table 8–21.) The surgical results, including the operative deaths that occur, are influenced by the presence of acute myocardial necrosis at surgery; by the presence of previous myocardial infarction with segmental abnormalities of left ventricular motion; by increased left ventricular end-diastolic volume and pressure; by impaired left ventricular function, such as a decreased ejection fraction; and by the number of procedures performed at one operation. When end-diastolic volume is increased (especially if the patient has cardiac failure) or if the ejection fraction is less than 35%, the operative mortality rate is higher. There is a progressive fall in mortality rate if the bypass is done after the first week. The mortality rate stabilizes at about 30–60 days. As a result, elective surgery is usually delayed at least 2 months following an acute myocardial infarction.

The availability of a skilled cardiac surgeon with a well-trained, efficient team and adequate diagnostic and therapeutic facilities is necessary if bypass surgery is performed for incapacitating angina in patients with good left ventricular function. Coronary angiograms of high quality are essential in preparation for coronary bypass surgery. The presence of severe disease is not sufficient to justify surgery; the patient

Table 8–21. Beneficial and adverse effects of coronary bypass surgery.

Beneficial Effects	Adverse Effects
Relief of angina in 85%	Immediate demise at operation
Improved exercise tolerance and left ventricular function in an unknown percentage	Morbidity associated with heart surgery, and high cost
	Intraoperative myocardial infarction
Increased survival rates in some patients (eg, those with left main disease or 3-vessel disease with easily induced ischemia and clinically high-risk subsets)	Progression of coronary disease in the native circulation
	Occlusion of the graft
	Worsening of left ventricular function in some
	No proof of prevention of myocardial infarction, premature death, or ventricular arrhythmias, except in left main coronary artery disease, 3-vessel disease, and high-risk subsets

must also have vessels that can be bypassed. Similarly, left ventricular function must be good enough so that the patient can survive surgery and the postoperative risks.

Complications of Coronary Bypass Surgery

The adverse results that have followed bypass surgery include the following:

(1) Intraoperative myocardial infarction in 5–10% of patients, manifested by new Q waves, the development of increased MB CPK, and positive pyrophosphate isotope scans.

(2) A surgical mortality rate of approximately 1–3%, which rises to 10% if additional procedures are required.

(3) Difficulty in finding a satisfactory distal segment for anastomosis preoperatively by means of coronary arteriography.

(4) Early (within 1 year) occlusion of about 20% of the grafts, often related to a relatively low blood flow at the time of the grafting.

(5) Progression of coronary disease postoperatively. Some patients are worse postoperatively, due in part to the so-called coronary steal syndrome and in part to the fact that progression of stenoses is greater in the proximal portion of bypassed arteries than in arteries that have been untouched.

(6) Late occlusion of bypass graft. If, in addition to progression of a partially stenosed artery, the graft applied distally to the stenosis becomes occluded, the patient is then worse off, develops more left ventricular dysfunction and more segmental contraction disorders, and may have more severe angina.

(7) Persistence of exercise-induced ventricular premature beats even when ventricular scars and ventricular aneurysms are resected.

(8) Decrease of collateral circulation that occurs after grafting and deterioration with respect to heart failure and chest pain over a period of years.

Late Consequences of Coronary Bypass Surgery

Despite unequivocal evidence of relief of pain following bypass surgery in 85% of patients with unacceptable angina pectoris, 15% continue to have substantial angina. Furthermore, recurrent late angina is now being reported more frequently. Studies in patients with recurrent symptoms after a period of years usually show closure of one or more grafts in about half and incomplete revascularization and progression of underlying atherosclerotic disease in the remainder. After 5 years, about half of operated patients will develop significant new lesions (Hamby, 1980).

Relief of Symptoms With Reoperation

Patients with recurrent or persistent chest pain after surgery should first be studied by exercise electrocardiography and thallium 201 to document the presence of myocardial ischemia and, if this is found to be present, referred for coronary arteriography and contrast ventriculograms. Reoperation (possibly coronary angioplasty—see below) is recommended if ischemia is documented and the coronary anatomy is favorable. A new noninvasive procedure to determine the patency of coronary bypass grafts is computerized tomography (CT scan), which correlates highly with coronary angiography (Brundage, 1983).

A second bypass operation for patients with recurrent angina after bypass surgery has a relatively low mortality rate (2–4%) but fails to relieve angina in about half of patients; about a third do not benefit from the second procedure (Brooks, 1979).

PERCUTANEOUS TRANSLUMINAL CORONARY ANGIOPLASTY

Percutaneous transluminal coronary angioplasty is a promising nonoperative approach to treatment of highly selected patients with angina pectoris uncontrolled by medication who would otherwise be candidates for coronary bypass surgery. The procedure has been greeted with considerable enthusiasm around the world and has been used in thousands of patients. The procedure is performed in the cardiac catheterization laboratory using techniques similar to those of coronary angiography; a cardiac surgeon, support team, and operating room must be available for backup. A balloon catheter is introduced into the stenotic portion of a coronary artery or a stenosed bypass graft and inflated with the aid of a pressure system to 4–8 atm. In successful cases, the pressure inflation depresses the atherosclerotic plaque and enlarges the lumen of the stenosed artery; the benefit can be demonstrated by repeat coronary arteriograms. The pressure gradient across the stenosis is greatly reduced, and, following a successful procedure, patients have relief of angina, increased exercise tolerance, and objective evidence of reduced ischemia during exercise as judged by thallium scans or radioangiography as well as improved left ventricular function. Successful dilation has been variously described as a 20–50% increase in the luminal diameter of the stenosis.

It is important to select patients who have significant symptoms and an angiographic lesion warranting bypass surgery. Ideally, the symptoms should be of relatively short duration and there should be proximal localized noncalcific stenosis exceeding 70% of the lumen of a single vessel. Results to date indicate successful dilation in approximately two-thirds of patients. Complications such as complete coronary occlusion or coronary dissection or other acute conditions requiring emergency bypass surgery occur in 5–10%; recurrent stenosis occurs in 20% (usually within approximately 3 months); successful second dilation is performed in about 80%; and long-lasting benefits occur in 75–85% of patients. The mortality rate is less than 1%. Results are best with discrete lesions of the proximal left anterior descending artery; less good with the right coronary artery; and least good with lesions of the left circumflex artery. Because of the early success with single-vessel disease, the procedure is now being performed in distal disease, 2-vessel disease, left main disease, occluded bypass grafts, and even in 3-vessel disease. As the procedure is used more extensively, the success rate will probably fall and complications will be reported more often. It is estimated that about 10% of patients who would otherwise be candidates for bypass surgery are suitable candidates for percutaneous transluminal coronary angioplasty (Grüntzig, 1982).

At present, patients having the procedure have had essentially normal left ventricular function; it remains to be seen whether dilation would be suitable in patients with more advanced left ventricular dysfunction. Ancillary measures such as anti-platelet aggregating drugs are used before the procedure and for several months afterward. Heparin is given during the procedure, and calcium entry-blocking agents are begun the day before and continued for several days or, if the patient has coronary spasm, for a longer period. Nitrates, given intravenously or by intracoronary injection, are used to provide maximum vasodilation and to reverse any spasm that might have been induced. In patients with acute myocardial ischemia, some centers are combining percutaneous transluminal coronary angioplasty and thrombolysis with streptokinase; others are adding coronary bypass surgery even if complications have not been induced. (See National Heart, Lung, and Blood Institute, 1984.)

REFERENCES

Overview of Coronary Heart Disease

Braunwald E (editor): *Heart Disease: A Textbook of Cardiovascular Medicine,* 2nd ed. Saunders, 1984.

McAlpine WA: *Heart and Coronary Arteries: An Anatomical Atlas for Clinical Diagnosis, Radiological Investigation, and Surgical Treatment.* Springer-Verlag, 1975.

Oliver MF (editor): *Coronary Heart Disease in Young Women.* Churchill Livingstone, 1978.

Robbins SL, Angell M: *Basic Pathology,* 2nd ed. Saunders, 1976.

Schaper W: *The Collateral Circulation of the Heart.* North-Holland, 1971.

Selzer A: *Principles and Practice of Clinical Cardiology,* 2nd ed. Saunders, 1983.

Soto B, Russell RO Jr, Moraski RE: *Radiographic Anatomy of the Coronary Arteries: An Atlas.* Futura, 1976.

Pathogenesis of Atherosclerotic Coronary Heart Disease

AHA Committee Report: Risk factors and coronary disease: A statement for physicians. *Circulation* 1980;**62:**449A.

AHA Nutrition Committee: Special report on rationale of the diet-heart statement of the American Heart Association. *Arteriosclerosis* 1982;**4:**177.

Bache RJ, Dymek DJ: Local and regional regulation of coronary vascular tone. *Prog Cardiovasc Dis* 1981;**24:**191.

Bilheimer DW et al: Genetics of the low density lipoprotein receptor: Diminished receptor activity in lymphocytes from heterozygotes with familial hypercholesterolemia. *J Clin Invest* 1978;**61:**678.

Blumgart HL, Zoll PM: Pathologic physiology of angina pectoris and acute myocardial infarction. *Circulation* 1960;**22:**301.

Brensike JF et al: Effects of therapy with cholestyramine on progression of coronary arteriosclerosis: Results of the NHLBI Type II Coronary Intervention Study. *Circulation* 1984;**69:**313.

Brown MS, Goldstein JL: Familial hypercholesterolemia: A genetic defect in the low-density lipoprotein receptor. *N Engl J Med* 1976;**294:**1386.

Brown MS, Goldstein JL: Familial hypercholesterolemia: Genetic, biochemical, and pathophysiological aspects. *Adv Intern Med* 1975;**20:**273.

Brown MS et al: Prenatal diagnosis of homozygous familial hypercholesterolaemia: Expression of a genetic receptor disease in utero. *Lancet* 1978;**1:**526.

Case RB et al: Type A behavior and survival after acute myocardial infarction. *N Engl J Med* 1985;**312:**737.

Castelli WP: Epidemiology of coronary heart disease: The Framingham Study. *Am J Med* 1984;**76:**4.

Crawford T, Dexter D, Teare RD: Coronary-artery pathology in sudden death from myocardial ischaemia. *Lancet* 1961;**1:**181.

Dawber TR, Kannel WB: An epidemiologic study of heart disease: The Framingham Study. *Nutr Rev* (Jan) 1958;**16:**1.

DeWood MA et al: Prevalence of total coronary occlusion during the early hours of transmural myocardial infarction. *N Engl J Med* 1980;**303:**897.

Dimsdale JE et al: Type A personality and extent of coronary atherosclerosis. *Am J Cardiol* 1978;**42:**583.

Duguid JB: Thrombosis as a factor in the pathogenesis of coronary atherosclerosis. *J Pathol* 1946;**58:**207.

Falk E: Plaque rupture with severe pre-existing stenosis precipitating coronary thrombosis: Characteristics of coronary atherosclerotic plaques underlying fatal occlusive thrombi. *Br Heart J* 1983;**50:**127.

Farquhar JW, Sokolow M: Response of serum lipids and lipoproteins of man to beta-sitosterol and safflower oil. *Circulation* 1958;**17:**890.

Folkow B: Role of sympathetic nervous system. Page 68 in: *Coronary Heart Disease and Physical Fitness.* Larson OA, Malmborg O (editors). Munksgaard, 1971.

Fozzard HA: Electrophysiology of the heart: The effects of ischemia. *Hosp Pract* (May) 1980;**15:**61.

Friedman M et al: Alteration of type A behavior and reduction in cardiac recurrences in postmyocardial infarction patients. *Am Heart J* 1984;**108:**237.

Fuller JH et al: Coronary-heart-disease risk and impaired glucose tolerance: The Whitehall Study. *Lancet* 1980;**2:**373.

Fuster V, Chesebro JH: Antithrombotic therapy: Role of platelet-inhibitor drugs. 2. Pharmacologic effects of platelet-inhibitor drugs (Second of 3 parts.) *Mayo Clin Proc* 1981;**56:**185.

Gillum RF (guest editor): Proceedings of the symposium on coronary heart disease in black populations. *Am Heart J* 1984;**108:**727.

Gofman JW, Young W, Tandy R: Ischemic heart disease, atherosclerosis and longevity. *Circulation* 1966;**34:**679.

Goldstein JL, Brown MS: Familial hypercholesterolemia. Pages 672–712 in: *The Metabolic Basis of Inherited Disease,* 5th ed. Stanbury JB et al (editors). McGraw-Hill, 1983.

Goldstein JL, Kita T, Brown MS: Defective lipoprotein receptors and atherosclerosis: Lessons from an animal counterpart of familial hypercholesterolemia. *N Engl J Med* 1983;**309**:288.

Goldstein JL et al: Hyperlipidemia in coronary heart disease: Lipid levels in 500 survivors of myocardial infarction. *J Clin Invest* 1973;**52**:1533.

Gordon DJ et al: Habitual physical activity and high-density lipoprotein cholesterol in men with primary hypercholesterolemia: The Lipid Research Clinics Coronary Primary Prevention Trial. *Circulation* 1983;**67**:512.

Hamby RI: *Clinical-Anatomical Correlates in Coronary Artery Disease.* Futura, 1979.

Hamby RI: Hereditary aspects of coronary artery disease. *Am Heart J* 1981;**101**:639.

Harrison DC (editor): Beta blockers and exercise: A symposium. *Am J Cardiol* 1985;**55**:1D. [Entire issue.]

Havel RJ, Goldstein JL, Brown MS: Lipoproteins and lipid transport. Pages 393–494 in: *Metabolic Control and Disease,* 8th ed. Bondy PK, Rosenberg LE (editors). Saunders, 1980.

Heiss G et al: Lipoprotein-cholesterol distributions in selected North American populations: The Lipid Research Clinics Program Prevalence Study. *Circulation* 1980;**61**:302.

Hubert HB et al: Obesity as an independent risk factor for cardiovascular disease: A 26-year follow-up of participants in the Framingham heart study. *Circulation* 1983;**67**:968.

James TN: *Anatomy of the Coronary Arteries.* Hoeber, 1961.

Jenkins CD: Recent evidence supporting psychologic and social risk factors for coronary disease. (2 parts.) *N Engl J Med* 1976;**294**:987, 1033.

Johnson KW, Payne GH: Report of a National Heart, Lung, and Blood Institute working conference on coronary heart disease in black populations. *Am Heart J* 1984;**108**:633.

Kane JP et al: Normalization of low-density-lipoprotein levels in heterozygous familial hypercholesterolemia with a combined drug regimen. *N Engl J Med* 1981;**304**:251.

Kannel WB, McGee D, Gordon T: A general cardiovascular risk profile: The Framingham Study. *Am J Cardiol* 1976;**38**:46.

Kannel WB, Wilson P, Blair SN: Epidemiological assessment of the role of physical activity and fitness in development of cardiovascular disease. *Am Heart J* 1985;**109**:876.

Kannel WB et al: Menopause and risk of cardiovascular disease: The Framingham Study. *Ann Intern Med* 1976;**85**:447.

Kannel WB et al: Optimal resources for primary prevention of atherosclerotic diseases. *Circulation* 1984;**70**:157A.

Klocke FJ: Measurements of coronary blood flow and degree of stenosis: Current clinical implications and continuing uncertainties. *J Am Coll Cardiol* 1983;**1**:31.

Kromhout D, Bosschieter EB, de Lezenne Coulander C: The inverse relation between fish consumption and 20-year mortality from coronary heart disease. *N Engl J Med* 1985;**312**:1205.

Kuo PT: Lipoproteins, platelets, and prostaglandins in atherosclerosis. *Am Heart J* 1981;**102**:949.

Leon AS: Physical activity levels and coronary heart disease: Analysis of epidemiologic and supporting studies. *Med Clin N Am* 1985;**69**:3.

Levy RI et al: The influence of changes in lipid values induced by cholestyramine and diet on progression of coronary artery disease: Results of the NHLBI type II coronary intervention study. *Circulation* 1984;**69**:325.

Lipid Research Clinics Program: The lipid research clinics coronary primary prevention trial results. 1. Reduction in incidence of coronary heart disease. 2. The relationship of reduction in incidence of coronary heart disease to cholesterol lowering. *JAMA* 1984;**251**:351, 365.

Lober PH: Pathogenesis of coronary sclerosis. *Arch Pathol* 1953;**55**:357.

Lown B, Graboys TB: Sudden death: An ancient problem newly perceived. *Cardiosvasc Med* 1977;**2**:219.

Mabuchi H et al: Homozygous familial hypercholesterolemia in Japan. *Am J Cardiol* 1978;**65**:290.

Mackay A et al: Ischaemic heart disease in young hypertensive women. *Br Heart J* 1980;**43**:80.

Maseri A: Pathogenetic mechanisms of angina pectoris: Expanding views. *Br Heart J* 1980;**43**:648.

Maseri A, Chierchia S: Coronary artery spasm: Demonstration, definition, diagnosis, and consequences. *Prog Cardiovasc Dis* 1982;**25**:169.

Maseri A, Chierchia S, Labbate A: Pathogenetic mechanisms underlying the clinical events associated with atherosclerotic heart disease. *Circulation* 1980;**62(6–Part 2)**:3.

Maseri A, Parodi O, Fox KM: Rational approach to the medical therapy of angina pectoris: The role of calcium antagonists. *Prog Cardiovasc Dis* 1983;**25**:269.

Mehta J: Platelets and prostaglandins in coronary artery disease. *JAMA* 1983;**249**:2818.

Morales AR, Romanelli R, Boucek RJ: The mural left anterior descending coronary artery, strenuous exercise and sudden death. *Circulation* 1980;**62**:230.

Morris JN et al: Vigorous exercise in leisure-time: Protection against coronary heart disease. *Lancet* 1980;**2**:1207.

Multiple Risk Factor Invervention Trial Research Group: Multiple risk factor intervention trial: Risk factor changes and mortality results. *JAMA* 1982;**248**:1465.

National Academy of Sciences Food and Nutrition Board: *Toward Healthful Diets.* National Research Council, 1980.

Patterson D, Slack J: Lipid abnormalities in male and female survivors of myocardial infarction and their first-degree relatives. *Lancet* 1972;**1**:393.

Pitt B et al: Prostaglandins and prostaglandin inhibitors in ischemic heart disease. *Ann Intern Med* 1983;**99**:83.

Pooling Project Research Group: Relationship of blood pressure, serum cholesterol, smoking habit, relative weight and ECG abnormalities to incidence of major coronary events: Final report of the Pooling Project. *J Chronic Dis* 1978;**31**:201.

Rechnitzer PA et al: Relation of exercise to the recurrence rate of myocardial infarction in men: Ontario Exercise Heart Collaborative Study. *Am J Cardiol* 1983;**51**:65.

Rissanen AM, Nikkilä EA: Aggregation of coronary risk factors in families of men with fatal and non-fatal coronary heart disease. *Br Heart J* 1979;**42**:373.

Robbins SL, Angell M: *Basic Pathology,* 2nd ed. Saunders, 1976.

Rosenman RH et al: Multivariate prediction of coronary heart disease during 8.5 years follow-up in the Western Collaborative Group Study. *Am J Cardiol* 1976;**37**:903.

Ross R: George Lyman Duff Memorial Lecture: Atherosclerosis: A problem of the biology of arterial wall cells and their interactions with blood components. *Arteriosclerosis* 1981;**1**:293.

Ross R, Glomset JA: The pathogenesis of atherosclerosis. (Part 1.) *N Engl J Med* 1976;**195**:369.

Royal College of General Practitioners' Oral Contraception Study: Further analyses of mortality in oral contraceptive users. *Lancet* 1981;**1**:541.

Ruderman NB, Haudenschild C: Diabetes as an atherogenic factor. *Prog Cardiovasc Dis* 1984;**26**:373.

Schaefer EJ, Levy RI: Pathogenesis and management of lipoprotein disorders. *N Engl J Med* 1985;**312**:1300.

Schmidt SB et al: Lipoprotein and apolipoprotein levels in angiographically defined coronary atherosclerosis. *Am J Cardiol* 1985;**55**:1459.

Schonfeld G: Disorders of lipid transport: Update, 1983. *Prog Cardiovasc Dis* 1983;**26**:89.

Schwartz SM, Ross R: Cellular proliferation in atherosclerosis and hypertension. *Prog Cardiovasc Dis* 1984;**26**:355.

Shaw LW: Effects of a prescribed supervised exercise program on mortality and cardiovascular morbidity in patients after a myocardial infarction: The National Exercise and Heart Disease Project. *Am J Cardiol* 1981;**48**:39.

Shekelle RB et al: Diet, serum cholesterol, and death from coronary heart disease: The Western Electric Study. *N Engl J Med* 1981;**304**:65.

Slack J: Risk factors in coronary heart disease. *Lancet* 1977;**1**:366.

Slack J: Risks of ischaemic heart disease in familial hyperlipoproteinaemic states. *Lancet* 1969;**2**:1380.

Slack J, Nevin NC: Hyperlipidaemic xanthomatoses. 1. Increased risk of death from ischaemic heart disease in first degree relatives of 53 patients with essential hyperlipidaemia and xanthomatosis. *J Med Genet* 1968;**5**:4.

Slone D et al: Risk of myocardial infarction in relation to current and discontinued use of oral contraceptives. *N Engl J Med* 1981;**305**:420.

Snow PJ et al: Coronary disease: A pathological study. *Br Heart J* 1955;**17**:503.

Solberg LA, Strong JP: Risk factors and atherosclerotic lesions: A review of autopsy studies. *Arteriosclerosis* 1983;**3**:187.

Spain DM, Bradess VA, Mohr C: Coronary atherosclerosis as a cause of unexpected and unexplained death. *JAMA* 1960;**174**:384.

Stamler J, Stamler R: Intervention for the prevention and control of hypertension and atherosclerotic diseases: United States and international experience. *Am J Med* 1984;**76**:13.

Stone NJ et al: Coronary artery disease in 116 kindred with familial type II hyperlipoproteinemia. *Circulation* 1974;**49**:476.

Swan HJC et al: Catheterization of the heart in man with use of a flow-directed balloon-tipped catheter. *N Engl J Med* 1970;**283**:447.

Symposium on high-density lipoproteins and coronary artery disease: Effects of diet, exercise, and pharmacologic intervention. *Am J Cardiol* 1983;**52(4)**:1B. [Entire issue.]

ten Kate LP et al: Familial aggregation of coronary heart disease and its relation to known genetic risk factors. *Am J Cardiol* 1982;**50**:945.

Vane JR: Prostaglandins and the cardiovascular system. *Br Heart J* 1983;**49**:405.

Waller BF, Palumbo PJ, Roberts WC: Status of the coronary arteries at necropsy in diabetes mellitus with onset after age 30 years: Analysis of 229 diabetic patients with and without clinical evidence of coronary heart disease and comparison to 183 control subjects. *Am J Med* 1980;**69**:498.

Weiss ES et al: Evaluation of myocardial metabolism and perfusion with positron-emitting radionuclides. *Prog Cardiovasc Dis* 1977;**20**:191.

Weiss SM: Coronary-prone behavior and coronary heart disease: A critical review. *Circulation* 1981;**63**:1199.

Weksler BB et al: Differential inhibition by aspirin of vascular and platelet prostaglandin synthesis in atherosclerotic patients. *N Engl J Med* 1983;**308**:800.

Latent Coronary Heart Disease

Astrand P: Quantification of exercise capability and evaluation of physical capacity in man. *Prog Cardiovasc Dis* 1976;**19**:51.

Froelicher VF: Exercise testing and training: Clinical applications. *J Am Coll Cardiol* 1983;**1**:114.

Goldman MJ: *Principles of Clinical Electrocardiography,* 12th ed. Lange, 1986.

Hjermann I et al: Effect of diet and smoking intervention on the incidence of coronary heart disease: Report from the Oslo Study Group of a randomised trial in healthy men. *Lancet* 1981;**2**:1303.

Rifkin RD, Parisi AF, Folland E: Coronary calcification in the diagnosis of coronary artery disease. *Am J Cardiol* 1979;**44**:141.

Robb GP, Seltzer F: Appraisal of the double two-step exercise test: A long-term follow-up study of 3325 men. *JAMA* 1975;**234**:722.

Sheffield LT, Roitman D: Stress testing methodology. *Prog Cardiovasc Dis* 1976;**19**:33.

Sudden Death

Bigger JT Jr, Weld FM: Drugs and sudden cardiac death. *Ann NY Acad Sci* 1982;**382**:229.

Cedres BL et al: Independent contribution of electrocardiographic abnormalities to risk of death from coronary heart disease, cardiovascular diseases and all causes: Findings of three Chicago epidemiologic studies. *Circulation* 1982;**65**:146.

Cobb LA, Werner JA, Trobaugh GB: Sudden cardiac death. 1. A decade's experience with out-of-hospital resuscitation. *Mod Concepts Cardiovasc Dis* 1980;**49**:31.

Cobb LA et al: Resuscitation from out-of-hospital ventricular fibrillation: 4 years follow-up. *Circulation* 1975;**52 (Suppl 3)**:III-223.

Davies MJ: Pathological view of sudden cardiac death. *Br Heart J* 1981;**45**:88.

DeSilva RA: Central nervous system risk factors for sudden cardiac death. *Ann NY Acad Sci* 1982;**382**:143.

Doyle JT et al: Factors related to suddenness of death from coronary disease: Combined Albany-Framingham Studies. *Am J Cardiol* 1976;**37**:1073.

Eisenberg MS, Hallstrom A, Bergner L: Long-term survival after out-of-hospital cardiac arrest. *N Engl J Med* 1982;**306**:1340.

Goldstein S et al: Characteristics of the resuscitated out-of-hospital cardiac arrest victim with coronary heart disease. *Circulation* 1981;**64**:977.

Greenberg HM, Dwyer EM Jr (editors): Sudden coronary death. *Ann NY Acad Sci* 1982;**382**:1. [Entire issue.]

Hypertension Detection and Follow-up Program Cooperative Group: Five-year findings of the Hypertension Detection and Follow-up Program: 1. Reduction in mortality of persons with high blood pressure, including mild hypertension. 2. Mortality by race, sex and age. *JAMA* 1979;**242**:2562, 2572.

James TN (chairman): 15th Bethesda Conference Report: Sudden cardiac death. *J Am Cardiol* 1985;**5(Suppl)**:1B.

Jelinek MV, Lohrbauer L, Lown B: Antiarrhythmic drug therapy for sporadic ventricular ectopic arrhythmias. *Circulation* 1974;**49**:659.

Josephson ME et al: Electrophysiologic and hemodynamic studies in patients resuscitated from cardiac arrest. *Am J Cardiol* 1980;**46**:948.

Kannel WB, Thomas HE Jr: Sudden coronary death: The Framingham Study. *Ann NY Acad Sci* 1982;**382**:3.

Kannel WB, Wilson P, Blair SN: Epidemiological assessment of the role of physical activity and fitness in development of cardiovascular disease. *Am Heart J* 1985;**109**:876.

Kuller LH: Sudden death: Definition and epidemiologic considerations. *Prog Cardiovasc Dis* 1980;**23**:1.

Lie JT, Titus JL: Pathology of the myocardium and the conduction system in sudden coronary death. *Circulation* 1975;**52(Suppl 3)**:III-41.

Lown B: Mental stress, arrhythmias and sudden death. *Am J Med* 1982;**72**:177.

Lown B: Sudden cardiac death: The major challenge confronting contemporary cardiology. *Am J Cardiol* 1979;**43**:313.

Lown B, Graboys TB: Sudden death: An ancient problem newly perceived. *Cardiovasc Med* 1977;**2**:219.

Lown B et al: Monitoring for serious arrhythmias and high risk of sudden death. *Circulation* 1975;**52(Suppl 3)**:III-189.

Mabuchi H et al: Reduction of serum cholesterol in heterozygous patients with familial hypercholesterolemia: Additive effects of compactin and cholestyramine. *N Engl J Med* 1983;**308**:609.

Miller DD et al: Clinical characteristics associated with sudden death in patients with variant angina. *Circulation* 1982;**66**:588.

Mirowski M et al: The automatic implantable defibrillator. *J Cardiovasc Med* 1982;**7**:498.

Mirowski M et al: Implantable automatic defibrillators: Their potential in prevention of sudden coronary death. *Ann NY Acad Sci* 1982;**382**:371.

Morady F et al: Electrophysiologic testing in the management of survivors of out-of-hospital cardiac arrest. *Am J Cardiol* 1983;**51**:85.

Myerburg RJ et al: Survivors of prehospital cardiac arrest. *JAMA* 1982;**247**:1485.

Myers A, Dewar HA: Circumstances attending 100 sudden deaths from coronary artery disease with coroner's necropsies. *Br Heart J* 1975;**37**:1133.

National Conference on Cardiopulmonary Resuscitation and Emergency Cardiac Care: Standards and guidelines for cardiopulmonary resuscitation (CPR) and emergency cardiac care (ECC). *JAMA* 1980;**244**:453.

Rabkin SW, Mathewson FAL, Tate RB: Relationship of ventricular ectopy in men without apparent heart disease to occurrence of ischemic heart disease and sudden death. *Am Heart J* 1981;**101**:135.

Ruberman W, Weinblatt E: Persistent risk of sudden death: Ventricular arrhythmia in MI survivors. *Primary Cardiol* 1983;**8**:33.

Rudikoff MT et al: Mechanisms of blood flow during cardiopulmonary resuscitation. *Circulation* 1980;**61**:345.

Smirk FH: R waves interrupting T waves. *Br Heart J* 1949;**11**:23.

Spain DM, Bradess VA, Mohr C: Coronary atherosclerosis as a cause of unexpected and unexplained death. *JAMA* 1960;**174**:384.

Stamler J: Sudden coronary death: Approaches to its prevention. *Med Clin North Am* 1976;**60**:245.

Thompson RG, Hallstrom AP, Cobb LA: Bystander-initiated cardiopulmonary resuscitation in management of ventricular fibrillation. *Ann Intern Med* 1979;**90**:737.

Weaver WD, Cobb LA, Hallstrom AP: Ambulatory arrhythmias in resuscitated victims of cardiac arrest. *Circulation* 1982;**66**:212.

Wellens HJ, Brugada P, Bär FW: The role of intraventricular conduction disorders in precipitating sudden death. *Ann NY Acad Sci* 1982;**382**:136.

Wilhelmsson C et al: Reduction of sudden deaths after myocardial infarction by treatment with alprenolol. *Lancet* 1974;**2**:1157.

Winkle RA: Clinical efficacy of antiarrhythmic drugs in prevention of sudden coronary death. *Ann NY Acad Sci* 1982;**382**:247.

Wolf S: Psychosocial forces in myocardial infarction and sudden death. *Circulation* 1969;**40(Suppl 4)**:IV-74.

Zipes DP, Gilmour RF Jr: Calcium antagonists and their potential role in the prevention of sudden coronary death. *Ann NY Acad Sci* 1982;**382**:258.

Angina Pectoris of Effort; Variant (Prinzmetal's) Angina (Coronary Spasm)

Bott-Silverman C, Heupler FA Jr: Natural history of pure coronary artery spasm in patients treated medically. *J Am Coll Cardiol* 1983;**2**:200.

Crawford MH, Amon KW, Vance WS: Exercise 2-dimensional echocardiography: Quantitation of left ventricular performance in patients with severe angina pectoris. *Am J Cardiol* 1983;**51**:1.

Epstein SE, Talbot TL: Dynamic coronary tone in precipitation, exacerbation and relief of angina pectoris. *Am J Cardiol* 1981;**48**:797.

Kannel WB, Feinleib M: Natural history of angina pectoris in the Framingham Study: Prognosis and treatment. *Am J Cardiol* 1972;**29**:154.

Krikler DM, Rowland E: Clinical value of calcium antagonists in treatment of cardiovascular disorders. *J Am Coll Cardiol* 1983;**1**:355.

Mark DB et al: Clinical characteristics and long-term survival of patients with variant angina. *Circulation* 1984;**69**:880.

Maseri A, Chierchia S: Coronary artery spasm: Demonstration, definition, diagnosis, and consequences. *Prog Cardiovasc Dis* 1982;**25**:169.

Mueller HS, Chahine RA: Interim report of multicenter double-blind, placebo-controlled studies of nifedipine in chronic stable angina. *Am J Med* 1981;**71**:645.

Prinzmetal M et al: Angina pectoris. 1. A variant form of angina pectoris. *Am J Med* 1959;**26**:375.

Reeder GS, Seward JB, Tajik AJ: The role of two-dimensional echocardiography in coronary artery disease: A critical appraisal. *Mayo Clin Proc* 1982;**57**:247.

Schroeder JS et al: Prevention of cardiovascular events in variant angina by long-term diltiazem therapy. *J Am Coll Cardiol* 1983;**1**:1507.

Stone PH, Goldschlager N: Left main coronary artery disease: Review and appraisal. *Cardiovasc Med* 1979;**4**:165.

Noninvasive & Invasive Studies

AHA Committee Report: Standards for cardiovascular exercise treatment programs. *Circulation* 1979;**59**:1084A.

AHA Special Report: Report of the Ad Hoc Committee on the Indications for Coronary Arteriography. *Circulation* 1977;**55**:969A.

AHS Subcommittee on Rehabilitation, Target Activity Group: Standards for adult exercise testing laboratories. *Circulation* 1979;**59**:421A.

Aldrich RF et al: Coronary calcification in the detection of coronary artery disease and comparison with electrocardiographic exercise testing. *Circulation* 1979;**59**:1113.

Berger BC et al: Effect of coronary collateral circulation on regional myocardial perfusion assessed with quantitative thallium-201 scintigraphy. *Am J Cardiol* 1980;**46**:365.

Berger HJ, Zaret BL: Nuclear cardiology. (2 parts.) *N Engl J Med* 1981;**305**:799, 855.

Block PJ, Popp RL: Echocardiography in coronary heart disease. *Cardiovasc Rev Rep* 1982;**3**:1675.

Bodenheimer MM et al: Comparative sensitivity of the exercise electrocardiogram, thallium imaging and stress radionuclide angiography to detect the presence and severity of coronary heart disease. *Circulation* 1979;**60**:1270.

Brody WR et al: Intravenous arteriography using digital subtraction techniques. *JAMA* 1982;**248**:671.

Brown BG, Bolson EL, Dodge HT: Arteriographic assessment of coronary atherosclerosis: Review of current methods, their limitations, and clinical applications. *Arteriosclerosis* 1982;**2**:2.

Brownell GL et al: Positron tomography and nuclear magnetic resonance imaging. *Science* 1982;**215**:619.

Bruce RA: Exercise testing for evaluation of ventricular function. *N Engl J Med* 1977;**296**:671.

Bruce RA: Exercise testing of patients with coronary heart disease. *Ann Clin Res* 1971;**3**:323.

Bruce RA et al: Enhanced risk assessment for primary coronary heart disease events by maximal exercise testing: 10 years' experience of Seattle Heart Watch. *J Am Coll Cardiol* 1983;**2**:565.

Bruschke AVG et al: The anatomic evolution of coronary artery disease demonstrated by coronary arteriography in 256 nonoperated patients. *Circulation* 1981;**63**:527.

Califf RM et al: Relationships among ventricular arrhythmias, coronary artery disease, and angiographic and electrocardiographic indicators of myocardial fibrosis. *Circulation* 1978;**57**:725.

Chaitman BR et al: Angiographic prevalence of high-risk coronary artery disease in patient subsets (CASS). *Circulation* 1981;**64**:360.

Chaitman BR et al: Clinical, angiographic, and hemodynamic findings in patients with anomalous origin of the coronary arteries. *Circulation* 1976;**53**:122.

Cohn K et al: Use of treadmill score to quantify ischemic response and predict extent of coronary disease. *Circulation* 1979;**59**:286.

Cosby RS et al: Clinicoarteriographic correlations in angina pectoris with and without myocardial infarction. *Am J Cardiol* 1979;**30**:472.

Crawford MH, Amon KW, Vance WS: Exercise 2-dimensional echocardiography: Quantitation of left ventricular performance in patients with severe angina pectoris. *Am J Cardiol* 1983;**51**:1.

Davis K et al: Complications of coronary angiography in the Collaborative Study of Coronary Artery Surgery (CASS). *Circulation* 1979;**59**:1105.

Dodge HT, Kennedy JW: Introduction: Twelfth Bethesda Conference: Noninvasive Technology in the Assessment of Ventricular Function. Sponsored by the American College of Cardiology, June 5 and 6, 1981, Heart House, Bethesda, Maryland. *Am J Cardiol* 1982;**49**:1309.

Edwards WD, Tajik AJ, Seward JB: Standardized nomenclature and anatomic basis for regional tomographic analysis of the heart. *Mayo Clin Proc* 1981;**56**:479.

Ellestad MH, Wan KC: Predictive implications of stress testing: Follow-up of 2700 subjects after maximum treadmill stress testing. *Circulation* 1975;**51**:363.

Epstein SE: Implications of probability analysis on the strategy used for noninvasive detection of coronary artery disease: Role of single or combined use of exercise electrocardiographic testing, radionuclide cineangiography and myocardial perfusion imaging. *Am J Cardiol* 1980;**46**:491.

Fuller CM et al: Exercise-induced coronary arterial spasm: Angiographic demonstration, documentation of ischemia by myocardial scintigraphy and results of pharmacologic intervention. *Am J Cardiol* 1980;**46**:500.

Goldberg HL et al: Digital subtraction intravenous left ventricular angiography: Comparison with conventional intraventricular angiography. *J Am Coll Cardiol* 1983;**1**:858.

Grossman W (editor): *Cardiac Catheterization and Angiography*, 2nd ed. Lea & Febiger, 1980.

Heupler FA Jr: Provocative testing for coronary arterial spasm: Risk, method and rationale. *Am J Cardiol* 1980;**46**:335.

Hollenberg M et al: Treadmill score quantifies electrocardiographic response to exercise and improves test accuracy and reproducibility. *Circulation* 1980;**61**:276.

Hutchins GM et al: Correlation of coronary arteriograms and left ventriculograms with postmortem studies. *Circulation* 1977;**56**:32.

Ideker RE et al: Evaluation of asynergy as an indicator of myocardial fibrosis. *Circulation* 1978;**57**:715.

Jengo JA et al: Evaluation of left ventricular function (ejection fraction and segmental wall motion) by single pass radioisotope angiography. *Circulation* 1978;**57**:326.

Johnson RA et al: Patterns of haemodynamic alteration during left ventricular ischaemia in man: Relation to angiographic extent of coronary artery disease. *Br Heart J* 1979;**41**:441.

Kaufman L et al: The potential impact of nuclear magnetic resonance imaging on cardiovascular diagnosis. *Circulation* 1983;**67**:251.

Libertson RR, Dinsmore RE, Fallon JT: Aberrant coronary artery origin from the aorta: Report of 18 patients, review of literature and delineation of natural history and management. *Circulation* 1979;**59**:748.

Maseri A, Chierchia S: Coronary artery spasm: Demonstration, definition, diagnosis, and consequences. *Prog Cardiovasc Dis* 1982;**25**:169.

Massie BM, Botvinick EH, Brundage BH: Correlation of thallium-201 scintigrams with coronary anatomy: Factors affecting region by region sensitivity. *Am J Cardiol* 1979;**44**:616.

McNeer JF et al: The role of the exercise test in the evaluation of patients for ischemic heart disease. *Circulation* 1978;**57**:64.

Michaelson SP et al: Recurrent myocardial infarction with normal coronary arteriography. *N Engl J Med* 1977;**297**:916.

Morganroth J, Pohost GM: Symposium: Two dimensional echocardiography versus cardiac nuclear imaging techniques. *Am J Cardiol* 1980;**46**:1093. [Entire issue.]

Nitter-Hauge S et al: Angiographic and risk factor characteristics of subjects with early onset ischaemic heart disease. *Br Heart J* 1981;**46**:325.

Phelps ME et al: Positron computed tomography for studies of myocardial and cerebral function. *Ann Intern Med* 1983;**98**:339.

Pridie RB et al: Coronary angiography: Review of 1500 consecutive cases. *Br Heart J* 1976;**38**:1200.

Proudfit W et al: Prognosis of 1000 young women studied by coronary angiography. *Circulation* 1981;**64**:1185.

Reeder GS, Seward JB, Tajik AJ: The role of two-dimensional echocardiography in coronary artery disease: A critical appraisal. *Mayo Clin Proc* 1982;**57**:247.

Schroeder JS et al: Provocation of coronary spasm with ergonovine maleate: New test with results in 57 patients undergoing coronary arteriography. *Am J Cardiol* 1977;**40**:487.

Schulze RA Jr et al: Coronary angiography and left ventriculography in survivors of transmural and nontransmural myocardial infarction. *Am J Med* 1978;**64**:108.

Selzer A: Transmural myocardial infarction with normal coronary arteriogram. *J Cardiovasc Med* 1980;**5**:595.

Sobel BE, Ter-Pogossian MM, Geltman EM: Positron-emission tomography in cardiac evaluation. *Hosp Pract* (Nov) 1981;**16**:93.

Stiles GL, Rosati RA, Wallace AG: Clinical relevance of exercise-induced S–T segment elevation. *Am J Cardiol* 1980;**46**:931.

Thomson PD, Kelemen MH: Hypotension accompanying the onset of exertional angina: A sign of severe compromise of left ventricular blood supply. *Circulation* 1975;**52**:28.

Weiner DA, McCabe CH, Ryan TJ: Identification of patients with left main and three vessel coronary disease with clinical and exercise test variables. *Am J Cardiol* 1980;**46**:21.

Treatment & Prognosis of Stable Angina

Abrams J: Nitroglycerin and long-acting nitrates in clinical practice. *Am J Med* 1983;**74**:85.

Abrams J, Roberts R (editors): First North American Conference on Nitroglycerin Therapy: Perspectives and mechanisms. *Am J Med* 1983;**74**:1. [Entire issue.]

Braunwald E: Mechanism of action of calcium channel–blocking agents. *N Engl J Med* 1982;**307**:1618.

Burggraf GW, Parker JO: Prognosis in coronary artery disease: Angiographic, hemodynamic and clinical factors. *Circulation* 1975;**51**:146.

Charlap S, Frishman WH: Comparative effects of verapamil and beta blockers in the therapy for patients with stable angina pectoris. *Cardiovasc Rev Rep* 1983;**4**:66.

Chatterjee K, Rouleau J-L, Parmley WW: Medical management of patients with angina: Has first-line management changed? *JAMA* 1984;**252**:1170.

Conley MJ et al: The prognostic spectrum of left main stenosis. *Circulation* 1978;**57**:947.

Conti CR et al: Nitrates for treatment of unstable angina pectoris and coronary vasospasm. *Am J Med* 1983;**74**:40.

Epstein SE et al: Strategy for evaluation and surgical treatment of the asymptomatic or mildly symptomatic patient with coronary artery disease. *Am J Cardiol* 1979;**45**:1015.

Frank CW, Weinblatt E, Shapiro S: Angina pectoris in men: Prognostic significance of selected medical factors. *Circulation* 1973;**47**:509.

Frishman WH: Drug therapy: Atenolol and timolol, two new systemic beta-adrenoreceptor antagonists. *N Engl J Med* 1982;**306**:1456.

Gold HK et al: Refractory angina pectoris: Follow-up after intraaortic balloon pumping and surgery. *Circulation* 1976;**54(Suppl 3)**:III-41.

Goldman GJ, Pichard AD: The natural history of coronary artery disease: Does medical therapy improve the prognosis? *Prog Cardiovasc Dis* 1983;**25**:513.

Gross H, Vaid AR, Cohen MV: Prognosis in patients rejected for coronary revascularization surgery. *Am J Med* 1978;**64**:9.

Hollenberg M, Go M: Clinical studies with transdermal nitroglycerin. *Am Heart J* 1984;**108**:223.

Karsh DL et al: Prolonged benefit of nitroglycerin ointment on exercise tolerance in patients with angina pectoris. *Am Heart J* 1978;**96**:587.

Kuo PT et al: Use of combined diet and colestipol in long-term (7–7½ years) treatment of patients with type II hyperlipoproteinemia. *Circulation* 1979;**59**:199.

Leren P: The effect of plasma cholesterol lowering diet in male survivors of myocardial infarction: A controlled clinical trial. *Acta Med Scand* [Suppl]1966;**446**:1.

Levy RI (editor): Hyperlipoproteinemia: Dietary and Pharmacologic Intervention: Proceedings of a Symposium. *Am J Med* 1983;**74(5A)**:1. [Entire issue.]

Markis JE et al: Sustained effect of orally administered isosorbide dinitrate on exercise performance of patients with angina pectoris. *Am J Cardiol* 1979;**43**:265.

Maseri A, Parodi Q, Fox KM: Rational approach to the medical therapy of angina pectoris: The role of calcium antagonists. *Prog Cardiovasc Dis* 1983;**25**:269.

McAllister RG Jr: Clinical pharmacology of slow channel blocking agents. *Prog Cardiovasc Dis* 1982;**25**:83.

McGregor M: Pathogenesis of angina pectoris and role of nitrates in relief of myocardial infarction. *Am J Med* 1983;**74**:21.

Michaelson SP et al: Recurrent myocardial infarction with normal coronary arteriography. *N Engl J Med* 1977; **297**:916.

Multiple Risk Factor Intervention Trial Research Group: Multiple risk factor intervention trial: Risk factor changes and mortality results. *JAMA* 1982;**248**:1465.

Packer M et al: Hemodynamic consequences of combined beta-adrenergic and slow calcium channel blockade in man. *Circulation* 1982;**65**:660.

Parmley WW: The combination of beta-adrenergic blocking agents and nitrates in the treatment of stable angina pectoris. *Cardiovasc Rev Rep* 1982;**3**:1425.

Peduzzi P, Hultgren HN: Effect of medical vs surgical treatment on symptoms in stable angina pectoris: The Veterans Administration Cooperative Study of Surgery for Coronary Arterial Occlusive Disease. *Circulation* 1979;**60**:888.

Podrid PJ, Graboys TB, Lown B: Prognosis of medically treated patients with coronary artery disease with profound ST segment depression during exercise testing. *N Engl J Med* 1981;**305**:1111.

Reeves TJ: Medical management of the patient with angina pectoris: An overview of the problem. *Circulation* 1982; **65(7–Part 2)**:3.

Robb GP, Seltzer F: Appraisal of the double two-step exercise test: A long-term follow-up study of 3325 men. *JAMA* 1975;**234**:722.

Rosati RA et al: Problems and advantages of an observational data base approach to evaluating the effect of therapy on outcome. *Circulation* 1982;**65(7–Part 2 Suppl)**:27.

Ruberman W et al: Ventricular premature complexes in prognosis of angina. *Circulation* 1980;**61**:1172.

Samuel P: Drug treatment of hyperlipidemia. *Am Heart J* 1980;**100**:573.

Schroeder JS, McAuley B, Ginsburg R: Diltiazem: A clinical and pharmacologic profile. *J Cardiovasc Med* 1983;**8**:41.

Selzer A: Transmural myocardial infarction with normal coronary arteriogram. *J Cardiovasc Med* 1980;**5**:595.

Severi S et al: Long-term prognosis of "variant" angina with medical treatment. *Am J Cardiol* 1980;**46**:226.

Sheldon WC et al: Surgical treatment of coronary artery disease: Pure graft operations, with a study of 741 patients followed 3-7 years. *Prog Cardiovasc Dis* 1975;**18**:237.

Singh BN: The pharmacology of slow-channel blocking drugs. *Cardiovasc Rev Rep* 1983;**4**:179.

Stamler J, Stamler R: Intervention for the prevention and control of hypertension and atherosclerotic diseases: United States and international experience. *Am J Med* 1984;**76**:13.

Thadani U et al: Oral isosorbide dinitrate in the treatment of angina pectoris: Dose-response relationship and duration of action during acute therapy. *Circulation* 1980;**62**:491.

Thompson RH: The clinical use of transdermal delivery devices with nitroglycerin. *Cardiovasc Rev Rep* 1983;**4**:91.

Waters DD et al: Provocative testing with ergonovine to assess the efficacy of treatment with nifedipine, diltiazem and verapamil in variant angina. *Am J Cardiol* 1981;**48**:123.

Winniford MD, Huxley RL, Hillis LD: Randomized, double-blind comparison of propranolol alone and a propranolol-verapamil combination in patients with severe angina of effort. *J Am Coll Cardiol* 1983;**1**:492.

Yasue H et al: Exertional angina pectoris caused by coronary arterial spasm: Effects of various drugs. *Am J Cardiol* 1979;**43**:647.

Zelis R, Flaim SF: Angina pectoris: Advances in medical therapy. *Primary Cardiol* 1983;**9**:107.

Unstable Angina Pectoris

Alison HW et al: Coronary anatomy and arteriography in patients with unstable angina pectoris. *Am J Cardiol* 1978;**41**:204.

Aroesty JM et al: Medically refractory unstable angina pectoris. 2. Hemodynamic and angiographic effects of intraaortic balloon counter pulsation. *Am J Cardiol* 1979;**45**:883.

Brown CA et al: Prospective study of medical and urgent surgical therapy in randomizable patients with unstable angina pectoris: Results of in-hospital and chronic mortality and morbidity. *Am Heart J* 1981;**102(6–Part 1)**:959.

Chierchia S et al: Impairment of myocardial perfusion and function during painless myocardial ischemia. *J Am Coll Cardiol* 1983;**3**:924.

Epstein SE (editor): Calcium-channel blockers: Present status and future directions. (Symposium.) *Am J Cardiol* 1985;**55**:1B. [Entire issue.]

Herling IM: Intravenous nitroglycerin: Clinical pharmacology and therapeutic considerations. *Am Heart J* 1984;**108**:141.

Jaffee AS et al: Abnormal technetium-99m pyrophosphate images in unstable angina: Ischemia versus infarction? *Am J Cardiol* 1979;**44**:1035.

Kaplan K et al: Intravenous nitroglycerin for the treatment of angina at rest unresponsive to standard nitrate therapy. *Am J Cardiol* 1983;**51**:694.

Langou RA et al: Surgical approach for patients with unstable angina pectoris: Role of the response to initial medical therapy and intraaortic balloon pumping in perioperative complications after aortocoronary bypass grafting. *Am J Cardiol* 1978;**42**:629.

Lewis HD Jr et al: Protective effects of aspirin against acute myocardial infarction and death in men with unstable angina: Results of a Veterans Administration Cooperative Study. *N Engl J Med* 1983;**309**:396.

Maseri A, Chierchia S: Coronary artery spasm. *Prog Cardiovasc Dis* 1982;**25**:169.

Maseri A, Parodi O, Fox KM: Rational approach to the medical therapy of angina pectoris: The role of calcium antagonists. *Prog Cardiovasc Dis* 1983;**25**:269.

Moses JW et al: Efficacy of nifedipine in rest angina refractory to propranolol and nitrates in patients with obstructive coronary artery disease. *Ann Intern Med* 1981;**94(4–Part 1)**:425.

Mulcahy R et al: Natural history and prognosis of unstable angina. *Am Heart J* 1985;**109**:753.

National Cooperative Study Group to Compare Surgical and Medical Therapy: Unstable angina pectoris. 2. In-hospital experience and initial follow-up results in patients with one, two and three vessel disease. *Am J Cardiol* 1978;**42**:839.

National Cooperative Study Group to Compare Surgical and Medical Therapy: Unstable angina pectoris. 3. Results in patients with S–T segment elevation during pain. *Am J Cardiol* 1980;**45**:819.

National Cooperative Study Group to Compare Surgical and Medical Therapy: Unstable angina pectoris. 4. Results in patients with left anterior descending coronary artery disease. *Am J Cardiol* 1981;**48**:517.

Plotnick GD et al: Cardiac catheterization in patients with unstable angina: Recent onset vs crescendo pattern. *JAMA* 1980;**244**:574.

Pugh B et al: Unstable angina pectoris: A randomized study of patients treated medically and surgically. *Am J Cardiol* 1978;**41**:1291.

Rafflenbeul W et al: Quantitative coronary arteriography: Coronary anatomy of patients with unstable angina pectoris reexamined 1 year after optimal medical therapy. *Am J Cardiol* 1979;**43**:699.

Rentrop KP et al: Effects of intracoronary streptokinase and intracoronary nitroglycerin infusion on coronary angiographic patterns and mortality in patients with acute myocardial infarction. *N Engl J Med* 1985;**311**:1457.

Roberts R, Sobel BE: Creatine kinase isoenzymes in the assessment of heart disease. *Am Heart J* 1978;**95**:521.

Victor MF et al: Unstable angina pectoris of new onset: A prospective clinical and arteriographic study of 75 patients. *Am J Cardiol* 1981;**47**:228.

Weintraub RM et al: Medically refractory unstable angina pectoris. 1. Long-term follow-up of patients undergoing intraaortic balloon counter-pulsation and operation. *Am J Cardiol* 1979;**45**:877.

Williams DO et al: Evaluation of the role of coronary angioplasty in patients with unstable angina pectoris. *Am Heart J* 1981;**102**:1.

Acute Myocardial Infarction

Alonso DR et al: Pathophysiology of cardiogenic shock: Quantification of myocardial necrosis, clinical, pathologic and electrocardiographic correlations. *Circulation* 1973;**48**:588.

Baigrie RS et al: The spectrum of right ventricular involvement in inferior wall myocardial infarction: A clinical, hemodynamic and noninvasive study. *J Am Coll Cardiol* 1983;**1**:1396.

Beller GA et al: Localization of radiolabeled cardiac myosin-specific antibody in myocardial infarcts: Comparison with technetium-99m stannous pyrophosphate. *Circulation* 1977;**55**:74.

Berger HJ, Gottschalk A, Zaret BL: Dual radionuclide study of acute myocardial infarction: Comparison of thallium-201 and technetium-99m stannous pyrophosphate imaging in man. *Ann Intern Med* 1978;**88**:145.

Bishop SP, White FC, Bloor CM: Regional myocardial blood flow during acute myocardial infarction in the conscious dog. *Circ Res* 1976;**38**:429.

Botvinick EH et al: Late prognostic value of scintigraphic parameters of acute myocardial infarction size in complicated myocardial infarction without heart failure. *Am J Cardiol* 1983;**51**:1045.

Boutefeu J et al: Aneurysms of the sinus of Valsalva: Report of seven cases and review of the literature. *Am J Med* 1978;**65**:18.

Bradbury EM et al: Nuclear magnetic resonance techniques in medicine. *Ann Intern Med* 1983;**98**:514.

Chatterjee K, Swan HJC: Hemodynamic profile of acute myocardial infarction. Chapter 6 in: *Myocardial Infarction.* Corday E, Swan HJC (editors). Williams & Wilkins, 1973.

DeWood MA et al: Prevalence of total coronary occlusion during the early hours of transmural myocardial infarction. *N Engl J Med* 1980;**303**:897.

Eaton LW et al: Regional cardiac dilatation after acute myocardial infarction: Recognition by two-dimensional echocardiography. N Engl J Med 1979;**300**:57.

Forrester JS, Diamond GA, Swan HJC: Correlative classification of clinical and hemodynamic function after acute myocardial infarction. Am J Cardiol 1977;**39**:137.

Gibson RS et al: Prediction of cardiac events after uncomplicated myocardial infarction: A prospective study comparing predischarge exercise thallium-201 scintigraphy and coronary angiography. Circulation 1983;**68**:321.

Gibson RS et al: Value of early two-dimensional echocardiography in patients with acute myocardial infarction. Am J Cardiol 1982;**49**:1110.

Han J: Mechanisms of ventricular arrhythmias associated with myocardial infarction. Am J Cardiol 1969;**24**:800.

Horie T et al: Coronary thrombosis in pathogenesis of acute myocardial infarction: Histopathological study of coronary arteries in 108 necropsied cases using serial section. Br Heart J 1978;**40**:153.

Khaja F et al: Intracoronary fibrinolytic therapy in acute myocardial infarction: Report of a prospective randomized trial. N Engl J Med 1983;**308**:1305.

Khaw BA et al: Specificity of localization of myosin-specific antibody fragments in experimental myocardial infarction. Circulation 1979;**60**:1527.

Klocke FJ: Measurements of coronary blood flow and degree of stenosis: Current clinical implications and continuing uncertainties. J Am Coll Cardiol 1983;**1**:31.

Kramer NE et al: Differentiation of posterior myocardial infarction from right ventricular hypertrophy and normal anterior loop by echocardiography. Circulation 1978;**58**:1057.

Kupper W et al: Left ventricular hemodynamics and function in acute myocardial infarction: Studies during the acute phase, convalescence and late recovery. Am J Cardiol 1977;**40**:900.

Leinbach RC: Right ventricular infarction. J Cardiovasc Med 1980;**5**:499.

Leren P: The effect of plasma cholesterol lowering diet in male survivors of myocardial infarction: A controlled clinical trial. Acta Med Scand [Suppl] 1966;**446**:1.

Liberthson RR et al: Atrial tachyarrhythmias in acute myocardial infarction. Am J Med 1976;**60**:956.

Lie KI et al: Observations on patients with primary ventricular fibrillation complicating acute myocardial infarction. Circulation 1975;**52**:755.

Lorell B et al: Right ventricular infarction: Clinical diagnosis and differentiation from cardiac tamponade and pericardial constriction. Am J Cardiol 1979;**43**:465.

Madias JE, Gorlin R: The myth of acute "mild" myocardial infarction. Ann Intern Med 1977;**86**:347.

Massie BM et al: Myocardial scintigraphy with technetium-99m stannous pyrophosphate: An insensitive test for nontransmural myocardial infarction. Am J Cardiol 1979;**43**:186.

Morris DC, Hurst JW, Logue RB: Myocardial infarction in young women. Am J Cardiol 1976;**38**:299.

Morrison J et al: Correlation of radionuclide estimates of myocardial infarction size and release of creatine kinase-MB in man. Circulation 1980;**62**:277.

Pantridge JF, Webb SW, Adgey AAJ: Arrhythmias in the first hours of acute myocardial infarction. Prog Cardiovasc Dis 1981;**23**:265.

Pape LA et al: Fatal pulmonary hemorrhage after use of the flow-directed balloon-tipped catheter. Ann Intern Med 1979;**90**:344.

Parmley WW: Hemodynamic monitoring in acute ischemic disease. Pages 105–120 in: Heart Failure. Fishman AP (editor). Hemisphere Publishing Corp.,1978.

Pell S, Fayerweather WE: Trends in the incidence of myocardial infarction and in associated mortality and morbidity in a large employed population, 1957–1983. N Engl J Med 1985;**312**:1005.

Reeder GS, Seward JB, Tajik AJ: The role of two-dimensional echocardiography in coronary artery disease. Mayo Clin Proc 1982;**57**:247.

Roberts R, Sobel BE: Creatine kinase isoenzymes in the assessment of heart disease. Am Heart J 1978;**95**:521.

Scheinman MM (editor): Cardiac Emergencies. Saunders, 1984.

Silverman KF et al: Value of early thallium-201 scintigraphy for predicting mortality in patients with acute myocardial infarction. Circulation 1980;**61**:996.

Sobel BE et al: Detection of remote myocardial infarction in patients with positron emission transaxial tomography and intravenous ^{11}C-palmitate. Circulation 1977; **55**:853.

Solomon H, Edwards A, Killip T: Prodromata in acute myocardial infarction. Circulation 1969;**40**:463.

Swan HJC et al: Catheterization of the heart in man with use of a flow-directed balloon-tipped catheter. N Engl J Med 1970;**283**:447.

Swan HJC et al: Hemodynamic spectrum of myocardial infarction and cardiogenic shock: A conceptual model. Circulation 1972;**45**:1097.

Tans AC, Lie KI, Durrer D: Clinical setting and prognostic significance of high degree atrioventricular block in acute inferior myocardial infarction. Am Heart J 1980;**99**:4.

Taylor GJ et al: Predictors of clinical course, coronary anatomy and left ventricular function after recovery from acute myocardial infarction. Circulation 1980;**62**:960.

Wackers FJT et al: Prevalence of right ventricular involvement in inferior wall infarction assessed with myocardial imaging with thallium-201 and technetium-99m pyrophosphate. Am J Cardiol 1978;**42**:358.

Warner RA et al: Electrocardiographic criteria for the diagnosis of combined inferior myocardial infarction and left anterior hemiblock. Am J Cardiol 1983;**51**;718.

Weiss ES et al: Evaluation of myocardial metabolism with perfusion with positron-emitting radionuclides. Prog Cardiovasc Dis 1977;**20**:191.

Willerson JT, Buja LM: Myocardial infarction—1983: State of the art. Clin Res 1983;**31**:364.

Wit AL, Bigger JT Jr: Possible electrophysiological mechanisms for lethal arrhythmias accompanying myocardial ischemia and infarction. Circulation 1975;**52**:96.

Course & Complications in Acute Myocardial Infarction

Asinger RW et al: Incidence of left-ventricular thrombosis after acute transmural myocardial infarction: Serial evaluation by two-dimensional echocardiography. N Engl J Med 1981;**305**:297.

Atkins JM et al: Ventricular conduction blocks and sudden death in acute myocardial infarction. N Engl J Med 1973;**288**:281.

Bates RJ et al: Cardiac rupture: Challenge in diagnosis and management. Am J Cardiol 1977;**40**:429.

Battler A et al: The initial chest x-ray in acute myocardial infarction: Prediction of early and late mortality and survival. Circulation 1980;**61**:1004.

Bedell SE et al: Survival after cardiopulmonary resuscitation in the hospital. *N Engl J Med* 1983;**309:**569.

Campbell RW, Murray A, Julian DG: Ventricular arrhythmias in first 12 hours of acute myocardial infarction: Natural history study. *Br Heart J* 1981;**46:**351.

Cohn LH: Surgical management of acute and chronic cardiac mechanical complications due to myocardial infarction. *Am Heart J* 1981;**102(6–Part 1):**1049.

Corbett JR et al: Left ventricular functional alterations at rest and during submaximal exercise in patients with recent myocardial infarction. *Am J Med* 1983;**74:**577.

DeSanctis RW, Block P, Hutter AM Jr: Tachyarrhythmias in myocardial infarction. *Circulation* 1972;**45:**681.

Dressler W, Leavitt SS: Pericarditis after acute myocardial infarction. *JAMA* 1960;**173:**1225.

Drobac M et al: Ventricular septal defect after myocardial infarction: Diagnosis by the 2-dimensional contrast echocardiography. *Circulation* 1983;**67:**335.

Ehrich DA et al: The hemodynamic response to intraaortic balloon counterpulsation in patients with cardiogenic shock complicating acute myocardial infarction. *Am Heart J* 1977;**93:**274.

Forrester JS, Nierenberg RJ: Cardiac abnormalities in acute myocardial infarction. *Primary Cardiol* (Feb) 1978;**4:**40.

Fraker TD, Wagner GS, Rosati RA: Extension of myocardial infarction: Incidence and prognosis. *Circulation* 1979;**60:**1126.

Gatewood RP Jr, Nanda NC: Differentiation of left ventricular pseudoaneurysm from true aneurysm with two dimensional echocardiography. *Am J Cardiol* 1980;**46:**869.

Grube E, Redel D, Janson R: Non-invasive diagnosis of a false left ventricular aneurysm by echocardiography and pulsed Doppler echocardiography. *Br Heart J* 1980;**43:**232.

Heikkilä J: Mitral incompetence as a complication of acute myocardial infarction. *Acta Med Scand* [*Suppl*] 1967;**475:**1. [Entire issue.]

Herfkens RJ, Brundage BH, Lipton MJ: Cardiovascular applications of computed tomography. *Cardiovasc Rev Rep* 1983;**4:**979.

Higgins CB et al: False aneurysms of the left ventricle: Identification of distinctive clinical, radiographic, and angiographic features. *Radiology* 1978;**127:**21.

Hill JD, Hampton JR, Mitchell JRA: A randomised trial of home-versus-hospital management for patients with suspected myocardial infarction. *Lancet* 1978;**1:**837.

Hossack KF, Bruce RA: Low-level treadmill testing after myocardial infarction: A guide to activity. *Primary Cardiol* (Feb) 1980;**6:**106.

Hutter AM Jr: Early hospital discharge after myocardial infarction. *N Engl J Med* 1973;**288:**1141.

Keating EC et al: Mural thrombi in myocardial infarctions. *Am J Med* 1983;**74:**989.

Kereiakes DJ, Ports TA: Intra-aortic balloon counterpulsation and the diagnosis and management of surgical complications of acute myocardial infarction. Chap 4, pp 75–88, in: *Cardiac Emergencies*. Scheinman MM (editor). Saunders, 1984.

Killip T: Arrhythmias in myocardial infarction. *Med Clin North Am* 1976;**60:**233.

Krauss KR, Hutter AM, DeSanctis RW: Acute coronary insufficiency: Course and follow-up. *Arch Intern Med* 1972;**129:**808.

Krone RJ et al: Low-level exercise testing after myocardial infarction: Usefulness in enhancing clinical risk stratification. *Circulation* 1985;**71:**80.

McNeer JF et al: Hospital discharge one week after acute myocardial infarction. *N Engl J Med* 1978;**298:**229.

Miller DH, Borer JS: Exercise testing early after myocardial infarction: Risks and benefits. *Am J Med* 1982;**72:**427.

Nishimura RA et al: Papillary muscle rupture complicating acute myocardial infarction: Analysis of 17 patients. *Am J Cardiol* 1983;**51:**373.

Ritter WS et al: Permanent pacing in patients with transient trifascicular block during acute myocardial infarction. *Am J Cardiol* 1976;**38:**207.

Ross J Jr: Hemodynamic changes in acute myocardial infarction. *Hosp Pract* (March) 1972;**7:**125.

Rotman M, Wagner GS, Wallace AG: Bradyarrhythmias in acute myocardial infarction. *Circulation* 1972;**45:**703.

Rude RE, Muller JE, Braunwald E: Efforts to limit the size of myocardial infarcts. *Ann Intern Med* 1981;**95:**736.

Scheidt S et al: Mechanical circulatory assistance with the intraaortic balloon pump and other counterpulsation devices. *Prog Cardiovasc Dis* 1982;**25:**55.

Scheinman MM, Gonzales RP: Fascicular block and acute myocardial infarction. *JAMA* 1980;**244:**2646.

Schuster EH, Bulkley BH: Early post-infarction angina: Ischemia at a distance and ischemia in the infarct zone. *N Engl J Med* 1981;**305:**1101.

Sorensen SG et al: Noninvasive detection of ventricular aneurysm by combined two-dimensional echocardiography and equilibrium radionuclide angiography. *Am Heart J* 1982;**104:**145.

Stratton JR et al: Detection of left ventricular thrombus by two-dimensional echocardiography: Sensitivity, specificity, and causes of uncertainty. *Circulation* 1982;**66:**156.

Swan HJC et al: Catheterization of the heart in man with use of a flow-directed balloon-tipped catheter. *N Engl J Med* 1970;**283:**447.

Taylor GJ et al: Predictors of clinical course, coronary anatomy and left ventricular function after recovery from acute myocardial infarction. *Circulation* 1980;**62:**960.

Taylor SH et al: A long-term prevention study with oxprenolol in coronary heart disease. *N Engl J Med* 1982;**307:**1293.

Weber KT et al: Identification of high risk subsets of acute myocardial infarction: Derived from the Myocardial Infarction Research Units Cooperative Study Data Bank. *Am J Cardiol* 1978;**41:**197.

Welin L, Vedin A, Wilhelmsson C: Characteristics, prevalence, and prognosis of postmyocardial infarction syndrome. *Br Heart J* 1983;**50:**140.

Prevention, Treatment, & Prognosis in Acute Myocardial Infarction; Thrombolysis

Aspirin Myocardial Infarction Study Research Group: A randomized, controlled trial of aspirin in persons recovered from myocardial infarction. *JAMA* 1980;**243:**661.

Braunwald E (chairman): The thrombolysis in myocardial infarction (TIMI) trial: Phase I findings. (Special report.) *N Engl J Med* 1985;**312:**932.

Bussmann WD et al: Reduction of CK and CK-MB indexes of infarct size by intravenous nitroglycerin. *Circulation* 1981;**63:**615.

Chatterjee K, Ports TA, Parmley WW: Nitroprusside: Its clinical pharmacology and application in acute heart failure. Pages 25–62 in: *Vasodilator Therapy for Cardiac Disorders*. Gould L, Reddy CV (editors). Futura, 1979.

Chatterjee K, Swan HJC: Hemodynamic profile of acute myocardial infarction. Chapter 6 in: *Myocardial Infarction*. Corday E, Swan HJC (editors). Williams & Wilkins, 1973.

Cohn JN et al: Effect of short-term infusion of sodium nitroprusside on mortality rate in acute myocardial infarction complicated by left ventricular failure: Results of a Veterans Administration Cooperative Study. *N Engl J Med* 1982;**306**:1129.

Curtis JJ et al: Intra-aortic balloon assist: Initial Mayo Clinic experience and current concepts. *Mayo Clin Proc* 1977; **52**:723.

DeBusk RF et al: Serial ambulatory electrocardiography and treadmill exercise testing after uncomplicated myocardial infarction. *Am J Cardiol* 1980;**45**:547.

DeWood MA et al: Prevalence of total coronary occlusion during the early hours of transmural myocardial infarction. *N Engl J Med* 1980;**303**:897.

Frishman WH, Furberg CD, Friedwald WT: Beta-adrenergic blockade for survivors of acute myocardial infarction. *N Engl J Med* 1984;**310**:830.

Furberg CD, Friedewald WT, Eberlein KA (editors): Proceedings of the workshop on implications of recent beta-blocker trials for post-myocardial infarction patients. *Circulation* 1983;**67**(6–Part 2):1. [Entire issue.]

Ganz Q: Intracoronary thrombolysis in acute myocardial infarction. *J Cardiovasc Med* 1982;**7**:169.

Ganz W et al: Intravenous streptokinase in evolving acute myocardial infarction. *Am J Cardiol* 1984;**53**:1209.

Gross H, Vaid AR, Cohen MV: Prognosis in patients rejected for coronary revascularization surgery. *Am J Med* 1978;**64**:9.

Health and Public Policy Committee, American College of Physicians: Thrombolysis for evolving myocardial infarction. *Ann Intern Med* 1985;**103**:463.

Hutter AM et al: Nontransmural myocardial infarction: Hospital and late clinical course of patients with that of matched patients with transmural anterior and transmural inferior myocardial infarction. *Am J Cardiol* 1981;**48**:595.

Hypertension Detection and Follow-Up Program Cooperative Group: Five-year findings of the Hypertension Detection and Follow-Up Program. 1. Reduction in mortality of persons with high blood pressure, including mild hypertension. 2. Mortality by race, sex and age. (2 parts.) *JAMA* 1979;**242**:2562, 2572.

Johnson SA et al: Treatment of cardiogenic shock in myocardial infarction by intraaortic balloon counterpulsation and surgery. *Am J Med* 1977;**62**:687.

Kennedy JW et al: The Western Washington randomized trial of intracoronary streptokinase in acute myocardial infarction: A 12-month follow-up report. *N Engl J Med* 1985;**312**:1073.

Laffel GL, Braunwald E: Thrombolytic therapy: A new strategy for the treatment of acute myocardial infarction. (Parts 1 and 2.) *N Engl J Med* 1984;**311**:710, 770.

Marmor A, Sobel BE, Roberts R: Factors presaging early recurrent myocardial infarction ("extension"). *Am J Cardiol* 1981;**48**:603.

Mason DT (editor): Papers from special symposium updating the current state of the art on streptokinase thrombolysis in acute myocardial infarction held in Atlanta, April 29, 1982. *Am Heart J* 1982;**104**:891. [Entire issue.]

Massie BM, Chatterjee K: Medical therapy for pump failure complicating acute myocardial infarction. Chap 2, pp 29–58, in: *Cardiac Emergencies*. Scheinmann MM (editor). Saunders, 1984.

Meizlish JL et al: Functional left ventricular aneurysm formation after acute anterior transmural myocardial infarction. *N Engl J Med* 1984;**311**:1001.

Moss AJ: The Multicenter Postinfarction Research Group: Risk stratification and survival after myocardial infarction. *N Engl J Med* 1983;**309**:331.

Namay DL et al: Effect of perioperative myocardial infarction on late survival in patients undergoing coronary artery bypass surgery. *Circulation* 1982;**65**:1066.

Raizner AE et al: Intracoronary thrombolytic therapy in acute myocardial infarction: A prospective, randomized, controlled atrial. *Am J Cardiol* 1985;**55**:301.

Ritter WS et al: Permanent pacing in patients with transient trifascicular block during acute myocardial infarction. *Am J Cardiol* 1976;**38**:207.

Roberts R et al: Effect of propranolol on myocardial-infarct size in a randomized blinded multicenter trial. *N Engl J Med* 1984;**311**:218.

Roberts WC (editor-in-chief): Symposium: Göteborg metoprolol trial in acute myocardial infarction. *Am J Cardiol* 1984;**53**:1D. [Entire issue.]

Sammel NL, O'Rourke MF: Arterial counterpulsation in continuing myocardial ischaemia after acute myocardial infarction. *Br Heart J* 1979;**42**:579.

Scheidt S et al: Mechanical circulatory assistance with the intraaortic balloon pump and other counterpulsation devices. *Prog Cardiovasc Dis* 1982;**25**:55.

Schlant RC et al: The natural history of coronary heart disease: Prognostic factors after recovery from myocardial infarction in 2789 men: The 5-year findings of the coronary drug project. *Circulation* 1982;**66**:401.

Schröder R: Intravenous short-term infusion of streptokinase in acute myocardial infarction. *Texas Heart Inst J* 1984;**11**:18.

Sivarajan ES et al: Treadmill test responses to an early exercise program after myocardial infarction: A randomized study. *Circulation* 1982;**65**:1420.

Smalling RW et al: Sustained improvement in left ventricular function and mortality by intracoronary streptokinase administration during evolving myocardial infarction. *Circulation* 1983;**68**:131.

Spann JF: Changing concepts of pathophysiology, prognosis, and therapy in acute myocardial infarction. *Am J Med* 1983;**74**:877.

Stampfer MJ et al: Effect of intravenous streptokinase on acute myocardial infarction. *N Engl J Med* 1982;**307**:1180.

Starling MR et al: Treadmill exercise tests predischarge and six weeks post-myocardial infarction to detect abnormalities of known prognostic value. *Ann Intern Med* 1981; **94**:721.

Tans AC, Lie KI, Durrer D: Clinical setting and prognostic significance of high degree atrioventricular block in acute inferior myocardial infarction. *Am Heart J* 1980;**99**:4.

Topol EJ et al: Hemodynamic benefit of atrial pacing in right ventricular myocardial infarction. *Ann Intern Med* 1982;**96**:594.

Vermeulen A, Lie KI, Durrer D: Effects of cardiac rehabilitation after myocardial infarction: Changes in coronary risk factors and long-term prognosis. *Am Heart J* 1983;**105**:798.

Verstraete M et al: Randomized trial of intravenous recombinant tissue-type plasminogen activator versus intravenous streptokinase in acute myocardial infarction. *Lancet* 1985;**1**:842.

Welin L, Vedin A, Wilhelmsson C: Characteristics, prevalence, and prognosis of postmyocardial infarction syndrome. *Br Heart J* 1983;**50**:140.

Wohl AJ et al: Cardiovascular function during early recovery from acute myocardial infarction. *Circulation* 1977;**56**:931.

Yusuf S, Lopez R, Sleight P: Heart rate and ectopic prematurity in relation to sustained ventricular arrhythmias. *Br Heart J* 1980;**44**:233.

Yusuf S et al: Beta blockade during and after myocardial

infarction: An overview of the randomized trials. *Prog Cardiovasc Dis* 1985;**27**:335.

Chronic (Established) Coronary Heart Disease

Åberg A et al: Declining trend in mortality after myocardial infarction. *Br Heart J* 1984;**51**:346.

AHA Committee Report: Statement on exercise. *Circulation* 1981;**64**:1327A.

Anturane Reinfarction Italian Study: Sulphinpyrazone in post-myocardial infarction. *Lancet* 1982;**1**:237.

Anturane Reinfarction Trial Research Group: Sulfinpyrazone in the prevention of sudden death after myocardial infarction. *N Engl J Med* 1980;**302**:250.

Aspirin Myocardial Infarction Study Research Group: A randomized, controlled trial of aspirin in persons recovered from myocardial infarction. *JAMA* 1980;**243**:661.

Berge KG, Canner PL, Hainline A: High-density lipoprotein cholesterol and prognosis after myocardial infarction. *Circulation* 1982;**66**:1176.

Berglund G et al: Coronary heart-disease after treatment of hypertension. *Lancet* 1978;**1**:1.

Beta-Blocker Heart Attack Study Group: The β-blocker heart attack trial. *JAMA* 1981;**246**:2073.

Bigger JT Jr et al: The relationships among ventricular arrhythmias, left ventricular dysfunction, and mortality in the 2 years after myocardial infarction. *Circulation* 1984;**69**:250.

Bonow RO et al: Exercise-induced ischemia in mildly symptomatic patients with coronary-artery disease and preserved left ventricular function. *N Engl J Med* 1984;**311**:1339.

Braunwald E: Treatment of the patient after myocardial infarction: The last decade and the next. (Editorial.) *N Engl J Med* 1980;**302**:290.

Brown MS, Goldstein JL: Lowering plasma cholesterol by raising LDL receptors. (Editorial.) *N Engl J Med* 1981;**305**:515.

Califf RM et al: Outcome in one-vessel coronary artery disease. *Circulation* 1983;**67**:283.

Case RB et al: Type A behavior and survival after acute myocardial infarction. *N Engl J Med* 1985;**312**:737.

Chatterjee K, Rouleau JL: Hemodynamic and metabolic effects of vasodilators, nitrates, hydralazine, prazosin, and captopril in chronic ischemic heart failure. *Acta Med Scand [Suppl]* 1981;**651**:295.

Council on Scientific Affairs: Physician-supervised exercise programs in rehabilitation of patients with coronary heart disease. *JAMA* 1981;**245**:1463.

Coronary Drug Project Research Group: Clofibrate and niacin in coronary heart disease. *JAMA* 1975;**231**:360.

DeBusk RF, Harrison DC: The clinical spectrum of papillary muscle disease. *N Engl J Med* 1969;**281**:1458.

Dunn RF et al: Comparison of thallium-201 scanning in idiopathic dilated cardiomyopathy and severe coronary artery disease. *Circulation* 1982;**66**:804.

Dwyer EM et al: Nonfatal cardiac events and recurrent infarction in the year after acute myocardial infarction. *J Am Coll Cardiol* 1984;**4**:695.

Dymond DS et al: Assessment of function of contractile segments in patients with left ventricular aneurysms by quantitative first pass radionuclide ventriculography. *Br Heart J* 1980;**43**:125.

Epstein SE, Palmeri ST, Patterson RE: Evaluation of patients after acute myocardial infarction: Indications for cardiac catheterization and surgical intervention. *N Engl J Med* 1982;**307**:1487.

Furberg CD, Friedwald WT, Eberlein KA (editors): Proceedings of the workshop on implications of recent beta-blocker trials for post-myocardial infarction patients. *Circulation* 1983;**67**:I-1. [Entire issue.]

Fuster V, Chesebro JH: Series on pharmacology in practice. X. Antithrombotic therapy: Role of platelet-inhibitor drugs. 2. Pharmacologic effects of platelet-inhibitor drugs. (Part 2 of 3 parts.) *Mayo Clin Proc* 1981;**56**:185.

Gibson RS et al: Prediction of cardiac events after uncomplicated myocardial infarction: A prospective study comparing predischarge exercise thallium-201 scintigraphy and coronary angiography. *Circulation* 1983;**68**:321.

Graham I et al: Natural history of coronary heart disease: A study of 586 men surviving an initial acute attack. *Am Heart J* 1983;**105**:249.

Grundy SM (chairman): NIH Consensus Development Conference Summary: Treatment of hypertriglyceridemia. *Arteriosclerosis* 1984;**4**:296.

Hammermeister KE, DeRouen TA, Dodge HT: Variables predictive of survival in patients with coronary disease: Selection by univariate and multivariate analyses from the clinical, electrocardiographic, exercise, arteriographic, and quantitative angiographic evaluations. *Circulation* 1979;**59**:421.

Havel RJ, Kane JP: Therapy of hyperlipidemic states. *Annu Rev Med* 1982;**33**:417.

Hjermann I et al: Effect of diet and smoking intervention on the incidence of coronary heart disease: Report from the Oslo Study Group of a randomized trial in healthy men. *Lancet* 1981;**2**:1303.

Hung J, Chaitman BR: Post-myocardial infarction stress tests: When? What do they show? *J Cardiovasc Med* 1984;**9**:417.

Hutter AM Jr et al: Nontransmural myocardial infarction: A comparison of hospital and late clinical course of patients with that of matched patients with transmural anterior and transmural inferior myocardial infarction. *Am J Cardiol* 1981;**48**:595.

Jamieson WR et al: Influence of ischemic heart disease on early and late mortality after surgery for peripheral occlusive vascular disease. *Circulation* 1982;**66(2–Part 2)**:I-92.

Jelinek MV, Lohrbauer L, Lown B: Antiarrhythmic drug therapy for sporadic ventricular ectopic arrhythmias. *Circulation* 1974;**49**:659.

Kallio V et al: Reduction in sudden deaths by a multifactorial intervention programme after acute myocardial infarction. *Lancet* 1979;**2**:1091.

Kannel WB, Sorlie P, McNamara PM: Prognosis after initial myocardial infarction: The Framingham Study. *Am J Cardiol* 1979;**44**:53.

Klocke FJ: Measurements of coronary blood flow and degree of stenosis: Current clinical implications and continuing uncertainties. *J Am Coll Cardiol* 1983;**1**:31.

Leren P: The effect of plasma cholesterol lowering diet in male survivors of myocardial infarction: A controlled clinical trial. *Acta Med Scand [Suppl]* 1966;**446**:1.

Lim JS, Proudfit WL, Sones FM: Left main coronary arterial obstruction: Long-term follow-up of 141 nonsurgical cases. *Am J Cardiol* 1975;**36**:131.

McLane M, Krop H, Mehta J: Psychosexual adjustment and counseling after myocardial infarction. *Ann Intern Med* 1980;**92**:514.

Marriott HJL: Transtelephonic ECG monitoring for the heart at risk. *Primary Cardiol* 1984;**10**:28.

Massie BM et al: Relationship of regional myocardial perfusion to segmental wall motion: A physiologic basis for understanding the presence and reversibility of asynergy. *Circulation* 1978;**58**:1154.

May GS et al: Secondary prevention after myocardial infarction: A review of short-term acute phase trials. *Prog Cardiovasc Dis* 1983;**25**:335.

Mock MB et al: Survival of medically treated patients in the coronary artery surgery study (CASS) registry. *Circulation* 1982;**66**:562.

Moss AJ: The Multicenter Postinfarction Research Group: Risk stratification and survival after myocardial infarction. *N Engl J Med* 1983;**309**:331.

Multiple Risk Factor Intervention Trial Research Group: Multiple risk factor intervention trial: Risk factor changes and mortality results. *JAMA* 1982;**248**:1465.

Mustard JF, Kinlough-Rathbone RL, Packham MA: Aspirin in the treatment of cardiovascular disease: A review. *Am J Med* 1983;**74**:43.

Myerburg RJ et al: Antiarrhythmic drug therapy in survivors of prehospital cardiac arrest: Comparison of effects on chronic ventricular arrhythmias and recurrent cardiac arrest. *Circulation* 1979;**59**:855.

Nitter-Hauge S et al: Studies of correlation between progression of coronary artery disease, as assessed by coronary arteriography, left ventricular end-diastolic pressure, ejection fraction, and employability. *Br Heart J* 1977;**39**:884.

Norwegian Multicenter Study Group: Timolol-induced reduction in mortality and reinfarction in patients surviving acute myocardial infarction. *N Engl J Med* 1981;**304**:801.

Oliver MF et al: Report of the Committee of Principal Investigators: WHO Cooperative Trial on primary prevention of ischaemic heart disease with clofibrate to lower serum cholesterol: Final mortality follow-up. *Lancet* 1984;**2**:600.

Pantely GA, Bristow JD: Ischemic cardiomyopathy. *Prog Cardiovasc Dis* 1984;**27**:95.

Pell S, D'Alonzo CA: Immediate mortality and 5-year survival of employed men with first myocardial infarction. *N Engl J Med* 1964;**270**:915.

Persantine-Aspirin Reinfarction Study Research Group: Persantine and aspirin in coronary heart disease. *Circulation* 1980;**62**:449.

Proceedings of the workshop on platelet-activity drugs in the secondary prevention of cardiovascular events. *Circulation* 1980;**62(6–Part 2)**:1. [Entire issue.]

Proudfit WL et al: Fifteen-year survival study of patients with coronary artery disease. *Circulation* 1983;**68**:986.

Pryor DB et al: An improving prognosis over time in medically treated patients with coronary artery disease. *Am J Cardiol* 1983;**52**:444.

Rechnitzer PA et al: Relation of exercise to the recurrence rate of myocardial infarction in men: Ontario Exercise Heart Collaborative Study. *Am J Cardiol* 1983;**51**:65.

Rosman HS, Goldstein S: Preventing mortality and morbidity after myocardial infarction. *J Cardiovasc Med* 1982;**7**:961.

Ruberman W et al: Ventricular premature beats and mortality after myocardial infarction. *N Engl J Med* 1977;**297**:750.

Ruberman W et al: Ventricular premature complexes in prognosis of angina. *Circulation* 1980;**61**:1172.

Ryan M, Lown B, Horn H: Comparison of ventricular ectopic activity during 24-hour monitoring and exercise testing in patients with coronary heart disease. *N Engl J Med* 1975;**292**:224.

Sami M et al: The prognostic significance of serial exercise testing after myocardial infarction. *Circulation* 1979; **60**:1238.

Sanz G et al: Determinants of prognosis in survivors of myocardial infarction: A prospective clinical angiographic study. *N Engl J Med* 1982;**306**:1065.

Schuster EH, Bulkley BH: Ischemic cardiomyopathy. *Am Heart J* 1980;**100**:506.

Shaw LW: Effects of a prescribed supervised exercise program on mortality and cardiovascular morbidity in patients after a myocardial infarction: The National Exercise and Heart Disease Project. *Am J Cardiol* 1981;**48**:39.

Sobel BE et al: Detection of remote myocardial infarction in patients with positron emission transaxial tomography and intravenous ^{11}C-palmitate. *Circulation* 1977;**55**:853.

Taylor GJ et al: Predictors of clinical course, coronary anatomy and left ventricular function after recovery from acute myocardial infarction. *Circulation* 1980;**62**:960.

Turi ZG, Braunwald E: The use of beta-blockers after myocardial infarction. *JAMA* 1983;**249**:2512.

Vedin JA, Wilhelmsson C, Werkö L: Chronic alprenolol treatment of patients with acute myocardial infarction after discharge from hospital: Effects on mortality and morbidity. *Acta Med Scand [Suppl]* 1975;**575**:1. [Entire issue.]

Veterans Administration Cooperative Study Group on Antihypertensive Agents: Effects of treatment on morbidity in hypertension. 2. Results in patients with diastolic blood pressure averaging 90 through 114 mm Hg. *JAMA* 1970; **213**:1143.

Visser CA et al: Echocardiographic-cineangiographic correlation in detecting left ventricular aneurysm: A prospective study of 422 patients. *Am J Cardiol* 1982;**50**:337.

Wenger NK: Early ambulation after acute myocardial infarction. *Primary Cardiol* (Sept) 1979;**5**:45.

Wenger NK (editor): *Exercise and the Heart*, 2nd ed. Davis, 1985.

Wenger NK: Rehabilitation of the coronary patient: Scope of the problem and responsibility of the primary care physician. *Cardiovasc Rev Rep* 1981;**2**:1249.

Wilhelmsen L, Vedin A, Wilhelmsson C: Beta blockade and sudden death following myocardial infarction. *Cardiovasc Med* 1978;**3**:557.

Coronary Heart Surgery

Barratt-Boyes BG et al: The results of surgical treatment of left ventricular aneurysms: An assessment of the risk factors affecting early and late mortality. *J Thorac Cardiovasc Surg* 1984;**87**:87.

Borer JS et al: Detection of left ventricular aneurysm and evaluation of effects of surgical repair: The role of radionuclide cineangiography. *Am J Cardiol* 1980;**45**:1103.

Braunwald E: Effects of coronary-artery bypass grafting on survival: Implications of the randomized coronary-artery surgery study. (Editorial.) *N Engl J Med* 1983;**309**:1181.

Braunwald E (chairman): The thrombolysis in myocardial infarction (TIMI) trial: Phase I findings. (Special report.) *N Engl J Med* 1985;**312**:932.

Brooks N et al: Reoperation for recurrent angina. *Br Heart J* 1979;**42**:333.

Brundage BH: Computed tomography: A new view of cardiovascular disease. *Primary Cardiol* 1983;**9**:57.

Campeau L et al: Loss of the improvement of angina between 1 and 7 years after aortocoronary bypass surgery: Correlations with changes in vein grafts and in coronary arteries. *Circulation* 1979;**60(2–Part 2)**:I-1.

CASS principal investigators and their associates: Coronary Artery Surgery Study (CASS): A randomized trial of coronary artery bypass surgery: Survival data. *Circulation* 1983;**68**:939.

Chaitman BR et al: Angiographic prevalence of high-risk coronary artery disease in patient subsets (CASS). *Circulation* 1981;**64**:360.

Chaitman BR et al: Effect of coronary bypass surgery on survival patterns in subsets of patients with left main coronary artery disease: Report of the Collaborative Study in Coronary Artery Surgery. *Am J Cardiol* 1981;**48**:765.

Cohen M, Packer M, Gorlin R: Indications for left ventricular aneurysmectomy. *Circulation* 1983;**67**:717.

Cosgrove DM, Loop FD, Sheldon WC: Results of myocardial revascularization: A 12-year experience. *Circulation* 1932;**65**(7–Part 2 Suppl):37.

Council on Scientific Affairs: Indications for aortocoronary bypass graft surgery, 1979. *JAMA* 1979;**242**:2709.

Cowley MJ, Vetrovec GW, Wolfgang TC: Efficacy of percutaneous transluminal coronary angioplasty: Technique, patient selection, salutary results, limitations and complications. *Am Heart J* 1981;**101**:272.

Detre K: Effect of bypass surgery on survival in patients in low-risk and high-risk subgroups delineated by the use of simple clinical variables. *Circulation* 1981;**63**:1329.

Dorros G et al: Percutaneous transluminal coronary angioplasty: Report of complications from the National Heart, Lung, and Blood Institute PTCA registry. *Circulation* 1983;**67**:723.

Douglas JS Jr et al: Percutaneous transluminal coronary angioplasty in patients with prior coronary bypass surgery. *J Am Coll Cardiol* 1983;**2**:745.

Epstein SE et al: Strategy for evaluation and surgical treatment of the asymptomatic or mildly symptomatic patient with coronary artery disease. *Am J Cardiol* 1979;**43**:1015.

European Coronary Surgery Study Group: Prospective randomised study of coronary artery bypass surgery in stable angina pectoris: Second interim report by the European Coronary Surgery Study Group. *Lancet* 1980;**2**:491.

Favaloro RG et al: Direct myocardial revascularization by saphenous vein graft. *Ann Thorac Surg* 1970;**10**:97.

Faxon DP et al: Determinants of successful percutaneous transluminal coronary angioplasty: Report from the National Heart, Lung and Blood Institute Registry. *Am Heart J* 1984;**108**:1019.

Fox AC, Glassman E, Isom OW: Surgically remediable complications of myocardial infarction. *Prog Cardiovasc Dis* 1979;**11**:461.

Gersh BJ et al: Coronary arteriography and coronary artery bypass surgery: Morbidity and mortality in patients ages 65 years or older: A report from the Coronary Artery Surgery Study. *Circulation* 1983;**67**:483.

Gibson RS et al: Prospective assessment of regional myocardial perfusion before and after coronary revascularization surgery by quantitative thallium-201 scintigraphy. *J Am Coll Cardiol* 1983;**3**:804.

Gross H, Vaid AR, Cohen MV: Prognosis in patients rejected for coronary revascularization surgery. *Am J Med* 1978;**64**:9.

Grüntzig A: Results from coronary angioplasty and implications for the future. *Am Heart J* 1982;**103**:779.

Grüntzig AR, Senning A, Siegenthaler WE: Nonoperative dilatation of coronary-artery stenosis: Percutaneous transluminal coronary angioplasty. *N Engl J Med* 1979;**301**:61.

Hall RJ et al: Coronary artery bypass: Long-term follow-up of 22,284 consecutive patients. *Circulation* 1983;**68**(3–Part 2):20.

Hamby RI et al: Recurrent angina after bypass surgery: Evaluation by early and late arteriography. *Am Heart J* 1980;**99**:607.

Hultgren HN et al: Unstable angina: Comparison of medical and surgical management. *Am J Cardiol* 1977;**39**:734.

Kent KM et al: Effects of coronary-artery bypass on global and regional left ventricular function during exercise. *N Engl J Med* 1978;**298**:1434.

Kent KM et al: Improved myocardial function during exercise after successful percutaneous transluminal coronary angioplasty. *N Engl J Med* 1982;**306**:441.

Kirklin JW, Blackstone EH, Rogers WJ: The plights of the invasive treatment of ischemic heart disease. *J Am Coll Cardiol* 1985;**5**:158.

Laird-Meeter K et al: Reoperation after aortocoronary bypass procedure: Results in 53 patients in a group of 1041 with consecutive first operations. *Br Heart J* 1983;**50**:157.

Lawrie GM et al: Clinical results of coronary bypass in 500 patients at least 10 years after operation. *Circulation* 1982;**66**(2–Part 2):I-1.

Lytle BW et al: Replacement of aortic valve combined with myocardial revascularization: Determinants of early and late risk for 500 patients, 1967–1981. *Circulation* 1983;**68**:1149.

McIntosh HD, Garcia JA: The first decade of aortocoronary bypass grafting, 1967–1977: A review. *Circulation* 1978;**57**:405.

McKay CR et al: Evaluation of early postoperative coronary artery bypass graft patency by contrast-enhanced computed tomography. *J Am Coll Cardiol* 1983;**2**:312.

Murphy ML et al: Treatment of chronic stable angina. *N Engl J Med* 1977;**297**:621.

Murray GC, Beller GA: Cardiac rehabilitation following coronary artery bypass surgery. *Am Heart J* 1983;**105**:1009.

National Heart, Lung, and Blood Institute: Proceedings of the National Heart, Lung, and Blood Institute Workshop on the outcome of percutaneous transluminal coronary angioplasty. *Am J Cardiol* 1984;**53**:1C. [Entire issue.]

NIH Reports: Consensus statement on scientific and clinical aspects of coronary artery bypass surgery. *J Cardiovasc Med* 1981;**6**:331.

Norris RM et al: Coronary surgery after recurrent myocardial infarction: Progress of a trial comparing surgical with nonsurgical management for asymptomatic patients with advanced coronary disease. *Circulation* 1981;**63**:785.

Ott DA et al: Improved cardiac function following left ventricular aneurysm resection. *Tex Heart Inst J* 1982;**9**:267.

Passamani E et al: A randomized trial of coronary artery bypass surgery: Survival of patients with a low ejection fraction. *N Engl J Med* 1985;**312**:1665.

Pigott JD et al: Late results of surgical and medical therapy for patients with coronary artery disease and depressed left ventricular function. *J Am Coll Cardiol* 1985;**5**:1036.

Rahimtoola SH et al: Ten-year survival after coronary bypass surgery for unstable angina. *N Engl J Med* 1983;**308**:676.

Rosati RA et al: Problems and advantages of an observational data base approach to evaluating the effect of therapy on outcome. *Circulation* 1982;**65**(7–Part 2 Suppl):27.

Sanders CA et al: Mechanical circulatory assistance: Current status and experience with combining circulatory assistance, emergency coronary angiography, and acute myocardial revascularization. *Circulation* 1972;**43**:1292.

Schaff HV et al: Survival and functional status after coronary artery bypass grafting: Results 10 to 12 years after surgery in 500 patients. *Circulation* 1983;**68**(3–Part 2):200.

Schroeder JS et al: Coronary bypass surgery for unstable angina pectoris: Long-term survival and function. *JAMA* 1977;**237**:2609.

Selzer A: Preventive intervention in coronary artery disease. *Primary Cardiol* 1983;**9**:14.

Selzer A, Gerbode F, Kerth WJ: Clinical, hemodynamic and surgical considerations of rupture of the ventricular septum after myocardial infarction. *Am Heart J* 1969;**78**:598.

Varnavskas E: Prospective randomized study of coronary artery bypass surgery in stable angina pectoris: A progress report on survival. *Circulation* 1982;**65**(7–Part 2):67.

Veterans Administration Cooperative Group for the Study of Surgery for Coronary Arterial Occlusive Disease: Veterans Administration Cooperative Study of Surgery for Coronary Arterial Occlusive Disease. 3. Methods and baseline characteristics, including experience with medical treatment. *Am J Cardiol* 1977;**40**:212.

Veterans Administration Coronary Artery Bypass Surgery Cooperative Study Group: Eleven year survival in the Veterans Administration randomized trial of coronary bypass surgery for stable angina. *N Engl J Med* 1984;**311**:1333.

Waldo AL et al: Diagnosis and treatment of arrhythmias during and following open heart surgery. *Med Clin North Am* 1984;**68**:1153.

Whalen RE et al: Survival of coronary artery disease patients with stable pain and normal left ventricular function treated medically or surgically at Duke University. *Circulation* 1982;**65**(7–Part 2 Suppl):49.

Winkle RA et al: Results of reoperation for unsuccessful coronary artery bypass surgery. *Circulation* 1975;**52**(**Suppl I**):I-61.

Zimmern SH et al: Total occlusion of the left main coronary artery: The Coronary Artery Surgery Study (CASS) experience. *Am J Cardiol* 1982;**49**:2003.

Systemic Hypertension 9

Definition

Essential or primary hypertension is sustained elevated arterial pressure of unknown cause—as contrasted with secondary hypertension, where the cause is known (see p 237). Most authorities consider hypertension to be present when the diastolic pressure consistently exceeds 100 mm Hg in a person over age 60 or consistently exceeds 90 mm Hg in a person under age 50. WHO criteria place the upper limits of normal at 160/95 mm Hg. The criteria for the diagnosis of hypertension are arbitrary, because the arterial pressure rises with age and varies from one occasion of measurement to another. The vascular complications of hypertension are thought to be due to the raised arterial pressure and associated atherosclerosis of major arterial circuits.

Hypertension is uncommon before age 20, although recent data suggest a higher frequency if one uses different criteria for children, such as pressure exceeding the 90th percentile for age. In young people, it is commonly caused by chronic glomerulonephritis, renal artery stenosis, pyelonephritis, or coarctation of the aorta.

Hypertension that has not demonstrably affected the heart is called hypertensive vascular disease. When left ventricular hypertrophy, heart failure, or coronary artery disease is present, "hypertensive cardiovascular disease" is the appropriate term.

Transient elevation of blood pressure caused by excitement, apprehension, or exertion and the purely systolic elevation of blood pressure in elderly people caused by loss of elasticity in their major arteries do not constitute hypertensive disease if the mean blood pressure is less than 107 mm Hg. The mean pressure as defined here is an approximation computed as follows:

Diastolic blood pressure + 1/3 pulse pressure = Mean pressure

However, systolic elevation is a significant disease reflecting atherosclerosis of the aorta, and the prognosis is therefore correspondingly less good. Treatment with antihypertensive agents has not been established as effective in decreasing the mortality rate in this group, and drugs must be used cautiously and in small doses to prevent hypotension and decreased cardiac output.

Hypertension is an important preventable cause of cardiovascular disease; prospective studies have shown that without treatment, hypertension greatly increases the incidence of cardiac failure, coronary heart disease with angina pectoris and myocardial infarction, hemorrhagic and thrombotic stroke, and renal failure. Epidemiologic studies have shown that only a small percentage of the population is receiving effective antihypertensive therapy; education of the physician and the patient is necessary to identify the patient with hypertension, to ensure adequate treatment, and to reinforce the concept that treatment is a lifelong process and that compliance with the treatment program is essential to an effective result. The prevention—as well as the reversibility—of hypertensive complications by antihypertensive therapy is a major public health concern.

Antihypertensive Drugs

The introduction of ganglionic blocking agents such as hexamethonium for the treatment of severe hypertension in 1950 was the beginning of a new era in the management of hypertension and showed for the first time that blood pressure could be lowered safely, that the elevated pressure was not essential for adequate perfusion of vital organs (as had been supposed), and that the dire consequences of the hypertension, such as the malignant phase, could be reversed or prevented. Rapid advances in the development and availability of various therapeutic agents have occurred in the last 30 years, and we now have many hypertensive drugs that act in various ways to control raised arterial pressure.

Etiology & Classification

A. Primary (Essential) Hypertension: Hypertension of undetermined cause.

B. Secondary Hypertension: Hypertension due to—

1. Renal disease—

a. Renal arterial disease (renal artery stenosis due to atherosclerosis or fibromuscular hyperplasia), aneurysm, embolism, and infarction.

b. Renal parenchymal disease (acute or chronic glomerulonephritis, pyelonephritis, polycystic kidney, tuberculosis of the kidney, pericapsular hemorrhage, and subsequent scarring from trauma).

c. Renal tumors (Wilms's tumor, renin-producing tumors).

d. Arteritis (polyarteritis nodosa, neurofibromatosis, and nonspecific).

2. Endocrine disorders—

a. Cushing's syndrome.

b. Acromegaly.

c. Primary aldosteronism.

d. Pheochromocytoma.

e. Desoxycorticosterone acetate and salt administration.

3. Coarctation of the aorta.

4. Enzymatic defects—

a. Enzymatic defect of 17β-hydroxylation, leading to amenorrhea due to overproduction of cortisol precursors.

b. Enzymatic defects of 11β-hydroxylation and 21-hydroxylation, with resulting infant virilism.

5. Neurologic disorders–Increased intracranial pressure from brain tumors or cardiovascular accident.

6. Drug-induced hypertension–

a. Prolonged administration of corticosteroids.

b. Excessive use of desoxycorticosterone and salts of 5α-fluoro compounds in the treatment of postural hypotension.

c. The use of amphetamines or excessive thyroxine.

d. Chronic licorice ingestion, producing pseudoaldosteronism.

e. Use of oral contraceptive agents.

7. Hypercalcemia from any cause.

8. Neurogenic, possibly psychogenic, disorders.

9. Deficiency of vasodilating tissue enzymes (speculative) (prostaglandins, bradykinin, renal medullary tissue).

PATHOPHYSIOLOGY

Mean arterial pressure is the product of the systemic vascular resistance and the mean cardiac output. As a result, either an increase in cardiac output or an increase in systemic vascular resistance—or both—can raise the blood pressure; both factors in this relationship are constantly changing throughout the course of a day. Blood pressure is not a static physiologic feature but a variable one in all individuals, both normal and hypertensive, from one occasion of measurement to another.

Normal Blood Pressure

Normal blood pressure is maintained by complex mechanisms made up of many interacting regulatory forces acting on cardiac output and peripheral resistance.

As one proceeds along the cardiovascular system from the cardiac "pump" to the capacitance vessels (the veins), the arterial pressure drop is greatest at the precapillary resistance vessels (the arterioles); it is chiefly the caliber of these vessels that controls the systemic vascular resistance (Fig 9–1).

Many homeostatic mechanisms of the body are brought into play to maintain the blood pressure within a normal range (Table 9–1). Functional and structural changes in the resistance vessels (arterioles) are brought about by many influences: increased smooth muscle contraction; baroreceptor reflexes sending afferent impulses to the medulla and hypothalamic centers; other influences on these centers resulting in efferent autonomic discharge; blood volume; humoral and neurogenic influences from the kidneys and endocrine organs; effects of the renin-angiotensin-aldosterone system; and local effects of prostaglandins, kinins, adenosine, serotonin, and the newly discovered atrial natriuretic factors. Intrinsic autoregulation also operates to control arteriolar caliber independently of sympathetic adrenergic stimuli (Bayliss, 1902; Cowley, 1980). Transient elevations of blood pressure due to physiologic decrease in the caliber of arterioles should not be confused with sustained or established hypertension. It is apparent, therefore, why such factors as anxiety, emotion, fear, noise, pain, anger, cold, an unfamiliar or threatening environment, exercise, or tachycardia can increase the arterial pressure either by increasing cardiac output or by raising the systemic vascular resistance through arteriolar vasoconstriction. The control systems influencing these various factors have both positive and negative feedback loops. The complex interrelationships of the factors have been analyzed by Guyton (1972) and others.

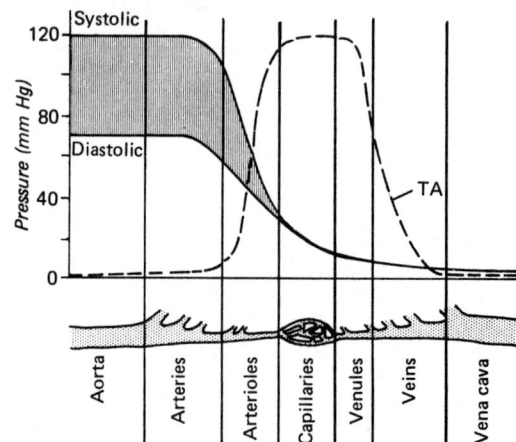

Figure 9–1. Diagram of the changes in pressure as blood flows through the systemic circulation. TA, total cross-sectional area of the vessels, which increases from 4.5 cm² in the aorta to 4500 cm² in the capillaries. (Modified and reproduced, with permission, from Ganong WF: *Review of Medical Physiology*, 12th ed. Lange, 1985.)

Pathophysiologic influences combating rises in blood pressure include (1) baroreceptor reflexes to the brain via the ninth and tenth cranial nerves from the carotid and aortic bodies, which decrease sympathetic adrenergic vasoconstriction when tension in the carotid body rises; and (2) local tissue factors such as the prostaglandins, which are naturally occurring unsaturated fatty acids that have potent and variable biologic activity.

As indicated in the discussion of atherosclerosis (see p 137 and Fig 8–7), the physiologic functions of prostaglandins (PG) and thromboxanes (TX) are the subject of active research. The vasodilating action of prostacyclin (PGI_2) and the vasoconstricting action of thromboxane (TXA_2), which modulate blood flow within the kidney and thereby influence blood pressure, are of considerable interest. Prostaglandins increase the release of renin and are involved in the regulation of glomerular filtration, renal blood flow, and the excretion of electrolytes. Fig 8–7 describes the pathway for biosynthesis and metabolism of pros-

Table 9–1. Factors contributing to increases in systolic and diastolic blood pressure. Mean arterial pressure = Cardiac output × Systemic arterial resistance.

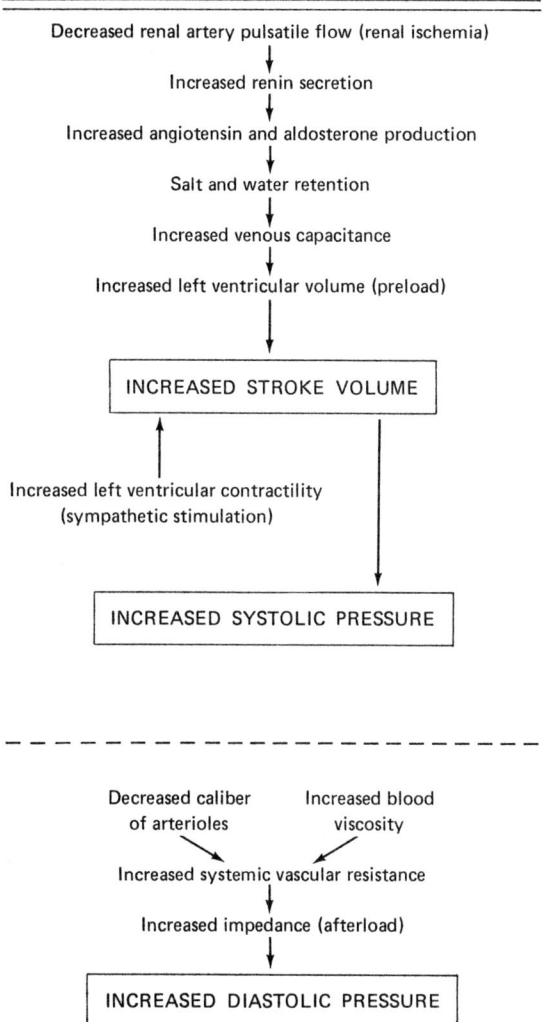

taglandins. Since interrelationships between the renin-angiotensin system, dietary sodium, blood volume, adrenergic neural stimuli, and adrenal steroids all influence the action of prostaglandins on blood pressure regulation, they may be important in the pathophysiology of hypertension (Levenson, 1982). Furthermore, bradykinin, local hormones from the adrenal medulla, and other peptides may also play a role.

It has been postulated that a decreased amount or availability of PGI_2 synthetase as a result of intimal damage (as in hypertension) tilts the balance of control forces toward the TXA_2 action on platelet clumping, which may then foster the development of thrombi and, subsequently, atherosclerotic plaques (Swartz, 1980; Moncada, 1982).

The apparent circadian rhythm of blood pressure in both normal subjects and hypertensive patients may be due to impulses from the central nervous system. As a rule, blood pressure is lowest during sleep and begins to rise immediately before or after awakening (Floras, 1981) (Fig 9–2). The role of circadian rhythm in the complications of hypertension is unknown.

Phases in the Development of Hypertension

Many patients with established hypertension have a past record of transiently raised pressures under usual conditions of measurement, sometimes associated with tachycardia and with evidences of emotional lability. Hemodynamic studies in such individuals with so-called early labile hypertension have shown that systemic vascular resistance is normal but cardiac output increased.

It is believed by some (Folkow, 1971) that increased cardiac output in the presence of normal systemic vascular resistance could, by autoregulation and increased myogenic contractions, decrease arteriolar caliber and thus protect the capillaries in the short term but ultimately induce structural changes in the arterioles. This may explain why in older people with established hypertension, cardiac output is normal and the hypertension is due to increased systemic vascular resistance. Arteriolar structural changes have been found in the kidneys of patients who have been examined at autopsy or by renal biopsy and are less severe in persons with early mild hypertension than in older people with more advanced disease.

In between the above 2 groups of patients are the early middle-aged individuals who may have both increased systemic vascular resistance and increased cardiac output.

A. Early Phase: In older patients with established hypertension, hemodynamic studies have demonstrated raised systemic vascular resistance and a normal cardiac index.

An early "labile phase" of hypertension with blood pressure fluctuating into the normal range (see p 256) is common in younger individuals, often resulting from increased cardiac output with or without increased systemic vascular resistance thought by some investigators to be due to excessive sympathetic adrenergic impulses arising in the central nervous system from the cortex, hypothalamus, or medullary cardiovascular centers. There can be no doubt that emotional factors cause neurohumoral discharge from the higher cortical centers and that this in turn increases sympathetic adrenergic excitation impulses and raises arterial pressure by vasoconstriction of the arterioles.

"Labile" hypertension is clearly related to age (see p 256) and is defined by Moeller (1959) as a blood pressure that is elevated (>140/90 mm Hg) when the patient enters the hospital but that falls to normal (<140/90 mm Hg) after a few days. Others characterize this as "borderline" hypertension. Sustained hypertension is that which is present on admission and also after a short hospital stay; normal blood pressure is that which is normal both on admission and after a few days in the hospital. The high fre-

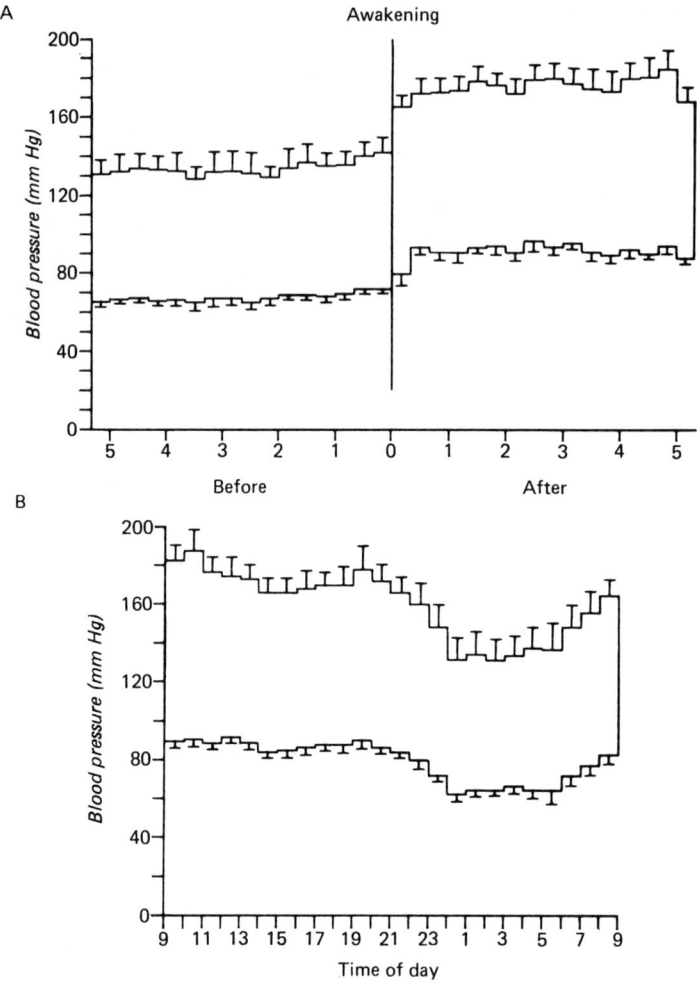

Figure 9–2. Mean systolic and diastolic pressures in 14 untreated hypertensive subjects. *A:* Data analyzed with respect to the moment of waking as recorded by the patients, in 20-minute intervals for a 5-hour period up to the moment of waking and for a 5-hour period subsequent to waking. *B:* Data analyzed in hourly intervals over the 24-hour period. (Redrawn and reproduced, with permission, from Floras JS et al: Arousal and the circadian rhythm of blood pressure. *Clin Sci Mol Med* 1978;**55** [Suppl 4]:395s.)

quency of "labile" hypertension as defined by these authors is noteworthy.

There are many problems in identifying patients with hypertension, including systematic biases and normal variability of the blood pressure. In the Charlottesville Blood-Pressure Survey, for example, 20% of over 12,000 adults were initially classified as hypertensive, yet after repeated blood pressure measurements only 9% were found to have sustained hypertension (Carey, 1976). The variability of the blood pressure, not only from one time of measurement to another but from beat to beat, was clearly shown by direct intra-arterial pressure recordings by Watson (1980). The major factors influencing variability are the level of pressure, the intensity of physical activity, and negative affect states. Systolic variability increases with progressive impairment of sinoaortic baroreflexes. Emotional states and the circumstances of measurement, whether in the physician's office, at work, at home, or during ambulatory recording, influence the diagnosis of hypertension.

B. Established Hypertension: The mechanism of the transition between transiently elevated pressures resulting from emotional factors and established hypertension resulting from structural arteriolar abnormalities is not determined. Folkow (1971) believes that periodic distention of smooth muscle by autoregulation may ultimately lead to structural changes. In older patients with established hypertension, hemodynamic studies have demonstrated raised systemic vascular resistance and a normal cardiac index. Emotional factors, which superimpose transient further rises of pressure on an individual with established hypertension, could understandably accelerate vascular complications. This hypothesis is supported by studies in spontaneously hypertensive rats that when exposed to disturbing situations such as noise or vibration, respond with further increases in blood pressure and, ultimately, an increase in vascular complications. One can infer, therefore, that social and psychologic factors operating on an individual who tolerates emotional stress poorly can aggravate an existing elevated blood pressure by superimposing arteriolar vasoconstriction on structural arteriolar changes. There is no conclusive evidence, however, that repetitive functional changes can be the sole cause of such structural abnormalities.

Pulse Pressure

Both systolic and diastolic pressure rise in the usual case of hypertension; the difference between them (the pulse pressure) depends not only upon age but upon whether the major component of the raised pressure is due to an increase in cardiac output or to peripheral resistance. Thus, a wide pulse pressure is most apt to occur in early labile hypertension of young people with a raised output or in the elderly person with perhaps only a slight increase in diastolic pressure but with a greater increase in systolic pressure owing to a less distensible aorta. Actuarial data indicate that both systolic and diastolic pressures are important with respect to mortality statistics, and it is often difficult to separate their effects because the correlation between them is so high, being on the order of $r = 0.7$.

Systolic Hypertension

Systolic hypertension is usually defined as a systolic pressure above 160 mm Hg and a diastolic pressure less than 90 mm Hg. It is most commonly seen in older patients. Various studies have demonstrated that the mortality rate in hypertensive patients is as closely related to systolic as to diastolic pressure, which means that the traditional emphasis on diastolic pressure is unwarranted. The mortality rate is probably increased, because most cases of purely systolic hypertension (omitting conditions such as complete atrioventricular block, severe bradycardia, arteriovenous fistulas, thyrotoxicosis, and aortic insufficiency) are due to decreased distensibility (increased rigidity) of the central aorta and its branches as a result of atherosclerosis. Atherosclerosis, being a generalized disorder, is apt to be present elsewhere if it occurs in the aorta, and so the mortality rate can be expected to be greater than in persons who do not have aortic atherosclerosis. Furthermore, the correlation coefficient between systolic and diastolic pressures is about 0.7, indicating that both indices usually are elevated together, so that a raised systolic pressure usually is associated with an increased diastolic pressure.

There are few data indicating the prognosis when systolic pressure exceeds 160 mm Hg and the diastolic is not merely below 95 mm Hg but below 70–75 mm Hg, so that the mean pressure is less than 107 mm Hg (upper limits of normal). A diastolic pressure of 90 mm Hg in association with a systolic pressure of 180 mm Hg, for example, would represent a mean pressure of 90 + 90/3, or 120 mm Hg, an elevated mean pressure. A systolic pressure of 180 mm Hg would require a diastolic pressure of 70–75 mm Hg in order to represent a normal mean pressure. Therefore, when the diastolic pressure is about 90 mm Hg, a raised systolic pressure represents a raised systemic vascular resistance as well as decreased elasticity of the aorta. The mean pressure is the best index of the significance of a dominantly or purely systolic elevation of blood pressure with respect to the diagnosis of essential hypertension. If systolic pressure is raised out of proportion to the diastolic pressure, the load on the left ventricle is increased, and cautious therapy with low doses of either a diuretic or a beta-adrenergic blocking agent or both may be indicated to decrease the work of the heart if cardiac symptoms are present. Younger patients with systolic pressures of 150 mm Hg or greater and diastolic pressures of 95 mm Hg or less show a hyperkinetic circulation with tachycardia and increased cardiac output, whereas older patients have a raised systemic vascular resistance but no increase in cardiac output. Older patients have a greater systemic vascular resistance than younger ones. Dominantly systolic hypertension (with diastolic pressures up to 95 mm Hg) should not be defined as purely systolic hypertension, because diastolic pressures of this magnitude with a systolic pressure that is elevated increase the mean arterial pressure but rarely increase the cardiac output. There are no studies describing the prognosis of patients with systolic hypertension with diastolic pressures sufficiently low to have normal mean pressures. The mean pressure in the older hypertensive patients of Adamopoulos (1975) was 112 ± 1 mm Hg (the average systolic pressure was 159 mm Hg; the average diastolic pressure, 88 mm Hg), in contrast to an average mean pressure of 95 mm Hg in the older normotensive group. The older hypertensive group had a higher mean pressure, so the difference in prognosis was not due strictly to the elevated systolic pressure. The authors recognize this and state that whether the patients with systolic hypertension were younger or older than 35 years of age, the diastolic pressures were always significantly higher than those of normotensive individuals, thereby raising the mean pressure.

Years ago, Wiggers (1939) demonstrated in an artificial circulation machine that decreasing the elasticity of the aorta but keeping cardiac output and peripheral resistance constant caused an increased systolic pressure, a decreased diastolic pressure, an increased pulse pressure, and an unchanged mean pressure. Decreasing aortic compliance after arteriolar caliber was decreased caused an increase in all 3 pressures (systolic, diastolic, and pulse). The diastolic pressure increase was less than when peripheral resistance alone was decreased.

The essential effect of aging consists of decreased elasticity and enlargement of the aorta. There are no adequate data describing the benefits or hazards of treating systolic blood pressure with a normal mean pressure in an older person. Because the raised systolic pressure "compensates" for the decreased aortic distensibility (compliance), antihypertensive drugs may cause a decreased cardiac output, with weakness or faintness resulting from decreased perfusion of the vital organs of the body. If medication is tried, it should be given cautiously and in low dosage, with careful observation of its effects.

If drugs are to be used, see the section on treatment of mild hypertension on p 258.

1. PATHOPHYSIOLOGY OF ESSENTIAL HYPERTENSION

The Role of the Central Nervous System

Although the factors regulating blood pressure are known, the cause of essential hypertension is by definition unestablished. The underlying cause is unknown also in many instances of hypertension associated with the disorders listed above in the section on etiology and classification. One theory that has many proponents is that the central nervous system, through its efferent autonomic discharges, increases cardiac output and that this induces contraction of the arteriolar muscle to prevent flooding the capillaries, thus increasing systemic vascular resistance and arterial pressure. The pressure changes also influence the kidney by the effects on the blood volume and the renin-angiotensin-aldosterone system. (See p 210 for the multiple factors involved in the regulation of blood pressure.) Oft-repeated smooth muscle contraction leads ultimately to structural changes in the arterioles, permanently increasing systemic vascular resistance.

The problem of identification of the mechanisms of primary and secondary hypertension is made more difficult by the fact that no matter what the initial mechanisms were that established hypertension, lesions in the arterioles and interlobular arteries in the kidney may lead to small vessel ("Goldblatt") disease, with persistent hypertension after the primary cause is removed (eg, renal artery stenosis, aldosteronism, pheochromocytoma, and nephrectomy for unilateral pyelonephritis). The mechanisms responsible for persistence of hypertension may differ from those responsible for initiation of it, eg, secondary vascular changes in the kidney or increased secretion of renin.

The Role of the Sympathetic Nervous System

The role of the sympathetic nervous system has been extensively studied, and the general conclusion is that abnormalities of the system are not the cause of primary (essential) hypertension, although there is some evidence showing increased sympathetic nervous system activity in borderline or mild hypertension. The raised cardiac output, heart rate, and ejection fraction seen in the so-called hyperkinetic circulation of young hypertensive individuals may be related to increased sympathetic stimuli to the heart.

In studies comparing normotensive subjects with hypertensive patients, the concentration of circulating plasma norepinephrine was sometimes found to be higher in hypertensive patients. However, this difference was not statistically significant, except in young hypertensive patients with hyperkinetic circulations (Goldstein, 1983; Lake, 1977). One difficulty in determining the role of plasma norepinephrine in hypertension is that concentrations are labile and vary with even mildly stressful procedures (eg, venipuncture), with changes in posture, and during exercise.

The Role of Baroreceptors

Pressoreceptors in the wall of a carotid artery or the carotid sinus and in the region of the aortic arch increase the rate of their firing when arterial pressure rises and reduce it when the pressure falls. Nervous impulses from these sensory receptors travel via the carotid sinus nerve or the vagus nerve to the cerebral medulla. The efferent pathway from the medullary centers is via the vagal and sympathetic nerves. The pressoreceptors are sensitive to mean pressure and to the rate of change of pressure and initiate an adrenergic reflex baroreceptor response that affects the blood pressure and heart rate (Fig 9–3).

There has been much speculation about the role of the baroreceptors in the pathogenesis of hypertension. Initial enthusiasm waned when it was found that denervation of the baroreceptors often did not produce neurogenic hypertension and that when it did, the increase in blood pressure was slight. Many authorities agreed with Guyton that the arterial baroreceptors were not responsible for long-term control of arterial pressure in humans. Ambulatory continuous intra-arterial pressures show marked discrepancies in variability between systolic and diastolic pressure; the higher the systolic pressure, the greater the variability, which may reflect poor baroreceptor reflex control in hypertension (Littler, 1978; Sleight, 1979).

The Role of Sodium

The etiologic importance of sodium intake in hypertension has been debated for years. Although there may be some individuals in whom increased sodium intake results in raised blood pressure (as it does in salt-sensitive Dahl rats), the general consensus is that most hypertensive patients are not salt-sensitive. Studies supporting this general conclusion have shown that (1) the mean urinary excretion of sodium, potassium, and water is not significantly different among normotensive, borderline, and hypertensive subjects (Ljungman, 1981; Omvik, 1983), nor is the relationship between arterial pressure and salt intake; (2) the blood pressure in hypertensive patients does not differ when they are on low-salt or high-salt diets (Ledingham, 1982); and (3) moderate restriction of sodium does not affect the blood pressure, but rigid restriction does, and this is not well tolerated by most patients.

Many factors other than dietary sodium may affect blood pressure. A genetic defect in the kidney's ability to excrete sodium has been postulated, but this theory

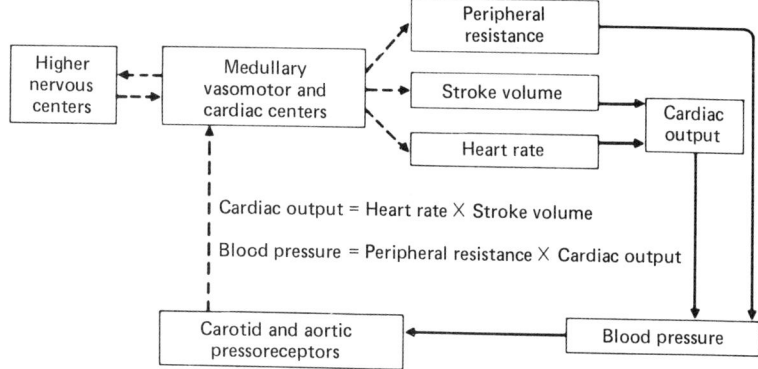

Figure 9–3. Blood pressure is sensed by the pressoreceptors, which send impulses to the central nervous system. The central nervous system sends impulses to motor fibers of the sympathetic and parasympathetic nervous system. When pressure at the receptor rises or falls, it is reflexly corrected by an alteration of heart rate, stroke volume, and peripheral resistance. Dotted lines indicate neural connections. (Reproduced, with permission, from Scher AM: Control of arterial blood pressure. Pages 146–169 in: *Physiology and Biophysics,* 20th ed. Vol 2. Ruch TC, Patton HD [editors]. Saunders, 1974.)

has not been generally accepted (de Wardener, 1982). Obese patients who consume a high-salt diet tend to have higher blood pressures because they also have higher caloric intakes. Although it has been shown that in some underdeveloped countries individuals who consume low-sodium diets do not show increased blood pressure corresponding to increased age, this may be due to factors other than dietary sodium.

The Role of the Renin-Angiotensin System

Renin, a proteolytic enzyme, is secreted by the juxtaglomerular cells surrounding the afferent arterioles near the vascular pole of the kidney in response to a "signal." It is hypothesized that the signal is related to stretch of the afferent arteriole or to decreased "effective" blood volume or to sodium content of the nearby macula densa of the distal tubule. Renin then acts on a substrate in the plasma (α_2-globulin), producing the decapeptide angiotensin I, which is then acted upon by a converting enzyme in the lung to form the octapeptide angiotensin II, which is a potent pressor substance. Angiotensin II, by an effect on the zona glomerulosa of the adrenal cortex, increases the secretion of aldosterone, which results in sodium and water retention by its characteristic action on the distal renal tubule, thus restoring blood volume. By negative feedback, the secretion of renin is then reduced until equilibrium results (Fig 9–4).

The complex factors affecting renin levels (Table 9–2 and Fig 9–4) and regulating renin release from the kidney may be important in hypertension, and there is considerable evidence supporting the importance of regulation by the nervous system and the autonomic sympathetic amines. The mechanisms regulating renin release can be classified as (1) intrarenal, which include (a) alteration of sensing by the afferent arteriole of changes in the renal perfusion pressure,

Table 9–2. Factors affecting renin levels.*

Decreased plasma renin activity (PRA)
   Expanded fluid volume
      Salt loads
      Mineralocorticoid excess
      Renal insufficiency
   Depression of sympathetic nervous system activity
      Autonomic dysfunction
      Treatment with adrenergic neuronal blockers: reserpine, methyldopa, guanethidine sulfate, clonidine hydrochloride
      Treatment with β-adrenergic blockers: propranolol hydrochloride
   Potassium loads
   Decreased ability to synthesize renin: renal disease

Increased PRA
   Shrunken fluid volume
      Salt deprivation or wastage
      Decreased effective plasma volume
         Diuretic therapy
         Chronic edematous states (cirrhosis, nephrosis)
         Upright posture
   Decreased renal perfusion
      Therapy with peripheral vasodilators: hydralazine hydrochloride, prazosin hydrochloride, diazoxide, sodium nitroprusside
      Renal ischemia (renovascular hypertension)
   Increased sympathetic nervous activity: exercise, stress, hyperthyroidism
   Hypokalemia
   Increased renin substrate
      Pregnancy
      Estrogen therapy
   Autonomous renin secretion: renin-producing tumors

Variable
   Spontaneous fluctuations and circadian rhythm
   Menstrual cycle

*Reproduced, with permission, from Kaplan NM: Renin profiles: The unfulfilled promises. *JAMA* 1977;**238**:611.

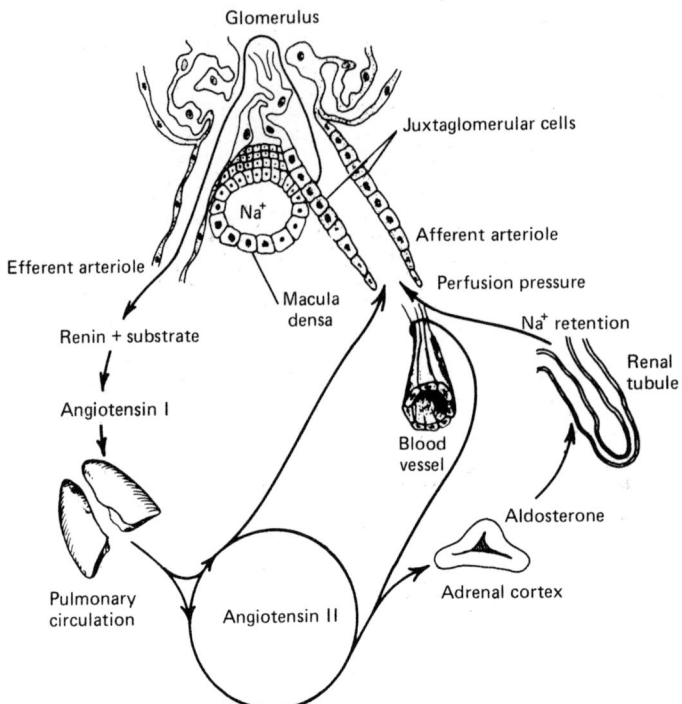

Figure 9-4. Feedback regulation of renin release. Several feedback loops are shown. An increase in angiotensin II concentration results in decreased renin secretion by increased sodium retention resulting in increased extracellular fluid volume; direct negative feedback; increased blood pressure through the central nervous system; increased blood pressure through direct systemic vasoconstriction; and direct sodium effects on the macula densa. (Reproduced, with permission, from the American Heart Association, Inc., Haber E: The role of renin in normal and pathological cardiovascular homeostasis. *Circulation* 1976;**54**:849.)

(b) the influence of the alleged sodium receptor in the macula densa, which senses changes in the sodium concentration in the distal tubule, and (c) prostaglandins; (2) autonomic factors, including the effects of catecholamines and nervous impulses via the renal nerves; and (3) humoral effects of electrolytes, vasopressin, angiotensin, and adrenergic impulses from the higher cerebral centers. Renin exists in the plasma in an inactive prorenin form and in an active renin form. The area postrema in the bulbar region is probably responsible for the centrally mediated neurogenic effects of angiotensin II. There is considerable evidence that the area postrema has an active function in central cardiovascular control, including regulation of the blood pressure. Electrical stimulation of this area increases sympathetic outflow in a fashion similar to what happens when angiotensin II is infused into the central arteries (Ferrario, 1979). Adrenergic beta blockers decrease active renin but may also increase the concentration of inactive prorenin; adrenergic impulses may therefore activate inactive renin. The interactions between the nervous system and the renin-angiotensin system are varied and interrelated.

Renin changes in hypertension are probably secondary to pressure changes.

In a random group of hypertensive patients on a normal sodium diet, about 20% will have low, 60% normal, and 20% high plasma renin, defined in different ways by different authorities.

Although Laragh and his associates (1974, 1976) believe that low-renin hypertension may be due to increased secretion of a mineralocorticoid that increases the extracellular and plasma blood volume which, by negative feedback, turns off renin production, the mineralocorticoid has not been identified (Ganguly, 1979). The Medical Research Council Unit in Glasgow did not find increased extracellular or plasma volume or increased total exchangeable sodium in low-renin hypertension. A study reported at an NIH conference concluded that hypertensive patients with low plasma renin do not have high-volume hypertension but rather a primary renal abnormality with decreased secretion of renin; they become relatively deficient in angiotensin II and aldosterone when they are subjected to diuresis. Other investigators find that when other risk factors are equivalent, complications may occur in low- as in normal-renin hypertension. Hypertensive patients with normal renin and vascular complications are apt to have, concomitantly, other risk factors, whereas patients whose risk factors are minimal have fewer complications despite the normal renin (Kaplan, 1975).

Determination of plasma renin in clinical practice is useful mainly to detect patients with curable secondary hypertension (Gifford, 1980).

Until the role of renin in prognosis and selection of therapy is established, we think it unwise to stop antihypertensive therapy that is controlling the blood pressure in order to determine the plasma renin unless one is searching for primary aldosteronism. Vigorous antihypertensive therapy is warranted in significant hypertension regardless of the level of the plasma renin.

Prospective studies to determine subsets of hypertension (low-, normal-, and high-renin types) and the response of renin to inhibitors of the renin-angiotensin system may lead to the use of "preferred" antihypertensive agents. Studies of agents that selectively inhibit the enzymatic conversion of angiotensin I to angiotensin II (teprotide, captopril, and enalapril) and of agents that competitively inhibit the action of angiotensin II on the receptor within the kidney (saralasin) have attempted to clarify the physiologic role of each component of the renin-angiotensin-aldosterone system. The system appears to play an important role in renovascular hypertension (see below) and in severe or accelerated hypertension, in which plasma renin is usually elevated and secondary hyperaldosteronism is sometimes seen. The inverse relationship between serum sodium and plasma renin results in elevated plasma renin activity with sodium or volume depletion, as during diuretic therapy. Chemical isolation and synthesis of renin and the availability of specific active and inactive renin antibodies will contribute to knowledge of renin release and its physiologic significance (Dzau, 1981).

The Role of Atrial Natriuretic Factors

Considerable interest has been aroused by the recent discovery of natriuretic factors derived from atrial cells. Injection of these substances induces a rapid increase in the urinary excretion of sodium and water and higher rates of glomerular filtration and renal blood flow. These findings suggest a possible role in the development of hypertension and uses in its treatment. Further data are awaited.

The Role of Social & Psychologic Factors

Adverse social and psychologic factors in hypertensive patients may set off adrenergic impulses from the central nervous system and cause increased vasoconstriction, superimposing further transient rises in pressure on established hypertension and gradually worsening the structural changes in the arterioles and the interlobular arteries of the kidney. This leads to higher blood pressures and consequent vascular abnormalities and complications.

There is no clear evidence that social or psychologic factors *cause* hypertension. Folkow's hypothesis—that emotional factors operating through the central nervous system cause smooth muscle contraction, arteriolar structural changes, and thus hypertension—has not been fully accepted. Adverse social and psychologic factors might accelerate hypertension by inducing substantial recurrent rises in pressure, thus increasing the load on the heart and precipitating left ventricular failure. In the presence of coronary disease, transient blood pressure elevations may precipitate cardiac arrhythmias and angina pectoris or may rupture a Charcot microaneurysm in one of the small penetrating arteries in the brain.

For this reason, attention to the social and psychologic aspects of the patient's life is an integral part of management of the hypertensive patient. One could say the same thing about every patient with heart disease, but the principle seems particularly applicable to the hypertensive patient.

2. PATHOPHYSIOLOGY OF SECONDARY HYPERTENSION

Secondary hypertension involves the following mechanisms, which will be discussed briefly now and amplified in the section dealing with secondary hypertension. Factors involved in essential hypertension may also be involved in secondary hypertension (see pp 214ff).

(1) Increased secretion of catecholamines, as in pheochromocytoma (see p 249).

(2) Increased release of renin, as in renal artery stenosis and acute glomerulonephritis (see also p 238).

(3) Sodium and blood volume. These components play a key role in hypertension, especially when associated with hypertensive renal diseases and renal failure. When sodium intake exceeds the kidney's ability to excrete sodium, blood pressure rises. Any sodium-retaining agent increases blood volume and makes the hypertension and renal failure worse. Blood pressure regulation depends on the interrelationship of factors that control blood volume and systemic vasoconstriction. Hypertension of chronic renal disease is primarily volume-dependent: it is due either to an absolute excess in extracellular volume or to a relatively reduced plasma volume in relation to the vascular capacity.

In renal failure, if a high-sodium diet is given, patients develop sodium and water retention that worsens the hypertension. The normal diet contains about 3–5 g (130–217 meq) of sodium.

Hypertension occurs in 80% of patients with chronic renal failure by the time they reach the end stage but may occur early or late. Hypertension accelerates the cardiovascular complications that are the major cause of death in dialysis and transplant patients. The appearance of hypertension in patients with impaired renal function rapidly worsens the renal failure, because patients develop sodium retention, especially if they are on a high-sodium diet. All patients with chronic renal disease must be monitored closely for hypertension so that it can be treated promptly, before irreversible renal damage occurs.

(4) Increased extracellular and plasma volume, as in primary aldosteronism, hypertension associated with

desoxycorticosterone acetate administration, acute glomerulonephritis, renoprival hypertension (hypertension in the absence of both kidneys), and renal failure.

(5) Reduced perfusion pressure proximal to the kidney, as in coarctation of the aorta, which may initiate increased secretion of renin.

(6) Unknown mechanisms, eg, chronic glomerulonephritis (some patients with uremia have normal blood pressure), chronic pyelonephritis, and vasculitis of the kidney in connective tissue disorders (Adamopoulous, 1975).

(7) Adrenocortical hormones may play a role in hypertension. (See p 246 for Cushing's disease and syndrome.) In earlier, mild hypertension, there may be a state of inappropriate hypermineralocorticoid activity associated with salt and arteriolar changes (Genest, 1977). The therapeutic benefit of a low-sodium diet and diuretic therapy and the role of the adrenal cortex in the regulation of sodium balance make it appear likely that the adrenal cortex has a significant role in the regulation of blood pressure.

EPIDEMIOLOGIC STUDIES OF THE PREVALENCE OF HYPERTENSION

Epidemiologic studies indicate that about 15–20% of adults in the USA have blood pressures above 160/95, the upper limits of normal according to WHO criteria. The percentage falls to 5% if a diastolic pressure of 105 mm Hg is used as the cutoff point. Insurance companies consider 140/90 to be the upper limits of normal; the Framingham epidemiologic study, published over the past 10–15 years, classified patients between 140/90 and 160/95 as borderline hypertensives. It should be appreciated that there is no sharp dividing line between normotension and hypertension; when one plots the blood pressure at different ages in a large healthy population, the distribution curve does not demonstrate 2 distinct populations. Hypertension is a quantitative deviation from normal (Pickering, 1968). As a result, the criteria for the diagnosis of hypertension must be regarded as arbitrary; this has caused confusion in the literature because different authors use different numbers to diagnose hypertension.

Prospective studies have shown that without treatment, hypertension greatly increases the incidence of cardiac failure, coronary heart disease, hemorrhagic and thrombotic stroke, renal failure, dissection of the aorta, and death. The morbid events have a higher incidence with increasing age, even in a treated group (VA Study, 1967, 1972). Preventing or reversing hypertensive complications by antihypertensive therapy is a major public health concern. This has led to intensive efforts to screen populations in various ways for the presence of hypertension. One must be cautious in extrapolating pressures under these unnatural conditions, because at least half will be found to be "normal" on subsequent examinations. Most "unaware" hypertensive individuals found in screening are of the "labile" type (Carey, 1976).

Age & Hypertension

Hypertension is regarded as uncommon before age 20, although recent data suggest that this view may not be completely justified, because physicians have used adult criteria to determine normality in adolescents. If one uses different criteria for children, secondary hypertension is often found in young hypertensive individuals; coarctation of the aorta, chronic glomerulonephritis, pyelonephritis, renal artery stenosis, endocrine disorders, and raised pressure from oral contraceptive agents must all be considered in this age group.

The mean blood pressure rises with age in most Western populations but not in all individuals in the population groups. In normal subjects, the greatest rise occurs between birth and age 20, when the average systolic pressure may increase from 80 to 120 mm Hg. There is then a slow increase in pressure until ages 35–46, when the slope of the rise becomes steeper and many individuals cross over into a range that is arbitrarily defined as high blood pressure (see below). The systolic pressure may then continue to rise more slowly, not only because of the factor of decreased compliance of the aorta with age but presumably also because of familial or genetic factors. The diastolic pressure follows the systolic rise up to about age 40, when the rise with age becomes less steep. Blood pressure distribution according to sex and age in the entire city of Bergen, Norway, has been tabulated by Humerfelt (1963), showing the 5th, 25th, 50th, 75th, and 95th percentiles for both systolic and diastolic pressures in both females and males.

The rise in pressure with age in various epidemiologic studies is greater in persons who gain the most weight (especially black women), in persons who have a family history of hypertension, and in persons who have personality or emotional factors that influence blood pressure. Plasma norepinephrine and plasma renin increase and decrease, respectively, with age. Cardiac output decreases with age in patients with systolic hypertension, whereas the systemic vascular resistance rises with age. The role of these various factors has not been adequately studied in populations that show a rise in pressure with age. About 30% of the rise in pressure with age is due to genetic factors and the remainder to environmental factors. The nature of the latter factors has not been precisely determined, but they could be "factors operating through the mind" (Pickering, 1968). The relative roles of genetic and environmental factors vary in different individuals.

Race & Hypertension

It is clear from a number of studies that the death rate from hypertension in blacks is considerably greater than that in whites, but this may be a function of access to treatment rather than an inherent susceptibility to hypertension, because in the VA Study (1967) black and white patients did equally well with treatment and equally badly in the untreated group. There are few data to indicate that the prognosis is worse in blacks than in whites with mild hypertension; the higher mortality rate from hypertension in blacks is to a great extent due to their greater likelihood of having severe hypertension with cardiac failure or malignant hypertension.

Mortality Rates Associated With Hypertension

Actuarial data gathered during the large insurance study of 1959 dealing with almost 4 million lives and 100,000 deaths—as well as the Framingham Study—show that the mortality rate rises with increasing blood pressure. There is no sharp dividing line below which the mortality rate is unaffected and above which it is increased (Fig 9–5) (Pickering, 1968). There are progressive excessive morbidity and mortality rates as blood pressure rises in the group studied by the insurance companies, especially in younger individuals. (The excess mortality rate is much lower in older subjects.) The physician should think not in terms of hypertension or normotension ("either/or") but of the actual level of the blood pressure, both systolic and diastolic, in relationship to age. Data from many sources show that age is a major factor in determining the importance of the degree of deviation that any pressure represents and is of prognostic significance at any given level of blood pressure. A systolic pressure of 160 mm Hg, for example, would be in the 95th or 98th percentile for a 25-year-old but in the 50th percentile for a 60-year-old. The actuarial data from insurance companies likewise show the importance of age and the much greater likelihood of a fatal outcome over a period of years in younger individuals as compared to older ones with similar pressures. The mortality rate is higher in males, perhaps because of the increased incidence of coronary disease (Fig 9–6).

CLINICAL FINDINGS

The clinical, laboratory, and radiologic findings relate to (1) the height of the blood pressure; (2) the involvement of "target organs" such as the heart, brain, kidneys, eyes, and peripheral arteries; (3) the presence of vascular complications such as cardiac failure, myocardial infarction, cerebral infarction, cerebral hemorrhage, atherosclerosis elsewhere, and dissection of the aorta; and (4) evidence of secondary "curable" hypertension.

Symptoms

Primary hypertension early in its course is usually an asymptomatic disorder compatible with well-being for many years. Vague symptoms of nonspecific headache, dizziness, fatigue, and pounding of the heart may be present in hypertensive patients (often only after patients learn that they have the condition) but are no more frequent than in some groups of patients with normotension. The frequency of vague symptoms that resemble those seen in psychoneurotic disorders has led investigators such as Ayman (1940) to conclude that these nonspecific symptoms in patients with mild hypertension are functional in origin and not organic. Screening of adult population groups often reveals the blood pressure to be elevated in vigorous subjects who have no symptoms whatever.

A. Headaches: When hypertension is more severe, especially if it is the accelerated variety (with rapid rise in pressure and hemorrhages or exudates in the fundi, considered premalignant; see p 232), throbbing suboccipital headaches, worse in the morning and subsiding during the day, are common. In malignant hypertension in association with visual disturbances, the headaches can be severe and most difficult to relieve except by reduction of the blood pressure. In contrast with the typical hypertensive headache, the usual tension headache is more apt to be frontal and nonthrobbing; the differentiation is often difficult.

B. Heart Failure: When left ventricular dilatation and early left ventricular failure occur in patients with compensatory cardiac hypertrophy, symptoms include progressively more severe dyspnea on exertion, paroxysmal nocturnal dyspnea, and orthopnea (see Chapter 10). If coronary heart disease is also present, as it commonly is, patients may complain of angina pectoris or may develop myocardial infarction. Left ventricular failure resulting from the combination of increased work of the left ventricle due to hypertension and associated coronary heart disease is frequent and makes precise distinction between causative factors difficult. Cardiac failure from modest elevations of blood pressure alone does not usually occur. When the raised blood pressure is greater, and particularly when it occurs abruptly, as in malignant hypertension, cardiac failure may occur in the absence of coronary

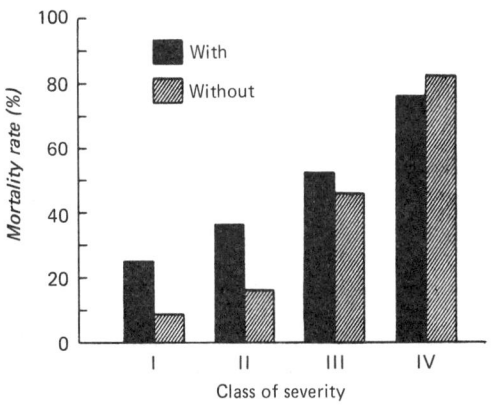

Figure 9–5. Mortality rates of hypertensive patients with and without atherosclerotic complications. Severity classes I–IV are described in the article and indicate progressively increasing severity of vascular complications. (Reproduced, with permission, from the American Heart Association, Inc., Sokolow M, Perloff D: The prognosis of essential hypertension treated conservatively. *Circulation* 1961;**23**:697.)

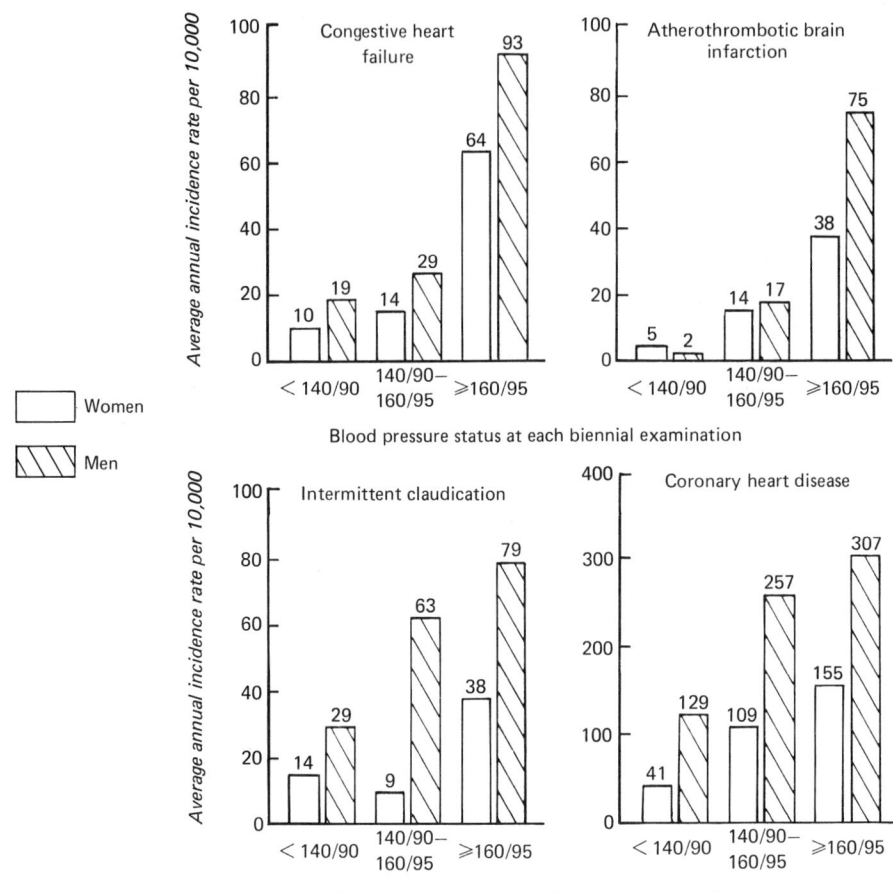

Figure 9-6. Average annual incidence of cardiovascular disease according to blood pressure status at each biennial examination, men and women 55–64, 16-year follow-up: Framingham Study. (Source: Framingham Monograph No. 26.) (Reproduced, with permission, from Kannel WB: Role of blood pressure in cardiovascular morbidity and mortality. *Prog Cardiovasc Dis* 1974;17:5.)

heart disease and is rapidly reversed when the blood pressure is lowered. Hypertensive patients with cardiac hypertrophy often develop symptoms and signs of cardiac failure if the sodium intake is abruptly increased, as with ingestion of baking soda, Alka-Seltzer, or a high-sodium diet; these patients often respond rapidly to treatment. Cardiac failure is an uncommon cause of death in the well-managed patient unless it follows the complications of myocardial infarction. Typical electrocardiographic examples of left ventricular hypertrophy and its reversal are illustrated in Fig 9–16.

C. Renal Symptoms: Although nephrosclerosis is a common finding on pathologic examination (by either necropsy or renal biopsy), renal failure is not common unless hypertension is accelerated, or malignant. Patients with severe hypertension may develop nocturia or, more rarely, intermittent hematuria. In nonaccelerated cases, renal blood flow and glomerular filtration rate may be somewhat decreased, but renal failure and azotemia are rare. If accelerated, or malignant, hypertension occurs, however, necrotic lesions in the arterioles and narrowed interlobular arteries may significantly decrease the renal blood flow and glomerular filtration rate; renal function may deteriorate rapidly over a period of weeks or months.

The most common cause of death in malignant hypertension is renal failure; determination of renal function is essential in all patients with hypertension, because as will be discussed in the section on prognosis, it is important to lower the blood pressure before renal failure has occurred.

D. Central Nervous System Symptoms: Older patients with hypertension and associated cerebral and carotid artery sclerosis may develop any of the clinical manifestations of atherosclerosis of the arteries and arterioles to the head that might be expected from the pathologic findings described above. Patients may develop severe headache, confusion, coma, convulsions, blurred vision, transient neurologic signs, ataxia, or neurologic deficit due to cerebral infarction or hemorrhage. If the blood pressure rises abruptly, acute cerebral symptoms may develop such as somnolence, coma, confusion, or convulsions, collectively known as hypertensive encephalopathy—presumably due to cerebral spasm and cerebral edema—and these may be quickly reversed with rapidly acting antihypertensive agents. More commonly, however, when these severe cerebral symptoms develop, a vascular accident has occurred rather than cerebral spasm and edema.

Acute interruption of the blood supply to a localized area of the brain causes a focal neurologic deficit (stroke). The most common type is thrombotic cerebral infarction; the least common is cerebral embolus; and intermediate in frequency is cerebral hemorrhage from rupture of a berry aneurysm or a Charcot-Bouchard microaneurysm of one of the small arteries of the brain. Impaired blood supply may be either intra- or extracranial and may occur at a wide variety of sites in any of the extracranial arteries, especially the internal carotid, the basilar, and the vestibular arteries. The intracranial sites for atherosclerosis are dominantly the middle cerebral artery and the circle of Willis (Fig 9–7).

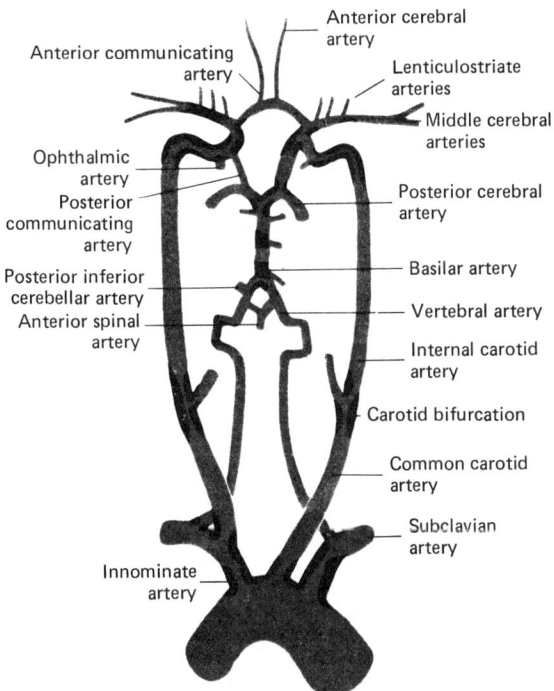

Figure 9–7. Major vascular lesions in stroke. Shown are the extracranial and intracranial arteries supplying blood to the brain as well as to the circle of Willis and its principal branches. The main locations of atherosclerosis of the cerebral vessels are the carotid bifurcation and takeoff of the branches from the aorta, innominate, and subclavian arteries. (Courtesy of Lawrence C McHenry, Jr, MD.) (Reproduced, with permission, from Cooper ES, West JW: Hypertension and stroke. *Cardiovasc Med* 1977;**2**:429.)

E. Claudication: When atherosclerosis involves the aorta and the arteries of the lower extremities, patients may present with intermittent claudication, and hypertension is only noted incidentally.

F. Chest Pain: Severe chest pain radiating to the back, followed by interruption of the arterial supply to the head, neck, back, and lower extremities, occurs after dissection of the aorta; in type I (p 234) involving the ascending aorta, aortic insufficiency may result. Hypertension may be noted only incidentally in patients who present with severe chest pain simulating acute myocardial infarction or acute aortic insufficiency.

As indicated under heart failure above, coronary heart disease frequently complicates hypertension. Patients may develop angina pectoris or myocardial infarction; chest pain may not be due to dissection of the aorta but to angina pectoris and myocardial ischemia.

Signs

The physical signs in hypertension are related to the underlying cause of the hypertension, its duration and severity, the blood pressure itself, the presence and degree of involvement of the target organs, and complications resulting from vascular involvement.

A. Blood Pressure: Varying levels of blood pressure on different occasions of measurement are almost the rule in hypertension (Hypertension Detection and Follow-Up Program Cooperative Group Study, 1982). Many patients with elevated pressures on the first examination had normal or lower pressures on subsequent ones.

The patient should be relaxed, comfortably warm, and unhurried, and the physician's routine should include allowing the patient to adjust to the examining room. The pressure must be taken in both arms to avoid discrepancies caused by atherosclerosis of the subclavian artery; the arm in which the pressure is to be taken on subsequent occasions should be noted.

The blood pressure should be taken with a mercury manometer or a well-calibrated aneroid manometer in both arms and in the legs, using a cuff at least 12 cm wide in most persons; a wide leg cuff (14–15 cm) must be used on the arm if the patient is obese or very muscular, with a large upper arm circumference. The cuff should be at least two-thirds as wide as the upper arm is long. Errors are frequently made in diagnosing hypertension if the cuff is too narrow and does not adequately compress the brachial artery. The basic principle is that a cuff which is too narrow for the size of the arm gives readings that are falsely high.

Accurate technique in taking the blood pressure is essential, and nurses, field workers, and others must be carefully instructed in placement of the rubber bag over the artery and the speed of inflation and deflation in measuring the pressure.

1. Home measurement and ambulatory blood pressure recordings–The patient or a member of the patient's family can be taught to take blood pressure readings at home. Systolic and diastolic pressures taken 3 or 4 times a day can be averaged into weekly mean pressures. Mean blood pressures so obtained are reliable not only in establishing the presence of hypertension but also in providing a baseline to evaluate treatment. Ambulatory blood pressure readings can be taken with portable self-recording equipment in order to eliminate the pressor effect of the physician and the medical environment. Mean ambulatory pressures lower than mean office pressures occurred in 85% of 675 untreated hypertensive patients. Mean ambulatory pressures averaged 13% lower than office pressures for the total population, with a wide scatter, even though the correlation coefficient of the 2 methods of measuring pressures is 0.67 (Sokolow, 1966). These ancillary techniques are usually needed only when raised pressures are mild to moderate (<180/105 mm Hg) and are not necessary when the pressures are considerably raised on 2 or 3 occasions but normal on others. Examples of the use of ambulatory blood pressure monitoring are shown in Figs 9–8 and 9–9. Table 9–3 shows office and ambulatory pressures related to severity of hypertension.

Even when office blood pressures are more than moderately raised, an occasional patient will have essentially normal readings at home when pressures are taken by someone other than a physician or when pressures are recorded by a portable apparatus. Prolonged recording with intra-arterial or automatic devices, especially during sleep, is valuable in assessing hypertension and may demonstrate a marked decrease in pressures in the early morning hours (Fig 9–2).

2. Variations in measurement–The body position of the patient is also important; when the patient sits, the diastolic pressure may increase over recumbent levels. The systolic pressure may stay the same or occasionally may fall slightly in the standing position, but it may increase in the sitting position. If the patient is hypovolemic as a result of administration of diuretics or has postural hypertension from antihypertensive agents interfering with adrenergic transmission, the systolic and diastolic pressures may be considerably lower in the sitting and standing positions than in recumbency. In autonomic insufficiency, postural hypotension is accompanied by little or no tachycardia, in contrast to the marked tachycardia that occurs in postural hypotension due to hypovolemia. Because of the transient rise in pressure that occurs with the stress of the examination in the sometimes threatening environment of the doctor's office, a raised pressure must be present on at least 3 different occasions of measurement before one considers the pressure to be representative. Sometimes the pressure is so variable that it is elevated on one occasion but well within the normal range on another; this may occur in 10–20% of individuals during any short period of time. It then becomes necessary to obtain frequent office, home, or ambulatory blood pressure readings over a period of weeks or even months or to have readings taken by a nurse in the office under relaxed circumstances without the doctor being present.

B. Signs in Target Organs: Particular emphasis should be placed on the following signs related to an

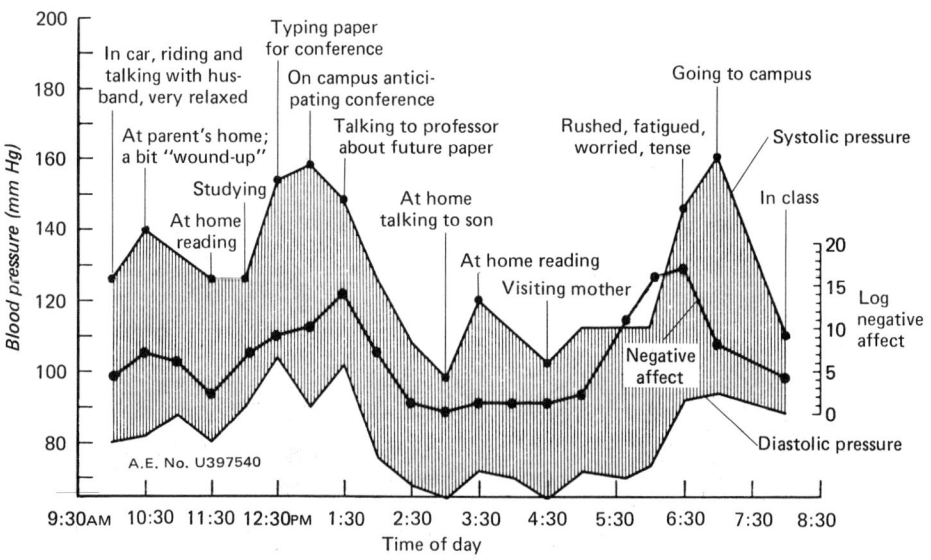

Figure 9–8. Serial blood pressure obtained with ambulatory blood pressure recordings correlated with patient's activities and emotions. The negative affect scale was derived from the patient's serial entries on an adjective checklist coincident with each blood pressure recording. The peak blood pressure readings, both systolic and diastolic, occurred when the patient was on the university campus where she returned after a lapse of many years in order to get her PhD. Each time that she was on the campus, the negative affect was greater. She admitted that she really did not want to get her PhD. (Reproduced, with permission, from Sokolow M et al: Preliminary studies relating portably recorded blood pressures to daily life events in patients with essential hypertension. *Bibl Psychiatr* 1970;**144**:164. S. Karger AG, Basel.)

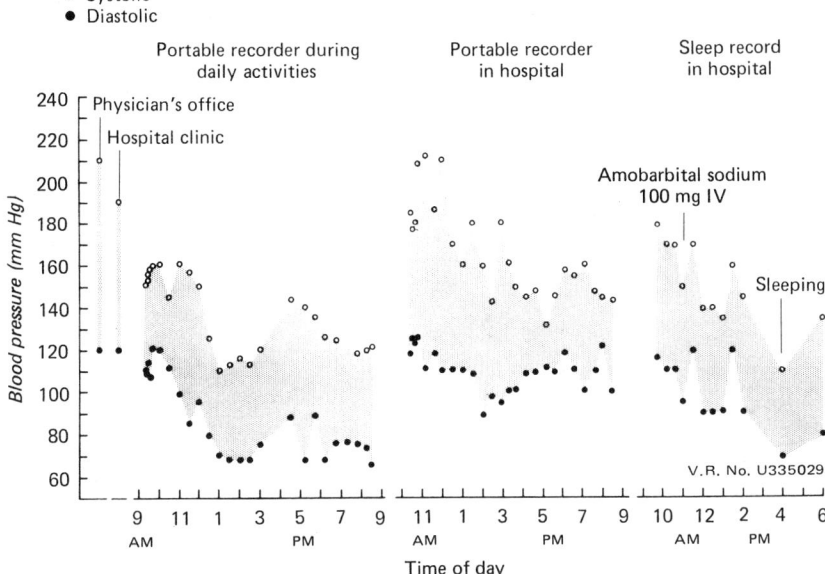

Figure 9-9. Ambulatory blood pressure recordings in a patient who had normal pressures during his daily activities but elevated pressures when in the hospital clinic. When he was put to sleep in the hospital with intravenous sodium amobarbital, his pressures were similar to those during his outside activities.

assessment of the presence and degree of involvement of the target organs affected by hypertension or by the presence or absence of vascular complications of hypertension.

1. Retinas—In examining the retinas one should note particularly the degree of narrowing or irregularity of the arterioles, the presence of arteriovenous defects ("nicking" or "nipping"), the presence of flame-shaped or circular hemorrhages or of fluffy cotton wool exudates, or the presence of papilledema with blurring of the temporal edge or elevation of the optic disk. Keith, Wagener, and Barker (1939) have classified the retinal changes (called Keith-Wagener [KW] changes) as follows:

KW I: Minimal arteriolar narrowing, irregularity of the lumen, and increased light reflex.

KW II: More marked narrowing with focal spasm, more

Table 9-3. Ambulatory and office mean systolic and diastolic blood pressures related to degree of severity of hypertensive complications.*

Class or Grade of Severity†	Overall Severity	Severity of Individual Complications		
		Ocular Funduscopic Abnormalities	Left Ventricular Hypertrophy	Cardiac Enlargement
Ambulatory pressures (mm Hg)				
0	137/82	139/83	147/89	155/94
I	150/91	152/92	161/99	
II	165/101	171/105	168/100	162/98
III	192/124	207/128	198/128	171/114
Office pressures (mm Hg)				
0	148/94	154/96	158/99	170/104
I	167/101	167/102	178/108	
II	181/112	183/113	187/111	181/110
III	206/125	237/131	220/129	177/116

*Reproduced, with permission, from the American Heart Association, Inc., Sokolow M et al: Relationship between the level of blood pressure measured casually and by portable recorders and severity of complications in essential hypertension. *Circulation* 1966;**34**:279.

†Classes of severity are graded 0–III depending on the presence and degree of changes in the fundi, ECG, chest film, and renal function. Class 0 denotes no abnormalities other than a raised blood pressure. (For further details see Sokolow & Perloff, 1961.)

marked irregularity, and arteriovenous nicking with changes in course and distention of the vein as it crosses the arteriole. The arteriole and the venule travel in the same sheath, and when there is thickening of the arteriole it compresses the venule.

KW III: In addition to the arteriolar changes noted previously, multiple flame-shaped hemorrhages and fluffy "cotton wool" exudates are scattered throughout the retinas (Fig 9–10). These are due to localized axon swellings and swollen nerve fibers in avascular areas. Hard, very small, sharply defined, translucent exudates are due to exudation in a different part of the retina, are of lesser significance, and do not indicate acute arteriolar damage.

KW IV: Any of the above with the addition of papilledema with blurring of the temporal side of the optic disk and elevation of the disk.

Caution should be exercised in interpreting blurring of the nasal edge of the disk as being due to papilledema. Old, healed papilledema in the absence of current elevation of the disk margins is often revealed by the presence of small collateral vessels crossing the edge of the disk.

Benign hypertension is the rule when KW I and KW II are present, whereas KW III and KW IV are associated with accelerated, or malignant, hypertension (Fig 9–10). When malignant hypertension develops abruptly with only a short history of hypertension, patients may have hemorrhages, exudates, or papilledema in the absence of arteriolar changes or arteriovenous nicking.

The Keith-Wagener classification has some deficiencies, particularly in the differentiation of hypertensive from atherosclerotic changes in KW I and II and in the interpretation of single hemorrhages and "hard" exudates. The 2 processes, hypertension and atherosclerosis, are independent entities, but hypertension accelerates atherosclerosis. When the arterioles are very narrowed and irregular and compress the venules, the findings are a combination of the 2 pathologic processes and are not due to hypertension alone; therefore, arteriovenous nicking indicates the presence of atherosclerosis and, by inference, a longer duration of the hypertensive process. The fundal changes of accelerated hypertension are an urgent indication for immediate and vigorous antihypertensive therapy.

Retinopathy is more common in diabetics who also have an elevated blood pressure, suggesting that control of the blood pressure may reduce the incidence of retinopathy in diabetics (Knowler, 1980).

2. Heart–Examination of the heart and blood vessels may reveal evidence of left ventricular hypertrophy, left ventricular failure, or involvement of the various arteries by atherosclerosis. Raised systemic vascular resistance increases the work of the left ventricle, and depending upon the stage of the disease, the heart may show concentric hypertrophy or combined hypertrophy and dilatation. The latter indicates inadequacy of compensatory hypertrophy and represents the earliest evidence of left ventricular failure.

Left ventricular wall thickness and left ventricular mass as determined by heart weight are the best signs of left ventricular hypertrophy. The upper limit of normal for left ventricular wall thickness is usually considered to be 1.5 cm, whereas heart weight is related to total body weight and is greater in men than in women. Heart weight exceeding 400 g is abnormal in either sex.

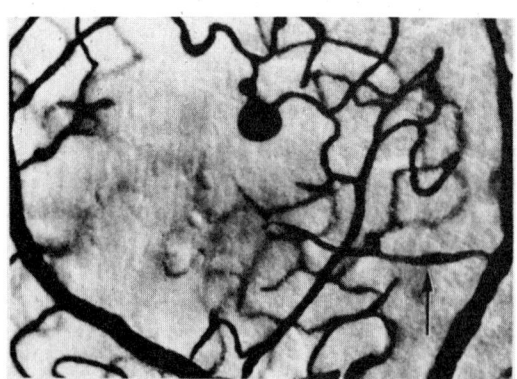 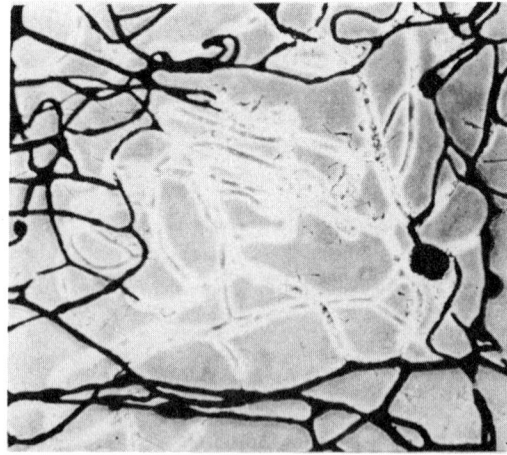

Figure 9–10. *Left:* Retina from a patient with malignant hypertensive retinopathy, showing a cotton wool spot. The capillaries within the affected area have failed to become injected, whereas the capillaries at the margin are dilated and show aneurysmal formation. Swollen nerve fibers may be seen in the avascular area. The terminal arteriole (arrow) showed hyalin lipid occlusion. (Injected with India ink; stain: oil red O; × 90.) *Right:* Retina from a patient with malignant hypertensive retinopathy, showing a cotton wool spot. The retina has been digested, revealing that capillaries are present within the uninjected zone; they appear patent and consist of simple basement membrane tubes without endothelial cells or pericytes. (Injected with India ink; × 130.) (Reproduced, with permission, from Ashton N: Pathophysiology of retinal cotton-wool spots. *Br Med Bull* 1970;**26**:143.)

As shown by Traube in the late 19th century, the best sign of left ventricular hypertrophy is a left ventricular heave, a localized sustained lift of the left ventricular impulse. Because concentric hypertrophy is the rule prior to dilatation and left ventricular failure, the heart is not displaced to the left unless cardiac failure is present. The decreased distensibility of the thick left ventricle commonly produces a presystolic gallop (S_4); this does not indicate cardiac failure but is a sign of decreased left ventricular compliance. The presence of a left ventricular heave and an S_4 indicates established left ventricular hypertrophy and usually long-standing disease.

If the patient has been untreated or inadequately treated with antihypertensive agents, there may be evidence of left and right heart failure with chronic passive congestion of the liver. The mechanisms leading to hypertensive heart failure are illustrated in Fig 9–11.

Although left ventricular hypertrophy is initially compensatory and beneficial following the development of hypertension with raised systemic vascular resistance, progressive left ventricular hypertrophy reaches a point at which the increased left ventricular mass no longer is able to compensate for the raised arterial pressure, so its contractile ability deteriorates, leading to the development of left ventricular failure.

Left ventricular hypertrophy occurs in spontaneously hypertensive rats and can be prevented and reversed if the elevated blood pressure is treated pharmacologically. Similarly, left ventricular hypertrophy may be prevented or reversed by antihypertensive therapy in humans with hypertension.

3. Arteries and veins–Hypertension induces arterial and arteriolar disease, predominantly in the arterioles and interlobular arteries of the kidney but also in the larger arteries of the body.

Early in the course of hypertensive disease, the arterioles and arteries are histologically normal, because the rise in pressure is due to functional vasoconstriction with decreased arteriolar caliber and not to struc-

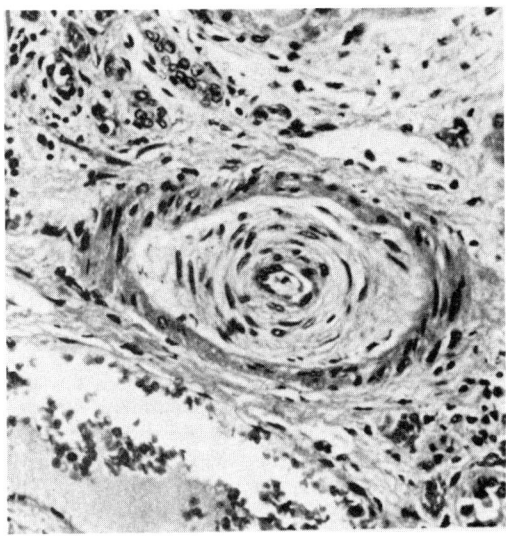

Figure 9–12. Cellular intimal hyperplasia (proliferative endarteritis or endarteritis fibrosa) in an interlobular renal artery (H&E; × 220). (Reproduced, with permission, from Kincaid-Smith P, McMichael J, Murphy EA: The clinical course and pathology of hypertension with papilloedema [malignant hypertension]. Q J Med 1958;27:117.)

tural change. Later on, the renal arterioles demonstrate medial hypertrophy and intimal fibrous thickening, resulting in a lower lumen-to-wall ratio and raising the systemic vascular resistance even at full vasodilatation. Arterioles throughout the body are affected to various degrees, but in almost all cases of established hypertension the renal arterioles show the structural changes known as nephrosclerosis (Fig 9–12).

The larger arteries are usually spared in established hypertension until atherosclerosis, an independent process accelerated by the hypertension, develops. When this occurs, the arterial lesions show no distinguishing feature that separates atherosclerosis

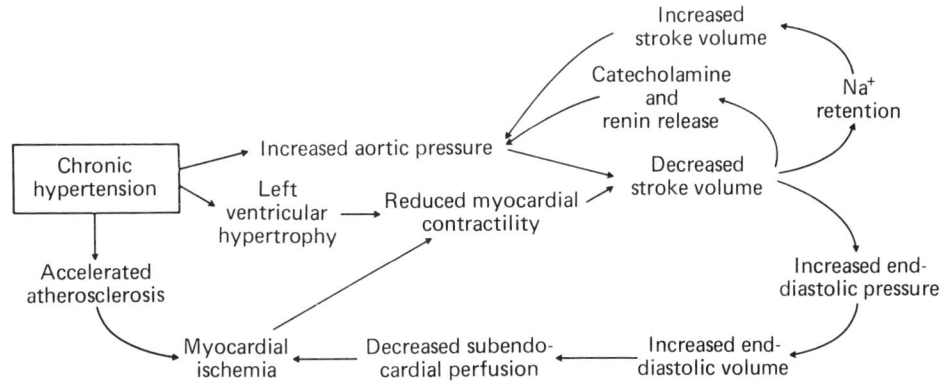

Figure 9–11. Some mechanisms initiated by hypertension that may lead to left ventricular decompensation. Vicious circles tend to aggravate the problem. (Redrawn and reproduced, with permission, from Cohn JN et al: Hypertension and the heart. Arch Intern Med 1974;133:969.)

accelerated by hypertension from atherosclerosis that develops independently of hypertension. The lesions may appear in the aorta, the coronary arteries, the arteries to the lower extremities, and the arteries of the neck and brain (Table 9–4).

Atherosclerosis of the aorta aggravates cystic medial necrosis, which is more common in hypertensive atherosclerotic disease, and patients may develop aortic dissection pathologically indistinguishable from cystic medial necrosis in Marfan's syndrome.

The jugular venous pulse is usually normal in the absence of right ventricular failure; the carotid pulses are usually normal in volume and upstroke unless the patient has coarctation of the aorta, in which case the carotid pulse is unusually prominent and jerky. The presence of bruits over the carotid should always be sought as a possible clue to the presence of atherosclerotic disease of the internal carotid arteries. The presence or absence of pulmonary rales is valuable in recognizing early left ventricular failure. If the failure is more obvious and more severe, pulsus alternans may be noted. Particular note should be made of the volume and character of all the pulses and their symmetry on the 2 sides. This serves not only to demonstrate coarctation of the aorta if the pulses of the lower extremities are weak and delayed as compared to those of the radials but also to provide a baseline in the event the patient develops chest pain, with variation in the various pulses suggesting aortic dissection. The presence or absence of bruits should be sought, especially over the femoral and popliteal arteries, to determine the presence of atherosclerosis of these vessels. Bruits should be sought in the epigastrium and in the flanks, since they may provide clues that suggest renovascular hypertension.

Coarctation of the aorta is strongly suggested by the presence of weak or delayed femoral pulses in comparison with the radial pulses, the presence of a basal systolic ejection murmur transmitted to the interscapular area, and palpable collateral intercostal arteries along the inferior rib margins and scapular borders. The carotid pulse is unusually prominent and jerky. Examination of the abdominal aorta may reveal an aneurysm as a complication of concomitant atherosclerosis. Careful palpation below each rib should be done in a search for pulsating intercostal arteries, which are prominent in coarctation of the aorta and serve as collateral vessels to arteries below the coarctated site. (See also p 251 and Chapter 11.)

4. Kidneys–Long-standing hypertension produces progressive renal nephrosclerosis with tubular atrophy, progressive scarring of the glomeruli, and slight shrinkage of the size of the kidney. Unless malignant hypertension supervenes, the clinical findings of renal failure are uncommon; however, the kidneys are somewhat small and granular, with a thin cortex.

When the hypertension is more severe or occurs rapidly, the interlobular arteries of the kidney become involved, and there may also be focal necrosis of the renal arterioles. This combination of abnormalities impairs renal blood flow and glomerular filtration rate, which in turn increases the secretion of renin and the production of angiotensin, further impairing renal function. This sequence of events is common in accelerated, or malignant, hypertension, in which fibrinoid necrosis of arterioles, especially of the kidney, occurs (Fig 9–13).

Polycystic kidneys are suspected if the kidneys are large and easily palpable, especially in the presence of long-standing hypertension, when the kidneys would be expected to be small.

5. Brain–In long-standing hypertension, so-called Charcot-Bouchard microaneurysms (Fig 9–14) may develop in the small arteries of the brain; rupture of these small aneurysms is responsible for cerebral hem-

Table 9–4. Coronary arteriosclerosis in hypertensive and nonhypertensive patients.*

Grade of Coronary Artery Disease (Left Artery)	Percentage of Patients in Each Grade	
	Hypertensives (152 Cases)	Nonhypertensives (146 Cases)
None	11.2	71.2
Slight to moderate	50.6	26.0
Severe	38.1	2.8
Thrombus	21.0	0

*Modified from Bell ET, Clawson BJ: Primary (essential) hypertension: A study of 420 cases. *Arch Pathol* 1928;5:939. Reproduced, with permission, from Heptinstall RH: Relation of hypertension to changes in the arteries. *Prog Cardiovasc Dis* 1974;17:25.

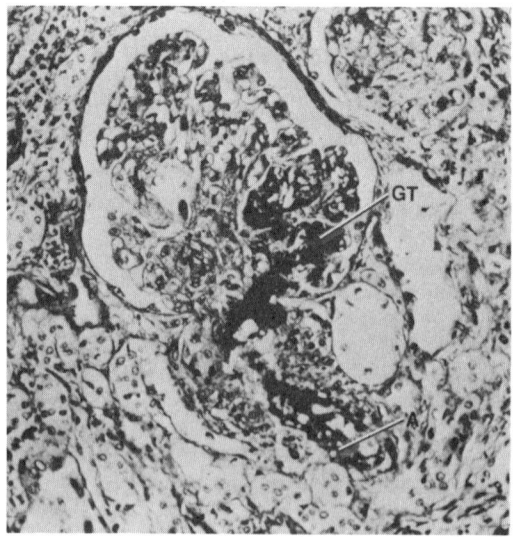

Figure 9–13. Fibrinoid necrosis in an afferent arteriole (A) extending into the glomerular tuft (GT) (Mallory's azo carmine; × 180). (Reproduced, with permission, from Kincaid-Smith P, McMichael J, Murphy EA: The clinical course and pathology of hypertension with papilloedema [malignant hypertension]. *Q J Med* 1958;27:117.)

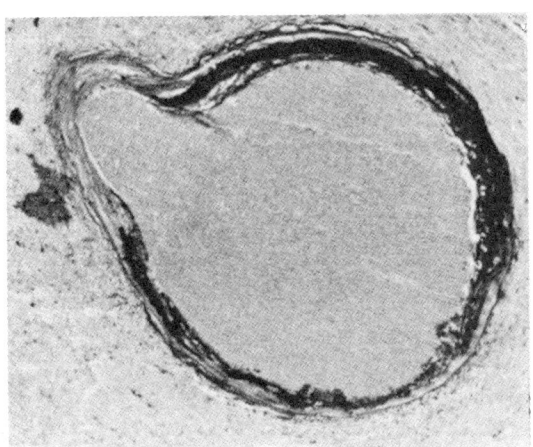

Figure 9-14. Cross section of microaneurysm showing plasma insudation of wall (PTAH; × 90). (Reproduced, with permission, from Russell RW: How does blood-pressure cause stroke? *Lancet* 1975;2:1283.)

orrhage that commonly interrupts the course of long-standing hypertension.

In addition to the microaneurysms, the brain may show atherosclerotic occlusion or thrombosis in the internal carotid, basilar, or vertebral artery system as well as thrombosis in the vessels of the circle of Willis. Cerebral infarction may then occur, although cerebral hemorrhage that may enter the cerebral ventricles may result from rupture of microaneurysms into the cerebral hemispheres. Cerebral infarction may become hemorrhagic if anticoagulants are used.

6. Central nervous system–Examination for evidence of residual neurologic deficit from previous cerebral infarction may be fruitful. There may be a positive Babinski or Hoffman reflex, hemiparesis, hemiplegia, or hemianopia. The presence of ataxia may indicate involvement of the posterior inferior cerebellar artery.

7. Endocrine dysfunction–The patient should be examined for signs suggesting any of several types of endocrine abnormalities. **Cushing's syndrome** is suspected if there is central trunk obesity, hirsutism, acne, purple striae, moon facies, and thin skin with ecchymoses. **Primary aldosteronism** is suggested by muscular weakness, hypoactive deep tendon reflexes, and diminished or absent vasomotor circulatory reflexes. **Pheochromocytoma** is suspected if an attack of headache, sweating, palpitations, and a markedly increased blood pressure is induced by an examination over the upper abdomen that presses on a tumor.

Laboratory Findings

Laboratory investigations are designed to determine the involvement of any of the target organs affected by hypertension and to recognize the presence of any evidence of secondary hypertension. (The diagnosis and details of secondary hypertension will be described later.)

A. Urinalysis: Urinalysis is usually normal until renal impairment occurs, when the specific gravity may become low and mild proteinuria may appear. In malignant hypertension there may be substantial proteinuria, approaching values suggesting nephrosis. A low fixed specific gravity suggests advanced renal parenchymal disease or the hypokalemic nephropathy of primary aldosteronism. The presence of granular or red cell casts and hematuria suggests glomerulonephritis. The presence of pyuria favors chronic pyelonephritis, but if advanced renal failure is present, the microscopic appearance of the urinary sediment is often not helpful in diagnosis. In connective tissue disorders, such as lupus erythematosus, the urine sediment may show red cells, white cells, and casts of all types at one time (Krupp, 1943).

A fresh, clean voided urine specimen should be examined for bacteria. If organisms are found, the specimen should be cultured and quantitative bacterial counts performed to establish the presence of chronic pyelonephritis. If no organisms are found but other features of the history are suggestive of urinary tract infection, cultures should be repeated, because the bacilluria in chronic pyelonephritis may be intermittent.

For details of the diagnosis of the secondary causes of hypertension, see pp 237 ff.

B. Blood Chemistry: In renal parenchymal disease, the serum creatinine and blood urea nitrogen are elevated, and anemia associated with advanced azotemia may be present. In aldosteronism, the blood urea nitrogen and serum creatinine are usually normal; renal function is not severely impaired, but the serum potassium is low, and serum sodium and bicarbonate are increased.

It usually is not necessary to do more sensitive renal function studies if the serum creatinine and blood urea nitrogen are normal; however, if the blood urea nitrogen approaches 20 mg/dL or the serum creatinine is 1.3 mg/dL or above, it is wise to determine the creatinine clearance as a measure of the glomerular filtration rate, because the latter may be reduced even though the serum creatinine may be within the normal range.

Electrocardiographic Findings

A. Left Ventricular Hypertrophy: The ECG is the most readily available specific method of establishing the presence of left ventricular hypertrophy, although left ventricular mass may precede electrocardiographic evidence of left ventricular hypertrophy (Dunn, 1977). The ECG is often abnormal when there is no left ventricular heave and when the chest x-ray shows no left ventricular enlargement. The ECG reflects hypertrophy and not dilatation, whereas the chest x-ray reveals enlargement rather than hypertrophy. The earliest electrocardiographic sign of left ventricular hypertrophy is increased voltage of the QRS complexes in the left ventricular leads. Increased amplitude (> 18 mm) of the R wave in lead X on orthogonal electrocardiography using the Frank lead system may be a better method than conventional electrocardiography in the recognition of early left ventricular hypertrophy. As hypertrophy continues, the T waves become of lower amplitude, and this change is followed by slight depression of the ST segment; later, the ST segment depression is more marked and associated with asymmetrically inverted T waves in the left ventricular leads. In the fully developed pattern, the left ventricular QRS voltage is high and the ST segment in these leads is depressed, with a convex contour followed by an asymmetrically inverted T wave. Table 9–5 gives the criteria for the diagnosis of left ventricular hypertrophy. Examples of the development and regression of the electrocardiographic changes in left ventricular hypertrophy are shown in Figs 9–15 and 9–16. Patients with increased left ventricular volume may not have the typical electrocardiographic signs of left ventricular hypertrophy, because dilatation of the left ventricle decreases the left ventricular QRS voltage. The maximum spatial QRS voltage and the R wave voltage in leads V_5 and V_6 were inversely correlated with the end-diastolic volume (Talbot, 1977).

Left ventricular echocardiography is the most sensitive aid in recognition of left ventricular hypertrophy in hypertension. Left ventricular wall thickness—the sum of the thickness of the ventricular septum and the posterior wall—correlates well with the spatial maximum QRS voltage (r = 0.67) and the sum of

Table 9–5. Criteria for diagnosis of left ventricular hypertrophy in adults over 30 years of age.

Standard limb leads
(1) Voltage $R_1 + S_3$ = 25 mm or more.
(2) RST_1 depressed 0.5 mm or more.
(3) T_1 flat, diphasic, or inverted, particularly when associated with (2) and a prominent R wave.
(4) T_2 and T_3 diphasic or inverted in the presence of tall R waves and findings in (2).
(5) T_3 greater than T_1 in the presence of left axis deviation and high voltage QRS complex in leads I and III.

Precordial leads
(1) $RV_5 + SV_1$ more than 35 mm.
(2) Tallest R + deepest S more than 45 mm.
(3) Voltage of R wave in V_5 or V_6 exceeds 26 mm.
(4) RST segment depressed more than 0.5 mm in V_4, V_5, or V_6.
(5) A flat, diphasic, or inverted T wave in leads V_{4-6} with normal R and small S waves and findings in (2).
(6) Ventricular activation time in V_5 or V_6 = 0.06 second or more, especially when associated with a tall R wave.

Unipolar limb leads
(1) RST segment depressed more than 0.5 mm in aVL or aVF.
(2) Flat, diphasic, or inverted T wave, with an R wave of 6 mm or more in aVL or aVF and findings in (1).
(3) Voltage of R wave in aVL exceeds 11 mm.
(4) Upright wave in aVR.

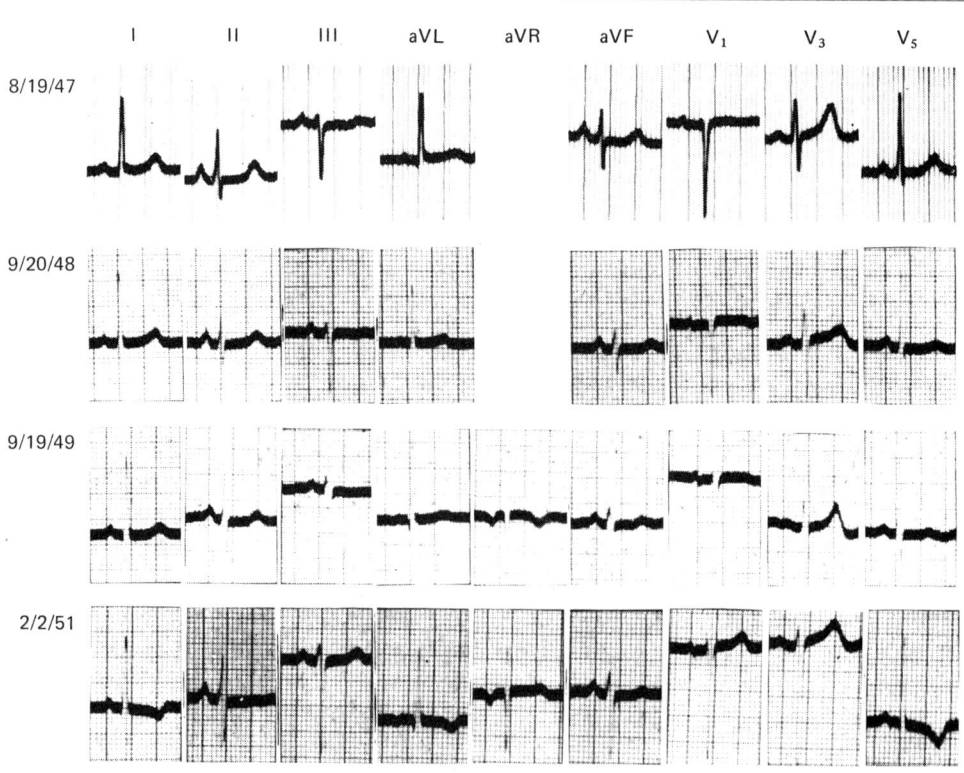

Figure 9–15. Progressive ST–T abnormalities in leads I, aVL, and V_5 between 1947 and 1951 in a 53-year-old woman. Serial chest x-rays showed no change in the size of the heart during this period. (Reproduced, with permission, from Grubschmidt HA, Sokolow M: The reliability of high voltage of the QRS complex as a diagnostic sign of left ventricular hypertrophy in adults. *Am Heart J* 1957;**54**:689.)

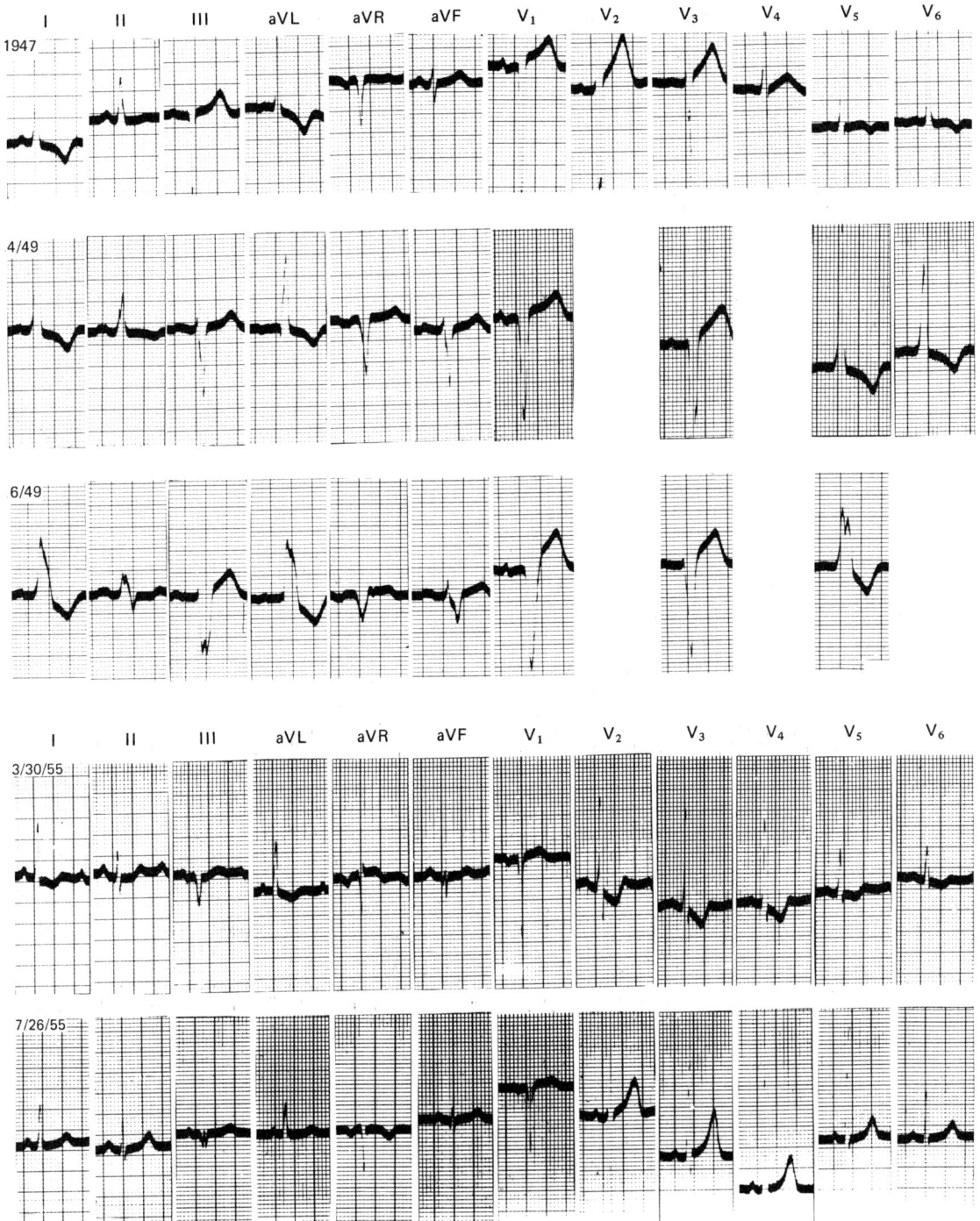

Figure 9–16. *Top:* Hypertensive cardiovascular disease and angina pectoris in a 73-year-old man. Cardiac enlargement +32%. Note progression from left ventricular hypertrophy to incomplete left bundle branch block to complete left bundle branch block with a wide monophasic QRS complex in lead I. *Bottom:* Malignant hypertension reversed to almost normotensive levels following unilateral nephrectomy in a 62-year-old man. Complete return of ST–T changes in leads V_{2-6} to normal in 4 months.

RV_5 and SV_1 (r = 0.85) (Toshima, 1977). There are significant correlations among various echocardiographic measurements, radiologic estimates of heart volume, and electrocardiographic evidence of left ventricular hypertrophy. The presence of left ventricular dilatation interferes with the echo measurement of left ventricular hypertrophy as well as with the diagnosis by electrocardiography.

B. Differentiation From Myocardial Infarction: The ST segment and T wave changes of left ventricular hypertrophy are in the same direction and are differentiated from myocardial ischemia (see Chapter 8), in which the ST segment when depressed is horizontally depressed and the T wave when inverted is symmetrically inverted with or without ST depression. The characteristic ST-T changes in left ventricular hypertrophy occur only to the left of the ventricular septum (the transitional zone), and the inverse of this pattern is present in leads to the right of the transitional zone, ie, in the right precordial leads the ST segment is elevated and there is a tall, asymmetrically elevated T wave. This is in contrast to myocardial ischemia (see Chapter 8), in which the ST and T abnormalities seen in the left ventricular leads (V_4–V_6) spread across the transitional zone and may involve V_2 and V_3 as well. The ECG may also reveal evidence of previous myocardial infarction or obvious evidence of myocardial ischemia with classic Q waves or ischemic ST segments. In patients with long-standing hypertension, especially if there have been multiple episodes of myocardial ischemia, peripheral left ventricular conduction defects may be present with slurred QRS complexes, usually with a QRS duration less than 0.12 second. Even with well-marked left ventricular hypertrophy, the frontal plane axis rarely exceeds −30 degrees; when the axis is farther to the left, in the range of −45 degrees, a left anterior hemiblock is superimposed and the axis change is not due to the left ventricular hypertrophy per se. Progressive abnormalities may include incomplete and complete left bundle branch block.

C. Effect of Drugs on ECG: It is important to know what medications the patient is receiving in order to evaluate the electrocardiographic pattern in hypertension. In hypertensive patients receiving diuretic agents with resultant hypokalemia, sagging nonspecific ST segments and prominent U waves may be present similar to those found in primary aldosteronism. If the patient has been receiving digitalis, the characteristic sagging ST segments of digitalis and the decreased QT interval due to shortening of the action potential may also be present.

X-Ray Findings

A. Plain Chest Film: The plain chest film may be completely normal despite well-marked hypertension if the concentric hypertrophy has not led to dilatation. The convex rounding of the left ventricle seen especially on the lateral views may allow the radiologist to suspect the presence of concentric hypertrophy, but it is not until left ventricular dilatation has occurred that enlargement of the left ventricle will be confirmed. The chest x-ray may show notching of the ribs in coarctation of the aorta, but this finding is rarely present before the late teen years. If there is left ventricular failure, pulmonary venous engorgement can be seen with or without diversion of blood to the upper lobes and pleural effusion. In the acute pulmonary edema of hypertension, there may be "bat's wing" densities or fluid in the interlobar spaces. The aortic knob may be enlarged and the descending aorta dilated out of proportion to the patient's age, suggesting the presence of associated aortic atherosclerosis. If the widening is excessive, chronic dissection of the aorta may be suspected; this may be confirmed by an aortogram. (For examples of chest x-rays, see Chapter 10, p 296.)

B. Intravenous Urograms: Excretory urography may provide important evidence of possible renal vascular or renal parenchymal disorders as causes of hypertension. In younger patients with severe hypertension, the presence of unilateral renal artery stenosis may be evidenced by late appearance, hyperconcentration, and late disappearance of the contrast media, and the involved kidney is usually smaller than its mate by more than 1.5 cm (see p 239).

If renovascular hypertension is suspected on the basis of the clinical picture, the presence of bruits, and the rapid sequence intravenous urographic findings, transfemoral aortography by the Seldinger technique is indicated in combination with differential renal vein renin studies only if renovascular surgery is contemplated (see p 242 for indications). Selective renal artery angiograms disclose the anatomic features of stenosis, but the functional significance of the stenosis must be determined by still another technique. The method now considered to be most reliable is the relative renal vein renin production on the 2 sides; the difference is considered significant when the renal vein renin concentration on the affected side is at least 1½ times the concentration measured on the opposite (unaffected) side. However, both false-positive and false-negative results occur, as determined by the benefits of surgery. (See p 241.) If differential renal vein renin cannot be determined, renal artery stenosis can be strongly suspected by the decrease in water and sodium, with increased osmolality and creatinine concentration on the affected side. If the selective renal arteriogram shows no lesion of the main renal artery but a suspected lesion in one of the branches, determination of renin production from different segments of the kidney may reveal a segmental lesion or renin-producing tumor (Schambelan, 1974).

COURSE & PROGNOSIS

Mild Hypertension

The average patient with mild to moderate hypertension is asymptomatic; the only abnormality is the rise in arterial pressure. The patient may complain of nonspecific headache or dizziness, but these have been shown to fluctuate with the emotional state and are unrelated to the height of the blood pressure in benign hypertension. Visual symptoms are absent or unrelated to the blood pressure.

Moderate Hypertension

Prognostic studies in untreated patients have shown that headaches and dizziness have no adverse prognostic significance unless they are associated with accelerated hypertension or with other evidence of neurologic disorder. When hypertension persists without treatment (as it almost always does), the patient may remain asymptomatic, but examination may reveal evidences of left ventricular hypertrophy as manifested by a left ventricular heave or electrocardiographic changes (see above). The retinal arterioles may become irregularly narrowed, and arteriovenous nicking with a KW II classification may develop. The development of vascular abnormalities such as left ventricular hypertrophy or retinal arteriolar changes presages the development of clinical events and is an adverse prognostic sign (Sokolow, 1961).

If there is no accelerated phase, the first symptoms may reflect the development of left ventricular failure, with dyspnea, orthopnea, and paroxysmal nocturnal dyspnea associated with pulmonary rales and x-ray evidence of pulmonary congestion.

The prognosis with respect to mortality in hypertension is related to the age, race, and sex; to the height of the blood pressure; to the initial abnormality of the fundi, ECG, and chest x-ray; and to the presence or absence of atherosclerotic complications when the patient is first seen. Figs 9–5, 9–17, and 9–18 illustrate the relationship of the mortality rate to these various factors. It should be emphasized that the mortality figures given refer to the experience in San Francisco, which is probably representative of the USA as a whole with respect to average cholesterol levels in middle-aged adults (about 240 mg/dL). The mortality rate is considerably lower in rural communities in Jamaica unless the blood pressure exceeds 180/110 (Ashcroft, 1978), perhaps in part because of the lower levels of serum cholesterol in these communities. Similar mortality data are found in some African countries where hypertension is relatively benign and does not increase the incidence of coronary disease. Both in Africa and in Jamaica, there is a low prevalence of other risk factors; acute coronary events are uncommon in these rural areas but more common in urban communities with more affluent patients.

Malignant Hypertension

Malignant hypertension is a syndrome characterized by a rapidly rising blood pressure (diastolic pressure usually in excess of 130 mm Hg) from any cause. The initial symptoms are usually severe suboccipital headaches, weakness, and visual disturbances, and the signs are papilledema, hemorrhages and exudates in the macular area, and gross hematuria (Table 9–6).

Unless effective antihypertensive therapy is given promptly, there may be severe visual loss associated

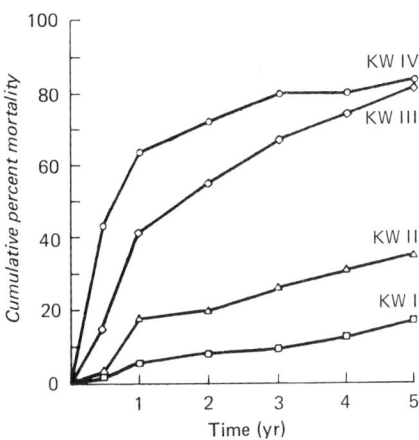

Figure 9–17. Relationship of mortality rate and initial fundal classification in hypertensive patients. (Reproduced, with permission, from the American Heart Association, Inc., Sokolow M, Perloff D: The prognosis of essential hypertension treated conservatively. *Circulation* 1961;**23**:697.)

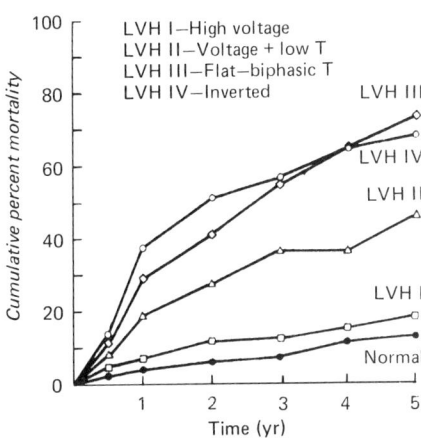

Figure 9–18. Relationship of mortality rate and initial degree of left ventricular hypertrophy (ECG) in hypertensive patients. (Reproduced, with permission, from the American Heart Association, Inc., Sokolow M, Perloff D: The prognosis of essential hypertension treated conservatively. *Circulation* 1961;**23**:697.)

with hemorrhage, exudates, and papilledema of the ocular fundi; and death due to uremia, heart failure, or cerebral hemorrhage usually occurs in less than 1 year. Pathologic changes are seen in the arterioles and in the small interlobular arteries (see Fig 9–13). The kidney is progressively destroyed by ischemic atrophy of the nephrons, with decrease in glomerular filtration rate and renal blood flow because of fibrinoid necrosis of the arterioles and cellular intimal proliferation of the interlobular arteries. Some patients with pathologically proved fibrinoid necrosis do not have pa-

Table 9–6. Symptoms marking onset of malignant phase of hypertension in 104 cases.*

Symptom	Number of Cases
Visual impairment	79
Acute headache	6
Gross hematuria	5
Visual impairment and gross hematuria	3
Acute cardiac failure	1
Gastrointestinal upset with nausea, vomiting, and epigastric pain	1
Undetermined due to vagueness of symptoms	9

*Reproduced, with permission, from Schottstaedt MF, Sokolow M: The natural history and course of hypertension with papilledema (malignant hypertension). Am Heart J 1953;45:331.

pilledema, but they usually have hemorrhages or exudates in the fundi. Prognostic studies have shown that the 3- to 5-year mortality rate is essentially indistinguishable in untreated patients with KW III fundi as compared to those with KW IV fundi; both represent accelerated hypertension.

The rapid rise in blood pressure may cause cardiac failure within 1–2 weeks and renal failure within a month. Examination of the retinas for evidence of accelerated hypertension is necessary in all hypertensive patients, because the early stages of the malignant phase may be essentially asymptomatic, although severe headache, acute visual disturbances, and gross hematuria are the usual presenting manifestations. Cardiac and renal failure may occur with great rapidity, and treatment to lower the blood pressure is urgent. Patients seen early with evidence of accelerated, or malignant, hypertension may have normal renal function and even absence of proteinuria. This rapidly progresses, however, to malignant hypertension with proteinuria and azotemia and then finally to renal failure. For this reason, treatment is essential before the development of renal failure.

Malignant hypertension is a quantitatively more severe form of hypertension, and prevention is far more effective than treatment of the established or advanced disease. Accelerated, or malignant, hypertension is rare in properly treated hypertensive patients.

If no treatment is given, the mortality rate in 1 year is 80% and in 2 years approaches 100%.

The importance of prevention of the malignant phase can be outlined as follows:

(1) Malignant hypertension is rare in the properly managed patient with benign hypertension (Smirk, 1963; Pickering, 1968).

(2) Adequate follow-up and education of the patient regarding compliance with therapy is essential. Stopping therapy in severe hypertension is hazardous.

(3) Early symptoms of accelerated disease (sudden onset of visual disturbances, severe headache, gross hematuria) should trigger therapeutic treatment.

(4) Prognosis of malignant hypertension is related to the degree of renal impairment existing when treatment began (Schottstaedt, 1952; Kincaid-Smith, 1958).

(5) Treatment of severe hypertension prevents the malignant phase; early treatment of the malignant phase prevents azotemia; treatment of azotemia without uremia prevents uremia. Rapid reduction of the blood pressure in malignant hypertension (see p 272) may induce cerebral ischemic complications; greatly elevated pressures should be reduced cautiously over a period of days and not to normal levels immediately.

(6) Mortality rate in the treatment of severe hypertension is related to the effectiveness with which the blood pressure was lowered (Farmer, 1963; Gifford, 1974; Perry, 1969; Doyle, 1975).

Development of Clinical Manifestations of Atherosclerosis

The patient may develop a symptom indicating atherosclerotic involvement in one of the major vessels. The most common is the development of angina pectoris or acute myocardial infarction, although the first manifestation may be intermittent claudication, transient ischemic cerebral attacks, or even cerebral infarction or cerebral hemorrhage.

Development of Cardiac Disease

A. Hypertensive Heart Failure: Because hypertension is the most common cause of heart failure and is the most important risk factor in accelerating coronary atherosclerosis, and because it is responsible for at least half of all deaths from heart failure and for almost all cases of cerebral hemorrhage, epidemiologists participating in the Framingham Study (Kannel, 1974) have stated that the most important means of preventing cardiovascular disease is to identify and treat hypertension before complications develop.

It is difficult to separate the effects of hypertension and coronary heart disease in causing heart failure when they coexist in the same patient. Cardiac failure is frequent, however, in young adults with coarctation of the aorta and hypertension who do not have coronary disease. The importance of treating the elevated blood pressure in such cases should be readily apparent.

Before the advent of antihypertensive therapy, heart failure was responsible for death in 25% of patients with hypertension. In a study of left ventricular failure, Bedford (1939) found that 80–85% of patients with paroxysmal dyspnea with or without angina or myocardial infarction had hypertension. Aortic valve disease was the third and least common cause of heart failure in the triad of hypertension, coronary heart disease, and aortic valve disease. The prognosis for life, once left ventricular failure with paroxysmal dyspnea or pulmonary edema occurred, was very poor. The average duration of life was 1 year, and one-third of the patients died within 6 months. Goldring and Chasis (1944), in a study of untreated hypertensive patients, found that 85% were dead within 3 years of the development of cardiac failure. (See Table 9–7.)

B. Effect of Hypertension on Coronary Disease: Coronary artery disease associated with hypertension is commonly present without development of

Table 9–7. Cause of death* in relation to initial severity of hypertension.†

Severity of Hypertension	Total Number Deaths	Cardiac Failure	"Hypertensive" Causes		Coronary Thrombosis	Cerebrovascular Accident	Aortic Dissection	Noncardiovascular Causes
			Uremia	Malignant Hypertension				
Classes I & II	32	2	0	1	8	11	0	10
Classes III & IV	121	19	9	17	25	41	3	7

*In an additional 8 patients, cause of death was unknown.
†Reproduced, with permission, from the American Heart Association, Inc., Sokolow M, Perloff D: The prognosis of essential hypertension treated conservatively. *Circulation* 1961;**23**:697.

hypertensive heart failure. The evidence supporting the role of hypertension in accelerating coronary heart disease has been corroborated by the pathologic data of Bell and Clawson and by the prospective studies of the Framingham group (see Chapter 8). Data from Bell and Clawson (1928) indicate that severe coronary disease was 10 times more common in an autopsied group of patients who had hypertension during life than in a normotensive group. Evidence of coronary disease during life was 7 times more common in the hypertensive group. They also showed a high correlation between the severity of atherosclerosis in the cerebral, carotid, and basilar-vertebral arteries and the systolic blood pressure.

Since the purely hypertensive complications of a raised pressure are prevented or reversed by antihypertensive therapy, the atherosclerotic complications predominate and are the most common cause of disability and death in treated hypertensive patients. Therefore, coronary heart disease in all of its manifestations, cerebral infarction, cerebral hemorrhage, and carotid and extremity atherosclerosis, although particularly prevalent in the hypertensive population, cannot be distinguished from the same manifestations in the nonhypertensive but atherosclerotic population.

Effect of Antihypertensive Therapy on Prognosis

The introduction of effective antihypertensive therapy has changed the picture dramatically. Table 9–8, from the Veterans Administration Cooperative Study, documents the considerable decrease in morbid events in the treated group as compared to the control, untreated group. Morbid events included hypertensive complications such as heart failure, cerebral hemorrhage, accelerated or malignant hypertension, or dissection of the aorta. Not only is heart failure reversed by antihypertensive therapy, but the development of heart failure during adequate therapy is rare, indicating the dominant role played by elevated blood pressure in the development of heart failure. At present, no more than 5% of all deaths in hypertensive patients receiving effective treatment are due to heart failure, although the combination of myocardial infarction and hypertension may lead to ischemic cardiomyopathy and heart failure. Eighty percent of patients with hypertensive heart failure treated by Smirk (1963) were leading unimpaired lives 2–7 years after treatment—in marked contrast to Goldring's (1944) data, which showed that only one-fourth of such patients survived for 3 years.

The rapid response of heart failure in hypertensive patients to antihypertensive therapy is much more striking than the response of heart failure to medical treatment in patients with coronary heart disease without hypertension who develop ischemic cardiomyopathy following myocardial infarction.

COMPLICATIONS

Most complications of hypertensive disease are discussed elsewhere (cardiac failure, p 287; malignant hypertension, p 231; hemorrhagic stroke, p 220; myocardial infarction, p 163; transient ischemic attacks, p 604; cerebral infarction, p 177). Aortic dissection

Table 9–8. Incidence of morbid events with respect to level of prerandomization blood pressure.*

Prerandomization Blood Pressure (mm Hg)	Control Group			Treated Group			Percent Effectiveness
	Patients Randomized	Patients With "Morbid Event"		Patients Randomized	Patients With "Morbid Event"		
		Number	Percent		Number	Percent	
Systolic < 165	98	15	15.3	108	10	9.3	40
Systolic 165+	96	41	42.7	78	12	15.4	64
Total	194	56		186	22		
Diastolic 90–104	84	21	25.0	86	14	16.3	35
Diastolic 105–114	110	35	31.8	100	8	8.0	75
Total	194	56		186	22		

*Reproduced, with permission, from Veterans Administration Cooperative Study Group on Antihypertensive Agents: Effects of treatment on morbidity in hypertension. *JAMA* 1970;**213**:1143. Copyright © American Medical Association.

is discussed below. In general, the presence of a significant complication warrants hospitalization so that patients can be given appropriate treatment for severe hypertension. Ancillary methods of treatment should not be neglected, such as digitalis in cardiac failure, anticoagulants and surgical correction of the carotid artery lesion in transient ischemic attacks, and, if necessary, surgery in aortic dissection. Treatment of the elevated blood pressure is usually of less importance than other approaches in patients with angina pectoris, myocardial infarction, or atherosclerosis of the legs with intermittent claudication. The pressure may be high in hemorrhagic stroke and hypertensive encephalopathy with neurologic deficit; these patients should have their blood pressure lowered cautiously, as described under malignant hypertension.

It has been shown that hypertension is the most important of the known risk factors for the development of cardiovascular disease. The vascular complications of hypertension are the consequences of raised arterial pressure and of the associated atherosclerosis of major arterial circuits. After a follow-up of 18 years, 105 cerebral infarctions occurred in the Framingham Study, only 10 of which occurred in normotensive persons. Hypertension is the most common and most important precursor of cerebral infarction in stroke (Kannel, 1974, 1976).

Hypertensive Encephalopathy

This syndrome results from a rapid, marked increase in blood pressure, causing increased vascular permeability and cerebral edema and resulting in an acute neurologic clinical state that may be rapidly reversible if treated early and vigorously but may develop into malignant hypertension if not managed properly. The patient complains of severe headache, confusion, impaired vision, restlessness, and perhaps focal neurologic signs and appears to have developed acute malignant hypertension. There may be cotton wool patches in the retina or early papilledema, and the differentiation from malignant hypertension may be difficult. Rapid but graduated reduction of blood pressure (see p 272) usually reverses the process before complications in the kidney and heart develop.

Dissection of the Aorta

One of the complications of hypertension that often is unrecognized, especially in pregnant women, is dissection of the aorta. Early diagnosis is most important in order to initiate treatment to lower the pressure. The current status of diagnosis and treatment is summarized by Wheat (1980) and Doroghazi (1981). Hypertension is the presumed cause in one-third of cases of proximal and two-thirds of cases of distal dissection (Slater, 1976). Cystic medial necrosis and arteriosclerosis are much less common causes. The onset is usually acute (90% of cases), with severe instantaneous chest pain radiating to the neck, jaw, back, or abdomen combined with evidence of varying or sequential obstruction of the branches of the aorta and diminished or absent pulses from the carotids to the femoral arteries. Neurologic symptoms and signs occur in about 15% of patients. In rare instances, the dissection is painless or relatively so. The diagnosis, location, and extent of the dissection can be established by supravalvular angiography, although it can be strongly suspected clinically and radiologically (Table 9–9 and Figs 9–19 and 9–20). If one records a widened aorta or a double echo in the aorta with an oscillating intimal flap in the presence of clinical evidence of aortic root dissection, the diagnosis can also be suspected on the basis of 2-dimensional echocardiography. Caution should be exercised before relying exclusively on the echocardiogram, because false-positive and false-negative characteristics are frequent. CT scans can demonstrate dissection, but until more evidence is available, supravalvular angiography is the method of choice to determine the presence, location, and extent of the dissection. The abrupt development of chest pain, aortic insufficiency, diminished or absent pulses, or the appearance of signs of "sympathectomy" on one side and of neurologic deficit with cerebral symptoms should make one think of dissection of the aorta. The pain may be differentiated from that of acute myocardial infarction by its instantaneous onset, its severity, the absence of central pulses, and the presence of hypertension despite pain or even shock. Aortic dissection has been classified as type I, which involves the proximal ascending aorta and aortic arch, at times extending distally to the iliac arteries; type II, which involves only the ascending aorta and is sometimes combined with type I and called proximal dissection; and type III, which involves only the distal aorta beyond the left subclavian artery. Types I and II may involve the aortic valve, causing aortic insufficiency and heart failure, and are more serious than type III. The pathogenesis of dissection is illustrated in Fig 9–21.

In type I and II (proximal) dissection the mortality rate is high, aortic insufficiency may occur, and the aorta may rupture into the pericardium or pleura; after immediate lowering of the blood pressure with parenteral antihypertensive agents and establishment of the diagnosis by supravalvular aortography, surgical treatment is recommended. Without treatment the

Table 9–9. Roentgenographic findings in aortic dissection.*

Abnormalities on Chest Roentgenogram	Dissection	
	Proximal (n = 45) Percent	Distal (n = 71) Percent
Definitely abnormal aortic contour	34	64
"Possibly" abnormal aorta	8	5
Normal chest roentgenogram	3	2
"Calcium" sign	0	10
Pleural effusion	2	9

*Reproduced, with permission, from Slater EE, DeSanctis RW: The clinical recognition of dissecting aortic aneurysm. Am J Med 1976;60:625.

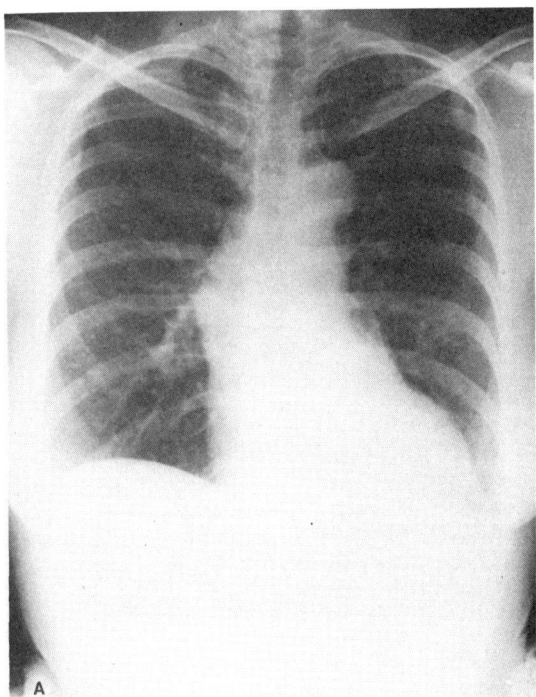
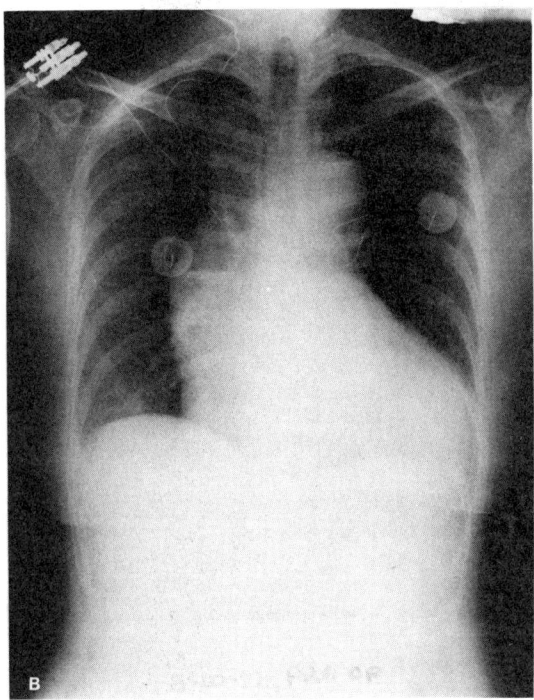
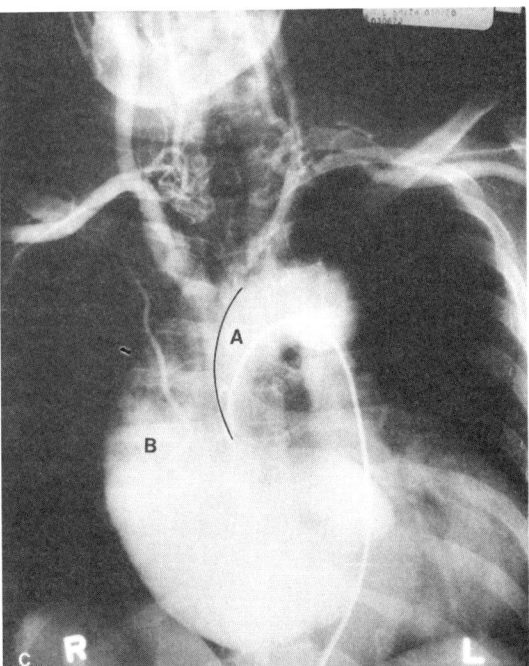
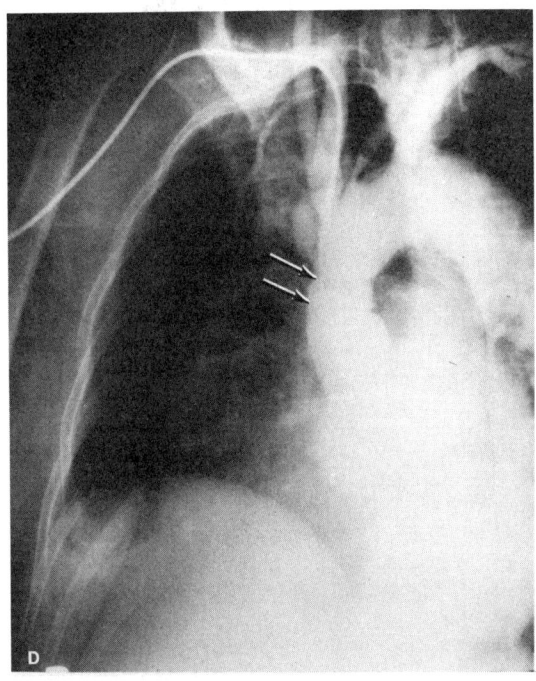

Figure 9–19. Dissection of the aorta in hypertension in a 52-year-old man with severe chest pain. *A:* 3/6/72—Plain chest film predissection showing dilated ascending aorta in asymptomatic patient. *B:* 3/10/72—Preoperative plain chest film postdissection after sudden severe chest pain showing massive dilatation of the ascending and descending aorta with striking changes since *A*. *C:* 3/7/72—Aortogram showing the true channel (A) and the aneurysmal sac (B), partially filled with contrast medium. The dark line shows the separation between the true and false channels. *D:* 3/28/72—Postoperative angiogram after resection of the ascending aorta and aneurysmal sac and insertion of a Dacron graft (see arrow) from the ascending aorta. Pathologic focal degeneration of media and intimal fibrosis.

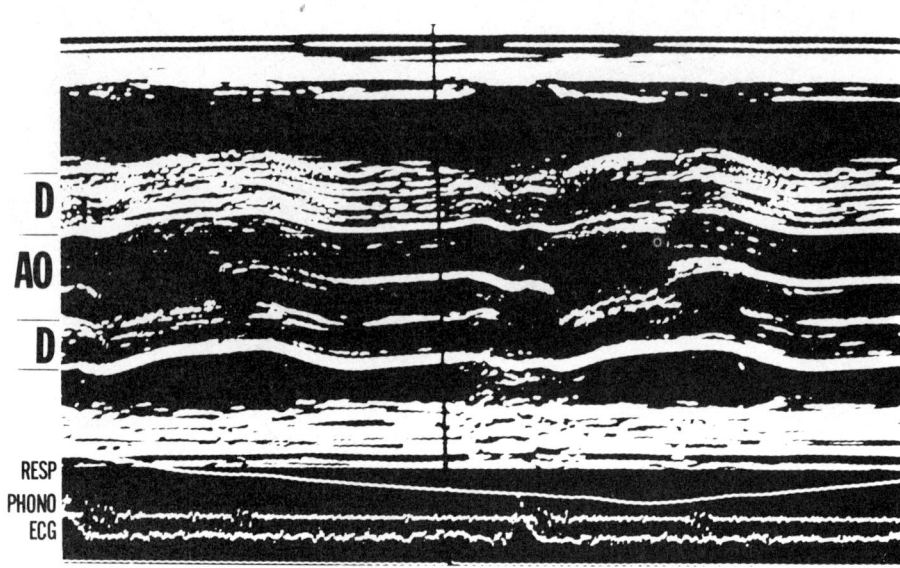

Figure 9–20. Aortic root echogram reveals marked parallel widening of both anterior and posterior walls. Aortic valve cusps are slender and show normal motion pattern. D, width of the dissecting hematoma; AO, aorta; RESP, respirations; PHONO, phonocardiogram; ECG, electrocardiogram. (Reproduced, with permission, from the American Heart Association, Inc., Nanda NC, Gramiak R, Shah PM: Diagnosis of aortic root dissection by echocardiography. *Circulation* 1973;**48**:506.)

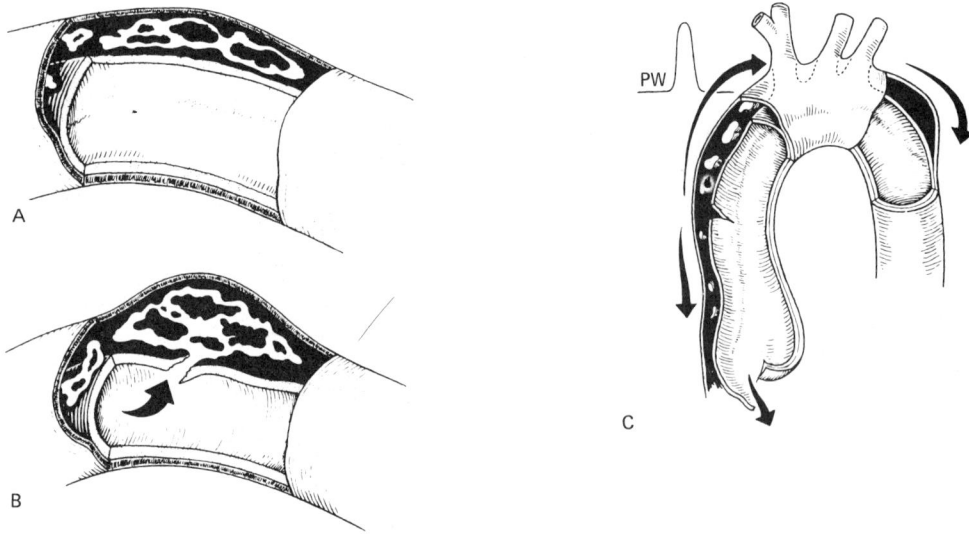

Figure 9–21. Diagrammatic representation of pathogenesis of aortic dissection. *A:* Cystic medial necrosis in the aortic wall sets the stage. *B:* Combined forces acting on the aortic wall result in the intimal tear, directing aortic bloodstream into the diseased media. *C:* Resulting dissecting hematoma is propagated by the pulse wave (PW) produced by each myocardial contraction. (Reproduced, with permission, from Wheat MW: Treatment of dissecting aneurysms of the aorta: Current status. *Prog Cardiovasc Dis* 1973;**16**:87.)

mortality rate is very high, but with modern surgical treatment survival may be as high as 75%.

Dissection involving the distal aorta (distal dissection) may be monitored in the intensive care unit and treated medically with drugs that both lower the arterial pressure and reduce the force and velocity of left ventricular ejection into the weakened aorta. Severe pain is relieved promptly once the arterial pressure has been reduced to the lowest possible level compatible with adequate perfusion of the vital circuits of the body. Intensive antihypertensive therapy includes (see also p 272) sodium nitroprusside or trimethaphan (Arfonad) infusion combined with beta-blocking agents; surgical treatment is reserved for the patient who fails to respond. When intensive intravenous hypotensive therapy is used, the renal output must be carefully monitored and not allowed to decrease below 20 or 30 mL/h.

The prognosis for untreated aortic dissection is poor (Fig 9–22). When the dissection is confined to the distal aorta, medical antihypertensive treatment permits most patients to survive without operation. In proximal aortic dissections, the prognosis is poor with medical treatment, because of the risks of aortic insufficiency, cardiac failure, rupture of the hematoma, or progression of the dissection, and surgical treatment is advised. The indications for prompt surgical therapy are summarized in Table 9–10. With surgical treatment of proximal dissections, the mortality rate has decreased from 80% in 2 weeks to 15–20%. Medical treatment should be continued even though dissection has been treated surgically, both in order to prevent a subsequent tear and to control the complications of hypertension.

Table 9–10. Specific complications requiring strong consideration for surgical therapy.*

Overwhelming aortic insufficiency
Progressive heart failure
Occlusion of major aortic branches
Progressive symptoms
Continuing dissection
Pain after hypertension is controlled
Uncontrolled bleeding into left side of chest
Hemopericardium and tamponade
Widening of mediastinum on x-ray study
Impending rupture as shown by x-ray study
   Shift of left border of descending aorta to the left
   Loss of sharpness of border of retrocardiac aortic shadow
   Hazy markings in left lower lung field
   Left pleural effusion
   Enlarging para-aortic mass
   Patchy infiltration or "ray"-like infiltration of adjacent lung field

*Modified slightly and reproduced, with permission, from Anagnostopoulos CE, Prabhakar MJS, Kittle CF: Aortic dissections and dissecting aneurysms. *Am J Cardiol* 1972;**30**:263.

DISEASES & DISORDERS ASSOCIATED WITH SECONDARY HYPERTENSION

In secondary hypertension there may be pathologic evidence of primary disease in the kidney, the endocrine glands, or the aorta. Adenoma of the zona glomerulosa of the adrenal cortex is the usual pathologic finding in primary aldosteronism, although bilateral adrenal hyperplasia may be noted in some instances. Cushing's disease is due to a tumor, often microscopic, of the basophilic or chromophobe cells of the anterior pituitary gland, causing increased secretion of ACTH, which stimulates the adrenal glands to secrete excess cortisol (see p 246). Less commonly, Cushing's syndrome may be due to a benign adenoma of the adrenal gland, an ectopic ACTH-producing tumor, or exogenous corticosteroid or ACTH therapy (see p 246). Unsuspected coarctation of the aorta may be found at autopsy. This is also true of unsuspected pheochromocytoma, which may originate in any part of the chromaffin system. Renal vascular stenosis is rarely overlooked at autopsy today because it is routine to examine the initial portion of the renal artery arising from the aorta. Pathologically, renal vascular stenosis may be due either to atherosclerosis of the proximal part of the renal artery or to fibromuscular hyperplasia with aneurysm formation in the more distal portions of the renal artery. Aneurysm, arteriovenous fistula, and other uncommon vascular anomalies may also be found.

A wide variety of systemic diseases may cause vasculitis that results in hypertension. The patholo-

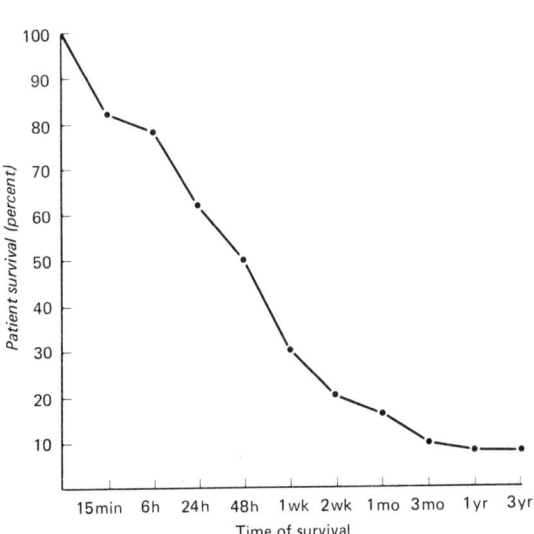

Figure 9–22. Graphic illustration of the length of survival of 963 patients with acute aortic dissection who were not treated. (Reproduced, with permission, from Wheat MW: Treatment of dissecting aneurysms of the aorta: Current status. *Prog Cardiovasc Dis* 1973;**16**:87; as modified from Anagnostopoulos CE, Prabhaker MJS, Kittle CF: Aortic dissections and dissecting aneurysms. *Am J Cardiol* 1972;**30**:263.)

gist, therefore, may find evidence of scleroderma, polyarteritis nodosa, lupus erythematosus, rheumatoid arthritis, or nonspecific arteritis. Disease of the brain (eg, brain tumor) is sometimes an unexpected finding as a cause of raised arterial pressure secondary to increased intracranial pressure or disease of the fourth ventricle.

In summary, the pathologic features may be predominantly in the arterioles, may extend to the small interlobular arteries of the kidney, or may involve the major arteries in the body with atherosclerosis, leading to the consequences that follow all varieties of atherosclerosis. In addition, there may be cardiac hypertrophy, cerebral hemorrhage, aortic dissection, and fundal changes or necrotizing lesions in the kidney following malignant hypertension.

Prevalence of Secondary Hypertension

The frequency of secondary hypertension in the hypertensive population at large has apparently been considerably overestimated, presumably because most of the reported studies have dealt with hospitalized patients. In a study of 686 randomly selected patients, 95% of cases of hypertension were due to primary hypertension, and the majority of the remaining 5% were due to renal parenchymal disease (Wilhelmsen, 1977). This finding of low frequency of secondary hypertension was supported by a study of over 26,000 patients from the Mayo Clinic in which the prevalence of surgically treatable secondary causes of hypertension was less than 0.05% per year; if patients whose diastolic pressures were 105 mm Hg or more were considered, the frequency of operations was tripled (Tucker, 1977). The vigor with which diagnostic investigations for secondary hypertension are carried out obviously influences the frequency with which it is found. A higher percentage of renal artery stenosis amenable to surgery was found at the Cleveland Clinic, probably because renal arteriograms were performed in a higher percentage of cases than at the Mayo Clinic (Gifford, 1977). Regardless of the precise figures, the data from these 2 series should emphasize to the practicing physician that surgically curable secondary hypertension is infrequent, especially if invasive procedures to rule out such conditions are being considered.

1. RENAL ARTERY STENOSIS

The most common cause of significant renal artery stenosis is atherosclerosis, followed by fibromuscular hyperplasia; small renal artery; small kidney; and miscellaneous lesions, including thrombosis, aneurysm, and fibrosis (Sokolow, 1966).

The vascular complications can often be managed by medical antihypertensive therapy in less severe cases. Operation is associated with significant morbidity and mortality rates in older people with atherosclerotic renal artery stenosis due to clinical atherosclerosis elsewhere in the vascular system. Furthermore, surgical or angioplastic relief of the obstruction does not always cure the hypertension even in patients whose renal artery stenosis has been proved by selective renal angiography and differential renal vein renin concentration. Significant improvement occurs in about 75% of patients with fibromuscular hyperplasia and about 50% of those with atherosclerotic renal artery stenosis.

A primary role for the renin-angiotensin system was strengthened when Gutmann (1973) demonstrated a marked increase in plasma renin within a few minutes after ligating the renal artery in a dog. Barger (1979) further established the role of the renin-angiotensin system by showing the marked change in blood pressure when converting enzyme inhibitors are given and then withdrawn in these experimental dogs. However, plasma renin has usually been normal in proved renal artery stenosis in humans, so other pathogenetic factors are clearly involved.

The kidney has been shown to produce antihypertensive factors that counteract the effects of constricting one renal artery in the dog. When the uninvolved kidney is removed, the rise in blood pressure is more brisk and more sustained, indicating that the normal kidney has an antihypertensive function. Antihypertensive medullary vasodilator lipid and tissue substances such as kinins and prostaglandins have been obtained from the kidney and may counteract the renin-angiotensin factors that elevate blood pressure (Muirhead, 1975). A decrease in prostaglandin E, prostacyclin, or kallikrein or an increase in bradykinin all have been considered possible pathogenetic factors. There may be a local homeostatic balance between agents that tend to increase arteriolar vasoconstriction and those that produce vasodilatation; this balance can be disturbed by a decrease in bradykinin or prostaglandins, and the result is vasoconstriction.

The complex hormonal action of angiotensin II and the role of long-term control of blood pressure or of sodium in the pathogenesis of renal hypertension are incompletely understood. Although the renin-angiotensin system seems to be an integral part of the problem, the characterization of the various converting enzymes and their inhibitors; the role of extrarenal renin; and the involvement of other humoral, neurogenic, and immunogenic factors need to be integrated (Bumpus, 1977).

Clinical Findings

There are no distinctive symptoms that separate primary from secondary hypertension due to renal artery stenosis. Factors that favor a diagnosis of renal vascular hypertension are a negative family history of hypertension, the presence of a systolic or diastolic epigastric bruit transmitted to the flanks, accelerated (malignant) hypertension, hypertension appearing for the first time after age 50, or significant x-ray findings (see below). Table 9–11 shows the comparative clinical characteristics of essential hypertension versus renovascular hypertension cured by surgery.

Table 9-11. Clinical characteristics of essential hypertension and renovascular hypertension cured by surgery.*†

	Essential Hypertension (Percent)	Renovascular Hypertension (Percent)
Duration of hypertension		
< 1 year	12	24
>10 years	15	6
Age at onset (> 50 years)	9	15
Family history of hypertension	71	46
Fundi, grade III or IV	7	15
Bruit		
Abdomen	6	46
Flank	1	12
Abdomen or flank	7	48
Blood urea nitrogen > 20 mg/dL	8	15
Serum K < 3.4 meq/L	8	16
Serum CO_2 > 30 meq/L	5	17
Urinary casts	9	20
Proteinuria (trace or more)	32	46

*Reproduced, with permission, from Maxwell MH: Cooperative study of renovascular hypertension: Current status. *Kidney Int [Suppl]* 1975;8:S153.
†Patients were matched (131 pairs) by age, sex, race, and diastolic blood pressure (from Maxwell).

A. X-Ray Findings:

1. Intravenous urogram—Rapid sequence intravenous urogram suggests renal artery stenosis if it shows one kidney to be shorter than the other by 1.5 cm or more, with delayed appearance, hyperconcentration, and delayed emptying of the contrast medium. The most reliable of these signs is delay in appearance of the contrast medium in the calices on one side. One- and 2-minute films should be obtained to look for the early delay in appearance time; in later films the disparity may be lost. The difference in size of the 2 kidneys is less helpful because occasionally there may be a difference of 1.5–2 cm in size of the 2 kidneys without other abnormality. Hyperconcentration is due to increased reabsorption of water from a proximal tubule with normal reabsorption of sodium. The reduced volume of fluid with a high sodium concentration reaching the distal tubule results in a relatively greater concentration of the contrast medium. Recognition of increased concentration is sometimes difficult because of differences in the anteroposterior depth of the 2 kidneys, and one should examine the 2 ureters for confirmation. Delayed uptake and excretion of radioisotopes on the affected side may be seen also in a triple radioisotope renogram (see p 242). Notching of the ureters is a helpful sign of increased collateral circulation that, as with arterial stenosis elsewhere, reflects a significant hemodynamic stenosis. Seventy to 80% of patients with renal artery stenosis have positive urologic signs on the rapid sequence intravenous urogram, but both false-positive and false-negative results are reported. A completely negative intravenous urogram suggests the probable absence of renovascular hypertension, but 20–25% of patients with proved renovascular hypertension have a negative intravenous urogram. Figs 9–23 and 9–24 show typical radiologic findings of renal artery stenosis. Atrophic or hypoplastic kidneys shown on the intravenous urogram are a special problem. The small size of a kidney on one side is more apt to be due to

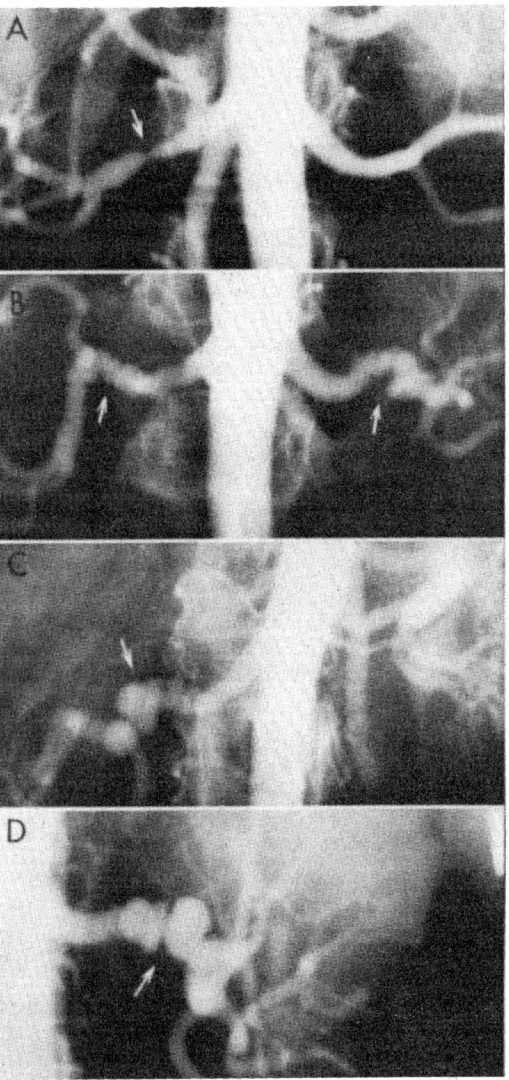

Figure 9–23. Examples of fibromuscular hyperplasia of the renal arteries. *A* and *D*, unilateral; *B* and *C*, bilateral. In *C*, the disease on the left is obscured by the tortuous overlapping vessel; upright arteriograms or studies with the patient in deep inspiration would have better defined the lesion on the left. In *B*, the pathologic changes extend into the branches of the main renal arteries, and in *C* and *D*, aneurysms are present. (Reproduced, with permission, from Palubinskas AJ, Perloff D, Wylie EJ: Curable hypertension due to renal artery lesions. *Radiologia Clinica* 1964;33:207. S Karger AG, Basel.)

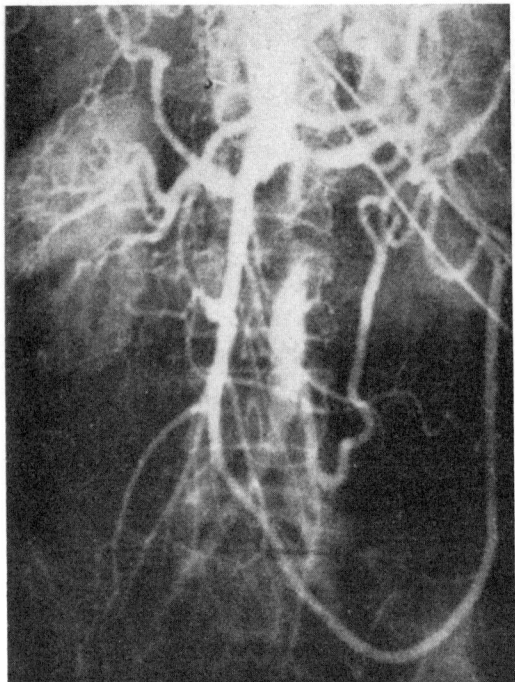

Figure 9–24. Aortogram of a 46-year-old woman; complete obstruction of the abdominal aorta and stenosis of the proximal portion of the left renal artery were found at operation to be due to atherosclerosis. (Reproduced, with permission from the American Heart Association, Inc., Perloff D et al: Hypertension secondary to renal artery occlusive disease. *Circulation* 1961;**24**:1286.)

Table 9–12. Urographic signs suggesting renovascular disease in hypertensive patients.*

Decreased renal size—disparity in renal pole-to-pole diameter of more than 1.5 cm.

Unilateral delay in appearance time of the contrast medium in the pelvic caliceal collecting system of the involved or more severely involved kidney in the early films.

Late hyperconcentration of contrast medium.

Ureteral notching suggesting the presence of pelvic-ureteral collateral vessels.

Delayed washout of pelvic caliceal contrast medium with diuresis.

Nonfunctioning kidney on excretory urogram, with normal retrograde pyelogram.

Defect in renal silhouette suggestive of segmental renal infarction.

*Reproduced, with permission, from Youngberg SP, Sheps SG, Strong CG: Management of the patient with renovascular hypertension. *Am Heart J* 1977;**94**:785.

a small or stenotic renal artery than to congenital atrophy or chronic pyelonephritis. If the renal vein renin determination indicates a lesion in the atrophic kidney, surgical treatment is indicated.

Despite the value of the rapid sequence intravenous urogram in the recognition of renovascular hypertension, one should not perform the procedure unless one is prepared to go further to establish the diagnosis by renal vein renin determinations and surgery if the studies show definitive abnormalities. The procedure should not be routinely done, because most patients have essential hypertension, not renal artery stenosis, and because of the length of time and the expense of the procedure. These same comments are even more pertinent in the case of determining differential renal vein renin, especially since the total number of patients who have surgically correctable hypertension is a very small percentage of the hypertensive population at large. Urographic signs suggesting renovascular disease in hypertensive patients are outlined in Table 9–12.

2. Renal angiogram—The indications for renal angiography are controversial. Hypertension developing for the first time after age 50 when there is reliable documentation of previously normal blood pressures or severe or malignant hypertension occurring in a patient of any age, especially if the patient is not known to have primary renal disease, requires a renal arteriogram to exclude surgically treatable disease. Other indications are shown in Table 9–13.

Table 9–13. Frequency of major occlusive renal artery disease in relation to clinical indications for arteriography.*

	Patients With Abnormal Arteriogram		Patients With Normal Arteriogram		Total Patients
	Number	Percent	Number	Percent	Cases
Aortoiliac atherosclerosis	60	73	22	27	82
Onset of hypertension over age 50	33	70	15	30	48
Epigastric bruit	108	64	59	36	167
KW III or IV fundi	28	52	26	48	54
Abnormal intravenous pyelogram	94	41	132	59	226
Recent onset of hypertension	70	40	101	60	171
Recent increase in hypertension	31	37	51	63	82
Onset of hypertension under age 20	7	13	46	87	53
Hypertension without other indications	4	10	35	90	39

*Reproduced, with permission, from Sokolow M et al: Current experiences with renovascular hypertension. Page 341 in: *Proceedings of the International Club on Arterial Hypertension.* Expansion Scientitique Francaise, 1966.

Younger individuals (under age 40), especially women, are more apt to have fibromuscular hyperplasia or some unusual renal vascular lesion other than atherosclerosis and are apt to have a less severe variety of hypertension. These patients deserve study with invasive techniques if they have an epigastric bruit and classic changes on the intravenous urogram, because the surgical mortality rate is low and complete cure of hypertension is possible.

B. Laboratory Findings:

1. Assessment of differential renal function (Howard or Stamey test)–Differential renal function measurement by the Howard or Stamey test is not often done today, having been replaced by differential renal vein renin determinations or by the vasodepressor response to angiotensin blockade. The substantial morbidity rate from catheterization of the ureters and the difficulty of accurate collection of specimens because of the long time involved for the study have made split function tests relatively uncommon except in hospitals in which renal vein renin levels or saralasin (an inhibitor of already formed angiotensin II) responses with or without moderate sodium depletion cannot be obtained, or when the differential renal vein renins are equivocal. Decreased glomerular filtrate and renal blood flow in renal artery stenosis causes a smaller volume of glomerular filtrate to enter the proximal tubule, resulting in the excretion from the affected side of a low volume of urine with a low sodium concentration but a high creatinine concentration and high osmolality.

2. Renal vein renin determination–It has long been postulated that hypertension due to renal ischemia results from increased secretion of renin. What has not been explained is why many patients with renovascular hypertension have normal plasma renin concentration, possibly due to dilution from the normal kidney. It has been shown that when the renal blood pressure was experimentally lowered in dogs, the renal vein renin increased within 1 minute and the arterial pressure rose within 5 minutes, showing the rapid response of the renin-angiotensin system in the regulation of arterial pressure (Haber, 1976). Whether the raised renin is the effect or the cause has not been established. Angiotensin-inhibiting agents also prevent the rise in blood pressure. Various studies have shown that a low plasma renin concentration argues against renovascular hypertension but a normal plasma renin concentration does not; a raised plasma renin level is often absent except in severe hypertension.

a. Differential renal vein renin levels–Much more helpful than single renal vein renins or plasma renin in determining the functional significance of renal artery stenosis is assessment of differential renal vein renin, with a ratio of at least 1.5:1, but preferably 2:1, representing a positive test. Blood from selected tributaries of the renal vein should be obtained to localize an area with an abnormally high renin content when segmental disease or renin-producing tumor is suspected. Schambelan (1973) has found abnormal amounts of renin from branches of the renal vein in segmental disease in which renin from the main renal vein was normal. Differential renal vein renin has been particularly valuable in predicting the results of surgical repair of renal artery stenosis, in contrast to renal arteriography, which displays the anatomic disease. Bookstein (1975), however, has shown that the arteriographic demonstration of collateral circulation, either periureteral collaterals with irregular narrowing of the ureter or tortuous collaterals within the kidney, is a good sign of a hemodynamically significant stenosis. When the renal vein renin concentration on one side is more than 1½–2 times that on the opposite side, 80–90% of patients benefit from surgical repair of the stenosis. About half of patients with equivalent renal vein renins on the 2 sides, in the presence of anatomically proved stenosis, benefit from surgery (Table 9–14). The variable results may be explained in various ways as follows: (1) one-fourth to one-third of patients with renovascular hypertension have bilateral lesions; (2) the methods of determining renal vein renin are not without defects; (3) renal vein renin is sometimes estimated without stimulation of renin release by depletion of sodium or upright posture; or (4) drugs that decrease renin release, such as propranolol or methyldopa, may not be stopped before the study, either because the physician fails to appreciate their importance or because the hypertension is so severe that the physician is reluctant to stop antihypertensive therapy.

b. Technical problems in prognosis–The technical problem of making certain of the location of the catheter may be pertinent in determining segmental disease. It is not known why 20% of operations in patients with a positive 1.5:1 differential renal vein renin ratio are failures or why 50% of operations in patients with an equivalent or lesser ratio are successful. Nevertheless, the combination of localized anatomic stenosis associated with collateral vessels on renal arteriography and an abnormal differential

Table 9–14. Operative outcome in hypertensive patients with and without lateralizing renal vein renin (RVR) ratios.*

	Summary of Literature Review (Kaufman, 1975)	Present Data	Total
Number of patients	412	56	468
Patients with lateralizing (1.4–2.5) RVR ratios			
Cured or improved	267	24	291
Failed	19	3	22
Patients without lateralizing RVR ratios			
Cured or improved	64	24	88
Failed	62	5	67

*Adapted and reproduced, with permission, from Stamey TA: Unilateral renal disease causing hypertension. *JAMA* 1976; **235**:2340; modified from Kaufman JJ: Progress in the diagnosis and management of renovascular hypertension. *Urol Digest* 1975;**14**:12.

renal vein renin ratio provides the best means of predicting surgical benefit.

These special invasive techniques should not be advised unless the patient's clinical status is such that surgical treatment can be recommended if the structural findings and functional studies are clear-cut. They should not be done in cases where manifestations of atherosclerotic disease elsewhere would be contraindications to operation.

3. Inhibitors of the renin-angiotensin system–Agents that either inhibit the generation of angiotensin II from angiotensin I (such as the converting enzyme inhibitors captropril or enalapril) or inhibit already formed angiotensin II (by their affinity for its receptor) have been used in an attempt not only to recognize renin-dependent hypertension due to renal artery stenosis but also to predict the results of surgery. These studies have been combined with renal vein renin comparisons between the 2 kidneys and with and without the use of furosemide. The results in various series have been conflicting; the depressor response to saralasin, renal vein renin differences, and plasma renal activity, alone or in combination, have not been as predictive as the early results implied. Failure of the blood pressure to return to normal or to be significantly diminished may occur despite all the so-called favorable test responses. It is clear that none of the tests are without error. The decision to operate must take all clinical factors into consideration, especially the duration and severity of hypertension and the congruence of various tests. Factors that influence plasma renin activity, such as sodium depletion or sympathetic nervous system activity, plus other factors that influence the tests have diminished the appeal of pharmacologic testing to predict surgical results.

C. Radioisotopic Kidney Studies: Isotopic renograms have been used by many physicians to evaluate the vascularity of each kidney in an effort to determine the presence of regional or localized renal ischemia that might cause renovascular hypertension. Double or triple isotopes have been used (such as the combination of chlormerodrin Hg 203, which shows scars and other renal parenchymal defects; technetium Tc99m, which allows recognition of reduced renal blood flow by diminished uptake of the isotope by the kidney; and iodohippurate I131, which reflects transit time through the kidney and reveals ischemia). Technical difficulties with the method and the frequency of false-positive and false-negative studies have minimized the value of radioactive scans in the diagnosis of renovascular hypertension, but the method is valuable in the follow-up of patients who have had renovascular surgery. Renal scans continue to be important in the diagnosis of renal tumors.

Treatment

Treatment consists of routine medical management as in essential hypertension (see pp 254, 258), surgery, or percutaneous transluminal angioplasty.

A. Surgical Treatment:
1. Selection of patients–As suggested above, the question of how far one should go to search for renal artery stenosis is controversial. Although the number of patients who have surgically correctable renal artery stenosis is small, the benefit to the few is great if they can be identified. Intravenous urography and search for renal artery stenosis by renal angiography, renal vein renin, and possibly angiotensin inhibitors are best confined to younger individuals with severe hypertension and minimal atherosclerosis elsewhere whose hypertension has appeared recently and to those in whom antihypertensive therapy has not been effective. Surgical treatment should be confined to patients with severe hypertension who have a functionally significant renovascular lesion, especially if renal function is unilaterally impaired. A report of revascularization in 100 consecutive patients with high-risk atherosclerotic renovascular disease had a surgical mortality rate of only 2%; 40% of the patients were cured, 51% were improved, and failure occurred in 9%. Postoperative serum creatinine was improved in most patients in whom surgery was performed to preserve renal function (Novick, 1981).

2. Repair of distal artery–As is true of atherosclerosis generally, disease may appear initially in any portion of the arterial circuit and not be demonstrable elsewhere. If the renal arterial lesion is distal, removal of the kidney with its peripheral arteries may allow repair of the distal artery and its branches while the kidney is being perfused, as it is when renal transplantation is underaken. In this way, it may be possible under direct vision to correct the abnormalities in the distal renal arteries while preserving the function of the kidney. The kidney can then be reanastomosed to the patient. Some brilliant results have followed this procedure. Nephrectomy is inadvisable in the presence of fibromuscular hyperplasia, since the disease is often bilateral or, even if not bilateral at the outset, may develop in a few years in the opposite kidney. This consideration is not so important in atherosclerotic disease if the kidney is atrophic and nonfunctioning and the disease unilateral.

B. Renal Percutaneous Transluminal Angioplasty: A newer form of treatment, renal percutaneous transluminal angioplasty, has been developed (Fig 9–25) and is gaining in popularity. Further experience is required to define the type of patient in whom balloon dilation is indicated and to further study its hemodynamic consequences. Enough information is at hand, however, to indicate that balloon dilation should be considered in proximal, localized, noncalcific, discrete renal artery stenosis, especially in patients in whom the surgical resection risk is considerable. The immediate results of transluminal angioplasty have been good, but the long-term benefits have been conflicting.

Prognosis
A. With Surgical Repair:
I. Patients with impaired renal function–Pa-

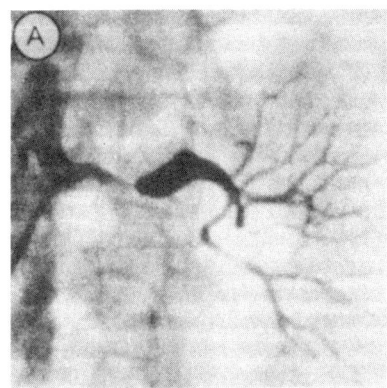

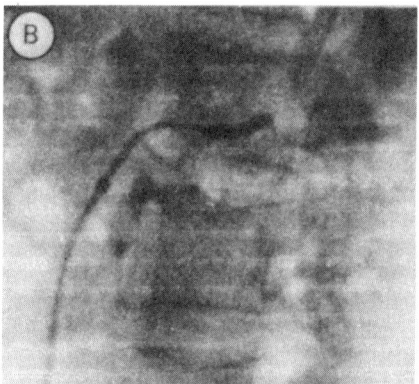

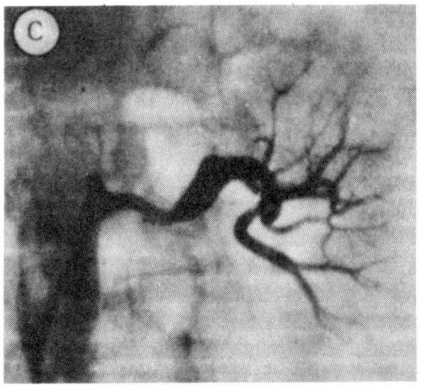

Figure 9–25. Selective renal arteriogram of the left renal artery. *A:* Renal artery before the dilation procedure, showing subtotal stenosis and poststenotic dilation. *B:* The distensible balloon segment of the dilation catheter is located in the renal artery stenosis and inflated with contrast material. *C:* After withdrawal of the dilation catheter, the renal artery shows moderate residual stenosis. (Reproduced, with permission, from Grüntzig A et al: Treatment of renovascular hypertension with percutaneous transluminal dilatation of a renal-artery stenosis. *Lancet* 1978;1:801.)

tients with impaired renal function are a particularly difficult group in which to judge the value of surgery. The results are less good when the creatinine clearance is less than 40 mL/min, but this may be due to accelerated hypertension with vascular necrosis or to bilateral disease. However, the prognosis of accelerated hypertension with impaired renal function is so poor that surgery or angioplasty may be considered if there is a significant stenotic lesion and increased renal vein renin on that side, especially if the patient fails to respond well to medical treatment.

Patients who have angina, a history of myocardial infarction, or extensive cerebral vascular disease have a 2–5% surgical mortality rate following the resection necessary for treatment of atherosclerotic renal artery stenosis; furthermore, the high postoperative incidence of neurologic deficit, myocardial ischemia or infarction, or arrhythmias engenders caution in advocating surgery in people with extensive vascular disease.

2. Results of surgical repair in general–The results of surgical treatment vary with the cause—being better when fibromuscular hyperplasia is present. Table 9–15 compares the results of surgical and medical treatment. About half of patients with atherosclerotic renovascular hypertension have diastolic pressures less than 100 mm Hg following surgical repair; the figure is closer to 75% in patients with fibromuscular hyperplasia. One-fourth to one-half of the patients, especially with atherosclerotic disease, require some antihypertensive therapy following surgical treatment.

The National Cooperative Study of Renovascular Hypertension (Maxwell, 1975) indicates that the best results are achieved in patients with the following clinical and historical prognostic indicators: clear-cut lateralization studies, severe hypertension of short duration, secondary aldosteronism, hypokalemia, a negative family history of hypertension, classic urographic findings, and a long systolic or diastolic bruit.

B. With Percutaneous Transluminal Angioplasty: Restenosis occurred in a substantial percentage of patients studied by Grim (1981), whereas excellent 2-year responses were reported by Mahler (1982). In the latter series, poststenotic renal artery pressure increased, the renal arteries were patent on angiograms, the blood pressure was lower or normal in almost all patients, and in the patients in whom restenosis occurred (one-fourth of the patients studied), repeat dilation was successful. Further long-term studies are obviously needed. The technique and current status of the procedure are summarized by Roberts (1982) and Sos (1983).

2. PRIMARY ALDOSTERONISM

Further experience has shown that primary aldosteronism is usually due to oversecretion of aldosterone by an adenoma of the adrenal (Fig 9–26), that

Table 9–15. Surgical and medical treatment of renal artery stenosis compared.*

A. Results of Surgical Treatment for Renal Artery Stenosis With Hypertension (100 Cases)

Status of Patients	Follow-Up Interval for Type of Stenosis Range and Mean (Years)					
	Atheromatous (37 Patients)			Fibromuscular (63 Patients)		
	1–6 (3.6)	5–10 (7.0)	7–12 (8.8)	1–8 (3.0)	5–12 (7.0)	7–14 (8.8)
Surviving	37	29	26	62	60	58
< 90 mm Hg diastolic blood pressure						
No medication	14	13	12	41	39	39
Mild medication	14	14	12	15	16	15
Taking sympatholytic agents	9	2	2	6	5	4

B. Results of Medical Treatment for Renal Artery Stenosis With Hypertension (114 Cases)

Status of Patients	Follow-Up Interval for Type of Stenosis Range and Mean (Years)					
	Atheromatous (44 Patients)			Fibromuscular (70 Patients)		
	1–8 (3.8)	5–12 (7.1)	7–14 (9.0)	1–8 (3.9)	5–12 (7.2)	7–14 (9.1)
Dead	3	16	27	0	5	12
Subjected to surgery	2	7	7	2	9	9
Surviving with medication	39	21	10	68	56	49
Blood pressure control usually < 100 mm Hg diastolic	33	15	9	59	48	43
Unsatisfactory blood pressure control	6	6	1	9	8	6

*Reproduced, with permission, from Hunt JC et al: Renal and renovascular hypertension: A reasoned approach to diagnosis and management. *Arch Intern Med* 1974;133:988.

it is a relatively uncommon (1–2%) cause of hypertension, that some patients (20–25%) have bilateral adrenal hyperplasia rather than adenoma (70–80%), and that these patients have a milder variety of aldosteronism (Biglieri, 1982; Bravo, 1983). Patients with primary adenoma excrete greater amounts of aldosterone in the urine and have lower plasma renin and serum potassium levels than do patients with aldosteronism secondary to bilateral adrenal hyperplasia (Biglieri, 1982). Aldosteronism itself is not the cause of the hypertension, because aldosterone levels may be much higher in conditions in which hypertension is absent, such as normal pregnancy, cirrhosis of the liver, and Addison's disease.

Adenomas may be relatively small (1–2 cm in diameter) and difficult to find at surgery, are golden yellow in appearance, and are associated with normal or hyperplastic adrenal tissue surrounding the tumor. This is in contrast to Cushing's syndrome, in which the gland surrounding a tumor is atrophic and the opposite adrenal may also be hypoplastic.

Clinical Findings

The clinical features of primary aldosteronism are often no different from those of essential hypertension; occasionally, symptoms related to potassium depletion, such as nocturia, polyuria, fatigue, or paresthesias, may dominate. One now rarely sees the paralysis due to extremely low potassium reported in the early literature. Aldosteronism is more frequent in women below age 40 years; hypertension is usually mild to moderate; retinopathy is usually grade I or grade II; and malignant hypertension is rare. Hypertensive complications, such as cardiac failure, are uncommon. If there is severe hypokalemic alkalosis, the patient may have autonomic insufficiency with postural hypotension without tachycardia. In suspected cases, the initial screening test is a determination of serum potassium.

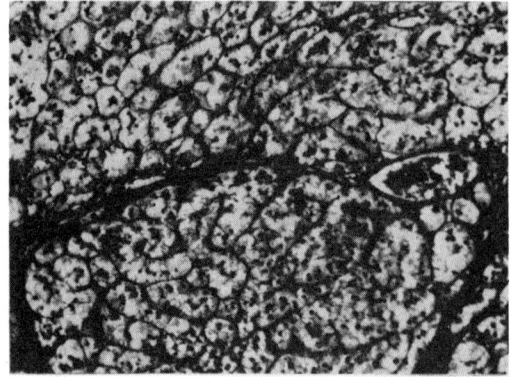

Figure 9–26. Adenoma of the adrenal gland showing clear cells and fibrous trabeculae. (Reproduced, with permission, from Nicholls MG et al: Primary aldosteronism: A study in contrasts. *Am J Med* 1975;59:334.)

A. Serum Potassium: If the serum potassium is consistently above 4 meq/L on a normal sodium intake, the likelihood of a primary aldosterone-producing adenoma is sufficiently remote that no further studies are probably indicated. The serum potassium may be normal if the patient is on a low-sodium diet, because potassium excretion at the sodium-potassium exchange site in the distal tubule is reduced; patients should therefore be on a normal-sodium diet before serum electrolytes are measured. If the serum potassium is less than 4 meq/L—and especially if it is less than 3.5 meq/L—the 24-hour urine potassium and serum potassium should be determined on a normal sodium diet of approximately 100–150 meq/d. In primary aldosterone-producing adenomas, serum potassium falls over a 5- to 10-day period if the patient has been placed on a high-sodium diet. If the 24-hour urine potassium exceeds 30 meq/L in the presence of a serum potassium less than 3.5 meq/L (especially if the serum potassium falls as a result of the high sodium intake), further biochemical studies such as plasma aldosterone and renin are indicated to exclude aldosteronism, because hypokalemia due to other causes such as decreased dietary intake or loss of potassium in the stool from diarrhea usually is associated with a decreased urinary potassium excretion to preserve body potassium stores. If primary aldosteronism accounts for the hypokalemia and increased potassium excretion in the urine, there also should be salt and water retention and increased extracellular and plasma volume, associated with decreased circulatory reflexes (bradycardia) and lack of hypertension overshoot following the Valsalva maneuver.

B. Evaluation of Low Serum Potassium in Hypertensive Patients: One of the difficult problems facing the physician is the hypertensive patient who has been receiving antihypertensive therapy, including oral diuretics, who presents with a low serum potassium. Oral diuretics increase the excretion of potassium, so it is common to find a low serum potassium in patients on diuretics, but this does not exclude the possible associated presence of primary aldosteronism. When potassium secretion is increased by diuretics, sodium is excreted as well, producing the combination of a low serum potassium and a low serum sodium between 130 and 135 meq/L. In addition, mild alkalosis with serum bicarbonate in the range of 25–32 meq/L is present. If the serum sodium, instead of being decreased, is increased—in the range of 144–149 meq/L—and if the serum bicarbonate is higher (in the range of 35–39 meq/L), the possibility of primary aldosteronism is increased in patients in whom the serum potassium is low. To exclude primary aldosteronism, Biglieri (1982) advises that biochemical and hormonal studies be done.

If the conclusion is that the patient has hyperplasia, and hypertension is only mild to moderate, the treatment of choice is with spironolactone, 300 mg/d in divided doses for 1 month followed by smaller doses, because adrenalectomy often does not cure the hypertension. If the patient has chemical findings suggesting adenoma, then other procedures such as adrenal and CT scans to localize the tumor should be done because the surgical results are sufficiently good to warrant the procedure.

C. Plasma Renin: Plasma renin should be decreased to nil or very low values in aldosteronism because the increased blood volume by negative feedback (see negative feedback loop in Fig 9–4) decreases renal renin secretion. If the plasma concentration is normal or high, primary aldosteronism is excluded as a cause of hypokalemia. A low plasma renin level is even more significant if it remains low following upright posture and the use of potent diuretics, which stimulate renin secretion in the normal individual but which may not do so in the presence of the hypervolemia of increased aldosterone production. If the plasma renin level remains low, especially after provocative maneuvers to increase it, plasma and urinary aldosterone values should be determined. Interpretation of the plasma renin concentration may be doubtful unless the conditions of testing are rigidly controlled. This is best done in the hospital and consists of control of sodium and potassium intake, avoidance of antihypertensive drugs, ambulation for 4 hours before the sample is taken, and sodium depletion with diuretics on the day of the test to make certain that plasma renin does not respond to these maneuvers and remains suppressed. These tests are done only in special laboratories that have facilities to measure the hormone accurately.

D. Plasma Aldosterone: Increased plasma aldosterone with clinical and laboratory evidence of excess aldosterone production may be due either to the presence of an isolated adrenal adenoma or to bilateral adrenal hyperplasia. Adenoma is suspected if the plasma aldosterone fails to increase in the upright posture, as it does in hyperplasia, or if an iodine 131 iodocholesterol scintiscan or a CT scan localizes a tumor in one of the adrenals.

Desoxycorticosterone has no effect on adenoma, ie, it does not suppress the production of aldosterone from the tumor, as it does in indeterminate aldosteronism (hyperplasia).

E. Adrenal Scan: Most cases of adrenal adenoma can be identified and localized by an adrenal scintiscan, or perhaps more definitively by CT scan. It is important to attempt to localize the adenoma so the surgeon will know which adrenal is involved.

F. Adrenal Vein Catheterization: If the biochemical studies strongly suggest aldosteronism but an adrenal scan or CT scan does not reveal the tumor (because it is <1 cm in diameter), or if the scans are equivocal, localization should be attempted by percutaneous adrenal vein catheterization via the femoral vein, with assays of aldosterone in the venous effluent of blood from both kidneys and from segments of each kidney. Estimate of cortisol should be made at the outset to be sure that the catheter is in the adrenal and not the renal vein. The tumor may be small (<1 cm), flattened, and difficult to find at surgery. Preoperative localization of the site of the tumor is of considerable help in finding the adenoma and avoiding adrenalectomy.

Adrenal vein catheterization by a skilled team, available now only in research centers (although physicians who perform renal vein catheterization can, with experience, catheterize adrenal veins), not only permits adrenal venous blood to be examined for aldosterone but also allows an adrenal venogram to be done if necessary. This is less desirable, because adrenal hemorrhage has occurred in some cases, and biochemical studies of venous effluent are preferred. In contrast to the 1.5:1 ratio of renal vein renin in the diagnosis of renovascular hypertension, the ratio of aldosterone in the 2 adrenal veins is closer to 5:1 or 10:1 when an adenoma is present in one adrenal (Melby, 1976). Catheterization of the left adrenal vein is easier than catheterization of the right because of the variable origin of the right adrenal vein. The combination of a positive adrenal isotope scan and positive adrenal vein characterization of an adenoma by aldosterone assay permits a positive diagnosis in 85–90% of patients with adenoma. Adrenal arteriography is done infrequently because of the difficulty of the procedure and because it does not allow differential adrenal vein sampling for aldosterone.

Treatment

If bilateral renal hyperplasia rather than adenoma is the cause, the patient should be treated with antihypertensive therapy including spironolactone (the aldosterone antagonist) rather than bilateral adrenalectomy, because of the high prevalence of persistent hypertension after surgery and the need for replacement therapy after adrenalectomy. Spironolactone usually corrects both the serum potassium and the hypertension. In adenoma, resection of the adrenal tumor promptly decreases aldosterone production and restores the serum potassium to normal, but hypertension is "cured" in only 60–70% of cases. Because of this relatively low "cure" rate in mild aldosteronism due to hyperplasia, when the blood pressure, serum potassium, and hypervolemia can be corrected by spironolactone, medical rather than surgical treatment can be advised.

Prognosis

Without surgery, however, the symptoms of adenoma can only be partially controlled by medical treatment, and surgical removal is required. The serum potassium usually falls to less than 2.5–3 meq/L after thiazide therapy in unsuspected cases of aldosteronism, leading to hypokalemic symptoms of fatigue, nocturia, arrhythmia, and nephropathy; these are corrected by spironolactone. Failure to control blood pressure leads to cardiac and cerebral complications found in other types of hypertension. Postural hypotension may be a problem because of a defect in circulatory reflexes not due to increased central blood volume.

3. SECONDARY ALDOSTERONISM

Secondary hyperaldosteronism is much more common than primary and is usually due to accelerated or severe hypertension, which, by reducing renal blood flow, initiates the production of angiotensin, which in turn increases the secretion of aldosterone. Patients with secondary aldosteronism are likely to have an elevated plasma renin as well, in contrast to the low plasma renin expected in primary aldosteronism. The serum potassium may be low in both secondary and primary aldosteronism, but the serum sodium is not elevated in secondary as it is in primary aldosteronism. The serum sodium is rarely less than 140 meq/dL in primary cases, and it may be as high as 155 meq/dL. When the blood pressure is reduced by antihypertensive agents such as thiazide diuretics (but not spironolactone), secondary aldosteronism is reduced, and the serum potassium may rise to normal even though the oral diuretics tend to increase the plasma renin. The "effective" blood volume is raised in both types of aldosteronism but is reduced in patients with cirrhosis of the liver or Addison's disease, conditions in which renin levels may be very high. Secondary aldosteronism may also occur in renal artery stenosis because of the increased secretion of renin, with resulting increased plasma and urinary aldosterone. The increased plasma renin is critical in separating the 2 varieties.

Treatment

Treatment is by vigorous antihypertensive therapy to lower the blood pressure, which then causes the secondary aldosteronism to disappear.

4. CUSHING'S DISEASE & SYNDROME

Cushing's syndrome is probably a more common cause of hypertension than primary aldosteronism. Although the terms Cushing's disease and Cushing's syndrome have been used interchangeably, they should be distinguished. The term Cushing's disease originally described a primary tumor of the anterior pituitary causing bilateral adrenal hyperplasia and hypercortisolism. Because the pituitary tumor often could not be identified, the oversecretion of cortisol and the bilateral adrenal hyperplasia were called Cushing's syndrome. It was subsequently learned that a benign adenoma of the adrenal and ectopic ACTH-producing tumors (eg, bronchogenic carcinoma) could also cause the ectopic hypercortisolism. Complicating the terminology even more is the syndrome simulating Cushing's disease, which is induced by exogenous administration of corticosteroids or ACTH for a wide variety of diseases.

The advent of microsurgery of the anterior pituitary has shown that most cases of overproduction of cortisol are due to a tumor (often microscopic) of the basophilic or chromophobic cells of the anterior pituitary or to an adenoma of the adrenal gland; idiopathic bilateral adrenal hyperplasia is now considered rare. It is speculated that some cases of Cushing's syndrome are hypothalamic in origin, with the anterior pituitary stimulated by excess hypothalamic-releasing factor.

Hypertension is a common accompaniment of Cushing's syndrome, although most patients present primarily to an endocrinologist because of a characteristic appearance with "moon" facies, central truncal obesity, muscular weakness, ecchymosis with thin skin, purple striae, increased acne, hirsutism, and perhaps osteoporosis. Hypertension may be mild or severe, but malignant hypertension is rare.

Clinical Findings

A. Symptoms and Signs: The diagnosis of Cushing's syndrome is suspected from the clinical features, but most patients with obesity, hirsutism, and round, bloated facies do not have Cushing's disease (Table 9–16).

B. Laboratory Findings: Because cortisol is increased several times above normal values, retention of sodium and water with increased extracellular fluid volume may occur. The pathogenesis of hypertension in Cushing's syndrome is not established but is probably due to increased salt and water retention associated with excess cortisol production, increased vascular responsiveness to pressor agents, or increased plasma renin substrate. The last may contribute to increased aldosterone production and superimpose a mineralocorticoid excess on the glucocorticoid excess. In pure cortisol excess, plasma renin and aldosterone are normal, as is the serum potassium.

Table 9–16. Common initial signs and differential diagnoses in Cushing's disease.*

Common Initial Signs	Differential Diagnoses
Rapid onset	
Facial edema	Hypothyroidism
Rapid weight gain	Nephritis or nephrosis
Renal colic	Allergic or cardiac edema
Amenorrhea with facial edema or rapid weight gain	Simple obesity
	Idiopathic renal calculi
Physical weakness	Psychoses
Mental disturbance	Collagen disease
Gradual onset	
Gradual weight gain	Simple obesity
Oligomenorrhea and hirsutism	Familial hirsutism; psychogenic amenorrhea
Diabetes mellitus	Diabetes mellitus
Hypertension	Essential hypertension
Mental or emotional changes	Psychosomatic conditions
Osteoporosis	Postmenopausal osteoporosis

Other differential diagnoses: hyperthyroidism, Guillain-Barré syndrome or diabetic neuropathy, hyperparathyroidism, peptic ulcer, polycythemia, purpuras, ovarian tumors.
*Reproduced, with permission, from Hurxthal LM, O'Sullivan JB: Cushing's syndrome: Clinical differential diagnosis and complications. *Ann Intern Med* 1959;**51**:1.

Both cortisol and ACTH levels are elevated in Cushing's disease with pituitary hypercortisolism; increased ACTH stimulates the adrenal cortex to secrete more cortisol. In addition, one can determine the morning plasma 17-hydroxycorticosteroid (17-OHCS) levels after suppression of ACTH by giving the patient 1 mg of dexamethasone and a sedative (phenobarbital, 100 mg, or flurazepam [Dalmane], 15–30 mg) at bedtime the night before. Normal individuals usually suppress the plasma 17-OHCS from the normal value of 10–20 μg/dL to less than 5 μg/dL, whereas patients with Cushing's disease rarely suppress from elevated values of 15–40 μg/dL to less than 10 μg/dL (Melby, 1976). Values of 5–10 μg/dL are borderline. Suppression of plasma cortisol by dexamethasone implies that the hypercortisolism is primary in the pituitary or in an ectopic ACTH-producing tumor and is not due to autonomous adrenal secretion. In Cushing's syndrome due to adrenal adenoma, increased cortisol production suppresses the hypothalamic-pituitary axis and reduces the level of ACTH. The diagnosis is further supported when plasma cortisol is not suppressible by dexamethasone.

The clinical and laboratory diagnosis of adrenocortical hypertension is summarized by Biglieri (1982). He discusses Cushing's syndrome, primary aldosteronism, and deoxycorticosterone-excess syndromes, such as 11β-hydroxylation deficiency and 17α-hydroxylation deficiency (Fig 9–27).

C. X-Ray Findings: The radiologic diagnosis of pituitary tumors is difficult, and in most cases standard skull films are normal. The use of tomography or CT scans may increase the frequency of suggestive findings, but even with contrast dye injections into the carotid artery the microadenomas have often been missed (Salassa, 1978).

Adrenal tumors are usually large and associated with atrophy of the surrounding as well as the contralateral adrenal. Preoperative lateralization of the tumor is not always successful, although it has been considerably improved by CT scan. If this fails, it is always necessary to expose and explore both adrenal glands. Sampling of blood from both adrenal veins and adrenal venography may be helpful in identifying the tumor, but the adrenal scan is simpler and should be employed first. If a carcinoma of the adrenal is suspected, arteriography may be helpful, because the tumor is vascular.

Treatment

Once the diagnosis of Cushing's disease is made and exogenous administration of corticosteroids or ACTH excluded, a search should be made for ectopic ACTH-producing tumors or an adrenal adenoma. If either of these tumors is identified (see diagnosis above), surgical resection is the treatment of choice. If neither is present and Cushing's disease is diagnosed, microresection of the tumor of the pituitary under microscopic visualization is now the preferred treatment. Irradiation of the anterior pituitary and cryosurgery, formerly used in treatment, have been superseded.

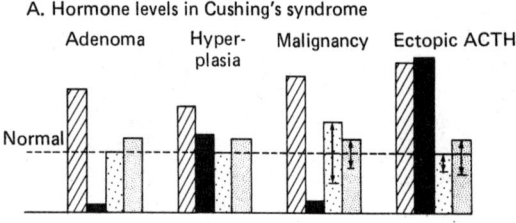

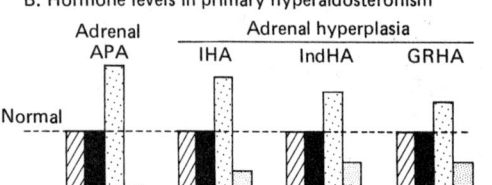

APA, aldosterone-producing adenoma; IHA, idiopathic hyperaldosteronism; IndHA, indeterminate hyperaldosteronism; GRHA, glucocorticoid-remediable hyperaldosteronism.

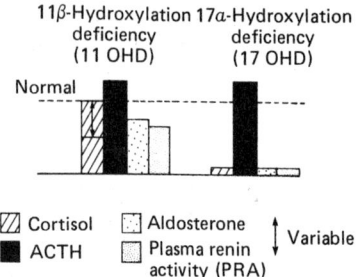

Figure 9–27. Hormone levels in Cushing's syndrome, primary hyperaldosteronism, and deoxycorticosterone-excess syndromes. (Modified and reproduced, with permission, from Biglieri EG, Lopez JM: Clinical and laboratory diagnosis of adrenocortical hypertension. *Cardiovasc Med* 1976;1:335.)

Transsphenoidal microresection of the pituitary under microscopic visualization is the preferred treatment in adults (Tyrrell, 1978), and the results have been very satisfactory, with a low ($\pm 1\%$) mortality rate and rare cases of permanent diabetes insipidus. The results of microsurgery in childhood Cushing's disease are not known, and most cases in this category have been "cured" with pituitary irradiation (Jennings, 1977).

Chemotherapy with cyproheptadine or mitotane with or without pituitary irradiation has been reported to have achieved favorable results in a few cases.

If ectopic ACTH-producing tumors cannot be resected, metyrapone can be tried in order to inhibit the synthesis of cortisol.

Prognosis

Without treatment, the symptoms and signs of the syndrome become progressively worse, although the hypertension may be controlled by antihypertensive therapy. If hypertension is overlooked because other findings dominate the clinical picture, complications of hypertension such as cardiac failure and cerebral or renal vascular disease may develop and may be the cause of death.

5. CONGENITAL ADRENAL HYPERPLASIA

The rare conditions causing congenital adrenal hyperplasia were not considered hypertensive disorders until recently. They are due to enzymatic defects in the synthesis of cortisol and are treated with cortisol.

17α-Hydroxylase Deficiency

Biglieri (1966, 1981, 1982) demonstrated in some patients with amenorrhea and hypertension a 17-hydroxylase deficiency that blocked the synthesis not only of cortisol from cholesterol and pregnenolone but also of androgens (androsterone) and estrogens (17-hydroxyprogesterone) by the adrenal gland. As a result, secondary sex characteristics failed to develop at puberty, and women presented with amenorrhea. By positive feedback, the decreased cortisol stimulates the pituitary gland to secrete excessive amounts of ACTH, which in turn stimulates the adrenal to produce increased deoxycorticosterone, causing mineralocorticoid excess with hypertension and hypokalemia.

Treatment with moderate doses of cortisol corrects the abnormality and diminishes excessive ACTH secretion and consequently the amount of deoxycorticosterone secreted, correcting the hypokalemia and hypertension.

21-Hydroxylase and 11β-Hydroxylase Deficiencies

Other known enzymatic defects causing decreased synthesis of cortisol are 21-hydroxylase and 11-hydroxylase deficiencies in congenital adrenal hyperplasia associated with virilism. In these cases, synthesis of the adrenal androgens is not blocked, and increased secretion of ACTH resulting from decreased cortisol stimulates further androgen synthesis, causing infant virilization, which is the presenting symptom. Excessive deoxycorticosterone causes hypertension and hypokalemia in 11β-hydroxylase deficiency, but in 21-hydroxylase deficiency, deoxycorticosterone is raised to a lesser degree and does not always cause hypertension and hypokalemia.

Treatment consists of oral cortisol, which by negative feedback halts the increased ACTH secretion, resulting in less androgen secretion and decreased virilism; the decreased deoxycorticosterone corrects the hypokalemia and hypertension.

6. PHEOCHROMOCYTOMA

Pheochromocytoma is a dramatic but rare tumor, only one or 2 cases a year being seen in the usual large general hospital. The tumor arises anywhere in the chromaffin system (the remnant of the fetal neural crest) that synthesizes epinephrine and norepinephrine. The overwhelming majority occur in the adrenal medulla, but these tumors may occur in chromaffin cells in the abdomen, the periaortic area, the organ of Zuckerkandl, and, rarely, in the thorax and bladder wall (Fig 9–28). They are often multiple and familial and rarely may be associated with other endocrinopathies such as Sipple's disease (multiple parathyroid adenomas) or Recklinghausen's disease (neurofibromatosis); most patients have no associated endocrinopathy. The tumor is usually benign, but about 10% are malignant and require treatment with radiation therapy and chemotherapy.

It is important to recognize pheochromocytoma promptly, because successful excision of the tumor is curative in almost all of the benign tumors and prevents the severe hypertensive crises that may cause myocardial infarction, fatal ventricular arrhythmias, or cerebral hemorrhage. A valuable review is presented by Manger (1977).

Tumors vary in the relative amounts of norepinephrine and epinephrine that they secrete, and the clinical signs may vary depending on which catecholamine is secreted.

Clinical Findings

A. Symptoms and Signs: The most typical clinical features are those associated with an abrupt surge of catecholamine secretion, causing pallor, sweating, palpitations, headache, and anxiety, usually all occurring together in association with an abrupt rise in systolic and diastolic pressure (Table 9–17).

1. Cause of attacks–The attacks may be spontaneous or precipitated by changes in posture, pressure on the abdomen, or procedures such as intravenous urograms. (*Note:* Intravenous phentolamine must be available for emergency use.) One or another of these symptoms may be present in anxiety attacks, and most patients referred with a diagnosis of possible pheochromocytoma have transient rises in pressure associated with anxiety. If epinephrine is the amine secreted, flushing rather than pallor is characteristic, and the patient is more tremulous. In rare instances, precursors of norepinephrine may be secreted, and hypotension has occasionally been found when dopamine is secreted in large amounts. The hypertension may be sustained or intermittent. In most cases it is sustained, with intermittent superimposed rises in conjunction with paroxysmal symptoms. Malignant hypertension may occur with papilledema, and this is seen relatively more frequently than in Cushing's syndrome or aldosteronism.

2. Symptoms during attack–The rise in blood pressure may be severe, and during attacks in young people, diastolic pressures of 150 mm Hg are not unusual. The high, abrupt rises in pressure may cause myocardial ischemia or infarction, ventricular

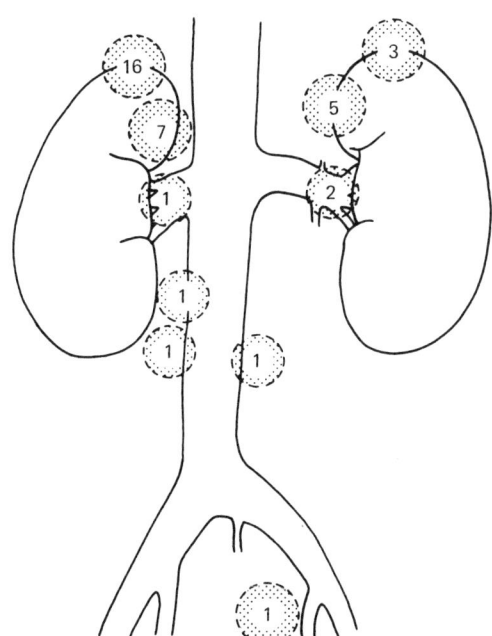

Figure 9–28. Illustration of the sites of occurrence of pheochromocytoma in 34 patients, with the number of tumors found at various locations indicated in the circles. (Adapted and reproduced, with permission, from Zelch JV, Meaney TF, Belhobek GH: Radiologic approach to the patient with suspected pheochromocytoma. *Radiology* 1974;**111**:279.)

Table 9–17. Symptoms in 100 patients with pheochromocytoma.*

Symptom	No.	Symptom	No.
Headache	80	Dizziness or faintness	8
Perspiration	71	Convulsions	5
Palpitation (with or without tachycardia)	64	Neck-shoulder pain	5
		Extremity pain	4
Pallor	42	Flank pain	4
Nausea (with or without vomiting)	42	Tinnitus	3
		Dysarthria	3
Tremor or trembling	31	Gagging	3
Weakness or exhaustion	28	Bradycardia (noted by patient)	3
Nervousness or anxiety	22		
Epigastric pain	22	Back pain	3
Chest pain	19	Coughing	1
Dyspnea	19	Yawning	1
Flushing or warmth	18	Syncope	1
Numbness or paresthesia	11	Unsteadiness	1
Blurring of vision	11	Hunger	1
Tightness in throat	8		

*Reproduced, with permission, from Thomas JE, Rooke ED, Kvale WF: The neurologist's experience with pheochromocytoma: A review of 100 cases. *JAMA* 1966;**197**:754. Copyright © American Medical Association.

arrhythmias, or cardiac failure; patients may present with one or more of these complications.

When pheochromocytoma occurs in the urinary bladder, the hypertensive crises may be induced by urination, or the patient may have asymptomatic hematuria. A review of 35 previously reported cases and a well-studied individual case are offered by Raper (1977).

B. Laboratory Findings: The laboratory diagnosis of pheochromocytoma in patients who have a characteristic history usually can be accomplished by assay of catecholamine excretion in the 24-hour urine specimen. Table 9–18 shows the normal range of catecholamine and metabolite concentrations in the urine and blood.

1. VMA determination–The spectrophotometric determination of vanillylmandelic acid (VMA), one of the products of catecholamine metabolism, is a screening test that is available in most laboratories. Clofibrate (Atromid-S) gives false-negative results, but the spectrophotometric assay is not affected by common foods such as bananas, coffee, or vanilla desserts which do affect the less precise and commonly used simple colorimetric test. Normal VMA excretion is less than 7 mg/24 h but may be 5–10 times this amount in pheochromocytoma. Methyldopa does not interfere with assay for VMA, but it does interfere with assay for total urinary catecholamine excretion.

2. Metanephrine and normetanephrine–More recently, determination of other metabolites, notably the combination of metanephrine and normetanephrine, on a single voided specimen has been shown to be simple and highly reliable, with the distinct advantage of not requiring a 24-hour specimen. The upper limits of normal for the assay are 1 μg/mg of creatinine in the urine. Single voided urine specimens from 500 hypertensive patients contained 0.351 ± 0.356 μg of metanephrine per milligram of creatinine, whereas in pheochromocytoma, spot specimens were almost always 5–10 μg/mg and sometimes many times more than this (Kaplan, 1977). Chlorpromazine produces falsely high readings, but no diet or obesity drugs or antihypertensive drugs interfere with the test. This assay may be positive when the VMA assay is negative, but the reverse is rarely true.

Accurate methods of determining plasma norepinephrine concentrations indicate that in patients with pheochromocytoma, levels of 2.5–5 μg/L occur, in contrast to the normal 0.25–1 μg/L. Most of the norepinephrine released at the adrenergic nerve ending is reabsorbed, metabolized, or taken up again by the axon terminal. That which escapes into the circulation, while much higher than normal, is only a small fraction of the amount that is released. The sudden release of norepinephrine into the circulation in hypertensive crises in patients with pheochromocytoma produces dramatic effects. In patients with brief episodes of catecholamine release, prolonged intra-arterial blood pressure recordings may establish the diagnosis by demonstrating short peaks of elevated pressure coincident with the episodic symptoms (Mancia, 1979). Not only is measurement of plasma norepinephrine a most useful diagnostic test, but plasma measurements at different venous sites may help localize the tumor.

3. Urine tests–Urinary assay of the free catecholamines norepinephrine and epinephrine is infrequently used in screening, since these substances are technically more difficult to measure and may be increased in the urine, causing false-positive results if the patient has been receiving bronchodilators, nasal sprays, or drugs such as tetracycline or chlorpromazine that produce urinary fluorescence. Methyldopa also interferes with the catecholamine test but not the VMA test. In the absence of interfering drugs, the plasma catecholamines, when abnormally high, are more sensitive than the urinary metabolites in the diagnosis of pheochromocytoma (Bravo, 1979).

4. Pharmacologic tests–Tests based on administration of drugs are rarely used today because they may cause both false-positive and false-negative results. *Histamine,* by inducing outpouring of catecholamines from the tumor, *may produce a hypertensive crisis* with arrhythmia, myocardial ischemia, or even death.

5. Other tests–The availability of the more specific chemical tests makes the provocative tests with histamine or glucagon unnecessary today except in those individuals with an otherwise suspicious history whose pressures are completely normal and in whom no attacks are observed over a period of weeks. In these patients, 0.01 mg of histamine may be used as a provocative measure to induce an attack.

Treatment

Because the increased secretion of catecholamines results in hypertension and reduction of the plasma volume in many instances, alpha-adrenergic blocking drugs combined with beta-adrenergic blocking agents

Table 9–18. Normal range of catecholamine and metabolite concentrations.*†

Urine
Catecholamines‡
Norepinephrine: 10–70 μg/24 h
Epinephrine: 0–20 μg/24 h
Normetanephrine and metanephrine: < 1.3 mg/24 h
Vanillylmandelic acid: 1.8–9.0 mg/24 h
Dopamine: < 200 μg/24 h
Blood
Catecholamines: < 1 μg/L
Adrenal medulla
Norepinephrine: 0.04–0.16 mg/g
Epinephrine: 0.22–0.84 mg/g

*Reproduced, with permission, from Melmon KL: Catecholamines and the adrenal medulla. Part 2, pages 283–322, in: *Textbook of Endocrinology,* 5th ed. Williams RH (editor). Saunders, 1974.

†Since the values obtained in different laboratories vary considerably, only a general range can be given.

‡In most patients with pheochromocytomas, total catecholamine excretion is > 300 μg/d.

in order to inhibit the peripheral actions of the catecholamines must be used regardless of the ultimate method of treatment (medical or surgical).

A. Medical Treatment: Give phentolamine (Regitine), 10–30 mg orally every 4–6 hours, or phenoxybenzamine (Dibenzyline), 10–50 mg orally twice daily, to control both blood pressure and blood volume before technical procedures that may cause marked rise or fall in pressure are done to localize the tumor (Fig 9–29).

Treatment of acute episodes. During such acute hypertensive episodes, patients should be given phentolamine, 1–5 mg intravenously every 5–10 minutes, until the pressure falls and is stabilized in order to avoid myocardial ischemia or arrhythmias. If the latter occurs or if there is severe tachycardia, 1–2 mg of propranolol can be given intravenously over a 10-minute period followed by 20 mg orally every 6 hours. When intravenous phentolamine is given, the patient is best placed in the Fowler position so that if excessive fall of pressure occurs, a shift to the supine position can be swiftly made. Dramatic abortion of attacks occurs with intravenous phentolamine, and the drug should be available for all diagnostic procedures that might liberate catecholamines and induce an attack.

B. Surgical Treatment: After the diagnosis of pheochromocytoma is made and surgery is contemplated, careful examination of the head and neck, chest fluoroscopy, chest x-rays, and intravenous urograms with tomography should be carried out. Inferior vena cava and adrenal venous venography with multiple venous sampling for catecholamine concentration are also used to determine the site of the tumor. Adrenal arteriography may be necessary, especially if the tumor is extrarenal; adrenal scans are less helpful when this is so.

After suitable preparation with alpha-adrenergic blocking agents (see above) to restore the blood volume and lower the blood pressure, as well as daily propranolol (10–40 mg 3 times daily) to control tachycardia and arrhythmias, surgical excision of the tumor is the treatment of choice. Before it was recognized that it was important to control the blood volume preoperatively, the intraoperative course was characterized by marked rises in pressure due to surgical manipulation, and a fall to hypotensive levels when the tumor was excised. Phentolamine (Regitine) should be available for immediate intravenous use for the former and norepinephrine and volume expanders for the latter.

Prognosis

As indicated above, acute hypertensive crises may precipitate ventricular arrhythmias and myocardial or cerebral ischemia or infarction. These are not prevented by the usual antihypertensive therapy, and patients with acute crises are therefore at considerable risk from these complications.

In patients with sustained hypertension without acute severe hypertensive episodes, conventional antihypertensive therapy may lower the blood pressure without affecting the basic mechanism of increased secretion of catecholamine.

7. COARCTATION OF THE AORTA
(See also Chapter 11.)

Coarctation in adults usually consists of a localized narrowing or constriction in the region of the ligamentum arteriosum and is often associated with a bicuspid aortic valve. The patient may present with hypertension or with a basal systolic ejection murmur that is crescendo-decrescendo when due to the bicuspid aortic valve or late systolic when it occurs at the coarcted site. Rarely, patients present with intermittent claudication of the legs. The patient is usually male, and coarctation can be suspected from the elevated blood pressure, the increased pulsations of the carotid arteries, and the delayed weak pulsations in the femoral arteries and in the arteries distal to them. If there is doubt about whether the pulses are weak and delayed in the legs, the blood pressure should be taken in the legs; if there is still doubt, direct intra-arterial pressures can be obtained in the brachial and in the femoral arteries before and after exercise. Exer-

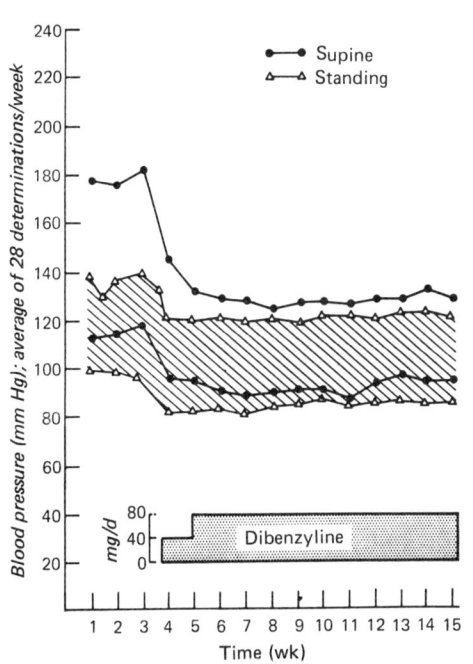

Figure 9–29. Response of the supine and standing blood pressure to treatment with phenoxybenzamine in a patient with malignant pheochromocytoma. Note that the marked orthostatic fall in blood pressure present in the pretreatment period is reduced after therapy is begun. (Reproduced, with permission, from Engelman K, Sjoerdsma A: Chronic medical therapy for pheochromocytoma: A report of 4 cases. *Ann Intern Med* 1964;**61**:231.)

cise aggravates the disparity between the pressures in the upper and lower extremities. If the patient is past puberty, pulsating collateral intercostal arteries below the margins of the ribs may be found. Coarctation varies in severity, but by early adult life the patient almost always has signs of left ventricular hypertrophy, both clinically and electrocardiographically, and the chest x-ray may show scalloping of the ribs as a result of the enlarged collateral intercostal arteries (see Chapter 11).

Surgical correction is required for all but the mildest cases of coarctation, and repair can usually be carried out safely in early childhood and even in infancy. The surgical mortality rate of repair of coarctation is less than 3%. The risk is higher if surgery is delayed until the 40s, when coronary heart disease may be superimposed and the sclerotic aorta is hard to repair. Recently, in a few cases in children, transluminal angioplasty has been attempted with some preliminary success. Further experience is required.

Prognosis

Without treatment, coarctation usually leads to death by the 40s, and the patient dies of cardiac failure, ruptured cerebral aneurysm, or aortic dissection.

The incidence of persistent hypertension following repair of a coarctation is now 5–10%. If surgery is delayed until late adult life, complications of the hypertension may still follow.

8. RENAL PARENCHYMAL LESIONS

Acute and chronic glomerulonephritis, chronic pyelonephritis, lupus erythematosus, polycystic kidney, and scarring from old trauma probably are the most common causes of secondary hypertension due to renal factors. Prior to the phase of renal failure, the diagnosis of acute glomerulonephritis can be strongly suspected from the history of poststreptococcal proteinuria, edema, or hypertension with associated hematuria and red cell casts. It can also be discovered by accidentally finding hematuria or proteinuria in a healthy young adult from a history of pyelonephritis or lupus erythematosus, or finding bacteria and white cells in the urine; by finding evidence of renal or ureteral stone; or by uncovering a family history of early death from uremia and hypertension due to polycystic kidneys. The presence of polycystic kidneys can be established by an intravenous urogram to demonstrate polycystic or large cystic kidneys. Urinalysis, urine culture, renal function studies, and serologic studies to rule out hyperparathyroidism, lupus erythematosus, or diabetes are helpful ancillary measures. Additional studies may include a retrograde urogram with determination of ureteral reflux during cytoscopy in patients with pyelonephritis, renal arteriograms, and renal biopsy. When renal failure has occurred, the urinary sediment and the degree of proteinuria may be similar in primary hypertension in the malignant phase and in chronic renal parenchymal disease.

The accelerated form of hypertension that occurs in the late stages of renal disease further aggravates renal function, and efforts to lower the blood pressure are essential regardless of the cause. Control of the high blood pressure prolongs life and delays the onset of renal failure; when the latter occurs, dialysis or renal transplantation (or both) is indicated.

9. HYPERTENSION DUE TO ORAL CONTRACEPTIVE AGENTS

It is becoming increasingly apparent that there is an association between the use of oral contraceptive agents and the development of hypertension. In many instances the rise in pressure is slight, but in a few patients severe or even malignant hypertension has resulted. There is some evidence that the individuals who develop hypertension have either a family history of hypertension or a history of preeclampsia-eclampsia. The rise in pressure is often gradual, and the incidence of hypertension is greater over a period of years than during the first 6 months of use of the agent.

The mechanism by which the oral contraceptive agents produce hypertension is not certain. The most generally accepted hypothesis is that it is caused by the considerable rise in renin substrate that follows the use of the estrogen-progesterone agents.

Oral contraceptive agents increase plasma renin and aldosterone as well as renin substrate. When hypertension is associated with a raised plasma aldosterone as well as a raised plasma renin, primary aldosteronism is excluded, but oral contraceptive agents must be considered in females. The combination of a low plasma renin, a high plasma aldosterone, and normal serum potassium in a hypertensive patient taking oral contraceptive agents virtually excludes the latter as likely causative agents. Screening of female hypertensives by determining plasma renin and aldosterone levels may make it unnecessary to stop the oral contraceptive agents for several months, as is otherwise necessary in order to determine this possible etiologic role in the hypertension.

A *rising* blood pressure, however, calls for cessation of the oral contraceptives and the use of an alternative method of contraception.

The Royal College of General Practitioners in England (1977) indicates that there is an increased mortality rate from circulatory diseases in women who have used oral contraception, with the risk increasing with age, smoking, the size of the estrogen dose, and the duration of use. The English study may be influenced by the large number of physicians and the small number of deaths in relation to the total number of women involved in the study. Further prospective studies are in progress, especially with agents that contain smaller amounts of estrogens.

Table 9-19. Incidence of polyarteritis in various organs at necropsy.*

	Incidence of Polyarteritis	
	Group With Lung Involvement (30 Cases) (%)	Group Without Lung Involvement (54 Cases) (%)
Lungs (pulmonary arteries)	47	0
Heart	60	35
Kidneys		
Glomerulitis	57	30
Renal polyarteritis	60	65
Stomach and intestines	40	30
Liver	37	54
Pancreas	17	39
Spleen	43	35
Brain	3	4
Periadrenal connective tissue	40	41
Voluntary muscle	33	20

*Reproduced, with permission, from Rose GA, Spencer H: Polyarteritis nodosa. Q J Med 1957;101(New Series 26):43.

10. CONNECTIVE TISSUE DISORDERS (Polyarteritis Nodosa, Lupus Erythematosus) (See also Chapter 20.)

Connective tissue disorders such as polyarteritis nodosa are often associated with vasculitis of the interlobular arteries and of the arterioles and are associated with hypertension in about half of cases. The hypertension may be severe and rarely may present with the malignant phase. The disease is often generalized, involving many body systems, and the hypertension may merely be part of a total systemic disease (Table 9-19).

Renovascular lesions are common in lupus erythematosus, but hypertension is much less common than in polyarteritis nodosa. Other forms of arteritis of nonspecific cause may also induce hypertension and subsequent renal failure when the lesions involve the kidney.

Treatment is with corticosteroids and conventional drug treatment for hypertension. Immunosuppressive drugs may be of value.

11. ACROMEGALY

Acromegaly is caused by excessive production of growth hormone by specific cells of the anterior pituitary gland. The disorder may be associated with hypertension, although other clinical and metabolic consequences are more common. Symptoms include early complaints of fatigue, paresthesias, amenorrhea, arthralgia, and headache. Later symptoms include increasing size of the hat, gloves, and shoes; visual disturbances that develop insidiously over a period of years; decreased libido; and excessive perspiration, with warm, moist hands. On examination, there may be progressive mandibular enlargement, as shown by serial photographs; large tongue; increased soft tissue over the heels, hands, and feet; widening spaces between the teeth; hypertension; and, sometimes, goiter. Radiologically, enlargement and ballooning of the sella turcica can be recognized. The hypertension is rarely severe, and treatment is directed at the acromegaly per se.

The diagnosis can be established by finding by immunoassay a high serum growth hormone level that falls below 2–5 ng/mL 1–2 hours after oral administration of 100 g of glucose. This is a useful screening test. About 10% of patients have a lower than expected serum growth hormone concentration, and in these patients abnormal growth hormone regulation by the hypothalamus is thought to be the cause. It is still not certain how many cases of acromegaly are due to an independent pituitary tumor and how many are due to abnormality of the hypothalamic growth hormone–releasing factor, which then induces pituitary hyperfunction. Contrast-enhanced CT scan may demonstrate an enlarged sella and a pituitary mass.

Treatment

Treatment now consists of microsurgery of the pituitary tumor, as in Cushing's disease. However, if the tumor is large, encroaching on the optic chiasm and the third ventricle, open surgical resection may be indicated. Irradiation of the pituitary is disappointing as judged by the fall in serum growth hormone, perhaps because the disease is far advanced before irradiation is undertaken. Serum concentrations above 15 ng/mL may persist for several years, and reoperation may be necessary. Chemotherapy with agents such as bromocriptine (5–20 mg 3 times daily), a semisynthetic ergot alkaloid that activates dopamine receptors in the brain, reducing growth hormone, is under investigation, but the effects are usually transient, and growth hormone levels rarely fall to normal values. Complete clinical remission is uncommon.

12. RECKLINGHAUSEN'S DISEASE (Neurofibromatosis)

The frequency of pheochromocytoma in this condition has been stressed in the literature, based on the frequency of Recklinghausen's disease in patients with pheochromocytoma. However, vascular lesions of the small- to medium-sized arteries with decreased or obliterated lumen, microaneurysm formation, and intimal proliferation are more common. The vascular lesions of neurofibromatosis are different from those of polyarteritis nodosa and do not show perivascular infiltration or necrosis. Differential renal vein renin may demonstrate increased renin production by a unilaterally involved kidney, especially one with aneurysms. Arteriography may demonstrate small aneurysms in various larger tributaries of the gastrointestinal tract, as can also be seen in polyarteritis. Hypertension can occur, as it may in any condition associated with renal arteritis, and the mechanism probably involves the renin-angiotensin system.

TREATMENT OF ESSENTIAL HYPERTENSION

One of the major advances in cardiology in the past 30 years has been the development and widespread use of effective antihypertensive agents. Before 1950, the only means of lowering blood pressure in patients with hypertension were a strict low-sodium diet, such as the rice-fruit diet of Kempner (1948), and sympathectomy. The diet was extremely difficult for most patients to follow, and sympathectomy was a major surgical procedure associated with a substantial morbidity rate and some deaths. The long-term benefits of sympathectomy were controversial; on balance, it was considered helpful in severe or malignant hypertension, but the operation was promptly abandoned when the ganglionic blocking agents became available.

Since 1950, when agents such as hexamethonium were introduced, a succession of effective compounds with different mechanisms of action have been developed that usually can be taken without seriously interfering with the patient's accustomed mode of life. The dramatic decrease in mortality rate—about 40% in the past 20 years—was most strikingly evident in the more severe varieties of hypertension and its complications. The effectiveness of the available drugs has made hypertension important by emphasizing the need to find the large numbers of people with unrecognized hypertension so that they can receive the benefit of therapy.

Hypertension per se should be treated because vascular abnormalities and their complications occur no matter whether raised blood pressure is primary or secondary. Any drug regimen that brings the blood pressure down into the normal range will prevent and reverse the malignant phase of hypertension, improve cardiac failure, decrease the mortality rate from dissection of the aorta, prevent hemorrhagic stroke, and prolong life (Tables 9–20 and 9–21). Many studies have shown that malignant hypertension, cardiac failure, and hemorrhagic stroke are rare in the properly treated hypertensive patient and that when malignant hypertension and cardiac failure develop in an untreated or inadequately treated hypertensive patient, lowering the blood pressure with effective agents will reverse these complications. Whether lowering the blood pressure will prevent late atherosclerotic complications such as cerebral infarction, coronary heart disease, or atherosclerosis of the peripheral vessels is still an unanswered question, although some studies suggest that treatment of hypertension decreases the incidence of clinical coronary disease (Berglund, 1978; Hypertension Detection Cooperative Group 1979, 1982). Fatal ischemic events just missed significance in the Australian trial (1980) in patients whose diastolic pressure was 100 mm Hg or greater ($p < 0.051$). Atherosclerosis develops over a period of years, and most of the therapeutic trials have been too short to demonstrate the effectiveness of therapy. The age of the patient when therapy was begun also influences the incidence of morbid events. In the VA Study (1972), 15% of the control group developed morbid events if under age 50, but 43% developed morbid events if they were over age 50. In the treated group, there was still a distinct disadvantage in the older group, but the incidence of morbid events was less than in the untreated group. Seven percent of those under age 50 and 18% of those 50 or over developed morbid events during the period of observation. Therapeutic trials are still under way in various parts of the world to test the hypothesis that effective antihypertensive therapy begun at a younger age and in milder hypertensive patients will decrease, delay, or prevent atherosclerosis, which is the leading cause of death in mild to moderate hypertension.

An 8-year follow-up study of the large Medical

Table 9–20. Percentages of hypertensive patients surviving 5 years according to the presence and severity of various complications.*

Complication of Hypertension	Grade of Severity of Complication			
	1	2	3	4
Retinopathy (all cases)	82	65	20	18
Retinopathy plus renal failure	43	24	23	11
Radiologic cardiac enlargement	79	51	35	0
Electrocardiographic abnormalities	82	55	34	28

*Reproduced, with permission, from the American Heart Association, Inc., Nagle R: The prognosis of hypertension. *Practitioner* (July) 1971;**207**:52. Modified from Sokolow M, Perloff D: The prognosis of essential hypertension treated conservatively. *Circulation* 1961;**23**:697.

Table 9–21. Effect of treatment on mortality rate and major cardiovascular complications. (After Veterans Administration Cooperative Study Group, 1970.)*

Diastolic Blood Pressure (mm Hg)	Placebo				Treated				Follow-Up Period (Years)
	No.	Deaths	Complications		No.	Deaths	Complications		
			No.	%			No.	%	
115–129	70	4	27	38.6	73	0	1	1.4	1.6
90–114	194	19	56	29	186	8	22	11.8	3.3

*Reproduced, with permission, from Nagle R: The prognosis of hypertension. *Practitioner* (July) 1971;**207**:52.

Research Council trial of the treatment of mild hypertension (diastolic pressure 90–109 mm Hg) showed that the incidence of coronary events was *not* reduced when results of treatment using a thiazide or propranolol were compared to results obtained with a placebo; the incidence of stroke, however, *was* reduced (Medical Research Council Working Party, 1985).

When to Treat Hypertension

Considerable care must be taken to establish the diagnosis of hypertension before instituting treatment, because treatment is usually a lifelong process. Treatment is rarely urgent in the absence of severe or accelerated hypertension.

As indicated previously, established hypertension must be differentiated from transient elevation of blood pressure caused by excitement, apprehension, exertion, or the systolic elevation of blood pressure that occurs in elderly people as a result of increased stiffness of the aorta or at any age as a result of a raised cardiac output, increased cardiac contraction, or increased stroke output from a slow ventricular rate.

The decision to start treatment is in many instances based on the individual physician's philosophic perception of the consequences of inaction. The premise underlying antihypertensive therapy is that lowering the blood pressure will decrease the likelihood of disability and death from vascular complications. There is no single point at which all physicians will agree that treatment is required. Furthermore, if the physician diagnoses hypertension on the basis of the blood pressure at a single visit, the diagnosis of hypertension will be in error regardless of how many pressures are obtained that day, because more than a third of individuals fail to sustain the elevated levels (Alderman, 1977; Carey, 1976). In addition, if one uses as a criterion diastolic pressures of 105 mm Hg or more, the prevalence of hypertension in the adult population would fall from 20% to about 5%.

Hypertension can be considered a continuum, progressing from (1) the earliest manifestations of transient occasional rises of blood pressure to (2) asymptomatic established hypertension without vascular abnormalities or complications through (3) the presence of vascular abnormalities alone without complications to (4) the presence of vascular complications and finally to (5) death. At what point along the continuum one decides to institute treatment depends on the philosophy and conviction of the physician that the benefits warrant the difficulties of lifelong treatment with antihypertensive agents.

Early Treatment

Some physicians are sufficiently concerned about the potential hazards of hypertension, for example, that they will begin treatment in a black male teenager if his blood pressure exceeds the 95th percentile for age, sex, and race—especially if he has a family history of hypertension. Others wait until hypertension is established and even then do not treat unless the diastolic pressure consistently exceeds 105 mm Hg in the office unless other circumstances suggest that the risk of vascular complications is great. This view is based on the Veterans Administration Study, a randomized study of approximately 400 hypertensive patients whose blood pressure elevation persisted in the hospital and who were found to be cooperative to therapy in an outpatient trial following hospitalization, half of whom were treated, half untreated (VA Study, 1970). The results (Table 9–22) unequivocally demonstrated the benefit of antihypertensive therapy in patients whose average office diastolic pressures

Table 9–22. Incidence of assessable events by age and diagnostic category in the VA Study.*

Diagnostic Category	< 50 C	< 50 T	50–59 C	50–59 T	60+ C	60+ T	Total Events C	Total Events T
Cerebrovascular accident	5	1	5	1	10	3	20	5
Congestive heart failure	1	0	1	0	9	0	11	0
Accelerated hypertension or renal damage	5	0	2	0	0	0	7	0
Coronary artery disease†	4	4	4	2	5	5	13	11
Atrial fibrillation	0	2	0	1	2	0	2	3
Aortic dissection	0	0	1	0	1	0	2	0
Other‡	0	0	1	0	0	3	1	3
Total morbid events	15	7	14	4	27	11	56	22
Diastolic > 124 mm Hg	15	0	3	0	2	0	20	0

Abbreviations: C = control group; T = treated group.
*Modified and reproduced, with permission, from the American Heart Association, Inc., Veterans Administration Cooperative Study Group on Antihypertensive Agents: Effects of treatment on morbidity in hypertension. 3. Influence of age, diastolic pressure, and prior cardiovascular disease; further analysis of side-effects. *Circulation* 1972; 45:991.
†Myocardial infarction or sudden death.
‡Includes in treated group one patient terminated because of hypotensive reactions, one death from ruptured atherosclerotic aneurysm, and one patient with second-degree heart block. Control group includes one patient with left bundle branch block.

equaled or exceeded 105 mm Hg. Vascular complications were 3 times as great in untreated as in treated patients.

The major dilemma regarding when drug treatment should be initiated concerns patients whose diastolic pressure is in the 90–100 mm Hg range (most hypertensives). Large therapeutic trials, including the VA Study, the Australian Therapeutic Trial, the Oslo Study, and the Hypertension Detection and Follow-Up Program Cooperative Group Study, found that patients in this group either had no decrease in cardiovascular morbidity or mortality rates or only a modest decrease. If the diastolic pressure is consistently less than 100 mm Hg, the patient should be observed closely and treated with nonpharmacologic methods (eg, weight reduction, limitation of sodium intake, measures to encourage relaxation) (p 258) unless there are significant risk factors for atherosclerosis. These risk factors include a family history of hypertension and its complications; black racial background, male sex, and age under 40 years; diabetes; hypercholesterolemia; or evidence of target organ damage. Treatment with antihypertensive drugs may be started if the diastolic blood pressure is less than 100 mm Hg and associated risk factors are present. If repeated observations indicate pressure exceeding 100 mm Hg, antihypertensive therapy should be started. All patients, whether or not they receive antihypertensive drugs, should be seen at least twice a year.

The younger the individual, the more significant is any given level of blood pressure, so that a pressure that might be in the 50th percentile in the sixth decade would be in the 90th or 95th percentile in an individual in the third decade, with a corresponding doubled or tripled mortality rate over a period of 20–30 years. Although it has not been proved that treating borderline hypertension prevents the development of atherosclerosis, the Framingham Study showed that the development of coronary disease is more frequent in borderline hypertensive than in normotensive individuals (see Fig 9–6). In a study (Berglund, 1978) in which 635 hypertensive men 47–54 years of age whose arterial pressure exceeded 175/115 mm Hg on 2 occasions were compared with a control group of 390 men who had this level of pressure on only one occasion and remained untreated for 4.3 years, the incidence of fatal and nonfatal coronary disease was significantly lower in the treated group (3.6% versus 6.9%) (Fig 9–30).

The term "borderline hypertension" is used by some authorities to mean diastolic pressures between 90 and 104 mm Hg, by others to mean pressures less than 160/95 but more than 140/90 mm Hg, and by still others to denote diastolic pressures that are sometimes 90–100 mm Hg and sometimes less than 90 mm Hg. The term "borderline hypertension" is most commonly used when average pressures are less than 160/100 mm Hg, associated with occasional normal readings; the term "mild hypertension" is used to mean average diastolic pressures between 90 and 104 mm Hg.

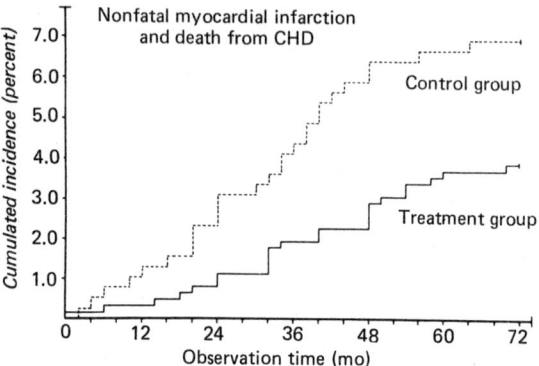

Figure 9–30. Cumulative incidence of nonfatal myocardial infarction and death from coronary heart disease (CHD) by life table analysis. (Reproduced, with permission, from Berglund G et al: Coronary heart-disease after treatment of hypertension. *Lancet* 1978;1:1.)

Significance of Vascular Complications

The development of vascular complications ("clinical events") is clearly related to the presence of prior vascular abnormalities (fundal or electrocardiographic abnormalities), even when comparable degrees of elevation of blood pressure are present. Insurance data and recordings of blood pressure have shown that for any given elevation of blood pressure the likelihood of cardiac failure and death is much greater when either left ventricular hypertrophy or abnormalities of the arterioles of the retina are present. For this reason, the presence of target organ damage warrants therapy in mild hypertension because the measured blood pressure at any given time may not be representative of the average value, which may be higher.

Evaluation of Blood Pressure

From the above, it follows that one should identify hypertension early in its course because it is often asymptomatic, because the first manifestation may be a complication, and because if it is not recognized until later, damage to the arterioles and arteries may have already occurred. Treatment should not be delayed until vascular complications have appeared. The first complication may be one that carries a high mortality rate, eg, cardiac failure, malignant hypertension, aortic dissection, or hemorrhagic stroke. These complications, unfortunately, are commonly seen in untreated hypertensives, especially in patients who have not had access to medical therapy or have discontinued therapy. For these reasons, vigorous efforts are now being made to make certain that the blood pressure is measured and recorded in every patient who enters the health care system for any reason. Public and voluntary health agencies have been encouraging widespread screening to identify asymptomatic hypertensive individuals; increased awareness of hypertension has resulted (Tuomilehto, 1980). As is true also of other types of screening (eg, glaucoma, diabetes), the purpose of this effort is not to make the diagnosis but to find people who need further evaluation. A high percentage of patients with elevated blood pressure in screened populations have normal pressures in the doctor's office. At least one-third of patients with initial diastolic pressures over 105–110 mm Hg will have pressures less than 90 mm Hg when readings are taken later. The current standards of what constitutes normal blood pressure are based on resting office pressures.

Even if the pressure is raised in the doctor's office, one must be certain that the elevated pressure is not transient. For example, one needs measurements on at least 3 separate occasions even if the diastolic pressure varies between 100 and 120 mm Hg. If diastolic pressures are so variable that they are 90–100 mm Hg on one occasion but less than 90 mm Hg on another occasion, it may be necessary to take 10, 20, or even 30 readings over a period of months before concluding that the patient is indeed an established hypertensive who needs lifelong therapy. Ten to 20% of patients at any given time may have variable pressures above or below whatever arbitrary line the physician regards as the upper limit of normal, above which treatment will be started; it is then necessary to use ancillary methods to try to obtain blood pressures under ordinary circumstances of the patient's life. As discussed previously, pressures can be taken by the patient or a family member at home, or by a nurse in the office in nonthreatening situations. Near-basal pressures utilizing sedation can be measured, as recommended by Smirk (1959) in New Zealand, and ambulatory pressures can be obtained semiautomatically by utilizing a portable blood pressure recorder. In almost 30% of cases, even patients with consistently elevated office pressures will have normal pressures after several days of hospitalization. The average drop in blood pressures in these patients is about 20–30 mm Hg depending on the age of the patient and the height of the pressure, but the significance of this difference is not known.

When the physician has taken an adequate number of readings under appropriate conditions and is convinced that this particular patient will benefit from treatment even after the potential side effects of the drug regimen have been considered, the patient must then be educated regarding the duration of treatment, and every responsible effort must be made to see to it that the patient continues in treatment indefinitely. In the VA Study (1975), hypertension returned, usually by 6 months, in 85% of patients in whom treatment was deliberately stopped (Fig 9–31).

The decision to begin antihypertensive therapy requires careful judgment and thorough discussion with the patient and should never be undertaken lightly. Antihypertensive therapy is a cooperative venture between the patient and the doctor, and agreement on a mutual objective at the outset increases the likelihood of patient compliance. Once begun, treatment should be continued without interruption, modified if necessary, along with treatment of other risk factors of atherosclerosis.

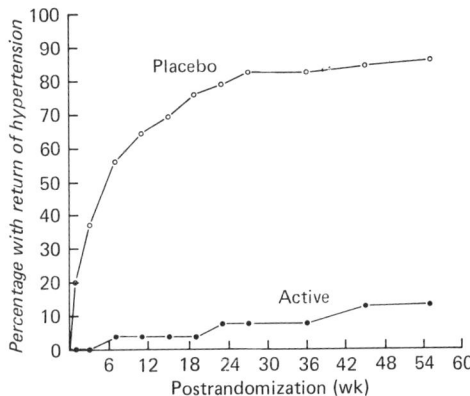

Figure 9–31. Cumulative percentage of patients attaining diastolic blood pressure of 95 mm Hg or higher on 2 successive clinic visits is shown on the ordinate. Time after randomization is shown on the abscissa. At 6 weeks after randomization, 51% of the placebo group demonstrated 95 mm Hg, and at 6 months 82% of the placebo group had reached this level. (Reproduced, with permission, from the American Heart Association, Inc., Veterans Administration Cooperative Study Group on Antihypertensive Agents: Return of elevated blood pressure after withdrawal of antihypertensive drugs. *Circulation* 1975;**51**:1107.)

Treat According to Severity

In the average patient with mild or moderate hypertension, it is preferable to begin slowly and gradually increase the dosage and potency of the therapeutic agents used; however, this is not adequate when the patient has accelerated hypertension, encephalopathy, cardiac failure, or similar urgent situations. The physician must estimate the urgency of the role of the elevated blood pressure and match the choice of drugs with the necessities of the situation. Even when it is urgent to lower the pressure quickly, one must not act precipitously and then have to retreat if the fall in pressure is excessive or if side effects occur.

In mild to moderate disease, one should begin with drugs of modest potency in low dosage given once or twice daily in order to avoid toxic side effects that might discourage the patient. The objective of treatment is to use as few agents as possible with the fewest possible side effects and to bring down the blood pressure and keep it down without interfering too much with the patient's life-style. Each drug must be used until the desired effect is achieved or until side effects prevent increased dosage. In the latter event, a new agent is added. The availability of a number of drugs with different mechanisms of action allows the physician to use trial and error to obtain an effective combination of agents with which the patient can live comfortably. Forcing the patient to accept unpleasant side effects usually leads to discouragement and noncompliance, especially if the patient is asymptomatic. The drugs are used orally except in compelling situations, when parenteral therapy is used in combination with oral therapy. (See below for details.)

1. BASIC PRINCIPLES OF TREATMENT

(1) Establish that persistent and not transient hypertension is present.

(2) Institute appropriate treatment of "curable" secondary causes of hypertension, if present.

(3) Evaluate the functional integrity or the degree and speed of involvement of target organs to estimate prognosis.

(4) Assess the need for treatment by the height of the arterial pressures taken in the office or home or while ambulatory and by the associated vascular complications.

(5) Assess the need for treatment in borderline or mild hypertension (diastolic pressure 90–104 mm Hg) in the light of adverse prognostic factors such as youth, male sex, positive family history, black race, and the presence of target organ damage. Also determine the presence of other risk factors known to influence atherosclerosis, eg, hypercholesterolemia, hypertriglyceridemia, cigarette smoking, diabetes, family history of atherosclerosis, personality disturbances, obesity. Decisions about therapeutic options such as the potency and mode of administration of drugs and whether to use one agent or a combination of agents are based upon the height of the arterial pressure and the urgency of the hypertensive complications, eg, cardiac failure, hypertensive encephalopathy and progression to malignant hypertension, aortic dissection, or hemorrhagic stroke.

(6) Begin treatment in mild to moderate hypertensive disease with an agent of moderate potency that is known to cause minimal side effects. Gradually increase the dose until the desired therapeutic effect is achieved or unpleasant side effects occur. If necessary, add another and then perhaps another agent until a combination of drugs is arrived at that gives an acceptable pressure with the fewest possible or least disturbing side effects.

(7) The aim is to achieve a standing office diastolic pressure less than 90 mm Hg or a systolic pressure less than 140 mm Hg. However, a pressure of 150/100 mm Hg is acceptable if untoward side effects make a lower pressure difficult to achieve, especially in patients with severe hypertension at the outset or in patients over age 70.

(8) Assess the patient's social, emotional, economic, and environmental problems in all cases, especially if the response to treatment is poor.

(9) Educate the patient and make treatment as convenient as possible to ensure compliance with long-term treatment.

(10) Treatment should be individualized, with minimal doses in frail, elderly people.

2. GENERAL THERAPEUTIC MEASURES

General measures such as diet, exercise, loss of weight in obesity, relaxation, modification of lifestyle, and attention to other risk factors should not be neglected in the care of the hypertensive patient.

Although the use of diuretic agents makes strict sodium restriction less important, a high sodium intake, either by the use of salt in the diet or by sodium-containing agents such as Alka-Seltzer, reduces the effectiveness of diuretic agents. The patient's sodium intake should be limited. There should be no added salt in the diet, and the patient should be advised to avoid very salty foods such as potato chips, bacon, soy sauce, etc. If the patient has carbohydrate intolerance, a prudent diet of modest carbohydrate and caloric restriction is advised; we encourage the patient to stay on this diet permanently. If the patient has hypercholesterolemia or hypertriglyceridemia, and especially if type IV hyperlipidemia is present as a result of increased carbohydrate or alcohol intake, reduced intake of these substances should be encouraged in order to reduce the serum triglycerides that may favor the development of coronary heart disease. In the presence of type II hypercholesterolemia, a reduced cholesterol intake is encouraged, and the patient is given drugs (colestipol or cholestyramine), as indicated in Chapter 8.

Weight reduction is recommended, not only because this may rarely reduce the blood pressure to normal but also because obesity aggravates and increases the likelihood of diabetes, marginally increases the likelihood of coronary heart disease, and interferes with the patient's sense of well-being.

Moderate physical activity is encouraged, not only for its effect on weight loss and general sense of well-being but also because moderate exercise decreases the systemic vascular resistance and seems beneficial, although there are scarce data to substantiate this. Advocates of physical exercise as a preventive measure against the development of acute myocardial infarction believe that physical conditioning increases the collateral circulation and decreases the likelihood of fatality if the patient does develop acute myocardial infarction.

Cigarette smoking may not only increase the likelihood of coronary heart disease but may also increase the likelihood of ventricular fibrillation and sudden death if the patient has concomitant coronary disease, as most hypertensives do. Hypertensive patients should stop smoking if possible.

There is no evidence that moderate amounts of alcohol, coffee, or tea are harmful to hypertensive patients; in fact, they may be helpful by virtue of their relaxant effects. Excessive use of alcohol, however, is undesirable because it increases the serum triglyceride concentration and because prolonged excessive use of alcohol may produce alcoholic cardiomyopathy. In a patient whose cardiac load is already increased by raised blood pressure, alcohol may favor the development of cardiac failure. The combination of hypertensive heart disease, coronary heart disease, and alcoholic cardiomyopathy is particularly ominous.

Relaxation, Meditation, or Biofeedback Therapy

Mental tranquility is always desirable. Over the years a variety of methods have been used to relax patients. Prior to the days of antihypertensive therapy, sedation, progressive relaxation, psychotherapy, frequent vacations, and attention to the environment were all used, but with only marginal benefit in the reduction of blood pressure. More recently, transcendental meditation, biofeedback, yoga, and other methods of relaxation have been explored in an effort to combat the environmental increase in systemic vascular resistance and cardiac output that occurs with the stresses of modern life. In a group of 20 hypertensive patients who received a professionally supervised program of transcendental meditation, no significant change in blood pressure occurred after 6 months (Pollack, 1977), although some subjects had a greater sense of well-being. There have been some reports that meditation lowered the blood pressure in a few patients. On the other hand, it should be appreciated that some forms of meditation in fact produce violent increases in blood pressure, such that one patient had "private thoughts" during meditation that raised his diastolic pressure to 170 mm Hg for several hours. We have been unimpressed by the reports of beneficial effects of biofeedback, and in the absence of data solidly demonstrating its value we rely on antihypertensive agents rather than on psychologic or nonpharmacologic methods as the primary therapy in treating hypertension. Psychologic methods such as relaxation therapy can be considered as auxiliary therapy.

3. DRUG TREATMENT

Drugs used in treating hypertension vary in dosage, potency, side effects, mechanism of action, and route of administration (oral or parenteral). The antihypertensive drugs available are summarized in Tables 9–23 and 9–24, and Table 9–25 reviews the adverse

Table 9–23. Oral treatment of hypertension (adult dosages).

	Tablet Size (mg)	Initial and Incremental Dose (mg)	Doses Per Day	Usual Oral Daily Dose (mg)	Interval Between Increment of Doses
Commonly used mild diuretics					
Hydrochlorothiazide (Hydrodiuril, Esidrix, Oretic)	25, 50, 100	25, 50	1–2	25–100	2 weeks
Chlorothiazide (Diuril)	250, 500	250, 500	1–2	250–1000	2 weeks
Bendroflumethiazide (Naturetin)	2.5, 5, 10	2.5	1–2	2.5–10	2 weeks
Chlorthalidone (Hygroton)	50, 100	50	1	50–100	2 weeks
Metolazone (Zaroxolyn)	2.5, 5, 10	2.5	1	2.5–10	2 weeks
Indapamide (Lozol)	2.5	2.5	1–2	2.5–5	2 weeks
Potassium-sparing diuretics					
Triamterene (Dyrenium)	50, 100	50	1–2	50–200	2 weeks
Spironolactone (Aldactone)	25	25	1–3	25–150	2 weeks
Amiloride (Moduretic)	5	5, 10	1	5–15	2 weeks
Potent diuretics					
Furosemide (Lasix)	20, 40	20–80	1–3	20–300	1 week
Ethacrynic acid (Edecrin)	25, 50	25, 50	1–3	25–200	1 week
Adrenergic inhibitors					
Reserpine (Serpasil)	0.05, 0.1, 0.25, 0.5, 1	0.05, 0.1	1	0.1–0.25	4 weeks
Guanethidine (Ismelin)	10, 25	10	1	10–200	1 week
Mecamylamine (Inversine)	2.5, 10	2.5	1–4	10–100	1 week
Pentolinium (Ansolysen)	20, 40, 100	20	1–4	80–200	1 week
Propranolol* (Inderal)	10, 40, 80	10	2–4	20–320	1 week
Vasodilators					
Prazosin (Minipress)	1, 2, 5 (capsules)	0.5–1	2–4	10–15	1 week
Hydralazine (Apresoline)	10, 25, 50, 100	10	2–4	100–200	1 week
Minoxidil (Loniten)	1, 5, 10	2.5	2–4	5–20	1 week
Captopril (Capoten)	25, 50, 100	6.25–12.5, 25	3	50–300	2 weeks
Nifedipine (Procardia)	10	5–10	2	20–40	1 week
Centrally acting alpha-adrenergic agonists					
Methyldopa (Aldomet)	125, 250, 500	250	2–4	500–2000	1 week
Clonidine (Catapres)	0.1, 0.2	0.1	1–2	0.1–0.6	1 week
Guanabenz (Wytensin)	4, 8	4	2	4–8	1 week

*The prototype of beta-adrenergic blocking drugs. See text for others.

Table 9-24. Parenteral treatment of hypertension (adult dosages).*

	How Supplied	Initial Dose and Route	Onset of Action	Duration of Action (Before Repeat Dose)
Adrenergic inhibitors				
Methyldopa (Aldomet)	250 mg/5 mL ampule	250–500 mg IV	2–4 hours	4–12 hours
Trimethaphan camsylate† (Arfonad)	500 mg/10 mL ampule	1–4 mg/min IV	Seconds to minutes	As long as infused
Reserpine (Serpasil)	5 mg/2 mL (also 10 mL) ampule	0.5–1 mg IM or IV bolus, slowly	2–6 hours	6–12 hours
Propranolol‡ (Inderal)	1 mg/mL ampule	1 mg IV bolus, slowly	Minutes	4–6 hours
Vasodilators				
Diazoxide† (Hyperstat)	300 mg/20 mL ampule	75–300 mg IV rapidly	1–5 minutes	5–12 hours
Hydralazine (Apresoline)	20 mg/mL ampule	10–20 mg IV or IM bolus, slowly	15–30 minutes	1–4 hours
Sodium nitroprusside§ (Nipride)	50 mg/5 mL vial	0.5–8 µg/min IV by infusion of 5% dextrose and water, not by direct injection	Immediate; can increase infusion rate every 5–10 minutes as needed	As long as infused
Diuretics				
Furosemide (Lasix)	20 mg/2 mL ampule	40–80 mg IV bolus	15–30 minutes	8–12 hours
Ethacrynate sodium (Edecrin)	50 mg/50 mL vial	50 mg IV bolus	15–30 minutes	8–12 hours

*Information regarding products, precautions, and methods of administration of all agents being given parenterally should be reviewed in the *Physicians' Desk Reference* prior to use in patients if the physician is not using the drugs frequently.
†Requires closely monitored supervision and titration for proper dose.
‡The prototype of beta-adrenergic blocking drugs. See text for others.
§Photosensitive—should be protected from light.

effects of these various agents. See p 269 for specific treatment protocols.

Oral Diuretic Agents

The thiazides are the prototype of this group of drugs, which act initially by depleting the body of sodium, potassium, and fluid volume and later by decreasing the systemic vascular resistance.

The sodium, potassium, chloride, and water losses may be substantial over the first few days and then tend to diminish. The 24-hour excretion after a standard dose of a thiazide diuretic is almost 100–200 meq of Na^+, 40–50 meq of K^+, 200 meq of Cl^-, and 1000–1500 mL of water. Early in the course of treatment, hypovolemia may be associated with dizziness, weakness, nausea, cramps, and postural hypotension; later, the plasma volume and extracellular volume return almost to normal (reduced to about 3–5%), and postural hypotension is uncommon. The dose-response curve of a given drug is such that maximum diuretic effects of the drugs occur with about 100 mg of hydrochlorothiazide or 500 mg of the more potent furosemide, given as single doses. Continued hypovolemia can be inferred from the slight increases in serum creatinine and uric acid that occur in most patients. Thiazides increase the tubular reabsorption of urate, and so the plasma uric acid rises. There is a difference of opinion about whether or when one should use drugs such as allopurinol (which decreases the formation of circulating uric acid). A major problem associated with the use of diuretics is hypokalemia, which tends to occur with many of the diuretic agents and is due to impaired reabsorption at the sodium-potassium exchange site, where aldosterone causes increased secretion of potassium and reabsorption of sodium.

The magnitude of the decrease in serum K^+ is variable but averages about 0.6 meq/L (10–15%) in patients receiving the usual daily dose of hydrochlorothiazide in 2 divided doses. It requires 60–80 meq/d of a 10% elixir of potassium chloride to raise the serum potassium to the pretreatment value (Schwartz, 1974). Total potassium in the body is usually low when the serum potassium is reduced, but many patients have a substantial loss of total body potassium with a normal serum potassium, because the correlation between serum potassium and total exchangeable potassium is only 0.4 (Liebman, 1959). The acid-base equilibrium influences the intra- and extracellular balance of potassium, and if there is a tendency to alkalosis, the serum potassium may fall. Table 9–26 shows the average serum electrolytes after 6–8 weeks of treatment with diuretics. In the VA Study (1967), the serum potassium levels on the initial and first and second annual examinations showed that most patients after 1–2 years had serum K^+ levels exceeding 3.5 meq/L but that 20% were between 2.5 and 3.5 meq/L. The electrolyte response to a diuretic is enhanced by bed rest; the urine volume and sodium excretion in normal individuals when they are in bed is of the same order of magnitude as when they are up and about receiving a diuretic. During bed rest, water and sodium excretion doubles, but K^+ excretion does not change. The increased absorption of uric

Table 9–25. Adverse effects of antihypertensive agents.

Diuretics	Nausea, muscle cramps, hypovolemia, hypokalemia, nitrogen retention (especially in the elderly), hyponatremia, hyperuricemia, hyperglycemia, rash.
Potassium-sparing diuretics	Hyperkalemia, gynecomastia, renal stones from triamterene.
Adrenergic inhibitors	
Methyldopa	Drowsiness, dry mouth, impotence, hepatitis, postural hypotension, hemolytic anemia, fever.
Reserpine	Somnolence, nasal congestion, nightmares, mental depression.
Guanethidine	Postural hypotension, diarrhea, retrograde ejaculation, weakness on exertion.
Propranolol and other beta-blocking agents	Bradycardia, left ventricular failure, asthma, Raynaud's syndrome, central nervous system symptoms, sodium retention.
Mecamylamine and trimethaphan	Postural hypotension, parasympathetic blockade with constipation and paralytic ileus, loss of visual accommodation.
Clonidine	Dry mouth, drowsiness, rebound hypertension if drug stopped abruptly.
Vasodilator agents	
Prazosin	Tachycardia, headache, postural weakness and hypotension, especially with initial large dose and if volume-depleted.
Hydralazine	Lupuslike syndrome, headache, tachycardia, angina.
Minoxidil	Tachycardia, hirsutism, headache, sodium retention.
Diazoxide	Hyperglycemia, tachycardia, angina, sodium retention.
Sodium nitroprusside	Excess hypotension, acute tubular necrosis, thiocyanate toxicity.
Captopril	Proteinuria, rash, hypotension, neutropenia.
Nifedipine	Hypotension, syncope.

acid in the proximal tubule leads to raised serum uric acid, which in individuals with a history of gout may cause acute gout that can be prevented by the use of probenecid or allopurinol. Infrequently, glucose reabsorption in the proximal tubule is also impaired, and patients with a susceptibility to diabetes may develop hyperglycemia. The average increase in fasting blood sugar after 2 years of diuretic therapy was found to be 9.6 mg/dL and appears to be related to potassium loss (Amery, 1978). Similar findings were noted after 14 years of therapy (Murphy, 1982); changes between 6 and 14 years were not striking. When thiazides were withdrawn for 7 months, the average reduction in fasting blood glucose was 10% and in the 2-hour postprandial value 25%.

The hemodynamic changes that occur during long-term diuretic therapy have been described by Lund-Johansen (1970). If the dosage of diuretics is excessive, the patient may develop severe hyponatremia and dehydration with hypovolemia, but this is uncommon if the thiazides and not the loop diuretics (eg, furosemide) are used in moderate doses. The potassium loss makes digitalis toxicity more likely, so that particular care must be taken to avoid hypokalemia if digitalis is used. Hypokalemia is more common when dietary potassium is low, sodium intake is high, and laxatives are used frequently. If the serum potassium falls below 3.5 meq/L on ordinary doses of thiazides, the possibility of primary hyperaldosteronism should be considered. If symptoms of hypokalemia develop (polyuria, nocturia, muscle weakness, and fatigue) or if digitalis is prescribed, potassium-sparing diuretics such as spironolactone, amiloride, or triamterene may be added to the thiazides or other diuretics such as chlorthalidone, furosemide, and metolazone, provided renal function is adequate and the patients do not take oral potassium supplements (see below). Spironolactone may induce gynecomastia by altering the peripheral metabolism of testosterone (Rose, 1977); triamterene may result in impaired renal function. This may be particularly important in patients over age 60. In a cooperative study in patients over 60 years of age who received both hydrochlorothiazide, 25 mg daily, and triamterene, 50 mg daily, there was a progressive rise in serum creatinine of 40–50% over a period of 3–5 years (Amery, 1978). The rise in serum creatinine correlated significantly with the fall in systolic blood pressure and with the rise in serum uric acid. Further studies are required to determine the hazards of triamterene in elderly patients. Patients should be given a high-potassium diet (Table 9–27) or liquid potassium supplements if they have hypokalemia with symptoms. (Enteric-coated potassium supplements should be avoided because of their propensity for producing

Table 9–26. Average serum electrolytes after 6–8 weeks' treatment with 50 mg hydrochlorothiazide or 100 mg ethacrynic acid daily.*

Treatment Group	Sodium (meq/L)	Potassium (meq/L)	Chloride (meq/L)	Bicarbonate (meq/L)	Urea (mg/dL)	Uric Acid (mg/dL)
Control	143.9	4.3	103.3	27.5	29.8	5.3
Hydrochlorothiazide	137.8	3.7	95.4	29.0	32.0	7.2
Ethacrynic acid	139.4	3.8	98.0	27.9	41.1 (31.8)†	7.0

*Reproduced, with permission, from Dollery CT, Parry EHO, Young DS: Diuretic and hypotensive properties of ethacrynic acid: A comparison with hydrochlorothiazide. *Lancet* 1964;1:947.
†This figure is the average after eliminating the results on one patient whose blood urea rose to 155 mg/dL on ethacrynic acid.

Table 9-27. Foods helpful in addition to normal diet to supplement potassium (K$^+$) intake.*

Quantities of foods to supply approximately 0.5 g (500 mg) (13 meq) of potassium (K$^+$)
- 1 cup tomato juice†
- 1 cup low-sodium tomato juice, prune juice
- 1¼ cups orange juice, tangerine juice, orange-grapefruit juice, grapefruit juice

- 1 medium-sized banana
- 7–8 dates
- 4 figs
- 7 large prunes
- ½ cup raisins (dark)
- 6 apricots (fresh)
- ½ cantaloupe

- 1 cup broccoli
- ¾ cup winter squash
- 10 brussels sprouts, cooked
- 1 large white potato
- 1 large sweet potato
- 1/3 cup lentils (dry)
- 1½ cups raw cauliflower

- 4 tbsp nonfat milk powder†
- 1½ cups nonfat milk†

*Courtesy of California Heart Association.
†High in potassium but also high in sodium.

ulceration of the small intestine.) Liquid potassium preparations are unpleasant to take. If hypokalemia occurs at levels of 3–3.5 meq/L, oral potassium supplements of 40–80 meq/d should be prescribed.

Oral diuretic agents should be considered a basic treatment of most hypertensive patients because they suffice in many cases to lower the pressure satisfactorily when used alone, although some authorities prefer to begin with beta-adrenergic blocking drugs because of the side effects from the diuretics. The average reduction in blood pressure with hydrochlorothiazide is about 20 mm Hg systolic and 10–15 mm Hg diastolic. There is a minimal postural effect. This is approximately the magnitude of the fall following the use of methyldopa, but the diuretics diminish the required dosage of other agents added to a therapeutic regimen or are additive to other drugs. For example, when hydrochlorothiazide is added to methyldopa, the average fall in blood pressure is greater than with either drug used alone and averages about 32 mm Hg systolic and 15 mm Hg diastolic. Furthermore, they counteract the sodium retention that occurs with other drugs such as the vasodilator agents and methyldopa. If oral diuretics are added to an already stabilized regimen because of sodium retention or excessive hypertension, the dose of the basic drug should be reduced about 50% before the diuretic is added to avoid excessive fall in pressure. When methyldopa is added after the full effect of a thiazide diuretic is achieved, not only are the systolic and diastolic pressures lower, but the reduction of the glomerular filtration rate and the renal blood flow are reversed toward normal. Plasma renin activity, which is increased by a diuretic, is increased only half as much when methyldopa is added. If the diuretic is added after the full effect of methyldopa is obtained, the glomerular filtration rate is reduced by about 15 mL/min, renal blood flow is reduced by about 20 mL/min, and the plasma renin activity doubles or triples.

Reserpine

Reserpine can be given orally, intramuscularly, or intravenously. It inhibits sympathetic nervous transmission by depleting the peripheral nerve endings of norepinephrine as well as by depleting the central stores in the cardiovascular centers in the medulla. Because of its central action, its main side effects are lethargy, fatigue, and, especially with larger doses, nightmares and depression. If depression is severe and the patient is suicidal, an alternative drug to reserpine should be employed; such severe reactions are rare when the daily dose does not exceed 0.1–0.2 mg/d. When combined with the oral diuretics or with hydralazine, reserpine is an effective hypotensive agent. Another unpleasant side effect is stuffy nose, which is difficult to control, although nose drops may be helpful. (Avoid those that are strong vasoconstrictors.) Reserpine increases gastric acidity, but this is rarely significant with the small oral doses that are used, and peptic ulcer is rare. A reported association between the use of reserpine and carcinoma of the breast in women was not confirmed by later investigations, and the FDA did not remove reserpine from the market as was briefly expected. Intramuscular or intravenous reserpine is reserved for hypertensive emergencies when the pressure must be reduced within hours, and therapy is most effective when combined with hydralazine in acute glomerulonephritis. Reserpine may cause somnolence and thus is not the drug of choice in patients with hypertensive encephalopathy or cerebral symptoms, because the action of the drug makes interpretation of the patient's progress more difficult. Nevertheless, it is a valuable drug and has the advantage of not requiring minute-to-minute titration as do some of the other parenteral agents (see below).

Methyldopa

Methyldopa can be given orally, intramuscularly, or intravenously.

Methyldopa acts by stimulating alpha-adrenergic receptors in the medulla, resulting in decreased sympathetic impulses to the heart and blood vessels and decreased serum norepinephrine. The central action is responsible for its major side effects of drowsiness and fatigue, so that individuals whose work involves mental activity may find the drug unsatisfactory. Systemic vascular resistance is decreased with time, but cardiac output and renal blood flow are not affected; thus, the drug is valuable in the presence of impaired renal function.

Methyldopa is considered by many nephrologists to be the drug of choice when hypertension complicates renal dialysis or renal failure. It decreases renin secretion and does not interfere with tests of the renin-angiotensin-aldosterone system, which is an advantage when investigators are reluctant to stop all antihypertensive therapy to determine the status of the renin-angiotensin system. Raised renin production that follows hypovolemia with oral diuretics can be neutralized by the use of methyldopa. The drug may cause fever (infrequently), a direct positive Coombs test, hemolytic anemia (rarely), hepatitis with jaundice (rarely), and impotence—the commonest cause of patient noncompliance with treatment. All of these adverse effects are reversible when the drug is stopped.

Methyldopa can be used intramuscularly or intravenously in severe hypertension, when hours or 1–2 days are sufficient to achieve satisfactory lowering of the pressure without the necessity for minute-to-minute monitoring. It is not as effective as some of the other parenteral agents (see below) but is a valuable adjunct in severe but not accelerated, or malignant, hypertension. Minoxidil may be preferable under these circumstances or if methyldopa is ineffective.

Beta-Adrenergic Blocking Agents

These agents reduce systolic and diastolic blood pressure by reducing the heart rate at rest and after exercise by about 25% and the cardiac index during exercise by about 15%; systemic vascular resistance shows no change or may rise slightly. Renal blood flow and the glomerular filtration rate may fall slightly. In addition to their beta-blocking activities, beta blockers decrease renin release.

The long-term hemodynamic effects of atenolol have been documented by Lund-Johansen (1979). The hemodynamic changes noted after 1 year remained essentially the same after 5 years.

Because beta-blocking drugs neutralize the reflex tachycardia and increase in cardiac output that follow vasodilator drugs, they are particularly effective when combined with diuretic and vasodilator drugs (Fig 9–32). They rarely may mask the tachycardia and sweating and other warning signs of hypoglycemia in diabetics receiving insulin, especially while these patients are fasting. Suitable precautions should be taken. Propranolol (or other beta blockers) may cause Raynaud's phenomenon in cold weather, bradycardia, asthma, hypotension, syncope, left ventricular failure, and occasionally central nervous system symptoms such as lethargy, depression, and intense dreams.

Some beta-adrenergic blocking drugs are cardioselective and do not produce bronchial constriction and thus may be helpful in patients with a history of chronic bronchitis or asthma. The pharmacologic characteristics are outlined in Table 9–28. Beneficial effects usually occur within about 2 weeks.

The approved beta-adrenergic blocking agents and their dosages are noted in Table 9–28. They should be started at a low dose and titrated to a well-tolerated effective one. Atenolol and nadolol may have significant clinical advantages in that they are effective with once-daily doses. Atenolol and metoprolol do not cross the blood-brain barrier and therefore result in fewer central nervous system side effects. All beta-adrenergic blocking agents have similar effects in the treatment of hypertension but differ with respect to dosage, duration of effect, lipid solubility and entry into the brain, intrinsic sympathomimetic activity, and cardioselectivity for β_1 receptors. A drug with intrinsic sympathomimetic activity and a weak agonist effect (eg, pindolol) may cause less bradycardia, but the beta-blocking effect is dominant. The other beta blockers approved by the FDA do not have intrinsic sympathomimetic activity; however, no convincing studies have shown any clinical advantage when a drug with intrinsic sympathomimetic activity is used in hypertension. All of the beta-adrenergic blocking drugs are more effective when combined with a diuretic.

The beta-adrenergic blocking drugs in moderate

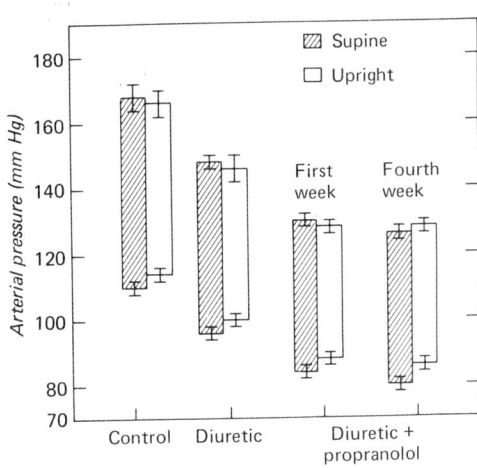

Figure 9–32. Time course of the fall in pressure and the magnitude of the hypotensive effects with addition of propranolol in 20 diuretic-treated patients with essential hypertension. Each paired column represents weekly averages of blood pressures with subjects supine and upright, measured at home twice daily (expressed as mean ± SE). Values attained with addition of propranolol are significantly different ($P < 0.001$) from control levels and from those during diuretic therapy alone. (Reproduced, with permission, from Bravo EL, Tarazi RC, Dustan HP: β-Adrenergic blockade in diuretic-treated patients with essential hypertension. N Engl J Med 1975;292:66.)

Table 9–28. Beta-adrenergic blocking drugs approved by FDA.

Agent	Cardio-selectivity	Half-Life (h)	Average Daily Dose (mg)
Propranolol	No	4–6	160–240 in 2–3 divided doses
Atenolol	Yes	6–9	50–100 once daily
Metoprolol	Yes	3–6	50–200 in 2 divided doses
Pindolol	No	3–5	5–10 in 2 divided doses
Timolol	No	4–6	10–30 in 2 divided doses
Nadolol	No	12–24	40–200 once daily

dosage produce an average fall of mean blood pressure of about 20 mm Hg (range, 10–40 mm Hg), and there is an increasing tendency, especially in Europe, to begin therapy with these drugs rather than with the diuretics. The major side effect if excessive doses are used is postural hypotension, although mental slowing and decrease in cardiac output may be significant, especially in patients with impending or actual left ventricular failure. It is not known whether the newer drugs also produce the cold hands and feet and disturbing dreams that occur with propranolol.

The absorption of propranolol from the gastrointestinal tract is highly variable, ranging from 10 to 80%. The plasma half-life is 4–5 hours. Therapeutic plasma levels are usually achieved with 160 mg/d (80 mg twice daily), but there is marked variation among patients. Following administration of propranolol, there is a rapid fall of plasma renin but a relatively slow fall in blood pressure, with no time relationship between the two. Furthermore, there has been no correlation between the efficacy of particular beta blockers in lowering plasma renin and their effect on blood pressure, thus throwing doubt on the concept that propranolol reduces hypertension by decreasing renin release, despite the fact that propranolol does, in fact, reduce plasma renin. Propranolol has a progressive action that may increase over a period of months.

A sequential antihypertensive regimen beginning with a beta blocker was used in a group of 188 patients by Bühler (1978). Fig 9–33 is a pie graph showing the percentage of patients whose pressures were returned to normal with the various therapies. The effect of beta blockers alone was quite striking.

Hydralazine

Hydralazine can be used orally, intramuscularly, or intravenously and acts directly on the smooth muscle of the arteriole, decreasing its contractility and thus decreasing systemic vascular resistance. The vasodilator effect with fall in pressure stimulates the baroreceptors to reflexly increase sympathetic discharge, with resulting tachycardia and raised cardiac output, which may cause side effects of palpitations, angina pectoris, and headache. These side effects can be prevented when beta-blocking drugs are given first or, less effectively, when reserpine, methyldopa, or guanethidine is used. Hydralazine fell out of favor in the early days of its use when it was given as the sole agent in doses of 600–800 mg/d; side effects were prominent, including a syndrome of arthritis, fever, positive LE cell preparations, and antinuclear antibody in the serum. These lupus erythematosus–like findings were usually temporary and only occurred with large doses or in patients who were "slow acetylators." Metabolic inactivation of hydralazine occurs by acetylation, ie, by the action of hepatic N-acetyltransferase. The activity of the enzyme is genetically determined, and some patients are slow and others are rapid acetylators. With any dose of the drug, slow acetylators have a higher plasma hydralazine concentration and run a greater risk of adverse effects than fast acetylators (Zacest, 1972). Such findings rarely occur with doses of less than 200 mg/d. Hydralazine can be used intramuscularly when a fall in blood pressure within 20–40 minutes is desired, especially when combined with parenteral reserpine in acute nephritis in children. It can also be given intermittently by injection to keep the pressure under control in severe hypertension until combined oral drug therapy has become effective.

Prazosin (Minipress)

Prazosin is a moderately effective vasodilator that relaxes smooth muscle by blocking alpha-adrenergic postsynaptic receptors (Lowenstein, 1979). Because its mechanism of action differs from hydralazine, the 2 drugs may be combined to lower the pressure if either of them alone is inadequate. Plasma volume increases in almost all patients, indicating the need for associated diuretic therapy (Koshy, 1977). The side effects are relatively minor but include postural hypotension, dizziness, fatigue, headache, drowsiness, and general lack of energy. Prazosin is supplied as 1-mg capsules for oral administration. The plasma concentration reaches a peak in about 3 hours, and the plasma half-life is 2–3 hours. It has approximately the same potency as methyldopa or hydralazine, plus the advantage of not increasing the heart rate, cardiac output, or plasma renin or decreasing the renal blood flow or glomerular filtration rate. By dilating both the arterial and venous circulations, prazosin is of particular value when hypertension is associated with

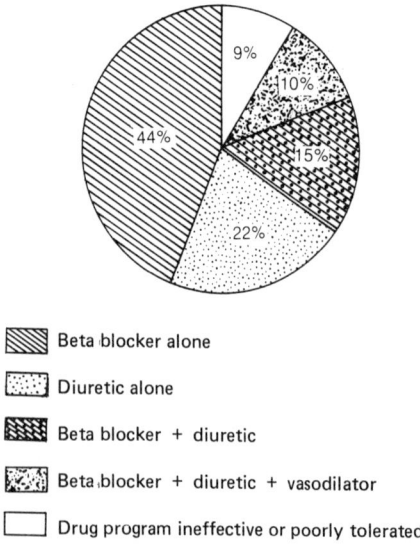

Figure 9–33. Efficacies of sequential antihypertensive regimens in 188 patients with essential hypertension. Blood efficacy is measured by diastolic blood pressure normalized to 95 mm Hg or less. (Reproduced, with permission, from Bühler FR, Bertel O, Lütold BE: Simplified and age-stratified antihypertensive therapy based on beta blockers. *Cardiovasc Med* 1978;3:135.)

cardiac failure or if diuretics or beta-adrenergic blocking agents cause side effects. Some authorities recommend prazosin as the initial drug. It may cause postural hypotension and collapse, especially if the patient is volume-depleted. The initial dose should be small, such as 0.5–1 mg at bedtime, gradually and slowly increased to tolerance depending upon the response of the patient (up to about 20 mg/d if necessary). Plasma volume is increased, and fluid retention may occur; if so, the drug should be used in combination with a diuretic as a second drug.

Guanethidine

Guanethidine is a potent agent that produces selective sympathetic blockade and inhibits transmission of adrenergic stimuli across peripheral nerve endings by impairing the release, and possibly the storage, of norepinephrine. Because it does not cross the blood-brain barrier, central nervous system symptoms such as occur with reserpine, methyldopa, and clonidine do not occur. It increases renin production. Its major side effects are postural and exercise hypotension, diarrhea, and retrograde ejaculation into the bladder. Postural hypotension results from interruption of the normal reflex autonomic vasoconstriction that occurs on standing, causing a fall in blood pressure; decreased venous return and cardiac output are due to unopposed parasympathetic action. The effectiveness of the drug should be determined with the patient in the standing position, especially after exercise, to avoid the syndrome of elevated pressures in the doctor's office and symptoms of fainting at home in the morning. The diarrhea can be distressing and is helped by small doses of ganglionic blocking agents such as mecamylamine or by cholinergic blocking drugs. Because of its potency, guanethidine is used when other combinations of agents have given unsatisfactory control of blood pressure. It is not often used by itself because of the resulting increased blood volume; its effectiveness is enhanced by combination with oral diuretics.

An unsatisfactory aspect of guanethidine therapy is its half-life of 5 days, the 3- to 5-day delay in the onset of its therapeutic effect, and the delay in subsidence of its hypotensive effect if too large a dose is given. On the other hand, its long duration of action allows the drug to be used once daily, which is helpful in securing patient compliance. The dose of the drug can be changed every 1–2 weeks. Tricyclic antidepressants and chlorpromazine compete with guanethidine for neuronal uptake and so diminish the hypotensive effect of guanethidine (Fann, 1971).

Clonidine

Clonidine acts by stimulating the alpha-adrenergic receptors in the medulla, decreasing sympathetic discharge to the arterioles, and lowering the blood pressure by decreasing the cardiac output and, to a lesser extent, the systemic vascular resistance. The drug crosses the blood-brain barrier, and patients may have fatigue and lethargy and also complain of dry mouth and hypotension. The drug also decreases renin release from the kidney, suggesting that the activation of an alpha-adrenergic receptor is also occurring in the kidney and perhaps other peripheral sites. However, renal blood flow and glomerular filtration rate do not change significantly (Houston, 1981). More than other antihypertensive compounds, it may cause a rebound vasoconstriction with hypertensive crises if it is stopped abruptly, so that patients must be warned against this eventuality. If the drug is to be stopped, it should be withdrawn gradually over a period of 3–5 days. The reality of the clinical withdrawal syndrome has been disputed (Whitsett, 1978). The average daily dose of clonidine required to decrease mean arterial pressure by 15 mm Hg varies from 0.5 to 0.6 mg/d. The dose ranges from 0.1 mg twice daily to 0.3 mg 3 times daily.

Guanabenz

Guanabenz is a new, centrally acting α_2-adrenergic agonist agent available in 4- and 8-mg tablets, which decreases the blood pressure by a mechanism similar to that of clonidine. The magnitude of the fall in blood pressure is similar to that of both clonidine and methyldopa. The heart rate and cardiac output are not affected; the side effects are similar to those of clonidine. Further data are required to compare the centrally acting drugs.

Minoxidil

Minoxidil is a potent oral agent that acts as a pure vasodilator, decreasing smooth muscle contractility of the arterioles and hence systemic vascular resistance (Pettinger, 1980). In common with other potent vasodilators, it causes reflex tachycardia and increased cardiac output, which then cause palpitations, headache, and angina. It also produces sodium retention.

Table 9–29. Adverse effects with vasodilators.*

Common to all
  (1) Reflex tachycardia, increased cardiac output
  (2) Angina, palpitations
  (3) Increased renin
  (4) Contraindicated in aortic dissection
  (5) Sodium and water retention
Hydralazine
  (1) Drug-induced lupus erythematosus
Diazoxide
  (1) Local burning
  (2) Hyperglycemia
  (3) Nausea and vomiting
Captopril
  (1) Maculopapular rash
  (2) Proteinuria
  (3) Neutropenia
  (4) Hypotension in salt-depleted patients
  (5) Alteration in taste
  (6) Use with caution in patients with impaired renal function

*Modified and reproduced, with permission, from Nies AS: Adverse reactions and interactions limiting the use of antihypertensive drugs. *Am J Med* 1975,58:495.

For all of these reasons, diuretics and beta-blocking agents such as propranolol or metoprolol are used whenever minoxidil is prescribed. Table 9–29 describes the adverse effects of vasodilators. About half of patients receiving minoxidil over a period of weeks develop hirsutism, which is particularly disturbing to women. Vigorous use of minoxidil in combination with large doses of furosemide and propranolol has proved very effective in the treatment of severe hypertension, especially in the presence of renal failure and when patients have failed to respond adequately to conventional antihypertensive medication (Mitchell, 1980). A typical chart showing the striking benefit of the addition of minoxidil to the regimen of a patient whose blood pressure was poorly controlled despite a combination of hydrochlorothiazide, methyldopa, propranolol, and hydralazine is shown in Fig 9–34. Fig 9–35 shows the dramatic effect of the addition of minoxidil to the medications of a patient receiving hydrochlorothiazide, propranolol, and hydralazine and the rapid increase in pulse rate when propranolol was stopped. As with other vasodilators, therefore, beta-adrenergic blocking agents should be added to the regimen when potent drugs such as minoxidil are used to prevent the subsequent reflex tachycardia. Another reason for adding beta-adrenergic blocking agents is to reverse the increase of plasma renin activity that follows the use of minoxidil.

Peak plasma levels occur rapidly within an hour after an oral dose, and the serum half-life, although said to be only 4 hours, allows a longer duration of action because the drug is bound in the vascular wall.

Minoxidil usually is begun in a dose of 2.5 mg and increased progressively up to 20, 30, or even 40 mg/d in resistant patients. Most of the severely ill hypertensives requiring minoxidil have elevated serum creatinine levels when the drug is begun, and 10–20% will require hemodialysis, at least temporarily. The

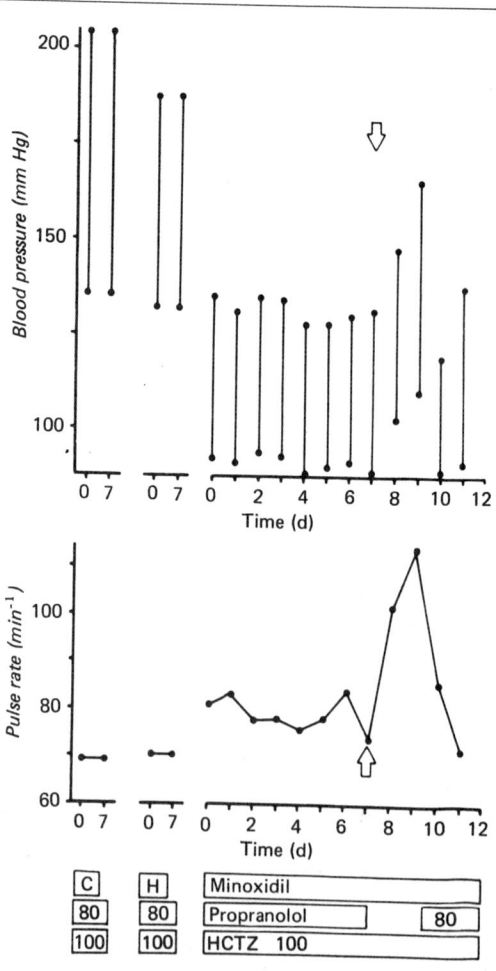

Figure 9–35. Blood pressure and heart rate data are summarized from one patient during the control period (C), the hydralazine period (H), and the minoxidil period. The effect of withdrawing propranolol (arrows) is shown by the increase in blood pressure and heart rate. HCTZ, hydrochlorothiazide. (Reproduced, with permission, from the American Heart Association, Inc., Gottlieb TB, Katz FH, Chidsey CA III: Combined therapy with vasodilator drugs and beta-adrenergic blockade in hypertension: A comparative study of minoxidil and hydralazine. *Circulation* 1972;**45**:571.)

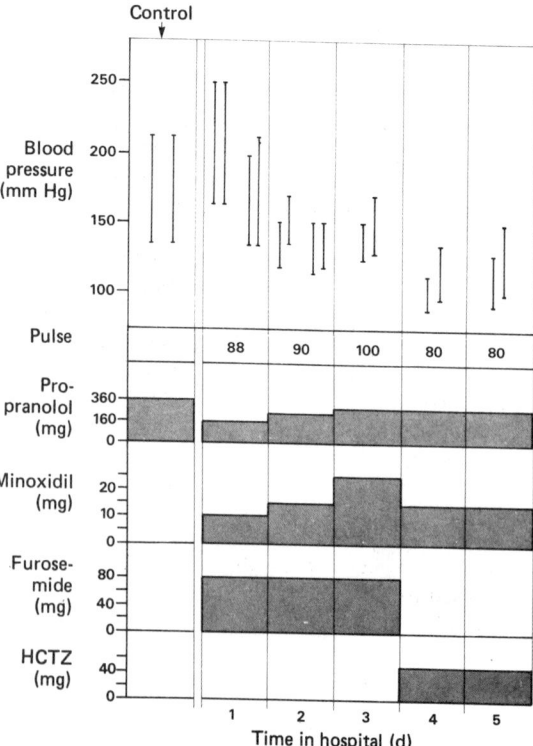

Figure 9–34. Successful treatment of hypertension with minoxidil following unsuccessful prehospital treatment with combined hydrochlorothiazide (HCTZ), methyldopa, propranolol, and hydralazine. (Courtesy of JA McChesney.)

main problem with the use of minoxidil is the development of fluid retention despite the use of diuretics, and at times patients develop pericardial effusion. Because of the impaired renal function, patients should receive furosemide rather than the thiazides to counteract the fluid retention. In a study of patients resistant to treatment with large doses of standard drugs, the mean doses of minoxidil, propranolol, and furosemide were 24.8, 708, and 53 mg/d, respectively. The main side effects were drowsiness, depression, vivid dreams, dry mouth, and hypertrichosis. Excessive hair growth was not dose-related (Dargie, 1977). In some of the patients, atenolol was given instead of propranolol in a dosage of 100 mg 2 or 3 times daily. Combination therapy controlled a group of severe hypertensives whose average presenting blood pressure was 223/139 mm Hg.

Combined Alpha- & Beta-Adrenergic Blocking Agents (Labetalol)

A combination that blocks both adrenergic systems may offer significant advantages in some patients. Alpha-receptor blockade counteracts the reflex increase in heart rate and cardiac output produced by other vasodilating agents such as hydralazine, but postural hypotension may occur. Labetalol can be used either orally (200–800 mg/d) or intravenously (50 mg) (Lund-Johansen, 1979). The oral dose must be titrated to the needs of the individual. Mean arterial blood pressure is reduced by about 20% and systemic vascular resistance by about 15%. If angina pectoris is present, it may be relieved, because the beta-blocking potency counteracts reflex tachycardia. The drug is now approved by the FDA, and further studies are awaited.

Diazoxide

Diazoxide is a parenteral vasodilator that acts directly on the smooth muscle of the arterioles. When given in a bolus intravenously, it lowers the blood pressure within minutes and lowers systemic vascular resistance about 25%, and the fall in pressure persists for many hours, with a gradual rise following the initial rapid fall in pressure. The hemodynamic effects also include an increase in heart rate of about 30 beats/min, increased cardiac index of 30–40%, and an increase in the left ventricular ejection rate of about 15%. Hypotension occurs infrequently, but if the situation is less urgent, one can use a smaller dose such as 75 mg instead of 300 mg and repeat the dose at intervals of 5–10 minutes until the desired antihypertensive effect is achieved. If diazoxide is used repeatedly, intravenous furosemide should be added to combat sodium and water retention (McDonald, 1977).

There is a dose-response relationship to the use of diazoxide in hypertensive children (Boerth, 1977). Fig 9–36 illustrates this. A dose of 2 mg/kg produces a fall in diastolic pressure of about 15 mm Hg, whereas 6 mg/kg produces an average fall of diastolic pressure of 40 mm Hg. A dose of 3 mg/kg decreases the diastolic pressure about 30 mm Hg, and this appears to

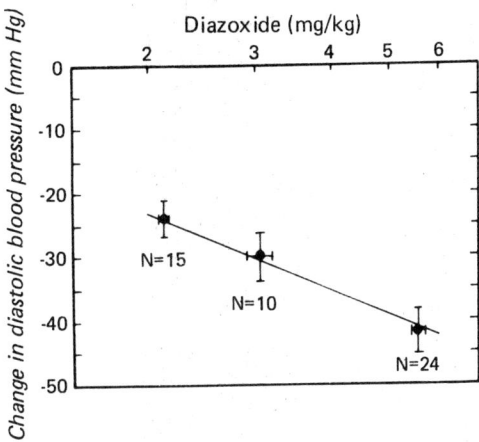

Figure 9–36. Log dose-response relation of diazoxide in hypertensive children. Symbols show mean dose and mean response for low-, middle-, and high-dose groups. N, number of responses in each group. Vertical brackets show standard error of the mean for responses in each dose group. Horizontal brackets show standard error of the mean for the doses in each dose group. (Reproduced, with permission, from the American Heart Association, Inc., Boerth RC, Long WR: Dose-response relation of diazoxide in children with hypertension. *Circulation* 1977;**56**:1062.)

be a reasonable dose to use in children. Table 9–30 describes other drugs used in the treatment of acute severe hypertension in children.

Diazoxide is valuable in hypertensive emergencies because of its effectiveness, because of its rapid onset and long duration of action, and because monitoring usually is required only for the first 15 or 20 minutes to make certain that excess hypotension has not occurred. Like hydralazine, it can be given intermittently in severe hypertension when potent oral therapy is being titrated. The major side effect, other than the possibility of excess hypotension, is hyperglycemia, and like other vasodilators, including hydralazine and minoxidil, it increases renin secretion. Despite this fact, all of the antihypertensive agents that increase renin secretion reverse the complications of hypertension, and increased renin production should not be considered a contraindication to the use of the drug. In some parts of the world, diazoxide is used orally in large doses with good effect on the blood pressure, but hyperglycemia prevents its continued use. It may be used for short periods to bring the pressure under control.

Ganglionic Blocking Agents

Ganglionic blocking agents such as trimethaphan camsylate (Arfonad), hexamethonium, pentolinium, and mecamylamine (Inversine) act by competing with acetylcholine at sympathetic ganglia and by blocking both parasympathetic and sympathetic outflow. As a result, their use has been sharply curtailed and superseded by other potent parenteral agents. An

Table 9-30. Pharmacologic therapy of acute severe hypertension in children.*

Drug	Administration	Starting Dose	Onset of Action (min)	Duration (h)	Mechanism
Reserpine	IM	0.07 mg/kg	60-120	4-6	Postganglionic depletion of catecholamines
Hydralazine hydrochloride	IM or IV	0.2 mg/kg	10-30	3-6	Vasodilation
Diazoxide	IV (push)	2-3 mg/kg	1-3	4-12	Vasodilation
Sodium nitroprusside	IV (infusion)	60 mg/L (0.03-0.5 mg/min)	½-1	Length of infusion	Vasodilation
Trimethaphan camsylate	IV (infusion)	1 g/L (1-10 mg/min)	½-1	Length of infusion	Sympathetic ganglionic blocker
Ethacrynic acid, furosemide	IV	0.5-1.0 mg/kg	10-20	2-4	Blocks tubular reabsorption of sodium and chloride, smooth muscle vasodilation

*Reproduced, with permission, from McLain LG: Therapy of acute severe hypertension in children. *JAMA* 1978;**239:**755.

exception to this is the use of trimethaphan for short periods (1-2 days) in the treatment of malignant (accelerated) hypertension or aortic dissection when it is desired to bring blood pressure under control in a matter of minutes. Hemodynamic observations in severe hypertension following the use of trimethaphan camsylate show a marked fall in arterial pressure, peripheral resistance, cardiac index, and left ventricular ejection rate, but a rise in heart rate (Bhatia, 1973). Unlike nitroprusside sodium, it acts in minutes rather than seconds. The drug should be given by continuous intravenous infusion under close monitoring in the coronary care or intensive care unit with the patient in the sitting position, so that if excess hypotension occurs the patient can lie down to counteract the hypotension.

Nitroprusside Sodium

This potent vasodilator is used almost exclusively in acute hypertensive emergencies or in acute cardiac failure with abnormal or elevated blood pressure. It acts directly on the smooth muscle of the arterioles and lowers the pressure within seconds. The drug is given by continuous dilute intravenous infusion by a constant infusion pump, and the dose is titrated to produce the desired effect (see Chapter 10 and Fig 10-16). As with trimethaphan, its use should be monitored to avoid excessive hypotension, which may lead to acute tubular necrosis of the kidney.

Experience with nitroprusside is still limited, but it may prove to be the treatment of choice in acute left ventricular failure with pulmonary edema and severe hypertension because, unlike other vasodilators such as hydralazine and minoxidil, it produces reflex tachycardia much less often and to a lesser degree. Why this is so with such a potent vasodilator is unclear, but the associated venodilating effect may be the explanation.

Nitroprusside is metabolized to thiocyanate, and if large doses of nitroprusside are used for more than a few days, thiocyanide levels may rise to toxic concentrations, producing side effects requiring cessation of the drug.

Inhibitors of Angiotensin

Saralasin is a competitive inhibitor of angiotensin II that must be given intravenously and has the disadvantage of being a partial agonist. It increases plasma bradykinin and causes excessive fall in blood pressure if the patient is sodium-depleted and tilted upright. When introduced clinically, saralasin was thought to predict which patients with renovascular hypertension would benefit from surgical intervention; false-positives and false-negatives have greatly limited its usefulness (see p 242).

Angiotensin-Converting Enzyme Inhibitors

Captopril and its analog enalapril are drugs that specifically inhibit the conversion of angiotensin I to angiotensin II. These drugs have been shown to effectively lower the blood pressure in hypertensive patients, regardless of the initial plasma renin levels. The long-term effects are not known, but in the studies reported, captopril in daily doses of 25-300 mg, often in combination with a diuretic or a beta-adrenergic blocking agent, lowered the pressure to normal or near normal, even in patients resistant to conventional treatment (Brunner, 1979; Bravo, 1979; Case, 1982). Captopril is absorbed quickly, and its effects persist for about 8 hours. Hemodynamically, the drug causes a fall in arterial pressure, a decrease in systemic vascular resistance, a slight rise in cardiac output, and some improvement in renal function. The fall in blood pressure may be considerable if patients are sodium-depleted or are receiving beta-adrenergic blocking drugs; the drug should be used with considerable caution in such circumstances.

The initial promising value of captopril in hypertension must be tempered by adverse reactions that have occurred in 1-15% of cases, consisting of a rash with or without fever, altered sense of taste, proteinuria, and rare cases of neutropenia. Granulocyte counts are required at least every 2 weeks for the first few months to detect possible neutropenia, which usually occurs within that time. Hyperkalemia may result when captopril is given to patients with severe hypertension and renal failure; the drug should be used with caution when renal function is impaired. Renal biopsy in some patients has shown glomerular membrane abnormalities, which persisted in a third of cases. A new oral converting enzyme inhibitor, enalapril ("MK-421"), is now undergoing investigational assessment. It is many times more potent than captopril. A single maintenance dose of 2.5–40 mg suppresses the development of angiotensin II for at least 24 hours; this is an advantage over captopril. Sodium retention, neutropenia, and proteinuria did not occur in early studies. Further studies are in progress.

Calcium Entry–Blocking Agents

Drugs in this category, such as nifedipine, verapamil, and diltiazem—especially the first—have been shown to be effective in hypertensive patients. They are potent vasodilators that are also valuable in coronary spasm (see p 147). They specifically inhibit the slow inflow of calcium ions into the myocardial cell plasma, where they inhibit excitation-contraction coupling, including vasodilatation and fall in blood pressure. Nifedipine, 10 mg orally every 8–12 hours (Guazzi, 1984), often combined with captopril, significantly reduces elevated blood pressure toward normal, reduces systemic vascular resistance, and increases cardiac output. No significant change in renal function occurs. In combination with beta blockers, nifedipine is particularly effective in patients with hypertension and angina (Opie, 1982; Frishman, 1982). Sublingual nifedipine (10 mg) has been effective in rapidly (30 min) lowering the blood pressure in hypertensive emergencies. Hypotension may occur. These drugs have not yet been approved by the FDA for the treatment of hypertension.

4. SUGGESTED DRUG PROTOCOLS

As indicated in the introductory paragraphs, the physician must first determine how urgent it is to lower the blood pressure and choose accordingly oral or parenteral treatment, the drugs and doses to be initiated, the frequency with which they should be repeated, and the speed with which the blood pressure should be brought under control. The physician must also balance the beneficial response of the blood pressure to treatment against side effects that may interfere with treatment and may require adjustment of dosage or change to a different therapeutic agent. Clinical judgment is required to decide when to be content with a moderate therapeutic response if side effects (such as lethargy or impotence with methyldopa) are disabling or when frequent medications cause difficulties in patient compliance. The costs of medications, visits to the physician, and laboratory tests to determine the effect on potassium, glucose, uric acid, or creatinine must also be considered. Treatment is empiric. By trial and error one arrives at the drug or combination of drugs that will lower the blood pressure while interfering as little as possible with the patient's life and work. Outpatient treatment is usually not urgent, so that therapy can be started slowly, utilizing one drug in low dosage, with a gradual increase to higher dosage or to additional more potent drugs.

The object of hypotensive therapy is to lower the blood pressure to 140/90 mm Hg or below for as much of the day as possible, consistent with the patient's cooperation and the absence of disabling side effects. With the exception of mild disease, good control is rarely achieved with a single drug. In older patients with impaired cerebral or coronary circulation in whom it is important to avoid excess hypotension or rapid changes in pressure, one should accept a diastolic pressure of 100 mm Hg if lowering the pressure produces further cerebral symptoms. In uncooperative patients with a poor compliance record, or in patients who find it difficult to take medication more than once or twice a day, the physician should accept partial control of the blood pressure if insisting on more frequent medication would cause the patient to abandon therapy altogether. The response to therapy should be determined not only by office pressure readings but by some variety of basal, home, or ambulatory recordings to obtain more representative pressures.

It is best to consider antihypertensive regimens as various steps, depending upon the responses of the patient.

Step 1:

In almost all mildly to moderately hypertensive patients except those who have a history of sensitivity to diuretics or a history of repeated attacks of gout from prior thiazide therapy, or diabetics who would require either a change of insulin therapy or a change to insulin therapy from other methods of diabetic control, initial therapy should be with one of the oral diuretics, either the short-acting mild diuretics (the thiazides) or the longer-acting mild diuretics (chlorthalidone or metolazone), or with beta-blocking agents (see p 263). Approximately 40% of patients with borderline or mild hypertension with diastolic pressures between 90 and 110 mm Hg will respond satisfactorily to diuretics alone. Since the need to lower the pressure is not urgent, thiazides should be begun in low dosage, such as 25–50 mg of hydrochlorothiazide once daily, the lower amount being used in patients who are elderly or are receiving digitalis or in those who have a clinical condition in which an unexpectedly large diuresis of water, sodium, and potassium would be precarious. The response to the thiazides begins to be evident within a few days, and by 2 weeks one can be fairly certain whether the dosage used is adequate. If not, it can be increased by increments of 25 mg up to a maximum single dose of 100 mg. Usually 50 mg once or twice a day is sufficient if diuretics alone are going to be effective in lowering the blood pressure. If the patient responds well to 50 mg of hydrochlorothiazide once or twice a day, for example, the dose can then be decreased to 25 mg once daily and perhaps to 25 mg every other day. The smaller doses may maintain the beneficial effects initially obtained by larger doses and decrease the urinary potassium loss. Since the average decrease in serum potassium with 50 mg of hydrochlorothiazide twice a day is about 0.6 meq/L, the loss can often be offset by increased oral intake of potassium in potassium-rich foods such as fruits and vegetables (see Table 9–27); or if the serum potassium falls below 3.5 meq/L and if the patient has symptoms from the hypokalemia, the physician can prescribe oral potassium chloride, 60 meq/d, in the absence of renal failure. Liquid potassium preparations are preferred but are sometimes poorly tolerated. One can use the matrix potassium Slow-K (Ciba); enteric-coated potassium tablets should not be used because of the frequency of ulcerations in the small bowel. If a month of oral diuretics does not lower the blood pressure to the desired level, one can then proceed to step 2 in treatment.

Step 2:

A variety of drugs are available that can be added to the thiazides. The second drug can be propranolol, atenolol, pindolol, metoprolol, nadolol, methyldopa, reserpine, clonidine, prazosin, hydralazine, captopril, or enalapril—each has its supporters. The choice often depends on the familiarity of the physician with the various drugs, but there are situations in which one drug or another is particularly desirable.

Beta-adrenergic blocking drugs are considered by many to be the best second drugs because they not only effectively lower the blood pressure but also decrease the plasma renin, the pulse rate, and the likelihood of arrhythmias or angina if the patient is receiving vasodilators or has concomitant coronary heart disease. However, propranolol cannot be used if the patient has a history of asthma or of Raynaud's phenomenon, incipient left ventricular failure, bradycardia, or ventricular conduction defects.

Propranolol should be begun in low dosage—10–20 mg once or twice a day—primarily to determine if any adverse effects will occur with its use. Propranolol may induce an attack of asthma or pulmonary edema; may cause bradycardia; may mask hypoglycemia in a diabetic patient taking insulin; and may produce central nervous system symptoms with excitement. Although the usual prescription calls for the drug to be taken 4 times daily, since the half-life is short (a matter of hours), the biologic effect may be more persistent. Many patients respond satisfactorily to twice-daily dosage. Infrequently, it is necessary to give more than 320 mg/d. **Metoprolol** can be started in an initial dose of 50 mg twice daily, increased as necessary, depending upon the patient's response, to 200 mg twice daily. Because it is cardioselective, it is preferred to propranolol in patients with chronic lung disease. Various other beta-blocking drugs have now been approved (atenolol, nadolol, pindolol); apart from (1) duration of action (atenolol and nadolol can be given once daily) and (2) lipophilic effect (atenolol and metoprolol are not lipid-soluble and do not cross the blood-brain barrier and thereby have fewer central nervous system effects), the antihypertensive effects are similar.

Methyldopa is moderately effective, but it produces lethargy and decreased mental acuity as well as impotence in men. There are very few data regarding the effect of methyldopa on sexual function in women. It is important to obtain accurate information regarding sexual function and activity in men prior to institution of therapy, because impotence, as well as other side effects, may occur with placebo medication and may not be due to the antihypertensive drug. An accurate history prior to starting therapy is helpful in interpreting the possible role of antihypertensive drugs in causing symptoms. Patients who require a high order of mental alertness at their jobs or patients in whom lethargy is a particularly unpleasant effect do poorly with methyldopa. On the other hand, if the patient is hyperactive, the sedative action of methyldopa is often beneficial. Postural hypotension is usually not too prominent with methyldopa, but it may be so in some cases. Methyldopa is begun in a dose of 250 mg once or twice daily; often this is sufficient to lower the pressure. As with propranolol, it is usually supposed to be taken 4 times daily, but patients often comply poorly with such frequent dosage, and many respond satisfactorily to 2 or 3 doses daily if they are going to respond to the drug at all. Although some patients respond to an increase of dosage to 2 g/d, this may produce more side effects and no more benefits than 1–1.5 g/d.

Reserpine, 0.05–0.1 mg once a day, is often effective as a second drug. It has the advantage of relaxing the patient and slowing the heart rate but the disadvantage that it may cause mental depression in susceptible individuals. Patients with a history of mental depression should not be given reserpine. The daily dose of reserpine should not exceed 0.25 mg/d and preferably not more than 0.1 mg/d. Reserpine is effective in once-daily dosage. When reserpine was discontinued because of reports of an association with carcinoma of the breast, it often took weeks to stabilize the patient equally well on methyldopa, propranolol, or even guanethidine. A combination of thiazides and reserpine is often effective, and when this is so, a total daily consumption of only 2–3 tablets is sufficient to control the hypertension.

Prazosin is a vasodilator that can be used if the patient is unable to take beta-adrenergic blocking agents, reserpine, or methyldopa because of the side effects mentioned above, and it can be substituted for hydralazine if this drug is ineffective or causes tachycardia (see below). It should be started in small doses, usually 0.5 mg or at most 1 mg at bedtime. A marked fall in pressure and collapse have been described when the drug is first begun. The first dose response can occur with doses of less than 2 mg, so the patient should be observed closely for this event. The patient is titrated with progressively increasing doses, as with all antihypertensive agents, and usually requires 2–5 mg 2 or 3 times daily for an effective response. As noted on p 264, prazosin can be used as a step 1 or 2 drug.

Clonidine has few enthusiastic supporters because it produces an unpleasantly dry mouth and lethargy. It can be started with 0.1 mg and increased to 0.2–0.4 mg 2 or 3 times a day, depending upon the response. It remains to be seen whether guanabenz, a centrally acting drug whose mechanism is similar to that of clonidine, will be tolerated better.

Hydralazine is an effective antihypertensive agent, especially when combined with propranolol or metoprolol, which neutralizes the headache and tachycardia that often follow the vasodilating action of hydralazine used alone. If propranolol, metoprolol, methyldopa, or reserpine is not used first, and hydralazine is used alone in full doses, patients often complain of severe headache and tachycardia, and if they have coronary heart disease they may develop angina pectoris. Reserpine and methyldopa are not as effective as propranolol or metoprolol in preventing the reflex tachycardia and palpitations, but they should be considered effective substitutes. In the VA studies (1967, 1970), a combination of thiazide, reserpine, and hydralazine showed convincing benefit to patients whose average diastolic pressure was 105 mm Hg or more.

Hydralazine has a plasma half-life of only a few hours, but its biologic action is longer because the drug becomes bound to smooth muscle of the blood vessels; twice-daily dosage is usually effective. It is begun with 10–25 mg once or twice a day, gradually increased at weekly intervals to 100 mg twice daily. Two hundred milligrams per day is usually the maximum dose that is used, because larger doses are associated with a lupus erythematosus–like syndrome with arthritis and a positive serum LE preparation. Hydralazine is metabolized by acetylation; the rate of acetylation is genetically determined, and patients vary in the rate of inactivation of the drug, with the rapid ones having a lower plasma concentration. Another reason for rarely exceeding 100 mg/dose is that hemodynamic studies in patients with chronic cardiac failure have shown that 50–75 mg of hydralazine effectively increases the cardiac output; therefore, this size dose is hemodynamically effective. A dose of 5–10 mg of hydralazine intramuscularly is effective in acute glomerulonephritis and in severe hypertension.

Captopril may be tried in patients not responding to the above drugs alone or combined, before minoxidil or guanethidine is used (see p 268). One should begin with a small dose such as 6.25 mg/d; final doses vary between 25 and 300 mg/d, usually combined with a diuretic or a beta-blocking agent. Side effects may be prominent and should be watched for. Repeated urinalyses for proteinuria and granulocyte counts for neutropenia should be performed during the first 3 months of therapy. Maculopapular rash, altered sense of taste, and possibly fever occur in 5–10% of patients and subside if the dose is lowered or with the passage of time. Further long-term studies are necessary before the exact role of captopril or its analog enalapril is established in the treatment of hypertension.

Calcium entry–blocking agents in the treatment of hypertension have been studied for only a short time. Considerable experience has been obtained with them, however, in the treatment of angina pectoris. Nifedipine is begun with 10 mg every 8 hours, verapamil with 40 mg, and diltiazem with 30 mg, increased as necessary. These drugs are particularly valuable if the patient has both hypertension and angina, because both peripheral and coronary vasodilatation occur. Verapamil is preferred if the patient has attacks of paroxysmal supraventricular tachycardia but is to be avoided if there are sinus or atrioventricular conduction defects or cardiac failure. The combination of beta-blocking agents and verapamil is to be used with caution in patients with impaired left ventricular function, especially if they have cardiac failure.

Sublingual or oral nifedipine capsules, 5–10 mg, may lower the blood pressure within 30 minutes with significant clinical improvement in emergencies, but possible hypotension is a concern; close observation is advised.

Step 3: Minoxidil

This is the most potent vasodilator and may reduce the blood pressure strikingly when all of the conventional drugs mentioned above fail to do so (Figs 9–34 and 9–35). It has the adverse effects shared by all vasodilator drugs, but sodium retention is more marked, and it has the unusual side effect of hirsutism, which limits its use in females. The drug is an extremely useful addition to the oral therapeutic protocol in severe hypertension, especially if there is beginning impairment of renal function. Minoxidil is begun in small doses of 2.5–5 mg/d and may be given 2–3 times daily, with gradually increasing titration to a maximum dosage of 20 mg/d. As seen in Fig 9–34, 10 mg/d lowered the diastolic blood pressure in a patient from 150 mm Hg to 115 mm Hg; 20 mg of minoxidil lowered the diastolic pressure to close to normal from a pretreatment value that persisted at 150 mm Hg despite full conventional therapy.

Step 4: Guanethidine

If the combination of drugs listed above fails to reduce the blood pressure to a satisfactory level, or if side effects prevent their effective use, guanethidine may be introduced. Guanethidine is a potent adrenergic blocking agent which can be used in increasing dosage but which requires close supervision because of frequent side effects. Postural hypotension is greater with guanethidine than with any of the other drugs. The patient may have the unpleasant experience of marked postural hypotension in the morning because of the vasodilatation resulting from being warm in bed, yet in the afternoon and evening have a blood pressure that is high and out of control. Guanethidine also produces unpredictable diarrhea, retrograde ejaculation into the bladder, and dizziness on exertion, especially in the morning. The postural hypotension and dizziness after exertion are not rapidly relieved by rest, especially if the exercise has been vigorous. Guanethidine is a very potent drug and has proved beneficial in many patients. It is begun in a dose of 10–20 mg orally that can be adjusted at weekly intervals because of its long half-life. This is convenient for outpatient therapy but is a disadvantage if overdosage occurs, because it takes 3–5 days for the drug effect to be eliminated when the drug is stopped. If guanethidine is used, reserpine and methyldopa usually add nothing to the therapeutic protocol except in unusual circumstances, because they all are adrenergic-depleting agents. However, diuretic therapy is a useful and important additive to guanethidine. It counteracts the sodium retention and allows a smaller daily dose of guanethidine.

Step 5:

About 90–95% of all patients with mild to moderately severe hypertension will be controlled by the drugs listed above. If the blood pressure is not controlled, one should suspect that the patient is not taking the medication or is taking too much sodium. Alternatively, there may be a substantial disparity between office and home readings, or the cuff of the blood pressure apparatus may be too narrow for the patient's arm. It is also possible that the malignant phase has supervened or that a new process such as pyelonephritis has occurred. A patient with renal impairment, cardiac failure, or hypertensive encephalopathy should be hospitalized. This removes the patient from the surrounding social and work environment, which may be contributing pressor influences interfering with the antihypertensive drugs, and also allows close monitoring of treatment of the blood pressure and, if necessary, the use of parenteral medication. Patients who have failed to respond to the full therapeutic regimen listed above, as well as patients who have acute hypertensive encephalopathy, malignant hypertension, acute pulmonary edema or severe cardiac failure, aortic dissection, hemorrhagic stroke with a markedly raised blood pressure, or episodic rises in pressure suggesting pheochromocytoma, should be hospitalized and given parenteral therapy (see Table 9–24).

TREATMENT OF MALIGNANT HYPERTENSION

The hallmark of malignant hypertension, as noted earlier, is papilledema; after the patient is hospitalized, the blood pressure should be lowered within hours or days depending upon the physician's estimate of the urgency of the clinical situation (see p 231). Some patients with malignant hypertension are critically ill, with diastolic pressures exceeding 150 mm Hg; their blood pressure should be lowered within hours. Other patients, early in the course of the malignant phase, may have much less commanding symptoms; therapy can then be given orally or parenterally but intermittently, with the objective of lowering the pressure within a few days.

The importance of prompt reduction of the pressure in patients with malignant hypertension is shown in Fig 9–37. Not only do the data demonstrate the great improvement in survival of patients with malignant hypertension given modern therapy (40% survival after 12 years, as compared to nil in the days before treatment was available), but they show that the improved survival occurs only in the cases of nonazotemic malignant hypertension in which the blood pressure is lowered before renal failure occurs. In patients with malignant hypertension in whom renal failure and azotemia were present when the patient was first treated, the 12-year survival rate was nil, although the 6-year survival rate was still 20%, in contrast to the average survival of 8 months in the days before modern therapy was possible. Dialysis treatment will probably improve the figures. One of our early cases, treated in 1951, is shown in Fig 9–38. This young man presented with severe headache uncontrolled by morphine, inability to read the headlines of the newspaper, marked vomiting associated with papilledema, and a diastolic pressure of 150 mm Hg. He failed to respond to symptomatic therapy in the hospital. He was then given hexamethonium subcutaneously in increasing doses, which lowered his blood pressure. The decrease in his headache, vomiting, and visual symptoms was dramatic and occurred in a matter of days. Papilledema, hemorrhages, and exudates disappeared within weeks, and he was seen in 1976 after a follow-up of 25 years with a normal blood pressure and normal renal function without antihypertensive therapy. This long remission is unique in our experience and was one of the early demonstrations of the importance of lowering blood pressure in malignant hypertension.

It should be appreciated that when the more potent drugs such as nitroprusside sodium and diazoxide are used, the blood pressure may be lowered in a matter of seconds or minutes, but the hazard of overstepping the mark and producing severe hypotension is also greater. Drugs that can be used in malignant hypertension and other hypertensive emergencies are listed in Table 9–24 along with route of administration, initial dose, time of onset, and duration of action. The choice of drugs depends upon the physician's own experience and the availability of second-to-second surveillance, as is necessary with infusions of nitroprusside sodium or trimethaphan. Both of these drugs should be given under the closest supervision, so that the patient can be placed in the recumbent position if hypotension develops. The rate of infusion

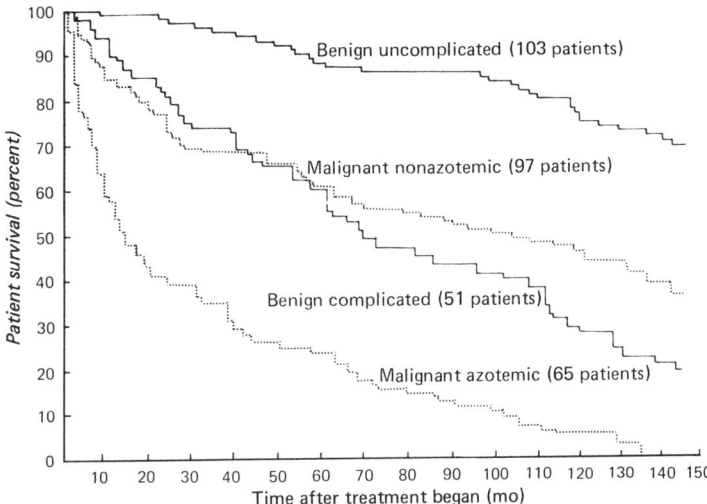

Figure 9–37. Percentage of surviving patients in each group for every month after inception of therapy. (Reproduced, with permission, from the American Heart Association, Inc., Perry HM Jr et al: Studies on the control of hypertension. 8. Mortality, morbidity, and remission during 12 years of intensive therapy. *Circulation* 1966;**33**:958.)

must be carefully titrated to avoid excessive hypotension and should be decreased as soon as possible after the blood pressure falls. One can then give intermittent intramuscular hydralazine or bolus injections of diazoxide. As soon as practicable, oral therapy should be given. If the clinical care facilities do not permit careful, moment-to-moment titration of the infusion in a coronary care or intensive care unit, it is safer to give boluses of diazoxide, 75–300 mg rapidly intravenously, which lowers the pressure in minutes but may last for hours. If the situation is less urgent, 5–20 mg of hydralazine intramuscularly or 1–5 mg of reserpine intramuscularly or intravenously can also be given intermittently and does not require as close supervision. Intramuscular hydralazine acts in 15–30 minutes and may persist for hours. Reserpine acts more slowly and may take several hours to lower blood pressure. As with all parenteral antihyperten-

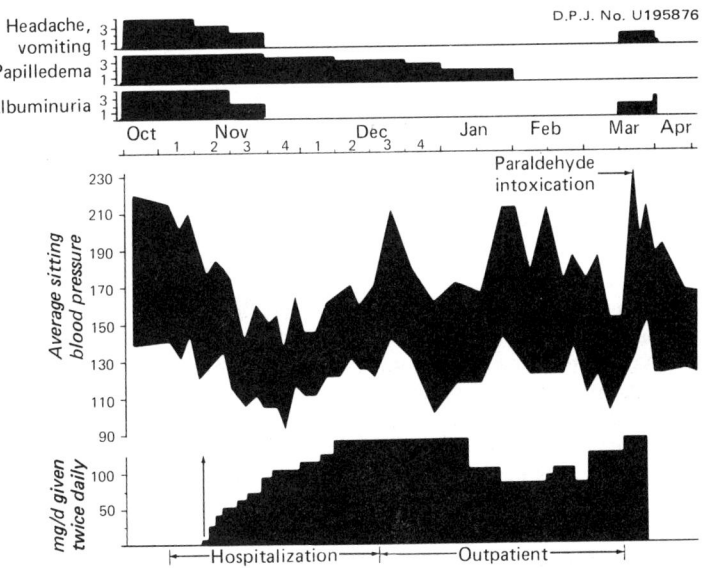

Figure 9–38. Essential hypertension with papilledema in a 23-year-old man. Hexamethonium treatment of malignant hypertension, 1951. (Reproduced, with permission, from Sokolow M, Schottstaedt MF: The management of malignant hypertension. *Ann Intern Med* 1953;**38**:647.)

sive drugs, hypotension may occur. For this reason, 1 mg rather than the previously recommended 2.5–5 mg is advised as the initial dose. Reserpine has the disadvantage of producing drowsiness and makes interpretation of cerebral symptoms more difficult. Methyldopa, 250–500 mg, can be given intramuscularly or intravenously, but this drug also takes 2–6 hours before its effect becomes obvious; and although it is effective in some patients, it may not lower the pressure in severe hypertensive emergencies.

In dissecting aorta, hemorrhagic stroke with high arterial pressure, and severe acute left ventricular failure, either sodium nitroprusside or trimethaphan is the drug of choice at the beginning, after which potent oral drugs can be substituted.

One should not lower the pressure to normal immediately, because this may produce neurologic deficit or oliguria; it is wiser to give smaller doses to lower the diastolic pressure to about 120 mm Hg and observe whether this pressure is tolerated without neurologic symptoms or evidence of decreased cardiac output with oliguria. The therapy can then be continued or increased to lower the pressure to 110 mm Hg diastolic for a day or 2 before gradually bringing it down to 100 mm Hg. It should be reemphasized that the great potency of the parenteral drugs is a distinct hazard. One should start with the smallest possible dose and increase the rate of infusion if needed. A modest fall in pressure is satisfactory at first; a greater fall can be achieved later after it is demonstrated that this can be tolerated without untoward symptoms.

The presence of impaired renal function should not deter the physician from lowering the pressure, although drugs such as guanethidine that decrease the cardiac output should be avoided if possible. In the presence of impaired renal function, thiazide diuretics are less effective, and furosemide should be used instead. Beta-blocking agents and oral vasodilators (hydralazine, prazosin, or minoxidil) are effective in the presence of impaired renal function and can be used alone or in combination after the blood pressure is brought under control with the parenteral therapy.

Principles of Management

(1) Prevent progression into the malignant phase by adequate treatment of underlying hypertension due to any cause.

(2) Treat as an emergency. Hospitalization and vigorous treatment are mandatory.

(3) Choose a mode of parenteral treatment appropriate to the speed of the desired effects: (1) seconds (sodium nitroprusside), (b) a few minutes (diazoxide, trimethaphan), (c) 20–40 minutes (hydralazine), (d) hours (reserpine, methyldopa, captopril, enalapril, minoxidil).

(4) Observe the patient closely, preferably in the coronary or intensive care unit; titrate the dosage of parenteral drugs carefully.

(5) Start with small doses if the patient is hypovolemic, is over age 60, or has vascular disease (angina, cerebral or extremity ischemic attacks).

(6) If one drug proves ineffective, add another rather than attempting massive doses of any one drug. Combined therapy is usually more effective and causes fewer side effects.

(7) Avoid dehydration and hypervolemia. The former causes extrarenal azotemia; the latter interferes with effective treatment, raises the blood pressure further, and causes heart failure.

(8) Start vigorous treatment at the first manifestation of accelerated hypertension, such as a diastolic pressure exceeding 130 mm Hg or hemorrhages or exudates in the fundi.

(9) Lower the blood pressure despite impaired renal function; use dialysis if necessary for relief of uremic symptoms or complications while acute arterial lesions heal as the blood pressure is lowered.

(10) Use vigorous antihypertensive treatment both orally and intravenously in combination with intermittent hemodialysis to control the blood pressure, even if the plasma renin level is high. Bilateral nephrectomy is rarely indicated.

(11) If the patient is overloaded with fluid, oliguric, and dyspneic, with pulmonary edema, dialyze to remove excess fluid and permit the antihypertensive agents to lower the blood pressure.

(12) Institute oral therapy as soon as possible—usually on the first or second day.

Renal Failure & Dialysis

If renal failure is present and the patient is receiving intermittent renal dialysis, therapy should be rigorous, with intermittent injections of diazoxide if needed to lower the pressure without decreasing the renal blood flow. If the patient's serum creatinine is less than 3 or 4 mg/dL, indicating moderate renal failure, and if the patient is not on dialysis and is not oliguric, vigorous oral therapy combined with diazoxide may prevent the need for hemodialysis. If the patient is receiving hemodialysis, lowering the pressure will often gradually reduce the required frequency of hemodialysis, so that patients who were having dialysis several times a week might need it only once every few weeks to several months. Renal dysfunction is greatly aggravated by severe hypertension, and lowering the blood pressure is an essential aspect of the treatment of renal failure, utilizing renal dialysis if necessary to control blood volume until the renal interlobular and arteriolar lesions can heal.

Follow-Up Evaluation

After the blood pressure is brought under control with potent parenteral medication, the beneficial antihypertensive effect can usually be maintained with more moderate oral therapy. Once the malignant phase is reversed by antihypertensive therapy, the patient often reverts to benign hypertension and can be controlled for years with a rather modest regimen of antihypertensive drugs. The serum creatinine, which may rise modestly during the first 2–3 weeks after antihypertensive therapy is begun, gradually falls, and 6 months later it is usually lower than when the patient was first seen with malignant hypertension. The impaired renal function persists, however, although the serum creatinine and creatinine clearance may stabilize at a low or moderately high level. The inability to completely restore renal function to normal, once it has reached a certain point of impairment, is the main reason why vigorous antihypertensive therapy should be given to patients with accelerated hypertension.

FOLLOW-UP THERAPY

The patient being treated with oral therapy of mild to moderate disease as well as the patient discharged from the hospital under treatment for severe or malignant hypertension should be seen approximately once a week as an outpatient until the situation is stabilized and an acceptable therapeutic program has been achieved. The frequency of visits can gradually be decreased, but in all but the mildest cases patients should be seen at intervals of 3–6 months even after they are well controlled to be certain that they are taking their medication and that the response to therapy is maintained. Circumstances in the patient's life, acute pyelonephritis, or unknown factors may worsen the hypertension even when the patient is on therapy. The patient must be encouraged to communicate with the physician whenever new or untoward symptoms appear and should be warned frequently against stopping medication without consulting the physician because of the danger of uncontrolled hypertension as well as the rebound effect that may occur when any antihypertensive agent is abruptly stopped. It is common for patients to run out of medication, and they often do not renew the prescription because they are free of symptoms and the drugs are not inexpensive. This problem should be anticipated and prevented by full discussion with frequent reinforcements. Failure of compliance with the physician's instructions is a persistent problem that must never be overlooked if the response to therapy seems not to be adequate (see below). Before assuming that antihypertensive therapy is inadequate—especially if the patient has previously been well controlled on the same medication—the possibility of noncompliance should be carefully considered. Ambulatory blood pressure recording with a semiautomatic apparatus (eg, Remler recorder) is reliable and may reveal better control of blood pressure than was thought from office readings alone. The prognosis for the development of vascular complications with target organ damage and for survival is better when ambulatory pressures are significantly lower than average office readings (Perloff, 1983) (Fig 9–39). In some cases, hospitalization may allow a more adequate estimate of the effectiveness of treatment and has the added advantage of removing the patient from a perhaps stressful environment that may be raising the blood pressure.

At each visit, the blood pressure should be determined and the patient questioned regarding medication, life events, and the appearance of new or untoward symptoms that may suggest a change in the course of the disease. Specific search should be made for any evidence of involvement or worsening of the target organs; in particular, examination of the fundi, heart, and peripheral vessels should be made at each visit. At approximately yearly intervals, repeat ECG, renal function studies, and chest x-rays are desirable. If the patient is taking oral diuretic agents, serum potassium, uric acid, plasma glucose, and serum creatinine should be measured every year. The effect of upright posture should be noted at each visit, not only with drugs that interfere with sympathetic transmission but also with oral diuretic agents, because postural hypotension may occur if hypovolemia is excessive. If the patient is receiving spironolactone or triamterene, serum potassium should be checked more frequently, and the ECG should be repeated frequently to exclude hyperkalemia; the patient must be repeatedly admonished not to take oral potassium agents. If renal function is impaired, these potassium-sparing drugs should not be used.

Serial assessment of left ventricular mass is helpful in determining response to treatment. There is a significant correlation between the fall in systolic pressure and the decrease in left ventricular mass index in treated patients as compared to controls studied by continuous intra-arterial ambulatory blood pressure monitoring (Rowlands, 1982).

Management of Patient Compliance

Studies on patients' compliance with the treatment program have shown that this is a difficult problem not entirely eliminated by free drugs, easy access to physicians, education of patients regarding their disease, and education of physicians to fortify their own understanding of the need for antihypertensive drug therapy. Frequent follow-up visits are a nuisance and an expense, take time away from work, and are often emotionally disturbing, so that patients tend to find excuses not to make or keep appointments. When patients are asked why they have not complied as urged and directed to do, common answers are, "I forgot," or "I feel all right," or "I ran out of pills and I don't like to be scolded." Perhaps more important and less well articulated is the attitude of the patient toward the physician or the clinic, especially in institutions in which physicians change frequently. In large clinics, a patient often has to wait several hours to see the physician, must then wait longer at the pharmacy to get the prescription filled or renewed, and then—all too often—has only a few minutes with the physician. Nurse assistants may help with this problem by making more time available for the patient, including a discussion of personal problems. A social worker can function in somewhat the same way by developing a relationship in which the patient feels free to discuss personal and socioeconomic problems, and clinical volunteers can often assist with the less severe or complicated cases. Every large clinic should provide some means whereby patients can get clear

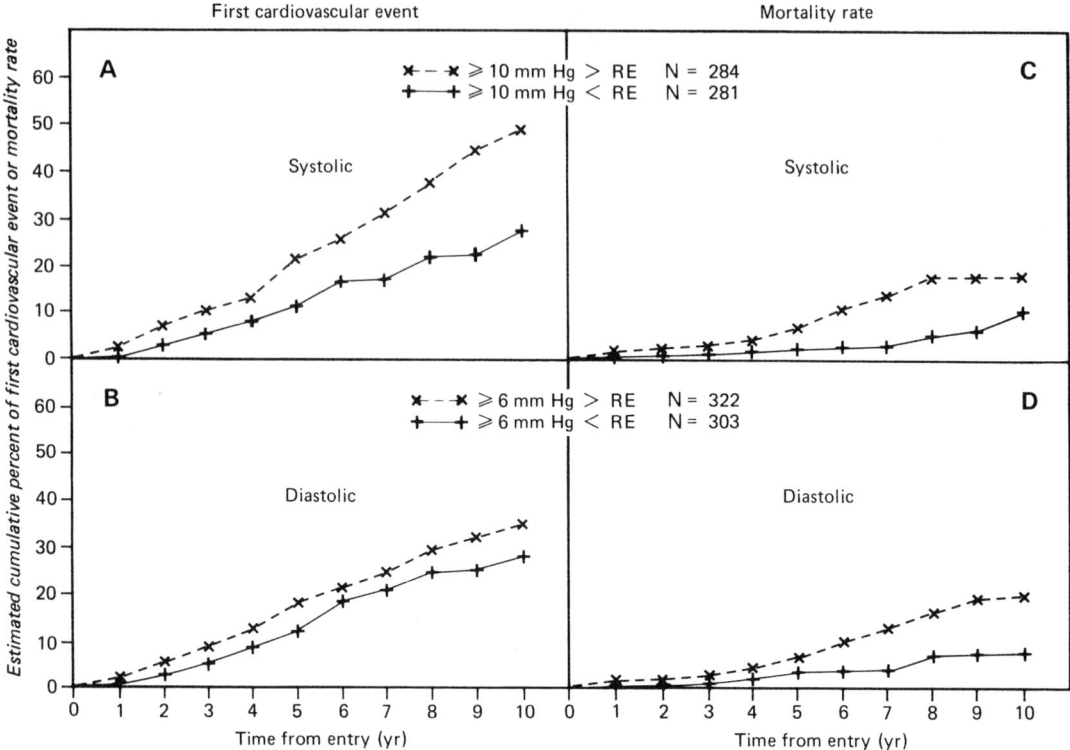

Figure 9-39. Estimated cumulative 10-year incidence of first clinical cardiovascular event *(A, B)* and cardiovascular mortality rate *(C, D)* among patients classified according to differences between observed and predicted blood pressures. The latter are derived from the regression equation (RE) for the regression of ambulatory on office pressures. $P = \leq 0.005$ for *A, B, C. D*. (Redrawn, modified, and reproduced, with permission, from Perloff D, Sokolow M, Cowan R: The prognostic value of ambulatory blood pressure. *JAMA* 1983;**249**:2792. Copyright © American Medical Association.)

answers to questions about their disease, the drugs, and their concerns. If the physician does not see the patient, an experienced clinical pharmacist should make a point of doing so and discussing the mechanism of action and problems concerning drugs, including possible interactions with drugs prescribed for other disorders. The physician, of course, should supervise this process and should know, for example, that tricyclic antidepressants neutralize the effect of guanethidine because both drugs compete for the same receptor sites.

A concerned physician who makes the patient an acknowledged partner in the therapeutic enterprise will have minimal problems with patient compliance.

As more and more hypertensive patients are identified and started in treatment, the load on the physician may become excessive, especially in large clinics. It appears to be well established now that nurse assistants, supervised closely by physicians, can do routine follow-up examinations for patients whose hypertension is adequately controlled. The nurse assistant can be taught to examine the fundi, listen to the heart for gallop rhythm, and examine for rales in the lungs and changes in the arterial pulses. Industrial nurses have also been used effectively in hypertension clinics in large factories. The use of nurse assistants in private practice has not been studied in sufficient detail to conclude whether this is desirable.

Continuation of Therapy If Blood Pressure Returns to Normal

This question has been studied by a number of investigators, and the general conclusion is that with infrequent exceptions, moderate to severe hypertension requires antihypertensive therapy for life because hypertension returns when the drugs are stopped. In cases of mild hypertension, on the other hand, after the blood pressure has been normal for several years, about 5-20% of patients remain normotensive when antihypertensive therapy is discontinued. A VA study (1975) (Fig 9-31) has indicated that there is a gradual recurrence of hypertension over a period of 3-9 months in 85% of patients with mild to moderate disease when antihypertensive therapy is stopped. More rarely, the pressure may begin to rise within the first month, especially if the patient has had severe disease before therapy is begun. If the pressure remains normal for 18 months to 2 years, the recurrence rate is very low.

The hazard of stopping therapy is that there may be a rebound phenomenon, with intense vasoconstriction, which may then be more difficult to reverse even if the same regimen used for successful control is restarted. Research groups who interrupt therapy for several weeks in order to perform renin, angiotensin, or steroid studies report that problems rarely occur when the drug is stopped for this short amount of time.

With the exception of stopping therapy for a short time to do specialized studies to exclude secondary hypertension, we ordinarily do not stop therapy. Once a diagnosis of hypertension has been established, patients require antihypertensive treatment for life. An attempt can be made to decrease dosage or the number of drugs prescribed, but rarely should therapy be stopped—even though 5–10% of patients remain normotensive for 1–2 years after all therapy is stopped. If the blood pressure is controlled at a low-normal level for 1 or 2 years, the size of the dose of the most potent agent that the patient is receiving can be decreased, especially if the patient has side effects which, while tolerated, are undesirable. This is done in slow, stepwise fashion. If the patient's pressure stays low for 6 months, we stop the most potent drug and then decrease the dose of the next most potent agent in similar fashion. If the blood pressure again remains normal for 6 months, we repeat the procedure with the remaining therapeutic agents. The likelihood of the blood pressure remaining normal is sufficiently small that if one attempts to stop therapy, close observation should be maintained to make certain that the patient does not have a high-pressure rebound. Patients should be informed about what is being done so that they will maintain close contact with the physician and not be lost to follow-up, only to return after months or years with severe complications of hypertension such as cardiac failure, malignant hypertension, or aortic dissection.

REFERENCES

Pathophysiology

Adamopoulos PN, Chrysanthakopoulis SG, Frohlich ED: Systolic hypertension: Nonhomogenous diseases. *Am J Cardiol* 1975;**36**:697.

Axelrod J: Catecholamines and hypertension. *Clin Sci Mol Med* 1976;**51**:415.

Barnes KL, Ferrario CM, Conomy JP: Comparison of the hemodynamic changes produced by electrical stimulation of the area postrema and nucleus tractus solitarii in the dog. *Circ Res* 1979;**45**:136.

Bayliss WM: On the local reactions of the arterial wall to changes of internal pressure. *J Physiol (Lond)* 1902;**28**:20.

Bell ET, Clawson BJ: Primary (essential) hypertension: A study of 420 cases. *Arch Pathol* 1928;**5**:939.

Benson H: Systemic hypertension and the relaxation response. *N Engl J Med* 1977;**296**:1152.

Brod J et al: Circulatory changes underlying blood pressure elevation during acute emotional stress (mental arithmetic) in normotensive and hypertensive subjects. *Clin Sci* 1959;**18**:269.

Byrom FB: Pathogenesis of hypertensive encephalopathy and its relation to the malignant phase of hypertension: Experimental evidence in the hypertensive rat. *Lancet* 1954;**2**:201.

Carey RM et al: The Charlottesville Blood-Pressure Survey: Value of repeated blood-pressure measurements to determine the prevalence of labile and sustained hypertension. *JAMA* 1976;**236**:847.

Cowley AW Jr (editor): Biochemical and neuroendocrine aspects of hypertension. *Hypertension* 1983;**5**:1. [Entire issue.]

Cowley AW Jr: The concept of autoregulation of total blood flow and its role in hypertension. *Am J Med* 1980;**68**:906.

Cryer PE: Physiology and pathophysiology of the human sympathoadrenal neuroendocrine system. *N Engl J Med* 1980;**303**:436.

Davis JO: Advances in our knowledge of the renin-angiotensin system. (Symposium.) *Fed Proc* 1977;**36**:1753.

de Wardener HE, MacGregor GA: The natriuretic hormone and essential hypertension. *Lancet* 1982;**1**:1450.

Dzau V et al: Monoclonal antibodies binding renal renin. *Hypertension* 1981;**3(Suppl 2)**:II-4.

Ferrario CM, Page IH: Current view concerning cardiac output in the genesis of experimental hypertension. *Circ Res* 1978;**43**:821.

Ferrario CM et al: Physiological and pharmacological characterization of the area postrema pressor pathways in the normal dog. *Hypertension* 1979;**1**:235.

Floras JS et al: Cuff and ambulatory blood pressure in subjects with essential hypertension. *Lancet* 1981;**2**:107.

Folkow B: Cardiovascular structural adaption: Its role in the initiation and maintenance of primary hypertension. (The Fourth Volhard Lecture.) *Clin Sci Mol Med* 1978;**55**:3s.

Folkow B: The haemodynamic consequences of adaptive structural changes of the resistance vessels in hypertension. *Clin Sci* 1971;**41**:1.

Ganguly A, Weinberger MH: Low renin hypertension: A current review of definitions and controversies. *Am Heart J* 1979;**98**:642.

Genest J, Koiw E, Kuchel O (editors): *Hypertension: Physiopathology and Treatment*. McGraw-Hill, 1977.

Gifford RW: Is the renin-sodium profile helpful in evaluating hypertension? *JAMA* 1980;**244**:35.

Goldblatt H, Lynch J, Hanzai R: Studies on experimental hypertension. 1. The production of persistent elevation of systolic blood pressure by means of renal ischemia. *J Exp Med* 1934;**59**:347.

Goldstein DS: Plasma catecholamines and essential hypertension: An analytical review. *Hypertension* 1983;**5**:86.

Gribbin B et al: Effect of age and high blood pressure on baroreflex sensitivity in man. *Circ Res* 1971;**29**:424.

Gross F, Dietz R: The significance of volume and cardiac output in the pathogenesis of hypertension. *Clin Sci* 1979;**57(Suppl 5)**:59s.

Guyton AC et al: Arterial pressure regulation: Overriding dominance of the kidneys in long-term regulation and in hypertension. *Am J Med* 1972;**52**:584.

Haber E: The role of renin in normal and pathological cardiovascular homeostasis. *Circulation* 1976;**54**:849.

Hamilton M et al: The aetiology of essential hypertension. 1. The arterial pressure in the general population. *Clin Sci* 1954;**13**:11.

Harris RE et al: Response to psychologic stress in persons who are potentially hypertensive. *Circulation* 1953;**7**:874.

Henry JP: Understanding the early pathophysiology of essential hypertension. *Geriatrics* 1976;**31**:59.

Kalis BL et al: Response to psychologic stress in patients with essential hypertension. *Am Heart J* 1957;**53**:572.

Kaplan NM: The prognostic implications of plasma renin in essential hypertension. *JAMA* 1975;**231**:167.

Keith NM, Wagener HP, Barker ND: Some different types of essential hypertension: Their course and prognosis. *Am J Med Sci* 1939;**197**:332.

Kincaid-Smith P, McMichael J, Murphy EA: The clinical course and pathology of hypertension with papilledema (malignant hypertension). *Q J Med* 1958;**27**:117.

Lake CR et al: Age-adjusted plasma norepinephrine levels are similar in normotensive and hypertensive subjects. *N Engl J Med* 1977;**296**:208.

Laragh JH (editor): *Laragh's Hypertension Manual.* Yorke Medical Books, 1974.

Laragh JH (editor): Symposium on hypertension. (2 parts.) *Am J Med* 1976;**60**:733 and **61**:721.

Ledingham JGG: Dietary salt and hypertension. *Cardiovasc Rev Rep* 1982;**3**:399.

Lee JB, Patak RV, Mookerjee BK: Renal prostaglandins and the regulation of blood pressure and sodium and water homeostasis. *Am J Med* 1976;**60**:798.

Levenson DJ, Simmons CE Jr, Brenner BM: Arachidonic acid metabolism, prostaglandins and the kidney. *Am J Med* 1982;**72**:354.

Liebman J, Edelman IS: Interrelations of plasma potassium concentrations, plasma sodium, arterial pH, and total exchangeable potassium. *J Clin Invest* 1959;**38**:2176.

Light KC, Obrist PA: Cardiovascular reactivity to behavioral stress in young males with and without marginally elevated causal systolic pressures: Comparison of clinic, home, and laboratory measures. *Hypertension* 1980;**2**:802.

Littler WA et al: The variability of arterial pressure. *Am Heart J* 1978;**95**:180.

Ljungman S et al: Sodium excretion and blood pressure. *Hypertension* 1981;**3**:318.

Marks LS, Maxwell MH, Kaufman JJ: Renin, sodium, and vasodepressor response to saralasin in renovascular and essential hypertension. *Ann Intern Med* 1977;**87**:176.

Masson GMC et al: Hypertensive vascular disease as a consequence of increased arterial pressure. *Am J Pathol* 1958;**38**:817.

McGiff JC: Kinins, renal function and blood pressure regulation. (Symposium.) *Fed Proc* 1976;**35**:172.

Mellander S, Johansson B: Control of resistance, exchange, and capacitance functions in the peripheral circulation. *Pharmacol Rev* 1968;**20**:117.

Moeller VJ, Heyder O: Die labile Blutdrucksteigerung. *Z Kreislaufforsch* 1959;**48**:413.

Moncada S: Prostacyclin and arterial wall biology. *Arteriosclerosis* 1982;**2**:193.

Muirhead EE: The antihypertensive function of the renal medulla. *Hosp Pract* (Jan) 1975;**10**:99.

Patel DJ et al: A control procedure for studies of blood pressure feedback in hypertension. *Cardiovasc Med* 1978;**3**:627.

Peart WS: Renin-angiotensin system. *N Engl J Med* 1975;**292**:302.

Pickering GP: Salt intake and essential hypertension. *Cardiovasc Rev Rep* 1980;**1**:13.

Pucak GJ (symposium chairman): Nutrition and blood pressure control: Current status of dietary factors and hypertension. (Symposium.) *Ann Intern Med* 1983;**98**:699.

Romero JC, Strong CG: Hypertension and the interrelated renal circulatory effects of prostaglandins and the renin-angiotensin system. *Mayo Clin Proc* 1977;**52**:462.

Ruskin A, Beard OW, Schaffer RL: "Blast hypertension": Elevated arterial pressures in the victims of the Texas City disaster. *Am J Med* 1948;**4**:228.

Russell RW: How does blood pressure cause stroke? *Lancet* 1975;**2**:1283.

Safar ME et al: Overhydration and renin in hypertensive patients with terminal renal failure: A hemodynamic study. *Clin Nephrol* 1975;**4**:183.

Scher AM: Control of arterial blood pressure. Pages 146–169 in: *Physiology and Biophysics,* 20th ed. Vol 2. Ruth TC, Patton HD (editors). Saunders, 1974.

Schwartz SM: Hypertension, endothelial injury, and atherosclerosis. *Cardiovasc Med* 1977;**2**:991.

Sleight P: Reflex control of the heart. *Am J Cardiol* 1979;**44**:889.

Strauer BE: Ventricular function and coronary hemodynamics in hypertensive heart disease. *Am J Cardiol* 1979;**44**:999.

Streeten DHP, Anderson GH Jr: Angiotensin blockade in hypertension. *Ann Intern Med* 1977;**86**:353.

Swartz SL et al: Captopril-induced changes in prostaglandin production: Relationship to vascular responses in normal man. *J Clin Invest* 1980;**65**:1257.

Tobian L et al: Prevention with thiazide of NaCl-induced hypertension in Dahl "S" rats: Evidence for a Na-retaining humoral agent in "S" rats. *Hypertension* 1979;**1**:316.

Vane JR, McGiff JC: Possible contributions of endogenous prostaglandins to the control of blood pressure. *Circ Res* 1975;**36(6-Suppl 1)**:I-68.

Watson RDS et al: Factors determining direct arterial pressure and its variability in hypertensive man. *Hypertension* 1980;**2**:333.

Weidmann P et al: Interrelations among blood pressure, blood volume, plasma renin activity and urinary catecholamines in benign essential hypertension. *Am J Med* 1977;**62**:209.

Wiggers CJ: *Physiology in Health and Disease,* 3rd ed. Lea & Febiger, 1939.

Williams GH: Angiotensin-dependent hypertension: Potential pitfalls in definition. *N Engl J Med* 1977;**296**:684.

Epidemiology

Aschroft MT, Desai P: Blood-pressure and mortality in a rural Jamaican community. *Lancet* 1978;**1**:1167.

Boe J, Humerfelt S, Werdevang F: The blood pressure in a population: Blood pressure readings and height and weight determinations in the adult population of the city of Bergen. *Acta Med Scand [Suppl]* 1957;**321**:1. [Entire issue.]

Build and Blood Pressure Study. Vol 1. Chicago: Society of Actuaries, 1959.

Carey RM et al: The Charlottesville Blood-Pressure Survey: Value of repeated blood-pressure measurements. *JAMA* 1976;**236**:847.

Ganong WF, Barbieri C: Neuroendocrine components in the regulation of renin secretion. Chap 9, p 231, in: *Frontiers in Neuroendocrinology.* Vol 7. Ganong WF, Martini L (editors). Raven Press, 1982.

Gibson G, Gibbons A: Hypertension among blacks: An annotated bibliography. *Hypertension* 1982;**4**:1. [Entire issue.]

Humerfelt SB: An epidemiological study of high blood pressure. *Acta Med Scand [Suppl]* 1963;**407**;1. [Entire issue.]

Kannel WB, McGee D, Gordon T: A general cardiovascular

risk profile: The Framingham Study. *Am J Cardiol* 1976;**38**:46.

Ledingham JGG: Dietary salt and hypertension. *Cardiovasc Rev Rep* 1982;**3**:399.

Lew EA: High blood pressure, other risk factors and longevity: The insurance viewpoint. *Am J Med* 1973;**55**:281.

Ljungman S et al: Sodium excretion and blood pressure. *Hypertension* 1981;**3**:318.

Messerli FH et al: Essential hypertension in black and white subjects: Hemodynamic findings and fluid retention. *Am J Med* 1979;**67**:27.

Mitchell JRA: Hypertension and arterial disease. *Br Heart J* 1971;**33**:122.

Needleman P et al: Atriopeptins as cardiac hormones. *Hypertension* 1985;**7**:469.

Okamoto K (editor): *Spontaneous Hypertension: Its Pathogenesis and Complications.* Igaku Shoin, Ltd, 1972.

Omvik P, Lund-Johansen P, Eide R: Sodium excretion and blood pressure in middle-aged men in the Sogn County: An intra- and interpopulation study. *J Hypertension* 1983;**1**:77.

Pickering G: *High Blood Pressure,* 2nd ed. Churchill, 1968.

Rabkin SW, Mathewson FA, Tate RB: Relationship of blood pressure in 20-39-year-old men to subsequent blood pressure and incidence of hypertension over a 30-year observation period. *Circulation* 1982;**65**:291.

Stamler J, Stamler R, Pullman TN (editors): *The Epidemiology of Hypertension.* Grune & Stratton, 1967.

US Department of Health, Education and Welfare, National Institutes of Health: *The National High Blood Pressure Education Program.* Department of Health, Education and Welfare Publication No. (NIH) 74–593, 1973.

Veterans Administration Cooperative Study Group on Antihypertensive Agents: Effects of treatment on morbidity in hypertension. 1. Results in patients with diastolic blood pressure averaging 115 through 129 mm Hg. *JAMA* 1967;**202**:1028.

Veterans Administration Cooperative Study Group on Antihypertensive Agents: Effects of treatment on morbidity in hypertension. 3. Influence of age, diastolic pressure, and prior cardiovascular disease; further analysis of side-effects. *Circulation* 1972;**45**:991.

Yamori Y, Lovenberg W, Freis ED (editors): *Prophylactic Approach to Hypertensive Diseases.* Vol 4 of: *Perspectives in Cardiovascular Research.* Raven Press, 1979.

Zinner SH, Levy PS, Kass EH: Familial aggregation of blood pressure in childhood. *N Engl J Med* 1971;**284**:401.

Clinical Features

Ayman D, Goldshine AD: Blood pressure determinations by patients with essential hypertension. 1. The difference between clinical and home readings before treatment. *Am J Med Sci* 1940;**200**:465.

Bevan AT, Honour AJ, Stott FH: Direct arterial pressure recording in unrestricted man. *Br Heart J* 1969;**31**:387.

Cole FM, Yates PO: Comparative incidence of cerebrovascular lesions in normotensive and hypertensive patients. *Neurology* 1968;**18**;255.

Cooper ES, West JW: Hypertension and stroke. *Cardiovasc Med* 1977;**2**:429.

des Combes BJ et al: Ambulatory blood pressure recordings: Reproducibility and unpredictability. *Hypertension* 1984;**6**:C110.

Finnerty FA Jr, Mattie EC, Finnerty FA III: Hypertension in the inner city. 1. Analysis of clinical dropouts. *Circulation* 1973;**47**:73.

Fitzgerald DJ et al: Accuracy and reliability of two indirect ambulatory blood pressure recorders: Remler M2000 and Cardiodyne Sphygmolog. *Br Heart J* 1982;**48**:472.

Freis ED: The clinical spectrum of essential hypertension. *Arch Intern Med* 1974;**133**:982.

Goldberg AD et al: Study of untreated hypertensive subjects by means of continuous intra-arterial blood pressure recordings. *Br Heart J* 1978;**40**:656.

Goldring W, Chasis H: *Hypertension and Hypertensive Disease.* Commonwealth Fund, 1944.

Graham JDP: High blood pressure after battle. *Lancet* 1945;**1**:239.

Heptinstall RH: Renal biopsies in hypertension. *Br Heart J* 1954;**16**:133.

Hodge JV, Dollery CT: Retinal soft exudates. *Q J Med* 1964;**33**:117.

The Hypertension Detection and Follow-Up Program Cooperative Group: Five-year findings of the Hypertension Detection and Follow-Up Program: 3. Reduction in stroke incidence among persons with high blood pressure. *JAMA* 1982;**247**:633.

Julius S: Borderline hypertension: Definitions and treatment. *Cardiovasc Med* 1976;**1**:77.

Kain HK, Hinman AT, Sokolow M: Arterial blood measurements with a portable recorder in hypertensive patients. 1. Variability and correlation with "casual" pressures. *Circulation* 1964;**30**:882.

Kannel WB: Role of blood pressure in the development of congestive heart failure. *N Engl J Med* 1972;**287**:782.

Kannel WB et al: Perspectives on systolic hypertension: The Framingham Study. *Circulation* 1980;**60**:1179.

Kaplan NM: *Clinical Hypertension,* 2nd ed. Williams & Wilkins, 1978.

Keith NM, Wagener HP, Barker ND: Some different types of essential hypertension: Their course and prognosis. *Am J Med Sci* 1939;**197**:332.

Kincaid-Smith P: Malignant hypertension. *Cardiovasc Rev Rep* 1980;**1**:42.

Kirkendall WM et al: Recommendation for human blood pressure determination by sphygmomanometer. *Circulation* 1967;**36**:981.

Knowler WC, Bennett PH, Ballintine EJ: Increased incidence of retinopathy in diabetics with elevated blood pressure: A six-year follow-up study in Pima Indians. *N Engl J Med* 1980;**302**:645.

Krupp MA: Urinary sediment in visceral angiitis (periarteritis nodosa, lupus erythematosus, Libman-Sachs disease): Quantitative study. *Arch Intern Med* 1943;**71**:54.

Laragh JH (editor): Symposium on hypertension. (2 parts.) *Am J Med* 1976;**60**:733 and **61**:721.

Littler WA, Honour AJ, Sleight P: Direct arterial pressure, pulse rate, and electrocardiogram during micturition and defecation in unrestricted man. *Am Heart J* 1973;**88**:205.

Londe S, Goldring D: High blood pressure in children: Problems and guidelines for evaluation and treatment. *Am J Cardiol* 1976;**37**:650.

Lund-Johansen P, Omvik P: Haemodynamic effects of nifedipine in essential hypertension at rest and during exercise. *J Hypertension* 1983;**1**:159.

National Heart, Lung and Blood Institute's Task Force on Blood Pressure Control in Children: Report of the Task Force on Blood Pressure Control in Children. *Pediatrics* 1977;**59**:797.

Perloff D, Sokolow M: The representative blood pressure: Usefulness of office, basal, home, and ambulatory readings. *Cardiovasc Med* 1978;**3**:655.

Pickering G: Hyperpiesia: High blood pressure without evident cause: Essential hypertension. *Br Med J* 1965;**2**:959.

Pickering G: *Hypertension,* 2nd ed. Churchill Livingstone, 1974.

Ramalho PS, Dollery CT: Hypertensive retinopathy: Caliber changes in retinal blood vessels following blood pressure reduction and inhalation of oxygen. *Circulation* 1968;**37**:580.

Reichek N et al: Anatomic validation of left ventricular mass estimates from clinical two-dimensional echocardiography: Initial results. *Circulation* 1983;**67**:348.

Romhilt DW, Estes EH Jr: A point score system for the ECG diagnosis of left ventricular hypertrophy. *Am Heart J* 1968;**75**:752.

Sandok BA, Whisman JP: Hypertension and the brain. *Arch Intern Med* 1974;**133**:947.

Sannerstedt R: Hemodynamic response to exercise in patients with arterial hypertension. *Acta Med Scand [Suppl]* 1966;**458**:1. [Entire issue.]

Schambelan M et al: Selective renal-vein sampling in hypertensive patients with segmental renal lesions. *N Engl J Med* 1974;**290**:1153.

Sheps SG, Kirkpatrick RA: Hypertension. *Mayo Clin Proc* 1975;**50**:709.

Smirk FH: *High Arterial Pressure.* Blackwell, 1957.

Sokolow M, Lyon TP: The ventricular complex in left ventricular hypertrophy as obtained by unipolar precordial and limb leads. *Am Heart J* 1949;**37**:161.

Sokolow M, Perloff D: The prognosis of essential hypertension treated conservatively. *Circulation* 1961;**23**:697.

Sokolow M et al: Preliminary studies relating portably recorded blood pressures to daily events in patients with essential hypertension. *Bibl Psychiatr* 1970;**144**:164.

Sokolow M et al: Relationship between level of blood pressure measured casually and by portable recorders and severity of complications in essential hypertension. *Circulation* 1966;**34**:279.

Talbot S et al: QRS voltage of the electrocardiogram and Frank vectorcardiogram in relation to ventricular volume. *Br Heart J* 1977;**39**:1109.

Toshima H, Koga Y, Kimura N: Correlations between electrocardiographic, vectorcardiographic, and echocardiographic findings in patients with left ventricular overload. *Am Heart J* 1977;**94**:547.

Woythaler JN et al: Accuracy of echocardiography versus electrocardiography in detecting left ventricular hypertrophy: Comparison with postmortem mass measurements. *J Am Coll Cardiol* 1983;**2**:305.

Course of the Disease & Prognosis

Aschroft MT, Desai P: Blood-pressure and mortality in a rural Jamaican community. *Lancet* 1978;**1**:1167.

Bechgaard P: The natural history of benign hypertension: 1000 hypertensive patients followed from 26–32 years. Page 357 in: *The Epidemiology of Hypertension.* Stamler J, Stamler R, Pullman TN (editors). Grune & Stratton, 1967.

Bedford DE: Left ventricular failure. *Lancet* 1939;**1**:1303.

Bell ET, Clawson BJ: Primary (essential) hypertension: A study of 420 cases. *Arch Pathol* 1928;**5**:939.

Breckenridge A, Dollery CT, Parry EHO: Prognosis of treated hypertension: Changes in life expectancy and causes of death between 1952 and 1967. *Q J Med* 1970;**39**:411.

Chalmers JP: Nervous system and hypertension: Review. *Clin Sci Mol Med* 1978;**55**:45s.

Dalen JE et al: Dissection of the aorta: Pathogenesis, diagnosis, and treatment. *Prog Cardiovasc Dis* 1980;**23**:237.

Doroghazi RM, Slater EE, DeSanctis RW: Medical therapy for aortic dissections. *J Cardiovasc Med* 1981;**6**:187.

Doyle AE: In: *The Pathophysiology and Management of Arterial Hypertension.* Berglund G, Hansson L, Werkö L (editors). AB Astra, 1975.

Dustan HP: Atherosclerosis complicating chronic hypertension. *Circulation* 1974;**50**:871.

Earnest IVF, Muhm JR, Sheedy PF II: Roentgenographic findings in thoracic aortic dissection. *Mayo Clin Proc* 1979;**54**:43.

Farmer RG, Gifford RW, Hines EA Jr: Effect of medical treatment on severe hypertension: Follow-up study of 161 patients with group three or group four hypertension. *Arch Intern Med* 1963;**112**:118.

Gifford RW Jr: Drug combinations as rational antihypertensive therapy. *Arch Intern Med* 1974;**133**:1053.

Goldring W, Chasis H: *Hypertension and Hypertensive Disease.* Commonwealth Fund, 1944.

Kannel WB: Role of blood pressure in cardiovascular morbidity and mortality. *Prog Cardiovasc Dis* 1974;**17**:5.

Keith NM, Wagener HP, Barker ND: Some different types of essential hypertension: Their course and prognosis. *Am J Med Sci* 1939;**197**:332.

Kincaid-Smith P, McMichael J, Murphy EA: The clinical course and pathology of hypertension with papilledema (malignant hypertension). *Q J Med* 1958;**27**:117.

Lund-Johansen P: Hemodynamics in essential hypertension: State of the art review. *Clin Sci* 1980;**59**:343s.

Maron BJ et al: Prognosis of surgically corrected coarctation of the aorta: A 20-year postoperative appraisal. *Circulation* 1973;**47**:119.

McCormack LJ et al: Effects of antihypertensive treatment in the evolution of renal lesions in malignant nephrosclerosis. *Am J Pathol* 1958;**34**:1011.

Moeller VJ, Heyder P: Die labile Blutdrucksteigerung. *Z Kreislaufforsch* 1959;**48**:413.

Perry M, Wessler S, Avioli LV: Survival of treated hypertensive patients. *JAMA* 1969;**210**:890.

Pickering G: *High Blood Pressure,* 2nd ed. Churchill, 1968.

Rabkin SW, Mathewson FAL, Tate RB: The relation of blood pressure to stroke prognosis. *Ann Intern Med* 1978;**89**:15.

Schottstaedt MF, Sokolow M: The natural history and course of hypertension with papilledema (malignant hypertension). *Am Heart J* 1952;**45**:331.

Shapiro LM, Beevers DG: Malignant hypertension: Cardiac structure and function at presentation and during therapy. *Br Heart J* 1983;**49**:477.

Shekelle RB, Ostfeld AM, Klawans HL Jr: Hypertension and risk of stroke in an elderly population. *Stroke* 1974;**5**:71.

Slater EE, DeSanctis RW: The clinical recognition of dissecting aortic aneurysm. *Am J Med* 1976;**60**:625.

Smirk FH, Veale AMO, Alstad K: Basal and supplemental blood pressures in relationship to life expectancy and hypertension symptomatology. *NZ Med J* 1959;**58**:711.

Smirk H, Hodge JV: Causes of death in treated hypertensive patients: Based on 82 deaths during 1959–61 among an average hypertensive population at risk of 518 persons. *Br Med J* 1963;**2**:1221.

Smuckler AL et al: Echocardiographic diagnosis of aortic root dissection by M-mode and two-dimensional techniques. *Am Heart J* 1982;**103**:897.

Sokolow M, Perloff D: The prognosis of essential hypertension treated conservatively. *Circulation* 1961;**23**:697.

Veterans Administration Cooperative Study Group on Antihypertensive Agents: Effects of treatment on morbidity in hypertension. 2. Results in patients with diastolic blood pressure averaging 90 through 114 mm Hg. *JAMA* 1970;**213**:1143.

Wheat MW Jr: Acute dissecting aneurysms of the aorta: Diagnosis and treatment—1979. *Am Heart J* 1980;**99**:373.

Secondary Hypertension

Anderson BG, Beierwaltes WH: Adrenal imaging with radioiodocholesterol in the diagnosis of adrenal disorders. *Adv Intern Med* 1974;**19**:327.

Atkinson RL et al: Acromegaly: Treatment by transsphenoidal microsurgery. *JAMA* 1975;**233**:1279.

Barger AC: The Goldblatt Memorial Lecture. Part 1: Experimental renovascular hypertension. *Hypertension* 1979;**1**:447.

Berson AS: NHLBI workshop on renovascular disease: Summary report and recommendations. *Hypertension* 1985;**7**:452.

Biglieri EG: Adrenocortical components in hypertension. *Cardiovasc Rev Rep* 1982;**3**:734.

Biglieri EG: Enzymatic disorders and hypertension. *Clin Endocrinol Metab* 1981;**10**:453.

Biglieri EG, McIlroy MB: Abnormalities of renal function and circulatory reflexes in primary aldosteronism. *Circulation* 1966;**33**:78.

Bookstein JJ, Walter JF: The role of abdominal radiography in hypertension secondary to renal or adrenal disease. *Med Clin North Am* 1975;**59**:169.

Bookstein JJ et al: Cooperative study of radiologic aspects of renovascular hypertension: Bilateral renovascular disease. *JAMA* 1977;**237**:1706.

Bravo EL, Gifford RW: Pheochromocytoma: Diagnosis, localization and management. *N Engl J Med* 1984;**311**:1298.

Bravo EL et al: The changing clinical spectrum of primary aldosteronism. *Am J Med* 1983;**74**:641.

Bravo EL et al: Circulating and urinary catecholamines in pheochromocytoma: Diagnostic and pathophysiologic implications. *N Engl J Med* 1979;**301**:682.

Bumpus FM, Khosla MC: Pathogenic factors involved in renovascular hypertension: State of the art. *Mayo Clin Proc* 1977;**52**:417.

Davis BA et al: Prevalence of renovascular hypertension in patients with grade III or IV hypertensive retinopathy. *N Engl J Med* 1979;**301**:1273.

Davis JO: Advances in our knowledge of the renin-angiotensin system. (Symposium.) *Fed Proc* 1977;**36**:1753.

Dunn FG et al: Pathophysiologic assessment of hypertensive heart disease with echocardiography. *Am J Cardiol* 1977;**39**:789.

Epstein AJ, Patel SK, Petasnick JP: Computerized tomography of the adrenal gland. *JAMA* 1979;**242**:2791.

Fregly MJ, Fregly MS (editors): *Oral Contraceptives and High Blood Pressure*. Dolphin Press, 1974.

Gabow PA, Ikle DW, Holmes JH: Polycystic kidney disease: Prospective analysis of nonazotemic patients and family members. *Ann Intern Med* 1984;**101**:238.

Gifford RW Jr: Curable causes of hypertension. (Correspondence.) *Mayo Clin Proc* 1977;**52**:827.

Gold EM: The Cushing syndromes: Changing views of diagnosis and treatment. *Ann Intern Med* 1979;**90**:829.

Goldfien A: Treatment of pheochromocytoma. *Mod Treat* 1966;**3**:1360.

Gordon DA, Hill FM, Ezrin C: Acromegaly: A review of 100 cases. *Can Med Assoc J* 1962;**87**:1106.

Grim CE et al: Percutaneous transluminal dilation in the treatment of renal vascular hypertension. *Ann Intern Med* 1981;**95**:439.

Grim CE et al: Sensitivity and specificity of screening tests for renal vascular hypertension. *Ann Intern Med* 1979;**91**:617.

Grüntzig A et al: Treatment of renovascular hypertension with percutaneous transluminal dilatation of a renal-artery stenosis. *Lancet* 1978;**1**:801.

Guerin CK et al: Computed tomographic scanning versus radioisotope imaging in adrenocortical diagnosis. *Am J Med* 1983;**75**:653.

Gutmann FD et al: Renal arterial pressure, renin secretion, and blood pressure control in trained dogs. *Am J Physiol* 1973;**224**:66.

Haber E: The role of renin in normal and pathological cardiovascular homeostasis. *Circulation* 1976;**54**:849.

Hodsman GP et al: Enalapril in treatment of hypertension with renal artery stenosis. *Am J Med* 1984;**77(2A Suppl)**:52.

Hogan MJ et al: Location of aldosterone-producing adenomas with ^{131}I-19-iodocholesterol. *N Engl J Med* 1976;**294**:410.

Hollenberg NK: Medical therapy of renovascular hypertension: Efficacy and safety of captopril in 269 patients. *Cardiovasc Rev Rep* 1983;**4**:852.

Hunt JC et al: Renal and renovascular hypertension: A reasoned approach to diagnosis and management. *Arch Intern Med* 1974;**133**:988.

Hurxthal IM, O'Sullivan JB: Cushing's syndrome: Clinical differential diagnosis and complications. *Ann Intern Med* 1959;**51**:1.

Jennings AS, Liddle GW, Orth DN: Results of treating childhood Cushing's disease with pituitary irradiation. *N Engl J Med* 1977;**297**:957.

Kaplan NM: The Goldblatt Memorial Lecture. Part 2: The role of the kidney in hypertension. *Hypertension* 1979;**1**:456.

Kaplan NM et al: Single-voided urine metanephrine assays in screening for pheochromocytoma. *Arch Intern Med* 1977;**137**:190.

Krieger DT: The central nervous system and Cushing's disease. *Med Clin North Am* 1978;**62**:261.

Krupp MA: Urinary sediment in visceral angiitis (periarteritis nodosa, lupus erythematosus, Libman-Sachs disease): Quantitative study. *Arch Intern Med* 1943;**71**:54.

Kuhlmann U et al: Renovascular hypertension: Treatment by percutaneous transluminal dilation. *Ann Intern Med* 1980;**92**:1.

Lessman RK et al: Renal artery embolism. *Ann Intern Med* 1978;**89**:477.

Mahler F et al: Lasting improvement of renovascular hypertension by transluminal dilatation of atherosclerotic and nonatherosclerotic renal artery stenoses: A follow-up study. *Circulation* 1982;**65**:611.

Mancia G et al: Prolonged intra-arterial blood-pressure recording in diagnosis of phaeochromocytoma. *Lancet* 1979;**2**:1193.

Manger WM, Gifford RW Jr: *Pheochromocytoma*. Springer, 1977.

Maxwell MH: Cooperative study of renovascular hypertension: Current status. *Kidney Int* 1975;**8(Suppl)**:153.

Maxwell MH et al: Predictive value of renin determinations in renal artery stenosis. *JAMA* 1977;**238**:2617.

Melby JC: Solving the adrenal lesions of primary aldosteronism. (Editorial.) *N Engl J Med* 1976;**294**:441.

Muirhead EE: The antihypertensive function of the renal medulla. *Hosp Pract* (Jan) 1975;**10**:99.

Novick AC et al: Diminished operative morbidity and mortality in renal revascularization. *JAMA* 1981;**246**:749.

Oparil S: Hypertension and oral contraceptives. *J Cardiovasc Med* 1981;**6**:381.

Palubinskas AJ, Perloff D, Wylie EJ: Curable hypertension due to renal artery lesions. *Radiol Clin (Basel)* 1964;**33**:207.

Parving H-H et al: Early aggressive antihypertensive treatment reduces rate of decline in kidney function in diabetic nephropathy. *Lancet* 1983;**1**:1175.

Perloff D, Schambelan M: Renovascular hypertension. *Clin Endocrinol Metab* 1981;**10**:513.

Perloff D et al: Hypertension secondary to renal artery occlusive disease. *Circulation* 1961;**24**:1286.

Raper AJ et al: Pheochromocytoma of the urinary bladder: A broad clinical spectrum. *Am J Cardiol* 1977;**40**:820.

Re R et al: Inhibition of angiotensin-converting enzyme for diagnosis of renal-artery stenosis. *N Engl J Med* 1978;**298**:582.

Roberts B, Ring EJ: Current status of percutaneous transluminal angioplasty. *Surg Clin North Am* 1982;**62**:357.

Royal College of General Practitioners' Oral Contraception Study: Mortality among oral-contraceptive users. *Lancet* 1977;**2**:727.

Salassa RM et al: Transsphenoidal removal of pituitary microadenoma in Cushing's disease. *Mayo Clin Proc* 1978;**53**:24.

Schambelan M et al: Role of renin and aldosterone in hypertension due to renin-secreting tumor. *Am J Med* 1973;**55**:86.

Sellars L, Shore AC, Wilkinson R: Renal vein renin studies in renovascular hypertension: Do they really help? *J Hypertension* 1985;**3**:177.

Sheps SG, Kincaid OW, Hunt JC: Serial renal function and angiographic observations in idiopathic fibrous and fibromuscular stenoses of the renal arteries. *Am J Cardiol* 1972;**30**:55.

Sokolow M et al: Current experiences with renovascular hypertension. Page 341 in: *Proceedings of the International Club on Arterial Hypertension.* Expansion Scientifique Française, 1966.

Sokolow M et al: Relationship between level of blood pressure measured casually and by portable recorders and severity of complications in essential hypertension. *Circulation* 1966;**34**:279.

Sos TA et al: Percutaneous transluminal renal angioplasty in renovascular hypertension due to atheroma or fibromuscular dysplasia. *N Engl J Med* 1983;**309**:274.

Stamey TA: Unilateral renal disease causing hypertension. *JAMA* 1976;**235**:2340.

Stewart BH et al: Localization of pheochromocytoma by computed tomography. *N Engl J Med* 1978;**299**:460.

Streeten DHP, Tomycz N, Anderson GH Jr: Reliability of screening methods for the diagnosis of primary aldosteronism. *Am J Med* 1979;**67**:403.

Thomas JE, Rooke ED, Kvale WF: The neurologist's experience with pheochromocytoma: A review of 100 cases. *JAMA* 1966;**197**:100.

Tucker RM, Labarthe DR: Frequency of surgical treatment for hypertension in adults at the Mayo Clinic from 1973 through 1975. *Mayo Clin Proc* 1977;**52**:549.

Tucker RM et al: Renovascular hypertension: Relationship of surgical curability to renin-angiotensin activity. *Mayo Clin Proc* 1978;**53**:373.

Tyrrell JB et al: Cushing's disease: Selective transsphenoidal resection of pituitary microadenomas. *N Engl J Med* 1978;**298**:753.

Weinberger MH et al: Primary aldosteronism: Diagnosis, localization, and treatment. *Ann Intern Med* 1979;**90**:386.

Wenting GH et al: Volume-pressure relationships during development of mineralocorticoid hypertension in man. *Circ Res* 1977;**40(5–Suppl 1)**:I-163.

White EA et al: Use of computed tomography in diagnosing the cause of primary aldosteronism. *N Engl J Med* 1980;**303**:1503.

Wilhelmsen L, Berglund G: Prevalence of primary and secondary hypertension. *Am Heart J* 1977;**94**:543.

Ying CY et al: Renal revascularization in the azotemic hypertensive patient resistant to therapy. *N Engl J Med* 1984;**311**:1070.

Youngberg SP, Sheps SG, Strong CG: Management of the patient with renovascular hypertension. *Am Heart J* 1977;**94**:785.

Treatment of Hypertension

Alderman MH: High blood pressure: Do we really know whom to treat and how? (Editorial.) *N Engl J Med* 1977;**296**:753.

Amery A et al: Antihypertensive therapy in patients above age 60 years: Fourth Interim Report of the European Working Party on High Blood Pressure in the Elderly (EWPHE). *Clin Sci Mol Med* 1978;**55**:263s.

Amery A et al: Mortality and morbidity results from the European Working Party on High Blood Pressure in the Elderly trial. *Lancet* 1985;**2**:1349.

Aoki VS, Wilson WR: Hydralazine and methyldopa in thiazide-treated hypertensive patients. *Am Heart J* 1970;**79**:798.

Australian therapeutic trial in mild hypertension: Report by the Management Committee. *Lancet* 1980;**1**:1261.

Baim DS et al: Evaluation of a new bipyridine inotropic agent—milrinone—in patients with severe congestive heart failure. *N Engl J Med* 1983;**309**:748.

Bauer JH, Brooks CS: The long-term effect of propranolol therapy on renal function. *Am J Med* 1979;**66**:405.

Beevers DG, Hamilton M, Harpur JE: The long-term treatment of hypertension with thiazide diuretics. *Postgrad Med J* 1971;**47**:639.

Beevers DG et al: Antihypertensive treatment and the course of established cerebral vascular disease. *Lancet* 1973;**1**:1407.

Berglund G, Andersson O: Beta-blockers or diuretics in hypertension? A six-year follow-up of blood pressure and metabolic side effects. *Lancet* 1981;**1**:744.

Berglund G et al: Coronary heart-disease after treatment of hypertension. *Lancet* 1978;**1**:1.

Bhatia SK, Frohlich ED: Hemodynamic comparison of agents useful in hypertensive emergencies. *Am Heart J* 1973;**85**:367.

Boerth RC, Long WR: Dose-response relation of diazoxide in children with hypertension. *Circulation* 1977;**56**:1062.

Bravo EL, Tarazi RC: Converting enzyme inhibition with an orally active compound in hypertensive man. *Hypertension* 1979;**1**:39.

Bravo EL, Tarazi RC, Dustan HP: β-Adrenergic blockade in diuretic-treated patients with essential hypertension. *N Engl J Med* 1975;**292**:66.

Brunner HR et al: Oral angiotensin-converting enzyme inhibitor in long-term treatment of hypertensive patients. *Ann Intern Med* 1979;**90**:19.

Bühler FR, Bertel O, Lütold BE: Simplified and age-stratified antihypertensive therapy based on beta blockers. *Cardiovasc Med* 1978;**3**:135.

Caldwell JR et al: The dropout problem in antihypertensive treatment: A pilot study of social and emotional factors influencing a patient's ability to follow antihypertensive treatment. *J Chronic Dis* 1970;**22**:579.

The Canadian Cooperative Study Group: A randomized trial

of aspirin and sulfinpyrazone in threatened stroke. *N Engl J Med* 1978;**299**:53.

Carey RM et al: The Charlottesville Blood-Pressure Survey: Value of repeated blood-pressure measurements to determine the prevalence of labile and sustained hypertension. *JAMA* 1976;**236**:847.

Case DB et al: Clinical experience with captopril in moderate to severe hypertension. *Cardiovasc Rev Rep* 1982;**3**:435.

Chalmers J et al: Effects of timolol and hydrochlorothiazide on blood-pressure and plasma renin activity: Double-blind factorial trial. *Lancet* 1976;**2**:328.

Clark AB, Dunn M: A nurse clinician's role in the management of hypertension. *Arch Intern Med* 1976;**136**:903.

Clarke E, Murphy EA: Neurological manifestations of malignant hypertension. *Br Med J* 1956;**2**:1319.

Cohn JN: Choice and rationale for vasodilators in the treatment of hypertension or relief of heart failure. *Cardiovasc Rev Rep* 1980;**1**:686.

Colucci WS: New developments in alpha-adrenergic receptor pharmacology: Implications for initial treatment of hypertension. *Am J Cardiol* 1983;**51**:639.

Colwill JM et al: Alpha-methyldopa and hydrochlorothiazide: A controlled study of their comparative effectiveness as antihypertensive agents. *N Engl J Med* 1964;**271**:696.

Connolly ME, Kersting F, Dollery CT: The clinical pharmacology of beta-adrenoceptor-blocking drugs. *Prog Cardiovasc Dis* 1976;**19**:203.

Dargie HJ, Dollery CT, Daniel J: Minoxidil in resistant hypertension. *Lancet* 1977;**2**:515.

Davies RO et al: Enalapril worldwide experience. *Am J Med* 1984;**77(Suppl 2A)**:23.

Davis JO: The pathogenesis of chronic renovascular hypertension. *Circ Res* 1977;**40**:439.

DeBono G et al: Acebutolol: Ten years of experience. *Am Heart J* 1985;**109**:1211.

DiCarlo L et al: Enalapril: A new angiotensin-converting enzyme inhibitor in chronic heart failure: Acute and chronic hemodynamic evaluations. *J Am Coll Cardiol* 1983;**2**:865.

Dollery CT, Emslie-Smith D, Milne MD: Clinical and pharmacological studies with guanethidine in the treatment of hypertension. *Lancet* 1960;**1**:381.

Dollery CT, Harrington M: Methyldopa in hypertension: Clinical and pharmacological studies. *Lancet* 1962;**1**:759.

Doroghazi RM et al: Long-term survival of patients with treated aortic dissection. *J Am Coll Cardiol* 1984;**3**:1026.

Douglas JG, Hollifield JW, Liddle GW: Treatment of low-renin essential hypertension: Comparison of spironolactone and a hydrochlorothiazide-triamterene combination. *JAMA* 1974;**227**:518.

Fagard R et al: Acute and chronic systemic and pulmonary hemodynamic effects of angiotensin converting enzyme inhibition with captopril in hypertensive patients. *Am J Cardiol* 1980;**46**:295.

Fagard R et al: Response of the systemic and pulmonary circulation to alpha- and beta-receptor blockade (labetalol) at rest and during exercise in hypertensive patients. *Circulation* 1979;**60**:1214.

Fann WE et al: Chlorpromazine reversal of the antihypertensive action of guanethidine. *Lancet* 1971;**2**:436.

Farmer RG, Gifford RW, Hines EA Jr: Effect of medical treatment on severe hypertension: Follow-up study of 161 patients with group three or group four hypertension. *Arch Intern Med* 1963;**112**:118.

Floras JS et al: Cardioselective and nonselective beta-adrenoceptor blocking drugs in hypertension: A comparison of their effect on blood pressure during mental and physical activity. *J Am Coll Cardiol* 1985;**6**:186.

Freis ED, Materson BJ, Flamenbaum W: Comparison of propranolol or hydrochlorothiazide alone for treatment of hypertension. 3. Evaluation of the renin-angiotensin system. *Am J Med* 1983;**74**:1029.

Frishman W: Beta-adrenoceptor antagonists: New drugs and new indications. *N Engl J Med* 1981;**305**:500.

Frishman W: Labetalol therapy in patients with systemic hypertension and angina pectoris: Effects of combined alpha and beta adrenoceptor blockade. *Am J Cardiol* 1981;**48**:917.

Frishman W et al: Comparison of oral propranolol and verapamil for combined systemic hypertension and angina pectoris: A placebo-controlled double-blind randomized crossover trial. *Am J Cardiol* 1982;**50**:1164.

Frohlich ED (editor): Calcium channel blockers: A new dimension in antihypertensive therapy. (Symposium). *Am J Med* 1984;**77(Suppl 2B)**:1. [Entire issue.]

Frohlich ED: New concepts in hypertension therapy. *Am J Med* 1984;**77(Suppl 4A)**:1. [Entire issue.]

Frohlich ED (guest editor): Role of calcium channel blockers in the management of hypertension. *Am J Med* 1985;**79**:1. [Entire issue.]

Fujita T et al: Hemodynamic and endocrine changes associated with captopril in diuretic-resistant hypertensive patients. *Am J Med* 1982;**73**:341.

Garrett BN, Kaplan NM: Clonidine in the treatment of hypertension. *J Cardiovasc Pharmacol* 1980;**2(Suppl 1)**:S61.

Gifford RW Jr: The HDFP, the JNC, and nonpharmacologic management of hypertension. *Mayo Clin Proc* 1980;**55**:651.

Gifford RW Jr: Managing hypertension: The Postgraduate Medicine Lecture. (3 parts.) *Postgrad Med* (March) 1977;**61**:153, 157, 162.

Gifford RW Jr, Tarazi RC: Resistant hypertension: Diagnosis and management. *Ann Intern Med* 1978;**88**:661.

Gottlieb TB, Katz FH, Chidsey CA III: Combined therapy with vasodilator drugs and beta-adrenergic blockade in hypertension: A comparative study of minoxidil and hydralazine. *Circulation* 1972;**45**:571.

Gross F (editor): *Antihypertensive Therapy: Principles and Practice*. Springer, 1966.

Guazzi MD et al: Calcium-channel blockade with nifedipine and angiotensin converting–enzyme inhibition with captopril in the therapy of patients with severe primary hypertension. *Circulation* 1984;**70**:279.

Harington M, Kincaid-Smith P, McMichael J: Results of treatment in malignant hypertension. *Br Med J* 1959;**2**:969.

Helgeland A: Treatment of mild hypertension: A five year controlled drug trial: The Oslo Study. *Am J Med* 1980;**69**:725.

Heptinstall RH et al: Does captopril cause renal damage in hypertensive patients? Report from the Captopril Collaborative Study Group. *Lancet* 1982;**1**:988.

Hickler RB: Mild hypertension: Implications and management. *Primary Cardiol* (Sept) 1980;**6**:41.

Holland OB et al: Synergistic effect of captopril with hydrochlorothiazide for the treatment of low-renin hypertensive black patients. *Hypertension* 1983;**5**:235.

Hoorntje SJ et al: Immune-complex glomerulopathy in patients treated with captopril. *Lancet* 1980;**1**:1212.

Houston MC: Clonidine hydrochloride: Review of pharmacologic and clinical aspects. *Prog Cardiovasc Dis* 1981;**23**:337.

Hua ASP et al: Studies with prazosin: A new effective hypertensive agent. 2. Two double-blind cross-over studies comparing the effects of prazosin and hydralazine. *Med J Aust* 1977;**2**:5.

The Hypertension Detection and Follow-Up Program Cooperative Group: Five-year findings of the Hypertension Detection and Follow-Up Program: Prevention and reversal of left ventricular hypertrophy with antihypertensive drug therapy. *Hypertension* 1985;**7**:105.

The Hypertension Detection and Follow-Up Program Cooperative Group: Five-year findings of the Hypertension Detection and Follow-Up Program: 1. Reduction in mortality of persons with high blood pressure, including mild hypertension. 2. Mortality by race, sex and age. (2 parts.) *JAMA* 1979;**242**:2562, 2572.

The Hypertension Detection and Follow-Up Program Cooperative Group: Variability of blood pressure and the results of screening in the Hypertension Detection and Follow-Up Program. *J Chronic Dis* 1978;**31**:651.

Ibrahim MM, Mossallam R: Clinical evaluation of atenolol in hypertensive patients. *Circulation* 1981;**64**:368.

Ibrahim MM et al: Electrocardiogram in evaluation of resistance to antihypertensive therapy. *Arch Intern Med* 1977;**137**:1125.

Isaac L: Clonidine in the central nervous system: Site and mechanism of hypotensive action. *J Cardiovasc Pharmacol* 1980;**2(Suppl 1)**:S5.

Joint National Committee on Detection, Evaluation and Treatment of High Blood Pressure: The 1984 report of the Joint National Committee on detection, evaluation, and treatment of high blood pressure. *Arch Intern Med* 1984;**144**:1045.

Kannel WB: Role of blood pressure in cardiovascular morbidity and mortality. *Prog Cardiovasc Dis* 1974;**17**:5.

Kaplan NM: Beta blockers in the treatment of hypertension. (2 parts.) *Primary Cardiol* (July) 1980;**6**:16 and (Aug) 1980;**6**:19.

Kaplan NM (guest editor): The increasing clinical value of beta blockers: Focus on nadolol. (Symposium.) *Am Heart J* 1984;**108**:1069. [Entire issue.]

Kaplan NM, Lowenstein J (guest editors): Symposium on first-line therapy for hypertension: Changing directions. *Am J Cardiol* 1984;**53**:1A. [Entire issue.]

Kaplan NM et al: Potassium supplementation in hypertensive patients with diuretic-induced hypokalemia. *N Engl J Med* 1985;**312**:746.

Kempner W: Treatment of hypertensive vascular disease with rice diet. *Am J Med* 1948;**4**:545.

Kincaid-Smith P: Management of severe hypertension. *Am J Cardiol* 1973;**32**:575.

Kincaid-Smith P, Bullen M, Mills J: Prolonged use of methyldopa in severe hypertension in pregnancy. *Br Med J* 1966;**1**:274.

Koch-Weser J: Drug therapy: Diazoxide. *N Engl J Med* 1976;**294**:1271.

Koch-Weser J: Drug therapy: Metoprolol. *N Engl J Med* 1979;**301**:698.

Koch-Weser J: Hydralazine. *N Engl J Med* 1976;**295**:320.

Koshy MC et al: Physiologic evaluation of a new antihypertensive agent: Prazosin HCl. *Circulation* 1977;**55**:533.

Kosman ME: Management of potassium problems during long-term diuretic therapy. *JAMA* 1974;**230**:743.

Liebman J, Edelman IS: Interrelations of plasma potassium concentrations, plasma sodium, arterial pH, and total exchangeable potassium. *J Clin Invest* 1959;**38**:2176.

Linas SL, Nies AS: Minoxidil. *Ann Intern Med* 1981;**94**:61.

Logan AG et al: Work-site treatment of hypertension by specially trained nurses. *Lancet* 1979;**1**:1175.

Lowenstein J: Clonidine. *Ann Intern Med* 1980;**92**:74.

Lowenstein J, Steele JM: Prazosin: Mechanism of action and role in antihypertensive therapy. *Cardiovasc Med* 1979;**4**:885.

Lund-Johansen P: Comparative haemodynamic effects of labetalol, timolol, prazosin, and the combination of tolamolol and prazosin. *Br J Clin Pharmacol* 1979;**8(Suppl 2)**:107s.

Lund-Johansen P: Hemodynamic changes in long-term diuretic therapy of essential hypertension: A comparative study of chlorthalidone, polythiazide and hydrochlorothiazide. *Acta Med Scand* 1970;**187**:509.

Lund-Johansen P: Hemodynamic consequences of long-term beta-blocker therapy: A 5-year follow-up study of atenolol. *J Cardiovasc Pharmacol* 1979;**1**:487.

Lund-Johansen P, Bakke OM: Haemodynamic effects and plasma concentrations of labetalol during long-term treatment of essential hypertension. *Br J Clin Pharmacol* 1979;**7**:169.

Mancia G et al: Methyldopa and neural control of circulation in essential hypertension. *Am J Cardiol* 1980;**45**:1237.

Mancia G et al: Twenty-four-hour hemodynamic profile during treatment of essential hypertension by once-a-day nadolol. *Hypertension* 1983;**5**:573.

Marzuk PM: Health and Public Policy Committee, American College of Physicians: Biofeedback for hypertension. *Ann Intern Med* 1985;**102**:709.

McAreavey D et al: "Third drug" trial: Comparative study of antihypertensive agents added to treatment when blood pressure remains uncontrolled by a beta blocker plus thiazide diuretic. *Br Med J* 1984;**288**:106.

McDonald WJ et al: Intravenous diazoxide therapy in hypertensive crisis. *Am J Cardiol* 1977;**40**:409.

McLain LG: Therapy of acute severe hypertension in children. *JAMA* 1978;**239**:755.

McLeay RAB et al: The effect of nifedipine on arterial pressure and reflex cardiac control. *Circulation* 1983;**67**:1084.

McMahon FG: Efficacy of an antihypertensive agent: Comparison of methyldopa and hydrochlorothiazide in combination and singly. *JAMA* 1975;**231**:155.

Medical Research Council Working Party: MRC trial of treatment of mild hypertension: Principal results. *Br Med J* 1985;**291**:97.

Miller DC et al: Independent determinants of operative mortality for patients with aortic dissections. *Circulation* 1984;**70(Suppl 1)**:I-153.

Mitchell HC, Graham RM, Pettinger WA: Renal function during long-term treatment of hypertension with minoxidil: Comparison of benign and malignant hypertension. *Ann Intern Med* 1980;**93**:676.

Mitchell JR, Arias L, Oates JA: Antagonism of the antihypertensive action of guanethidine sulfate by desipramine hydrochloride. *JAMA* 1967;**202**:973.

Morgan TO: Diuretics: Basic clinical pharmacology and therapeutic use. *Drugs* 1978;**15**:151.

Morgan TO: Basic clinical pharmacology and therapeutic use. *Drugs* 1978;**15**:151.

Moyer JH et al: The effect of treatment on the vascular deterioration associated with hypertension, with particular emphasis on renal function. *Am J Med* 1958;**24**:177.

Mroczek WJ, Davidov ME: A randomized clinical trial of clonidine and propranolol in hypertensive patients receiving a diuretic and a vasodilator. *Curr Ther Res* 1978;**23**:294.

Mroczek WJ et al: The value of aggressive therapy in the hypertensive patient with azotemia. *Circulation* 1969;**40**:893.

Murphy MB, Dollery C (guest editors): Calcium antagonists in the treatment of hypertension. (Symposium.) *Hypertension* 1983;**5(Suppl 2)**:II-1. [Entire issue.]

Murphy MB et al: Glucose intolerance in hypertensive patients treated with diuretics: A fourteen-year follow-up. *Lancet* 1982;**2**:1293.

Myers MG, de Champlain J: Effects of atenolol and hydrochlorothiazide on blood pressure and plasma catecholamines in essential hypertension. *Hypertension* 1983;**5**:591.

Nattel S, Rangno RE, Van Loon G: Mechanism of propranolol withdrawal phenomena. *Circulation* 1979;**59**:1158.

Nies AS: Adverse reaction and interactions limiting the use of antihypertensive drugs. *Am J Med* 1975;**58**:495.

Ochs HR et al: Spironolactone. *Am Heart J* 1978;**96**:389.

O'Malley K, O'Brien E: Management of hypertension in the elderly. *N Engl J Med* 1980;**302**:1397.

Opie LH, Jee L, White D: Antihypertensive effects of nifedipine combined with cardioselective beta-adrenergic receptor antagonism by atenolol. *Am Heart J* 1982;**104**:606.

Patel DJ et al: A control procedure for studies of blood pressure feedback in hypertension. *Cardiovasc Med* 1978;**3**:627.

Perloff D: Hypertensive emergencies. Chap 9, pp 181–201, in: *Cardiac Emergencies*. Scheinmann MM (editor). Saunders, 1984.

Perloff D, Sokolow M, Cowan R: The prognostic value of ambulatory blood pressures. *JAMA* 1983;**249**:2792.

Perry HM Jr: The management of malignant hypertension. *Drug Ther* (Oct) 1971;**1**:33.

Perry HM Jr et al: Studies on the control of hypertension. 8. Mortality, morbidity, and remission during 12 years of intensive therapy. *Circulation* 1966;**33**:958.

Pettinger WA: Minoxidil and the treatment of severe hypertension. *N Engl J Med* 1980;**303**:922.

Pettinger WA, Mitchell HC, Güllner H-G: Clonidine and the vasodilating beta blocker antihypertensive drug interaction. *Clin Pharmacol Ther* 1977;**22**:164.

Pickering G: Reversibility of malignant hypertension. *Lancet* 1971;**1**:413.

Pickering TG et al: What is the role of ambulatory blood pressure monitoring in the management of hypertensive patients? *Hypertension* 1985;**7**:171.

Pollack AA et al: Limitations of transcendental meditation in the treatment of essential hypertension. *Lancet* 1977;**1**:71.

Prichard BNC: β-Adrenergic receptor blockade in hypertension: Past, present, and future. *Br J Clin Pharmacol* 1978;**5**:379.

Ram CVS, Kaplan NM: Individual titration of diazoxide dosage in the treatment of severe hypertension. *Am J Cardiol* 1979;**43**:627.

Reichgott MJ: Problems of sexual function in patients with hypertension. *Cardiovasc Med* 1979;**4**:149.

Reid JL, Dean CR, Jones DH: Central actions of antihypertensive drugs. *Cardiovasc Med* 1977;**2**:1185.

Reisin E et al: Effect of weight loss without salt restriction on the reduction of blood pressure in overweight hypertensive patients. *N Engl J Med* 1978;**298**:1.

Richards AM et al: Renal, haemodynamic, and hormonal effects of human alpha atrial natriuretic peptides in healthy volunteers. *Lancet* 1985;**1**:545.

Rose LI et al: Pathophysiology of spironolactone-induced gynecomastia. *Ann Intern Med* 1977;**87**:398.

Rowlands DB et al: Assessment of left-ventricular mass and its response to antihypertensive treatment. *Lancet* 1982;**1**:467.

Sackett DL et al: Randomised clinical trial of strategies for improving medication compliance in primary hypertension. *Lancet* 1975;**1**:1205.

Samuelsson O et al: Predictors of cardiovascular morbidity in treated hypertension: Results from the primary preventive trial in Göteborg, Sweden. *J Hypertension* 1985;**3**:167.

Sassano P et al: Antihypertensive effect of enalapril as first-step treatment of mild and moderate uncomplicated essential hypertension: Evaluation by two methods of blood pressure measurement. *Am J Med* 1984;**77(Suppl 2A)**:18.

Schalekamp MADH et al: Hemodynamic effects of captopril in essential and renovascular hypertension: Correlations with plasma renin. *Cardiovasc Rev Rep* 1982;**3**:651.

Schirger A, Sheps SG: Prazosin: New hypertensive agent: A double-blind crossover study in the treatment of hypertension. *JAMA* 1977;**237**:989.

Schwartz AB, Swartz CD: Dosage of potassium chloride elixir to correct thiazide-induced hypokalemia. *JAMA* 1974;**230**:702.

Shapiro AP: Behavior modification: Can it control hypertension? *J Cardiovasc Med* 1980;**5**:1075.

Shea S et al: Treatment of hypertension and its effect on cardiovascular risk factors: Data from the Framingham Heart Study. *Circulation* 1985;**71**:22.

Singh BN, Ellrodt G, Peter CT: Verapamil: A review of its pharmacologic properties and therapeutic use. *Drugs* 1978;**15**:169.

Smirk FH, Veale AMO, Alstad K: Basal and supplemental blood pressures in relationship to life expectancy and hypertension symptomatology. *NZ Med J* 1959;**58**:711.

Smith WM: Treatment of mild hypertension: Results of a 10-year intervention trial. *Circ Res* 1977;**40(5-Suppl 1)**:I-98.

Smith WM et al: Cooperative clinical trial of alpha-methyldopa III: Double-blind control comparison of alpha-methyldopa and chlorothiazide and chlorothiazide and rauwolfia. *Ann Intern Med* 1966;**65**:657.

Sokolow M, Perloff D: The choice of drugs and the management of essential hypertension. *Prog Cardiovasc Dis* 1965;**8**:253.

Sokolow M, Perloff D: The prognosis of essential hypertension treated conservatively. *Circulation* 1961;**23**:697.

Sokolow M, Schottstaedt MF: The management of malignant hypertension. *Ann Intern Med* 1953;**38**:647.

Steptoe A: Psychological methods in treatment of hypertension: A review. *Br Heart J* 1977;**39**:587.

Stokes GS, Oates HF: Prazosin: New alpha-adrenergic blocking agent in treatment of hypertension. *Cardiovasc Med* 1978;**3**:41.

Stokes GS, Oates HF, MacCarthy EP: Antihypertensive therapy: New pharmacological approaches. *Am Heart J* 1980;**100**:741.

Strandberg I et al: Acetylator phenotype in patients with hydralazine-induced lupoid syndrome. *Acta Med Scand* 1976;**200**:367.

Swartz SL et al: Converting enzyme inhibition in essential hypertension: The hypotensive response does not reflect only reduced angiotensin II formation. *Hypertension* 1979;**1**:106.

Taguchi J, Freis ED: Partial reduction of blood pressure and prevention of complications in hypertension. *N Engl J Med* 1974;**291**:239.

Tarazi RC: Long-term effective antihypertensive therapy. *Ann Intern Med* 1980;**93**:772.

Tarazi RC (editor): Symposium on the heart in hypertension. *Am J Cardiol* 1979;**44**:845.

Textor SC et al: Hyperkalemia in azotemic patients during

angiotensin-converting enzyme inhibition and aldosterone reduction with captopril. *Am J Med* 1982;**73:**719.

Tinker JH, Michenfelder JD: Sodium nitroprusside: Pharmacology, toxicology, and therapeutics. *Anesthesiology* 1976;**45:**340.

Tuomilehto J et al: Community programme for control of hypertension in North Karelia, Finland. *Lancet* 1980;**2:**900.

VanZwieten PA: The central action of antihypertensive drugs, mediated via central α-receptors. *J Pharm Pharmacol* 1973;**25:**89.

Venkata C, Ram S, Engelman K: Abrupt discontinuation of clonidine therapy. *JAMA* 1979;**242:**2104.

Vesey CJ, Cole PV, Simpson PJ: Cyanide and thiocyanate concentrations following sodium nitroprusside infusion in man. *Br J Anaesth* 1976;**48:**651.

Veterans Administration Cooperative Study Group on Antihypertensive Agents: Comparison of prazosin with hydralazine in patients receiving hydrochlorothiazide: A randomized, double-blind clinical trial. *Circulation* 1981;**64:**772.

Veterans Administration Cooperative Study Group on Antihypertensive Agents: Comparison of propranolol and hydrochlorothiazide for the initial treatment of hypertension. 1. Results of short-term titration with emphasis on racial differences in response. 2. Results of long-term therapy. *JAMA* 1982;**248:**1996, 2004.

Veterans Administration Cooperative Study Group on Antihypertensive Agents: Effects of treatment on morbidity in hypertension: Effect on the electrocardiogram. *Circulation* 1973;**48:**481.

Veterans Administration Cooperative Study Group on Antihypertensive Agents: Effects of treatment on morbidity in hypertension. 1. Results in patients with diastolic blood pressures averaging 115 through 129 mm Hg. *JAMA* 1967;**202:**1028.

Veterans Administration Cooperative Study Group on Antihypertensive Agents: Effects of treatment on morbidity in hypertension. 2. Results in patients with diastolic blood pressures averaging 90 through 114 mm Hg. *JAMA* 1970;**213:**1143.

Veterans Administration Cooperative Study Group on Antihypertensive Agents: Effects of treatment on morbidity in hypertension. 3. Influence of age, diastolic pressure, and prior cardiovascular disease; further analysis of side-effects. *Circulation* 1972;**45:**991.

Veterans Administration Cooperative Study Group on Antihypertensive Agents: Multiclinic controlled trial of bethanidine and guanethidine in severe hypertension. *Circulation* 1977;**55:**519.

Veterans Administration Cooperative Study Group on Antihypertensive Agents: Propranolol in the treatment of essential hypertension. *JAMA* 1977;**237:**2303.

Veterans Administration Cooperative Study Group on Antihypertensive Agents: Return of elevated blood pressure after withdrawal of antihypertensive drugs. *Circulation* 1975;**51:**1107.

Veterans Administration Medical Centers: Low doses *v* standard dose of reserpine. *JAMA* 1982;**248:**2471.

Walker JM, Beevers DG: Mild hypertension: To treat or not to treat? *Drugs* 1979;**18:**312.

Whitsett TL et al: Abrupt cessation of clonidine administration: A prospective study. *Am J Cardiol* 1978;**41:**1285.

Wilburn RL, Blaufuss A, Bennett CM: Long-term treatment of severe hypertension with minoxidil, propranolol and furosemide. *Circulation* 1975;**52:**706.

Wilkinson PR: Potassium changes during diuretic therapy. *Cardiovasc Med* 1978;**3:**181.

Wilson GM: Diuretics. *Practitioner* 1968;**200:**39.

Woods JW, Blythe WB, Huffines WD: Management of malignant hypertension complicated by renal insufficiency. *N Engl J Med* 1974;**291:**10.

Woosley RL, Nies AS: Guanethidine. *N Engl J Med* 1976;**295:**1053.

Woosley RL et al: Effect of acetylator phenotype on the rate at which procainamide induces antinuclear antibodies and the lupus syndrome. *N Engl J Med* 1978;**298:**1157.

Zacest R, Gilmore E, Koch-Weser J: Treatment of essential hypertension with combined vasodilatation and beta-adrenergic blockade. *N Engl J Med* 1972;**286:**617.

Cardiac Failure 10

DEFINITIONS

Cardiac failure can be broadly defined as a state in which the heart fails to meet the varying oxygen and metabolic needs of the body under differing circumstances, or a state in which cardiac output (the ability of the heart to pump blood) is reduced relative to the metabolic demands of the body, assuming the existence of adequate venous return. The definition is arbitrary and controversial, because the phenomena of heart failure are complex and incompletely understood.

Cardiac failure may be present in the resting state or may appear only with excessive stress. It is easily recognized in its later stages, when symptoms and signs due to pulmonary or systemic venous congestion, increased ventricular volume and diastolic pressure, and decreased cardiac output are present.

In patients with heart disease, transient cardiac failure may be induced by any of the acute precipitating events (arrhythmias, respiratory infection, etc) listed below. When the precipitating event subsides with time or is cured by appropriate treatment, the patient's cardiac status may return to its previous asymptomatic state.

It should be obvious that the diagnosis of cardiac failure, like that of any other disease, depends upon its definition, which varies with different authorities. The distinction must be maintained between the presence of heart disease and the presence of cardiac failure, and the latter should be perceived as a continuum from (1) recognition of the presence of cardiac disease, to (2) a preclinical phase in which hemodynamic abnormalities but not symptoms may be present, and finally to (3) an overt clinical phase in which it is obvious to all that cardiac failure is present.

The heart fails ("decompensates") when various compensatory mechanisms are excessive (salt and water retention and increased systemic vascular resistance) or when cardiac hypertrophy, raised atrial pressure, ventricular dilatation, and increased force of contraction (see below) are inadequate to maintain the function of a diseased heart whose work load has been increased.

Initially, either the left or, less commonly, the right ventricle may fail; ultimately, however, especially after salt and water retention occurs, combined left and right failure is the rule (congestive failure).

CAUSES OF HEART FAILURE

The causes of ventricular failure can be summarized as follows:
(1) Intrinsic myocardial disease: Coronary heart disease, cardiomyopathy, infiltrative diseases such as hemochromatosis, amyloidosis, sarcoidosis, and myocarditis.
(2) Excess work load:
 (a) Increased resistance to ejection (pressure load): Hypertension, stenosis of aortic or pulmonary valves, hypertrophic cardiomyopathy.
 (b) Increased stroke volume (volume load): Aortic insufficiency, mitral insufficiency, tricuspid insufficiency, congenital left-to-right shunts.
 (c) Increased body demands ("high-output failure"): Thyrotoxicosis, anemia, pregnancy, arteriovenous fistula.
(3) Iatrogenic myocardial damage:
 (a) Drugs such as doxorubicin (Adriamycin) or disopyramide.
 (b) Radiation therapy for mediastinal tumors or Hodgkin's disease.

Factors precipitating failure. In at least half of cases, demonstrable precipitating disease or factors that increase the work load of the heart are present, and these factors should be sought in every patient with cardiac failure. They include arrhythmias, respiratory infection, myocardial infarction, pulmonary embolism, rheumatic carditis, thyrotoxicosis, anemia, excessive salt intake, corticosteroid administration, pregnancy, and excessive or rapid administration of parenteral fluids. Fever may aggravate failure (as in acute myocardial infarction) but does not cause it de novo.

Heart failure may occur in patients with normally functioning hearts that are subjected to excessive loads. The clearest example of this is systemic arteriovenous fistula. Even in otherwise healthy young people, a large fistula can produce heart failure; in older people, thyrotoxicosis, severe anemia, beriberi, or Paget's disease of bone may cause heart failure even though cardiac output is high.

HEMODYNAMIC & PATHOPHYSIOLOGIC FEATURES OF HEART FAILURE

Compensatory Mechanisms

The compensatory mechanisms by which the heart responds to an increased load include the following:
(1) concentric hypertrophy (hypertrophy without di-

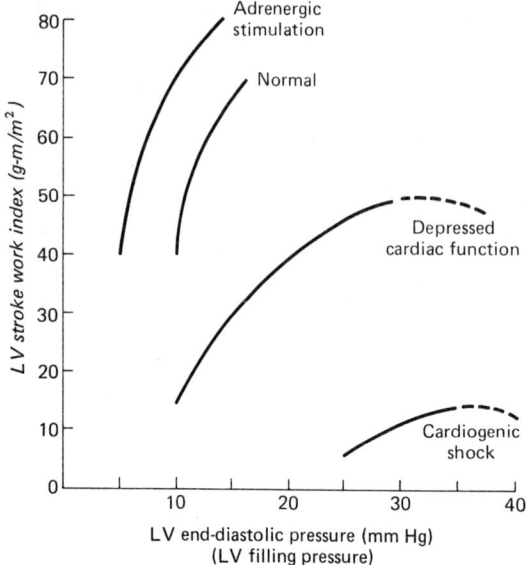

Figure 10–1. Family of Frank-Starling curves showing relation of force of contraction (left ventricular stroke work index) to fiber length or pressure (left ventricular end-diastolic pressure or filling pressure). (Modified and reproduced, with permission, from Swan HJC, Parmley WW: Congestive heart failure. Chapter 10 in: *Pathologic Physiology: Mechanisms of Disease*, 5th ed. Sodeman WA Jr, Sodeman WA [editors]. Saunders, 1974.)

latation), which provides larger contractile cells; (2) increased fiber length or dilatation, which increases the force of contraction, as shown by the Frank-Starling law (Fig 10–1); and (3) increased sympathetic nervous system activity, by which the force of contraction is increased at any fiber length without increasing the filling pressure, the renin-angiotensin-aldosterone system is stimulated, and the systemic vascular resistance is raised.

A. Hypertrophy and Compliance: Concentric hypertrophy is most apt to occur when the load placed on the heart is due to increased resistance to ejection with increased impedance, characteristically seen in aortic stenosis and hypertension. Early in the course of the disease, the only cardiac abnormality that can be identified is left ventricular hypertrophy, recognized both clinically and by echocardiography and electrocardiography (Fig 10–2). The increased thickness causes a decrease in the distensibility, or compliance, of the left ventricle, so that diastolic filling is slowed and the left ventricular end-diastolic pressure is raised, with a normal left ventricular volume; the raised filling pressure is required to augment left ventricular output in accordance with the Frank-Starling principle. The raised left ventricular end-diastolic pressure does not necessarily imply ventricular failure but occurs whenever compliance is decreased, as in the cardiac states noted above or in hypertrophic or infiltrative cardiomyopathy. It also occurs early in acute myocardial infarction, when the infarcted area becomes stiff and less distensible. Later—eg, in patients with hypertension or aortic stenosis—when left ventricular volume increases (because cardiac hypertrophy and more forceful contraction alone are insufficient to compensate), the left ventricular end-diastolic pressure rises even further, and left ventricular failure occurs.

B. Increased Stroke Volume and Failure: When the increased cardiac load is due to increased stroke volume, typically represented by aortic insufficiency, the increased stretch increases fiber length and so increases the force of left ventricular contraction as demonstrated by the Frank-Starling principle. As the stretch increases, left ventricular volume increases, as can be demonstrated by enlargement of the heart on the plain film of the chest or the echocardiogram or by left ventricular angiography. In these circumstances, distensibility is not decreased, and it is common to find an increased left ventricular volume with normal left ventricular end-diastolic pressure and normal or increased cardiac output. When left ventricular performance declines in the later stages of this type of lesion (as well as in so-called congestive cardiomyopathy), the ejection fraction falls from its normal value of 60–70% and may be as low as 10–20% in very severe failure. The ejection fraction is best determined by left ventricular angiography, although echocardiography provides an estimate. In general, patients tolerate increased volume load better than increased resistance load even though left ventricular wall tension and myocardial oxygen consumption increase when the heart is dilated and enlarged (law of Laplace). (See p 20 and Fig 1–27 for definition and details.)

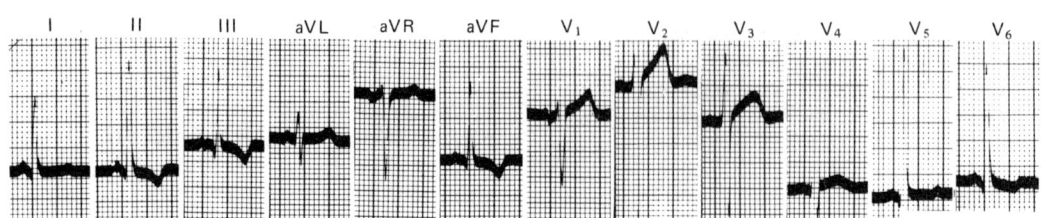

Figure 10–2. An example of moderate left ventricular hypertrophy in a vertically placed heart in a 28-year-old man with coarctation of the aorta. Note the tall R and diphasic to inverted T waves in leads V_6, II, III, and aVF.

C. Increased Sympathetic Stimulation: Increased sympathetic stimulation can be demonstrated in patients with cardiac failure by increased levels of catecholamines in blood and urine and by depletion of norepinephrine in cardiac tissue, notably atrial appendages removed at operation. Several investigators have demonstrated the importance of the sympathetic nervous system in improving cardiac contractility in cardiac failure and have noted its exhaustion in failure (Fig 10–1). Beta-adrenergic blocking agents, by decreasing the sympathetic drive to the heart, may worsen or precipitate ventricular failure. Raised systemic vascular resistance that results from compensatory increased sympathetic stimulation may be excessive; the enhanced afterload is the basis for using vasodilators in therapy (see p 314).

Hemodynamic Indices

The derived indices used in this chapter are discussed in Chapter 4.

Pathophysiology of Decompensation

Early in the course of various cardiac diseases, the compensatory mechanisms are adequate to maintain a normal cardiac output and normal intracardiac pressures at rest and after exercise. Hypertrophy may be recognized on the ECG, echocardiogram, or plain chest film. Compensated heart disease becomes "decompensated" as ventricular volume and filling pressures of the respective ventricles increase, although a raised filling pressure may be due to decreased compliance rather than to ventricular failure early in the course of the disease. As the filling pressure increases, pulmonary venous congestion occurs as the raised left atrial pressure is transmitted backward. This leads to interstitial and then alveolar edema of the lungs, resulting in symptoms of left ventricular failure, with dyspnea, exertional cough, orthopnea, paroxysmal nocturnal dyspnea, and pulmonary edema when the disease involves the left ventricle. Raised venous pressure, hepatomegaly, dependent edema, and ascites occur when failure involves the right ventricle (congestive or right ventricular failure). Cardiac output may be normal at this phase, especially at rest, but may be decreased on exercise; as the cardiac output on exercise diminishes, tachycardia occurs and thus increases the minute cardiac output when the stroke volume cannot increase adequately. The arteriovenous oxygen difference widens as blood flow to nonessential vascular systems decreases. When the ventricular filling pressure is increased—especially when ventricular compliance is decreased—atrial hypertrophy increases the force of atrial systole and thereby aids filling; loss of this so-called "atrial kick" can decrease the cardiac output when atrial fibrillation occurs.

High-Output Failure
(See also p 294.)

Although cardiac failure is usually associated with low cardiac output, especially with exercise, it may occur when output is greater than normal, because the heart cannot maintain the high output necessitated by the underlying cause. Tissue demands for oxygen may require increased cardiac output; this may occur in severe anemia, acute beriberi, thyrotoxicosis, Paget's disease, and large arteriovenous fistula or during extreme exertion in hot, humid climates. Systemic vascular resistance is decreased in these conditions, although the high output in thyrotoxicosis is probably due also to a combination of the effects of thyroxin and catecholamines on the heart. Greatly decreased systemic vascular resistance causes large amounts of blood to pass from the arteries to the veins, increasing the venous return and hence the cardiac output. Vasodilatation initially decreases arterial blood volume and causes the kidney to activate the renin-angiotensin system; this results in renin release and increased aldosterone production, causing salt and water retention and blood volume expansion. Pulmonary and systemic venous congestion follows, resulting in the clinical syndrome of heart failure. Management of the condition is that of the underlying cause (eg, arteriovenous fistula) (see also pp 294–295).

The hemodynamic effects of high-output states vary considerably with the underlying state of the myocardium. Thus, a relatively minor "high-output" factor such as anemia may be of much greater importance in an older patient with degenerative heart disease than in a younger person. In addition, the "high-output" load may increase the demand of oxygen by the myocardium relative to supply and cause anginal pain rather than heart failure.

PATHOPHYSIOLOGIC MECHANISMS OF SALT & WATER RETENTION

Increased sodium and water retention secondary to aldosterone production (see Fig 9–4) leads to an increase in blood volume, which, by raising the hydrostatic pressure in the capillaries, leads first to interstitial edema and then to transudation of fluid into tissues that have decreased tissue pressure, such as the subcutaneous tissues. As a result, edema of the ankles and lower extremities occurs when the patient is ambulatory and edema of the sacrum when the patient is recumbent. Symptoms such as dyspnea and edema are aggravated by salt and water retention and are reversed by the use of diuretics and low-sodium diets.

If sodium is restricted, moderate water intake does not add to sodium retention, as it does with free sodium intake. Water intake need not be restricted if sodium intake is (Fig 10–3), unless dilutional hyponatremia is present.

CLINICAL FINDINGS

When a patient with any type of heart disease—congenital, valvular, hypertensive, coronary, meta-

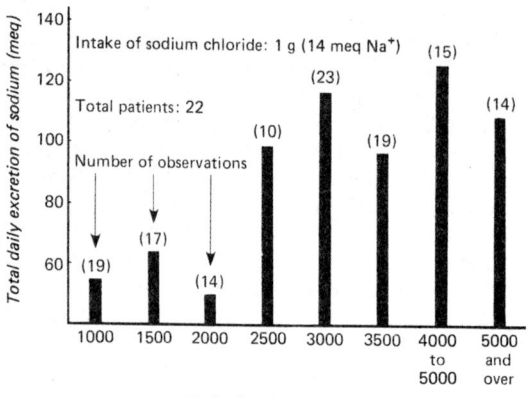

Figure 10-3. When sodium intake is low (approximately 14 meq), the total daily excretion increases when daily fluid intake increases. (Reproduced, with permission, from Gorham LW et al: The relative importance of dietary sodium chloride and water intake in cardiac edema. *Ann Intern Med* 1947;27:575.)

Table 10-1. Criteria for diagnosis of congestive heart failure (left and right).*†

Major criteria
   Paroxysmal nocturnal dyspnea or orthopnea
   Dyspnea and cough on exertion
   Neck vein distention
   Rales
   Cardiomegaly
   Acute pulmonary edema
   S_3 gallop
   Increased venous pressure > 16 cm water
   Hydrothorax
Minor criteria
   Ankle edema
   Night cough
   Hepatomegaly
   Pleural effusion
   Vital capacity reduced by one-third from maximum
   Tachycardia (rate of ≥ 120/min)
Major or minor criterion
   Weight loss ≥ 4.5 kg in 5 days in response to treatment

*Adapted and reproduced, with permission, from McKee PA et al: The natural history of congestive heart failure: The Framingham Study. *N Engl J Med* 1971;285:1441.
†For establishing a definite diagnosis of congestive heart failure, 2 major or one major and 2 minor criteria must be present concurrently.

bolic, etc—develops symptoms and signs of cardiac failure, the findings are usually not specific for any particular etiologic category. Symptoms and signs of pulmonary or systemic venous congestion, increased cardiac volume, and diastolic pressure combined with decreased cardiac output, raised venous pressure, and evidences of salt and water retention clearly indicate that cardiac failure has occurred. In patients with congenital heart disease, pulmonary heart disease, endocarditis involving the valves on the right side, right ventricular infarction, primary pulmonary hypertension, or obstructive diseases of the lungs, raised venous pressure, enlarged tender liver, and systemic edema indicate that cardiac disease has progressed to right-sided congestive failure. This is also true when pulmonary hypertension complicates mitral stenosis, and right heart failure and tricuspid regurgitation follow. Right heart failure is the rule in congenital heart disease, although there are a variety of congenital lesions such as patent ductus arteriosus, coarctation of the aorta, ventricular septal defect, and tricuspid atresia in which the excess load is on the left ventricle, which may ultimately fail. These conditions are all discussed in greater detail elsewhere in this book.

The criteria for diagnosis of congestive heart failure are listed in Table 10-1.

Left Ventricular Failure

Left ventricular failure is most commonly due to coronary heart disease, dilated cardiomyopathy, hypertension, or valvular heart disease, usually aortic valvular disease. Less common causes are mitral valve disease, hypertrophic cardiomyopathy, left-to-right shunts, and congenital heart lesions. Idiopathic infective endocarditis or that occurring as a complication of valvular disease may lead to left ventricular failure. Cardiac failure may also occur in various connective tissue disorders, thyrotoxicosis, severe anemia, arteriovenous fistula, myocarditis, beriberi, and myocardial involvement by tumors or granulomas.

Left ventricular failure may occur acutely with fluid overload, as may happen with too rapid infusion of large amounts of blood or saline in patients with minimal evidence of left ventricular failure prior to infusion. Ventricular or atrial arrhythmias associated with a rapid ventricular rate, severe anemia, acute leukemia, or abrupt slowing of the ventricular rate, as in atrioventricular block, may abruptly result in left ventricular failure. Drugs such as beta-adrenergic blockers, disopyramide, and verapamil, especially in combination, have a negative inotropic effect and may cause left ventricular failure by removing sympathetic drive to the heart. These drugs should be used with caution in patients with incipient left ventricular failure.

A. Symptoms:

1. Dyspnea—Both by reflex action and by increased work of breathing, the increased fluid in the tissue spaces causes dyspnea, at first on effort and then at rest. The work of breathing is greater because of the increased stiffness of the lungs, and the patient is aware of difficulty in breathing. Transudation of fluid into the alveoli superimposes cough on dyspnea of effort, and this combination is suggestive of left ventricular failure. The symptoms are usually progressive, and the earliest manifestation is shortness of breath on exertion that previously caused no difficulty. As pulmonary engorgement progresses, less and less activity brings on dyspnea and cough, until both are present even when the patient is at rest.

2. Orthopnea–Shortness of breath in recumbency that is promptly relieved by propping up the head or trunk is precipitated by the increase in pulmonary engorgement that occurs in the recumbent position. When the pulmonary blood volume is thus increased, the patient characteristically goes to sleep without difficulty but awakens several hours later with dyspnea (paroxysmal nocturnal dyspnea). The mechanism is believed to be increased pulmonary blood volume associated with recumbency and the "autotransfusion" of fluid accumulated in the lower half of the body during upright posture.

3. Paroxysmal nocturnal dyspnea–Paroxysmal nocturnal dyspnea with cough usually develops in a setting of progressive dyspnea on exertion and orthopnea, but it may appear at any time and may be the first manifestation of left ventricular failure in severe hypertension, aortic stenosis or insufficiency, or myocardial infarction. It also occurs in patients with tight mitral stenosis, but in this condition it is due to pulmonary venous congestion from obstruction at the mitral valve rather than left ventricular failure. Paroxysmal nocturnal dyspnea or cough may be associated with inspiratory and expiratory wheezing due to bronchospasm (so-called cardiac asthma). Depending upon the amount of fluid that accumulates in the lungs, the patient with paroxysmal nocturnal dyspnea may awaken with dyspnea that lasts only a few minutes and is relieved by sitting or standing, or the dyspnea may progress rapidly into an alarming episode of pulmonary edema.

4. Acute pulmonary edema–Acute pulmonary edema resulting from gross transudation of fluid into the alveoli due to the rapidly rising pulmonary capillary pressure causes the patient to sit up in bed gasping for breath; the patient is also cold, pale, anxious, and sweating profusely. The patient may become cyanotic, cough up frothy white or pink sputum, and be fearful of imminent death. Patients may ignore progressive dyspnea on exertion, but they rarely ignore acute pulmonary edema. Most attacks subside gradually in 1–3 hours, possibly because of the upright position as well as the progressive decrease in cardiac output. In some instances, the left ventricle rapidly weakens, leading to shock and death. Left atrial pressure has been shown to rise to 50 or 60 mm Hg during episodes of pulmonary edema.

Heroin administration is one of the common causes of pulmonary edema; the mechanism of action is presumably increased capillary permeability. This results in arterial hypoxemia and acidosis, which can be quite marked. The arterial P_{O_2} is usually less than 40 mm Hg in the presence of pulmonary edema, and the pH hovers around 7.15.

5. Interpretation of dyspnea–When dyspnea on exertion is the only symptom, its interpretation is often difficult, especially when the patient is obese and in poor physical condition (see Chapter 2).

a. Patients in poor physical condition almost never have orthopnea or paroxysmal nocturnal dyspnea, and the dyspnea is rarely progressive over a short period of time as it is when left ventricular failure develops in aortic stenosis or coronary disease.

b. Pulmonary causes of dyspnea such as chronic bronchitis, pulmonary fibrosis, and asthmatic bronchitis are more difficult to differentiate because the wheezing of left ventricular failure due to bronchospasm may simulate that of asthma. However, the patient with chronic lung disease usually gives a history of smoking, long-standing cough, or sputum production and frequent episodes of purulent bronchitis in winter. Cough is often present in the absence of dyspnea.

c. Moderate to severe anemia may also produce exertional dyspnea.

d. Advanced age, debility, extreme obesity, ascites due to any cause, abdominal distention due to gastrointestinal disease, or advanced stages of pregnancy may produce orthopnea in the absence of heart disease.

e. Neurocirculatory asthenia–(See p 613.) Patients with neurocirculatory asthenia or anxiety states with psychophysiologic cardiovascular reactions may suffer from sighing respirations simulating dyspnea.

6. Fatigue–Exertional fatigue and weakness due to reduced cardiac output are late symptoms and disappear promptly with rest. Severe fatigue rather than dyspnea is the chief complaint of patients with mitral stenosis who have developed pulmonary hypertension and low cardiac output.

7. Nocturia as a symptom of edema–Nocturia may represent excretion of edema fluid accumulated during the day and increased renal perfusion in the recumbent position; it reflects the decreased work of the heart at rest and often the effects of diuretics given during the day. It may also be due to noncardiac causes.

B. Signs: Evidence of the primary disease responsible for the failure, eg, hypertension or aortic stenosis, is almost always present. In some instances of severe failure due to aortic stenosis, the murmur may be absent or difficult to hear because of the decreased velocity of ejection and reduced cardiac output.

Evidence of so-called primary disease is at times misleading. For example, because of the compensatory systemic vasoconstriction that occurs in any condition with reduced cardiac output via the baroreceptor mechanism, blood pressure may be modestly raised in patients with cardiac failure due to any cause; one should therefore be cautious in defining the disease as hypertensive heart failure unless the blood pressure remains elevated after the failure is relieved by treatment.

1. Enlargement of heart–In the presence of symptoms of cardiac failure, hypertrophy or dilatation of the left ventricle is usually found on examination and confirmed by evidence of left ventricular hypertrophy on the ECG and left ventricular enlargement on the x-ray or echocardiogram.

2. Ventricular heave–The best clinical sign of left ventricular hypertrophy is a left ventricular heave at the apex of the heart. The heave is a localized, sustained, systolic outward motion of the left ventricular impulse that differs from the hyperdynamic left ventricular impulse of exertion, anxiety, or regurgitant valve disease and from the right ventricular heave of right ventricular hypertrophy. The latter is more diffuse, is felt over the center of the chest, and causes apical retraction rather than a lift during systole.

3. Third heart sound–(See Chapter 3.) When there is increased left ventricular volume, an exaggerated third heart sound is often heard as ventricular filling occurs during the rapid inflow phase.

4. Fourth heart sound–Decreased compliance of the left ventricle with resultant hypertrophy of the left atrium causes a fourth heart sound or atrial gallop that may be felt or seen and is also manifested by a large *a* wave in the jugular venous pulse or in the apexcardiogram.

5. Rales–Rales in the lungs may be absent at rest and even early in the episode of nocturnal dyspnea, when transudation occurs into the tissue spaces and not into the alveoli. Later, however, when alveolar fluid appears, the rales are loud and generalized; frothy, bubbling fluid may be obvious all over the lungs. Pleural effusion may occur (see p 294).

6. Cheyne-Stokes respiration–Cheyne-Stokes respiration is commonly seen in advanced cardiac failure (see Chapter 3).

7. Tachycardia–As the stroke volume decreases, tachycardia compensates to increase the minute cardiac output; it is usually present in cardiac failure.

8. Pulsus alternans–(See Chapter 3.)

C. Electrocardiographic and Chest X-Ray Findings: The ECG is usually more sensitive than the chest x-ray but less sensitive than 2-dimensional echocardiograms in demonstrating chamber hypertrophy, but the ECG may be normal or minimally abnormal when the chest x-ray shows concentric left ventricular hypertrophy and dilatation of the proximal aorta in aortic stenosis. When dilatation predominates over hypertrophy, the chest x-ray may show enlargement, whereas the ECG may show little or no abnormality. The ECG also may be confusing, with nonspecific manifestations of associated effects of treatment with digitalis or diuretics (hypokalemia) or with superimposed coronary disease. An apparent discrepancy in the specific chamber that is hypertrophied or enlarged on the chest x-ray as compared to the ECG usually means that both chambers are involved, although the ECG is less likely to give an erroneous picture when the abnormality is clear-cut.

D. Echocardiographic Findings: Echocardiography is both sensitive and specific for an increased left ventricular mass. A valuable sign of severe left ventricular failure is a wide E point separation between excursion of the anterior mitral valve leaflet and the ventricular septum (Massie, 1977). Fig 10–4 illustrates the normal case, in which there is no separation at all.

Right Ventricular Failure

Right ventricular failure is usually secondary to chronic left ventricular failure but may occur alone. The most common causes of right ventricular failure are tight mitral stenosis with pulmonary hypertension, pulmonary valve stenosis, cor pulmonale due to chronic lung disease, primary pulmonary hypertension with tricuspid insufficiency, right ventricular infarction, and other congenital diseases such as Eisenmenger's complex, and pulmonary hypertensive ventricular or atrial septal defects. Tricuspid valve disease may produce the same systemic venous congestion, but like mitral stenosis, the congestion is due to obstruction at the tricuspid valve and not to right ventricular failure unless there is an associated obstruction higher up, such as mitral stenosis. Rare causes are involvement of the pulmonary and tricuspid valves by carcinoid or infective endocarditis.

A. Symptoms: The dominant symptoms of right ventricular failure are those of systemic venous

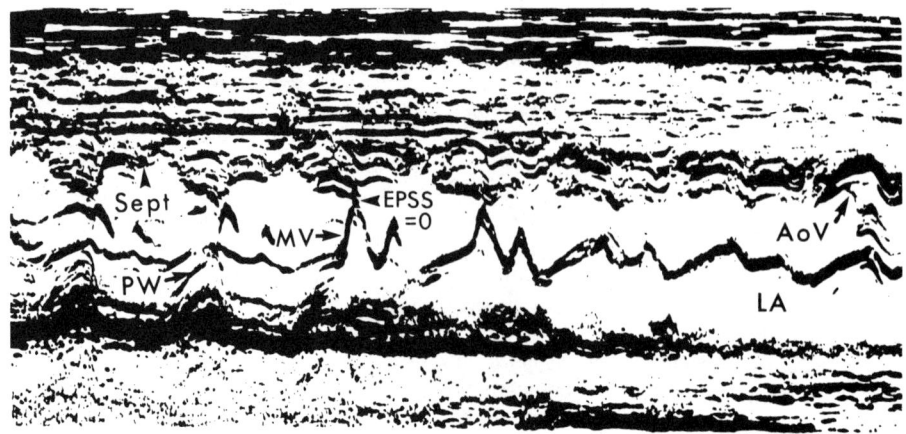

Figure 10–4. Normal echocardiogram showing E point separation (EPSS) = 0. Sept, septum; PW, posterior wall; MV, mitral valve; AoV, aortic valve; LA, left atrium. (Reproduced, with permission, from Massie BM et al: Mitral-septal separation: A new echocardiographic index of left ventricular function. *Am J Cardiol* 1977;**39**:1008.)

congestion—in contrast to left ventricular failure, in which symptoms of pulmonary venous congestion predominate. Pulmonary symptoms are rare unless there is associated left ventricular failure or unless right ventricular failure is due to chronic lung disease. Paroxysmal nocturnal dyspnea is uncommon.

1. Fatigue–The patient may complain of fatigue as cardiac output is reduced.

2. Dependent edema–Edema of the ankles may occur when the patient is up and about; edema of the sacrum, flanks, and thighs when in bed.

3. Liver engorgement–If right ventricular failure occurs rapidly, as when atrial fibrillation develops in tight mitral stenosis, congestion of the liver with distention of its capsule may result, causing right upper quadrant pain which has often been confused with that of cholecystitis or other abdominal disease.

4. Anorexia and bloating–Hepatic and visceral engorgement secondary to the raised venous pressure may cause anorexia, bloating, and other nonspecific gastrointestinal symptoms.

B. Signs: Evidence of the underlying disease is usually found when specifically sought, although special investigations may be necessary.

1. Right ventricular hypertrophy–In primary right ventricular failure, right ventricular hypertrophy can be diagnosed on the basis of right ventricular heave and right atrial gallop rhythm by auscultation.

2. Right ventricular heave–A right ventricular heave over the lower central chest, right atrial gallop rhythm, a loud pulmonary second sound at the base of the heart, and increased jugular venous pressure with systolic pulsations of tricuspid insufficiency are usually present.

3. Right atrial gallop–A right S_3 is often heard, especially when right ventricular failure is due to increased resistance to right ventricular outflow, as in pulmonary stenosis or pulmonary hypertension.

4. Murmurs–If the underlying disease is congenital or valvular, characteristic murmurs will be heard, although in some patients with Eisenmenger's syndrome with severe pulmonary hypertension and a balanced shunt flow, no murmurs may be heard—as is true also in primary pulmonary hypertension and chronic lung disease.

5. Chronic pulmonary signs–If right ventricular failure is secondary to chronic lung disease, there will be evidence of decreased distensibility of the lungs, rales, rhonchi, wheezes, and signs of chronic bronchitis.

6. Jugular pulse–The jugular venous pulse will not only demonstrate the pulsating systolic wave of tricuspid insufficiency (which may also be palpated over the liver, with systolic expansion of the liver); there may also be prominent presystolic *a* waves when there is decreased compliance of the right ventricle and raised right atrial pressure. In pulmonary stenosis with right ventricular failure and in tricuspid stenosis, *a* waves are also prominent. The venous pressure rises further when right upper quadrant pressure is exerted by the physician, and the right atrial pressure may be raised as much as 5 mm Hg by this maneuver (hepatojugular reflux). The systolic jugular venous pulse of tricuspid insufficiency is often associated with a pansystolic murmur over the xiphoid, often accentuated

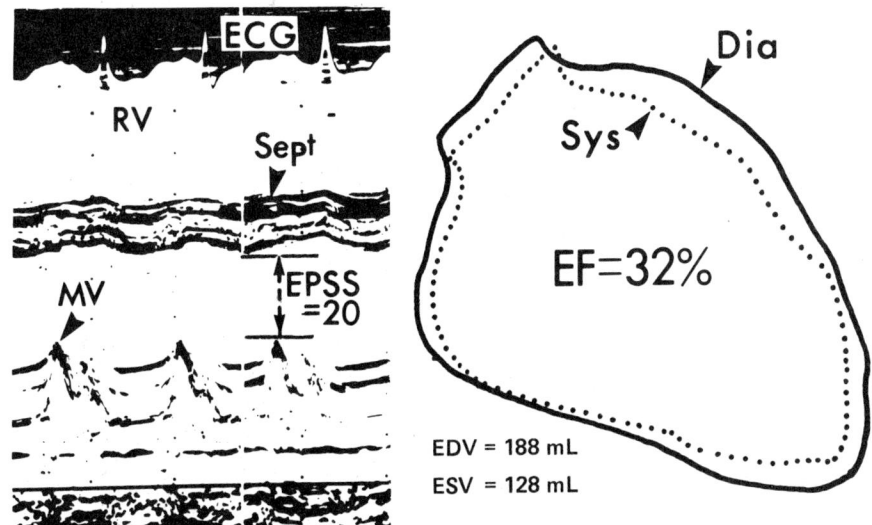

Figure 10–5. Echocardiogram of patient with alcoholic cardiomyopathy demonstrating a decreased ejection fraction of 32%, a large end-diastolic volume, and a wide separation between the anterior portion of the mitral valve leaflet and the ventricular septum. EF, ejection fraction; EDV, end-diastolic volume; ESV, end-systolic volume; MV, mitral valve; RV, right ventricle; Sept, septum; EPSS, end (E) point of mitral valve separated from septum; Sys, systole; Dia, diastole. (Reproduced, with permission, from Massie BM et al: Mitral-septal separation: A new echocardiographic index of left ventricular function. *Am J Cardiol* 1977;**39**:1008.)

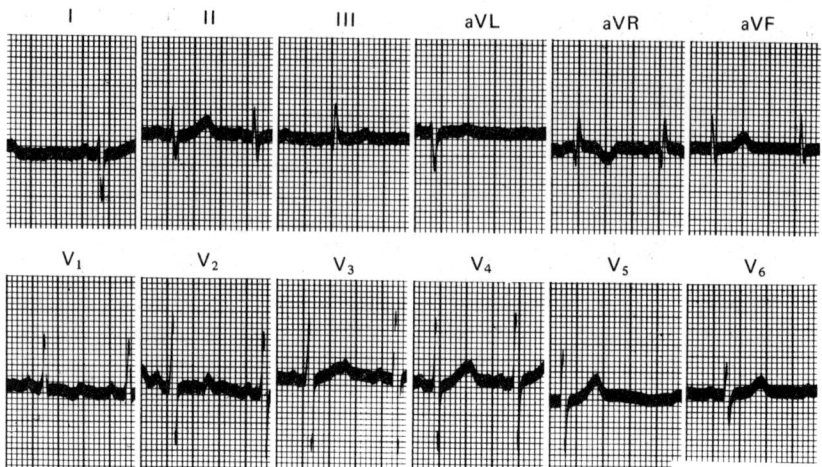

Figure 10–6. Pulmonary stenosis in a 7-year-old girl with right ventricular pressure of 43/0 mm Hg and pulmonary artery pressure of 15/5 mm Hg. The ECG shows typical marked right ventricular hypertrophy despite the moderate rise in right ventricular pressure. Note the monophasic tall R wave in V_1, a relatively smaller R wave in V_6, and a prominent S wave in V_6 and right axis deviation.

by inspiration and associated with a right atrial gallop that is also louder on inspiration.

7. Pulmonary second sound–The pulmonary second sound is accentuated if there is pulmonary hypertension but may be absent in severe pulmonary stenosis and fainter, with a wider split from A_2, if pulmonary stenosis is mild to moderate.

8. Pitting edema–Pitting edema of the ankles, lower extremities, and back is found in established right ventricular failure. Initially, the dependent edema caused by right heart failure usually subsides overnight. Eventually, it fails to subside with initial bed rest and may even increase during recumbency.

9. Ascites–Ascites is rarely prominent unless right ventricular failure has been neglected or obstructive lesions such as constrictive pericarditis, tricuspid stenosis, or cardiac tamponade are present. In constrictive pericarditis, the jugular venous pressure is raised, but there is no clinical evidence of tricuspid insufficiency; in fact, the dominant wave seen in the neck may be a prominent y descent.

10. Hydrothorax (pleural and pericardial effusion)–Hydrothorax is common in congestive heart failure, occurring in about a third of severe cases. It is more common in right than in left ventricular failure and more apt to occur in the right pleural space than in the left; bilateral hydrothorax is less common. Some authorities believe that isolated left hydrothorax should make one consider other conditions such as pulmonary infarction, but well-documented isolated left hydrothorax has often been reported. Fluid may accumulate in any serous cavity (eg, the pericardial and peritoneal cavities—the latter more apt to result from tricuspid stenosis or constrictive pericarditis). Rapid changes in the heart shadow should make one think of pericardial effusion rather than cardiac enlargement.

The mechanism of hydrothorax is not clearly understood. It is a result of systemic venous hypertension but is rare in acute pulmonary edema. It may also occur when swelling of the liver leads to engorged lymphatics, which may penetrate the diaphragm en route to the thoracic duct.

C. Electrocardiographic Findings:

1. Left ventricular pattern–If the ECG shows dominant left ventricular hypertrophy (Fig 10–2), it is likely that right ventricular failure is not the primary disorder but is secondary to left-sided failure.

2. Right ventricular pattern–Right ventricular hypertrophy is almost always found in congenital heart disease (eg, pulmonary stenosis) (Fig 10–6), although combined hypertrophy may be found when ventricular septal defect produces cardiac failure. Right ventricular hypertrophy is also marked in primary pulmonary hypertension or pulmonary hypertensive mitral stenosis (Fig 10–7), but the pattern of right ventricular hypertrophy is usually slight in clinically significant chronic cor pulmonale.

3. Right axis deviation and right ventricular hypertrophy–See Figs 11–15 and 11–19.

4. P waves–Prominent P waves in leads II and III and a dominant peaked anterior P wave in V_1 and V_2 indicate right atrial hypertrophy, which is often a clue to the presence of chronic cor pulmonale—in contrast to mitral stenosis, in which the P waves are wide and slurred and posteriorly (negatively) directed in V_1, indicating left atrial hypertrophy.

High-Output Failure
(See also p 289.)

Arteriovenous fistula is an uncommon cause of heart failure and may be congenital or acquired. The congenital variety may be due to congenital arteriovenous angioma, often involving a limb. Acquired fistulas are due to trauma (including surgical trauma),

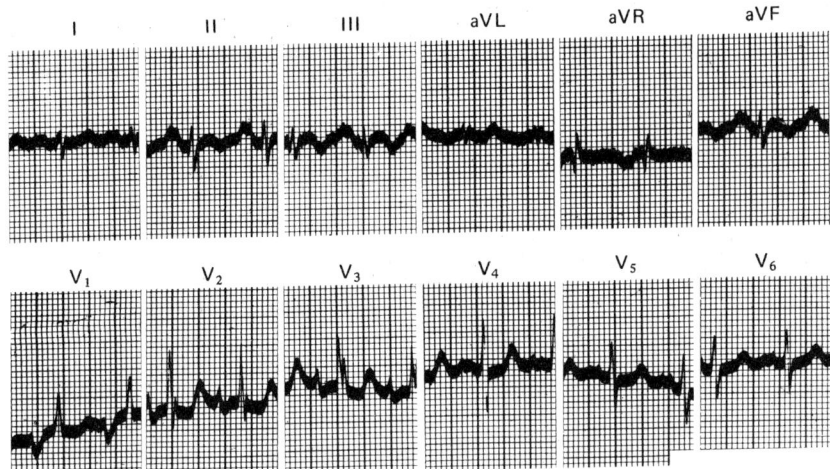

Figure 10-7. Progressive pulmonary venous congestion of 7 years' duration in a 39-year-old man with mitral stenosis and a recent femoral embolus. The ECG shows marked left atrial hypertrophy in association with right ventricular hypertrophy, indicating that the patient has mitral stenosis rather than congenital heart disease, in which right atrial hypertrophy would be expected, with anteriorly rather than posteriorly directed P waves. Note the monophasic tall R in V_1, a relatively small R in V_6, and a prominent S wave in V_6. Note also the slurred P wave, which is inverted and directed posteriorly in V_1, indicating left atrial hypertrophy.

usually involving the larger arteries of the limbs. They may be visceral (eg, following nephrectomy) or musculoskeletal (eg, after laminectomy). The condition may be insidious, and the fistula may not be clinically obvious.

Arteriovenous fistulas are created surgically in patients with renal disease in order to facilitate hemodialysis. Although such arteriovenous shunts are well tolerated by patients with normal hearts, they may cause heart failure in older patients with associated heart lesions. In high-output failure due to other causes such as severe anemia, Paget's disease of bone, thyrotoxicosis, or beriberi, the factor responsible for the failure is usually less obvious.

A. Symptoms: Dyspnea on exertion, edema of the ankles, and fatigue are indistinguishable from the same symptoms occurring in other patients with heart failure.

B. Signs: It is the physical signs of high-output failure that provide the clue to diagnosis. The cardinal sign is tachycardia that is disproportionate to the degree of failure and associated with a hyperdynamic cardiac impulse and clinical evidence of cardiac enlargement. Venous pressure is often elevated, and the pulse pressure is widened. A systolic ejection murmur may be heard at the base, resulting from increased stroke volume. In large arteriovenous fistulas, occlusion increases peripheral resistance, raises systemic arterial pressure, and causes a reflex bradycardia via the baroreceptor reflexes (Branham's sign). If this sign is positive, the fistula is large enough to be a potential cause of heart failure; however, a negative sign does not exclude arteriovenous fistula as a cause of failure. A hidden fistula should be searched for in any case of unexplained heart failure when a large heart and tachycardia are present. Examination of the patient should include listening for bruits over the abdomen, extremities, and back. If the fistula is in a limb, the extremity may be larger than normal and warm and may show marked varicosities. Infection of the fistula may lead to infective endocarditis.

C. Radiologic and Electrocardiographic Findings: Cardiac enlargement is usually seen on the chest x-ray, and the ECG may show evidence of left ventricular hypertrophy.

Acute Heart Failure

When cardiac failure is acute, the clinical picture is different in different disorders and will be described in the respective sections dealing with specific causes of acute failure.

RADIOLOGIC EXAMINATION OF THE HEART

Plain Film

Posteroanterior and lateral views of the chest may provide the first evidence of cardiac failure.

A. Heart Shadow: The film is usually abnormal, with hypertrophy and enlargement of the involved chamber, although the heart may not be enlarged if the patient has concentric hypertrophy (as in aortic stenosis or hypertension) or coronary heart disease.

B. Pulmonary Congestion: As the resistance of the lower lobe pulmonary arteries increases in left ventricular failure or in the pulmonary venous congestion of mitral stenosis, blood flows to the arteries with lower resistance, resulting in redistribution of fluid to the upper lobes (Figs 10–8 to 10–10), as can be seen on the plain film when the left atrial pressure rises to 20–25 mm Hg. In the presence of pulmonary hyper-

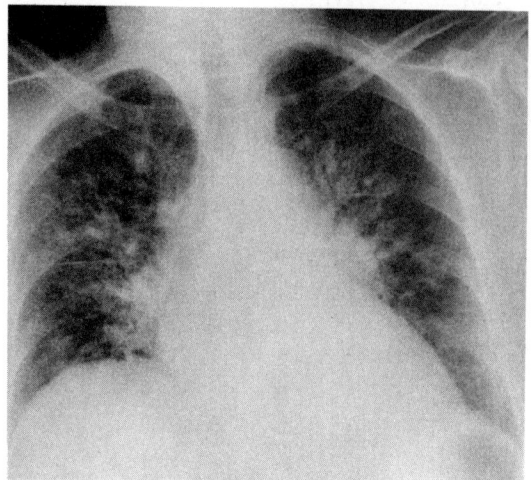

Figure 10–8. Posteroanterior chest x-ray in a man with acute pulmonary edema due to left ventricular failure. Note the bat's wing density, cardiac enlargement, increased flow to upper lobes, and pulmonary venous congestion.

tension, the pulmonary artery is dilated; and in severe pulmonary hypertension, especially primary pulmonary hypertension, there may be enlargement of the main and central pulmonary arteries, with abrupt cutoff in the caliber of the more peripheral pulmonary arteries. The pulmonary venous engorgement that occurs in right ventricular failure is absent, and there is no evidence of redistribution of blood, with widening of the pulmonary arteries of the upper lobes as compared to the lower, such as occurs in left ventricular failure. Attention to the pulmonary pattern, therefore, may be helpful in confirming chamber enlargement and in distinguishing left and right ventricular failure.

When fluid accumulates in the interlobular septa, horizontal Kerley B lines at the angles of the lateral lower lobes can be seen that reflect such fluid. Fluid may be localized in the interlobular spaces, simulating a tumor mass.

Attempts have been made to estimate left atrial pressure on the basis of signs of pulmonary venous congestion on the plain film, but the reliability of this method is only about 60%, chiefly because of the lag in appearance and disappearance of the findings in the chest film.

C. Pleural Effusion: In chronic left ventricular failure with raised pulmonary venous pressure, there may be right- or left-sided pleural effusion, usually the former. Right-sided effusions are usually due to right heart failure.

D. Calcification: Calcification of the mitral or aortic valve or in the pericardium or coronary arteries may be the clue to diagnosis.

E. Aorta: Examination of the aorta is often rewarding. If it is diffusely dilated, it suggests hypertensive disease; but if only the proximal aorta is dilated, especially if it can be seen within the heart shadow, it strongly suggests aortic stenosis. Fine eggshell calcification of the proximal aorta suggests syphilis (see Chapter 20); if the aorta is widely dilated proximally and in the arch but not distally, the question of dissection must be resolved by further studies. A local-

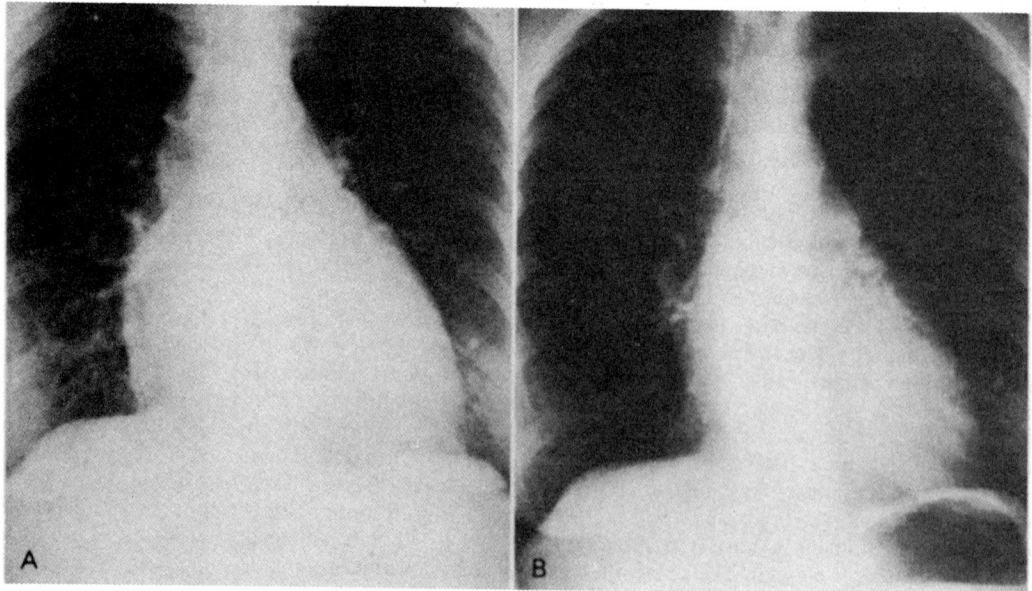

Figure 10–9. Enlarged heart and pulmonary venous congestion in a patient with high-output cardiac failure due to an end-to-side cephalic vein–radial artery fistula *(A)* before and *(B)* after banding of the vein. One month after banding, the heart has become smaller, and pulmonary venous congestion has improved. (Reproduced, with permission, from Anderson CB et al: Cardiac failure and upper extremity arteriovenous dialysis fistulas. *Arch Intern Med* 1976;**136**:292.)

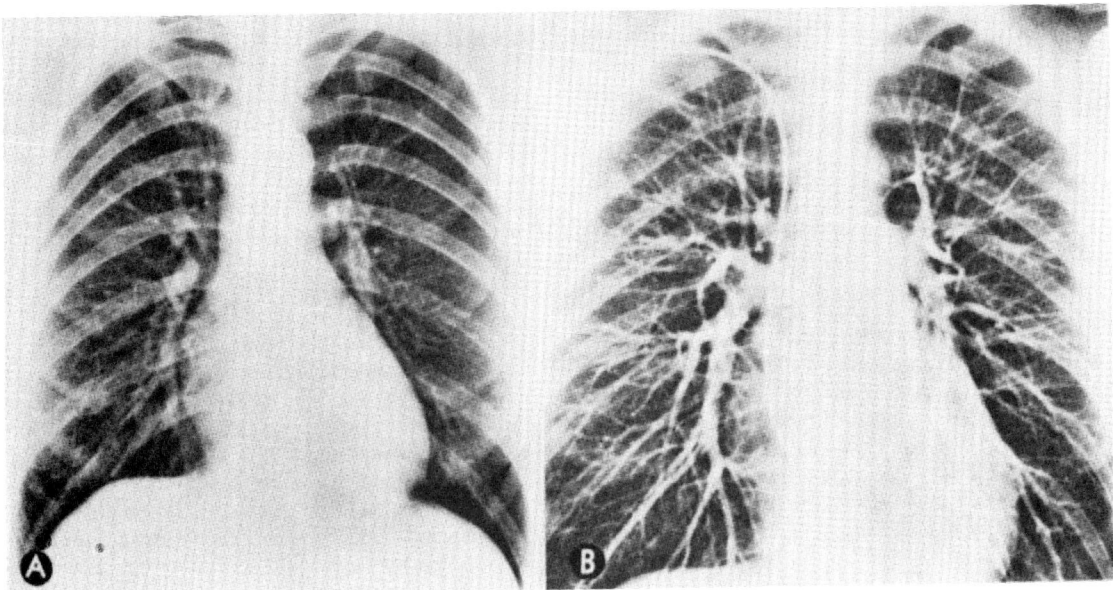

Figure 10–10. Chest x-rays and pulmonary arterial angiograms demonstrating that the vessels to the upper lobes are larger and more numerous than those to the lower lobes with hilar indistinction. *A:* Chest x-ray. *B:* Pulmonary arterial angiogram. (Reproduced, with permission, from Turner AF, Lau FYK, Jacobson G: A method for the estimation of pulmonary venous and arterial pressures from the routine chest roentgenogram. *Am J Roentgenol* 1972;116:1.)

ized aneurysm may also be demonstrated. The aorta may be small, with atrial septal defect or mitral stenosis because of decreased left ventricular flow. All of the congenital anomalies that may affect the aorta or its branches may be seen.

F. Rib Notching: Notching of the ribs may be the first sign of coarctation of the aorta in a patient with hypertension (see Chapter 11).

G. Left Atrial Study: Careful study of the left atrium is often helpful. Disproportionate left atrial enlargement, as in mitral stenosis or mitral regurgitation, may lead to a search for calcification of the mitral valve, echocardiographic studies, and careful physical examination. With left ventricular enlargement, the left atrium may be enlarged proportionately.

H. Other Findings: Chest films often show unexpected findings such as acute inflammatory disease of the lungs, pneumothorax, malignant tumors, or hilar nodes of lymphoma or sarcoidosis. In patients presenting with severe dyspnea, carcinomatous lymphatic spread in the lungs may occasionally lead to the diagnosis of carcinoma of the stomach or other organs.

LABORATORY FINDINGS

Red and white cell counts, hemoglobin, packed cell volume, and sedimentation rate are normal in uncomplicated heart failure. Polycythemia may occur in chronic cor pulmonale (see Chapter 19). Urinalysis often discloses significant proteinuria and granular casts. The blood urea nitrogen may be elevated because of reduced renal blood flow, but the urine specific gravity is high in the absence of primary renal disease. Serum sodium, potassium, chloride, and HCO_3^- are within normal limits in the usual case of congestive heart failure before diuretics are used. Specific tests should be made for any suspected unusual causes of heart failure, such as thyrotoxicosis, infective endocarditis, syphilis, connective tissue disease, and pheochromocytoma.

DIFFERENTIAL DIAGNOSIS

Cardiac failure must be distinguished from all conditions associated with dyspnea, cough, pulmonary venous congestion, venous pressure elevation, decreased cardiac output, cardiac enlargement, or peripheral edema. These clinical findings occur in a wide variety of conditions that can be conveniently discussed in groups, as in the following paragraphs.

Noncardiac & Nonthoracic Conditions Simulating Cardiac Failure

Examples include the dyspnea and fatigue of obesity, of sedentary individuals, and of emotional states with hyperventilation, and the edema that occurs as a result of thrombophlebitis or prolonged sitting in people with varicose veins. In these conditions, there are usually no objective signs of heart disease such as significant murmurs, friction rub, gallop rhythm, cardiac enlargement, or raised venous pressure. Cardiac diagnostic procedures—noninvasive or invasive—reveal no abnormalities of the cardiovascular system. At times these symptoms and signs from noncardiac causes occur in patients with known cardiac disease. As indicated in the introductory paragraphs, the presence of cardiac disease does not imply that all of the patient's symptoms and signs are due to cardiac failure.

Cardiac failure must be diagnosed on the basis of symptoms and signs combined with noninvasive and invasive techniques discussed in this chapter.

Lung Disease & Acute Respiratory Tract Infections Presenting With Respiratory Symptoms

These entities are discussed in Chapter 19. Right heart failure may occur in chronic lung disease (cor pulmonale), but many patients with chronic lung disease with chronic bronchitis, emphysema, etc, have dyspnea and cough for many years without abnormality of the heart. Patients with acute respiratory symptoms may have acute infections of the bronchi or lungs associated with fever and other symptoms and signs of acute illness. The differential diagnosis, including clinical and pulmonary function studies, is discussed in Chapter 19. Most helpful in chronic lung disease is the long history of chronic cough and sputum production, dyspnea, and wheezing, combined with clinical findings of poor lung expansion and chronic wheezes and rales. A history of cigarette smoking or of repeated respiratory infections in the absence of cardiac enlargement and the presence of gallop rhythm, ventricular heaves, or raised venous pressure are most helpful. Venous pressure becomes elevated when cardiac failure complicates chronic lung disease, but pulmonary symptoms are present for many years without this objective finding. Pulmonary function studies aid in the diagnosis of specific chronic lung diseases, and hemodynamic studies reveal increases of pressure in the pulmonary artery and the right heart with no abnormality in the left heart. When the 2 conditions coexist, the differentiation may be difficult.

Massive Pulmonary Embolism

Pulmonary embolism may produce symptoms similar to those of cardiac failure, or acute right ventricular failure may follow (1) massive pulmonary embolism with the development of acute pulmonary infarction, as noted on chest x-ray, or (2) pulmonary hypertension associated with signs of acute right ventricular overload, with physical signs of pulmonary hypertension and evidence on the ECG of right ventricular dilatation rather than systemic venous congestion (Sokolow, 1940). More precise diagnosis is provided by the combination of chest x-ray, pulmonary radioisotope scan, and pulmonary angiography (see Pulmonary Embolism, p 312).

Diseases of the Pericardium & Myocardium

Pericarditis and myocarditis due to various causes are discussed at length in Chapters 18 and 17, respectively. The most important distinguishing feature is raised left ventricular filling pressure relative to the right side, indicating that the disease is due to congestive cardiomyopathy with cardiac failure. Echocardiography is helpful in recognizing and quantifying the presence of pericardial effusion, which may not be suspected clinically, although findings of pericarditis such as pericardial friction rub can be diagnostic.

TREATMENT OF CARDIAC FAILURE

Cardiac failure may be of any degree of severity ranging from mild to moderate evidence of left ventricular failure, with increasing dyspnea on accustomed effort, to an emergency characterized by severe pulmonary edema, markedly reduced cardiac output, and an urgent threat to life (as in acute myocardial infarction or infective endocarditis with acute valvular insufficiency). Treatment therefore varies from a calm, conservative approach with nonurgent methods to urgent emergency measures depending upon the judgment of the physician.

The objectives of treatment are to remove the cause, increase the force and efficiency of myocardial contraction, decrease abnormal raised systemic vascular resistance, and reduce the abnormal retention of sodium and water. The patient shares a significant responsibility in the management of the disease, because treatment is long-term and involves restriction in diet and activity and the reliable use of cardiac drugs.

Identify, treat, and if possible eliminate the factor precipitating the cardiac failure, eg, infection (especially respiratory), pulmonary infarction, overexertion, increased sodium intake, medication, arrhythmias, particularly with rapid ventricular rates (eg, atrial fibrillation), myocardial infarction, and anemia.

The principles governing the treatment of cardiac failure are outlined in Table 10–2 and will be elaborated below.

Table 10–2. Principles of treatment of cardiac failure. These are discussed in sequence in the text that follows.

---

1. Make certain the diagnosis is correct and estimate the urgency of the need for therapeutic measures.
2. Reduce the energy requirement of the heart.
3. Reduce sodium intake unless diuretics have been given.
4. Consider and treat disturbances of rhythm.
5. Provide adequate but not excessive diuresis.
6. Identify and treat unsuspected acute myocardial processes.
7. Determine the presence of surgically treatable conditions that increase the mechanical load on the heart or interfere with left ventricular function.
8. Identify and treat precipitating factors in cardiac failure.
9. Digitalize adequately.
10. Treat systemic diseases that affect the heart.
11. Obtain a history of the use of cardiac depressant or damaging drugs and adjust or stop.
12. Mechanically remove fluid accumulations.
13. Treat with vasodilators in severe or refractory cardiac failure. Add inotropic agents if necessary.

1. VERIFY THE DIAGNOSIS & ESTIMATE THE URGENCY OF TREATMENT

Dyspnea, edema, fatigue, and other findings may not be due to cardiac failure even in patients with known heart disease. Careful questioning, taking into account the patient's intelligence, cooperation, understanding of language, and the possible effects of statements or diagnoses made by previous physicians, is always required.

The urgent treatment of pulmonary edema is discussed on p 319.

2. REDUCE THE ENERGY REQUIREMENT OF THE HEART

This is achieved by restricting physical and psychologic activity. Even modest activity induces sodium retention, tachycardia, and increased oxygen demands.

Rest

Physical and mental rest may be the most important aspect of treatment of early cardiac failure when cardiac reserves are reduced because compensatory mechanisms are beginning to falter and compensated heart disease is starting to "decompensate." The patient may be asymptomatic and have sufficient cardiac reserve to supply tissue oxygen needs at rest but not when stress is imposed. Many patients with mild cardiac failure improve dramatically with no treatment other than rest in bed, although if failure is more severe, other forms of therapy may be required. Rest not only decreases the work of the heart; recumbency decreases the stimulus to aldosterone production induced by erect posture, and sodium diuresis may result. About one-third of patients with left ventricular failure will respond with sodium and water diuresis and recover from cardiac failure with bed rest alone.

The duration of the period of physical and mental rest depends upon the severity of the heart failure, the age of the patient, and the cause of the underlying heart disease leading to failure, but even in the mildest cases the physician usually errs in allowing the patient to resume activity too early. For example, the patient in unequivocal left ventricular failure should be treated as though a small myocardial infarction has occurred and should have at least 2 or 3 weeks of rest, with gradual return to ambulatory status. Rest is preferably in the hospital but can be at home if failure is not severe, because the danger of ventricular arrhythmia is less than in acute myocardial infarction. In older patients, prolonged rest is associated with an increased risk of other problems (eg, thromboses, weakness, postural hypotension), and one should provide rest but not necessarily in bed. The use of a comfortable chair is equally effective, and short periods of walking decrease the likelihood of phlebothrombosis. Attention to the domestic, economic, and social situation of the patient is important; it obviously does no good to prescribe bed rest or rest in a chair if the patient has to do the marketing, cook and clean house, and care for the family. Social service agencies, home care assistance programs, and mobilization of all family resources are often helpful. A major flaw in treatment is an insufficient period of rest before the patient returns to the accustomed routine of stressful activities.

Reassurance

Dyspnea due to cardiac failure is a frightening experience. A reassuring and realistically optimistic attitude on the part of the physician and the judicious use of sedatives are important features of management.

3. DECREASE SODIUM INTAKE (Unless Diuretics Have Been Given)

Sodium in any form aggravates the peripheral manifestations of cardiac failure. Sodium excretion in patients with cardiac failure is usually decreased, and if the failure is severe it may be markedly decreased. When diuretics are used in adequate doses, strict sodium restriction is usually not necessary unless cardiac failure is severe or the patient has severe sodium retention such as occurs in chronic constrictive pericarditis. It is usually sufficient to avoid added salt in the diet, but patients must be warned about the sodium content of medications such as Alka-Seltzer or baking soda and foods high in sodium such as potato chips, pretzels, salted nuts, etc. Severe cardiac failure has occurred in patients ingesting large amounts of baking soda who thought they were taking a low-sodium diet, and also in patients who drink "softened" water. Booklets made available by local chapters of the American Heart Association give the sodium contents of common foods and should be distributed to patients at risk. The severity of sodium restriction should be adjusted according to the severity of cardiac failure and the effectiveness of diuretic therapy.

4. CORRECT ARRHYTHMIAS

Intermittent disturbances of rhythm may include paroxysmal atrial fibrillation or flutter, frequent ventricular premature beats or ventricular tachycardia, complete atrioventricular block, junctional rhythms due to digitalis toxicity, and sick sinus syndrome. Either rapid or slow heart rates may be deleterious. Rapid heart rates decrease diastolic filling time and impair coronary perfusion and may produce myocardial ischemia, decreasing the total cardiac output when stroke volume cannot be increased. An irregular rapid ventricular rate is more harmful than a regular rate, because systolic ejection is more profoundly disturbed by the irregular ventricular filling and subsequent response. When the ventricular rate is slow and the stroke output cannot be increased sufficiently to maintain an adequate minute volume output, patients may develop cardiac failure as well as impaired cerebral perfusion independently of episodes of syncope or Stokes-Adams attack.

The prevention and treatment of arrhythmias and of atrioventricular block may be crucial in the management of cardiac failure and are discussed at length in Chapters 14 and 15. Disturbances in rhythm and conduction may not be fully appreciated, because they may be paroxysmal or nocturnal. In patients with paroxysmal nocturnal dyspnea, the precipitating role of the arrhythmia may not be recognized without continuous monitoring of the ECG. With slow ventricular rates, artificial endocardial pacemakers may be required to induce a more rapid rate.

5. DIURETIC THERAPY

Physiology & Pharmacology

One of the spectacular advances in the past 40 years in the treatment of cardiac failure has been the development of diuretic agents, culminating in the introduction of the oral thiazide diuretics in 1957. About 40% of patients with cardiac failure will fail to respond to bed rest and digitalis and will require diuretic therapy to overcome the hypervolemia of cardiac failure.

A. Sodium Reabsorption in Cardiac Failure: Although the major physiologic event in cardiac failure is loss of the pumping action of the heart, failure of this function leads to hemodynamic changes in the kidneys, resulting in secondary retention of salt and water due to increased aldosterone secretion and other less well defined causes, which in turn leads to the congestive phenomena of the lungs and extremities that we call left and right heart failure, respectively. Although cardiac output is maintained adequately at rest in many patients as cardiac disease progresses, there comes a time when additional stresses such as exercise, emotional stress, or tachycardia fail to elicit an adequate increase in cardiac output, resulting in renal hemodynamic changes leading to increased renal tubular reabsorption of sodium. Renal tubular reabsorption of sodium is an important mechanism in regulation of isotonicity and volume of the extracellular fluids. The kidney responds to decreased cardiac output, especially with stress, by increased retention of sodium and water. This may be lifesaving in the event of hemorrhage but is deleterious in the presence of cardiac failure, causing pulmonary and systemic venous congestion and many of the more distressing clinical symptoms and signs of cardiac failure.

B. Mercurial Diuretics: For many years, mercurial diuretics were the physician's major resource in the diuretic treatment of left ventricular failure, but they have been abandoned in favor of modern oral diuretics.

C. Rational Use of Diuretic Therapy: The rational use of diuretic therapy (the increased excretion of sodium and water) requires a knowledge of the physiology of the nephron and of the sites in the nephron where sodium is filtered, reabsorbed, and exchanged for potassium (Fig 10–11). Sodium is filtered at the glomerulus, where it enters the proximal renal tubule as part of the protein-free ultrafiltrate fluid that begins its passage down the renal tubule. Drugs such as aminophylline and digoxin that increase the glomerular filtration rate may promote sodium excretion in the urine by increasing the amount of sodium filtered at the glomerulus. Mercurial diuretics act primarily on the proximal tubule (where 70% of the filtered sodium is normally reabsorbed), decreasing the reabsorption of sodium, but may also act on the distal tubule. The more potent, newer "loop" diuretics, such as furosemide and ethacrynic acid, act on the ascending limb of the loop of Henle, where sodium without water is reabsorbed. These so-called loop diuretics prevent reabsorption of sodium in the loop of Henle, with the result that the tubular fluid proceeding distally contains almost all of the sodium filtered at the glomerulus (except for that reabsorbed in the proximal tubule), thus causing diuresis of sodium and water. The thiazide diuretics have their site of action at the beginning of the distal convoluted tubule following the end of the ascending limb of the loop of Henle (see Fig 10–11) and decrease the reabsorption of sodium, thus increasing the excretion of sodium and water (diuresis). However, because the amount of sodium reabsorbed at this site is less than that reabsorbed more proximally in the ascending limb of the loop of Henle, the thiazide diuretics are less potent than the loop diuretics. The tubular fluid containing sodium then proceeds down the distal convoluted tubule to the so-called sodium-potassium exchange site at the end of the tubule, which is under the influence of aldosterone. The amount of potassium exchanged for sodium depends upon the amount of sodium in the tubular fluid delivered to this distal tubular site; it is greater when the sodium in the diet is high or when decreased reabsorption of sodium follows the use of thiazide or loop diuretics. As a result, a drug that prevents reabsorption of sodium as it passes along the tubule increases the excretion of potassium as well as sodium, and loss of both ions is the physiologic result of the diuretic agents. Increased diuresis of sodium is what is desired; increased diuresis of potassium is not desired and may produce hypokalemia—usually mild, with serum potassium infrequently below 3 meq/L.

D. Excessive Sodium Loss With Diuresis: The increased sodium and water retention resulting from decreased cardiac output and consequently decreased glomerular filtration rate in cardiac failure can be counteracted by the diuretic agents. However, with large doses of diuretic agents (especially the potent loop diuretics), when the amount of generalized edema due to salt and water retention is great, diuresis may be excessive, ie, the patient may lose such large quantities of salt and water in a matter of days that sodium depletion and hypovolemia replace sodium retention and hypervolemia. The patient may then become lethargic and sleepy, have postural hypotension and muscle cramps, and become severely ill. The physician must then liberalize the sodium intake and stop

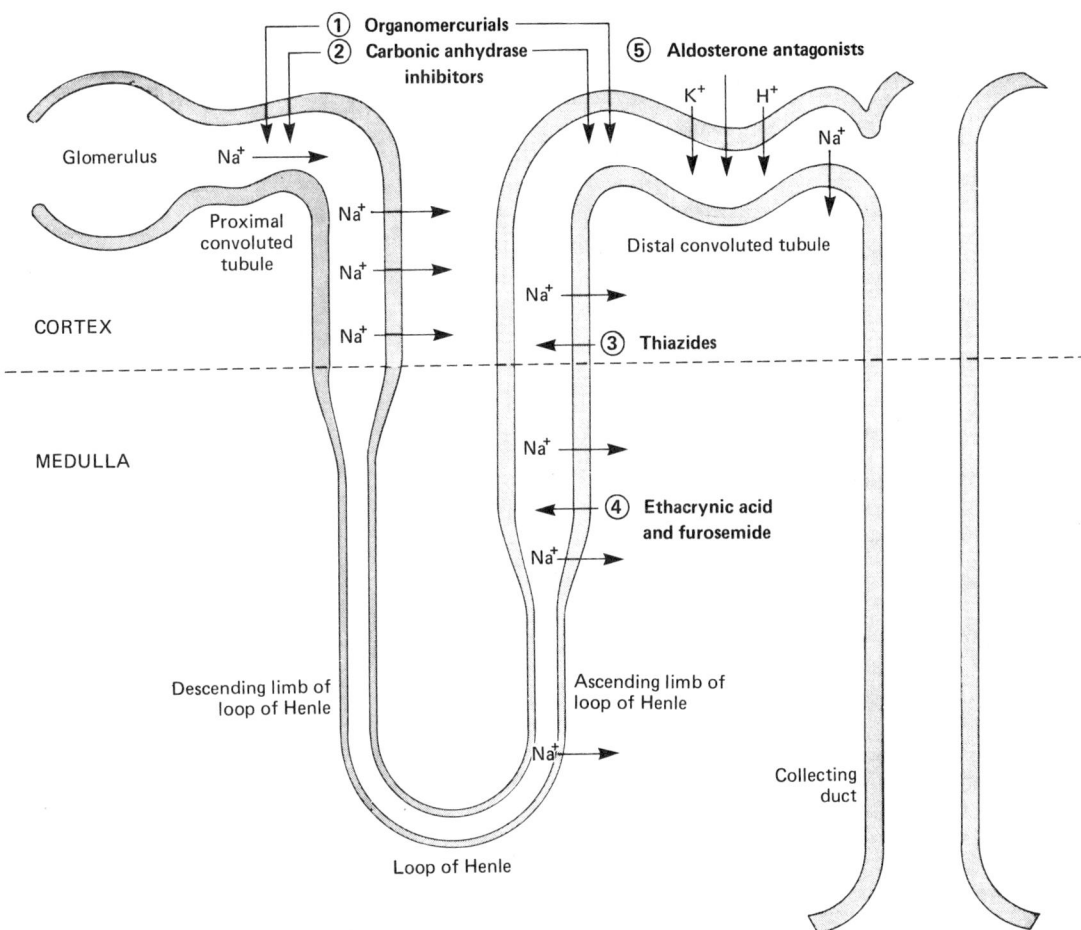

Figure 10–11. Sites of sodium reabsorption in the nephron and of action of different diuretics and carbonic anhydrase inhibitors. The mercurials (1) are carbonic anhydrase inhibitors (2) that act in the proximal or distal tubule to inhibit sodium reabsorption. Thiazides (3) act in the ascending limb of the loop of Henle, preventing sodium reabsorption and interfering with dilution. Ethacrynic acid and furosemide (4) also block sodium reabsorption. Aldosterone antagonists (5) prevent potassium excretion and increase sodium excretion. (Adapted and reproduced, with permission, from Laragh JH: Diuretics in the management of congestive heart failure. Hosp Pract [Nov] 1970;5:43; and Wilson GM: Diuretics. Practitioner 1968;200:39.)

the diuretics until a balance has been restored. To prevent excessive hypovolemia, diuresis should be started with milder diuretics in small doses—eg, hydrochlorothiazide, 50 mg daily (or 25 mg in an older patient)—and the dose increased only when it is certain that diuresis is not adequate with the smaller dose.

E. Counteracting Potassium Loss: In patients in whom significant hypokalemia results from the diuretic therapy, a high-potassium diet containing fresh fruits and vegetables, especially bananas, oranges, tomato juice, and other foods shown in Table 9–27, is helpful. The average fall in serum potassium in patients receiving 50 mg of hydrochlorothiazide twice daily was 0.62 meq/L. A daily potassium supplement of 60 meq 10% KCl elixir was required to restore the original level in most patients (Schwartz, 1974). If the serum potassium is still low, agents such as spironolactone—which is a competitive antagonist of aldosterone—or amiloride or triamterene—neither of which is an aldosterone antagonist—can be used to decrease the amount of potassium exchanged for sodium at the distal sodium-potassium exchange site. Spironolactone by itself is a weak sodium diuretic, but when given in combination with other diuretics it decreases the loss of potassium and so prevents hypokalemia. If, however, the patient has impaired renal function with oliguria or is receiving potassium supplements, serum potassium may rise progressively and hyperkalemia, with resulting severe cardiac conduction defects, may follow. In the presence of normal urine output and normal renal function, spironolactone rarely produces hyperkalemia because of the built-in defense system whereby an increase in serum potassium increases the secretion of aldosterone. However, if spironolactone or triamterene is used, serum potassium must be monitored frequently and frequent ECGs obtained so that an early rise in serum potassium or the appearance of high peaked T waves will not be missed. When the serum potassium increases to 5 or 6 meq/L, the drugs should be stopped; levels over 8 meq/L are extremely dangerous and must be avoided because of the cardiac effects. Because oral potassium supplements are unpleasant to take and only marginally improve the low serum potassium resulting from use of diuretics, the administration of spironolactone, amiloride, or triamterene in combination with other diuretics to prevent hypokalemia and in accordance with the specified precautions is becoming more widespread.

Renal stones and possibly interstitial renal changes have developed in patients receiving triamterene; further study is required to determine the effect of the drug on the kidney.

Clinical Use of Diuretics

The prototype class of oral diuretic agents is the thiazide group of drugs typified by chlorothiazide and hydrochlorothiazide (see Chapter 9 for additional details about drugs and dosages).

A. Indications for Oral Diuretics:

1. Treatment of mild edema–When edema is minimal or the evidence of left ventricular failure is slight, bed rest and sodium restriction may be adequate to effect diuresis.

2. Treatment of more severe failure–When cardiac failure is more severe, diuretic therapy is needed unless absolute bed rest and restriction of sodium intake to 200–300 mg/d are ordered. These restrictions on activity and diet are undesirable, and most patients with cardiac failure are not given strict low-sodium diets. Moderate restriction of sodium (no added salt in the diet) and small doses of a diuretic will usually reverse the salt and water retention that occurs with moderate cardiac failure.

B. Drugs and Dosages:

1. Thiazide diuretics–The initial dose of the thiazide diuretics is 25–50 mg of hydrochlorothiazide once daily, increased to 50 mg twice daily or to 100 mg once or twice daily if diuresis is inadequate. The dose-response characteristics of the thiazides are such that the maximum response occurs at a dosage of 100 mg, and therefore, no single dose larger than 100 mg should be given. When the thiazides are given orally, the onset of action is about 1 hour, the peak effect is reached in about 4 hours, and the duration of action varies, sometimes extending into the next 24-hour period. The drug should be given intermittently (every other day or 2–3 times a week if possible) to allow for restoration of losses of potassium and sodium; if the patient can be held at a steady dry weight without symptoms with a diuretic given twice a week, side effects are rare. Long-acting diuretics (chlorthalidone, metolazone) are discussed in Chapter 9.

2. Loop diuretics (furosemide, ethacrynic acid, bumetanide)–If cardiac failure is severe or renal failure is present and if diuresis does not occur with the use of moderately potent drugs such as the thiazides, the more potent loop diuretics can be used. These agents act on the ascending loop of Henle and will cause continued excretion of sodium when doses of up to 500 mg are given. Effectiveness depends on the size of the individual dose rather than the total daily dose. Furosemide and ethacrynic acid can be started at 40 mg/d and bumetanide at 0.5–1 mg/d. The dose can be gradually increased and then given twice daily if necessary, depending upon the severity of heart failure and the presence of renal failure. Oral loop diuretics have the same onset of action, peak effect, and duration of action as the oral thiazides (see above). When loop diuretics are given intravenously, as in the management of acute pulmonary edema, there may be significant diuresis within 15–30 minutes.

3. Spironolactone, amiloride, and triamterene–These diuretics counteract the action of aldosterone at the distal tubule Na^+-K^+ exchange site (spironolactone by competitive antagonism). They rarely are used alone but are combined with thiazide or loop diuretics to diminish potassium loss. They should not be used in the presence of oliguria or renal failure because of the hazard of hyperkalemia (see Chapter 9). Acetazolamide, acidifying drugs, aminophylline, and osmotic diuretics are rarely useful in cardiac failure.

Toxicity of Diuretics

In addition to sodium depletion and hypokalemia (discussed above), chronic hypovolemia produced by the diuretics as well as by direct action of the diuretics on the renal tubule may result in 20–30% increases of serum creatinine and uric acid and occasionally of plasma or serum glucose. Patients with a history of gout may develop acute gouty arthritis, and the dosage of thiazides must be reduced or the patient must be given a uricosuric drug such as probenecid. Diabetes mellitus is rarely induced in individuals with no history of the disease, but in patients with diabetes, hyperglycemia induced by diuretics may require increasing doses of insulin. The slight increases in serum creatinine, uric acid, and serum glucose and the associated hypokalemia usually cause no symptoms and are reversible when the agents are discontinued. The long-term hazards of these biochemical changes are not known, especially in patients with underlying impairment of renal function; however, there have been no reports of their deleterious effects on the kidney or other organs, even after almost 20 years of use.

Metabolic Alkalosis

Additional electrolyte and water disturbances that may occur in patients with cardiac failure treated with diuretic agents include hypokalemic and hypochloremic alkalosis. An increase in serum bicarbonate compensates for the loss of chloride and hydrogen ions, because both hydrogen and potassium are exchanged in the distal tubule for sodium. Chloride and potassium replacement can be accomplished with potassium chloride.

Dilutional Hyponatremia

Dilutional hyponatremia may occur in treated cardiac failure, especially when water intake is increased. In contrast to patients who develop depletional hyponatremia due to sodium depletion resulting from excessive diuresis, patients with dilutional hyponatremia (although they may have equivalent degrees of hyponatremia, sometimes to as low as 110 meq/L) continue to have generalized edema despite low serum sodium. Edelman (1958) and Maffly (1961) clarified this picture in a series of experiments showing that the edema almost always occurred in association with an increase in total body sodium and that edema in the presence of hyponatremia indicated an excess of body water rather than a depletion of body sodium. Edelman concluded that the serum sodium concentration served as a means of estimating the osmolality of the body fluids and reflected the total body solute/body water ratio. The use of hypertonic saline, which is valuable in depletional hyponatremia, may worsen cardiac failure in dilutional hyponatremia because the total body sodium is already increased. The patient may be ill, thirsty, and weak, and treatment consists of decreasing the water intake to about 500–700 mL/d and giving furosemide if necessary. As excess body water is lost through the skin and lungs, the balance between sodium and water is restored and the serum sodium gradually rises.

In depletional hyponatremia, the specific gravity of the urine is usually high; in dilutional hyponatremia, urine specific gravity it is low because of decreased solute excretion.

Caution With Diuretic Therapy

Diuretic therapy should be used with caution in patients who are receiving digitalis, because hypokalemia increases the hazard of digitalis toxicity. Diuretics should be used intermittently whenever possible and in the smallest effective dose, and digitalis should be given cautiously, with frequent observations including determinations of serum digitalis levels. Not only may hypokalemia and digitalis interact to increase digitalis toxicity, but the sicker cardiac patients may have decreased appetite and take less potassium in their diet, aggravating the situation. In these circumstances, small doses of spironolactone can be added if oliguria or renal failure is not present; patients should be observed for the hyperkalemia that may then result. Hirsutism and enlarged breasts, which can be very painful, may also occur. In the presence of renal failure, the loop diuretics are effective, whereas the thiazides are not; spironolactone should be avoided, especially if there is oliguria with renal failure. The loop diuretics are not recommended for the treatment of moderate cardiac failure if adequate diuresis can be achieved with the milder diuretics such as the thiazides, but one should not hesitate to use them if the thiazides fail.

6. IDENTIFY & TREAT UNSUSPECTED OR UNRECOGNIZED ACUTE MYOCARDIAL DISORDERS

The principal examples are listed in Chapter 17. The cause of cardiac failure is often unsuspected unless one specifically seeks it out by using appropriate investigative techniques. Acute dyspnea may mask the chest discomfort of acute myocardial infarction. The fever of infective endocarditis may be low-grade and intermittent. Murmurs may be minimal, and preexisting cardiac disease may be unsuspected, especially in drug addicts. Acute nephritis with salt and water retention may be entirely unsuspected unless one examines the urine, takes the blood pressure, and *thinks* of the possibility. Acute pericardial effusion must be distinguished from cardiac dilatation not only because unrecognized tamponade may be life-threatening but also because the cause of the effusion must be determined and specific therapy given as needed. (For further details see Chapters 9, 15, 16, 17, and 20.)

7. TREAT OPERABLE CONDITIONS THAT INCREASE THE LOAD ON THE HEART OR INTERFERE WITH LEFT VENTRICULAR FUNCTION

This should be done after maximal improvement has been achieved on medical treatment. Obviously, emergency situations must always be dealt with first, but the ideal management of cardiac failure is to identify and remove the cause of ventricular dysfunction if that is possible. Medical treatment is a temporizing measure that does not reach the underlying cause. Operative procedures may also be palliative but in many instances can be semicurative and result in dramatic improvement.

Conditions potentially treatable by means of operation should be evaluated while the patient is responding to bed rest and medical treatment. (See other chapters for surgical treatment of individual diseases.)

8. TREAT EXTRACARDIAC FACTORS

Extracardiac factors that increase the work of the heart include fever; anemia; acid-base, electrolyte, and endocrine abnormalities; hypoxia; and obesity, among many others. These factors increase the heart rate and myocardial oxygen demand; may decrease coronary blood flow and produce myocardial ischemia; may lead to the development of cardiac arrhythmias, with resulting impairment of coronary perfusion and production of myocardial ischemia; and may

Table 10-3. Cardiac glycoside preparations: Average adult doses and routes of administration.*

Glycoside and Preparations Available	Dose Digitalizing	Dose Maintenance	Rapid Method of Administration	Speed; Maximum Action and Duration
Parenteral preparations				
Deslanoside (Cedilanid-D), 2- and 4-mL ampules, 0.4 and 0.8 mg	8 mL (1.6 mg)	0.2–0.4 mg (1–2 mL)	1.2 mg (6 mL) IV or IM and follow with 0.2–0.4 mg (1–2 mL) IV or IM every 3–4 hours until effect is obtained.	1–2 hours; duration, 3–6 days.
Digitoxin (dilute before use), 1- and 2-mL ampules, 0.2 and 0.4 mg	1.2 mg (6 mL)	0.05–0.2 mg	0.6 mg (3 mL) IV or IM followed by 0.2–0.4 mg every 4–6 hours until 1.2 mg has been given.	3–8 hours; duration, 14–21 days.
Digoxin (Lanoxin), 2-mL ampules, 0.25 mg/mL	1.5 mg (6 mL)	0.125–0.75 mg (1–3 mL)	0.5–1 mg (2–4 mL) IV and 0.25–0.5 mg (1–2 mL) in 3–4 hours; then 0.25 mg (1 mL) every 3–4 hours until effect is obtained.	1–2 hours; duration, 3–6 days.
Oral preparations				
Digitalis, tablets, 0.03, 0.06, and 0.1 g	1–1.5 g	0.05–0.2 g	0.6 g stat; 0.4 g in 6–8 hours; 0.2 g every 6 hours for 2–3 doses; then 0.1 g twice daily until effect is obtained.	6–8 hours; duration, 18–21 days.
Digitoxin, tablets, 0.1, 0.15, and 0.2 mg	1.2 mg	0.05–0.2 mg	0.6 mg stat; repeat in 12 hours, and then 0.2 mg twice daily until effect is obtained.	6–8 hours; duration, 14–21 days.
Digitoxin, tablets, 0.25 and 0.5 mg	1.5–3 mg	0.125–0.5 mg	1 mg stat and then 0.25–0.5 mg every 6 hours until effect is obtained.	4–6 hours; duration, 2–6 days.
Gitalin (Gitaligin), tablets, 0.5 mg	4–6 mg	0.5 mg	1 mg 3 times on first day followed by 0.5 mg every 6 hours until effect is obtained.	4–6 hours; duration, 8–14 days.

*Check manufacturers' descriptive literature. Dosage sizes of tablets and ampules change from time to time.

aggravate or induce toxicity from therapeutic agents such as digitalis when hypokalemia is present. Cardiac failure induced by such extracardiac factors should be treated in accordance with the principles outlined in this chapter. At the same time, the underlying extracardiac factors should also be treated with appropriate measures.

9. DIGITALIS*

In addition to rest, diuretics, management of arrhythmias, and the other approaches discussed above, treatment with digitalis should be started.

Digitalis has been one of the major medical resources in the treatment of cardiac failure. There are a wide variety of digitalislike preparations, but digitalis is the generic term for any compound containing a steroid glycoside ring, a lactone ring, and a sugar residue. Differences in the sugar residues of various compounds influence their absorption, potency, and duration of action (see Tables 10–3 and 10–4). In recent years, digitalis leaf and digitoxin have been used less frequently than digoxin, the former because it is poorly absorbed and the latter because of its long duration of action. The purified glycosides with shorter duration of action, such as digoxin, are overwhelmingly the digitalis preparations most frequently used in the USA, and the same applies to similar preparations, perhaps with different names, used in other parts of the world. In Table 10–3 are listed the dosages and methods of administration of glycoside preparations (both oral and parenteral) that are available for clinical use. Table 10–4 lists the average doses of digitalis drugs given orally for digitalization and maintenance, according to degree of urgency. Effective maintenance dosage may differ as much as 5-fold from patient to patient because of individual variation in response.

Although newer inotropic agents and vasodilators (see below) are being used with greater frequency in patients with cardiac failure, digitalis compounds have the advantages of many years of experience and well-established effectiveness, both in the presence of sinus rhythm and in atrial fibrillation. Digitalis is most effective in patients with chronic cardiac failure and is less effective in patients with acute cardiac failure, acute myocardial infarction, severe primary cardiomyopathy, acute rheumatic carditis, and chronic lung disease. The value of digitalis in chronic cardiac failure with sinus rhythm has been controversial, and some authors have not found it efficacious. Withdrawal and readministration of digitalis, however, have often demonstrated improved hemodynamics (Sokolow, 1942; Arnold, 1980). Lee (1982) found digitalis effective in about half the patients with severe chronic cardiac failure and sinus rhythm. It is rarely effective in acute failure such as occurs in acute myocardial infarction. Digoxin is more effective in patients with atrial fibrillation, because it decreases atrioventricular conduction and slows the ventricular rate in addition to its direct inotropic action.

*See p 318 for newer inotropic agents.

Table 10–4. Average adult dosages of digitalis drugs given orally to digitalize and then to maintain digitalization, according to degree of urgency. Maintenance dosages are only averages and may be varied according to individual patient response.

Urgency	Drug	Dosage
Moderate	Digitalis leaf	0.4 g every 8 hours for 3 doses, then 0.1 g/d.
	Digitoxin	0.4 mg every 8 hours for 3 doses, then 0.1 mg/d.
	Digoxin	0.5 mg every 8 hours for 3 doses, then 0.25 mg once daily.
Intermediate	Digitalis leaf	0.2 g 3 times daily for 2 days or 0.1 g 4 times daily for 3 days, then 0.1 g/d.
	Digitoxin	0.2 mg 3 times daily for 2 days, then 0.1 mg/d.
	Digoxin	0.5 mg twice daily for 2 days or 0.25 mg 3 times daily for 3 days, then 0.25 mg once daily.
Least	Digitalis leaf	0.1 g 3 times daily for 4–5 days, then 0.1 g/d.
	Digitoxin	0.1 mg 3 times daily for 4–6 days, then 0.1 mg/d.
	Digoxin	0.25 mg twice daily for 4–6 days, then 0.25 mg once daily.

Indications for Administration
(See also Chapter 15.)

(1) Cardiac failure with sinus rhythm or atrial fibrillation.

(2) Atrial fibrillation or flutter with a rapid ventricular rate.

(3) Supraventricular paroxysmal tachycardia.

(4) Prevention of paroxysmal atrial or junctional arrhythmias in patients in whom quinidine has failed or is not tolerated.

(5) As maintenance therapy to prevent recurrence of cardiac failure in patients who have received digitalis initially for cardiac failure.

Mechanism of Action

The use of beta-adrenergic blocking agents does not interfere with the inotropic action of digitalis, and this apparently rules out the sympathetic nervous system as the mediator of its inotropic effect. Digitalis is bound to sites on the membrane of heart muscle cells, where it may affect the net uptake of potassium, sodium, and calcium. Increased availability of calcium ions, enhancing cardiac contraction, is thought to be the basic mechanism by which digitalis acts to increase the force and velocity of contraction.

Digitalis has a potent electrophysiologic action that results in increased automaticity of the secondary pacemakers in the atrioventricular nodal junction, in the atrioventricular nodal–His bundle junction, and in secondary pacemakers throughout the Purkinje system responsible for the ectopic rhythms that are a sign of digitalis toxicity. In addition, digitalis decreases impulse conduction in the heart, which is desirable in patients with atrial fibrillation but undesirable when it leads to reentry phenomena and paroxysmal atrial arrhythmias. Digitalis slows conduction velocity by increasing the refractory period of both specialized and ordinary cells, and when this occurs in the atrioventricular node it is of special benefit to patients with atrial fibrillation because it slows the ventricular rate. Digitalis increases the automaticity of cells by increasing the rate of spontaneous diastolic depolarization (phase 4; see Chapter 14), and in larger doses it decreases the slope of initial rapid depolarization (phase 0) and decreases the magnitude and shortens the duration of the action potential.

Pathophysiologic & Hemodynamic Effects

The effects of digitalis described above on the isolated cardiac muscle fiber in vitro must be distinguished from the clinical effects in the patient with cardiac failure or myocardial ischemia. Hemodynamic studies in patients who are in manifest heart failure have shown that digitalis increases cardiac output, decreases right atrial and peripheral venous pressure, decreases the filling pressure of the left ventricle, and increases the urinary excretion of sodium and water, thereby correcting some of the hemodynamic and metabolic abnormalities in cardiac failure. These clinical effects are not uniform, however, and digitalis is less effective in the presence of acute myocarditis, myocardial ischemia, high output cardiac failure, pulmonary or systemic venous congestion resulting from mechanical defects, and some cases of diffuse extensive primary cardiomyopathy or ischemic cardiomyopathy. It is possible that the stage of hemodynamic alteration in cardiac failure affects the response to digitalis and that this may explain the minimal hemodynamic benefit seen in some patients. Digitalis is more effective in the presence of atrial fibrillation with a rapid ventricular rate, because its ability to block conduction through the atrioventricular node decreases the ventricular rate and improves coronary perfusion. Better ventricular filling during diastole decreases left atrial pressure and pulmonary venous congestion. The effect of slowing the ventricular rate is particularly advantageous in the presence of obstructive lesions such as mitral stenosis.

Pharmacokinetics

A. Effect of Drug: As is true of all drugs, the various digitalis preparations may have different clinical effects depending upon the rate of absorption, the amount of body fluid in which the drug is distributed, its bioavailability, the renal function, the rate of metabolic degradation, thyroid function, and the mode of excretion—all of which may differ in different patients, so that no one dosage schedule is suitable for all patients. The bioavailability of digitalis—the amount absorbed and available to the body—was recognized as a cause of unpredictable blood levels and clinical effectiveness. The result has been that the FDA now includes dissolution rates as a part of the criteria for acceptance of all digoxin and other preparations. All digoxin and other preparations must now meet these requirements, and it is anticipated that bioavailability will not be a problem in the future.

B. Physiologic Factors: A number of studies have been published on the kinetics of digoxin and other digitalis preparations (Doherty, 1978; Smith, 1984). Absorption rates vary with the speed of dissolution of the tablets and are enhanced by sluggish gastrointestinal motility and hypothyroidism and decreased by the concomitant use of nonabsorbable drugs or antacids; they are increased by hyperthyroidism and the use of elixir as compared to tablet digoxin preparations. In patients with normal renal function, the mean half-life of digoxin is about 36 hours, but the range is wide and the standard deviation is about 8 hours. (The half-life is the time required for the digoxin in the body to decrease by 50%.) In contrast, the half-life of digitoxin is 4–6 days. The renal excretion of digoxin depends on the glomerular filtration rate; the dose of drug must be decreased in patients with impaired renal function and reduced glomerular filtration rate to prevent accumulation with high serum levels and toxicity. Fig 10–12 relates the blood urea nitrogen level to the clearance of digoxin, reflecting the delayed clearance in the presence of poor renal function.

Radioisotope studies have shown that when digoxin is given to patients who have not received digitalis in the past few days, a daily dose leads to a steady-state serum digoxin level in 6–9 days. If renal function is normal, a loading or saturation dose—once thought to be essential—is now considered unnecessary unless rapid digitalization is desired. A daily dose of digoxin given for 4–5 "half-lives" of digoxin results in a steady-state plateau of serum digoxin even if the dose is continued indefinitely. The drug is bound tightly to the tissues and so is not removed by dialysis or by open heart bypass procedures.

C. Digoxin Levels Affected by Dosage: About three-fourths of an oral dose of digoxin is absorbed from the gastrointestinal tract, and patients who have reached a steady state with daily maintenance doses of the drug achieve a new peak within 3 hours of administration of the next oral dose of digoxin, with the level beginning to rise within an hour. Because about one-third of the body stores of digoxin is excreted daily (assuming that renal function is normal) and because the half-life of digoxin is about 1½ days, the effects of digoxin will be dissipated in 4–5 days (4–5 half-lives) after the drug is stopped. The serum digoxin levels fall to zero in a week, but this may not adequately reflect the total loss of digoxin from the body, since ST–T abnormalities caused by digitalis may persist for as long as 3 weeks after the drug has been stopped.

Serum Digoxin Levels

Radioimmunoassay techniques have permitted accurate and reliable measurement of serum digoxin and digitoxin levels (Table 10–5), which can be correlated with the dose of the drug and the clinical effects (Smith, 1973). Serum digitoxin levels are 5–15 times greater than serum digoxin levels. Mixtures of different digitalis glycosides cannot be evaluated by radioimmunoassay. Age, renal function, thyroid status, and interference with absorption by noncardiac drugs have all been shown to influence the serum digoxin level. The average serum digoxin levels 7–10 days following a daily dose average approximately

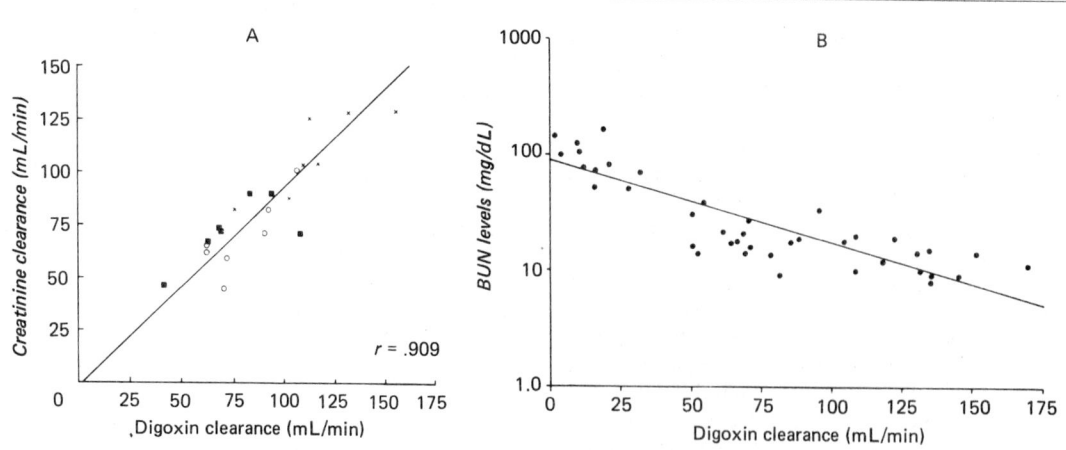

Figure 10–12. *A:* Relationship of creatinine clearance to digoxin clearance in donors before (x) and after (o) unilateral nephrectomy and in recipients (■) of these kidneys. The correlation coefficient, $r = 0.909$, is highly significant. (Reproduced, with permission, from Doherty JE, Flanigan WJ, Dalrymple GV: Tritiated digoxin. 17. Excretion and turnover times in normal donors before and after nephrectomy and in the paired recipient of the kidney after transplantation. *Am J Cardiol* 1972;**29**:470.) *B:* Relationship of blood urea nitrogen (BUN) to the clearance of digoxin. The higher the BUN level, the lower the digoxin clearance. (Reproduced, with permission, from Doherty JE: Digitalis glycosides: Pharmacokinetics and their clinical implications. *Ann Intern Med* 1973;**79**:229.)

Table 10–5. Digoxin and digitoxin serum levels.*†

	Serum Levels (ng/mL)	
	Therapeutic	Toxic
Digoxin	0.5–2.5	3+
Digitoxin	20–35	45+

*Reproduced, with permission, from Doherty JE: Digitalis glycosides: Pharmacokinetics and their clinical implications. Ann Intern Med 1973;**79**:229.
†Significant overlap may occur in electrolyte (K^+, Mg^{2+}) imbalance, thyroid disease, myocardial infarction, and hypoxia.

0.8, 1, and 1.4 ng/mL as the daily dose is increased from 0.125 mg to 0.25 mg and 0.5 mg/d (Marcus, 1975). The average levels in each group of patients receiving the respective maintenance dose are associated with a large standard deviation, indicating a considerable overlap between daily dose and blood level in different patients. In general, levels under 2 ng/mL are not likely to be associated with digitalis toxicity, whereas levels greater than 3 ng/mL are quite likely to be associated with toxic effects. Judgment is required in attempting to use the serum level as an isolated indication of toxicity (Smith, 1984). The factor most often neglected in patients receiving digitalis who develop digitalis toxicity is renal function. In patients with renal failure the half-life of digoxin is prolonged, resulting in toxic serum levels unless smaller doses of the drug are given (Fig 10–12). Thyroid abnormalities, electrolyte and acid-base balance, the severity and nature of the underlying heart disease, the patient's age and renal function, and the patient's compliance with therapy are other important factors. Serum levels must be interpreted in the light of all of the factors that might influence toxicity, including interactions with other drugs the patient may be taking. Quinidine is particularly important in this regard. When quinidine was given to patients receiving digoxin, the serum digoxin levels approximately doubled. The mean volume of distribution and the rate of renal clearance of digoxin are reduced during quinidine administration (Smith, 1984). Serum digoxin levels must be interpreted with caution in the presence of abnormalities of serum potassium. Elevated serum levels and manifestations of digitalis toxicity are apt to occur when ordinary doses of digoxin are given to patients with low serum potassium (see p 311). Serum levels are particularly helpful in patients who are unable to give a clear clinical history, especially of preceding digitalis administration, and in patients who fail to respond to the drug or seem to become toxic with only average doses of digoxin. Serum levels should be obtained roughly 6–8 hours after the last dose (Smith, 1984).

When serum levels are unusually low following average doses of digoxin (less than 0.5 ng/mL), the possibility of patient noncompliance must be considered or the possibility that the medication is not being taken as specifically instructed.

Administration of Digoxin
(See also Tables 10–3 and 10–4.)

A. Average Situation: As noted above, in the average patient with mild to moderate cardiac failure in whom digitalization is not urgent, digoxin can be given orally in an average maintenance dose of 0.25 mg/d. If the patient is old or has impaired renal function, hypothyroidism, or hypokalemia, the dose should be halved, eg, 0.125 mg/d. No saturation or loading dose is required. If after 7–10 days a therapeutic effect has not been obtained (relief of cardiac failure, slowing of the ventricular rate, diuresis and weight loss), serum digoxin levels should be measured to be certain that the patient is absorbing or taking the drug and that an adequate serum level has been achieved. If the serum level is low (< 0.8–1.2 ng/mL) and clinical improvement has not occurred, the daily dose can be increased to 0.375 mg/d for 7–10 days and the serum digoxin level again determined. If the level is still low, the maintenance dose can be increased to 0.5 mg/d. Some patients require 0.75 mg/d to produce clinical benefit without toxicity. In rare instances, even larger doses have been given, but these reports are suspect in the light of recent data on bioavailability (see above). In general, when digitalis is given, all other factors that might have a bearing on digitalis toxicity (hypokalemia, ischemia, hypoxia) should be stabilized so that a maintenance dose can be established that will be safe over a prolonged period.

If the clinical situation is more urgent, with increasing dyspnea and orthopnea, give 0.25 or 0.5 mg of digoxin every 6 hours until 1.5 mg has been given and then maintain the level with 0.25 mg every 8–12 hours until the appearance of evidence of therapeutic benefit or toxicity or until serum digoxin levels exceed 2.5–3 ng/mL. If satisfactory blood levels following a proper dose are not accompanied by adequate therapeutic effect, the dose should not be increased but the situation reassessed and other forms of treatment used (see below). As already noted, the clinical response to digitalis is not uniformly good, especially in severe cardiac failure or when failure is due to extracardiac, mechanical, or inflammatory causes. About 20% of patients given digoxin in general hospitals develop signs of toxicity, perhaps because they continue to receive progressive increments of digoxin after failing to respond to usually adequate doses.

B. More Urgent Situation: When it is necessary to obtain a digitalis effect within hours, as in pulmonary edema; or when symptomatic atrial fibrillation occurs postoperatively; or in the presence of mitral stenosis; or when the rapid ventricular rate produces dyspnea, angina, or cerebral impairment, intravenous therapy can be given, eg, digoxin, one-third to one-half of the total (1–1.5 mg) digitalizing dose every 2–4 hours, decreasing the dose by half when the ventricular rate begins to slow. At that time, oral digoxin therapy should then be instituted to avoid toxicity, which is more likely to occur when frequent doses of digoxin are administered intravenously.

Criteria of Adequate Digitalization

Digitalis is administered until a therapeutic effect is achieved (eg, relief of cardiac failure or slowing of the ventricular rate in atrial fibrillation) or until anorexia or arrhythmia appears (the earliest toxic effect). In congestive failure with normal sinus rhythm, digitalization is adequate (1) if diuresis with weight loss and loss of edema fluid occurs; (2) if cardiac size is decreased as the increased force and velocity of contraction improve the cardiac output and decrease cardiac dilatation; (3) if the jugular venous pressure and circulation time return toward normal; (4) if sinus tachycardia decreases (if the increase was due to cardiac failure); (5) if an engorged, tender liver becomes smaller and nontender; and (6) if symptoms of congestive failure subside or disappear. In atrial fibrillation, slowing of the ventricular rate to less than 80/min after mild exercise such as 5 or 6 sit-ups is usually sufficient evidence that digitalis is blocking atrial impulses in the atrioventricular node.

The most characteristic changes on the ECG following administration of digitalis are depressed sagging ST segments in a direction opposite to that of the major QRS deflection in the lead involved. This causes depressed sagging ST segments in the left ventricular leads and reciprocal elevated "reversed sagging" ST changes in the right arm lead (Figs 10–13 and 10–14). Later, especially if the serum levels are higher, the PR interval may be prolonged as partial atrioventricular block develops and the QT interval shortens as the duration of the action potential decreases. ST–T changes cannot be used as criteria of digitalis toxicity but merely of digitalis effect because they do not correlate positively with toxic symptoms or other manifestations such as arrhythmia; furthermore, they may persist after the serum levels fall to zero. Typical ST–T changes are helpful, however, in alerting the physician to the possibility that the patient has been receiving digitalis without knowing it.

Digitalis Toxicity

A detailed discussion of digitalis toxicity and an extensive bibliography can be found in Smith (1984).

A. Symptoms and Signs; Electrocardiographic Changes: In patients with cardiac failure who are otherwise in a relatively stable state, the first manifestation of digitalis toxicity is usually anorexia or mild nausea. To detect this change one must obtain a clear history of appetite before beginning digitalis therapy. If the patient is seen before each dose and the drug stopped when anorexia or mild nausea develops, more important manifestations of toxicity can be avoided, and the gastrointestinal symptoms will subside in 24 hours.

The most common important myocardial manifestation of digitalis toxicity is cardiac arrhythmia that results from enhanced automaticity and decreased conduction in the specialized automatic cells in the atria and ventricles and in the atrioventricular node. The combination leads to reentry as well as ectopic rhythms (Table 10–6). Ventricular premature beats are the most common arrhythmia occurring as a result of digitalis overdosage, but they do not usually progress to ventricular tachycardia or fibrillation unless early warnings are ignored, large doses are used, or high serum levels result from impaired renal function or other factors previously discussed.

Paroxysmal atrial tachycardia with block is probably the next most common arrhythmia; the pacemaker focus of the atrial arrhythmia is often the junc-

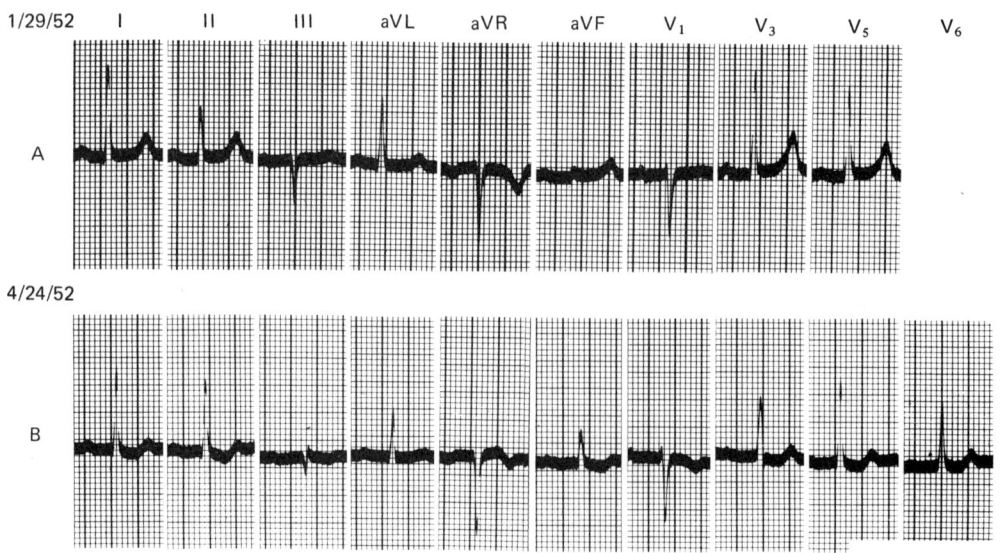

Figure 10–13. Typical sagging ST–T changes resulting from digitalis administration in a 52-year-old woman. Tracing A on 1/29/52 shows slight left ventricular hypertrophy and no ST abnormalities. The patient was digitalized on 2/12/52 and given digitalis leaf, 0.1 g 3 times daily. Tracing B on 4/24/52 shows typical ST sagging.

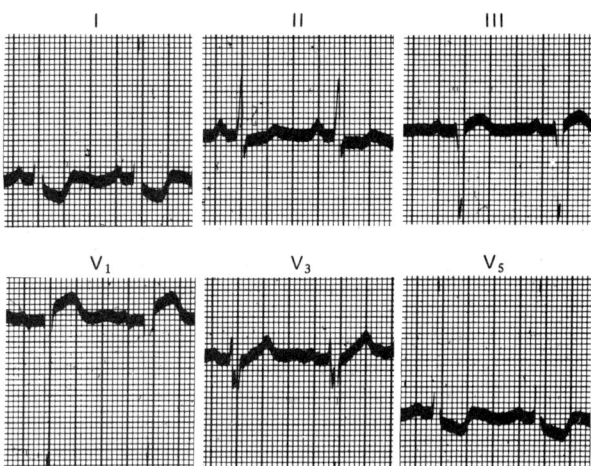

Figure 10-14. ST changes in a 56-year-old woman with left ventricular hypertrophy given digitalis. The patient had hypertensive cardiac failure. The sagging ST segments are superimposed on left ventricular hypertrophy. Note the sagging ST segments in leads I and V_6, with a relatively short QT interval.

Table 10-6. Frequency of various digitalis-induced arrhythmias in 10 series with a total of 631 patients.*

	Number of Series	Number of Arrhythmias	
Ventricular arrhythmias		470 (71%)	
Ventricular premature beats			420
Bigeminy	9		150
Multifocal	4		121
Not specified	4		79
Other (frequent, unifocal, occasional, etc)	3		70
Ventricular tachycardia	7		50
Atrioventricular block		194 (29%)	
First-degree	7		87
Second-degree	10		58
Wenckebach	3		4
Third-degree	6		37
Unspecified	2		12
Atrial arrhythmias		177 (26%)	
Atrial fibrillation	9		80
With slow rate	2		21
Paroxysmal atrial tachycardia with block	7		59
Atrial premature beats	4		27
Atrial flutter	4		11
Sinoatrial arrhythmias		85 (13%)	
Sinus tachycardia	3		29
Sinus bradycardia	4		27
With nodal escape	1		11
Sinus arrest	2		11
Sinoatrial block	3		7
Wandering pacemaker	3		11
Atrioventricular dissociation	4	65 (9.8%)	
Atrioventricular nodal arrhythmias		47 (7%)	
Nodal tachycardia			32
Nodal rhythm	2		11
Nodal premature beats	1		4

*Reproduced, with permission, from Fisch C: Treatment of arrhythmias due to digitalis. *J Indiana State Med Assoc* 1967;**60**:146.

tional tissue at the atrial-atrioventricular nodal junction. This arrhythmia is rarely seen in the absence of associated diuretic therapy with hypokalemia—in contrast to the ventricular arrhythmias and atrioventricular block that occur even when diuretics are not used (Fig 15–3).

Atrioventricular block is the third most common disturbance in rhythm in digitalis toxicity, and this is directly related to decreased conduction in the atrioventricular node, which is a cardinal electrophysiologic effect of digitalis. The atrioventricular block is usually slight, consisting only of prolongation of the PR interval, but in more severe toxicity, complete atrioventricular block may occur (Fig 10–15A and B). Digitalis also slows conduction in the sinoatrial node, and sinoatrial block with a shift in the pacemaker to the atrioventricular junction or to the lower atrium may result; digitalis excess must always be considered when sinoatrial abnormalities are present. Atrioventricular dissociation (see Chapter 14), with the atria and ventricles beating independently, is commonly the result of digitalis excess and is due to a combination of atrioventricular block and enhanced pacemaker activity in the junctional regions proximal or distal to the atrioventricular node. The atrioventricular dissociation may be intermittent, owing to a combination of only a partial defect in conduction and the fortuitous occurrence of P waves when the ventricles are not refractory. Atrioventricular dissociation may be due to acceleration of a subsidiary pacemaker in the junctional region even when the dominant sinus pacemaker is not unduly depressed or atrioventricular block present. So-called nonparoxysmal atrioventricular junctional tachycardia due to enhanced acceleration of the junctional pacemaker can occur with or without complete atrioventricular dissociation by chance capture of the ventricles, since atrioventricular block is not present.

B. Influence of Cardiac Disease on Arrhythmias: The extent and type of the underlying cardiac disease influence the likelihood of development of toxicity from digitalis. A person with no heart disease may ingest large doses of digitalis in a suicide attempt without dying or developing severe ventricular arrhythmias, yet patients with severe cardiomyopathy and cardiac failure may develop ventricular arrhythmias with only average doses of digoxin, especially if the drug is given intravenously. Changing conditions during the course of the cardiac illness may precipitate digitalis toxicity even if the dose of the drug is unchanged. These include hypokalemia resulting from diuretic therapy, hypoxia, and decreases in renal function that may follow hypovolemia or decreased cardiac output. Toxicity may therefore occur not because the drug is given incorrectly or in excessive doses but because there are other factors that must be recognized and managed.

C. Cardiac Disease Producing Arrhythmias: Cardiac arrhythmias in patients with cardiac failure do not always imply digitalis toxicity but may occur even when digitalis is not given. This is particularly true in heart failure associated with coronary heart disease, when ventricular arrhythmias may be the composite result of (1) localized ischemia; (2) variable and disproportionate duration of action potentials in adjacent fibers, with disparate refractory periods; and (3) variable conduction because of patchy myocardial fibrosis, leading to reentry or ectopic arrhythmias. The presence of arrhythmia, therefore, must not be assumed to be due to digitalis toxicity, especially at the onset of digitalis administration or if the patient is on a stable maintenance dose of digitalis when first seen.

Cardiac arrhythmias often disappear when cardiac failure is appropriately treated. Clinical judgment based on experience and careful analysis of all of the clinical findings, including serum digoxin levels, may warrant the conclusion that cardiac failure and not digitalis excess is the cause of the arrhythmia. If the reverse is the case and digitalis toxicity is strongly suspected and confirmed by serum digoxin levels, digitalis and diuretics must be stopped and the patient observed closely. If renal function is adequate and the serum potassium level is normal, digitalis-induced arrhythmias usually subside within 2–3 days.

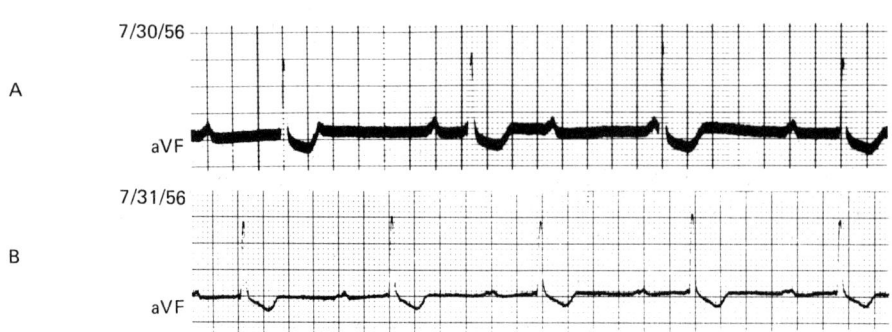

Figure 10–15. *A:* Complete atrioventricular block due to digitalis toxicity in a 60-year-old man given potassium chloride, 10 g orally daily. *B:* Partial atrioventricular block with PR interval of 0.4 second in 24 hours.

Treatment of Digitalis Toxicity

A. Initial Measures: The obvious initial step is to stop digitalis and diuretics and identify and treat conditions that increase the likelihood of digitalis toxicity: hypokalemia, hypoxia, myocardial ischemia, hypovolemia, and impaired renal function. It is usually sufficient to stop the digitalis and diuretics and observe the patient closely if there are no life-threatening arrhythmias with rapid ventricular rates, such as ventricular tachycardia or multifocal ventricular premature beats occurring early in diastole, or if these arrhythmias do not induce myocardial ischemia or hypotension or make the cardiac failure worse. If rapid ventricular arrhythmias induce severe hemodynamic abnormalities or threaten ventricular fibrillation, intravenous potassium should be infused (*not* by bolus injection) at a rate of 10–20 meq/h unless the patient has hyperkalemia or severely impaired renal function. A common method is to give 50–100 meq/L of potassium chloride in 5% dextrose or saline at a slow rate of 0.25–0.35 meq/min. If the situation is less urgent, potassium can be given orally in a dosage not to exceed 80 meq in 4–6 hours.

B. Alternative Measures: If potassium is ineffective or cannot be used, the most effective drug is phenytoin or propranolol (or its equivalent), with quinidine or lidocaine in reserve. The dosages are phenytoin, 3–5 mg/kg intravenously; or propranolol, 0.5–2 mg, at a rate of 0.5 mg/min repeated in 1–2 hours intravenously; or quinidine gluconate, 0.8 g in 500 mL dextrose, 1 mL/min; or lidocaine, 1 mg/kg every 1–5 minutes followed by an infusion of 0.5–2 mg/min.

C. Monitoring of ECG With Potassium: When potassium is given by infusion, the ECG should be monitored continuously and serum potassium levels determined. Oral therapy should be given when the infusion is stopped. The need for potassium is less urgent in the presence of atrioventricular block, and in such circumstances the drug should be used intravenously with considerable caution.

D. Temporary Pacemaker: If complete atrioventricular block is present with a slow ventricular rate—and especially if it is associated with an accelerated junctional tachycardia—a temporary endocardial pacemaker should be introduced prior to the use of drugs that depress escape pacemakers to avoid ventricular standstill and a Stokes-Adams attack.

E. Electric Cardioversion: Great caution must be exercised in the use of electric cardioversion in the presence of ectopic rhythms that may be due to digitalis toxicity, whether atrial or ventricular. Digitalis enhances the susceptibility of the myocardium to electric shock, and ventricular fibrillation may result. If the arrhythmia is life-threatening, atrial pacing with overdrive suppression of the ectopic foci is probably the treatment of choice if intravenous drug therapy as outlined above is ineffective.

F. Digitalis Antibodies: A promising new treatment for severe digitalis toxicity is the injection of digoxin-specific Fab antibody fragments. Dramatic improvement occurred in some patients in a multicenter trial (Wenger, 1985).

Prevention of Toxicity

Prevention of toxicity is obviously superior to treatment of toxicity. Digitalis toxicity is *least* in the following circumstances: (1) when the drug is used in patients in whom hypokalemia, hypoxia, and other factors influencing the half-life of the drug and hence its serum level are known and treated before the drug is used; (2) when digoxin is used in the smallest maintenance dose likely to be effective in the light of the total clinical picture; (3) when the patient during digitalization is seen daily prior to the next dose and early manifestations of toxicity are carefully sought; (4) when rapid digitalization and rapid diuretic therapy are avoided unless the clinical situation is urgent; and (5) when oral rather than parenteral preparations are used unless the indications for parenteral therapy are clear.

10. TREAT SYSTEMIC DISEASES AFFECTING THE HEART

Myxedema

Myxedema may result in a large "quiet" heart (poor pulsations), with myocardial dilatation and edema between the fibers, or pericardial effusion or a mixture of both. Myxedema is a slowly progressive disease with subtle signs that may be missed, such as slow speech, hoarse voice, and cold dry skin. Specific treatment with thyroxine is curative (see Chapter 17). In older patients, it is best to begin with very small doses and then gradually increase the dosage.

Hyperthyroidism

Hyperthyroidism may not be obvious, especially in the apathetic form in older people, but can be suspected from the "salmon skin" of increased blood flow, alert movements despite cardiac disability, and sinus tachycardia or paroxysmal atrial fibrillation. Diagnosis is not difficult, and treatment with radioiodine or antithyroid drugs (eg, propylthiouracil) is usually effective.

Cardiac failure is uncommon in younger people with thyrotoxicosis; more commonly, the increased secretion of thyroxine unmasks preexisting cardiac disease, usually coronary heart disease, and is more common in patients over 40 years of age. As a result, the response to treatment with radioiodine or thyroidectomy is not as dramatic as the treatment of myxedema heart with thyroxine; nevertheless, substantial benefits accrue from treatment of the hyperthyroidism (see Chapter 17).

Connective Tissue Disorders

Lupus erythematosus and other disorders in this group should be specifically sought because the acute vasculitis and hypertension often respond to corticosteroid therapy.

Pericardial Effusion

This must be considered because tamponade may occur, although it is not common.

Thiamine Deficiency

Beriberi heart disease is uncommon except in chronic alcoholics who eat poorly and in inhabitants of areas where famine is severe. In patients with borderline thiamine nutritional status, cardiac failure may develop when food intake is abruptly reduced or if an increased requirement for thiamine develops, such as in a febrile illness. In this situation, the patient may become abruptly breathless, and cardiac dilatation may develop, with warm extremities and evidence of high output failure. Large doses of thiamine abruptly reverse the process; within 1–2 weeks the patient may be asymptomatic, with a heart of normal size.

When chronic thiamine deficiency has resulted in chronic cardiac failure, cardiac output is reduced rather than increased, and there is no evidence of increased flow to the extremities; the clinical picture resembles that of the low output state which occurs in congestive cardiomyopathy due to alcohol. Thiamine deficiency is diagnosed by a history of inadequate thiamine intake, increased demand for thiamine (eg, fever), or a long history of high alcohol intake, and the diagnosis is confirmed by decreased urinary excretion of thiamine before and after intravenous injection of the vitamin. The response to thiamine and conventional cardiac therapy (rest, digitalis, diuretics) at this stage is slow and incomplete.

Anemia

Severe anemia, whether from blood loss, blood dyscrasias, or acute leukemia, may result in cardiac dilatation, with evidence of generalized cardiac failure such as systemic and pulmonary venous congestion, functional regurgitation of the mitral and tricuspid valves, and rarely, if the anemia is quite severe, dilatation of the aortic ring associated with an aortic diastolic murmur. Less severe anemia can produce or aggravate cardiac failure if the patient has underlying heart disease of any kind—coronary, hypertensive, or rheumatic; the decreased oxygen-carrying capacity of the hemoglobin and the increased cardiac output demanded by the anemia may precipitate cardiac failure. When anemia develops slowly, as in untreated pernicious anemia, it may be quite severe before dyspnea or other evidence of cardiac failure develops. It is of interest that when Minot was doing his pioneer work on the use of liver (orally or by crude extract) in pernicious anemia, he found dyspnea to be the cardinal indication for stopping the experiment and giving blood transfusions.

When blood is given for severe anemia, especially in the presence of cardiac failure, the patient should be closely monitored by inspection of the venous pulse, by examination of the lung bases for rales, and by auscultation for the development of gallop rhythm. The patient should be recumbent during the infusion of blood so that if fluid overload results in pulmonary edema with acute dyspnea, the patient can sit up, abruptly decreasing the pulmonary blood volume. Blood should be given slowly. If the patient needs only red cells and not plasma, then red cell mass rather than whole blood should be given if possible.

Inadvertent Rapid Administration of Sodium

The principles outlined above pertaining to administration of blood apply as well to infusions containing sodium. Acute pulmonary venous congestion and left ventricular failure may develop postoperatively in patients without intrinsic cardiac disease if intravenous saline is given too rapidly, as may happen in patients with borderline compensation or chronic cardiac disease in whom intravenous saline is given for any reason. Saline solution should be given slowly and with the same precautions as when blood is given, and the physician should consider whether dextrose and water or 0.5 N saline would serve as well.

Diseases Being Treated With Adrenal Corticosteroids

Corticosteroid therapy, especially with sodium-retaining steroids such as 9α-fluorinated compounds for postural hypotension due to autonomic insufficiency, may lead to salt retention and hypertension, increasing both the load on the heart and the extracellular volume, which may in turn lead to cardiac failure. Parenteral corticosteroids sometimes given for arthritis may unobtrusively cause iatrogenic Cushing's syndrome, with hypertension, salt and water retention, and left ventricular failure, especially in patients with underlying heart disease.

Polycythemia Vera

This is an uncommon cause of cardiac failure. The increased circulating red cell mass increases blood viscosity and impairs coronary perfusion. The diagnosis is suggested by the high red blood cell count and confirmed by the finding of a high total red cell mass with normal oxygen saturation, thus excluding chronic lung disease and secondary polycythemia.

Pulmonary Embolism

Pulmonary emboli often precipitate congestive heart failure in patients with heart disease, and the abrupt development of cardiac failure in a patient with known heart disease should prompt a search for unsuspected pulmonary emboli. Recurrent pulmonary emboli—even very small ones—may over a period of months or years cause diffuse obstructive pulmonary arterial disease and severe pulmonary hypertension. The episodes may not have been recognized, and the presenting picture is of primary pulmonary hypertension with right ventricular hypertrophy and right ventricular failure. If recurrent pulmonary emboli are recognized, anticoagulant therapy or appropriate venous ligation may prevent recurrent episodes and pulmonary hypertension.

11. WITHDRAW OFFENDING DRUGS AFFECTING THE HEART

Obtain a history of the use of medications that may cause cardiac damage or depression (see Chapter 17). Excessive sedation may not be obvious in patients taking several drugs, and some may not even know what drugs they are receiving.

Beta-Adrenergic Blocking Drugs

These compounds are probably the most frequent offenders because they are given for a wide variety of disorders, such as arrhythmias, angina, hypertension, and hypertrophic cardiomyopathy; when given to patients with incipient left ventricular failure, they may produce florid ventricular failure in hours or days. Inappropriate use of beta-adrenergic blocking drugs must be considered in every patient with cardiac failure, particularly when the onset is abrupt.

Quinidine

Quinidine has a negative inotropic action, but cardiac failure is likely to be induced only in patients with chronic cardiac disease and atrial fibrillation who are not given digitalis before quinidine. In this circumstance, the ventricular rate may rise to 150/min or more, resulting in cardiac failure as decreased diastolic filling impairs coronary perfusion. Cardiac failure was the most common manifestation of quinidine "toxicity" in the early days of its use, when digitalis was not given first, but it is now quite rare. Quinidine in toxic doses may produce ventricular arrhythmias, especially when combined with rapidly acting digitalis preparations in combination with a diuretic agent, but this is not cardiac failure per se.

Calcium Entry-Blocking Drugs

Verapamil is the calcium-blocker with the greatest negative inotropic action, diltiazem has less effect, and nifedipine has the least effect. Cardiac failure may worsen if verapamil is used, especially in combination with disopyramide or beta-adrenergic blocking drugs.

Antileukemic Agents

Daunorubicin or doxorubicin (Adriamycin) may produce cardiomyopathy and cardiac failure, especially when given in combination with other cytotoxic agents. This toxic effect is dose-related (± 500 mg) and associated with manifestations of cardiac toxicity such as changes on the ECG prior to the development of cardiac failure (see Chapter 17).

Disopyramide

This antiarrhythmic agent has a substantial negative inotropic action. About half of patients who have previously been in cardiac failure will have a recurrence when disopyramide is used. This does not occur in patients with no history of cardiac failure.

Emetine

Emetine given for amebiasis may produce electrocardiographic evidence of myocardial toxicity, but cardiac failure is rare.

Corticosteroids

See Chapter 17.

Spironolactone

In patients with impaired renal function who are receiving spironolactone, especially those who are taking potassium salts as well, hyperkalemia may develop, with resulting cardiac conduction defects and idioventricular rhythms that may induce cardiac failure. Conduction defects, however, are more common.

Digitalis

Digitalis may produce ectopic rhythms by increasing automaticity and favoring reentry arrhythmias, which may lead to cardiac failure. Similarly, it may uncommonly produce complete atrioventricular block, and the slow ventricular rate in patients with borderline compensation may result in cardiac failure.

Phenothiazines & Tricyclic Antidepressants That Have a "Quinidinelike" Action

These drugs may cause arrhythmias and cardiac failure, especially if underlying heart disease is present and failure is precipitated by the arrhythmias.

12. CONTROL ASCITES & EFFUSIONS

Thoracocentesis and abdominal paracentesis are not often required today because of the potency of the newer diuretics such as furosemide. However, large amounts of fluid in the pleural and abdominal cavities may cause severe distress, and fluid retained in cavities under increased pressure may itself, by uncertain mechanisms, trigger retention of salt and water. Removing the fluid mechanically not only makes the patient more comfortable by relieving dyspnea and abdominal distress but may also induce sodium diuresis.

The problem is more complex when cardiac failure and renal failure coexist. Some patients with renal insufficiency may be unable to conserve sodium (obligatory renal loss) and will suffer hypovolemia and dehydration, which exacerbate renal failure. Restricting sodium or giving diuretics is beneficial for cardiac failure but worsens renal failure. Conversely, if patients with combined renal and cardiac failure are given increased amounts of sodium and water to combat dehydration, overcome spontaneous sodium loss, and restore blood volume, the manifestations of cardiac failure may increase, and the patient may develop acute dyspnea with left ventricular failure or exaggerated systemic venous congestion with edema. A middle course of modest sodium restriction is safest.

13. VASODILATORS IN THE TREATMENT OF CARDIAC FAILURE

An important advance in the treatment of heart disease has been the use of vasodilators (to decrease the raised systemic vascular resistance) in the treatment of severe cardiac failure that responds inadequately to conventional therapy as outlined above. Patients with severe chronic failure require repeated hospitalizations and vigorous diuresis, leading to chronic weakness and electrolyte abnormality. The results of vasodilators have been impressive and at times dramatic.

Vasodilators were first used in severe heart failure during acute myocardial infarction or cardiomyopathy, with the response monitored in the coronary care unit (see Chapter 8). Patients with left ventricular failure and cardiogenic shock who have low cardiac output and a high left ventricular filling pressure (> 20 mm Hg) often improve when impedance to left ventricular output, elevated peripheral resistance, or afterload is reduced by vasodilator therapy. The striking benefit from intravenous nitroprusside, illustrated in Fig 10–16, led to the use of other vasodilators. The acute short-term benefits (decreased left ventricular filling pressure and increased cardiac output) followed by diuresis and clinical improvement also occur with chronic oral therapy (Cohn, 1977; Chatterjee, 1983).

Hemodynamic studies have shown that some vasodilators (hydralazine, minoxidil, calcium entry–blocking drugs) act directly on the smooth muscle of the arterioles, decreasing the afterload. Nitrates decrease the preload by dilating the venous capacitance bed. Prazosin and trimazosin reduce the afterload by blocking postsynaptic alpha-adrenergic receptors. Captopril and enalapril (so-called converting enzyme inhibitors) may inhibit the conversion of angiotensin I to angiotensin II. Vasodilator drugs may act at sites other than their dominant one, eg, nitrates may also decrease afterload; prazosin decreases preload as well as afterload; converting enzyme inhibitors decrease both preload and afterload. The choice of vasodilators depends on whether the predominant hemodynamic abnormality is raised left ventricular filling pressure or decreased cardiac output. Drugs that predominantly decrease preload are valuable in the former instance; those that decrease afterload are best in the latter instance. Vasodilators should be used cautiously if the arterial pressure is low. These agents can be given in combination with positive inotropic agents (see p 318).

Fig 10–17 shows the beneficial hemodynamic

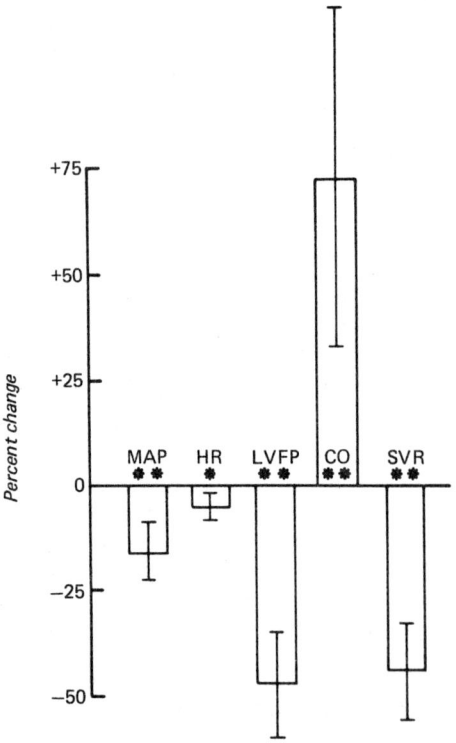

Figure 10–16. Average percentage change from control values during intravenous infusion of sodium nitroprusside in 18 patients with intractable heart failure. Vertical lines represent the standard error of the mean. MAP, mean arterial pressure; HR, heart rate; LVFP, left ventricular filling pressure; CO, cardiac output; SVR, systemic vascular resistance. **$P < 0.001$; *$P < 0.01$. (Reproduced, with permission, from Guiha NH et al: Treatment of refractory heart failure with infusion of nitroprusside. *N Engl J Med* 1974;**291**:587.)

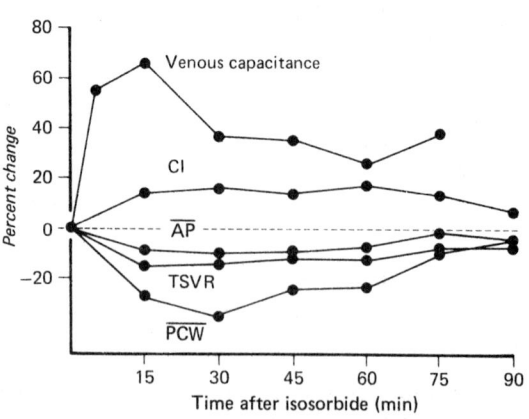

Figure 10–17. Effect of isosorbide dinitrate on 5 hemodynamic parameters over the course of 90 minutes. These data represent the mean percentage change from control values in 12 patients. A substantial increase in venous capacitance is seen at 5 min, with peak effect at 15 min. All other hemodynamic parameters have peak effect at 15–30 min. After 75 min, these effects are markedly reduced. AP, mean arterial blood pressure; CI, cardiac index; PCW, mean pulmonary capillary wedge pressure; TSVR, total systemic vascular resistance. (Reproduced, with permission, from Gray R et al: Hemodynamic and metabolic effects of isosorbide dinitrate in chronic congestive heart failure. *Am Heart J* 1975;**90**:346.)

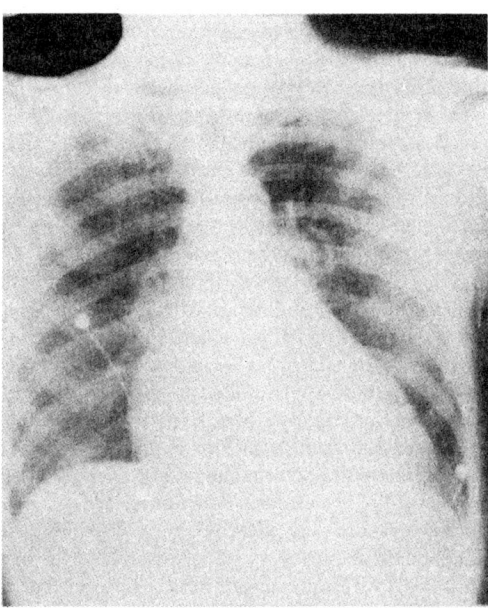 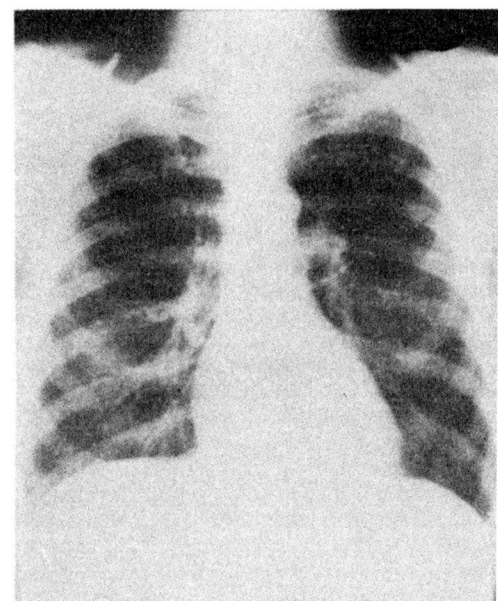

Figure 10–18. Marked decrease in size of the cardiac shadow followed 8 months of oral nitrate therapy in a patient with severe left ventricular failure. (Reproduced, with permission, from Cohn JN et al: Chronic vasodilator therapy in the management of cardiogenic shock and intractable left ventricular failure. *Ann Intern Med* 1974;81:777.)

effects of isosorbide dinitrate; there is a marked increase in venous capacitance and a more modest rise in cardiac index. Decrease in cardiac size demonstrated by x-ray (Fig 10–18) substantiates further the long-term benefit of oral nitrate therapy in severe cardiac failure. Fig 10–19 indicates that nitroglycerin ointment is also effective; transdermal slow-release patches are often preferred to the ointment (see p 316).

Vasodilator therapy in mitral and aortic incompetence reduces the regurgitant flow, improves the systolic emptying of the left ventricle, and thus increases the forward ejection fraction. Decreased left ventricular size reduces left ventricular wall tension and so improves left ventricular performance. This may benefit patients with mitral and aortic regurgitation and cardiac failure.

In Fig 10–20, the effects of vasodilator drugs are projected onto the family of Frank-Starling curves after adrenergic stimulation and in shock. It can be seen that the combination of nitrates and hydralazine (decreasing both preload and afterload) is more effective than either alone in decreasing left ventricular filling pressure and increasing the cardiac index and stroke work index (Massie, 1977).

Drugs, Dosages, & Routes of Administration
(See also Table 10–7.)

A. Sodium Nitroprusside (Nipride): Sodium nitroprusside is supplied as a powder in vials containing 50 mg for intravenous use. Solutions with 500–1000 mL of dextrose in water must be prepared immediately before administration, should not be given after 4 hours, and should be given alone without other

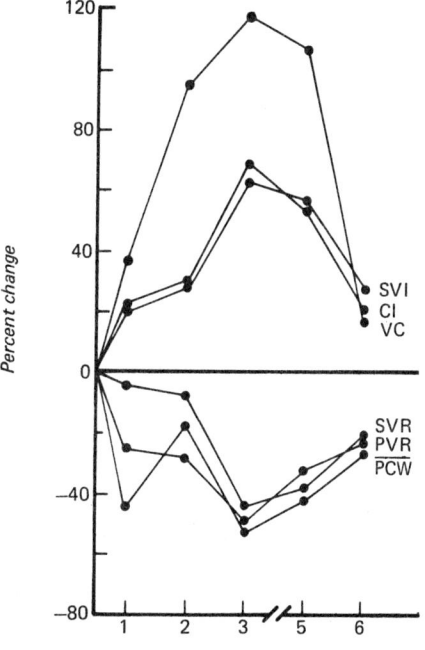

Figure 10–19. Hemodynamic changes after application of nitroglycerin ointment to the skin of a patient with severe mitral regurgitation. CI, cardiac index; PCW, mean pulmonary capillary wedge pressure; PVR, pulmonary vascular resistance; SVI, stroke volume index; SVR, systemic vascular resistance; VC, venous capacitance. (Reproduced, with permission, from Taylor WR et al: Hemodynamic effects of nitroglycerin ointment in congestive heart failure. *Am J Cardiol* 1976;38:469.)

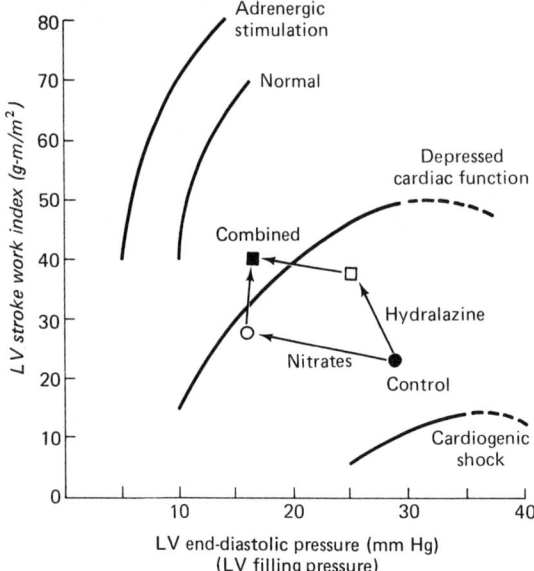

Figure 10–20. Effect of nitrates and hydralazine, alone and combined, on left ventricular performance in 12 patients with severe chronic cardiac failure projected onto the family of Frank-Starling left ventricular performance curves of Fig 10–1. (Adapted and reproduced, with permission, from Massie B et al: Hemodynamic advantage of combined oral hydralazine and nonparenteral nitrates in the vasodilator therapy of chronic heart failure. *Am J Cardiol* 1977;**40**:794.)

medication. The intravenous solution should be wrapped in aluminum foil to protect it from light and given by microdrip regulator to allow precise measurement of the rate of flow. Some patients respond much more sensitively over a wide range of flow (16–200 μg/min), and the drip rate must be individualized accordingly. Side effects of nausea and sweating occur if blood pressure is lowered too rapidly, because the drug works in seconds. Administration of sodium nitroprusside is begun at a rate of 16 μg/min and the infusion rate increased at intervals of 3–5 minutes until the pulmonary capillary wedge pressure is reduced to normal or becomes stable—provided the systolic blood pressure remains above 100 mm Hg.

B. Intravenous Nitroglycerin: Intravenous nitroglycerin is begun at a rate of 5 μg/min and is increased by 5-μg increments. The same precautions about systolic pressure apply as with sodium nitroprusside. The average maximal rate of infusion is about 50 μg/min.

Intravenous vasodilator therapy for acute disease should only be given when patients can be monitored closely (as in the coronary care unit) and hypotension can be avoided or treated. If sodium nitroprusside is used for prolonged periods, serum thiocyanate levels should be monitored to avoid toxicity. Thiocyanate is a metabolite of sodium nitroprusside, and toxicity from elevated levels of this compound (300 nmol/dL) may occur (Vesey, 1976).

Abrupt cessation of intravenous nitroprusside may cause a rebound rise in left ventricular filling pressure and a fall in cardiac output. It is best to reduce the rate of infusion slowly and add oral vasodilators when it is decided to stop intravenous nitroprusside.

C. Isosorbide Dinitrate: Give 10–40 mg orally or 5–15 mg sublingually every 4–6 hours. This drug is an effective agent in improving left ventricular performance at rest and with moderate exercise, but not at maximum exercise (Franciosa, 1979).

D. Topical Nitrates (Nitroglycerin Ointment [Nitrol] and Transdermal Nitrates): Nitroglycerin ointment (Fig 10–19) is usually applied to the skin of the abdomen, and the dose is determined by the size of the ointment strip applied to the skin. The beginning dose is usually 15 mg, or about 3.8 cm (1½ in) of the ointment strip. This is particularly valuable in patients with nocturnal angina or dyspnea, because the duration of action is 3–6 hours. Left ventricular filling pressure decreases by about one-third and cardiac index increases by about one-fourth in patients with heart failure managed in this way. Use of transdermal nitroglycerin, 5–30 mg in a slow-release patch, may supersede use of topical ointment because the patch is easier to use and is effective for 8–12 hours, whereas the ointment is effective for only 4–6 hours.

E. Hydralazine, Prazosin, and Minoxidil: (See Chapter 9.) Begin with 25 mg, 0.5–1 mg, and 2.5 mg, respectively, and gradually increase the dose, depending on the patient's response, to 25–75 mg, 2.5–10 mg, and 5–20 mg, 3 times daily, respectively. Hydralazine has proved effective for both short- and long-term treatment of chronic cardiac failure. The larger the heart in chronic cardiac failure, the better the response to hydralazine (Packer, 1980). Long-term alpha-receptor blockade with trimazosin (50–300 mg 3 times daily) has improved exercise ability and hemodynamics for a year (Weber, 1980).

F. Other Agents: Alpha-adrenergic blocking agents such as phentolamine (Regitine) can be infused intravenously at a rate of 10–40 mg/kg/min, or the drug can be used orally as for pheochromocytoma in a dosage of 50 mg 4 times daily (see pp 250–251). The left ventricular filling pressure can be reduced by a decrease in venous return and controlled hypotension by the monitored infusion of trimethaphan (Arfonad). The drug can be given as 0.5% solution (500 mg in 1 L of 5% glucose in water) by infusion pump and the dose adjusted so as not to lower the systolic pressure below 90 mm Hg.

G. Combined Preload After Treatment: A combination of nitrates and hydralazine is more effective than either alone, as demonstrated in Fig 10–20. The same is true when nitrates are combined with prazosin or when captopril is combined with hydralazine (Massie, 1983). In cases of severe failure, left ventricular performance may be effectively augmented by a combination of sodium nitroprusside infusion and infusion of an inotropic agent such as dobutamine (see p 318) or by a combination of dopamine and intravenous nitroglycerin (Loeb, 1983) (Fig 10–21). The effects of dopamine on pulmonary wedge pressure (increased

Table 10-7. More commonly used vasodilators.*

Drug	Mechanism	Route of Administration	Dose	Onset of Action	Usual Frequency of Administration	Side Effects
Nitroglycerin and nitrates	Direct vasodilator	IV, sublingual, oral, cutaneous	Wide range	Minutes	Variable	Headache, postural hypotension.
Hydralazine	Direct vasodilator	IV, IM, oral	IV and IM, 5–20 mg; oral, 25–300 mg	10–20 min even when given IV	IV and IM, variable; oral, every 6–8 h	Lupuslike syndrome, hyperkinetic circulation that may provoke ischemia; volume expansion; blood dyscrasias.
Prazosin	Alpha-adrenergic blockade	Oral	1–5 mg	0.5–2 h	Every 6–8 h	In hypertension, first-dose postural hypotension or syncope; palpitations, weakness, lassitude, tachyphylaxis in congestive heart failure.
Captopril	Converting enzyme inhibitor	Oral	Usually 25–100 mg	0.5–1.5 h	Every 8 h	Possible hypotension during acute therapy if sodium depletion is present; pruritic rash, proteinuria, rare leukopenia have been reported.
Minoxidil	Direct vasodilator	Oral	1–20 mg	1–2 h	Every 12 h	Marked fluid retention and volume expansion may be especially detrimental in congestive heart failure; hirsutism; pericardial effusions.
Nitroprusside	Direct vasodilator	IV	Start 0.5–1 μg/kg/min and titrate; only rarely, >10 μg/kg/min	Immediate	IV infusion; half-life 3–5 min	Sudden hypotension; thiocyanate and cyanide toxicity; symptoms related to sudden blood pressure reduction.
Phentolamine	Alpha blockade (? beta stimulation)	IV	IV, 0.1–2 mg/min and titrate for response; oral, 50 mg	Minutes	IV infusion	Oral form used mainly for pheochromocytoma; both forms may cause tachycardia, possibly a beta effect.
Trimethaphan	Ganglionic blockade	IV	Start 1–2 mg/min and titrate	Immediate	IV infusion	Sudden hypotension; potential tachyphylaxis after 48-hour infusion; general effects of ganglionic blockade.
Diazoxide	Direct vasodilator	IV	300 mg bolus; 50–75 mg minibolus	Immediate to minutes	Variable	Sudden hypotension may provoke angina, arrhythmias, CNS symptoms; possible hyperglycemia or fluid retention.

*Modified and reproduced, with permission, from Cody RJ: Choice and rationale for vasodilator therapy in hypertension and chronic congestive heart failure. *Cardiovasc Rev Rep* 1982;3:217.

pressure) are counteracted by the effects of nitroglycerin, which decreases pressure.

H. Converting Enzyme Inhibitors (Captopril): The angiotensin converting enzyme inhibitor captopril has been given orally in the treatment of acute and chronic cardiac failure to reduce systemic vascular resistance and plasma aldosterone levels. The drug reduces preload and afterload, maintains renal function, increases the cardiac index, and decreases the left ventricular filling pressure and diastolic volume (Kramer, 1983). *Caution* must be exercised because some patients have developed hypotension, proteinuria, rash, and leukopenia after daily doses of 25–150 mg of the drug. Renal biopsy in some of these patients with proteinuria has shown glomerular membrane nephropathy. More data are required to determine the frequency and severity of these untoward effects.

Newer converting enzyme inhibitors such as enalapril are undergoing clinical trial. Enalapril has the advantage of being more potent, has a longer duration of action, and does not have the toxic manifestations of captopril (Baim, 1983; DiCarlo, 1983).

I. Calcium Entry–Blocking Agents: Nifedipine, which has been discussed in the section on treatment of angina pectoris and coronary spasm (see p 157), is a more powerful vasodilator than verapamil; it seems promising (Elkayam, 1983). In this study, a single dose of 20–40 mg decreased systemic vascular resistance and increased the cardiac index but had no significant effect on left ventricular filling pressure in

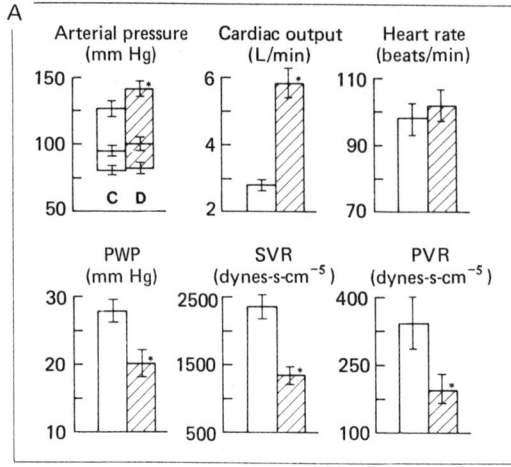 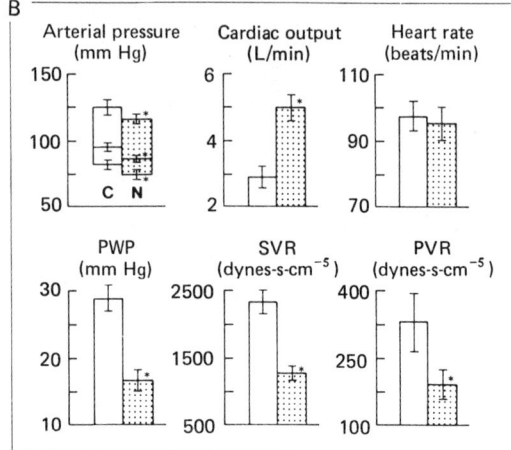

Figure 10–21. Hemodynamic response to dobutamine infusion *(A)* and to nitroprusside *(B)* in 12 cases of severe heart failure. C, control period; D, dobutamine; N, nitroprusside. Note marked increase in cardiac output, with only slight increase in systolic arterial pressure and decrease in pulmonary wedge pressure (PWP). Systemic vascular resistance (SVR) and pulmonary vascular resistance (PVR) decrease. (Reproduced, with permission, from Cohn JN, Franciosa JA: Selection of vasodilator, inotropic, or combined therapy for the management of heart failure. *Am J Med* 1978;**65**:181.)

---

patients with severe chronic heart failure. Intravenous diltiazem has beneficial hemodynamic effects in severe heart failure, but significant hypotension may occur (Walsh, 1984).

14. INOTROPIC AGENTS IN THE TREATMENT OF CARDIAC FAILURE WITH LOW-OUTPUT STATE

Experience in coronary care units and intensive care units has shown that patients with acute myocardial infarction in cardiac failure with low-output states as well as patients recovering from open heart surgery with low-output states often benefit from inotropic agents other than digitalis. Norepinephrine, isoproterenol, dobutamine (Leier, 1983), and dopamine have been used and are discussed in Chapter 8. The choice of drugs depends upon the status of the hemodynamic variables at the time, and as with the vasodilator agents, it is desirable to monitor these variables prior to treatment. Arterial pressure, left ventricular filling pressure, and cardiac output are the essential parameters to be monitored.

Norepinephrine & Isoproterenol

If the left ventricular filling pressure and cardiac index are within the normal range (LVFP, 12–15 mm Hg; CI [CO/m^2], 2.5–3.5 L/min/m^2) and hypotension is the dominant presenting clinical feature, a drug such as norepinephrine, which acts chiefly as a peripheral vasoconstrictor, can be used. If the left ventricular filling pressure is on the high side (> 15 mm Hg), norepinephrine may further increase the filling pressure and lead to pulmonary edema. Similarly, if the patient has moderate hypovolemia, continued use of vasopressor drugs such as norepinephrine will aggravate hypovolemia by disproportionate increase in venous constriction as compared to arteriolar constriction, with subsequent loss of fluid into the interstitial tissues. Isoproterenol, by producing vasodilatation, may aggravate hypotension, although it has a positive inotropic action; and if hypotension is not present, it may simultaneously decrease left ventricular filling pressure and increase cardiac output. On the other hand, it may induce ventricular premature beats and increase heart rate and myocardial oxygen consumption. As a result, coronary perfusion may be decreased following stimulation of the heart by isoproterenol.

Dopamine & Dobutamine

Dopamine hydrochloride (Intropin) and dobutamine (Dobutrex) (a relatively cardiospecific beta-adrenergic agent) have been found to be useful in the treatment of cardiac failure, decreasing both preload and afterload, neither of which occurs after digitalis therapy (Goldstein, 1980; Leier, 1983). Dopamine is the immediate precursor in the synthesis of norepinephrine and has the advantage that while it may increase cardiac output and decrease left ventricular filling pressure in low output cardiac failure, it does so without decreasing renal blood flow. Sodium and water diuresis, therefore, may be enhanced, and when dopamine is used in conjunction with diuretics, the patient with cardiac failure may improve. The effects of dopamine depend upon its dose; because it is a beta-adrenergic agonist, it may produce tachycardia and ventricular arrhythmia as the dose is increased. In larger doses it also stimulates alpha-adrenergic receptors, and a raised blood pressure may result, whereas dobutamine does not have this effect. In smaller dosages (< 10 µg/kg/min), dopamine usually does not cause tachycardia or raise the arterial pressure. As with vasodilator agents, dopamine should be started at a low rate of infusion, eg, 2–4 μg/kg/min, while the hemodynamic parameters are being monitored. The flow should be adjusted as with vasodilator agents, depending upon the hemodynamic response.

Dobutamine can be given at a rate of 10 μg/kg/min and, like dopamine, can be combined with intravenous nitroprusside or nitroglycerin in critical situations. The infusion must be adjusted depending upon the clinical and hemodynamic response (Stoner, 1977; Leier, 1983). Dobutamine is a derivative of dopamine and has a striking effect on increasing the cardiac output, with only a slight increase in the heart rate and a moderate increase in the mean blood pressure and without important side effects. Other β_1 agonists (eg, pirbuterol) as well as β_2 agonists (prenalterol and salbutamol) are undergoing therapeutic trial in congestive heart failure (Mifune, 1982; Wahr, 1984).

Experience with dopamine and dobutamine is limited, and further studies are required regarding not only their benefits but also their possible harmful effects. Digital ischemia with cyanosis and pain may occur as a result of vasoconstriction due to alpha-adrenergic stimulation from dopamine. Treatment consists of alpha-adrenergic blockade, such as the use of chlorpromazine intravenously. In a typical case, a 10-mg intravenous loading dose followed by an infusion at a rate of 0.6 mg/min (7.3 μg/kg/min) was given by Valdes (1976), with reversal of the digital ischemia within minutes. Other alpha-adrenergic blockers (eg, phentolamine, 50 mg) may be used alternatively.

Low cardiac output is common in the immediate period following cardiopulmonary bypass, and inotropic agents such as dopamine, dobutamine, and epinephrine may increase the cardiac index significantly. In one series, dopamine increased the mean cardiac index 50% (Steen, 1978).

Amrinone & Milrinone

Amrinone is a synthetic positive inotropic drug used orally in dosages of 50–300 mg (Wynne, 1984). It increases cardiac index, left ventricular ejection fraction, and effective renal plasma flow and decreases systemic vascular resistance. Despite its effectiveness in refractory cardiac failure, clinical use has been restricted because of the development of thrombocytopenia in about 20% of patients. Milrinone, an analog of amrinone, is more potent; has some vasodilator effects as well as its dominant inotropic effects; and, to date, has not caused thrombocytopenia. It has a short half-life and must be given daily in multiple doses (Wynne, 1984).

Glucagon

Glucagon, which has a variable and limited inotropic effect in therapeutic doses, has been largely superseded by the other inotropic agents.

15. INTRA-AORTIC BALLOON COUNTERPULSATION

This is discussed in Chapter 7.

16. EMERGENCY TREATMENT OF SEVERE HEART FAILURE OR ACUTE PULMONARY EDEMA

Severe heart failure or acute pulmonary edema is often a grave emergency, and treatment varies depending upon the cause and severity. For example, in a mild attack, morphine and rest in bed in the sitting position alone may suffice, although intravenous diuretics (see below) may also be required. Acute pulmonary edema may be treated with sublingual nitroglycerin, beginning with 0.4–0.6 mg and repeating the dose every 10 minutes if necessary (Bussman, 1978), or with sublingual nifedipine, 10 mg. See also Chapters 8, 9, and 12. Blood pressure should be monitored to recognize and avoid hypotension. If the attack is due to ventricular tachycardia or to atrial fibrillation with a rapid ventricular rate and the patient has severe dyspnea or pulmonary edema, cardioversion should be instituted without delay.

Intravenous nitroglycerin is the treatment of choice in acute severe left ventricular failure with pulmonary edema and severe dyspnea (as in myocardial infarction), when the wedge pressure may be high but the cardiac output is essentially normal. When the cardiac output is reduced in the presence of a high wedge pressure, intravenous nitroprusside is preferable because it dilates both arterioles and venules, whereas intravenous nitroglycerin is primarily a venodilator.

A patient who fails to respond to bed rest, digitalis, and diuretics in the hospital—and antihypertensive therapy if hypertensive—should be monitored in a critical care unit. Continuous monitoring of the ECG and intra-arterial blood pressures is required, and a flow-directed catheter should be introduced to allow intracardiac pressures and cardiac output to be intermittently observed, ie, pulmonary artery diastolic pressure or preferably pulmonary capillary wedge pressure, cardiac output by the thermodilution method, and arterial blood gases. Special nursing care is required for continuous close observation.

The patient is sedated with morphine, 5–10 mg intravenously, and placed in the sitting position, which decreases the venous return to the heart—the equivalent of venesection—and may allow an increase in cardiac output. Intravenous furosemide is given in a dosage of 40–80 mg, and oxygen with a face mask in high concentration (40–60%) and a high flow rate (6–8 L/min). Improvement should occur within an hour. Morphine relieves anxiety, depresses pulmonary reflexes, and induces sleep. Relief from forceful respiration decreases the negative intrathoracic pressure and the venous return to the heart. Oxygen relieves hypoxia and dyspnea and decreases pulmonary capillary permeability. Positive pressure breathing for short periods may be of great value, especially if there is respiratory acidosis with impaired ventilation. Positive pressure breathing improves ventilation, removes CO_2, and decreases venous return to the heart. If the patient has severe impairment of cardiac output, positive pressure breathing should be used with caution because the cardiac output may fall further. If the patient has acute bronchospasm, aminophylline, 0.25–0.5 g infused slowly intravenously, is often helpful. In addition to decreasing the bronchospasm, it may increase the glomerular filtration rate, renal blood flow, and cardiac output as well as the urinary excretion of sodium and water.

If the patient is still dyspneic or has episodic increases in dyspnea and fails to respond to the treatment given above, parenteral vasodilator agents should be added. If the situation is critical and systolic pressure exceeds 100 mm Hg, an infusion of sodium nitroprusside titrated to the response of the patient, beginning with 8–16 µg/min, can be started (see above and Chapter 8). Intravenous nitroglycerin can also be used (see above), depending on the cardiac output and systemic vascular resistance. If the situation is less critical, isosorbide dinitrate, 5–15 mg sublingually or 10–40 mg orally, can be used, and if the systolic pressure is not decreased below 100 mm Hg, sublingual nitroglycerin, 0.3–0.6 mg, or sublingual nifedipine, 10 mg, can be given. This is often of considerable value in acute pulmonary edema associated with hypertension. If the vasodilators just mentioned are not effective in relieving the dyspnea, one can add hydralazine, 50–75 mg orally or 2.5–10 mg intramuscularly, to dilate the arteriolar bed. The combination of nitrates *and* hydralazine produces both venous and arteriolar dilatation and is more effective than either drug used alone (Fig 10–20). If the patient has acute hypertensive heart failure, minoxidil, 2.5 mg, should be started, repeated in 6 hours, and the patient then reevaluated in the sitting or standing position— and the drug repeated if necessary and if tolerated without hypotension. Rotating soft rubber tourniquets are rarely used today because the agents mentioned previously are sufficient to reduce the venous flow to the heart and improve the stroke volume, whereas tourniquets decrease the filling pressure but not the cardiac index. If tourniquets are used, they should be applied with sufficient pressure to obstruct the venous but not the arterial flow and should be rotated every 15 minutes. The tourniquets should be removed gradually as the attack subsides. Venesection is infrequently used today unless the patient has acute pulmonary edema secondary to rapid intravenous infusion of sodium-containing fluids. Removal of 300–500 mL of blood is the most direct way of reducing the venous return to the heart and may strikingly increase cardiac output and decrease right atrial and peripheral venous pressure in low output cardiac failure. It should not be used if anemia is present.

If the patient remains critically ill, intra-aortic balloon counterpulsation may be added to decrease the work of the heart, as discussed in Chapter 7. Intra-aortic balloon counterpulsation is used earlier and more aggressively today than it was prior to 1974, especially in patients with acute myocardial infarction, and survival has been increased at least 2-fold, although intra-aortic balloon counterpulsation can be used in any case of severe chronic cardiac failure. Most of the patients who receive this therapy have cardiogenic shock following acute myocardial infarction (Kereiakes, 1984). A multicenter study indicated that the major complication rate is about 8%. Survival is now approximately 65% (McEnany, 1977; Scheidt, 1982).

If ventilation is impaired and acidosis is present, tracheal intubation may be helpful and further decrease the work of the heart.

If the patient does not promptly respond to the aggressive therapy described above, one should consider potentially curable causes of congestive heart failure that may require specific treatment directed at the cause, such as severe aortic stenosis, acute valvular insufficiency from infective endocarditis, severe mitral or pulmonary stenosis, severe thyrotoxicosis or myxedema heart disease, pericardial effusion, and the other conditions mentioned earlier in this chapter.

17. CARDIAC TRANSPLANTATION

Cardiac transplantation is still being performed, mainly at Stanford University, the University of Virginia, and some centers in England. The procedure has been difficult usually because of (1) legal complications in declaring a donor dead; (2) the large number of staff required for complex laboratory procedures, care, and intensive patient follow-up; (3) the high rate of complications (eg, rejection episodes requiring intensive immunosuppressive therapy for indefinite periods; severe, often fatal, infections); and (4) the relatively high mortality rate during the first year.

Because of improved selection of recipients, improved management techniques, and the use of cyclosporine, the 1-year survival rate is now approximately 65% and the 5-year rate about 40% (Pennock, 1982). Most patients surviving for 5 years have been successfully rehabilitated socially. Infection is the major cause of death.

It is difficult to accurately predict that a patient has irremediable heart disease, especially with the availability of newer medical and surgical methods of treatment (eg, more potent loop diuretics, vasodilator therapy, more potent isotropic agents, intra-aortic balloon assist devices, and left ventricular aneurysmectomy). Bedside monitoring with Swan-Ganz catheters allows more rigorous therapy than was previously safe.

The selection of patients suitable for cardiac transplantation has been narrowed to *exclude* patients over age 50 with a history of recent pulmonary embolism, pulmonary hypertension, or sepsis or with preformed antibodies against tissues of the prospective donor (Lower, 1976).

Improved management includes use of serial endomyocardial biopsies for more precise diagnosis of rejection and for guidance of treatment. Use of immunosuppressive agents (eg, cyclosporine), prednisone, and rabbit antihuman globulin has also contributed to improved survival rates.

The effort required is massive for a relatively small number of patients, but continued research may lead to simpler methods of management of patients who have undergone transplantations until a better method of treatment can be devised for the patient with otherwise unmanageable far-advanced disease.

PROGNOSIS

The overall prognosis of congestive, or cardiac, failure, while considerably improved in recent years because of the therapeutic advances discussed in the foregoing pages—especially the availability of oral diuretics, vasodilators, inotropic agents, and surgical and medical treatment of underlying causes—remains poor because treatment is often delayed until cardiac failure is far-advanced, ie, because treatable conditions such as hypertensive heart failure and valvular heart disease with heart failure are not recognized and treated early. At times, however, the basic cause (eg, ischemic cardiomyopathy or dilated cardiomyopathy) cannot be reversed, and treatment is therefore only palliative (Franciosa, 1983; Wilson, 1983).

REFERENCES

Definition & Causes

Braunwald E, Mock MB, Watson JT (editors): *Congestive Heart Failure: Current Research and Clinical Application.* Grune & Stratton, 1982.

Kannell WB et al: Role of blood pressure in the development of congestive heart failure: The Framingham Study. *N Engl J Med* 1972;**287**:781.

Hemodynamics & Pathophysiology

Aberman A, Fulop M: The metabolic and respiratory acidosis of acute pulmonary edema. *Ann Intern Med* 1972;**76**:173.

Ahearn DJ, Maher JF: Heart failure as a complication of hemodialysis arteriovenous fistula. *Ann Intern Med* 1972;**77**:201.

Bolen JL, Alderman EL: Hemodynamic consequences of afterload reduction in patients with chronic aortic regurgitation. *Circulation* 1976;**53**:879.

Braunwald E: Determinants and assessment of cardiac function. *N Engl J Med* 1977;**296**:86.

Cannon PJ: The kidney in heart failure. *N Engl J Med* 1977;**296**:26.

Curtiss C et al: Role of the renin-angiotensin system in the systemic vasoconstriction of chronic congestive heart failure. *Circulation* 1978;**58**:763.

Davis JO: The mechanisms of salt and water retention in cardiac failure. *Hosp Pract* (Oct) 1970;**5**:63.

Dodge HT: Hemodynamic aspects of cardiac failure. *Hosp Pract* (Jan) 1971;**6**:91.

Faxon DP et al: Central and peripheral hemodynamic effects of angiotensin inhibition in patients with refractory congestive heart failure. *Circulation* 1980;**61**:925.

Frand UI, Shim CS, Williams MH Jr: Heroin-induced pulmonary edema: Sequential studies of pulmonary function. *Ann Intern Med* 1972;**77**:29.

Guyton AC, Jones CE, Coleman TG: *Circulatory Physiology: Cardiac Output and Its Regulation,* 2nd ed. Saunders, 1973.

Leithe ME et al: Relationship between central hemodynamics and regional blood flow in normal subjects and in patients with congestive heart failure. *Circulation* 1984;**69**:57.

Maddox DE et al: Regional ejection fraction: A quantitative radionuclide index of regional left ventricular performance. *Circulation* 1979;**59**:1001.

Mitchell JH, Wallace AG, Skinner NS Jr: Intrinsic effects of heart rate on left ventricular performance. *Am J Physiol* 1963;**205**:41.

Parmley WW, Talbot L: Heart as a pump. Pages 429–460 in: *Handbook of Physiology—The Cardiovascular System I.* American Physiological Society, 1979.

Staub NC: The pathogenesis of pulmonary edema. *Prog Cardiovasc Dis* 1980;**23**:53.

Stein L et al: Pulmonary edema during volume infusion. *Circulation* 1975;**52**:483.

Clinical Findings

Artman M, Parrish MD, Graham TP Jr: Congestive heart failure in childhood and adolescence: Recognition and management. *Am Heart J* 1983;**105**:471.

Bedford DE: Left ventricular failure. *Lancet* 1939;**1**:1303.

Gould L, Lyon AF: Pulsus alternans: An early manifestation of left ventricular dysfunction. *Angiology* 1968;**19**:103.

Graettinger JS, Parsons RL, Campbell JA: Correlation of clinical and hemodynamic studies in patients with mild and severe anemia with and without congestive failure. *Ann Intern Med* 1963;**58**:617.

Kronenberg MW et al: Evaluation of left ventricular performance using digital subtraction angiography. *Am J Cardiol* 1983;**51**:837.

Massie B et al: Mitral-septal separation: A new echocardiographic index of left ventricular function. *Am J Cardiol* 1977;**39**:1008.

Popp RL: M mode echocardiographic assessment of left ventricular function. *Am J Cardiol* 1982;**49**:1312.

Rackow EC et al: Relationship of colloid osmotic pressure and pulmonary capillary pressure to pulmonary edema. *Cardiovasc Med* 1978;**3**:407.

Sokolow M, Katz LN, Muscovitz AN: The electrocardiogram in pulmonary embolism. *Am Heart J* 1940;**19**:166.

Wahr DW, Wang YS, Schiller NB: Left ventricular volumes determined by two-dimensional echocardiography in a normal adult population. *J Am Coll Cardiol* 1983;**1**:863.

Wayne KS: Positive end-expiratory pressure (PEEP) ventilation: A review of mechanisms and actions. *JAMA* 1976;**236**:1394.

Treatment

Armstrong PW, Armstrong JA, Marks GS: Pharmacokinetic-hemodynamic studies of nitroglycerin ointment in congestive heart failure. *Am J Cardiol* 1980;**46:**670.

Arnold SB et al: Long-term digitalis therapy improves left ventricular function in heart failure. *N Engl J Med* 1980;**303:**1443.

Baim DS et al: Evaluation of a new bipyridine inotropic agent—milrinone—in patients with severe congestive heart failure. *N Engl J Med* 1983;**309:**748.

Bank N: Physiological basis of diuretic action. *Annu Rev Med* 1968;**19:**103.

Bussmann WD, Schupp D: Effect of sublingual nitroglycerin in emergency treatment of severe pulmonary edema. *Am J Cardiol* 1978;**41:**931.

Captopril Multicenter Research Group: A placebo-controlled trial of captopril in refractory chronic congestive heart failure. *J Am Coll Cardiol* 1983;**2:**755.

Chatterjee K, Parmley WW: Vasodilator therapy for acute myocardial infarction and chronic congestive heart failure. *J Am Coll Cardiol* 1983;**1:**133.

Chatterjee K et al: (The Captopril Multicenter Research Group): A cooperative multicenter study of captopril in congestive heart failure: Hemodynamic effects and long term response. *Am Heart J* 1985;**110:**439.

Cody RJ: Choice and rationale for vasodilator therapy in hypertension and chronic congestive heart failure. *Cardiovasc Rev Rep* 1982;**3:**217.

Cohn JN (chairman): New concepts in the mechanisms and treatment of congestive heart failure. *Am J Cardiol* 1985;**55:**1A. [Entire issue.]

Cohn JN (editor): A symposium: Role of nitrates in congestive heart failure. *Am J Cardiol* 1985;**56:**1A. [Entire issue.]

Cohn JN, Franciosa JA: Selection of vasodilator, inotropic or combined therapy for the management of heart failure. *Am J Med* 1978;**65:**181.

Cohn JN, Franciosa JA: Vasodilator therapy of cardiac failure. (2 parts.) *N Engl J Med* 1977;**297:**27, 254.

DiCarlo L et al: Enalapril: A new angiotensin-converting enzyme inhibitor in chronic heart failure: Acute and chronic hemodynamic evaluations. *J Am Coll Cardiol* 1983;**2:**865.

Doherty JE et al: Clinical pharmacokinetics of digitalis glycosides. *Prog Cardiovasc Dis* 1978;**21:**141.

Dzau VJ et al: Sustained effectiveness of converting-enzyme inhibition in patients with severe congestive heart failure. *N Engl J Med* 1980;**320:**1373.

Edelman IS et al: Interrelations between serum sodium concentration, serum osmolarity and total exchangeable potassium and total body water. *J Clin Invest* 1958;**37:**1236.

Elkayam U et al: Acute hemodynamic effect of oral nifedipine in severe chronic congestive heart failure. *Am J Cardiol* 1983;**52:**1041.

Fisch CL (guest editor): William Withering: An account of the foxglove and some of its medical uses 1785–1985. *J Am Coll Cardiol* 1985;**5(Suppl A):**1A. [Entire issue.]

Fisch LC, Knoebel S: Digitalis cardiotoxicity. *J Am Coll Cardiol* 1985;**5(Suppl A):**91A.

Forrester JS, Waters DD: Hospital treatment of congestive heart failure: Management according to hemodynamic profile. *Am J Med* 1978;**65:**173.

Franciosa JA, Cohn JN: Effect of isosorbide dinitrate on response to submaximal and maximal exercise in patients with congestive heart failure. *Am J Cardiol* 1979;**43:**1009.

Franciosa JA, Wilen MM, Jordan RA: Effects of enalapril, a new angiotensin-converting enzyme inhibitor, in a controlled trial in heart failure. *J Am Coll Cardiol* 1985;**5:**101.

Franciosa JA et al: Minoxidil in patients with chronic left heart failure: Contrasting hemodynamic and clinical effects in a controlled trial. *Circulation* 1984;**70:**63.

Gavras H: Hypertension and congestive heart failure: Benefits of converting enzyme inhibition (captopril). *J Am Coll Cardiol* 1983;**2–Part 1):**518.

Goldstein RA, Passamani ER, Roberts R: A comparison of digoxin and dobutamine in patients with acute infarction and cardiac failure. *N Engl J Med* 1980;**303:**846.

Gorlin R: Congestive heart failure: Current approach. *Primary Cardiol* (Jan) 1980;**6:**84.

Gottlieb TB, Thomas RC, Chidsey CA: Pharmacokinetic studies of minoxidil. *Clin Pharmacol Ther* 1972;**13:**436.

Guiha NH et al: Treatment of refractory heart failure with infusion of nitroprusside. *N Engl J Med* 1974;**291:**587.

Henning RJ, Shubin H, Weil MH: Afterload reduction with phentolamine in patients with acute pulmonary edema. *Am J Med* 1977;**63:**568.

Howarth S, McMichael J, Sharpey-Schafer EP: Effects of venesection in low output heart failure. *Clin Sci* 1946;**6:**41.

Jamieson SW et al: Combined heart and lung transplantation. *Lancet* 1983;**1:**1130.

Kereiakes DJ, Ports TA: Intra-aortic balloon counterpulsation and the diagnosis and management of surgical complications of acute myocardial infarction. Chap 4, pp 75–88, in: *Cardiac Emergencies*. Scheinman MM (editor). Saunders, 1984.

Kramer BL, Massie BM, Topic N: Controlled trial of captopril in chronic heart failure: A rest and exercise hemodynamic study. *Circulation* 1983;**67:**807.

Leahey EB Jr et al: The effect of quinidine and other oral antiarrhythmic drugs on serum digoxin: A prospective study. *Ann Intern Med* 1980;**92:**605.

Lee DC et al: Heart failure in outpatients: A randomized trial of digoxin versus placebo. *N Engl J Med* 1982;**306:**699.

Leier CV, Unverferth DVL: Dobutamine. *Ann Intern Med* 1983;**99:**490.

LeJemtel TH et al: Systemic and regional hemodynamic effects of captopril and milrinone administered alone and concomitantly in patients with heart failure. *Circulation* 1985;**72:**364.

Loeb HS et al: Beneficial effects of dopamine combined with intravenous nitroglycerin on hemodynamics in patients with severe left ventricular failure. *Circulation* 1983;**68:**813.

Lower RR et al: Clinical observations on cardiac transplantation. *Transplant Proc* 1976;**8:**9.

McEnany T et al: Clinical experience with intra-aortic balloon pump support in 710 patients. *Circulation* 1977;**56:**249.

Maffly RH, Edelman IS: The role of sodium, potassium, and water in the hypo-osmotic states of heart failure. *Prog Cardiovasc Dis* 1961;**4:**88.

Marcus FI: Digitalis pharmacokinetics and metabolism. *Am J Med* 1975;**58:**452.

Massie B et al: Hemodynamic advantage of combined administration of hydralazine orally and nitrates nonparenterally in the vasodilator therapy of chronic heart failure. *Am J Cardiol* 1977;**40:**794.

Massie BM et al: Hemodynamic responses to combined therapy with captopril and hydralazine in patients with severe heart failure. *J Am Coll Cardiol* 1983;**2:**338.

Massie BM et al: Long-term oral administration of amrinone for congestive heart failure: Lack of efficacy in a multicenter controlled trial. *Circulation* 1985;**71:**963.

Massie BM et al: Long-term vasodilator therapy for heart failure: Clinical response and its relationship to hemodynamic measurements. *Circulation* 1981;**63:**269.

Materson BJ (moderator): Proceedings of a symposium on indapanide: A new indoline diuretic agent. April 23–24, 1982, Atlanta. *Am Heart J* 1983;**106**:(1–Part 2):183. [Entire issue.]

Mifune J et al: Hemodynamic effects of salbutamol, an oral long-acting beta-stimulant, in patients with congestive heart failure. *Am Heart J* 1982;**104**:1011.

Miller RR et al: Afterload reduction therapy with nitroprusside in severe aortic regurgitation: Improved cardiac performance and reduced regurgitant volume. *Am J Cardiol* 1976;**38**:564.

Miller RR et al: Combined dopamine and nitroprusside therapy in congestive heart failure: Greater augmentation of cardiac performance by addition of inotropic stimulation to afterload reduction. *Circulation* 1977;**55**:881.

Miller RR et al: Differential systemic arterial and venous actions and consequent cardiac effects of vasodilator drugs. *Prog Cardiovasc Dis* 1982;**24**:353.

Mungall DR et al: Effects of quinidine on serum digoxin concentration: A prospective study. *Ann Intern Med* 1980;**93**:689.

Olivari MT et al: Hemodynamic and hormonal response to transdermal nitroglycerin in normal subjects and in patients with congestive heart failure. *J Am Coll Cardiol* 1983;**2**:872.

Packer M: Vasodilator and inotropic therapy for severe chronic heart failure: Passion and skepticism. *J Am Coll Cardiol* 1983;**2**:841.

Packer M et al: Importance of left ventricular chamber size in determining the response to hydralazine in severe chronic heart failure. *N Engl J Med* 1980;**303**:250.

Packer M et al: Rebound hemodynamic events after the abrupt withdrawal of nitroprusside in patients with severe chronic heart failure. *N Engl J Med* 1979;**301**:1193.

Pennock JL et al: Cardiac transplantation in perspective for the future: Survival, complications, rehabilitation, and cost. *J Thorac Cardiovasc Surg* 1982;**83**:168.

Risler T et al: The effect of altered renal perfusion pressure on clearance of digoxin. *Circulation* 1980;**61**:521.

Scheidt S et al: Mechanical circulatory assistance with the intra-aortic balloon pump and other counterpulsation devices. *Prog Cardiovasc Dis* 1982;**25**:55.

Schwartz AB, Swartz CD: Dosage of potassium chloride elixir to correct thiazide-induced hypokalemia. *JAMA* 1974;**230**:702.

Smirk FH et al: The treatment of hypertensive heart failure and of hypertensive cardiac overload by blood pressure reduction. *Am J Cardiol* 1958;**1**:143.

Smith TW: Digitalis toxicity: Epidemiology and clinical use of serum concentration measurements. *Am J Med* 1975;**58**:470.

Smith TW, Haber E: Digitalis. (4 parts.) *N Engl J Med* 1973;**289**:945, 1010, 1063, 1125.

Smith TW et al: Digitalis glycosides: Mechanisms and manifestations of toxicity. (3 parts.) *Prog Cardiovasc Dis* 1984;**26**:413, 495; **27**:21.

Sokolow M et al: Digitalis in the prevention of recurrent cardiac failure in patients with sinus rhythm. *Ann Intern Med* 1942;**16**:427.

Steen PA et al: Efficacy of dopamine, dobutamine, and epinephrine during emergence from cardiopulmonary bypass in man. *Circulation* 1978;**57**:378.

Stemple DR, Kleiman JH, Harrison DC: Combined nitroprusside-dopamine therapy in severe chronic congestive heart failure: Dose-related hemodynamic advantages over single drug infusions. *Am J Cardiol* 1978;**42**:267.

Stoner JD III, Bolen JL, Harrison DC: Comparison of dobutamine and dopamine in treatment of severe heart failure. *Br Heart J* 1977;**39**:536.

Sturm JT et al: Treatment of postoperative low output syndrome with intra-aortic balloon pumping: Experience with 419 patients. *Am J Cardiol* 1980;**45**:1038.

Swedberg K et al: Beneficial effects of long-term beta-blockade in congestive cardiomyopathy. *Br Heart J* 1980; **44**:117.

Taylor WR et al: Hemodynamic effects of nitroglycerin ointment in congestive heart failure. *Am J Cardiol* 1976; **38**:469.

Tinker JH, Michenfelder JD: Sodium nitroprusside: Pharmacology, toxicology and therapeutics. *Anesthesiology* 1976; **45**:340.

Valdes ME: Post-dopamine ischemia treated with chlorpromazine. *N Engl J Med* 1976;**295**:1081.

Vesey CJ, Cole PV, Simpson PJ: Cyanide and thiocyanate concentrations following sodium nitroprusside infusion in man. *Br J Anaesth* 1976;**48**:651.

Wahr DW et al: Intravenous and oral prenalterol in congestive heart failure. *Am J Med* 1984;**76**:999.

Walker WG et al: Topics in clinical medicine: A symposium on uses and complications of diuretic therapy. *Johns Hopkins Med J* 1976;**121**:194.

Walsh RW et al: Beneficial hemodynamic effects of intravenous and oral diltiazem in severe congestive heart failure. *J Am Coll Cardiol* 1984;**3**:1044.

Weber KT et al: Long-term vasodilator therapy with trimazosin in chronic cardiac failure. *N Engl J Med* 1980;**303**:242.

Wenger TL et al: Treatment of 63 severely digitalis-toxic patients with digoxin-specific antibody fragments. *J Am Coll Cardiol* 1985;**5**(Suppl A):118A.

Wynne J, Braunwald E: New treatment for congestive heart failure: Amrinone and milrinone. *J Cardiovasc Med* 1984;**9**:393.

Prognosis

DiBianco R et al: Oral amrinone for the treatment of chronic congestive heart failure: Results of a multicenter randomized double-blind and placebo-controlled withdrawal study. *J Am Coll Cardiol* 1984;**4**:855.

Franciosa JA et al: Survival in men with severe chronic left ventricular failure due to either coronary heart disease or idiopathic dilated cardiomyopathy. *Am J Cardiol* 1983;**51**:831.

McGuire LB, O'Brien WM, Nolan SP: Patient survival and instrument performance with permanent cardiac pacing. *JAMA* 1977;**237**:558.

Wilson JR et al: Prognosis in severe heart failure: Relation to hemodynamic measurements and ventricular ectopic activity. *J Am Coll Cardiol* 1983;**2**:403.

11 Congenital Heart Disease (With Special Reference to Adult Cardiology)

Congenital heart disease represents the largest share of pediatric cardiologic practice. Increasing emphasis has been placed on investigation and treatment of younger patients with congenital heart lesions. Neonatal cardiology, which differs significantly from adult cardiology, is a subject of great current interest. Although it is reasonable to equate congenital heart disease in older children (6 years and over) with that seen in adults, it is not possible to devise a single description of the characteristics of congenital heart disease encompassing neonatal, infant, and adult disease. This chapter is confined to the clinical picture of congenital lesions as seen in adults and older children and does not purport to describe congenital heart disease as seen in infants.

Surgically Modified Disease

Because of the earlier diagnosis and more widespread and earlier surgical treatment, fewer patients with unmodified congenital heart lesions are now being seen in adult cardiology clinics. In their place, survivors of corrective and palliative surgical procedures are becoming the adult patients with congenital heart disease most commonly seen by cardiologists. These patients present new, iatrogenically modified, "unnatural" forms of heart disease.

The operative mortality rate has fallen dramatically in the more than 25–40 years since definitive cardiac surgery first became available for a number of congenital heart lesions, eg, coarctation of the aorta, patent ductus arteriosus, and atrial septal defect. Lesions that usually resulted in death in the fourth and fifth decades no longer carry a poor prognosis. Most of the operations performed in the early days of cardiac surgery involved adult or adolescent patients, and a number of survivors have already enjoyed life spans in excess of those expected in untreated cases.

Follow-up of patients treated surgically during infancy and childhood shows good results, but these patients are still young. Long-term follow-up over 20 years or more indicates that while many show considerable clinical improvement and often are symptom-free, few patients, other than those with patent ductus arteriosus or atrial septal defect treated in infancy or childhood, are completely normal. The problems being encountered are dealt with under the headings of the different lesions.

The types of operations performed have changed from year to year, and we anticipate seeing a wide spectrum of modified congenital heart disease in the next decade. In the past, patients with Fallot's tetralogy who had had palliative surgery (Blalock-Taussig, Potts, or Waterston operations) were the commonest examples of iatrogenically modified disease. In the 1980s we are seeing patients with other cyanotic lesions such as transposition of the great arteries, truncus arteriosus, and tricuspid atresia in addition to patients with Fallot's tetralogy who have had "total correction" of their lesions. Mention is made of patients with these modified forms of disease under the heading of each lesion.

Causes of Congenital Heart Disease

The basic causes of congenital heart disease, which occurs in about 0.9% of live births, are unknown. In Western countries, the diagnosis is usually made in the first 5 years of life. The same spectrum of congenital lesions is seen in all parts of the world, and congenital abnormalities in other systems are seen in only about a third of cases. This pattern of involvement of the heart alone suggests that disturbances in the complex embryologic development of the heart account for most of the lesions. Congenital lesions are not confined to humans and are seen in virtually all mammals.

Classification of Congenital Heart Disease

A classification based on embryologic studies has limited use for adult patients. The clinical classification used in this book gives an indication of the relative frequency with which lesions are encountered after puberty.

Not all forms of congenital heart disease are described in this chapter. The commonest abnormality—bicuspid aortic valve—which occurs in about 2% of the population, is most relevant to aortic valve disease and is described in Chapter 13. Similarly, congenital mitral valve lesions are described with other forms of mitral disease in Chapter 12, and hypertrophic obstructive cardiomyopathy is dealt with in Chapter 17, along with other types of cardiomyopathy. Rare congenital conditions that mimic valvular disease, such as cor triatriatum and sinus of Valsalva aneurysm, are also described in the valve disease chapters. Acquired ventricular septal defect is described under coronary artery disease in Chapter 8 rather than under ventricular septal defect.

The possible combinations of different forms of congenital heart lesions—eg, atrial septal defect plus ventricular septal defect, or Fallot's tetralogy plus atrial septal defect—are legion, and they will be mentioned only in passing. Each heading in the classification covers a number of forms of disease that differ in severity, anatomic detail, and pathophysiology.

ATRIAL SEPTAL DEFECT

Atrial septal defect is the commonest and most important congenital heart lesion the cardiologist is likely to encounter in adults.

Anatomic Types

The clinical syndrome of atrial septal defect covers a wide range of lesions that are often clinically indistinguishable. The anatomic sites of the different types of defects are shown in diagrammatic form in Fig 11–1. The commonest form—ostium secundum defect—involves the center of the atrial septum in the area of the fossa ovalis. The next most common—ostium primum defect—involves the lower part of the septum above the atrioventricular valves. The valves themselves are not infrequently cleft, giving rise to incompetence of the mitral or tricuspid valves. An even more extensive form of the defect results in a complete endocardial cushion defect, in which there is also a ventricular septal defect and a common atrioventricular canal. This defect is seen in about 20% of persons with Down's syndrome. A third form of defect involves the upper part of the septum and is known as sinus venosus defect. It is rare and often associated with partial anomalous pulmonary venous drainage, usually drainage of the right upper lobe into the superior vena cava. A persistent left-sided superior vena cava and anomalous venous drainage into the coronary sinus or right atrium may occur. In most cases with anomalous venous drainage, there is also an atrial defect.

Partial or complete unilateral anomalous pulmonary venous drainage to the inferior vena cava gives rise to a radiologic picture known as the **scimitar vein syndrome.** It is associated with thoracic abnormalities involving the lungs and chest wall. The patient is often asymptomatic, and the lesion is detected on chest radiography. Echocardiography is helpful in diagnosis. If the abnormal drainage is above the diaphragm, the results of surgery are better than if the vein enters below the diaphragm.

Cardinal Features & Pathogenesis

The essential feature of atrial septal defect is a left-to-right shunt of arterialized blood into the right atrium that produces a high tricuspid flow and increased blood flow to the lungs, with a normal pulmonary arterial pressure. The severity of the lesion depends in part only on the size of the defect, which can limit the size of the shunt. Atrial septal defect is often not diagnosed in infancy or childhood. At birth, the right and left ventricles are equal in size and thickness, and right-to-left shunt via a patent foramen ovale can normally occur. Whenever an atrial septal defect is present, however, left-to-right shunting is minimal at birth. With the normal decrease in pulmonary vascular resistance that follows birth, the right ventricle becomes more compliant. It then fills more readily than the left ventricle, and as a result, left-to-right shunting becomes apparent. Most atrial septal defects are large enough (2 × 2 cm or more) to equalize pressures between the right and the left atrium. Thus, the magnitude of the left-to-right shunt depends mainly on the filling characteristics of the right and left ventricles. In most cases (85%) in which the diagnosis can be made, the left-to-right shunt is at least equal to the left ventricular output, so that pulmonary flow is more than twice systemic flow. The increased pulmonary flow is readily accepted by the pulmonary circulation, so that pulmonary arterial pressure is usually low. The presence of anomalous venous drainage does not affect the clinical picture, but the presence of associated mitral or tricuspid incompetence or a complete endocardial cushion defect makes the lesion more severe.

Clinical Findings

A. Symptoms and Signs: The diagnosis of atrial septal defect is easily missed, and the examiner must maintain a high index of suspicion if all cases are to be recognized.

About half of patients with atrial septal defect are asymptomatic when the diagnosis is made. Symptoms develop in 60% of patients by age 30. The lesion is often noted in early adult life, either on routine physical examination or (more often) on a chest x-ray. The commonest presenting symptom is dyspnea on exertion (65%), followed by palpitations due to atrial arrhythmia (20%), and chest pain, which is usually not anginal in nature. A spurious past history of rheumatic fever may be present (5%). In about 20% of adult cases, the diagnosis of atrial septal defect presents some difficulty, either because the patient is middle-aged and the possibility of a congenital lesion is not considered or because the clinical picture is atypical. In about half of these cases, the patient is in right heart failure when first seen and edema and ascites tend to be more prominent than dyspnea.

Patients with Marfan's syndrome or other skeletal abnormalities (eg, Ehlers-Danlos syndrome or arachnodactyly) may also have atrial septal defects.

1. Cardiac signs–The physical signs depend on the magnitude of pulmonary blood flow. Increased right ventricular stroke volume produces a hyperdynamic right ventricular impulse with a visible and palpable pulse over the pulmonary artery in the second or third left intercostal space. A pulmonary systolic ejection murmur is almost always present because of increased flow through the pulmonary valve, but the murmur is often slight. The first heart sound is often loud because the tricuspid valve closes from a wide open position with right ventricular systole. There is relative tricuspid stenosis with atrial septal defect because the diastolic flow across the tricuspid valve is usually twice the normal value or more. In addition to the loud tricuspid first sound, there is often a right-sided third sound and a tricuspid diastolic murmur that becomes louder during inspiration. The presence

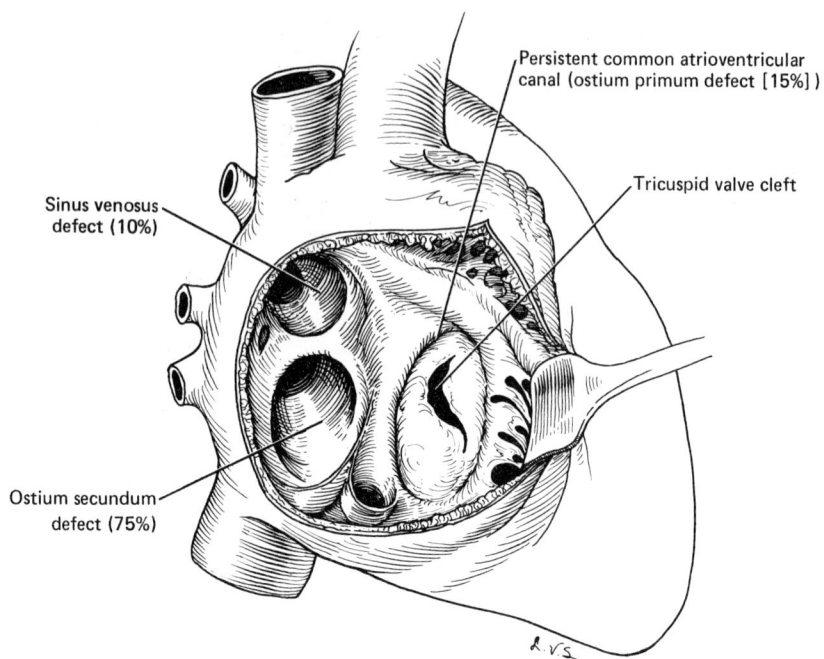

Anatomic features of atrial septal defects.

Cardinal features: *Left-to-right shunt into right atrium; high tricuspid flow; increased pulmonary blood flow; normal pulmonary arterial pressure.*

Variable factors: *Size of defect; size of shunt; anomalous venous drainage with sinus venosus defect; valve clefts with ostium primum defect.*

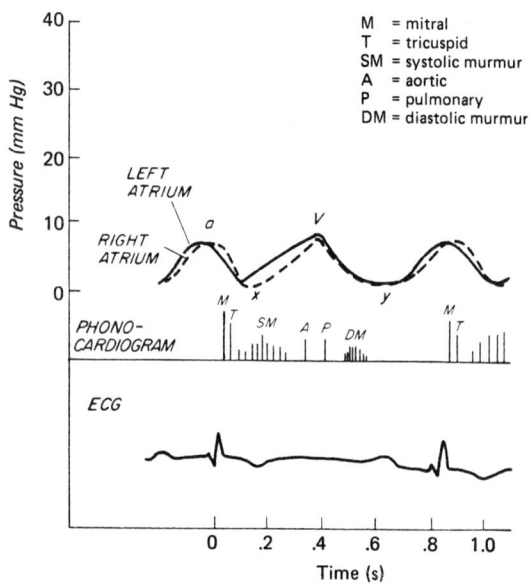

Diagram showing auscultatory and hemodynamic features of atrial septal defect.

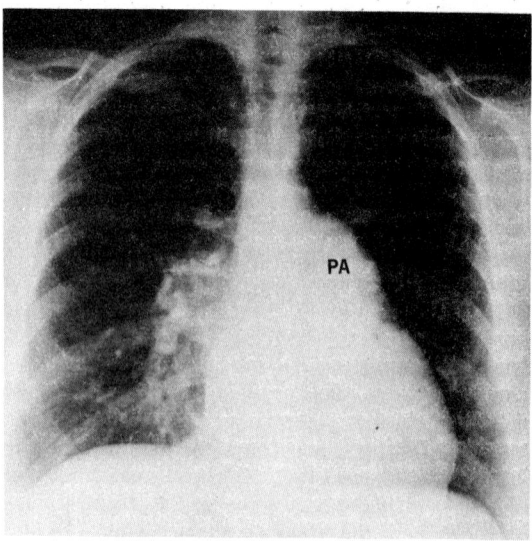

Chest x-ray of a patient with an ostium secundum atrial septal defect. The heart is large, with a prominent pulmonary artery (PA) and a small aorta.

Figure 11–1. Atrial septal defect. Structures enlarged: right atrium, right ventricle, pulmonary artery, and left atrium. Note small left ventricle and aorta.

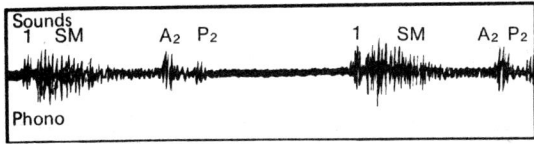

Figure 11–2. Ejection murmur (SM) and widely split second sound recorded at the upper left sternal border in a patient with atrial septal defect. (Courtesy of Roche Laboratories Division of Hoffman-La Roche, Inc.)

of a midsystolic click suggests associated mitral valve prolapse.

2. Second heart sound–The second heart sound is widely split in patients with atrial septal defect. The normal widening of the split with inspiration does not occur (Fig 11–2).

3. Ostium primum defects–In patients with ostium primum defects there may also be a hyperdynamic left ventricular impulse and a pansystolic apical murmur if mitral incompetence is present. Tricuspid incompetence is a lesion that also occurs with ostium primum defects, giving a pansystolic murmur that is best heard at the left lower sternal border. Incompetence of the atrioventricular valves can also occur in ostium secundum defects, especially when heart failure develops.

4. Pulse–The pulse is of small amplitude, and the venous pressure is normal. Atrial fibrillation commonly develops after age 40, and other varieties of atrial arrhythmia are also seen.

B. Electrocardiographic Findings: The ECG demonstrates a right ventricular conduction defect in 90% of individuals with an atrial septal defect (Fig 11–3). Because of late depolarization of the hypertrophied right ventricular outflow tract, the terminal portion of the QRS complex will be oriented anteriorly (producing an rsR' in V_1 and rightward (producing a permanent S in lead I). In 80% of patients the duration of the QRS complex is less than 0.12 second. Although the ECG has the appearance of an incomplete or complete right bundle branch block, the conduction delay is not located in the main right bundle system but rather peripherally in the myocardium.

In the 10% of patients in whom the ECG is normal, the diagnosis is more difficult. Left axis deviation in a patient with a right ventricular conduction defect (Fig 11–4) is strongly suggestive of ostium primum defect, but a normal or rightward axis does not rule out such a defect. If pulmonary hypertension develops, there will almost certainly be evidence of progressive right ventricular hypertrophy on the ECG. The presence of a tall secondary R wave in patients with conduction defects has been taken as evidence of right ventricular hypertrophy, but this sign may be due solely to the conduction defect.

C. X-Ray Findings: The chest x-ray is of great importance in the diagnosis of atrial septal defect. The heart is usually enlarged in proportion to the pulmonary blood flow, and the main pulmonary artery and its branches are dilated and stand out in contrast to the aorta, which looks small (Fig 11–1). The right atrium is more prominent in this lesion than in any other except Ebstein's malformation, and the right ventricle is also enlarged. A persistent left-sided superior vena cava is common in sinus venosus defects and can be seen on the chest x-ray (Fig 11–5).

Pulmonary plethora with increased lung markings due to enlarged pulmonary arteries and veins is common. These signs are due to increased pulmonary blood flow and are nonspecific. They are more common in atrial septal defect than in other types of left-to-right shunt because the pulmonary blood flow is so often large in this lesion.

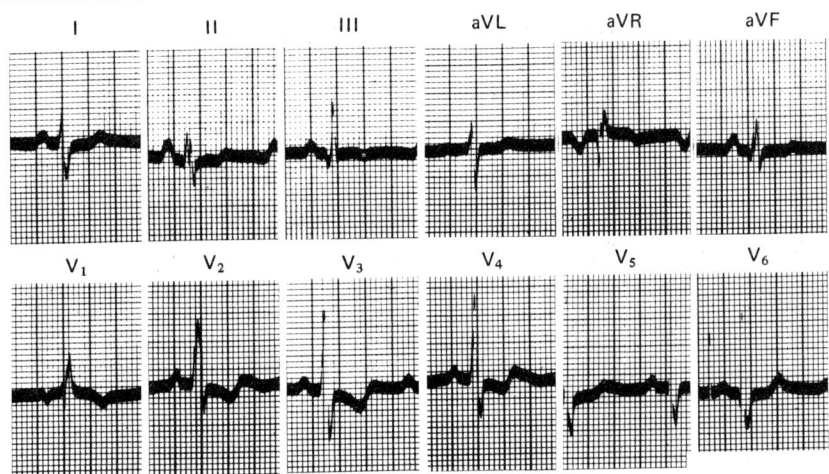

Figure 11–3. ECG from a 23-year-old woman with atrial septal defect proved by catheter. Widely split second sound and short systolic murmur at the base on phonocardiogram. Incomplete right bundle branch block with rsR' in lead V_1. Right ventricular pressure 35/0.

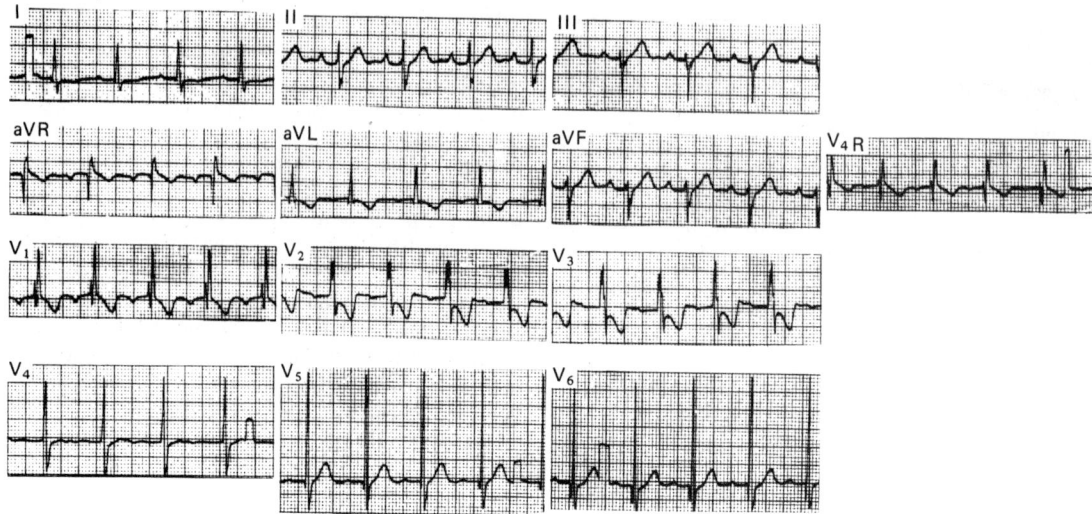

Figure 11–4. ECG of a patient with ostium primum defect showing left axis deviation and right bundle branch block. (Reproduced, with permission, from Chung EK: *Electrocardiography.* Harper & Row, 1974.)

D. Special Investigations: Although echocardiography and phonocardiography are often useful in the diagnosis of atrial septal defect, cardiac catheterization is essential for confirmation of the diagnosis.

1. Noninvasive techniques–

a. Echocardiography can be used to detect reduced or paradoxic movement of the ventricular septum as well as increased right ventricular size. These signs are indicative of increased right ventricular stroke volume, which suggests but does not specifically establish a diagnosis of atrial septal defect. Tricuspid or pulmonary incompetence can also cause this sign. Echocardiography is also helpful in comparing and detecting mitral and tricuspid valve motion (Fig 11–6). In atrial septal defect, the increased tricuspid flow causes increased excursion of valve leaflets. Echocardiography can distinguish between left and right ventricular enlargement in patients with large hearts.

Atrial septal defects are not well seen in the conventional 2-dimensional echographic views. A subcostal approach intersects the atrial septum at a more favorable angle and improves the rate of recognition of defects. While ostium primum defects can always be detected and 90% of secundum defects show up, special views and extra care are needed if sinus venosus defects are to be detected. An associated left-sided superior vena cava is readily detected by echocardiography. Combination of 2-dimensional echocardiography with Doppler studies can provide an estimate of the pulmonary-to-systemic flow ratio that correlates closely with values obtained at cardiac catheterization.

The presence of an interatrial communication can usually be established by contrast echocardiography. Forceful injection of saline containing microbubbles into the right atrium can often cause temporary right-to-left shunting and passage of the highly reflective bubbles into the left heart and aorta is readily detected. This technique can also demonstrate right-to-left shunting through a foramen ovale, especially in combination with the release of Valsalva's maneuver. Persistence of a patent foramen ovale is found in about 20% of normal adults at autopsy.

b. Radionuclear studies can be used to estimate the size of the left-to-right shunt. First-pass radioangiography with ^{99m}Tc, injected as a bolus and detected with a gamma camera, generates a time-activity curve, and computer-based deconvolution of the curve pro-

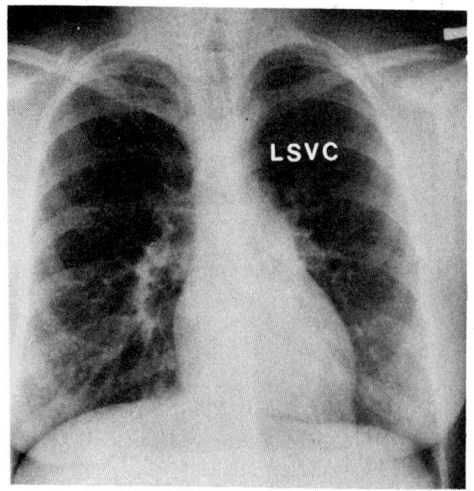

Figure 11–5. Chest x-ray of a 19-year-old woman with sinus venosus atrial septal defect with anomalous pulmonary venous drainage and a persistent left-sided superior vena cava (LSVC).

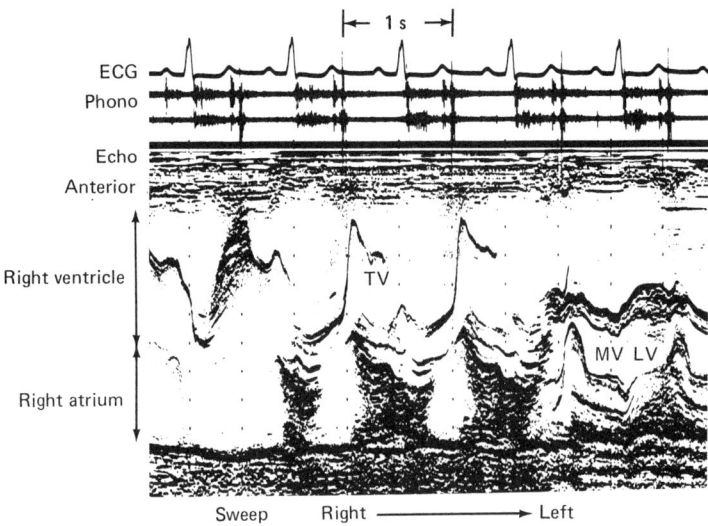

Figure 11-6. Echocardiogram showing sweep from tricuspid valve (TV) to mitral valve (MV) in a patient with atrial septal defect. The right ventricular chamber is larger than the left ventricular chamber. (Courtesy of NB Schiller.)

vides a measure of the pulmonary-to-systemic flow ratio. Gated cardiac pool scanning can also be used to measure the right ventricular ejection fraction.

2. Invasive techniques—

a. Cardiac catheterization is used in atrial septal defect to measure pulmonary and systemic blood pressure and flow and to pass the catheter through the atrial septal defect into the left atrium and ventricle. When the catheterization is performed using an arm vein, the left atrium should be entered in 85% of cases and the left ventricle in about 60%. The chances of passing the catheter across an atrial defect are better if the study is performed using a leg vein, but the pulmonary artery is more difficult to enter using the leg approach. The left and right atrial mean pressures usually appear to be equal, and the pressure difference across the defect is small and occurs mainly late in systole, before the v wave, as shown in Fig 11-7.

b. Pulmonary flow measurement—Pulmonary arterial oxygen saturation gives a rough indication of the size of pulmonary blood flow. Values between 80 and 85% indicate slightly increased flow; 85-90%, moderate increase; and over 90%, a large flow. The accuracy of pulmonary flow measurements falls as the size of the left-to-right shunt increases. The pulmonary arteriovenous oxygen difference becomes smaller, with the result that small errors in the measurement of oxygen content have a large effect on the calculated pulmonary flow.

c. Systemic flow measurement— Systemic output cannot be accurately measured in atrial septal defect because mixed venous oxygen content is difficult to measure. Some appropriately adjusted average value for superior and inferior vena caval oxygen contents must be selected to use as a value for a mixed venous sample. It is conventionally assumed that the inferior vena caval flow is twice that of the superior vena cava, and mixed venous oxygen content is considered to be one-third of the superior vena caval content plus two-thirds of the inferior vena caval content. Systemic blood flow tends to vary with age in patients with atrial septal defect. It is normal in young persons and decreases with age as atrial fibrillation and heart failure become more prevalent. The increase in pulmonary to systemic flow ratio with age is due as much to a decrease in systemic flow as to an increase

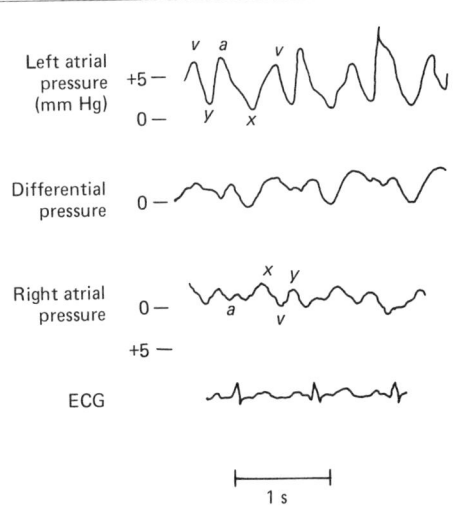

Figure 11-7. Simultaneous left and right atrial and differential pressure across an atrial septal defect. The pressure difference across the defect is greatest before the v wave. The right atrial pressure tracing is inverted because it is recorded by a differential manometer.

in pulmonary flow. The ratio of pulmonary to systemic flow is generally considered to be the best overall indication of the hemodynamic significance of an atrial septal defect.

d. Complete anatomic diagnosis of atrial septal defect cannot be established with certainty in all cases. Unexpected anomalies of pulmonary venous return may be overlooked. Recognition of ostium primum defects is important, since mitral valve surgery may be needed in addition to surgical closure of the defect. Left ventricular angiography is the best means of diagnosing this lesion. A "gooseneck" deformity of the left ventricular outflow tract is seen on a posteroanterior view of the ventricle (Fig 11–8).

e. Intracardiac pressure measurements in atrial septal defect are an important procedure, but the accuracy of tracings is poor because the hyperdynamic right ventricular contractions associated with the high flow tend to cause marked catheter fling. Right-sided pressures are usually lower than expected. Pressure differences between the right ventricle and the pulmonary artery are found in patients with markedly increased flow and in patients with associated pulmonary stenosis. If the patient presents with signs of an atrial defect, the pressure difference across the pulmonary valve is almost always less than 50 mm Hg, and surgically important pulmonary stenosis is not present.

f. Pulmonary vascular resistance should be measured in all patients with atrial septal defect. It is normally less than 2 mm Hg/L/min. It tends to be slightly raised (up to 3.5 mm Hg/L/min) in older patients with large shunts. A marked increase in resistance (7.5 mm Hg/L/min or more) constitutes a possible contraindication to surgery, and the decision whether or not to close the defect may be difficult. Right and left atrial pressures may be raised in older patients in whom heart failure has occurred, but values over 15 mm Hg are uncommon when the 2 atria are in free communication. In small defects there may be a detectable mean pressure difference between the 2 atria. A raised left atrial pressure with a significant pressure difference between the 2 atria indicates associated mitral disease. This may be either congenital, as in ostium primum lesions, or acquired, as in Lutembacher's syndrome, where it is presumably rheumatic in origin.

Differential Diagnosis

A. Rheumatic Heart Disease: Atrial septal defect is likely to be misdiagnosed as rheumatic mitral valve disease with mixed mitral stenosis and incompetence. The combination of cardiac enlargement, systolic and diastolic murmurs arising at the atrioventricular valves, and atrial fibrillation in a middle-aged woman can easily be mistaken for a rheumatic lesion, and pulmonary plethora due to increased blood flow can be confused in the chest x-ray with pulmonary congestion. If there is no rsR' pattern on the ECG, the possibility of a congenital lesion may not be considered until cardiac catheterization reveals a high pulmonary arterial oxygen saturation. The presence of a large heart with only mild symptoms and the patient's ability to easily tolerate the onset of atrial fibrillation should suggest the possibility of an atrial defect.

B. Other Lesions: Small atrial septal defects may be confused with a normal heart picture, especially in the presence of pectus excavatum, which tends to cause systolic and even diastolic murmurs and to make the heart look large on posteroanterior view. Idiopathic dilatation of the pulmonary artery may also lead to confusion. It causes a systolic ejection murmur, a widely split second heart sound, and a large main pulmonary artery on the chest x-ray, and it is often associated with an rsR' pattern in lead V_1 of the ECG.

Complications

A. Pulmonary Vascular Disease: Pulmonary vascular disease is the most important complication of atrial septal defect. In patients with ostium secundum defects, it is always acquired rather than congenital. In patients with ostium primum or sinus venosus defects with anomalous venous drainage, the congenital form of pulmonary hypertension (Eisenmenger's syndrome) occurs, in which a raised pulmonary vascular resistance is present in infancy or childhood and does not develop in later life (see p 349). Acquired pulmonary hypertension is due to the long-term effects of increased pulmonary blood flow on the pulmonary vascular bed, and pulmonary thromboembolism may initiate or aggravate the condition, especially in pregnancy. The incidence of this form of pulmonary hypertension, sometimes called acquired Eisenmenger's syndrome, is decreasing with earlier and more accurate diagnosis of congenital heart dis-

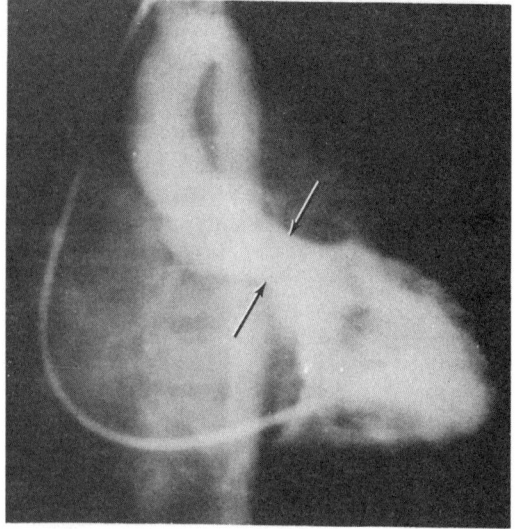

Figure 11–8. Left ventricular angiogram in a patient with ostium primum defect showing "gooseneck" deformity of the left ventricular outflow tract. (Courtesy of E Carlsson.)

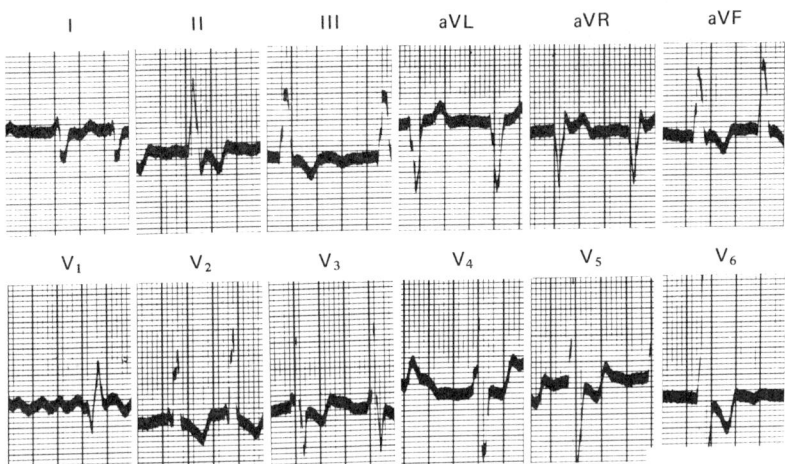

Figure 11–9. ECG of a 56-year-old woman with severe cardiac failure, pulmonary hypertension, and large atrial septal defect proved at autopsy. Tracing shows atrial fibrillation, right ventricular hypertrophy, and right ventricular conduction delay.

ease, but it still occurs in about 5% of cases. This complication is not inevitable, and patients with atrial septal defect who have been recatheterized after an interval of up to 20 years usually show no significant increase in pulmonary vascular resistance.

1. Symptoms and signs of pulmonary vascular disease–Increased dyspnea or cyanosis on exertion and intolerance of altitude are the commonest presenting symptoms. The patient may develop cyanosis and clubbing of the fingers, and polycythemia and increase in hematocrit are almost invariably found. There is usually a large *a* wave in the jugular venous pulse, and the heart is almost always greatly enlarged, with a prominent right ventricular heave. A pulmonary ejection click and a loud pulmonary valve closure sound are heard, and the second sound is closely split. The ECG shows right ventricular hypertrophy and often atrial fibrillation (Fig 11–9). Chest x-ray confirms cardiac enlargement and usually shows marked enlargement of the central pulmonary arteries. There is a progressive increase in the heart size and also in the size of the pulmonary arteries (Fig 11–10).

2. Cardiac catheterization–Cardiac catheterization shows pulmonary arterial hypertension and a pulmonary blood flow that is normal or only slightly increased. Right-to-left shunting may be present at

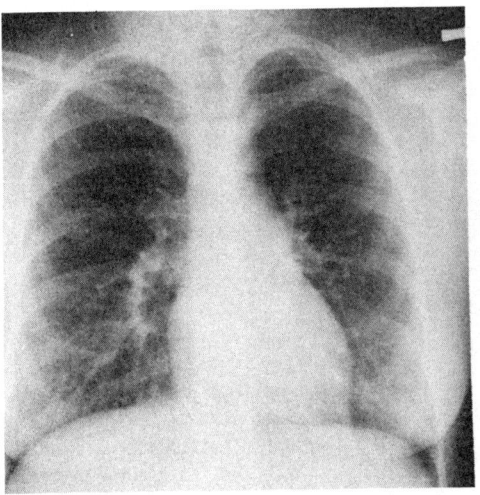 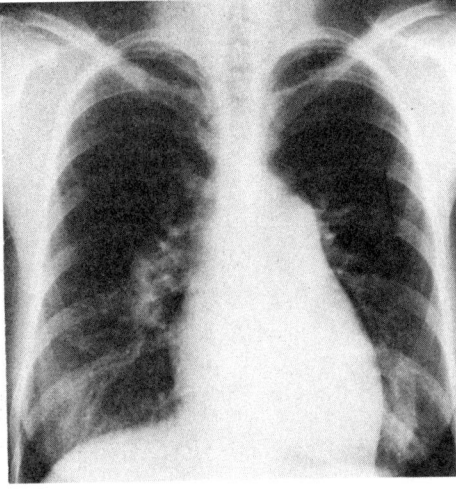

Figure 11–10. Serial chest x-rays taken 4 years apart in a 19-year-old patient with an atrial septal defect (sinus venosus) and systemic lupus erythematosus in whom severe pulmonary vascular disease developed. Heart size increased, and pulmonary arterial enlargement became more prominent.

rest, with an arterial saturation of 85–95%, or desaturation may develop during exercise. Accurate measurement of pulmonary vascular resistance, plus study of the effects of vasodilator drugs such as tolazoline (Priscoline) or acetylcholine plus oxygen breathing, is needed to decide whether surgery is warranted. Closure of the defect is likely to be successful when the pulmonary vascular resistance does not exceed 7.5 mm Hg/L/min. The magnitude of the left-to-right shunt is a factor of almost equal importance. If the pulmonary blood flow is increased, closing the defect can reduce the load on pulmonary circulation and reverse or halt the progress of pulmonary vascular disease. Surgery in advanced cases has a high mortality rate, and the results are poor because the "safety valve" of an actual or potential right-to-left shunt is removed.

B. Heart Failure: Heart failure is the other, almost equally important complication of atrial septal defect (Fig 11–11). It is usually seen in association with atrial fibrillation and is directly related to the age of the patient and the presence of a lesion interfering with filling of the left ventricle. In the natural course of atrial septal defect that is not surgically treated, heart failure probably occurs with almost the same frequency as shunt reversal due to pulmonary hypertension.

C. Atrial Arrhythmias: Atrial fibrillation and other atrial arrhythmias are almost inevitable, especially atrial fibrillation after age 40 in the absence of surgical treatment. These arrhythmias are also related to the severity of the lesion and are less common in patients with small shunts. Restoration of sinus rhythm should be postponed until after surgery in most cases, since the arrhythmia is well tolerated.

D. Other Complications: Infective endocarditis is rare in atrial septal defect. Patients with ostium primum defects are more prone to develop this complication than are those with other atrial septal defects, presumably because of valvular involvement. Mitral valve disease is an associated lesion rather than a complication. The lesion is usually mild in younger patients but tends to be more severe and readily produces congestive heart failure by reducing systemic flow and increasing the left-to-right shunt.

Treatment

Surgery is the treatment of choice in patients with atrial septal defect. Timing of the operation, the technique involved, and possible contraindications must be discussed by the surgeon and the patient.

A. Closure of Defect: Closure of atrial defects is now always carried out under direct vision during cardiopulmonary bypass. Ostium secundum defects can usually be sutured directly; the insertion of patches and baffles is likely to be needed only in ostium primum and sinus venosus defects. Although surgery almost always reduces the size of an atrial defect, residual defects may be overlooked, or the lesion may recur if stitches tear out postoperatively. Such complications are rare with open repair.

B. Relocation of Pulmonary Veins: Relocation of pulmonary veins is needed in patients with partial anomalous venous drainage. The atrial septal defect can often be sutured in such a way as to provide a tunnel through which the anomalous venous flow can be redirected without actually transecting the anomalous vein.

C. Mitral Incompetence: Suture of valve clefts, especially in the mitral valve, is the treatment of choice in younger patients. Mitral valve replacement is reserved for older patients.

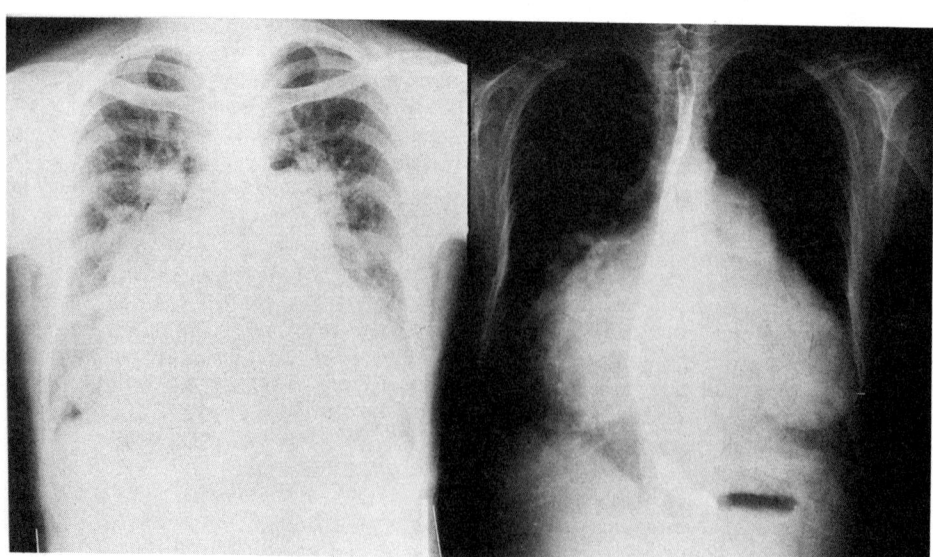

Figure 11–11. Chest x-ray with overpenetrated view and barium-filled esophagus in a patient with atrial septal defect in heart failure.

Indications & Contraindications to Surgery

Surgery is indicated in all patients with a pulmonary-to-systemic flow ratio of 2:1 or more. Smaller defects can safely be left open, especially when there is a significant pressure difference across the defect. Age is no bar to surgery. Since the operation "cures" the patient, it is recommended for asymptomatic persons. If heart failure develops, the patient should receive medical treatment with digitalis and diuretics, and surgical correction should be undertaken when the patient's condition has stabilized. A good response to medical therapy does not eliminate the need for operation. Severe pulmonary vascular disease with shunt reversal is the principal contraindication to surgery. The results of operation and the mortality rate (around 10%) are significantly worse than in patients with low resistance, in whom the mortality rate should be less than 1%. An attempt to restore sinus rhythm should be made about 6 weeks after operation in any patient with atrial fibrillation or flutter in whom arrhythmia persists.

Prognosis

The prognosis in atrial septal defect is good even without surgical treatment, and if operation is performed before symptoms develop, the patient should have a normal life expectancy. Patients with small defects who do not develop associated degenerative or atherosclerotic lesions in middle life may live long enough to die of another cause. The possibility of increasing left-to-right shunting with increasing age, the development of atrial fibrillation, and left ventricular disease are generally sufficient causes to advise surgery without waiting for signs of deteriorating cardiac function. The prognosis in ostium secundum lesions is better than that in ostium primum defects, and the development of pulmonary hypertension greatly worsens the prognosis.

Long-Term Results in Operated Cases

The long-term results after atrial septal defect closure are better than those after any other intracardiac operation. Since closure under direct vision became the rule, incomplete closure has become rare. Heart size may not return to normal if a large defect has been closed after puberty. The second heart sound may remain split and a systolic murmur may persist in spite of closure of the defect. The murmur may be either ejection in nature, arising from the pulmonary valve, or late or pansystolic due to associated mitral disease. The rsR' pattern usually persists in the ECG, and the pulmonary arteries remain large on the chest x-ray.

Right ventricular function does not always return to normal, especially in patients in whom closure of the defect is carried out in adult life. Atrial arrhythmias usually persist or recur in older patients. Most patients are symptom-free, and longevity has been shown to be increased in patients in whom operation is performed later in life.

PULMONARY STENOSIS

All forms of obstruction to blood flow to the lungs associated with an intact ventricular septum are included under this heading. Thus, patients with valvular stenosis, infundibular stenosis, and pulmonary artery stenosis of all degrees of severity are included, while Fallot's tetralogy and more complex lesions in which obstruction to the flow of blood to the lungs is associated with ventricular septal defect are described elsewhere.

Cardinal Features & Pathogenesis

The cardinal features of pulmonary stenosis include reduction in pulmonary blood flow, right ventricular hypertrophy, and a murmur at the site of obstruction. Among the variable factors that may be operating, the severity of obstruction influences the pulmonary blood flow and the extent of hypertrophy. Other factors are the site of obstruction (valvular, infundibular, or in the pulmonary artery) and the patency of the foramen ovale, which determines the presence of reversed interatrial shunt.

Various combinations of obstructive lesions are possible, and the severity of the obstruction varies. The principal load is on the right ventricle. The pulmonary artery is often dilated as a result of disturbance of flow due to the stenotic valve (poststenotic dilatation). In severe cases, a patent foramen ovale may permit right-to-left shunting at the atrial level. Pulmonary stenosis is the second most common form of congenital heart disease in adults mainly because this category includes patients with hemodynamically insignificant lesions. Two-thirds of adult cases are mild, and many could be classified as examples of idiopathic dilatation of the pulmonary artery. The spectrum of cases as shown in Fig 11–12 is wide, both because of differences in severity and because of varying sites of obstruction.

Clinical Findings

A. Symptoms: Hemodynamically insignificant or mild pulmonary stenosis does not cause significant symptoms. If a murmur has been detected, during the course of physical examination, the patient may be abnormally aware of the heart and develop noncardiac pain.

1. Dyspnea–Dyspnea is the commonest presenting symptom in patients with moderate or severe pulmonary stenosis. Its origin is obscure, and the conventional explanation of cardiac dyspnea—pulmonary congestion and reduced lung compliance—is not applicable. Patients with pulmonary stenosis tend to hyperventilate during exercise, and inadequate perfusion of the exercising muscles is thought to provoke reflex ventilatory stimulation.

2. Dizziness and faintness on exertion, palpitations, and chest pain–These may rarely be the presenting symptoms in severe cases of pulmonary stenosis. The chest pain may be indistinguishable from that of angina of effort, and the fainting attacks are

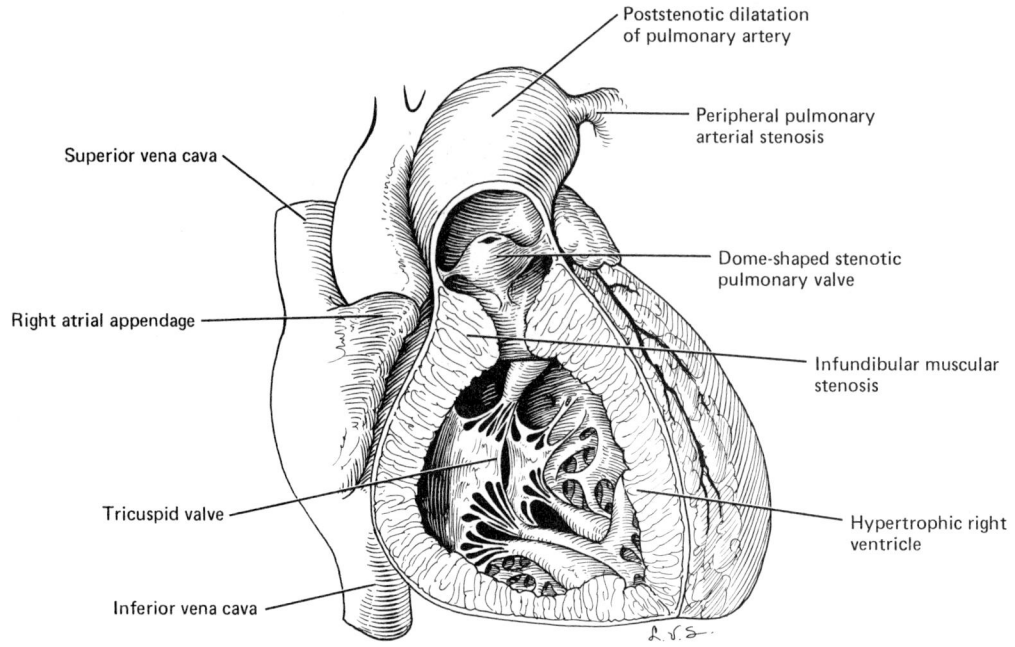

Anatomic features of pulmonary stenosis.

Cardinal features: *Reduction in pulmonary blood flow; right ventricular hypertrophy; murmur at the site of obstruction.*

Variable factors: *Severity of obstruction; site of obstruction: valvular, infundibular, or in pulmonary artery; patency of foramen ovale determines reversed interatrial shunt.*

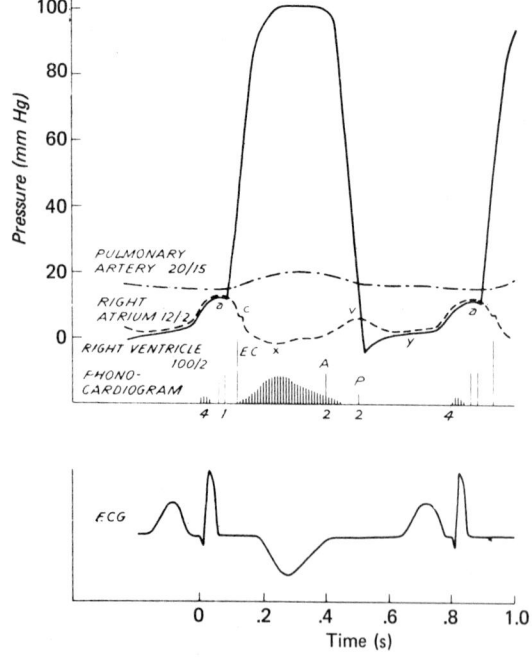

Diagram showing auscultatory and hemodynamic features of pulmonary stenosis. EC, ejection click. (Other abbreviations are explained in Fig 11–1.)

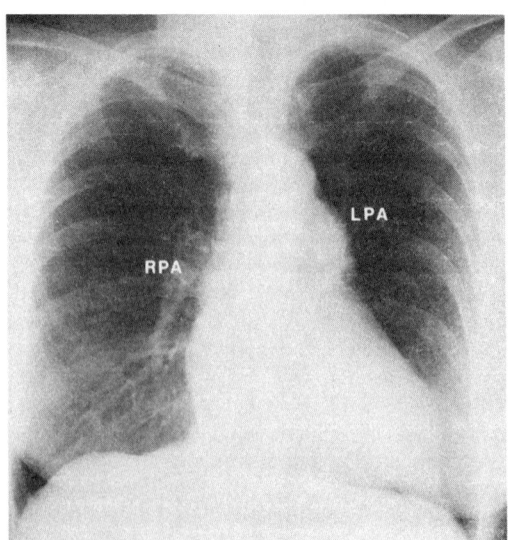

Chest x-ray of a patient with severe pulmonary stenosis showing large left pulmonary artery.

Figure 11–12. Pulmonary stenosis. Structures enlarged: right ventricle and sometimes pulmonary artery (poststenotic dilatation).

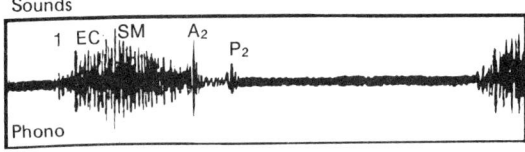

Figure 11-13. Typical phonocardiogram (recorded in third left interspace) in valvular pulmonary stenosis showing ejection click (EC), ejection murmur (SM), and late soft P_2. (Courtesy of Roche Laboratories Division of Hoffman-La Roche, Inc.)

similar to the syncope on unaccustomed effort that occurs in patients with severe aortic stenosis.

3. Right heart failure–Right heart failure often occurs in early adult life in severe cases, and if the patient has not been seen previously, the diagnosis may be difficult when the patient presents in right heart failure with an extremely low cardiac output and little or no murmur.

Female patients with Turner's syndrome characterized by 45 rather than 46 chromosomes—or male patients with Noonan's syndrome—may have pulmonary stenosis. Amenorrhea in females, hypertelorism, webbing of the neck, and short stature are seen in these syndromes. Pulmonary artery stenosis is one of the lesions commonly associated with maternal rubella.

Cyanosis is seen only in severe cases. It may be peripheral and due to low cardiac output, or central and due to arterial desaturation as a result of reversed interatrial shunt through a patent foramen ovale. In this case, it may be associated with clubbing of the fingers and polycythemia.

B. Physical Signs: The pulse is of small amplitude, and there is a giant *a* wave in the jugular venous pulse in severe cases. A right ventricular substernal heave is felt in moderate and severe cases.

A systolic murmur is always present except in moribund patients. In cases of valvular stenosis, the duration of the murmur is a function of the severity of the lesion. In mild cases of valvular stenosis, the murmur is short and diamond-shaped on the tracing.

It is preceded by an ejection click (Fig 11–13). If the obstruction is infundibular, the murmur is longer and more like the pansystolic murmur of ventricular septal defect. In pulmonary artery stenosis, the murmur peaks later and resembles the murmur of coarctation of the aorta. The loudness and timing of the pulmonary valve closure sound are valuable clues to the severity of valvular stenotic lesions. In mild cases the second sound is normally or widely split, and the split moves normally with respiration. In moderately severe lesions the pulmonary closure sound is delayed, occurring up to 0.1 second after aortic closure. It is also diminished in intensity because pulmonary blood flow tends to be low, but it still moves with inspiration (Fig 11–14). In severe cases the pulmonary valve closure sound is inaudible, and even aortic closure may not be heard because the sound is buried in the long pulmonary systolic murmur that results from prolonged contraction of the overloaded right ventricle. Pulmonary diastolic murmurs are uncommon before surgery, but pulmonary incompetence not infrequently follows valvotomy. In pulmonary artery stenosis the auscultatory findings can be confused with those of pulmonary hypertension because pulmonary valve closure is usually loud and often palpable and the second sound is often split.

C. Electrocardiographic Findings: Right ventricular hypertrophy in pulmonary stenosis is proportionate to the severity of the obstruction to right ventricular outflow. In mild cases the ECG shows only slight right ventricular dominance, whereas at the other end of the spectrum, severe pulmonary stenosis produces some of the most striking examples of right ventricular hypertrophy (Fig 11–15). Tall peaked P waves seen in severe cases are evidence of right atrial enlargement, and right bundle branch block sometimes occurs.

D. X-Ray Findings: The heart is of normal size in mild cases. Even in moderate to severe cases, cardiac enlargement may be absent because hypertrophy of the right ventricle occurs at the expense of the cavity of the ventricle. If the patient develops right ventricular failure, however, cardiac enlargement involving the right ventricle and right atrium always occurs. The main pulmonary artery and left pulmo-

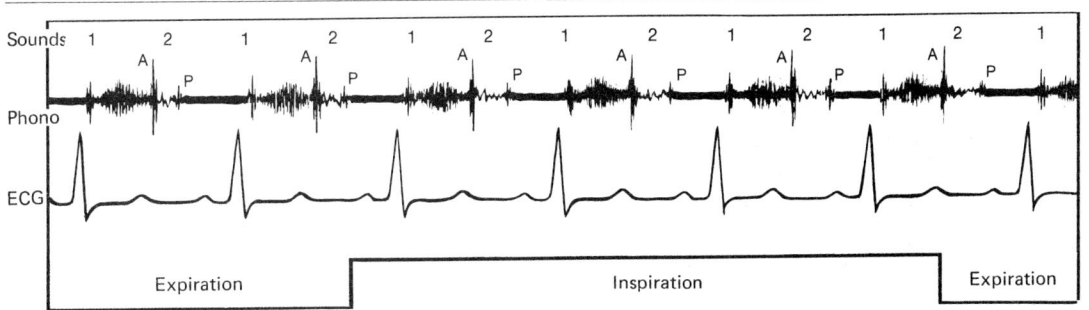

Figure 11-14. Phonocardiogram showing ejection murmur and soft late P_2—later still on inspiration—in pulmonary stenosis. (Courtesy of Roche Laboratories Division of Hoffman-La Roche, Inc.)

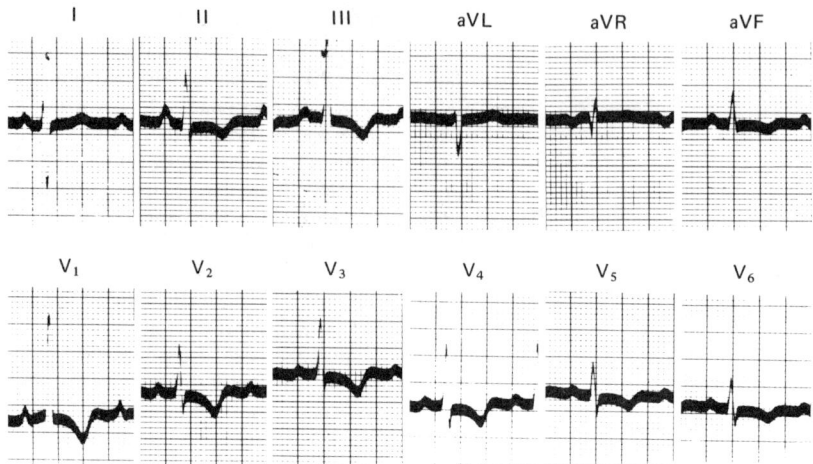

Figure 11-15. ECG of 25-year-old woman with pulmonary stenosis, patent interatrial septum, and cyanosis. Right ventricle, 1.5 cm; left ventricle, 1.1 cm. Normal coronary arteries. The tracing shows severe right ventricular hypertrophy.

nary artery are commonly enlarged when the lesion is valvular. Poststenotic dilatation does not involve the right pulmonary artery, which is smaller and lies lower in the chest than the left pulmonary artery, as shown in Fig 11–12. Pulmonary arterial dilatation is unrelated to the severity of stenosis, and in cases with insignificant lesions, the main pulmonary artery may be markedly dilated. In such cases a diagnosis of idiopathic dilatation of the pulmonary artery is sometimes made, and it is not clear if a distinction can or should be made between hemodynamically insignificant pulmonary stenosis and idiopathic dilatation of the pulmonary artery. Both lesions are equally benign and are seldom if ever associated with symptoms. In infundibular lesions the pulmonary artery is not dilated. If the obstruction is severe, the configuration of the heart resembles that seen in Fallot's tetralogy with infundibular obstruction (see p 338). If the obstruction is in the pulmonary arteries, the main pulmonary artery is usually dilated. In any severe obstructive lesion the pulmonary blood flow is reduced, and the lung markings are abnormally sparse.

E. Special Investigations:

1. Noninvasive techniques–Phonocardiography can be useful in establishing the timing and intensity of the pulmonary valve closure sound and demonstrating the length of the murmur. In severe cases, phonocardiography often makes it easier to detect that aortic valve closure is buried in a long systolic murmur.

Echocardiography is not always helpful in identifying the site of obstruction in pulmonary stenosis or in assessing its severity. The pulmonary valve is the most difficult valve to examine echographically, and the thickness of the valve does not always indicate the severity of the obstruction.

2. Invasive techniques–The definitive technique for diagnosis and assessment of severity of pulmonary stenosis is cardiac catheterization. Measurement of pulmonary arterial and right ventricular pressures and pulmonary blood flow is needed to establish the diagnosis and severity of the stenosis. The anatomic site of the stenosis can usually be established by drawing the catheter from the pulmonary artery to the right atrium through the right ventricle and closely following the pressure changes. A sample tracing of pulmonary arterial and right ventricular pressures is shown in Fig 11–16. In patients with high infundibular lesions and those with both valvular and infundibular stenosis, angiography may be needed to establish the site of obstruction. Angiography is also valuable in differentiating pulmonary stenosis from Fallot's tetralogy.

Differential Diagnosis

The differential diagnosis of pulmonary stenosis depends on the severity of the lesion and on the anatomic level of the stenosis.

A. Atrial Septal Defect: Mild valvular lesions can resemble or be associated with an atrial septal defect. The systolic murmur and widely split second sound are common to both lesions.

B. Ventricular Septal Defect: Infundibular stenosis may be confused with a small ventricular septal defect because both lesions have a loud, long systolic murmur, best heard to the left of the sternum.

C. Pulmonary Hypertension: Pulmonary artery stenosis tends to be confused with primary pulmonary hypertension or with Eisenmenger's syndrome. The pressure in the main pulmonary artery is raised in these conditions, and the loud second heart sound and evidence of right ventricular overload are common to all of them. Cardiac catheterization is necessary to establish the diagnosis.

D. Fallot's Tetralogy: When the pulmonary stenosis is moderate or severe and at the valvular or infundibular level, Fallot's tetralogy is the most important differential diagnosis. The ready fall in arterial oxygen saturation with exercise or amyl nitrite

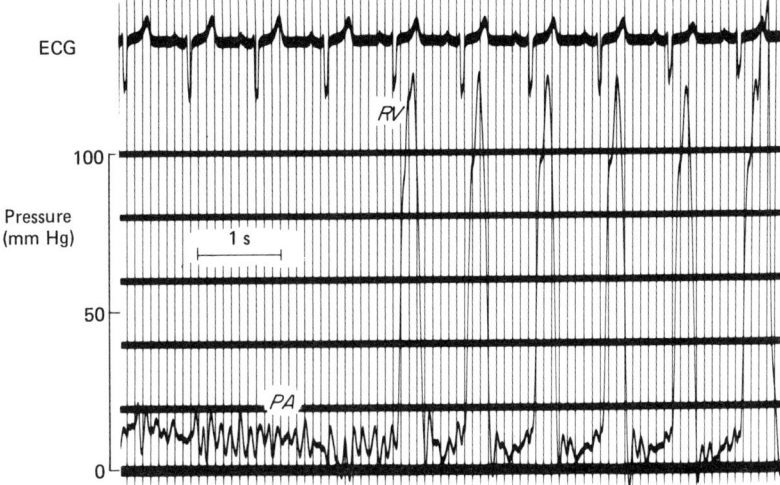

Figure 11-16. Pressure tracing showing withdrawal of a catheter across a stenotic pulmonary valve. PA, pulmonary artery; RV, right ventricle.

inhalation is perhaps the clearest point suggesting a diagnosis of Fallot's tetralogy.

Complications

A. Right Heart Failure: Right heart failure is an important late complication of moderate or severe pulmonary stenosis. It almost inevitably occurs immediately after surgical treatment of the lesion, and the postoperative course in adult patients is often difficult.

B. Infective Endocarditis: Infective endocarditis occurs in under 5% of cases of pulmonary stenosis and has a good prognosis because valvular damage is seldom severe.

C. Valvular Calcification and Incompetence: Valvular calcification and incompetence can occur with advancing age and are more likely after valvotomy.

D. Pulmonary Thrombosis and Embolism: Pulmonary thrombosis and embolism tend to occur in severe cases in which pulmonary blood flow is reduced. They may cause an increase in pulmonary vascular resistance in older patients. If this is the case, surgical relief of the stenosis does not bring complete relief.

Treatment

Insignificant and mild lesions run a benign course. An example of a chest x-ray that was indistinguishable from another taken 30 years later is shown in Fig 11-17. No treatment is needed, but the patient should be followed and seen at intervals. Antibiotic prophylaxis (see Chapter 16) for the prevention of endocarditis is necessary in both idiopathic dilatation of the pulmonary artery and mild pulmonary stenosis, even though this complication is rare.

Surgery is recommended when the pressure difference between the right ventricle and the pulmonary artery is more than 60 mm Hg, with a normal pulmonary blood flow. With pressure differences in the range of 40–60 mm Hg, other considerations such as heart size, age, and associated lesions influence the decision for or against surgery.

Valvular lesions are more amenable to surgical treatment than are infundibular or supravalvular lesions. Pulmonary artery stenoses may be multiple and so far distal that they are inaccessible. Surgical treatment of valvular stenosis may not relieve the obstruction to right ventricular outflow because bands of hypertrophied muscle in the outflow tract may form a sec-

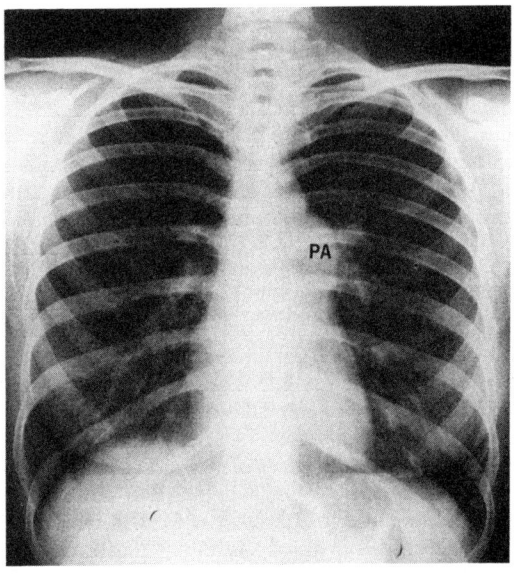

Figure 11-17. Chest x-ray of a 28-year-old woman with a dilated pulmonary artery (PA). Another chest x-ray taken 30 years later showed no change in the size of the heart or the pulmonary artery.

ondary obstruction, which persists when the primary valvular lesion is relieved.

Percutaneous balloon valvuloplasty, using the technique devised by Gruentzig (Grüntzig) (see Chapter 6), has recently been introduced. A balloon 4 cm long is inflated in the valve for about 10 seconds on several occasions. No ill effects have been reported, and success, as measured by reduction in right ventricular pressure and increase in pulmonary artery pressure with no change in cardiac output, is consistently reported. A similar technique can be used in pulmonary artery stenosis.

Prognosis

The prognosis in pulmonary stenosis is directly related to the severity of the lesion. The surgical mortality rate is negligibly low in moderate lesions but rises to about 10% when right ventricular pressure is at or above systemic level. The truly long-term (30- to 40-year) prognosis of patients operated on in infancy and childhood has yet to be determined.

Long-Term Problems in Operated Cases

Failure to resect sufficient muscle may result in residual obstruction; or conversely, excessive resection may weaken the outflow tract of the right ventricle and lead to aneurysm formation. Right ventricular failure is the commonest long-term problem in patients with pulmonary stenosis and may occur as a result of incomplete relief of obstruction or the long-term effects of surgically produced pulmonary incompetence. Calcification of the pulmonary valve may occur with time, and since surgical treatment usually consists of opening up a dome-shaped valve that bears no cusps, the valve is inevitably abnormal after operation. If the analogy between congenital aortic stenosis and congenital pulmonary stenosis is appropriate, it is likely that pulmonary valve replacement will be needed in later life, especially if valvular calcification occurs.

FALLOT'S TETRALOGY

Cardinal Features & Pathogenesis

The cardinal features of Fallot's tetralogy (Fig 11–18) are right ventricular hypertrophy, large ventricular septal defect, right ventricular outflow obstruction, and overriding aorta.

The ventricular septal defect is high in the membranous portion of the septum and large enough to equalize the pressures in the right and left ventricles. The right ventricular obstruction can be either valvular or infundibular or both, and the overriding of the aorta results in ejection of some right ventricular blood directly into the aorta. In some cases, an equivalent form of lesion occurs in which both great vessels arise from the right ventricle, a condition termed double outlet right ventricle. The principal variable determining the severity of Fallot's tetralogy is the degree of right ventricular outflow obstruction. The site (valvular, infundibular, or both) of obstruction and the degree of overriding of the aorta play little part in determining the size of the pulmonary blood flow (the principal variable is outflow obstruction) because the right and left ventricular pressures are kept equal by the large ventricular defect.

The spectrum of cases of Fallot's tetralogy ranges from cases of pulmonary atresia in which no blood passes through the pulmonary valve to patients with low, moderate, and high pulmonary blood flow. In the mildest cases of pulmonary stenosis there is even a left-to-right shunt through the ventricular defect, and the pulmonary-to-systemic blood flow ratio may be more than 2:1. Physicians disagree about the appropriateness of the term Fallot's tetralogy for patients with mild pulmonary stenosis, who are said to have acyanotic Fallot's tetralogy. However, the hemodynamic picture in patients with ventricular septal defect large enough to equalize pressures in the 2 ventricles conforms sufficiently to the definition to make the use of the term Fallot's tetralogy acceptable. The most characteristic feature of the condition is the marked drop in arterial oxygen saturation that occurs with exercise. This is not seen in patients with smaller ventricular defects; for these patients the term ventricular septal defect with pulmonary stenosis is appropriate.

The overall heart size in Fallot's tetralogy varies with the severity of the lesion. In the severest cases the heart is not enlarged; in fact, it may be smaller than normal. The aorta is usually large and may be right-sided. The right ventricle, although hypertrophied, is not large unless there is a left-to-right shunt. There may be poststenotic dilatation of the pulmonary artery if the right ventricular obstruction is at the valve. The left pulmonary artery may be absent in Fallot's tetralogy, but this abnormality, like a right-sided aortic arch, may occur independently.

Clinical Findings

A. Symptoms:

1. Cyanosis at birth–In all but its mildest forms Fallot's tetralogy is detectable at birth when cyanosis (blue baby) is noted. Cyanosis on exercise always occurs, but clubbing of the fingers is not seen in milder cases.

2. Dyspnea–Patients with Fallot's tetralogy are always disabled by dyspnea. Some patients say that they are not short of breath, perhaps because they have never experienced normal exercise tolerance, and sometimes it is not until after the lesion has been treated surgically that they realize how short of breath they actually were.

3. Squatting–Adopting the squatting position for relief of dyspnea after exercise is almost pathognomonic of Fallot's tetralogy in children. The mechanisms underlying the relief obtained from squatting are described in Chapter 2.

4. Other symptoms–Chest pain, arrhythmia, and congestive heart failure are rare in Fallot's tetralogy but are more commonly seen in adults than in chil-

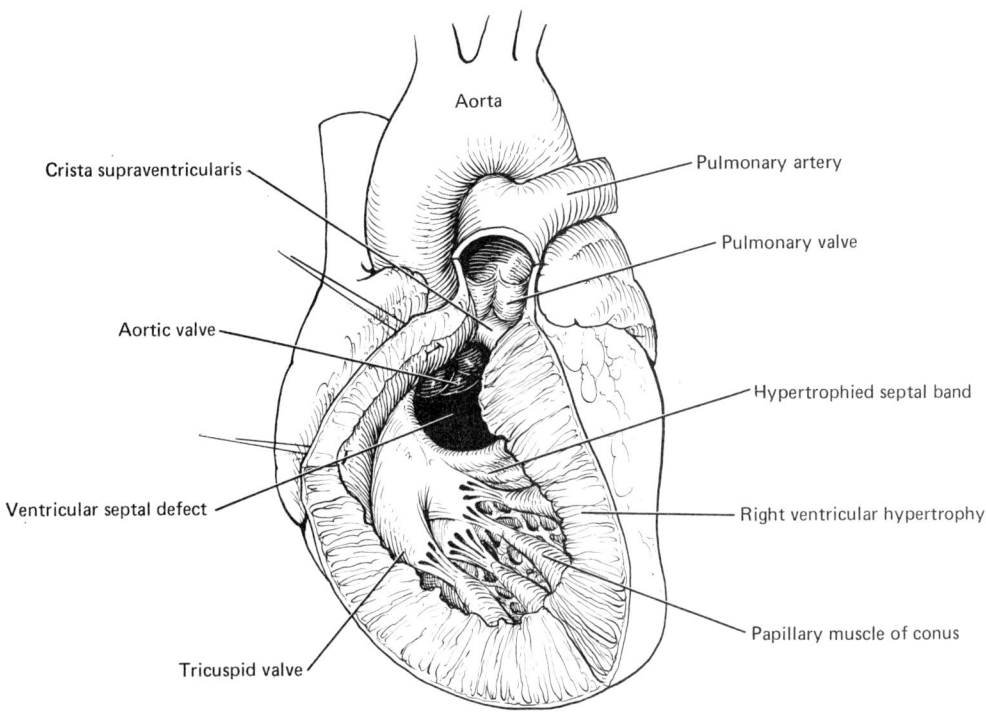

Anatomic features of Fallot's tetralogy. (Reproduced, with permission, from Way LW [editor]: *Current Surgical Diagnosis & Treatment,* 7th ed. Lange, 1985.)

Cardinal features: *Right ventricular hypertrophy; large ventricular septal defect; right ventricular outflow obstruction; overriding aorta.*

Variable factors: *Severity of right ventricular outflow obstruction determines size of shunt and pulmonary blood flow; site of obstruction: valvular or infundibular or both.*

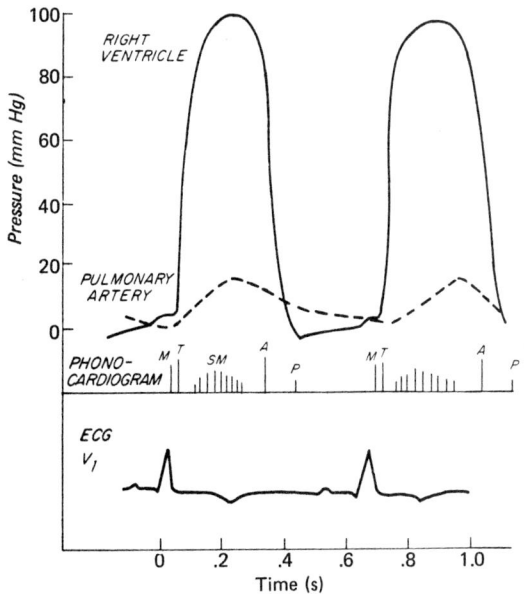

Diagram showing auscultatory and hemodynamic features of Fallot's tetralogy. (Abbreviations are explained in Fig 11–1.)

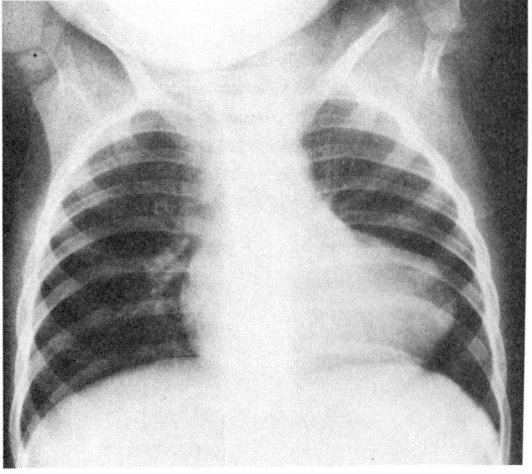

Chest x-ray of a child with Fallot's tetralogy showing a boot-shaped heart (coeur en sabot). (Courtesy of G Gamsu.)

Figure 11–18. Fallot's tetralogy. Structures enlarged: none in severe cases. Large aorta. Large right ventricle in mild cases.

dren. Because the right ventricle never generates a systolic pressure higher than the systemic arterial pressure, the clinical picture is different from that of severe pulmonary stenosis, in which a right ventricular pressure above systemic level can cause chest pain and right heart failure.

B. Attacks of Faintness: In some severe cases, especially with infundibular stenosis, the patient is subject to attacks of faintness and cyanosis. The patient seldom presents with these features initially, but they tend to occur later in the course of the disease. The mechanism of these attacks is infundibular muscular spasm, which reduces pulmonary blood flow. The right-to-left shunt increases, and the patient becomes progressively more hypoxic. Death may occur in the attack, but more commonly the right ventricular muscle itself becomes hypoxic and dilates, relieving the condition. These attacks rarely persist into adult life and respond to treatment with propranolol in 80% of cases.

C. Variability of Symptoms: The characteristic hemodynamic feature of Fallot's tetralogy is the shunting of blood across the ventricular septal defect dependent on the relative resistance of the systemic and pulmonary circulation. Because the resistance to blood flow to the lungs—the pulmonary stenosis—is usually fixed, the systemic resistance is of great importance. Systemic vasodilatation due to muscular exercise, arterial hypoxia, fever, pregnancy, and increased environmental temperature tends to increase or produce right-to-left shunting. As a result, the clinical status of patients with Fallot's tetralogy tends to be unstable and varies from day to day with the weather and the patient's activity and environment.

D. Physical Signs: The physical signs of Fallot's tetralogy vary widely according to the severity of the lesion.

The pulse is of normal volume because the systemic output is well maintained. The venous pressure is normal, with at most a small *a* wave visible in the neck.

The heart is quiet, with little right ventricular heave in severe cases. In milder cases with left-to-right shunts, there is a larger, more hyperdynamic right ventricle. The intensity and length of the murmur arising from right ventricular outflow obstruction vary with the severity of the lesion. In pulmonary atresia or with severe pulmonary stenosis, the pulmonary blood flow may be so small that there is no pulmonary systolic ejection murmur. In such cases an almost continuous murmur due to collateral bronchial blood flow may be heard, especially over the back. In mild acyanotic cases the murmur is long and loud. It may be pansystolic and arise from the ventricular septal defect in patients with a left-to-right shunt. Since the outflow obstruction is always severe enough to raise the right ventricular pressure to systemic levels, the pulmonary valve closure sound is usually inaudible. However, it can be detected by phonocardiography.

E. Electrocardiographic Findings: The ECG always shows some evidence of right ventricular hypertrophy in Fallot's tetralogy (Fig 11–19), but the changes may be surprisingly mild. In milder cases with a left-to-right shunt, there may be evidence of biventricular hypertrophy. P waves are seldom abnormal, and gross right ventricular hypertrophy of the type found in severe pulmonary stenosis is not seen. Left ventricular hypertrophy only occurs in patients with a large, palliative, surgically produced left-to-right shunt.

F. X-Ray Findings: The size of the heart on the chest x-ray is inversely related to the severity of the lesion.

1. Severe lesions–With severe pulmonary stenosis and reduced pulmonary blood flow, the left atrium and left ventricle are small; as a consequence, the overall heart size is reduced. The combination of right ventricular hypertrophy and infundibular ste-

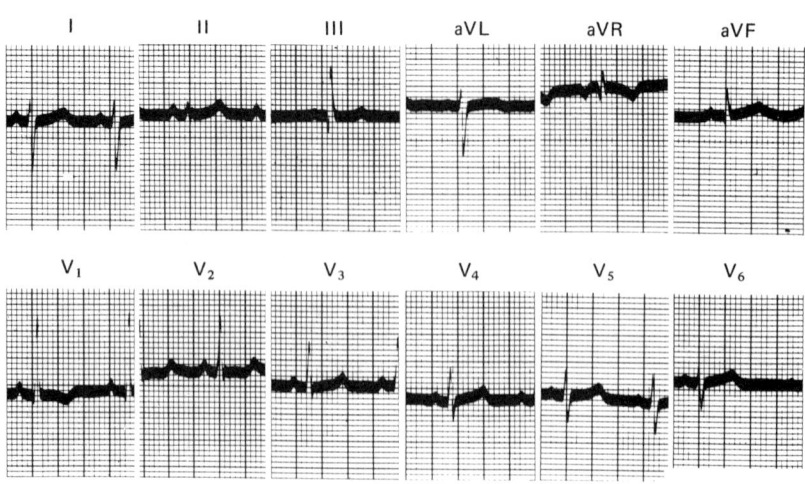

Figure 11–19. ECG of 7-year-old boy with tetralogy of Fallot showing right ventricular hypertrophy.

nosis gives the classic "coeur en sabot" (boot-shaped heart) radiologic picture, with the apex pointing upward and to the left (Fig 11–18). In severe cases, especially those with pulmonary atresia, increased bronchial collateral blood flow may give rise to a reticulated pattern of blood vessels in the lungs.

2. Milder lesions–In milder, acyanotic cases and those with valvular stenosis, the heart shadow is larger, and poststenotic dilatation of the pulmonary artery is seen. In some cases with infundibular stenosis, the heart shadow may appear surprisingly normal, as shown in Fig 11–20. Normal lung fields or even pulmonary plethora is seen in the milder cases.

The finding of a right-sided aortic arch (Fig 11–21) is independent of the severity of the lesion.

G. Special Investigations:
1. Noninvasive techniques–

a. Hematocrit–The degree of polycythemia, as shown by the hematocrit, varies with the degree of arterial hypoxia and thus with the severity of the lesion. Hematocrit levels as high as 75–80% are seen, especially in adults.

b. Echocardiography–M mode echocardiographic examination of the heart is of particular value in establishing the diagnosis of Fallot's tetralogy. By starting at a site intersecting the ventricular septum and pointing the ultrasound beam progressively upward toward the root of the aorta, it is possible to determine the presence and extent of overriding of the aorta and to see the break in continuity of the echoes that represent the ventricular septal defect (Fig 11–22). This noninvasive examination can thus distinguish between Fallot's tetralogy and pulmonary stenosis with intact ventricular septum. However, the actual diagnosis of Fallot's tetralogy by echocardiography cannot be made with absolute certainty because a similar form of over-

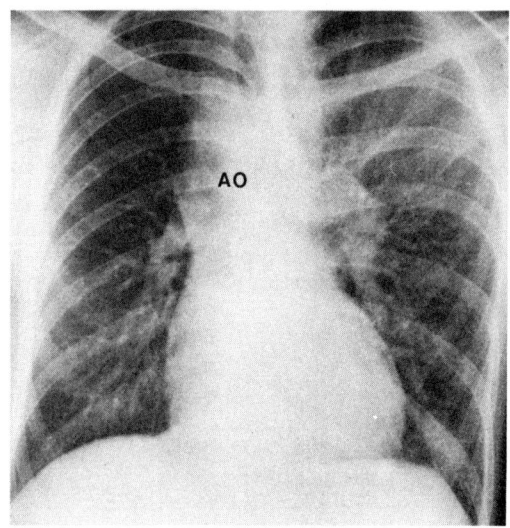

Figure 11–21. Chest x-ray of a man with Fallot's tetralogy with a Blalock-Taussig anastomosis. The aorta (AO) is right-sided.

riding of the aorta is seen in Eisenmenger's complex (see p 349), in which pulmonary hypertension rather than pulmonary stenosis is present.

2. Invasive techniques–Cardiac catheterization is always indicated before any surgical operation in patients with Fallot's tetralogy. The aim of the study is to measure the pulmonary arterial pressure and show that the right ventricular and aortic pressures are the same. In more than half of cases, these aims can be accomplished by right heart catheterization that passes the catheter through the ventricular septal defect into the aorta as well as into the pulmonary artery. In patients who have had palliative shunt operations, it is also important to determine the patency of the anastomosis that was produced. This may require retrograde arterial catheterization.

Angiographic demonstration of right ventricular outflow obstruction, aortic anatomy, and the ventricular septal defect should also be carried out routinely.

The average mean right atrial pressure was 6 mm Hg in 20 patients with Fallot's tetralogy age 15–53 (mean age, 33). The arterial oxygen saturation at rest averaged 90%, and the hematocrit was 55%.

Now that complete correction of Fallot's tetralogy is routine, the anatomy of the coronary circulation has become important to the surgeon. The commonest anomalies of the coronary circulation, seen in about 10% of cases, are the presence of a single coronary ostium from which the whole coronary arterial system arises and the origin of the anterior descending branch from the right coronary artery rather than the left. A large conus branch is often present, and congenital aneurysms of the coronary arteries may be seen.

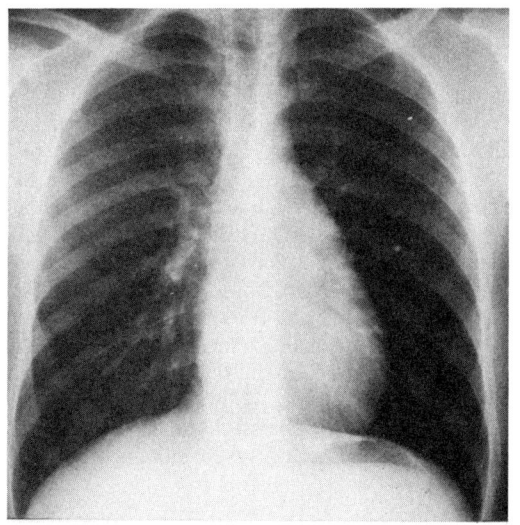

Figure 11–20. Chest x-ray of a 16-year-old boy with mild Fallot's tetralogy. The cardiac silhouette is almost normal in size and shape.

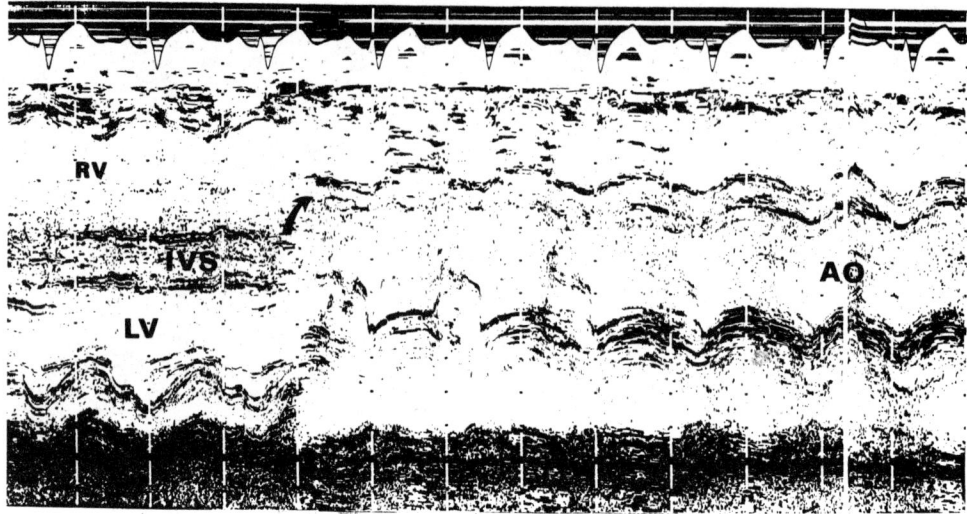

Figure 11–22. Echocardiogram showing aorta overriding ventricular septum in a patient with Fallot's tetralogy. RV, right ventricle; IVS, interventricular septum; LV, left ventricle; AO, aorta. (Courtesy of NB Schiller.)

Differential Diagnosis

Fallot's tetralogy must be distinguished from pulmonary stenosis with reversed interatrial shunt. It is not always possible to make the distinction on clinical grounds, and cardiac catheterization is often necessary to make the correct diagnosis. It may sometimes be difficult to distinguish Fallot's tetralogy from Eisenmenger's complex (ventricular septal defect with pulmonary hypertension), especially when Fallot's tetralogy is mild and there is a bidirectional shunt.

Complications

Progressive polycythemia may lead to cerebral or pulmonary thrombosis. Cerebral embolism or abscess formation is sometimes seen as a result of paradoxic embolization from the right heart through the shunt. Infective endocarditis can occur at the site of the ventricular septal defect in mild cases, or on the pulmonary valve, or in both places. It is occasionally seen both before and after palliative surgery. Right heart failure with edema and raised venous pressure is rare except after surgery.

Prevention

Antibiotic prophylaxis (see Chapter 16) for the prevention of endocarditis is necessary both before and after operation.

Surgical Treatment

A. Palliative Surgery: Palliative surgery to increase the blood flow to the lungs by producing an anastomosis between the subclavian and pulmonary arteries (Blalock-Taussig operation) or the aorta and the pulmonary artery (Potts operation) was introduced over 30 years ago with dramatic results. Patients with severe forms of Fallot's tetralogy benefited greatly from these operations, which resulted in lessening of cyanosis and marked improvement in exercise tolerance. Curative surgery, with complete repair of the defect, is now the treatment of choice.

B. Complete Repair: Complete repair is always indicated in adult patients. If the patient has reached adult life without surgery, the lesion is likely to be relatively mild, and complete correction should be comparatively easy, since the pulmonary vascular bed, left atrium, and left ventricle are probably capable of accepting a normal right ventricular output. The mortality rate of complete repair in adult patients is about 10%.

C. Complete Repair Following Palliative Surgery: If the patient has previously had a Blalock-Taussig or Potts operation, complete repair is still indicated. The operation may be more difficult because the shunt must be identified and closed, and the right ventricular outflow tract may be hypoplastic, or an aneurysm may have developed at the site of the anastomosis. Any patient with symptoms severe enough to have warranted palliative surgery in childhood would probably not have survived to adulthood without operation. A decision about the timing of complete operative repair is difficult, because the patient may be reasonably stable, leading a sheltered life, and unwilling to submit to a second life-threatening cardiac operation. It is important to follow such patients closely and to be alert to the possible development of pulmonary vascular disease, even though this is quite uncommon.

Prognosis

The prognosis in untreated Fallot's tetralogy is poor, and only patients with mild lesions survive to adult life without surgery. The condition is not a static one, since progressive infundibular hypertrophy may develop and decrease the blood flow to the lungs. At the same time, the right-to-left shunt through the ventricular septal defect can increase, leading to cyanosis, clubbing, and polycythemia. Fallot's tetralogy is a severe condition, and even in its mild form the pulmonary stenosis must be considered severe because right ventricular pressure equals systemic pressure. The course is not necessarily uncomplicated in patients who have had a palliative shunt operation in childhood. Infective endarteritis may develop in the shunt. Blalock-Taussig shunts between the subclavian and pulmonary arteries may close off with time, or the patient may "outgrow" the shunt, and cyanosis may recur. In patients with Potts's shunt from the aorta to the pulmonary artery, the pulmonary blood flow is more likely to be too large than too small. Left ventricular enlargement, increased pulmonary blood flow, aortic incompetence, pulmonary hypertension, and right heart failure may occur.

Long-Term Results in Operated Cases

The improvement in symptoms resulting from complete correction—or even palliative surgery—in Fallot's tetralogy is usually so dramatic that the patient is able to "lead a normal life." Though symptom-free, such patients often show considerable residual abnormalities. A residual systolic murmur may be present because of right-sided obstruction at the infundibular or valvular level. A diastolic murmur of pulmonary incompetence or aortic incompetence may develop, and cardiac catheterization usually shows some evidence of abnormality, especially during exercise studies. Conduction abnormalities and arrhythmias may cause sudden unexpected death years after an otherwise satisfactory repair, especially in older patients. If an attempted complete correction is only partially successful, recatheterization and reoperation are indicated, because pulmonary hypertension, with a large left-to-right shunt through an open ventricular defect, may develop rapidly and lead to right heart failure or a permanent increase in pulmonary vascular resistance.

In spite of these problems, the 8-year actuarial survival rate is now over 95% (Katz, 1982), and those who underwent surgery after age 20 had most complications.

VENTRICULAR SEPTAL DEFECT

The anatomic presence of a ventricular septal defect is probably the commonest congenital cardiac defect present at birth. Only about 10% of cases of adult congenital heart disease, however, have a ventricular septal defect without any associated lesion.

Cardinal Features

The cardinal features of ventricular septal defect (Fig 11-23) are left-to-right shunt into the right ventricle, increased pulmonary blood flow, and usually a low pulmonary artery pressure. Variable features are the size of the defect (large or small), the site of the defect (membranous or muscular), and the presence or absence of associated aortic incompetence. Only a small number of ventricular defects occur in the muscular part of the septum, and these may be multiple. The size and site of the ventricular defect determine the size of the left-to-right shunt, which in turn determines the clinical picture. Associated aortic incompetence, seen only with defects in the membranous septum, causes further left ventricular enlargement. A left-to-right shunt at the ventricular level produces an increased flow through the left atrium, left ventricle, and right ventricle. The right atrium is the only chamber through which flow is normal.

The clinical spectrum of cases is wide, varying from maladie de Roger, in which a loud murmur and thrill are the only detectable abnormalities, to defects large enough to cause moderate pulmonary hypertension and large left-to-right shunts.

Clinical Findings

A. Symptoms and Signs: Symptoms in patients with ventricular septal defect depend on the size of the defect and the age of the patient. Small shunts cause no significant hemodynamic effects and are compatible with a normal life expectancy. Larger defects, with pulmonary to systemic flow ratios of 1.5:1 or more, may cause dyspnea after age 30, and large defects with flow ratios of 3:1 or more are rare but are usually associated with dyspnea on exertion. There is usually a history of a heart murmur present since birth.

The physical signs of ventricular septal defect are dominated by the loud pansystolic murmur and thrill that are present in the third and fourth left intercostal spaces inside the apex. In more than half of adult cases, these are the only abnormal physical signs. In patients with larger shunts, the pulse is jerky, resembling a miniature water-hammer pulse, and the cardiac impulse is hyperdynamic. The increased force of left ventricular contraction, which is associated with ejection of an increased stroke volume out through the aorta and also into the low-pressure right ventricle, causes a hemodynamic pattern similar to that seen in mitral incompetence.

The increased pulmonary blood flow causes increased flow through the mitral valve, which produces a third heart sound and a short diastolic flow murmur resulting from relative mitral stenosis.

B. Electrocardiographic Findings: The ECG is normal in more than half of adult cases. In patients with large left-to-right shunts there is evidence of mild biventricular overload, with both tall R waves and deep S waves over the transitional zone leads, together with Q waves in the left ventricular leads. These findings are illustrated in Fig 11-24.

C. X-Ray Findings: The chest x-ray shows a normal cardiac configuration if the shunt is small. Cardiac enlargement is proportionate to the size of the shunt. Since large left-to-right shunts are rare in adults,

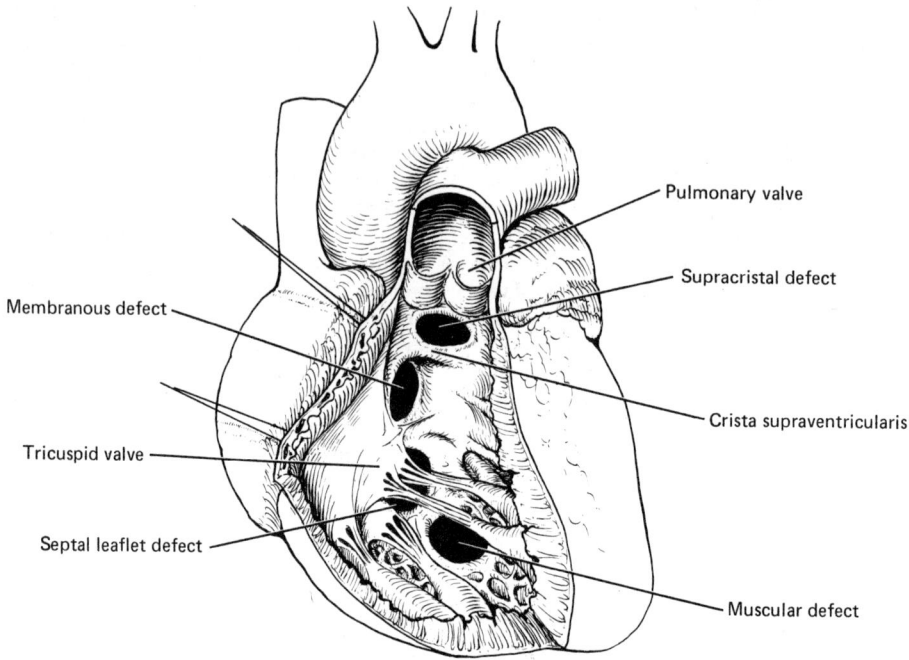

Anatomic location of ventricular septal defects. (Reproduced, with permission, from Way LW [editor]: *Current Surgical Diagnosis & Treatment,* 7th ed. Lange, 1985.)

Cardinal features: Left-to-right shunt into right ventricle; increased pulmonary blood flow; pulmonary arterial pressure usually low.

Variable factors: Size of defect; site of defect: membranous or muscular; associated aortic incompetence.

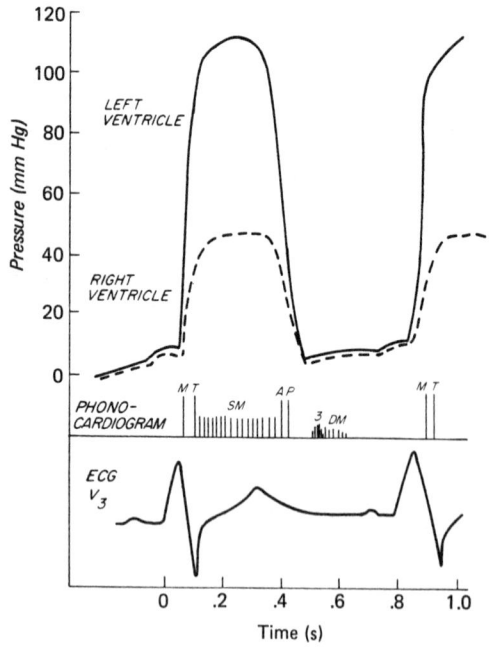

Diagram showing auscultatory and hemodynamic features of ventricular septal defect. (Abbreviations are explained in Fig 11–1.)

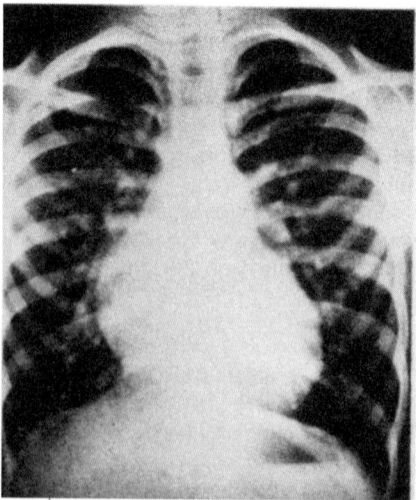

Dilatation of the pulmonary artery and pulmonary plethora in a case of ventricular septal defect. (Reproduced, with permission, from Wood P: *Diseases of the Heart and Circulation,* 3rd ed. Lippincott, 1968.)

Figure 11–23. Ventricular septal defect. Structures enlarged: left atrium, left ventricle, and right ventricle.

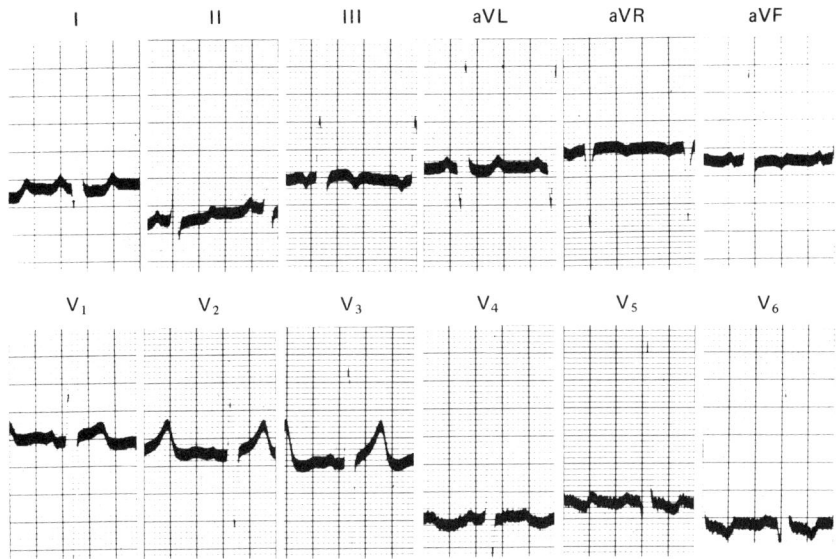

Figure 11–24. ECG of a 21-year-old man with ventricular septal defect proved by catheter; right ventricular pressure is 39/6.

increased heart size, which typically involves the left atrium, both ventricles, and the pulmonary artery, is not often seen. Left atrial appendage enlargement is not seen in ventricular septal defect, even when the left atrium is enlarged.

D. Special Investigations:

1. Noninvasive techniques–Echocardiography is particularly helpful in differential diagnosis. Although ventricular septal defect may be confused with certain conditions on physical examination, echocardiography reveals distinguishing features of these disorders, which include mitral incompetence, hypertrophic cardiomyopathy, infundibular stenosis, and ostium primum defects with mitral incompetence.

2. Invasive techniques–Cardiac catheterization is indicated to confirm the diagnosis, especially if surgical treatment is contemplated. In patients with small defects, a left-to-right shunt may not be detectable from blood samples taken from the right heart chambers, and right-sided pressures are usually normal. The absence of the large *v* wave of mitral incompetence in the wedge pressure tracings and the results of angiography, either with pulmonary arterial injection or with left ventricular injection of contrast material, will almost always establish the diagnosis. In some centers, qualitative detection of small left-to-right shunts of the type encountered in ventricular septal defect is performed using indicator gases such as hydrogen introduced via the lungs. The early appearance of hydrogen in the right ventricle following the start of inhalation of the gas is detected with a platinum catheter tip electrode. The practical value of such methods is not great, because a shunt which cannot be discovered from oxygen content differences and which needs a hydrogen electrode for its detection is of no surgical significance, and even the smallest defect needs antibiotic prophylaxis to prevent infective endocarditis. In patients with larger shunts, the wedge pressure and pulmonary arterial pressure may be increased. Measurement of pulmonary vascular resistance is always important; values of more than 7.5 mm Hg/L/min are seldom seen in patients with large shunts.

Differential Diagnosis

Ventricular septal defect is readily confused on physical examination with mitral incompetence, infundibular stenosis, ostium primum defects with cleft mitral valves, and hypertrophic obstructive cardiomyopathy. All these lesions can cause a loud pansystolic murmur and thrill in the left chest. Although the differential diagnosis is relatively easy in cases of severe defect, it is more difficult in patients with milder lesions, especially those in whom the murmur is the only abnormality. The almost inevitably severe left ventricular hypertrophy seen on the ECG in obstructive cardiomyopathy should serve to distinguish that lesion, but cardiac catheterization is generally indicated to confirm the diagnosis, even though echocardiography, which displays the ventricular septum and the mitral valve so readily, can be most helpful.

Complications

Infective endocarditis is the principal complication of ventricular septal defect. It occurs on the right ventricular wall at the point at which the jet stream of the shunt impinges on the endocardium. Since the infection is initially confined to the right heart and no valve is involved, the prognosis with treatment is good. Endocarditis occurs in about 5% of cases of uncomplicated ventricular septal defects and may recur.

Aortic incompetence occasionally occurs as an associated lesion. It is usually due to prolapse of an aortic valve cusp. It gives rise to a long diastolic murmur that, in conjunction with the pansystolic murmur of the ventricular defect, gives an almost continuous murmur. The aortic incompetence is usually moderate or severe and may develop as the patient grows. In some cases, prolapse of an aortic valve cusp may occlude the defect and abolish the shunt.

Heart failure, acquired pulmonary hypertension, and atrial arrhythmias are all much less common than in atrial septal defect, because so few patients with large ventricular defects are seen in adult life. Systemic hypertension and coronary atherosclerosis may occur in older patients but do not cause the severe problems seen in patients with atrial septal defects, because the size of the left-to-right shunt is limited by the size of the defect and is relatively uninfluenced by the compliance of either ventricle.

Treatment

A. Medical Treatment: The need for antibiotic prophylaxis (see Chapter 16) and acute awareness of the possibility of infective endocarditis are important points to remember in treating patients with ventricular septal defect.

B. Surgical Treatment: Closure of the defect is indicated if the pulmonary/systemic flow ratio is 2:1 or greater. In patients with smaller shunts, closure of the defect is sometimes advised in order to prevent the occurrence or recurrence of endocarditis and to "cure" the patient. The hazards of not operating on a ventricular defect are much less than those involved in leaving an atrial defect unclosed, but since the mortality rate is almost negligible in uncomplicated cases, more of the smaller defects are now surgically treated after it has become apparent that the defect is not going to close spontaneously. Spontaneous closure usually occurs before puberty.

Prognosis

The prognosis in uncomplicated ventricular septal defect in adults is good. Few patients have defects large enough to cause serious hemodynamic problems, and those few who have been recatheterized after 10 years of follow-up have shown no significant change in their status. The incidence of endocarditis has been negligible in those patients who have been followed.

Long-Term Results in Operated Cases

Infants with ventricular septal defects large enough to cause heart failure and pulmonary hypertension in the first 5 years of life have been treated surgically for 20 years or more. Increasing numbers of these patients are now being seen in adult cardiology clinics. Pansystolic murmurs due to residual ventricular defects are not uncommon, but the defects are seldom sufficient to warrant reoperation. Residual pulmonary hypertension is less likely in those operated in the first 2 years of life, and left ventricular function is usually within normal limits, with resting pulmonary capillary wedge pressures at the upper limit of normal.

Aortic incompetence may persist or develop after surgery and is often progressive. Right bundle branch block is common, even after closure of the defect via the transatrial route, and right ventricular function is usually abnormal as assessed by radionuclear methods. Heart block, ventricular arrhythmias, and sudden death are seen, even in patients with good hemodynamic results. Pulmonary vascular disease is not usually reversed, and many asymptomatic patients have high pulmonary arterial pressures and residual septal defects.

PATENT DUCTUS ARTERIOSUS

Persistent patency of the ductus arteriosus is the prime example of a congenital heart lesion resulting from persistence of the normal fetal circulation. It is a common finding in infants whose mothers had rubella during pregnancy.

Cardinal Features

Patent ductus arteriosus is the commonest form of aortopulmonary communication. The shunt is from the aorta at a point just distal to the left subclavian artery into the left pulmonary artery, as shown in Fig 11–25. Aortopulmonary window, in which there is a large communication between the proximal aorta and the main pulmonary artery, is a much rarer lesion that is clinically indistinguishable. The size of the aortopulmonary communication determines the size of the left-to-right shunt.

Patent ductus arteriosus results in an increased flow through the left atrium and left ventricle and also through the aorta and pulmonary artery. Since there is not an increased flow through the right heart, the lesion loads only the left heart.

Patent ductus arteriosus is more than twice as common in females as in males, and the diagnosis is now usually made in infancy or childhood.

Clinical Features

A. Symptoms and Signs: In hemodynamically insignificant lesions, which constitute more than half of adult cases, the patient is asymptomatic. A murmur has sometimes been present since birth, but more commonly the diagnosis is made later in childhood. A false history of rheumatic fever is present in about 10% of cases. The principal symptom is dyspnea on exertion, with palpitation and chest pain much less frequently seen.

The only abnormality in more than half of cases is the typical "machinery" murmur, heard high in the left chest below the clavicle. It is loudest at the time of the second heart sound, as shown in Fig 11–25. The murmur is not necessarily continuous in infancy and may be mainly systolic up to age 5, perhaps

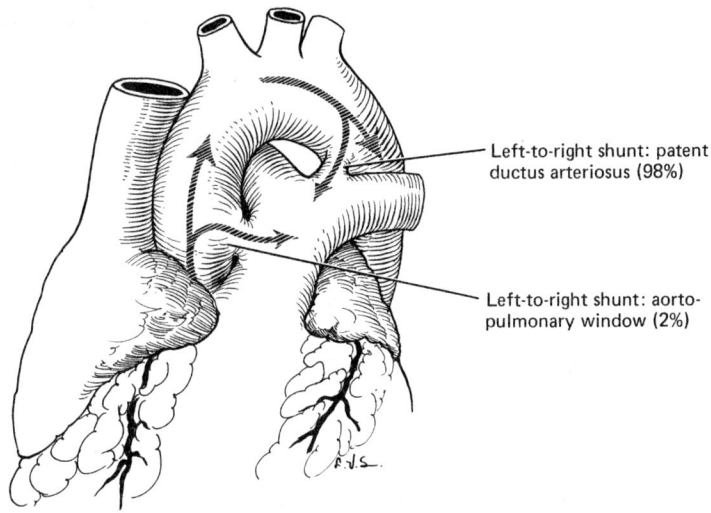

Anatomic sites of aortopulmonary defects.

Cardinal features: *Ductus distal to left subclavian artery; aortopulmonary window near root of aorta; left-to-right shunt; pulmonary arterial pressure usually low in patent ductus arteriosus.*

Variable factors: *Size of communication; size of left-to-right shunt.*

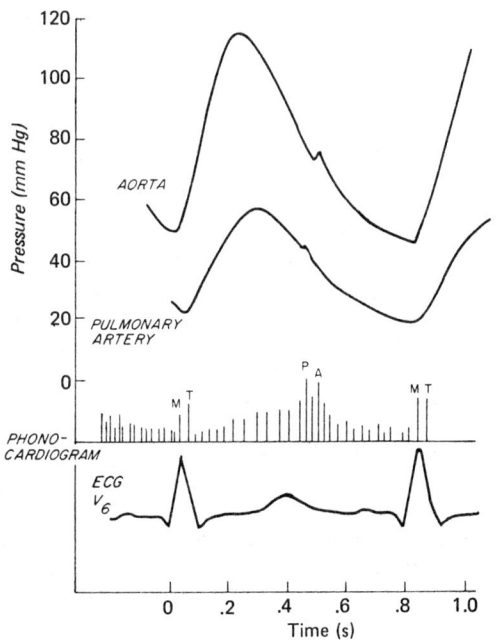

Diagram showing auscultatory and hemodynamic features of patent ductus arteriosus. The continuous murmur is loudest at the time of the second heart sound. (Abbreviations are explained in Fig 11–1.)

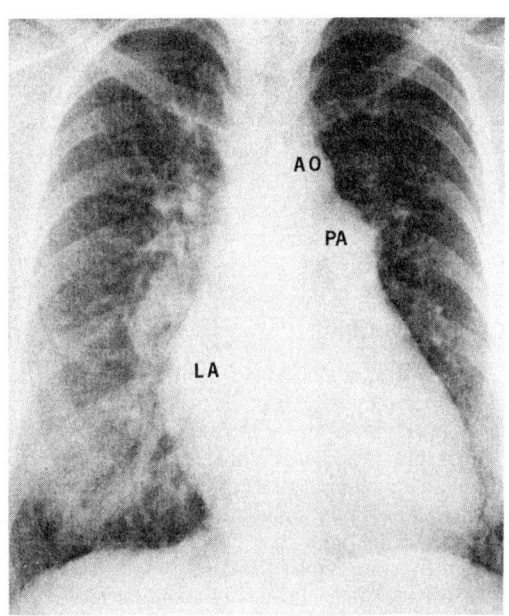

Chest x-ray of a patient with a large patent ductus arteriosus. The aorta (AO), pulmonary artery (PA), and left atrium (LA) are enlarged.

Figure 11–25. Patent ductus arteriosus and aortopulmonary window. Structures enlarged: left atrium and ventricle, aorta, and pulmonary artery.

because the pressure difference between the aorta and pulmonary artery is less at this time. In patients with large left-to-right shunts, cardiac enlargement and a prominent hyperdynamic left ventricular impulse are found. In patients with the largest shunts, a wide pulse pressure and a collapsing pulse are seen because of the large left ventricular stroke volume and the rapid runoff of aortic blood into the low-pressure pulmonary circulation. Palpable pulmonary valve closure, reversed splitting of the second heart sound, and a diastolic murmur of relative mitral stenosis are found in patients with large shunts. All of these features are seen in aortopulmonary window; the only distinguishing feature—a murmur heard low down in the third or fourth left interspace—is not a reliable indication of the diagnosis.

B. Electrocardiographic Findings: Left ventricular hypertrophy in patent ductus arteriosus is related to the size of the shunt. It is absent in hemodynamically insignificant lesions and may be severe with large shunts.

C. X-Ray Findings: The heart is of normal size when the shunt is small. A prominent pulmonary artery shadow running up to a large aortic knob is the most distinguishing radiologic sign of patent ductus arteriosus. Pulmonary plethora with left atrial and left ventricular enlargement and a large ascending aorta are seen in patients with large shunts (Fig 11–25). The ductus may calcify in later life.

D. Special Investigations: Two-dimensional echocardiography from the suprasternal notch provides the best noninvasive view of the ductus. Cardiac catheterization is indicated to confirm the presence of a left-to-right shunt at pulmonary arterial level and to measure the pulmonary and systemic pressure and flow. In right heart catheterization the aorta can occasionally be entered via the ductus in patients with large shunts. The characteristic position of the catheter is shown in Fig 11–26, and its passage down the descending aorta leaves no doubt about the diagnosis. Measurement of the pulmonary/systemic flow ratio is the best means of establishing the hemodynamic severity of the lesion. Ratios of 2:1 or more are found in moderate and severe lesions.

Because of the increasing availability of left heart catheterization, it has become customary to make absolutely certain of the site of the shunt by retrograde aortography. An injection of contrast material into the aortic arch with the patient in the left anterior oblique position will fill the pulmonary artery and outline the ductus. Aortopulmonary windows can also be demonstrated by aortography, thus pointing out the difference between these 2 otherwise similar lesions.

Differential Diagnosis

Patent ductus arteriosus can only be differentiated from aortopulmonary window by cardiac catheterization and angiography. The other lesions that have to be distinguished are those causing continuous or near-continuous murmurs. A venous hum gives a continuous bruit heard above the clavicle that is abolished

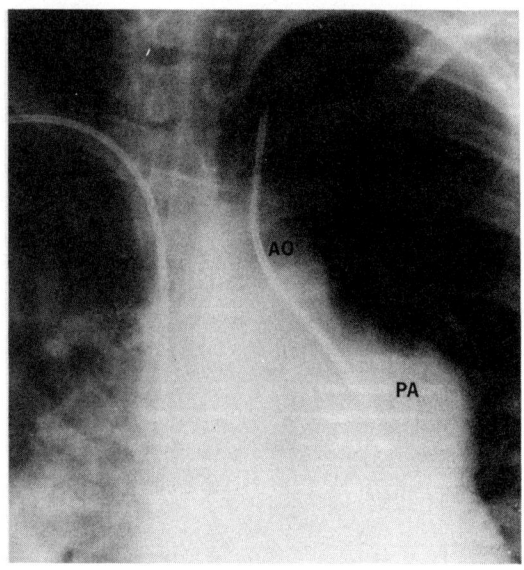

Figure 11–26. Chest x-ray showing the position of a cardiac catheter passing through a patent ductus arteriosus from the pulmonary artery (PA) to the aorta (AO).

by pressing on the veins at the root of the neck to interfere with blood flow. The bruit is caused by local narrowing of the vein and is often influenced by posture. Aortic valve disease and ventricular septal defect with aortic incompetence cause murmurs that may be continuous but show 2 peaks, one in mid systole and the other in early diastole. The murmurs of pulmonary artery stenosis and increased collateral bronchial blood flow start late in systole and peak before the second sound. The murmur of coronary arteriovenous fistula is probably the one most readily confused with patent ductus. It is truly continuous, and the fact that it is best heard at the left lower sternal border rather than in the second left interspace may be the only distinguishing feature.

Complications

Infective endarteritis is an important but infrequent complication. The infection occurs where the jet of aortic blood impinges on the wall of the pulmonary artery.

The left recurrent laryngeal nerve runs in close proximity to the ductus. It may be subjected to pressure or cut at surgery, causing hoarseness.

Acquired pulmonary hypertension with increase in pulmonary vascular resistance rarely occurs in patients with large left-to-right shunts. In most patients with pulmonary hypertension, the raised resistance is present from birth or early infancy (see Eisenmenger's syndrome).

Treatment

Surgical ligation and division of a patent ductus arteriosus is recommended in all patients with left-to-right shunt in whom the diagnosis is confirmed. The operative mortality rate is negligible if the shunt is small. In patients with small shunts, the operation is the simplest type of cardiac surgery and does not require cardiopulmonary bypass. In older patients and those with large left-to-right shunts, the aortopulmonary communication is short and friable and may be calcified. The aortic wall may tear easily, and surgical closure can be extremely difficult, even with cardiopulmonary bypass. In such cases the mortality rate rises to about 10%. It is important for the physician to divide the ductus at surgery rather than simply tie it.

Prognosis

The prognosis is good in mild cases. Surgery is performed to make the patient "normal" and is usually purely prophylactic in hemodynamically insignificant lesions. Endarteritis seldom threatens life, and it is only in the rare patient with a huge left-to-right shunt that life expectancy is less than normal.

Long-Term Results in Operated Cases

The long-term results in operated patients with patent ductus arteriosus are better than those with any other congenital heart lesion. Since the operation is extracardiac, conduction defects and arrhythmias are rare. The only important problem is recurrence of left-to-right shunt; it occurs in about 10% of cases in which division is not performed. If left-to-right shunt recurs several years after ligation, the acquired shunt lesion is much less well tolerated than the congenital shunt.

EISENMENGER'S SYNDROME

The term Eisenmenger's syndrome is used to describe pulmonary hypertension with reversed shunt. By definition, the pulmonary hypertension does not develop in the course of the disease but is seen on initial examination and has been present from birth or early infancy or childhood. The pathogenesis of the pulmonary vascular obstruction is poorly understood.

Cardinal Features

The pulmonary arterial pressure is at or near systemic level, and the shunt is either bidirectional or right-to-left. The pulmonary vascular resistance is raised to more than 7.5 mm Hg/L/min and is often in the same range as the systemic vascular resistance. The principal variable is the level at which the shunt takes place. In Eisenmenger's complex, which is the prototype of the lesion, the location is the ventricle, as shown in Fig 11–27. Because Eisenmenger's original patient had a ventricular defect, the term Eisenmenger's complex is used to indicate the ventricular nature of the defect, as opposed to the more general term Eisenmenger's syndrome, in which the defect may be at any level. The shunt may be at the aortopulmonary, atrioventricular, atrial, or ostium primum level, but it is never solely at the level of an ostium secundum atrial defect. Complex congenital lesions such as truncus arteriosus, transposition of the great arteries, single atrium or ventricle, or total anomalous venous drainage may be associated with the pulmonary hypertension.

It is thought that the Eisenmenger reaction, which is the development of severe pulmonary vascular disease, may occur in any form of congenital heart disease in which a large pulmonary blood flow or raised left atrial pressure is present in fetal, neonatal, or infant life. Clues to the mechanism of development of this form of pulmonary hypertension must be sought in the neonatal period. In adult patients, the pulmonary vascular disease of Eisenmenger's syndrome is severe enough to rule out closure of the defect or defects.

The right ventricle and pulmonary artery are almost always enlarged in Eisenmenger's syndrome. The other chambers that may be enlarged depend on the site of the associated lesion or lesions.

Acquired Pulmonary Hypertension (Eisenmenger Reaction)

Pulmonary hypertension develops after puberty in some patients, usually those with large left-to-right shunts due to ostium secundum atrial septal defects. In these cases the term "atrial septal defect with pulmonary hypertension" or "acquired Eisenmenger syndrome" has been used. In extremely rare cases, pulmonary hypertension develops after puberty in patients with other lesions, eg, ventricular septal defect or patent ductus arteriosus. Acquired pulmonary hypertension tends to progress more rapidly than the pulmonary vascular lesions seen in the Eisenmenger complex.

Use of the Term Eisenmenger's Syndrome

Because the clinical features vary little with the site of lesions and the signs of pulmonary hypertension are dominant, it is convenient to group together under the heading Eisenmenger's syndrome all patients with cardiac defects associated with pulmonary hypertension that has been present since early life. The clinical course of the patient is also independent of the exact anatomic nature of the defect and depends instead on the pulmonary hypertension. In practice, the exact anatomic nature of the lesion in adults with Eisenmenger's syndrome remains unproved until autopsy, and associated lesions such as a ventricular defect in addition to a patent ductus arteriosus and an ostium secundum atrial defect can be present without changing the clinical picture.

Eisenmenger's syndrome accounts for about 7% of cases of adult congenital heart disease and is seen more commonly in females than in males. In about one-third of cases, ventricular septal defect is the only lesion that is associated with the pulmonary hypertension.

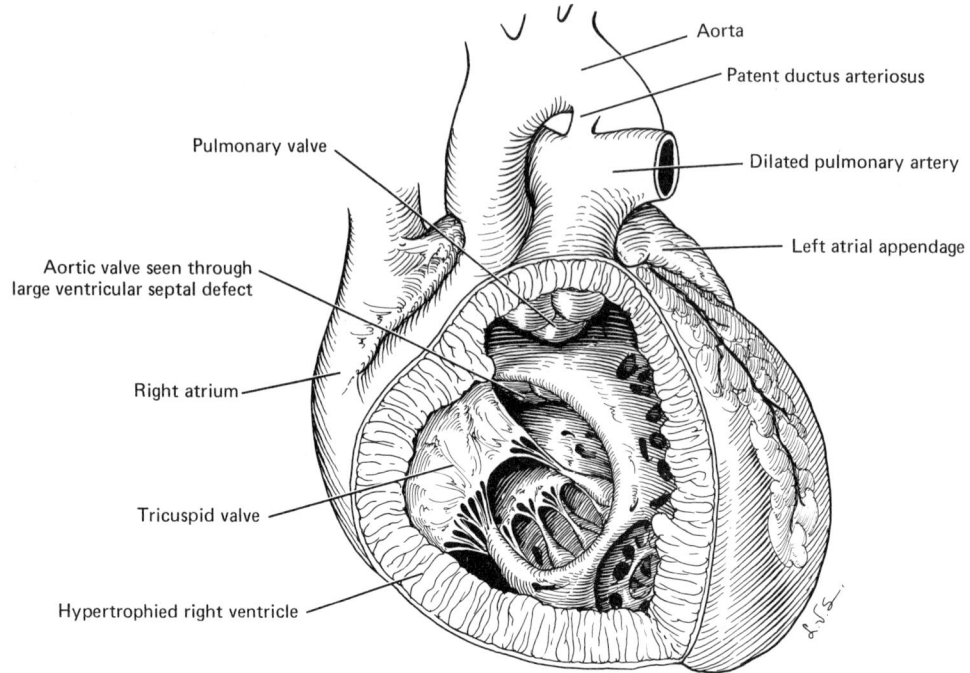

Anatomic features of Eisenmenger's complex.

Cardinal features: *Pulmonary hypertension at systemic level; communication(s) between right and left heart; bidirectional or right-to-left shunt; raised pulmonary vascular resistance.*

Variable factors: *Site of communication: Ventricle (Eisenmenger's complex), patent ductus arteriosus, aortopulmonary window, ostium primum defect, atrioventricular canal, truncus arteriosus transposition, single atrium, single ventricle, total anomalous venous drainage. Not present in ostium secundum defect.*

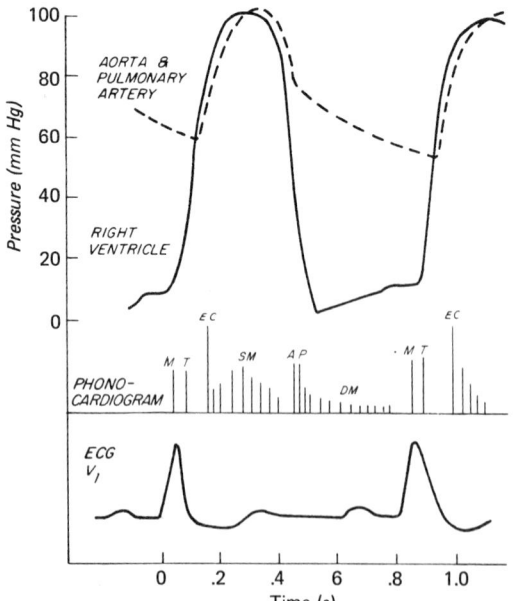

Diagram showing auscultatory and hemodynamic features of Eisenmenger's complex. EC, ejection click. (Other abbreviations are explained in Fig 11–1.)

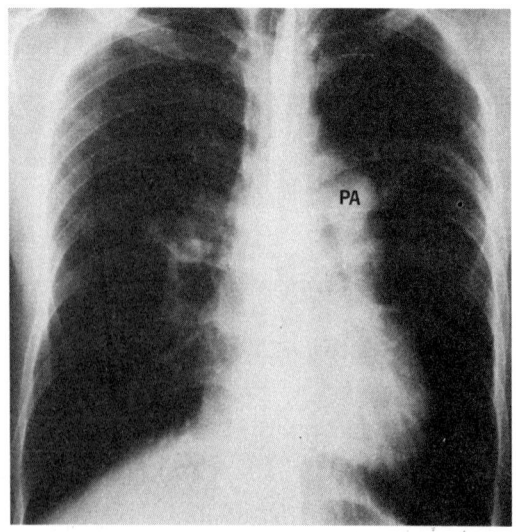

Chest x-ray of a patient with Eisenmenger's syndrome showing small heart and large pulmonary artery (PA) with oligemic lungs.

Figure 11–27. Eisenmenger's syndrome. Structures enlarged: right ventricle, right atrium, and pulmonary artery.

Clinical Findings

A. Symptoms and Signs: Patients with Eisenmenger's syndrome are invariably disabled by dyspnea. A murmur or cyanosis is often said to have been present from infancy, and the absence of any history of severe illness in infancy or childhood is striking. Pneumonia, heart failure, feeding problems, and susceptibility to infection, which are common manifestations of large left-to-right shunts in infancy, are not encountered in retrospective reviews of the history of adults with Eisenmenger's syndrome. Whereas dyspnea is invariably present regardless of age, hemoptysis, palpitation, chest pain, and fainting attacks may be seen in adolescence and young adult life. Pregnancy is poorly tolerated, and spontaneous abortion is common.

The physical signs are those of pulmonary hypertension. Cyanosis and clubbing of the fingers may be present, and there is often a prominent *a* wave in the jugular venous pulse. There may be "differential" cyanosis in patients with a reversed shunt through a patent ductus arteriosus. The shunted blood passes preferentially to the lower part of the body via the ductus and descending aorta. Thus, there may be cyanosis and clubbing of the toes when the hands—especially the right hand—are pink and show no clubbing of the fingers. The difference is best seen when the systemic circulation has been subject to vasodilatation, eg, after a hot shower or bath.

The heart is usually not much enlarged and is often quiet. A right ventricular heave may be present, and pulmonary valve closure is often palpable. There is usually a systolic ejection click, followed by a short systolic ejection murmur over the pulmonary artery and a loud single second heart sound. An early diastolic murmur of pulmonary incompetence is common, and the clearest examples of this murmur (Graham Steell murmur) are encountered in Eisenmenger's syndrome. Signs of congestive heart failure are seldom seen, but progressive cyanosis and polycythemia are common.

B. Electrocardiographic Findings: The ECG in patients with Eisenmenger's syndrome always shows right ventricular hypertrophy (Fig 11–28). In patients with atrioventricular canal defects, left axis deviation may be present even when pulmonary vascular resistance is markedly raised.

C. X-Ray Findings: The main trunk and branches of the pulmonary artery are large, but the heart is usually only slightly enlarged (Fig 11–27). Evidence of slight pulmonary plethora may be present, and the sparseness of the peripheral pulmonary vessels may be difficult to recognize.

D. Special Investigations:

1. **Noninvasive techniques**–Following the level of the hematocrit is useful in assessing the progress of the disease. Echocardiography is helpful in determining the site of the shunt lesion.

2. **Invasive techniques**–

a. **Cardiac catheterization** is always required to establish the diagnosis and show that pulmonary arterial pressure is raised and that pulmonary vascular resistance is at about the same level as systemic resistance. A left-to-right shunt may be detectable from analysis of the oxygen content of samples of blood obtained from the right heart chambers, and the catheter may cross a septal defect at catheterization. When the defect is at the atrioventricular level, pulmonary arterial pressure may be less than systemic pressure.

b. **Wedge pressure** measurement is of great importance, since it is always possible that the patient has a curable lesion that can be identified in this way. The abruptly tapering peripheral pulmonary arteries of patients with Eisenmenger's syndrome may not permit the wedging of a conventional cardiac catheter. In such cases, a Swan-Ganz balloon catheter should

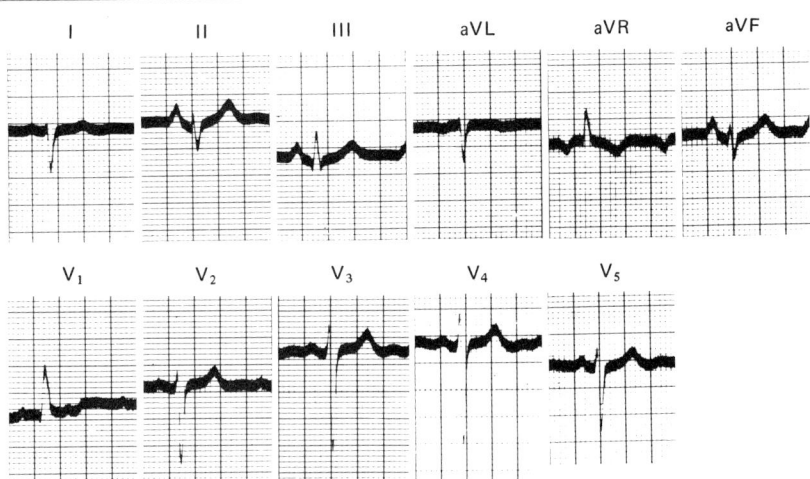

Figure 11–28. ECG of a 30-year-old man with Eisenmenger's syndrome showing right ventricular hypertrophy.

be used, and the pressure in the pulmonary artery distal to the inflated balloon should be taken as an indirect measure of the pulmonary venous pressure.

Differential Diagnosis

Eisenmenger's syndrome must be distinguished from pulmonary hypertension due to acquired lesions that raise left atrial pressure. Tight mitral stenosis is by far the commonest of these lesions, but rare lesions such as left atrial myxoma, cor triatriatum, and sclerosing mediastinitis with pulmonary venous obstruction may occur. Primary (idiopathic) and thromboembolic pulmonary hypertension should also be excluded because such conditions carry a worse prognosis than Eisenmenger's syndrome. The history of a murmur and cyanosis dating back to infancy is of great help in identifying congenital lesions but is not always available. In some patients with severe acquired pulmonary hypertension, opening of the foramen ovale may cause right-to-left shunting and lead to an erroneous diagnosis of a congenital lesion. Pulmonary artery stenosis may also be a possible cause of the physical signs of increased pressure in the main pulmonary artery.

Complications

When patients with Eisenmenger's syndrome are recatheterized after 10–20 years, it is remarkable how few changes are found in the hemodynamic status of the patient. Similarly, clinical findings show little change occurring between adolescence and the third and fourth decades. Complications of progressive polycythemia, pulmonary thromboembolism, and pulmonary infarction tend to become more frequent with the passage of time, and serious hemorrhage from plexiform angiomatous lesions in the pulmonary arterial bed may be fatal. Infective endocarditis is rare, and atrial arrhythmias are uncommon.

Treatment

A. Medical Treatment: Anticoagulant therapy and phlebotomy are recommended but have not been shown to have any significant effects on the course of the disease.

B. Surgical Treatment: The surgical closure of intracardiac or extracardiac (ductus or aortopulmonary window) defects in patients with Eisenmenger's syndrome is contraindicated. It removes the "safety valve" of a right-to-left shunt and tends to convert the patient's status to that associated with primary pulmonary hypertension. If the patient survives the operation, right heart failure and early death are likely to follow.

In some cases it is difficult to be sure that the pulmonary vascular resistance is indeed so high that surgical correction of the defect is out of the question. In patients with obvious cyanosis and pulmonary vascular resistance at or near the level of systemic resistance, there is no question of surgical correction, but in some cases there is still some left-to-right shunt, the pulmonary arterial pressure may not be as high as the systemic (as in a patient with an atrioventricular defect), and the possibility exists that surgery might be helpful. The outlook is best in patients with aortopulmonary defects, especially patent ductus arteriosus, and worst in cases with ventricular septal defect. Heart-lung transplantation offers new hope in the treatment of Eisenmenger's syndrome. The patients are young, and the possibility of treating the heart and lung lesions with a single operation is attractive. This form of therapy is still in the experimental stage.

Prognosis

Life expectancy is significantly reduced in patients with Eisenmenger's syndrome, and few patients in their 40s and 50s are seen by physicians. The course of the disease is not one of steady progression, as in primary pulmonary hypertension, and in a sheltered environment patients can live for 20 years or more with surprisingly little disability or evidence of progression.

Long-Term Results in Operated Cases

Operation to close intracardiac defects is contraindicated in patients with Eisenmenger's syndrome and, if performed, is associated with a high immediate mortality rate.

COARCTATION OF THE AORTA

Cardinal Features & Pathogenesis

This obstructive aortic lesion, which is characteristically associated with hypertension in the upper half of the body, with lower pressure in the legs, is usually diagnosed in childhood. The obstruction almost invariably is in the aortic isthmus just distal to the origin of the left subclavian artery and at the level where the ductus arteriosus joins the descending aorta, as shown in Fig 11–29. The obstruction may rarely be at other sites in the aorta. There is usually poststenotic dilatation of the aorta distal to the site of obstruction. Collateral vessels develop that tend to bypass the obstruction. The principal variables in the lesion are the severity of the obstruction, which varies from complete aortic atresia to slight narrowing, and the size of the collateral vessels. These can be so large that a minimal pressure difference is present between the ascending and descending aorta in a patient with complete aortic obstruction at the site of coarctation.

In coarctation of the aorta, the left ventricle is hypertrophied and enlarged in proportion to the severity of the lesion. The proximal aorta is distended, and there is poststenotic dilatation of the aorta distal to the obstruction.

Coarctation of the aorta is associated with a number of other left-sided congenital lesions, namely bicuspid aortic valve, patent ductus arteriosus, aortic stenosis or incompetence, ventricular septal defect, mitral stenosis, aortic or mitral atresia, and other hypoplastic left heart syndromes. Coarctation of the aorta represents about 5% of cases of adult congenital

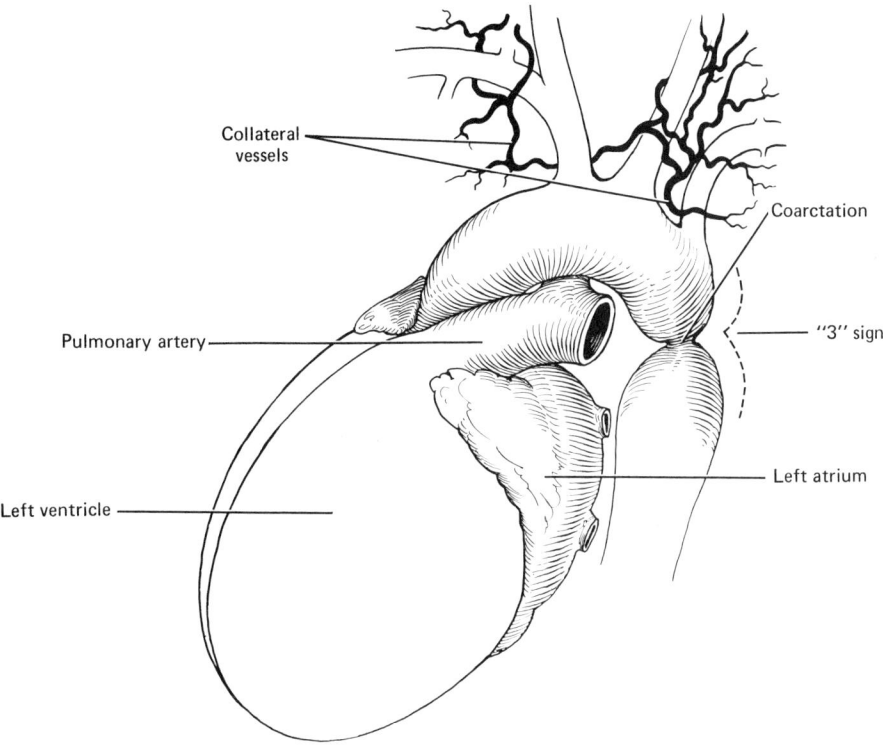

Anatomic features of coarctation of the aorta.

Cardinal features: *Obstruction distal to left subclavian artery; high pressure in proximal aorta; pressure drop across obstruction; poststenotic dilatation.*

Variable factors: *Severity of obstruction; size of collateral vessels; site in acquired lesions.*

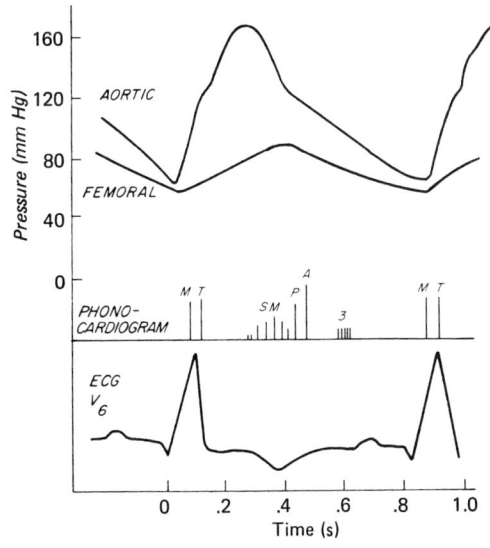

Diagram showing auscultatory and hemodynamic features of coarctation of the aorta. (Abbreviations are explained in Fig 11–1.)

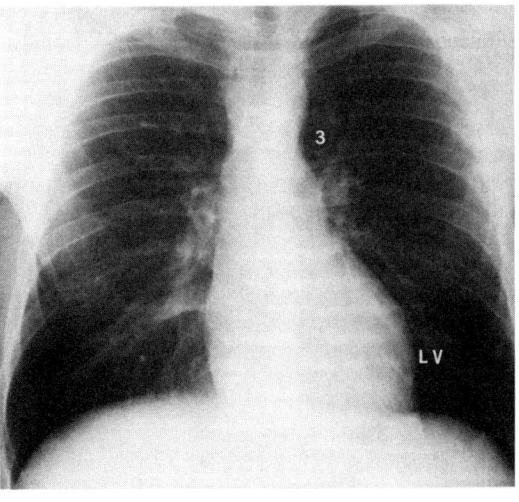

Chest x-ray of 19-year-old man with coarctation of the aorta showing "3" sign and slight left ventricular (LV) prominence.

Figure 11–29. Coarctation of the aorta. Structures enlarged: left ventricle, proximal aorta. Distal aorta: postenotic dilatation.

heart disease and is more common in males than in females by a factor of more than 2:1. Some clinically insignificant narrowing of the aorta at the isthmus of the aorta is common, even in the absence of hypertension. This should not be emphasized, however, and the use of the term pseudocoarctation to describe such a condition is not endorsed.

Clinical Findings

A. Symptoms and Signs: Coarctation of the aorta produces few symptoms. The lesion is usually discovered by finding an abnormally high blood pressure or a systolic murmur. Dyspnea on exertion, headache, and throbbing in the head are sometimes seen. In older, untreated cases, intermittent claudication may occur. Left heart failure, with pulmonary congestion and edema, occurs late in the disease, even in cases presenting in adult life.

The diagnosis of coarctation of the aorta can be readily made on physical examination. The carotid arteries show well-marked, bounding pulsations resulting from the forceful ejection of the left ventricular stroke volume into the reduced capacity of the arterial bed. There is usually a prominent pulsation in the suprasternal notch. The level of arterial pressure varies considerably with the age of the patient, being higher in older persons. The pulse pressure in the arms is wide, whereas that in the legs is reduced. The femoral pulses may be absent in severe cases; if they are present, the characteristic sign of delay between the timing of the upstrokes of the radial and femoral pulses should be sought. The examiner should first locate the femoral pulse with one hand and then palpate the radial pulse to detect and time the difference between the arrival of the 2 waves. The pulses are synchronous in subjects with normal hearts, whereas delays of 0.1 second are readily discernible in patients with coarctation. Collateral vessels are often present on the back. They are best detected by feeling the intercostal arteries under the ribs and the enlarged arteries around the scapula as the patient bends forward.

B. Cardiac Signs: The heart is often enlarged, with a prominent left ventricular heave. Two varieties of murmur in coarctation of the aorta can usually be distinguished. One arises from the aortic obstruction and is late systolic in timing and ejection in type. The other type is longer and more continuous and arises from the collateral vessels. Both are heard best in the back. The aortic valve closure sound is loud, and a third heart sound and a short delayed diastolic murmur arising from the mitral valve are occasionally heard.

C. Hemodynamic Findings: In coarctation of the aorta, the left ventricle pumps into a restricted arterial bed. This accounts for the high arterial pressure and pulse pressure seen in the upper extremities. However, the hemodynamics of coarctation are not as simple as they seem, and mechanical factors cannot account for all the findings. There may be disproportionate left ventricular hypertrophy and unexplained high resting cardiac output. The hypertension cannot be entirely explained on mechanical grounds, and a renal component has been suggested.

D. Electrocardiographic Findings: Some degree of left ventricular hypertrophy is present in all but the mildest cases. The electrocardiographic changes may be out of proportion to the level of arterial pressure. This suggests that aortic stenosis or left ventricular disease may also be present. Left bundle branch block is sometimes seen in older patients, and atrial fibrillation may occur.

E. X-Ray Findings: The characteristic radiologic sign is the so-called "3" sign in the region of the aortic knob. It is shown in Fig 11-29. The upper half of the 3 is formed by the left subclavian artery and the lower half by the poststenotic dilatation of the aorta below the coarctation. Rib notching is another radiologic sign closely associated with coarctation. It is caused by the large collateral intercostal arteries that erode the inferior surfaces of the ribs. The sign, which may be absent in childhood, is not invariably present in adults and is more significant in the outer portions of the ribs, 10 cm or more from the costovertebral junction. Left ventricular enlargement with prominence of the ascending aorta is seen in most cases.

F. Special Investigations: Patients with coarctation of the aorta present such a clear clinical picture that many are referred for surgical treatment without the need for special investigation. However, it is becoming more common to recommend measurement of the pressure difference across the obstruction (Fig 11-30), together with systemic cardiac output. The resistance offered by the involved segment cannot be measured because the volume of blood flowing across the obstruction is unknown. Aortography is often performed, but the outline of the lesion is often seen just as well on a plain x-ray.

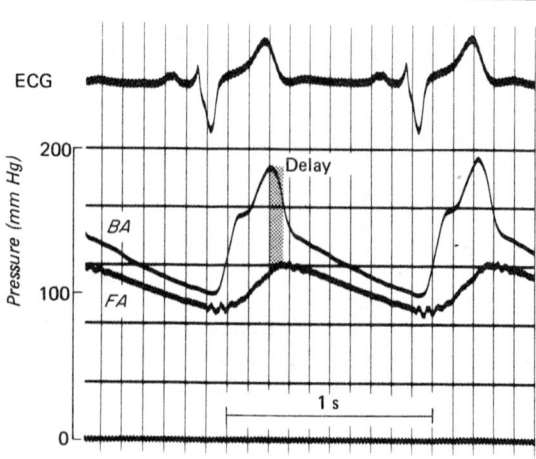

Figure 11-30. Pressure tracings above (BA) and below (FA) the site of obstruction in a patient with coarctation of the aorta. The delay of the peak systolic wave is indicated.

Differential Diagnosis

Coarctation of the aorta enters into the differential diagnosis of systemic hypertension (see Chapter 9). Minor forms of the lesion without systemic hypertension cause more problems in diagnosis, and when aortic stenosis or marked dilatation of the ascending aorta coexists, coarctation may be difficult to detect. Acquired forms of coarctation may occasionally cause problems in diagnosis. The aorta may rupture as a result of trauma.

Aortic obstruction due to arteritis (see Chapter 20) is another acquired lesion that can be confused with coarctation.

Complications

Subarachnoid hemorrhage due to rupture of a congenital aneurysm in the circle of Willis, aortic rupture, and left ventricular failure were the common causes of death before surgical treatment became available. Infective endarteritis may occur at the site of coarctation. In this case, emboli are confined to the lower parts of the body.

Treatment

If the lesion is hemodynamically significant, surgical resection of the coarcted area should always be recommended. In most cases, the ends of the cut aorta can be sutured without the insertion of a graft. Although the operation is relatively easy in childhood, it can be extremely difficult in older patients with larger collateral vessels and friable aortic tissue. Reoperation to deal with an inadequate previous repair presents serious problems. The mortality rate is higher in older patients, being approximately 10% in patients over age 30.

In patients with severe lesions, the sudden increase in perfusion pressure, especially of the gut and other abdominal organs, results in an acute postoperative rise in blood pressure and an arterial lesion that histologically resembles the arteritis of malignant hypertension or polyarteritis nodosa. Abdominal pain may be severe enough to warrant exploratory laparotomy. Antihypertensive medication and expectant treatment are all that is required, and the lesions are short-lived. Paraplegia is another rare complication of surgery. Interference with the blood supply to the spinal cord at operation is responsible. This complication can also occur in patients who have not been operated on.

Nonsurgical treatment using percutaneous balloon dilation has been recently introduced for the relief of coarctation. It has been shown to be effective even in adult patients. This approach may increase the frequency of the peculiar form of arteritis seen after relief of coarctation of the aorta.

Prognosis

The prognosis in coarctation of the aorta is good when surgical treatment is performed in childhood. Blood pressure does not always return to normal, especially if the lesion is not corrected until adult life, and left ventricular hypertrophy may persist. The later development of aortic incompetence or stenosis (which occurs when the bicuspid aortic valve, so commonly associated with coarctation, calcifies in middle life) tends to worsen the prognosis.

Long-Term Results in Operated Cases

Persistent hypertension in the upper part of the body is the most important long-term problem. It occurs most commonly in 2 groups of patients: those in whom surgery is performed in the first year of life, and those in whom repair is delayed until after the age of 30. The incidence of postoperative hypertension increases with the patient's age at operation after the first year of life. Patients show a tendency to develop hypertension later in life, and only 20% of patients followed for 25 years or more were free of complications and had normal blood pressure.

Congestive heart failure, like persistent hypertension, is more likely to occur in older patients in whom operation was performed in adult life. Cerebrovascular accidents are also correlated with postoperative hypertension and represent a significant problem, occurring in about 5% of operated patients.

A bicuspid aortic valve is commonly associated with coarctation of the aorta. Thus, valvular calcification with an aortic systolic murmur and the development of aortic valve disease in middle age are to be expected. Infective endocarditis also remains a problem, and penicillin prophylaxis for major dental work is still required in operated patients.

EBSTEIN'S MALFORMATION

This rare congenital malformation is illustrated in Fig 11-31 and represents about 1% of cases of adult congenital heart disease.

The basic abnormality is downward displacement of the tricuspid valve, with atrialization of a large part of the right ventricle. The principal variable is the presence or absence of an associated ostium secundum atrial septal defect. The atrialized portion of the ventricle hinders rather than helps the forward flow of blood, and the tricuspid valve is congenitally incompetent. The lesion is remarkably well tolerated and was first recognized clinically in a cyanotic form in patients who also had an atrial septal defect. More acyanotic cases without atrial defects have come to be recognized, and it now appears that the lesion probably occurs more commonly *without* an atrial defect. Pulmonary blood flow is reduced, especially when right-to-left shunting through an atrial defect is present.

Clinical Findings

A. Symptoms and Signs: Dyspnea and fatigue are the commonest presenting symptoms. Atrial arrhythmias commonly cause palpitations, and right heart failure occurs with increasing age. The pulse is of small amplitude, and the venous pressure is usually raised in adult patients. Atrial fibrillation is usually

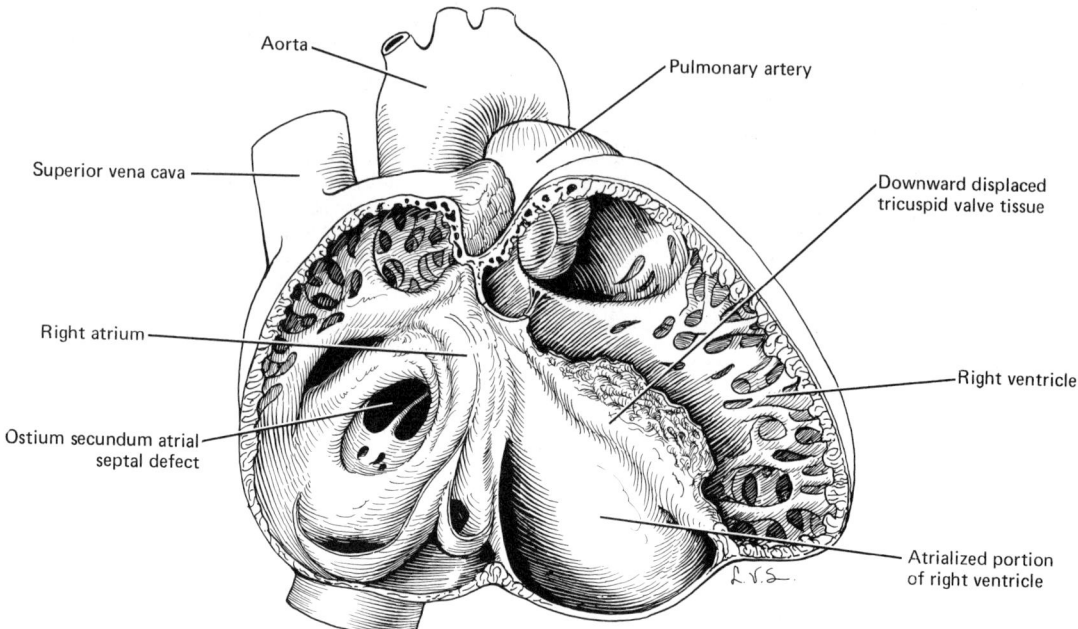

Figure 11–31. Anatomic features of Ebstein's malformation. (Redrawn from the illustrations of Dr Frank H Netter, as printed in: *Heart.* Vol 5 of: *CIBA Collection of Medical Illustrations.* CIBA Pharmaceutical Company, 1969.)

present after age 20. The heart is quiet, with distant heart sounds. There is usually a systolic murmur of tricuspid origin and wide splitting of the second heart sound. A short scratchy diastolic murmur or third heart sound arising from the tricuspid valve is usually heard at the left sternal edge. The murmurs tend to increase in intensity during inspiration.

B. Electrocardiographic Findings: The ECG usually shows incomplete or complete right bundle branch block and a low voltage. Preexcitation (Wolff-Parkinson-White syndrome) is seen in about 20% of cases.

C. X-Ray Findings: The heart is large, with a well-defined border because its excursions are small. The lungs are oligemic, and the pulmonary artery is not enlarged (Fig 11–32). The cardiac enlargement is all right-sided.

D. Special Investigations:

1. Noninvasive techniques–Echocardiography reveals delayed closure of the tricuspid valve coinciding with an early systolic click. There is rightward rotation of the heart, large excursions of the tricuspid valve, and downward displacement of the entire valve mechanism. These findings are not specific and reflect marked right heart dilatation. More specific changes are seen on 2-dimensional studies, in which the abnormal position of the tricuspid valve is more clearly seen.

2. Invasive techniques–Cardiac catheterization is indicated to confirm the diagnosis. Right-sided pressures are all about the same level, and it is difficult to tell from the pressure tracings whether the catheter is in the pulmonary artery, the distal right ventricle, the proximal right ventricle, the right atrium, or the superior vena cava.

Intracardiac electrocardiography has been advocated as the definitive diagnostic test (Fig 11–33). The finding of right atrial pressure tracings at a level in the right heart at which the intracardiac ECG shows a right ventricular electrogram is said to be diagnostic,

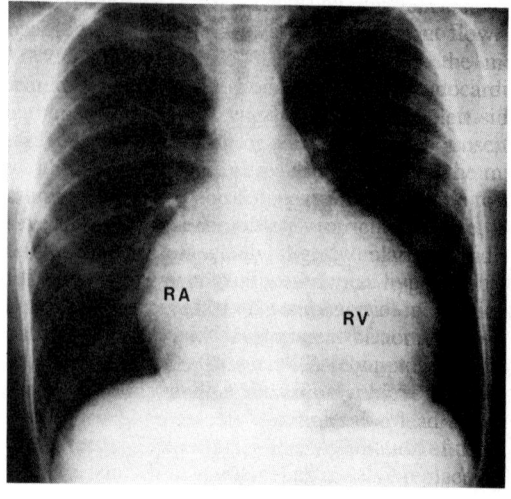

Figure 11–32. Chest x-ray showing cardiac enlargement involving the right atrium (RA) and right ventricle (RV) in a patient with Ebstein's malformation.

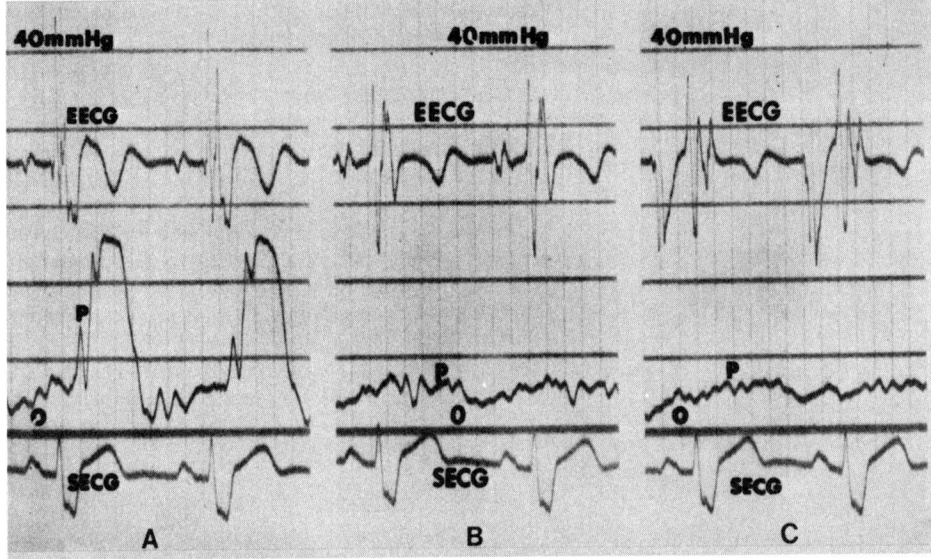

Figure 11-33. Simultaneous endocardial ECG (EECG), pressure tracing (P), and surface ECG (SECG) in a patient with Ebstein's malformation. In *A*, the catheter is in the right ventricle. In *B*, the catheter has been withdrawn to a position in which the EECG shows a ventricular complex but the pressure is atrial (atrialized ventricle). In *C*, the catheter is in the true atrium (atrial EECG and atrial pressure). (Courtesy of EH Botvinick.)

but there is some disagreement about the specificity of the finding.

Differential Diagnosis

Massive cardiac enlargement due to pericardial disease can usually be distinguished on the basis of the history. The cardiac enlargement will have developed recently, whereas in Ebstein's malformation there is a long history of heart disease. Severe right heart failure in patients with congenital pulmonary stenosis may produce a somewhat similar picture, and advanced rheumatic tricuspid valve disease can be recognized and ruled out because there will almost certainly be some associated mitral valve disease.

Complications

Atrial arrhythmias and right heart failure are sufficiently common to be considered as part of the disease rather than as complications.

Treatment

Plication of the right atrium, eliminating the atrialized portion of the ventricle, has been advocated. The operation is palliative rather than curative and is certainly not indicated in mild forms of the condition. More recently, tricuspid valve replacement has been advocated. The results of surgical treatment are generally poor, but the possibility of surgical ablation of accessory atrioventricular pathways must be kept in mind. If the patient has preexcitation and control of arrhythmia is a problem, surgery may be indicated for a dual purpose. Epicardial mapping is necessary, and the results of cutting accessory pathways are good when the pathway has been clearly identified (see Chapter 14).

Prognosis

Patients with Ebstein's malformation have a reduced life expectancy and seldom reach age 50. Persons with milder forms of the disease can have an almost normal life span.

MORE COMPLEX & COMBINED CONGENITAL HEART LESIONS

1. TRANSPOSITION OF THE GREAT ARTERIES

In transposition of the great arteries, the aorta rises from the right ventricle and the pulmonary artery from the left ventricle. If the infant is to survive, there must be some form of septal defect to permit circulation of the blood. The pulmonary blood flow is usually increased in infants with this lesion, and only those who have large septal defects and who develop a raised pulmonary vascular resistance survive without surgery (Fig 11-34).

If transposition of the great arteries is associated with pulmonary stenosis, the pulmonary vascular bed may be protected and the patient may present with a clinical picture resembling Fallot's tetralogy and benefit from a palliative Blalock-Taussig operation. If transposition is associated with tricuspid atresia, that lesion dominates the clinical picture (see p 359).

Transposition of the great arteries with increased

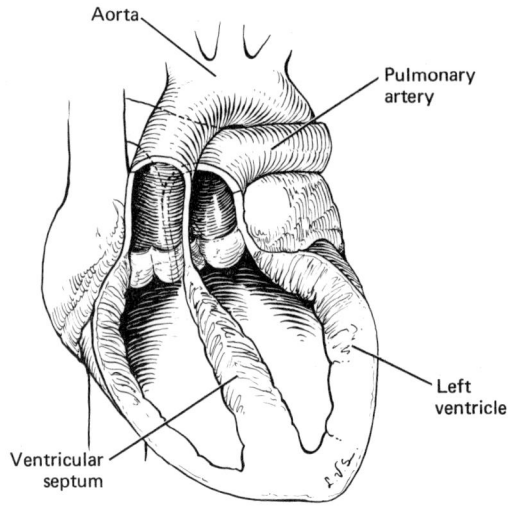

Figure 11-34. Typical transposition of the great arteries. The aorta arises from the morphologic right ventricle and is anterior to and slightly to the right of the pulmonary artery, which originates from the morphologic left ventricle. (Reproduced, with permission, from Way LW [editor]: *Current Surgical Diagnosis & Treatment*, 7th ed. Lange, 1985.)

pulmonary blood flow is a relatively common lesion in infancy, and most patients die within the first year unless treated surgically. In early infancy, the patient's condition may deteriorate when the ductus arteriosus closes. In such cases, the surgical creation of an atrial septal defect (Blalock-Hanlon operation) was first advocated. Subsequently, either the Baffes procedure, to reposition the atrial septum to make the right pulmonary veins drain into the right (systemic) ventricle and direct the inferior vena cava into the left atrium, or the Edwards procedure, to relocate the right pulmonary veins, was used as a palliative operation to improve the mixing of pulmonary and systemic blood. A more successful palliative procedure has been the Rashkind procedure—the "noninvasive" creation or enlargement of an atrial septal defect. A balloon catheter is passed into the left atrium and, after inflation, pulled forcefully back into the right atrium, tearing the septum. The procedure is surprisingly well tolerated.

The development of Mustard's operation for the correction of transposition has led to the increased survival of patients. The operation consists of excision of the atrial septum and insertion of a baffle made of pericardial tissue, which is sewn into the atrium to redirect the pulmonary venous flow to the mitral valve and the systemic venous return to the tricuspid valve.

The long-term results of this operation are just beginning to be appreciated, and as yet few patients have reached adult life. Their clinical status is far from normal, and problems often arise from failure of the baffle to grow. Baffle leaks are relatively uncommon, but obstruction to venous return from either the lungs or the systemic circulation (superior rather than inferior vena cava) is not uncommon, and second operations may be needed. Pulmonary hypertension with raised pulmonary vascular resistance is particularly important, because pulmonary hypertension has often been present before surgery, and the tendency for pulmonary venous return to become impeded causes further increase in pulmonary arterial pressure.

The extensive atrial surgery tends to disrupt the conduction system, and supraventricular arrhythmias (tachycardia or bradycardia) are common. Sudden death has been reported and has been attributed to arrhythmia. The ability of the embryologic right ventricle to support the systemic circulation has been questioned, but this does not seem to be a problem in the absence of obstructive lesions.

2. CORRECTED TRANSPOSITION

In corrected transposition, the aorta arises from the embryonic right ventricle, whereas the pulmonary artery arises from the embryonic left ventricle. The term "corrected" indicates that unlike the situation in transposition of the great arteries, the systemic venous return goes to the lungs and the pulmonary venous blood passes to the aorta. The atrioventricular valves are transposed so that the venous "tricuspid" valve is mitral in shape, and the systemic "mitral" valve has 3 cusps (Fig 11-35). The morphology of the ventricle can be accurately determined by 2-dimensional echocardiography. The abnormality can be associated with almost any form of congenital heart disease, but ventricular septal defect and complete heart block are the lesions most commonly seen. The exact positions of the great vessels in relation to one another can vary, but the aorta is commonly on the left and in front of the pulmonary artery. The lesion can be seen in adult life and is presumably compatible with a normal life span if it is the sole abnormality. Problems may occur during cardiac catheterization because it is difficult to enter the pulmonary artery. In such cases a Swan-Ganz balloon catheter will often float through the right ventricle and enter the pulmonary artery, making it possible to record the pulmonary arterial pressure, which is of clinical importance. Surgical treatment of other defects in patients with this lesion was for many years made difficult and dangerous by the fact that the right coronary artery often runs across the outflow tract of the right ventricle, over the usual site of ventriculotomy. Now that septal defects can be closed by a transatrial approach, operations on patients with corrected transposition have become less dangerous, but coronary arteriography should be performed in patients in whom surgery is contemplated. The long-term problems in surgically treated cases mainly stem from conduction defects and arrhythmias.

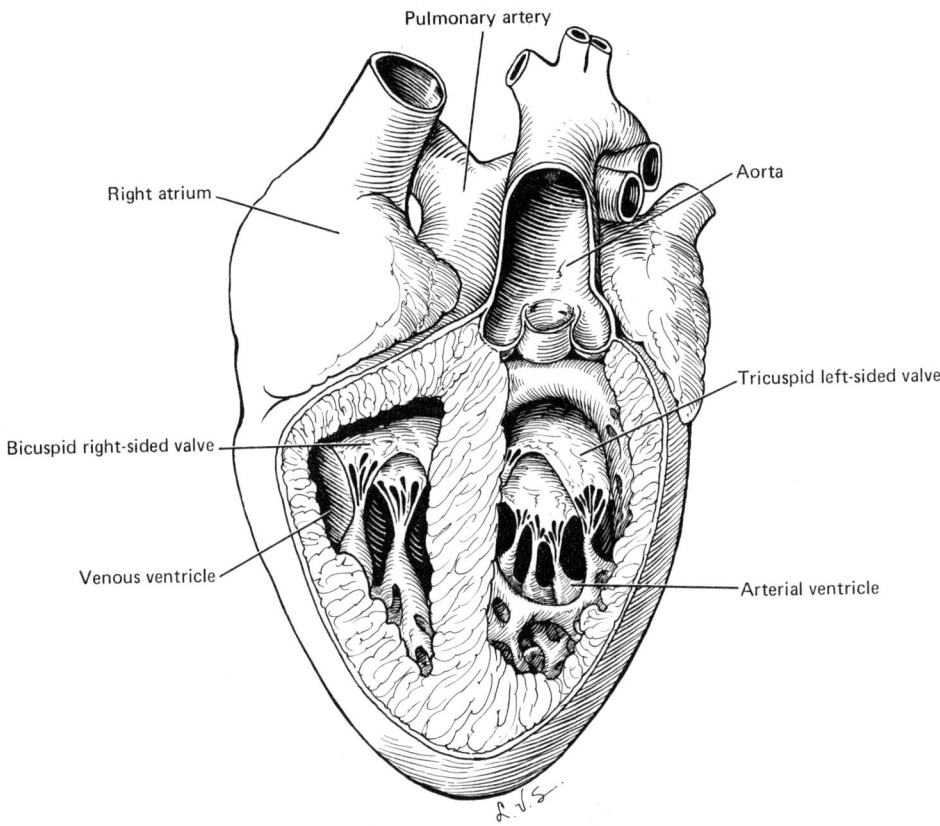

Figure 11-35. Drawing showing anatomic features of corrected transposition. The aorta arises in front and to the left of the pulmonary artery, but the great vessels are connected to the appropriate ventricles (aorta to arterial ventricle; pulmonary to venous ventricle). The right-sided atrioventricular valve is bicuspid (mitral); the left-sided atrioventricular valve has 3 cusps. (Redrawn from the illustration of Dr Frank H Netter, as printed in: *Heart.* Vol 5 of: *CIBA Collection of Medical Illustrations.* CIBA Pharmaceutical Company, 1969.)

3. TRUNCUS ARTERIOSUS

In truncus arteriosus the blood vessels supplying blood to the lungs arise from the aorta (Fig 11-36). A ventricular septal defect is always part of this lesion. The level of pulmonary flow and pulmonary vascular resistance varies. Almost all patients who survive infancy have a raised pulmonary vascular resistance. The exact origin of the vessels supplying the lungs varies and has been used to classify patients into 4 types. This classification does not greatly influence the clinical picture, except that type IV, in which the blood supply to the lungs arises from bronchial vessels, is really pulmonary atresia and best considered to be a severe form of Fallot's tetralogy. In many cases, there is a common outflow valve with more than 3 cusps. This valve tends to be incompetent and causes a loud immediate diastolic murmur. The lesion can now be treated surgically by the Rastelli procedure provided that pulmonary vascular resistance is not too high. A plastic right ventricular prosthesis is interposed between the right atrium and the pulmonary arteries, which are removed from the aorta and sutured to the prosthesis. The ventricular defect is closed, and although the result is not a normal heart, the outcome is more favorable than was formerly the case.

The long-term results of the surgical treatment of truncus arteriosus are just beginning to be appreciated. Calcification and obstruction in the prosthesis may occur, and residual pulmonary hypertension is often a problem.

4. TRICUSPID ATRESIA

In cases of atresia of the tricuspid valve, there must be an atrial defect through which all the systemic venous return reaches the left heart (Fig 11-37). As a result, there is left ventricular hypertrophy that shows up clearly on the ECG as left ventricular dominance because the right ventricle is absent or not functional. Various associated lesions, especially transposition of the great arteries, may be present, and the origin of blood flow to the lungs is the principal variable. There may be associated pulmonary atresia with reduced pulmonary blood flow, or there may be a ventricular

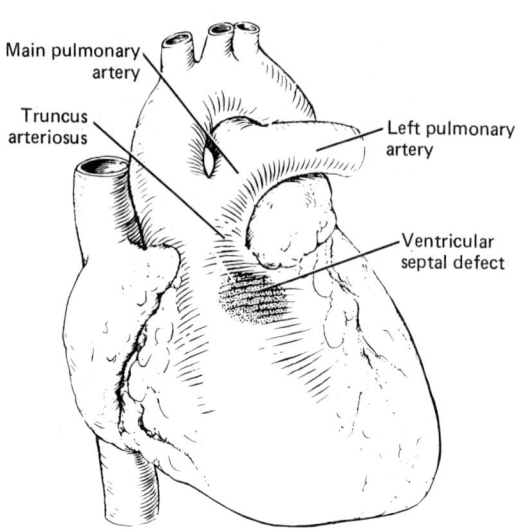

Figure 11-36. Truncus arteriosus. The main pulmonary artery arises from the truncus arteriosus downstream to the truncal semilunar valve. A ventricular septal defect is always present. (Modified and reproduced, with permission, from Way LW [editor]: *Current Surgical Diagnosis & Treatment,* 7th ed. Lange, 1985.)

septal defect through which an increased pulmonary blood flow reaches the lungs. If pulmonary atresia is present and blood flow is reduced, a palliative Blalock-Taussig shunt may increase the pulmonary blood flow and increase the patient's life span. In rare cases, the tricuspid atresia is not complete, and there is a small underdeveloped right ventricle. In such patients the characteristic finding of the lesion (left ventricular hypertrophy on the ECG) is still present. Increasingly effective palliation by means of Glenn's operation, anastomosing the superior vena cava to the right pulmonary artery, has increased the number of patients reaching adult life. Correction by Fontan's procedure involves connecting the superior vena cava to the right pulmonary artery and directing the inferior vena caval flow via a valved conduit to the left pulmonary artery and closing the atrial defect. This operation is now being carried out in older patients who have had palliative surgery. The indications for this further surgery are not yet clear, and long-term results are not available.

5. TOTAL ANOMALOUS PULMONARY VENOUS DRAINAGE

In this lesion all the blood returning from the lungs enters the right heart (Fig 11-38). There must of necessity be an atrial septal defect. The principal variable is the route taken by the pulmonary venous return,

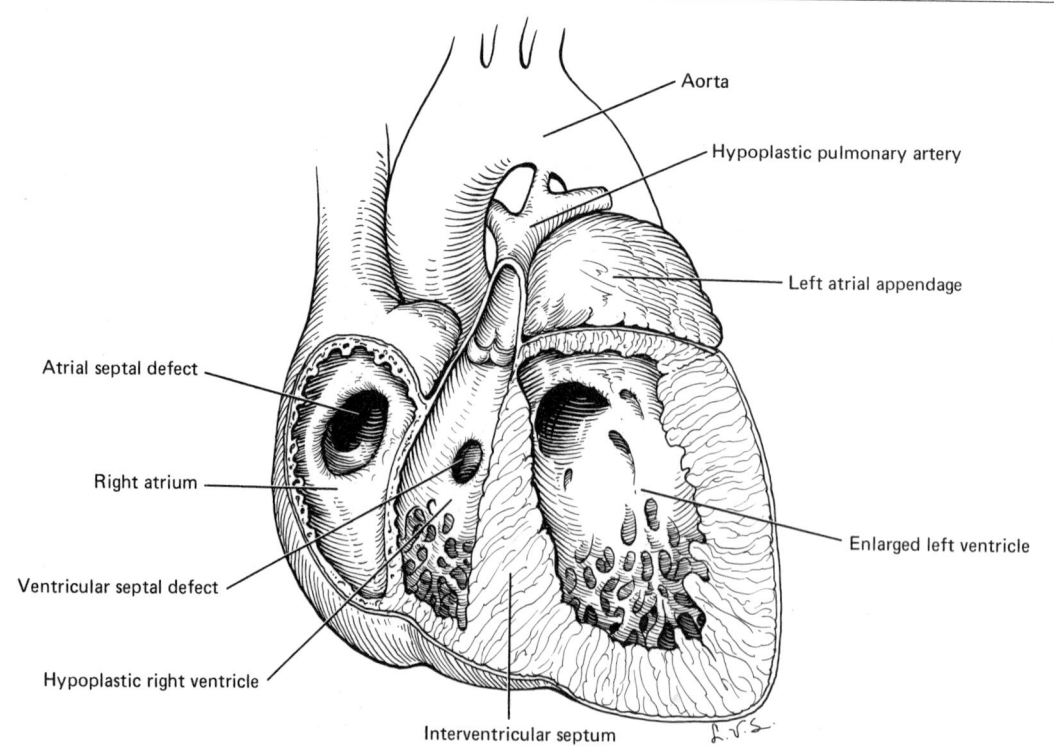

Figure 11-37. Tricuspid atresia, right-sided view.

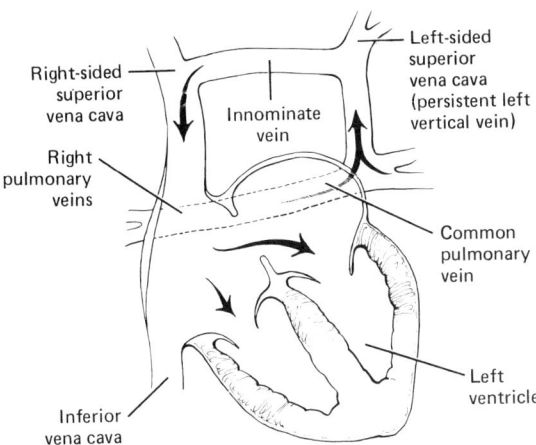

Figure 11-38. Common type of total anomalous pulmonary venous connection. The pulmonary veins connect to a persistent left-sided superior vena cava (left vertical vein), the innominate vein, and the right superior vena cava. (Reproduced, with permission, from Way LW [editor]: *Current Surgical Diagnosis & Treatment,* 7th ed. Lange, 1985.)

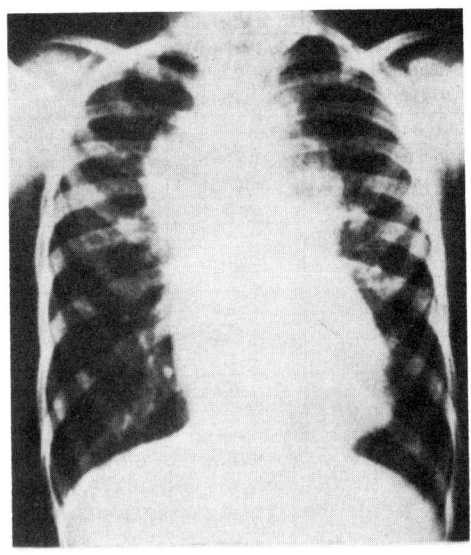

Figure 11-39. Chest x-ray showing typical "snowman" appearance owing to total anomalous pulmonary venous drainage into left innominate vein. (Reproduced, with permission, from Wood P: *Diseases of the Heart and Circulation,* 3rd ed. Lippincott, 1968.)

which is most commonly via a left-sided superior vena cava to the innominate vein and thence to the right atrium via the superior vena cava. The other common pattern seen in infancy is via the inferior vena cava below the diaphragm. More rarely, other patterns of venous return are seen. The pulmonary blood flow and blood pressure vary, and the pulmonary venous return may be obstructed, leading to pulmonary venous congestion and edema. The variety of the lesion most commonly seen in older children is the pattern involving the innominate vein. The venous return is free, and there is usually raised pulmonary vascular resistance. In this lesion there is a characteristic chest x-ray picture called "snowman heart." The upper circular shadow is the anomalous venous pathway that lies above the lower circular shadow formed by the rest of the heart (Fig 11-39).

Correction of the lesion in infancy, before severe pulmonary vascular disease has developed, offers the best hope. Patients reaching adult life almost inevitably have too high a pulmonary vascular resistance to warrant surgery.

CONGENITAL CONDUCTION DEFECTS

Congenital defects of the cardiac conduction system are described in Chapter 14. The most important are the Wolff-Parkinson-White syndrome and congenital complete atrioventricular block. Both lesions usually occur without associated congenital defects, but the former may be seen in association with Ebstein's anomaly and the latter with corrected transposition and ventricular septal defect. Conduction defects and arrhythmias are commonly a problem both early and late after extensive surgery for congenital heart disease.

CONGENITAL ABNORMALITIES OF THE CORONARY CIRCULATION

Anomalies of the coronary circulation are seen either alone or in association with other lesions. The origin of the left coronary artery from the pulmonary artery is perhaps the most important (Fig 11-40). In this lesion, the blood flow through the anomalous vessel is into the pulmonary artery, and a left-to-right shunt is seen. There is usually an electrocardiographic pattern of severe myocardial ischemia or infarction. Ligation of the abnormal vessel at the pulmonary artery level benefits the patient but does not cure the condition. Reanastomosis of the vessel to the aorta is the treatment of choice.

In some cases the coronary arteries arise from abnormal sites, often from the wrong sinus of Valsalva. In other cases the coronary vessel may appear to become kinked as it follows its abnormal course. The lesion is occasionally found at autopsy in young persons who die suddenly; ventricular arrhythmia is believed to be the immediate cause of death.

Coronary arteriovenous fistulas are seen both as isolated lesions and in association with other lesions. The coronary arteries arise appropriately from the sinuses of Valsalva, and vessels enter a fistulous area,

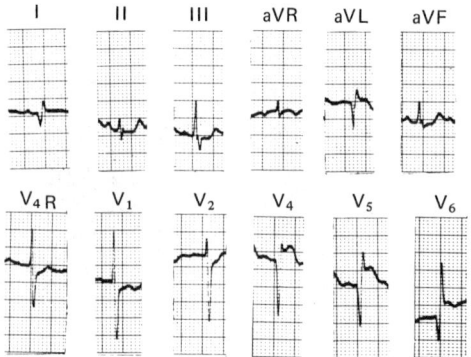

Figure 11–40. Representative ECG leads from a patient with anomalous left coronary artery originating from the aorta showing a current of injury pattern in the anterolateral left ventricular wall. (Reproduced, with permission, from Askenazi J, Nadas AS: Anomalous left coronary artery originating from the aorta. *Circulation* 1976;**51**:976.)

usually draining into the right atrium, right ventricle, or coronary sinus. The right coronary artery is more frequently involved than the left, and the patient presents with a continuous murmur over the lower precordium in a position unlike that seen with patent ductus arteriosus. The fistula flow is often not sufficient to cause significant increase in pulmonary blood flow, and the diagnosis is usually made by angiography.

ABNORMAL POSITION OF THE HEART

Cause of Abnormal Position of the Heart; Associated Conditions

Displacement of the heart interferes with physical examination more than it impairs function of the heart. Abnormalities on the ECG and chest x-ray due to displacement of the heart are also confusing and often suggest more serious abnormalities than are actually present. Abnormal position of the heart may be due to congenital abnormalities, as in dextrocardia, or absence of the left pericardium. It may be due to lung disease, which either pushes or pulls the heart and mediastinal contents to one side, or to abnormalities of the thoracic cage, which may be congenital or acquired. There may be associated congenital abnormalities in the heart itself, especially when chest deformity is congenital. Chest deformity also occurs as a result of congenital heart disease. Cardiac hypertrophy in children with a soft cartilaginous thorax tends to produce a bulge in the left upper chest, which is seen well in ventricular septal defect. The developing thorax becomes fixed in its abnormal shape, and the deformity persists into adult life. The heart itself may be normally situated, but the great vessels may be abnormal, as in right-sided aortic arch or absence of the left pulmonary artery, which may occur as isolated lesions or with Fallot's tetralogy. A left-sided superior vena cava may persist, either alone or with a right superior vena cava, and the inferior vena cava may enter the right atrium in an abnormal position. These lesions are seen with atrial septal defects but can also occur alone.

Dextrocardia

The heart may be situated in the right side of the chest either because of mirror image dextrocardia or because it is displaced from its normal left-sided position. Dextrocardia is usually associated with complete situs inversus involving the abdominal viscera; it is also found with other congenital heart anomalies. There may be isolated dextrocardia with a normal position of the abdominal viscera (situs solitus). In this case, associated cardiac malformations are extremely common. The position of the atria is best determined from the ECG. If the atrial positions are reversed, the P wave is negative in leads I and aVL, with a positive wave in aVR. The position of the atria coincides with the position of the viscera, so that with few exceptions the positions of the stomach and liver give an accurate indication of the atrial position. Electrocardiography and 2-dimensional echocardiography give the best indication of the position of the ventricles, and 2-dimensional echo is also an effective means of determining the positions of the great vessels.

Displacement Due to Abnormalities of the Thoracic Cage

Displacement of the heart due to pectus excavatum and kyphoscoliosis may cause physical findings suggestive of heart disease. Since associated congenital heart lesions are common, the diagnosis is often difficult. Depression of the sternum may be associated

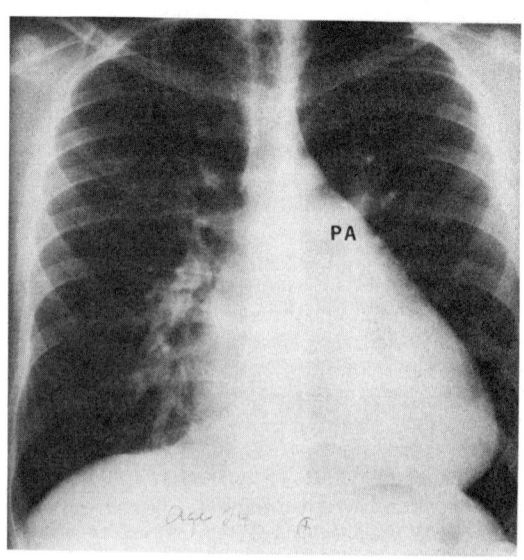

Figure 11–41. Posteroanterior chest x-ray of a patient with pectus excavatum and atrial septal defect. The pulmonary artery (PA) is prominent, and the heart appears to be greatly enlarged.

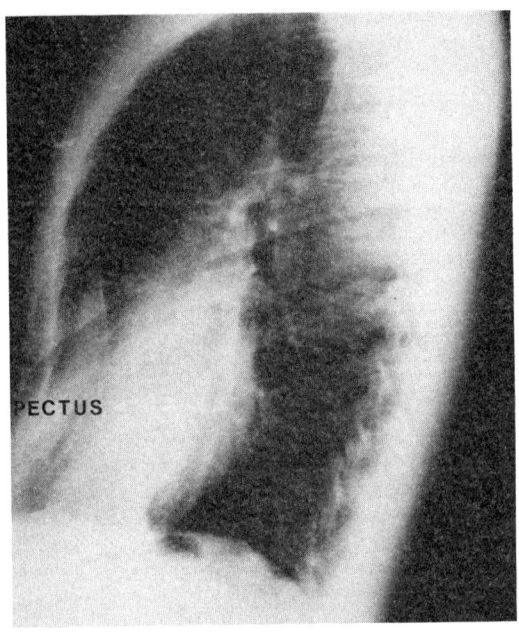

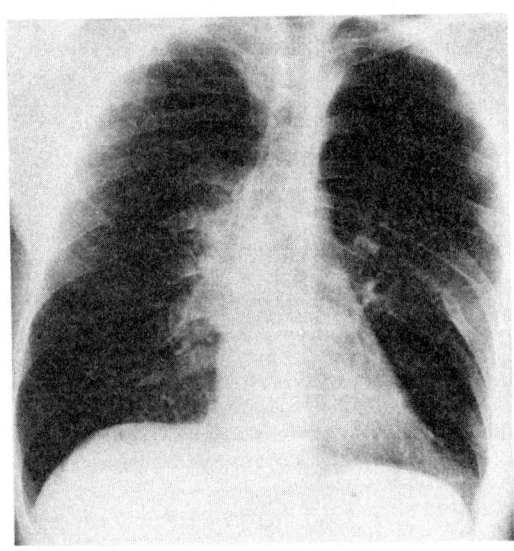

Figure 11–42. Lateral chest x-ray of a patient with pectus excavatum and atrial septal defect. The depression of the sternum (pectus) can be seen. The heart does not appear to be enlarged on this view (compare with Fig 11–41).

Figure 11–43. Chest x-ray of a patient with kyphoscoliosis showing rotation of the heart toward the right anterior oblique position. (Courtesy of G Gamsu.)

with abnormalities of the position of the thoracic spine. These abnormalities narrow the anteroposterior diameter of the thorax. In this case, the heart may appear enlarged on the posteroanterior view and narrowed on the lateral view. Systolic ejection murmurs, wide splitting of the second sound, and even diastolic murmurs can occur. The ECG may show an incomplete right bundle branch block, and the large cardiac shadow on the posteroanterior view with a prominent right ventricular outflow tract may suggest atrial septal defect. In some cases, atrial septal defect is actually present, as in Figs 11–41 and 11–42. In kyphoscoliosis (Fig 11–43), the heart is often rotated, usually toward a right anterior oblique position. The outflow tract is thus abnormally prominent. The ECG shows clockwise rotation of the heart as a result of cardiac displacement, and it is often difficult to be sure that the heart is normal. Patients with chest deformity not infrequently complain of symptoms similar to those of effort syndrome, eg, dyspnea, palpitations, sweating, fatigue, noncardiac pain, and nervousness. In the large majority of cases, there is no underlying heart disease and no specific cardiac treatment is indicated. If the chest deformity is severe, operation may be indicated for cosmetic repair of pectus excavatum. Orthopedic treatment of kyphoscoliosis should not be influenced by cardiac considerations.

REFERENCES

General

Ashby DW et al: The Holt-Oram syndrome: Associated skeletal and cardiac abnormalities. *Q J Med* 1969;**151**:267.

Auerback ML, Sokolow M: Phonocardiography in acyanotic congenital heart disease. *Pediatrics* 1959;**24**:1026.

Baffes TG: New method for surgical correction of transposition of the aorta and pulmonary artery. *Surg Gynecol Obstet* 1956;**102**:227.

Blalock A, Hanlon CR: The surgical treatment of complete transposition of the aorta and pulmonary artery. *Surg Gynecol Obstet* 1950;**90**:1.

Botvinick EH, Schiller NB: The complementary roles of M-mode echocardiography and scintigraphy in the evaluation of adults with suspected left-to-right shunts: Additional observations on the role of two-dimensional echocardiography. *Circulation* 1980;**62**:1070.

Brown OR et al: Aortic root dilatation and mitral valve prolapse in Marfan's syndrome: An echocardiographic study. *Circulation* 1975;**52**:651.

Campbell M: Congenital complete heart block. *Br Heart J* 1943;**5**:15.

Case RB et al: Anomalous origin of the left coronary artery: The physiologic defect and suggested surgical treatment. *Circulation* 1958;**17**:1062.

Collett RW, Edwards JE: Persistent truncus arteriosus: A classification according to anatomic types. *Surg Clin North Am* 1949;**29**:1245.

Davia JE et al: Anomalous left coronary artery origin from the right coronary sinus. *Am Heart J* 1984;**108**:165.

Donaldson RM et al: Management of cardiovascular complications in Marfan syndrome. *Lancet* 1980;**2**:1178.

Edwards WS, Bargeron LM Jr: The superiority of the Glenn operation for tricuspid atresia in infancy and childhood. *J Thorac Cardiovasc Surg* 1968;**55**:60.

Edwards WS, Bargeron LM, Lyons C: Repositioning of right pulmonary veins in transposition of the great vessels. *JAMA* 1964;**188**:522.

Engle MA, Diaz S: Key references: Long-term results of surgery for congenital heart disease. 1. Surgery of specific anomalies. *Circulation* 1982;**65**:415.

Engle MA, Diaz S: Key references: Long-term results of surgery for congenital heart disease. 2. Surgery of specific anomalies (continued), surgical procedures and devices, and surgical techniques. *Circulation* 1982;**65**:634.

Fontan F, Baudet E: Surgical repair of tricuspid atresia. *Thorax* 1971;**26**:240.

Fontan F et al: Repair of tricuspid atresia: Surgical considerations and results. *Circulation* 1974;**50(Suppl 3)**:72.

Glenn WWL, Brown M, Whittemore R: Circulatory bypass of the right side of the heart: Cava-pulmonary artery shunt–indications and results. Pages 345–357 in: *The Heart and Circulation in the Newborn Infant*. Grune & Stratton, 1966.

Gomes MMR et al: Total anomalous pulmonary venous connection. *J Thorac Cardiovasc Surg* 1970;**60**:116.

Hoffman JI, Christianson R: Congenital heart disease in a cohort of 19,502 births with long-term follow-up. *Am J Cardiol* 1978;**42**:641.

Holt AR, Oram S: Familial heart disease with skeletal malformations. *Br Heart J* 1960;**22**:236.

Keith JD, Rowe RD, Vlad P: *Heart Disease in Infancy and Childhood*, 3rd ed. Macmillan, 1978.

Kidd BSL, Keith JD (editors): *The Natural History and Progress in Treatment of Congenital Heart Defects*. Thomas, 1971.

Kimbiris D et al: Anomalous aortic origin of coronary arteries. *Circulation* 1978;**58**:606.

Leatham A: *Auscultation of the Heart and Phonocardiography*, 2nd ed. Churchill Livingstone, 1975.

Lev M et al: Single (primitive) ventricle. *Circulation* 1969;**39**:577.

Marfan AB: Un cas de déformation congenitale des quatre membres, plus prononcée aux extremités, caracterisée par l'allongement des os avec un certain degré d'amincissement. *Bull Soc Med Paris* 1896;**13**:220.

McGoon DC, Rastelli GC, Ongley PA: An operation for the correction of truncus arteriosus. *JAMA* 1968;**205**:59.

McNamara DG, Latson LA: Long term follow-up of patients with malformations for which definitive surgical repair has been available for 25 years or more. *Am J Cardiol* 1982;**50**:560.

Morrow AG et al: Successful surgical repair of a ruptured aneurysm of the sinus of Valsalva. *Circulation* 1957;**16**:533.

Moss AJ: What every primary physician should know about the postoperative cardiac patient. *Pediatrics* 1979;**63**:320.

Moss AJ, Adams FH, Emmanouilides GC (editors): *Heart Disease in Infants, Children and Adolescents*, 2nd ed. Williams & Wilkins, 1977.

Mustard WT et al: The surgical management of transposition of the great vessels. *J Thorac Cardiovasc Surg* 1964;**48**:953.

Newfeld EA et al: Pulmonary vascular disease in transposition of the great vessels and intact ventricular septum. *Circulation* 1979;**59**:525.

Noonan JA: Association of congenital heart disease with syndromes or other defect. *Pediatr Clin North Am* 1978;**25**:797.

Patterson W et al: Tricuspid atresia in adults. *Am J Cardiol* 1982;**49**:141.

Perloff JK: *The Clinical Recognition of Congenital Heart Disease*. Saunders, 1970.

Perloff JK: Pediatric congenital cardiac becomes a postoperative adult: The changing population of congenital heart disease. *Circulation* 1973;**47**:606.

Rashkind WJ, Miller WM: Creation of an atrial septal defect without thoracotomy: A palliative approach to complete transposition of the great arteries. *JAMA* 1966;**196**:992.

Rastelli GC, McGoon DC, Wallace RB: Anatomic correction of the great arteries with ventricular septal defect and subpulmonary stenosis. *Cardiovasc Surg* 1969;**58**:545.

Rigby ML, Shinebourne EA: The aetiology and epidemiology of congenital heart disease. In: *Scientific Foundations of Cardiology*. Sleight P, Jones JV (editors). Heinemann, 1983.

Rippe JM et al: Mitral valve prolapse in adults with congenital heart disease. *Am Heart J* 1979;**97**:561.

Roberts WC: Cardiac valvular residua and sequelae after operation for congenital heart disease. *Am Heart J* 1983;**106**:1181.

Rudolph AM: *Congenital Diseases of the Heart*. Year Book, 1974.

Rudolph AM (editor): *Pediatrics*, 17th ed. Appleton-Century-Crofts, 1982.

Schiller NB, Snider AR: Echocardiography in congenital heart disease. *Circulation* 1981;**63**:461.

Somerville J: Congenital heart disease: Changes in form and function. *Br Heart J* 1979;**41**:1.

Taussig HB: World survey of the common cardiac malformations: Developmental error or genetic variant? *Am J Cardiol* 1982;**50**:544.

Taussig HB, Bing RJ: Complete transposition of the aorta and a levoposition of the pulmonary artery. *Am Heart J* 1949;**37**:551.

Trusler GA, Mustard WT: Palliative and reparative procedures for transposition of the great arteries: Current review. *Ann Thorac Surg* 1974;**17**:410.

Vetter VL, Horowitz LN: Electrophysiologic residua and sequelae of surgery for congenital heart defects. *Am J Cardiol* 1982;**50**:588.

Atrial Septal Defect

Andersen M et al: The natural history of small atrial septal defects: Long-term follow-up with serial heart catheterizations. *Am Heart J* 1976;**92**:302.

Baron MG et al: Endocardial cushion defects: Specific diagnosis by angiocardiography. *Am J Cardiol* 1964;**13**:162.

Bedford DE, Papp C, Parkinson J: Atrial septal defect. *Br Heart J* 1941;**3**:37.

Bedford DE et al: Atrial septal defect and its surgical treatment. *Lancet* 1957;**1**:1255.

Besterman EMM: Atrial septal defect with pulmonary hypertension. *Br Heart J* 1961;**23**:587.

Bourdillon PDV, Foale RA, Rickards AF: Identification of atrial septal defects by cross-sectional contrast echocardiography. *Br Heart J* 1980;**44**:401.

Brandenburg RO et al: Clinical follow-up study of paroxysmal supraventricular tachyarrhythmias after operative repair of a secundum type atrial septal defect in adults. *Am J Cardiol* 1983;**51**:273.

Carabello BA et al: Normal left ventricular systolic function in adults with atrial septal defect and left heart failure. *Am J Cardiol* 1982;**49**:1868.

Davies LG, Fotiades B: Sinus arrhythmia: Observations in atrial septal defect and normal subjects. *Br Heart J* 1960;**22**:301.

Dexter L: Atrial septal defect. *Br Heart J* 1956;**18**:209.

Egeblad H et al: Non-invasive diagnosis in clinically suspected atrial septal defect of secundum or sinus venosus type: Value of combining chest x-ray, phonocardiography, and M-mode echocardiography. *Br Heart J* 1980;**44**:317.

Gault JH et al: Atrial septal defect in patients over the age of forty years: Clinical and hemodynamic studies and the effects of operation. *Circulation* 1968;**37**:261.

Gerbode F et al: Endocardial cushion defects. *Ann Surg* 1967;**166**:486.

Hagen PT et al: Incidence and size of patent foramen ovale during the first 10 decades of life: An autopsy study of 965 normal hearts. *Mayo Clin Proc* 1984;**59**:17.

Hurwitz RA et al: Current value of radionuclide angiocardiography for shunt quantification and management in patients with secundum atrial septal defect. *Am Heart J* 1982;**103**:421.

Hynes JK et al: Partial atrioventricular canal defect in elderly patients (aged 60 years or older). *Am J Cardiol* 1982;**50**:59.

Kitabatake A et al: Noninvasive evaluation of the ratio of pulmonary to systemic flow in atrial septal defect by duplex Doppler echocardiography. *Circulation* 1984;**69**:73.

Leatham A, Gray I: Auscultatory and phonocardiographic signs of atrial septal defect. *Br Heart J* 1956;**18**:193.

Liberthson RR et al: Right ventricular function in adult atrial septal defect. *Am J Cardiol* 1981;**47**:56.

Lynch JJ et al: Prevalence of right-to-left atrial shunting in a healthy population: Detection by Valsalva maneuver contrast echocardiography. *Am J Cardiol* 1984;**53**:1478.

Oakley D et al: Scimitar vein syndrome: Report of nine new cases. *Am Heart J* 1984;**107**:596.

Schapira JN et al: Single and two dimensional echocardiographic features of the interatrial septum in normal subjects and patients with an atrial septal defect. *Am J Cardiol* 1979;**43**:816.

Sellers RD et al: Secundum type atrial septal defects: Results with 275 patients. *Surgery* 1966;**59**:155.

Shub C et al: Sensitivity of two-dimensional echocardiography in the direct visualization of atrial septal defect utilizing the subcostal approach: Experience with 154 patients. *J Am Coll Cardiol* 1983;**2**:127.

Sutton MGS, Tajik AJ, McGoon DC: Atrial septal defect in patients ages 60 years or older: Operative results and long-term postoperative follow-up. *Circulation* 1981;**64**:402.

Pulmonary Stenosis

Abrahams DG, Wood P: Pulmonary stenosis with normal aortic root. *Br Heart J* 1951;**13**:519.

Brock RC: Pulmonary valvulotomy for the relief of congenital pulmonary stenosis. *Br Med J* 1948;**1**:1121.

Edwards BS et al: Morphologic changes in the pulmonary arteries after percutaneous balloon angioplasty for pulmonary arterial stenosis. *Circulation* 1985;**71**:195.

Greene DG et al: Pure congenital pulmonary stenosis and idiopathic congenital dilatation of the pulmonary artery. *Am J Med* 1949;**6**:24.

Hultgren HN et al: The ejection click of valvular pulmonic stenosis. *Circulation* 1969;**40**:631.

Kan JS et al: Percutaneous transluminal balloon valvuloplasty for pulmonary valve stenosis. *Circulation* 1984;**69**:554.

Lababidi Z, Wu JR: Percutaneous balloon pulmonary valvuloplasty. *Am J Cardiol* 1983;**52**:560.

Moller I, Weenevold A, Lyngborg KE: The natural history of pulmonary stenosis: Long-term follow-up with serial heart catheterizations. *Cardiology* 1973;**58**:193.

Nadas AS: Pulmonic stenosis: Indications for surgery in children and adults. *N Engl J Med* 1972;**287**:1196.

Tetralogy of Fallot

Abraham KA: Tetralogy of Fallot in adults: A report on 147 patients. *Am J Med* 1979;**66**:811.

Bertranou EG et al: Life expectancy without surgery in tetralogy of Fallot. *Am J Cardiol* 1978;**42**:458.

Blalock A, Taussig HB: The surgical treatment of malformations of the heart in which there is pulmonary stenosis or pulmonary atresia. *JAMA* 1945;**128**:189.

Caldwell RL et al: Right ventricular outflow tract assessment by cross-sectional echocardiography in tetralogy of Fallot. *Circulation* 1979;**59**:395.

Capelli H et al: Aortic regurgitation in tetrad of Fallot and pulmonary atresia. *Am J Cardiol* 1982;**49**:1979.

Chiariello L et al: Intracardiac repair of tetralogy of Fallot: 5 year review of 403 patients. *J Thorac Cardiovasc Surg* 1975;**70**:529.

Crawford DW, Simpson E, McIlroy MB: Cardio-pulmonary function in Fallot's tetralogy after palliative shunting operations. *Am Heart J* 1967;**74**:4.

Dabizzi RP et al: Distribution and anomalies of coronary arteries in tetralogy of Fallot. *Circulation* 1980;**61**:95.

Deanfield JE et al: Ventricular arrhythmia in unrepaired and repaired tetralogy of Fallot. *Br Heart J* 1984;**52**:77.

DiSessa TG: Two dimensional echocardiographic characteristics of double outlet right ventricle. *Am J Cardiol* 1979;**44**:1146.

Emanuel RW, Pattinson JN: Absence of the left pulmonary artery in Fallot's tetralogy. *Br Heart J* 1956;**18**:289.

Fallot A: Contribution a l'anatomie pathologique de la maladie bleue (cyanose cardiaque). *Marseilles Med* 1888;**25**:77.

Fuster V et al: Long-term evaluation (12 to 22 years) of open heart surgery for tetralogy of Fallot. *Am J Cardiol* 1980;**46**:635.

Garson A Jr, Gillette PC, McNamara DG: Propranolol: The preferred palliation for tetralogy of Fallot. *Am J Cardiol* 1981;**47**:1098.

Hu DCK et al: Total correction of tetralogy of Fallot at 40 years and older: Long-term follow-up. *J Am Coll Cardiol* 1985;**5**:40.

Katz NM: Late survival and symptoms after repair of tetralogy of Fallot. *Circulation* 1982;**65**:403.

Kirklin JW, Karp RB: *The Tetralogy of Fallot From a Surgical Viewpoint.* Saunders, 1970.

Kirklin JW et al: Routine primary repair vs two-stage repair of tetralogy of Fallot. *Circulation* 1979;**60**:373.

Murphy JD et al: Hemodynamic results after intracardiac repair of tetralogy of Fallot by deep hypothermia and cardiopulmonary bypass. *Circulation* 1980;**62(2–Part 2)**: I-168.

Pacifico AD, Kirklin JW, Blackstone EH: Surgical management of pulmonary stenosis in tetralogy of Fallot. *J Thorac Cardiovasc Surg* 1977;**74**:382.

Partridge JB, Fiddler GI: Cineangiocardiography in tetralogy of Fallot. *Br Heart J* 1981;**45**:112.

Potts WJ, Smith S, Gibson S: Anastomosis of the aorta to a pulmonary artery. *JAMA* 1946;**132**:627.

Reduto LA et al: Radionuclide assessment of right and left ventricular exercise reserve after total correction of tetralogy of Fallot. *Am J Cardiol* 1980;**45**:1013.

Scott WC et al: Aneurysmal degeneration of Blalock-Taussig shunts: Identification and surgical treatment options. *J Am Coll Cardiol* 1984;**3**:1277.

Starr A, Bonchek LI, Sunderland CO: Total correction of tetralogy of Fallot in infancy. *J Thorac Cardiovasc Surg* 1973;**65**:45.

Tofler OB: The pulmonary component of the second heart sound in Fallot's tetralogy. *Br Heart J* 1963;**25**:509.

Vick GW III, Serwer GA: Echocardiographic evaluation of the postoperative tetralogy of Fallot patient. *Circulation* 1978;**58**:842.

Waterston DJ: Lecem Fallotovy tetralogie u zeti do jednoho roko veku. *Rozhl Chir* 1962;**41**:181.

Ventricular Septal Defect

Allwork SP: Maladie du Roger 1879: A new translation for the centenary. *Am Heart J* 1979;**98**:307.

Blake RS et al: Conduction defects, ventricular arrhythmias, and late death after surgical closure of ventricular septal defect. *Br Heart J* 1982;**47**:305.

Corone P et al: Natural history of ventricular septal defect: A study involving 790 cases. *Circulation* 1977;**55**:908.

Hoffman JIE: Natural history of congenital heart disease: Problems of its assessment with special reference to ventricular septal defects. *Circulation* 1968;**37**:97.

Jablonsky G et al: Rest and exercise ventricular function in adults with congenital ventricular septal defects. *Am J Cardiol* 1983;**51**:293.

Keck EWO: Ventricular septal defect with aortic insufficiency. *Circulation* 1963;**27**:203.

Leatham A, Segal B: Auscultatory and phonocardiographic signs of ventricular septal defect with left-to-right shunt. *Circulation* 1962;**25**:318.

Otterstad JE, Nitter-Hauge S, Myrhe E: Isolated ventricular septal defect in adults: Clinical and hemodynamic findings. *Br Heart J* 1983;**50**:343.

Otterstad JE, Simensen S. Erikssen J: Hemodynamic findings at rest and during supine exercise in adults with isolated uncomplicated ventricular septal defect. *Circulation* 1985;**71**:650.

Somerville J, Brandao A, Ross DN: Aortic regurgitation with ventricular septal defect. *Circulation* 1970;**41**:317.

Soto B et al: Classification of ventricular septal defects. *Br Heart J* 1980;**43**:332.

Patent Ductus Arteriosus

Campbell M: Natural history of persistent ductus arteriosus. *Br Heart J* 1968;**30**:4.

Gross RE: Complete division for the patent ductus arteriosus. *J Thorac Cardiovasc Surg* 1947;**16**:314.

Jones JC: Twenty-five years' experience with the surgery of patent ductus arteriosus. *J Thorac Cardiovasc Surg* 1965;**50**:149.

Marquis RM et al: Persistence of ductus arteriosus with left to right shunt in older patients. *Br Heart J* 1982;**48**:469.

Neill C, Mounsey P: Auscultation in patent ductus arteriosus. *Br Heart J* 1958;**20**:61.

Silone ED et al: Oral prostaglandin E_2 in ductus-dependent pulmonary circulation. *Circulation* 1981;**63**:682.

Eisenmenger's Syndrome

Dammann JF, Ferenz C: The significance of the pulmonary vascular bed in congenital heart disease. *Am Heart J* 1956;**52**:210.

Dexter L: Pulmonary vascular disease in acquired and congenital heart disease. *Arch Intern Med* 1979;**139**:922.

Edwards JE: Functional pathology of the pulmonary vascular tree in congenital heart disease. *Circulation* 1957;**15**:164.

Eisenmenger V: Die angeborenen Defecte der Kammerscheidwand des Herzens. *A Klin Med* 1897;**32(Suppl 1)**.

Ellis FH et al: Patent ductus arteriosus with pulmonary hypertension: An analysis of cases treated surgically. *J Thorac Cardiovasc Surg* 1956;**31**:268.

Hoffman JE, Rudolph AM, Heymann MA: Pulmonary vascular disease with congenital heart lesions: Pathologic features and causes. *Circulation* 1981;**64**:873.

Kimball KG, McIlroy MB: Pulmonary hypertension in patients with congenital heart disease. *Am J Med* 1966;**41**:883.

Muller WH Jr, Dammann JF Jr: The treatment of certain congenital malformations of the heart by the creation of pulmonic stenosis to reduce pulmonary hypertension and excessive pulmonary blood flow. *Surg Gynecol Obstet* 1952;**95**:213.

Steell G: The murmur of high pressure in the pulmonary artery. *Med Chron* 1888;**9**:182.

Sutton G, Harris A, Leatham A: Second heart sound in pulmonary hypertension. *Br Heart J* 1968;**30**:743.

Warnes CA et al: Eisenmenger ventricular septal defect with prolonged survival. *Am J Cardiol* 1984;**54**:460.

Whitaker W et al: Patent ductus arteriosus with pulmonary hypertension. *Br Heart J* 1955;**17**:121.

Wood P: The Eisenmenger syndrome. (2 parts.) *Br Med J* 1958;**2**:701, 755.

Wood P: Pulmonary hypertension. *Br Med Bull* 1952;**8**:348.

Coarctation of the Aorta

Brewer LA III et al: Spinal cord complications following surgery for coarctation of the aorta. *J Thorac Cardiovasc Surg* 1972;**64**:368.

Clarkson PM et al: Results after repair of coarctation of the aorta beyond infancy: A 10 to 28 year follow-up with particular reference to late systemic hypertension. *Am J Cardiol* 1983;**51**:1481.

Crafoord C, Nylin G: Congenital coarctation of the aorta and its surgical treatment. *J Thorac Cardiovasc Surg* 1945;**14**:347.

Dock W: Erosion of ribs in coarctation of the aorta: A note on the history of pathognomic sign. *Br Heart J* 1948;**10**:148.

Earley A et al: Blood pressure and effect of exercise in children before and after surgical correction of coarctation of the aorta. *Br Heart J* 1980;**44**:411.

Freed MD et al: Exercise-induced hypertension after surgical repair of coarctation of the aorta. *Am J Cardiol* 1979;**43**:253.

Lababidi Z et al: Balloon coarctation angioplasty in an adult. *Am J Cardiol* 1984;**54**:350.

Liberthson RR et al: Coarctation of the aorta: Review of 234 patients and clarification of management problems. *Am J Cardiol* 1979;**43**:835.

Rytand DA: The renal factor in arterial hypertension with coarctation of the aorta. *J Clin Invest* 1938;**17**:391.

Schuster SR, Gross RE: Surgery for coarctation of the aorta: A review of 500 cases. *J Thorac Cardiovasc Surg* 1962;**43**:54.

Verska JJ, DeQuattro V, Wooley MM: Coarctation of the aorta: The abdominal pain syndrome and paradoxical hypertension. *J Thorac Cardiovasc Surg* 1969;**58**:746.

Ebstein's Malformation

Crews TL et al: Auscultatory and phonocardiographic findings in Ebstein's anomaly: Correlation of first heart sound with ultrasonic records of tricuspid valve movement. *Br Heart J* 1972;**34**:681.

Ebstein W: Ueber einen sehr seltenen Fall von Insufficienz der Valvula tricuspidalis bedingt durch eine angeborene bochgradige Missbildung derselben. *Arch Anat Physiol* 1866;**238**.

Gussenhoven WJ et al: Echocardiographic criteria for Ebstein's anomaly of tricuspid valve. *Br Heart J* 1980;**43**:31.

Watson H: Natural history of Ebstein's anomaly of the tricuspid valve in childhood and adolescence: An international co-operative study of 505 cases. *Br Heart J* 1974;**36**:417.

Abnormal Positions of the Heart

Bergofsky EH et al: Cardiorespiratory failure in kyphoscoliosis. *Medicine* 1959;**38**:263.

McIlroy MB, Bates DV: Respiratory function after pneumonectomy. *Thorax* 1956;**11**:303.

Rao PS: Dextrocardia: Systematic approach to differential diagnosis. *Am Heart J* 1981;**102**:389.

12

Valvular Heart Disease; Mitral Valve Disease

In this book we have used a clinical classification of valvular disease based on physical signs. Both mitral and aortic valve disease have been dealt with under the main headings of stenosis and incompetence, with a separate description of mixed stenosis and incompetence of the mitral valve. Pulmonary valve disease has already been dealt with under congenital heart disease (Chapter 11), and tricuspid valve disease and multiple valve involvement are described in Chapter 13, together with the clinical pictures seen after surgical treatment. Arbitrary decisions about classification have of necessity been made for the sake of clarity and to take account of differences in the severity, acuteness, and etiology of the disease processes in different patients.

Etiology

Rheumatic heart disease has for centuries been the commonest and most important cause of valvular heart disease. Rheumatic endocarditis occurring in the course of rheumatic fever (see p 533) was responsible until recently for the vast majority of cases of mitral valve disease and for about half of cases of aortic valve disease. It is only in the last 25 years that this picture has changed. Improved housing conditions, reduction in the size of families—with less overcrowding—and widespread use of penicillin to treat tonsillitis and reduce the incidence of recurrences of rheumatic fever have probably been responsible for the decline in incidence of rheumatic heart disease in the Western world. Rheumatic heart disease is still an important problem in many parts of the world, however. In tropical and subtropical countries, rheumatic fever occurs earlier in life and runs a more florid course (possibly because of frequent recurrence), with more frequent and more severe cardiac muscle involvement. More valves are involved at an earlier age, and purely mechanical lesions, such as mitral stenosis with little or no residual myocardial damage, are less common.

Natural History

A. Chronic Valvular Lesions: Chronic valvular lesions tend to have a long course. Impairment of cardiac function may be detected when the patient is asymptomatic. There is not necessarily a direct relationship between the severity of symptoms and the degree of functional impairment of cardiac performance, and the varying responses to disease make it virtually impossible to correlate a given degree of disability with a certain severity of valvular abnormality.

1. Effects of myocardial disease–Emphasis on the importance of the severity of the valvular lesion in valvular disease has varied. Before the advent of cardiac surgery for the relief of valvular disease, cardiologists felt that the state of the myocardium was the most significant factor. After cardiac surgery became widely available, myocardial function was considered to be of secondary importance. In actuality, both the severity of the lesion and the degree of myocardial dysfunction are important, and these factors are synergistic in their relation to each other. Thus, myocardial disease causes cardiac dilation, thereby exaggerating the effects of valvular disease by increasing the severity of the effects of incompetence on the heart. Similarly, valvular disease augments the effects of myocardial disease by increasing the load on diseased heart muscle.

2. Causes of progression–The natural history and course of chronic valvular disease are long and difficult to follow. It is not easy to predict the course, nor is it clear how much of the progression is due to actual worsening of the anatomic lesion caused by the original valvular damage. A valve that is the site of an anatomic lesion is subject to abnormal mechanical stress and premature degenerative changes. Such changes as sclerosis, fibrosis, and calcification influence the progress of valvular lesions regardless of the original cause of the lesion.

B. Acute Valvular Lesions: The clinical picture in patients with acute valvular lesions is different from that seen in classic chronic lesions associated with rheumatic fever. Pure valvular incompetence rather than stenosis is an example of the classic acute lesion. It has become increasingly important to distinguish the clinical features of an acute lesion—which develops over a period of minutes, days, or weeks—from the more readily recognized effects of chronic valvular lesions. Acute lesions are relatively rare (10%), and their importance depends on their severity. If the patient survives the onset of an acute lesion, compensatory responses to increased cardiac load occur, leading to hypertrophy or dilation of the appropriate chambers. Such a lesion becomes chronic in about 1 year. In acute severe valvular lesions, the heart tolerates the extra load poorly. The lungs carry the brunt of the disease, and some of the cardiac manifestations associated with chronic valvular lesions may not appear for several weeks.

MITRAL VALVE DISEASE

Rheumatic heart disease is the commonest cause of mitral valve disease. Acute clinical manifestations of rheumatic fever are detected in only about half of patients who subsequently develop mitral valve disease. The presence or absence of a history of rheumatic fever makes no difference in the course of the disease or in its clinical, hemodynamic, or pathologic findings. In patients who have no history of rheumatic fever, it is generally assumed that a subclinical attack without overt signs of cardiac or joint involvement was responsible for the valvular lesion.

Classification of Mitral Valve Disease

The classification of mitral valve disease is shown in Table 12–1.

Mitral valve disease has been classified somewhat arbitrarily into 3 types: mitral stenosis, mixed mitral stenosis and incompetence, and mitral incompetence. The classification depends primarily on the physical findings rather than the history, although the history and course of the disease vary in the different lesions.

Development of Rheumatic Mitral Lesions

A past history of rheumatic fever is present in about half of patients with mitral valve disease. It is least common in patients with acute mitral incompetence (15%), more common in chronic mitral incompetence (20%) and mitral stenosis (50%), and commonest in mixed mitral stenosis and incompetence (70%). The physical signs of rheumatic mitral valve lesions develop at different times after an acute attack of rheumatic fever. In the case of mitral incompetence or mixed mitral stenosis and incompetence, murmurs are usually audible during or shortly after the acute attack. In mitral stenosis, signs of rheumatic mitral valve lesions develop after several years. In all but the most severe cases, physical signs precede symptoms by many years. A murmur is usually present by age 20, and since the majority of patients are women, pregnancy constitutes an important form of stress in the course of a disease that may last for 20–30 years. More severe cases of mitral stenosis cannot withstand the stress of pregnancy, but it is remarkable that many women who present in their 40s and 50s with mitral stenosis and pulmonary hypertension have had several pregnancies without difficulty.

Cause of Mitral Valve Disease

Rheumatic heart disease is, in effect, the sole cause of all mitral valve disease except mitral incompetence. Even in cases of mitral incompetence, however, rheumatic fever probably accounts for half of chronic lesions. Rheumatic heart disease is much more common in women than in men; the female:male ratio of 9:1 in mitral stenosis falls to 3:1 in mixed mitral stenosis and incompetence and 1:1 in mitral incompetence. The only nonrheumatic causes of mitral stenosis or mixed stenosis and incompetence are congenital heart disease and hypertrophic cardiomyopathy. Congenital heart disease is rare, being encountered in less than 1% of adult cases.

MITRAL STENOSIS

The cardinal features of mitral stenosis are shown in Fig 12–1. In mitral stenosis, rheumatic endocarditis scars the mitral valve and commonly causes fusion of the commissures and matting of the chordae tendineae, which interfere with the opening of the valve. The left atrium bears the brunt of the load, and the extent to which it dilates depends on its internal pressure and the state of the atrial myocardium. With time, calcification of the mitral valve renders it less mobile. In some patients with tight mitral stenosis, pulmonary vascular resistance rises because the pulmonary arteriolar smooth muscle responds to the increase in pulmonary venous pressure by vasoconstriction. Severe pulmonary vascular lesions with markedly raised pulmonary vascular resistance (> 7.5 mm Hg/L/min) are virtually limited to severe mitral stenosis; lesser increases in resistance are seen in other forms of mitral disease. When pulmonary vascular resistance rises, the course of mitral stenosis is altered; the brunt of the load is transferred from the left atrium to the right ventricle, and right ventricular failure eventually occurs if the stenosis is not relieved.

Onset of Atrial Fibrillation

In patients without pulmonary hypertension, atrial fibrillation almost always develops with the passage of time. Even if pulmonary hypertension is present, 30% of patients develop atrial fibrillation early in the course of the disease. Atrial fibrillation is most closely correlated with age, but it also depends on left atrial pressure and the severity of involvement of the left atrium in the rheumatic process.

Clinical Findings

A. Symptoms:

1. Dyspnea–The commonest presenting symptom (80%) in patients with mitral stenosis is shortness of breath on exertion. In women with severe lesions,

Table 12–1. Classification of mitral valve disease.

Mitral stenosis
  (1) With low pulmonary vascular resistance
  (2) With pulmonary hypertension
Mixed mitral stenosis and incompetence
Mitral incompetence (regurgitation, insufficiency)
  (1) Hemodynamically insignificant lesions ("click-murmur syndrome," mitral valve prolapse)
  (2) Hemodynamically significant lesions
    (a) Acute
    (b) Chronic

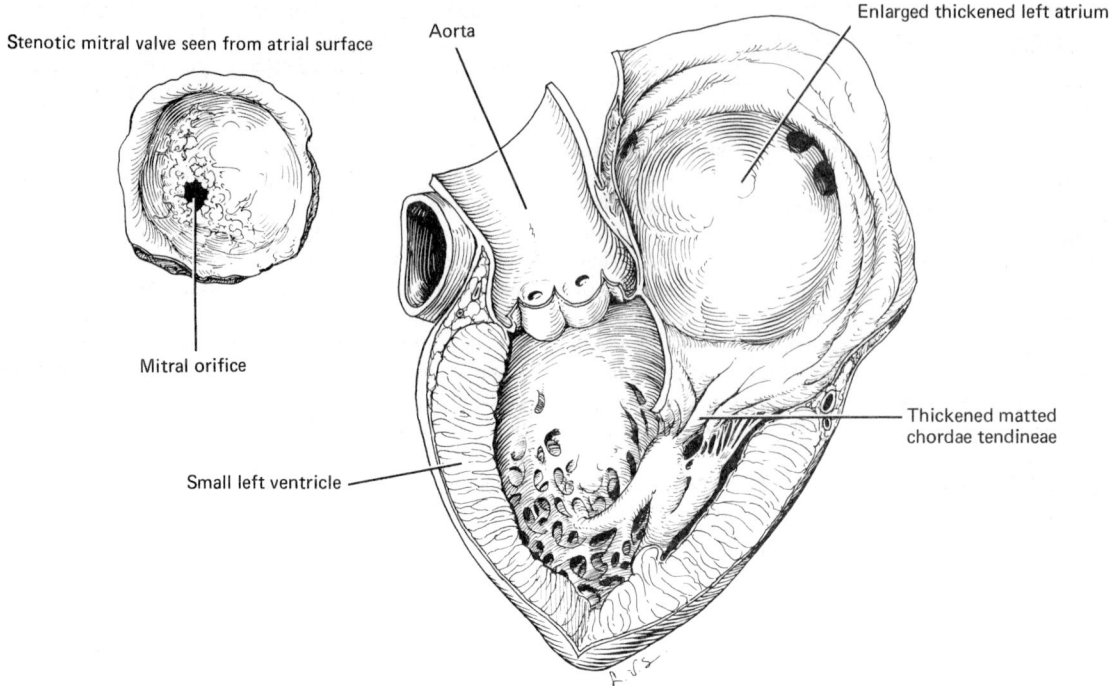

Drawing of left heart in left anterior oblique view showing anatomic features of mitral stenosis.

Cardinal features: *Thickening and fusion of mitral valve cusps; raised left atrial pressure; left atrial enlargement.*

Variable factors: *Severity of obstruction; severity of rheumatic myocarditis; level of pulmonary vascular resistance.*

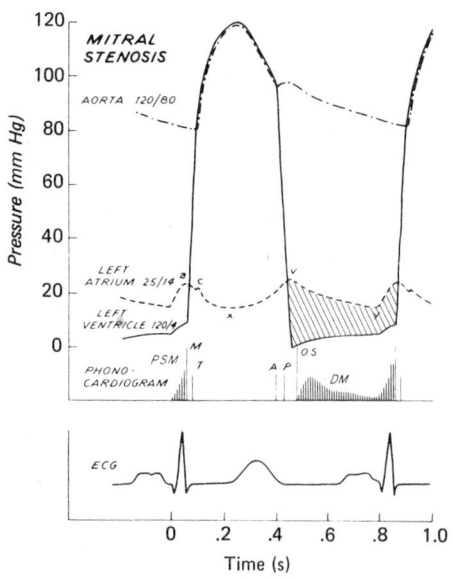

Diagram showing auscultatory and hemodynamic features of mitral stenosis. PSM, presystolic murmur; OS, opening snap. (Other abbreviations are explained in Fig 11–1.)

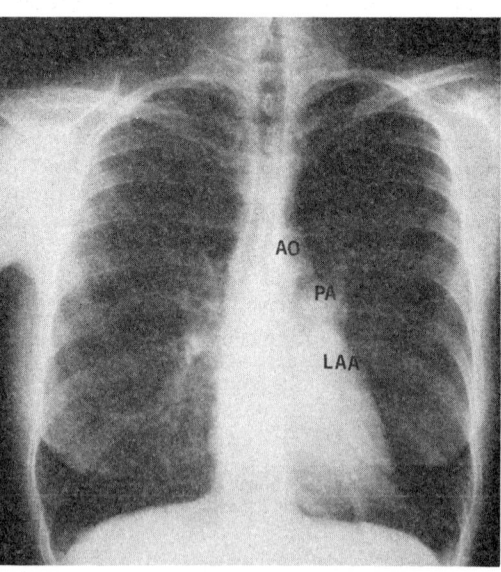

Chest x-ray of a patient with mitral stenosis showing left atrial appendage (LAA) enlargement. PA, pulmonary artery; AO, aorta.

Figure 12–1. Mitral stenosis. Structures enlarged: left atrium. Note small left ventricle. (Redrawn from the illustrations of Dr Frank H Netter, as printed in: *Heart.* Vol 5 of: *CIBA Collection of Medical Illustrations.* CIBA Pharmaceutical Company, 1969.)

this is usually noticed in early adult life (age 20–30), while the patient is still in sinus rhythm, perhaps during pregnancy. The dyspnea is due to pulmonary congestion that results from a rise in left atrial pressure associated with an increase in heart rate and a decrease in left atrial emptying time. The increased stiffness of the lungs increases the work of breathing, and the fall in cardiac output resulting from mitral valve obstruction leads to an increase in heart rate that further aggravates the congestion. Any factor that increases the heart rate is likely to aggravate dyspnea in mitral stenosis; anxiety, anemia, exposure to high altitude, pregnancy, thyrotoxicosis, and atrial arrhythmia are poorly tolerated. The onset of atrial fibrillation in a patient with significant mitral stenosis virtually always provokes dyspnea. In milder cases there may have been no dyspnea prior to the onset of arrhythmia, but in most instances the onset of atrial fibrillation exacerbates dyspnea rather than provoking it for the first time. Conversely, when a patient believed to have significant mitral stenosis develops atrial fibrillation without experiencing dyspnea, the diagnosis is in doubt and the lesion is at most mild.

2. Paroxysmal nocturnal dyspnea–The dyspnea in patients with mitral stenosis may be severe enough to progress to episodes of acute pulmonary edema, especially in the presence of some additional stress. Increased heart rate due to anxiety, atrial arrhythmia, fever due to intercurrent infection, excessive salt intake, or unaccustomed exertion should be sought.

3. Hemoptysis–Hemoptysis is the second most common presenting symptom in mitral stenosis. There may be frank pulmonary hemorrhage from rupture of a pulmonary vein; frothy pink, blood-tinged sputum in pulmonary edema; or hemoptysis resulting from pulmonary infarction. Hemoptysis is seen in patients with raised pulmonary vascular resistance and in those with pulmonary congestion.

4. Systemic embolism–Presenting symptoms due to systemic embolism are infrequent in patients with mitral stenosis. Embolism is more common after atrial fibrillation has occurred and tends to occur later in the disease.

5. Palpitations–Palpitations are rarely the chief complaint. Any arrhythmia is likely to provoke dyspnea, and the patient will usually complain of dyspnea rather than palpitations.

6. Symptoms in patients with raised pulmonary vascular resistance–Fatigue, coldness of the extremities, abdominal discomfort, and swelling of the abdomen and ankles are symptoms of right heart involvement. They suggest the presence of severe pulmonary hypertension and raised pulmonary vascular resistance with a low cardiac output and are thus indicative of severe mitral stenosis. Symptoms of right heart involvement can also occur in patients with associated organic involvement of the tricuspid valve. Chest pain that is indistinguishable from angina pectoris is occasionally noted in the presence of raised pulmonary vascular resistance or pulmonary embolism.

7. Episodic symptoms–Confusion in diagnosis sometimes occurs when the patient's symptoms are episodic. In this case arrhythmia should be suspected, and 24-hour monitoring of the ECG is indicated.

B. Signs: The physical signs in patients with mitral stenosis vary with the severity of the valvular lesion and also with the amount of increase in pulmonary vascular resistance. The classic signs of mitral stenosis develop early in the natural course of the condition and can usually be noted before symptoms develop. However, the patient may have to engage in exercise in order to elicit the signs. In classic mitral stenosis, the pulse is normal or small in amplitude, and the blood pressure and systemic venous pressure are normal.

1. Loud first heart sound–The heart is not enlarged, and on palpation there is an obvious localized tapping cardiac impulse. This represents the vibrations from the loud first heart sound that result from closure of the mitral valve (closing snap). There may also be a diastolic thrill with presystolic accentuation felt at the apex and a palpable opening snap felt at the base of the heart.

2. Opening snap–On auscultation the first sound is loud, and the second sound is followed by a loud opening snap that is high-pitched and widely transmitted but heard best to the left of the sternum, near the base of the heart.

3. Diastolic murmur with presystolic accentuation–The characteristic finding in predominant mitral stenosis is a long, loud, rumbling mitral diastolic murmur with presystolic accentuation due to atrial systole (Fig 12–2). The murmur is often best heard in a localized area about 2.5 cm in diameter located at the apex of the heart. The patient should lie on the left side after exercise, and the physician should use the bell of the stethoscope and light pressure on the chest. The murmur may be absent in mid diastole in mild cases but still show presystolic accentuation (Fig 12–3).

4. S_2–OS interval–The time elapsing between the aortic valve closure sound and the opening snap is roughly related to left atrial pressure. If left atrial pressure is high, the valve will open early because

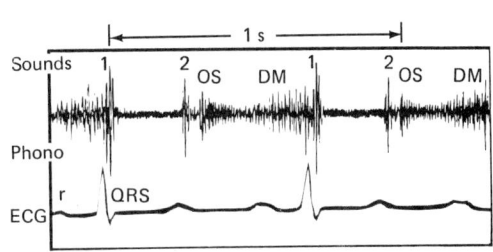

Figure 12–2. Typical phonocardiogram in mitral stenosis showing loud first sound and opening snap (OS), followed by long diastolic rumbling murmur (DM) with presystolic accentuation. (Courtesy of Roche Laboratories Division of Hoffman-La Roche, Inc.)

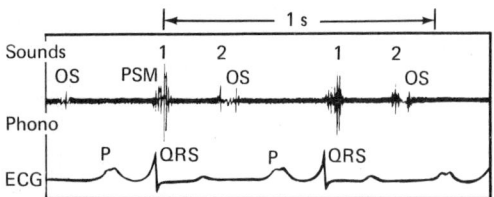

Figure 12–3. Phonocardiogram of loud first sound in mitral stenosis. Note presystolic murmur (PSM) and opening snap (OS) with no diastolic murmur following the snap. (Courtesy of Roche Laboratories Division of Hoffman-La Roche, Inc.)

left atrial pressure soon comes to exceed left ventricular pressure. Conversely, if left atrial pressure is low, a longer time will elapse before left atrial pressure exceeds left ventricular pressure and filling starts.

There is not infrequently a mitral systolic murmur in pure mitral stenosis. A long, rumbling diastolic murmur with presystolic accentuation during atrial contraction is the definitive auscultatory sign of mitral stenosis, and the presence of a presystolic (atrial systolic) murmur excludes a diagnosis of significant mitral incompetence. Thus, even though hemodynamically insignificant mitral incompetence is mild, it may cause a loud systolic murmur. This should not be construed as evidence of significant mitral incompetence when a patient has none of the other signs of mitral incompetence but some of the signs of mitral stenosis. The murmur may be due to tricuspid incompetence.

5. Signs in the presence of atrial fibrillation–When the patient develops atrial fibrillation, the presystolic murmur disappears. The heart rate becomes irregular, and after the heart rate has been slowed by digitalis therapy it becomes important to listen for the length of the diastolic murmur during the longest diastolic pauses. In patients with predominant mitral stenosis, the murmur should persist until the end of diastole even in cardiac cycles lasting 1 second. A shorter murmur suggests either mixed mitral stenosis and incompetence or raised pulmonary vascular resistance. It is the length of the diastolic murmur and not the fact that it lasts until the next first heart sound that is important in the determination of the severity of mitral stenosis.

6. Pulmonary signs–Rales at the bases of the lungs are commonly found in mitral stenosis, but their absence does not exclude the possibility of pulmonary congestion or even edema. The patient is often orthopneic because the lungs become more congested when the patient is in a supine position, the respiratory rate increases as the lungs become stiffer, and the patient becomes breathless.

7. Signs in the presence of pulmonary hypertension–When pulmonary vascular resistance is markedly raised (> 7.5 mm Hg/L/min), the physical signs of mitral stenosis tend to be different. The patient usually has a low cardiac output and is often thin, with peripheral cyanosis, cool extremities, and a pulse of small volume. Dilated veins on the cheeks combined with peripheral cyanosis give rise to a "mitral facies" that is also seen in other patients with a chronically low cardiac output. Systemic venous pressure is likely to be raised, with a prominent a wave visible in the jugular pulse if sinus rhythm is present. The heart may be enlarged, with a right ventricular substernal impulse. The auscultatory signs of mitral stenosis tend to be less florid than those in patients with low pulmonary vascular resistance because the cardiac output is lower. In about one-third of cases, either reduction in the cardiac output or valvular calcification modifies the classic physical signs, making the diagnosis difficult. Calcification of the valve may eliminate the opening snap but should not affect the murmur. Low output may eliminate the murmur but should not affect the snap. Calcification of the mitral valve does not always affect the physical signs, and more than half of patients with valvular calcification have an opening snap. There is often a pulmonary systolic ejection click and a short pulmonary systolic murmur in addition to a loud pulmonary valve closure sound.

a. Pulmonary incompetence–Pulmonary incompetence secondary to pulmonary hypertension may cause an immediate diastolic murmur at the base of the heart (Graham Steell murmur). In practice, associated hemodynamically insignificant aortic incompetence is a more common cause of such a basal murmur.

b. Tricuspid incompetence–Pansystolic murmurs are common in patients with pulmonary hypertension and are usually due to secondary tricuspid incompetence, as shown by increased systemic venous pressure, a prominent v wave in the neck, and increased intensity of the murmur during inspiration. When right ventricular failure occurs, the right side of the heart may become so large that it occupies the whole front of the chest.

8. Signs in the presence of low output–In severely ill patients, the mitral diastolic murmur may vary in intensity because of changes in cardiac output or heart rate. The fact that one observer has heard the murmur and another has not should not be discounted, and repeated examinations may be helpful. A mitral diastolic murmur that is ordinarily inaudible may be heard by listening in the axilla, with the patient lying on the left side.

9. Assessment of severity from physical signs–Assessment of the severity of mitral stenosis based on physical signs is not of sufficient accuracy to be clinically valid. Patients with varying degrees of stenosis can all show fully developed classic physical signs.

C. Electrocardiographic Findings: The ECG is of little help in diagnosing or assessing the severity of predominant mitral stenosis with low pulmonary vascular resistance. A broad, notched, posteriorly oriented P wave (P mitrale) is usually all that is present. If right ventricular hypertrophy is present, pulmonary vascular resistance is almost certainly raised. Evidence of right ventricular hypertrophy on the ECG is seen in 75% of patients whose pulmonary vascular resistance is over 7.5 mm Hg/L/min. The absence of right ventricular hypertrophy on the ECG does not rule out severe pulmonary hypertension, but some signs are usually present, and the progressive development of changes on the ECG is an important clue to the diagnosis of raised pulmonary vascular resistance. Evidence of left ventricular hypertrophy on the ECG suggests a diagnosis of systemic hypertension, aortic valve disease, or rheumatic myocardial disease rather than mitral incompetence.

D. X-Ray Findings: In predominant mitral stenosis with normal pulmonary vascular resistance, the overall heart size may be normal, as shown in Fig 12–1. The left atrium is enlarged, and the left atrial appendage is usually visible on the left cardiac border. The pulmonary artery is not greatly enlarged unless pulmonary arterial pressure is over 45 mm Hg. Minor enlargement of the pulmonary artery contributes to straightening of the left cardiac border when the pulmonary artery pressure is lower. The left main bronchus may be elevated and lie more horizontally than normally. With moderate left atrial enlargement, the right border of the left atrium produces a double density on the right.

1. Pulmonary changes–The chest x-ray is useful in assessing the degree of pulmonary congestion. The most characteristic finding is the presence of Kerley's B lines, as shown in Fig 12–4. These are thickened interlobular septa that are usually seen at the outer edges of the lungs at the bases. They are evidence of chronic pulmonary congestion and are almost invariably associated with significantly increased pulmonary venous pressure. Diffuse pulmonary fibrosis in patients without evidence of heart disease occasionally causes Kerley's B lines. The pattern of pulmonary congestion in mitral valve disease is influenced by the effects of gravity. The bases of the lungs occupy the lowest position in the chest whether the patient is standing or supine. The level of the pulmonary venous and arterial pressures is therefore highest at the bases of the lungs.

2. Pulmonary hypertension–The response of pulmonary blood vessels to increased pressure is hypertrophy of their walls; consequently, pulmonary vascular disease is most marked at the base of the lungs. As the pulmonary arterioles thicken and develop an increased resistance to blood flow, redistribution of pulmonary blood flow occurs. As a result, the veins of the upper lobe of the lung become more prominent, and the lower lobes receive a smaller proportion of pulmonary blood flow. "Pruning" of the pulmonary arterial tree appears first at the base and later spreads to involve the entire lung. Occasionally, passive pulmonary venous congestion with intra-alveolar hemorrhage causes hemosiderosis, giving rise to a diffuse mottled pattern on the chest x-ray.

3. Ventricular enlargement–When the heart is enlarged, it is not always easy to decide on purely radiologic grounds whether the right ventricle (Fig 12–5) or the left ventricle (Fig 12–10) is enlarged.

E. Special Investigations:

1. Noninvasive techniques–The mitral valve is one of the structures that registers most clearly and consistently on echocardiography. The movements of the valve during systole and diastole and the effects of atrial contraction can usually be clearly discerned. Echocardiography is thus especially helpful in the diagnosis and clinical assessment of patients with mitral stenosis. The valve is thickened and less mobile than

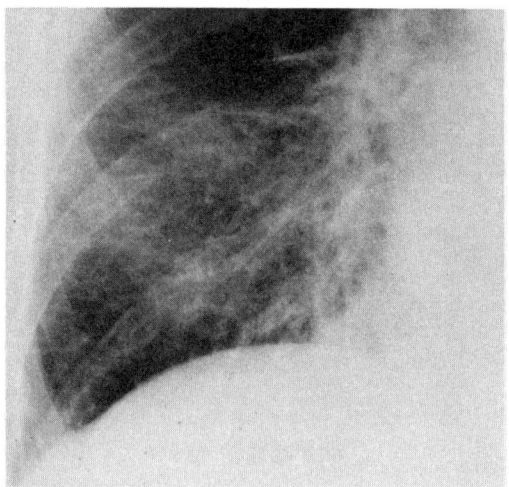

Figure 12–4. Close-up of chest x-ray of base of right lung of patient with mitral stenosis showing Kerley's B lines.

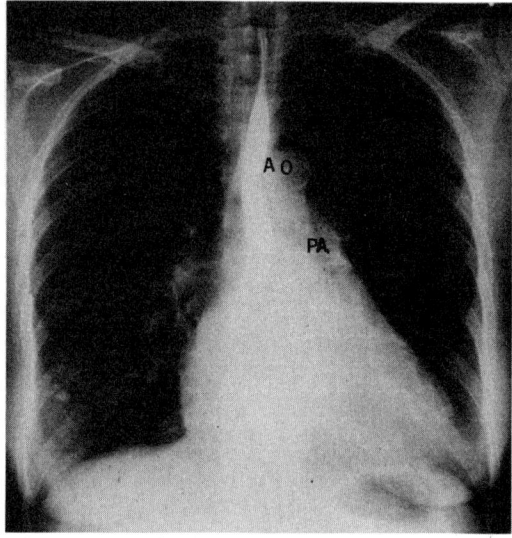

Figure 12–5. Chest x-ray of a 60-year-old woman with cardiac enlargement resulting from mitral stenosis with pulmonary hypertension. Ventricular enlargement is right-sided. AO, aorta; PA, pulmonary artery.

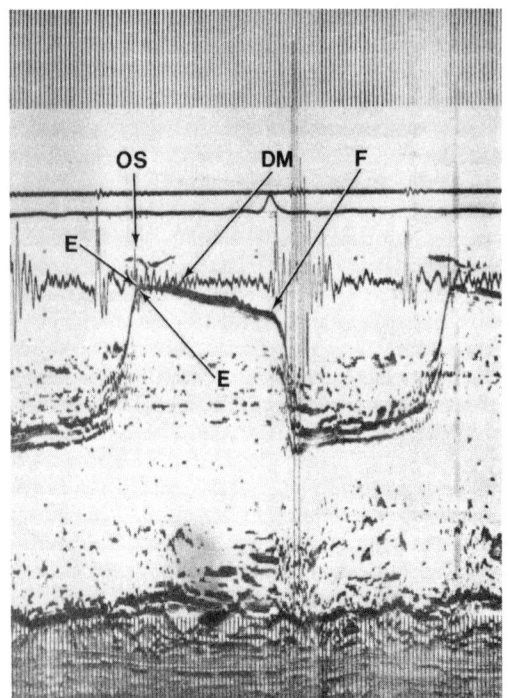

Figure 12–6. Echocardiogram showing slow diastolic posterior motion of stenotic mitral valve. Atrial fibrillation is present. OS, opening snap; E, E point on mitral valve echo; F, F point on mitral valve echo; DM, diastolic murmur. (Courtesy of NB Schiller.)

normally in patients with mitral stenosis, as shown in Fig 12–6. The thickened adherent mitral valve leaflets move together; and, while anterior valve motion may be less than normal, the posterior leaflet may in some cases move more than normally. Measurement of the mitral valve slope gives some indication of the severity of stenosis. The valve slope is the rate of change in the position of the fused mitral valve cusps that occurs as the valve closes during diastole. It is measured by drawing a straight line through the echo tracing and calculating the E → F slope in mm/s. The normal E → F slope of 80 mm/s or more falls to about 20 mm/s in mitral stenosis, and the values obtained in different patients correlate significantly with the mitral valve area calculated from data obtained during cardiac catheterization. The measurement is not completely specific, since slow posterior valve motion is also seen in patients with extremely low cardiac output. However, it may be valuable in following the course of the disease, since the effect of operation on the mitral valve slope can be clearly demonstrated (Fig 12–7).

Two-dimensional echocardiography is also valuable in assessment of the severity of mitral stenosis. An idea of the diastolic dimensions of the mitral valve orifice can usually be obtained in short-axis views. The valve area measured by this means has been shown to correlate significantly with measurements made at cardiac catheterization.

Doppler blood velocity recordings from the mitral valve orifice can be obtained with a transducer aimed from the apex of the heart toward the mitral valve.

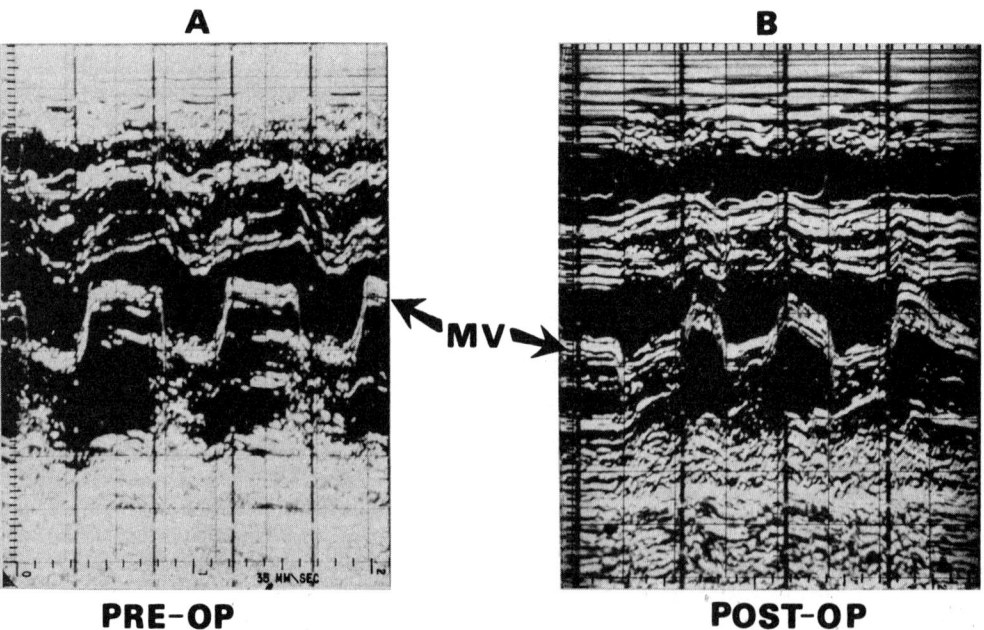

Figure 12–7. Preoperative *(A)* and postoperative *(B)* echocardiograms showing mitral valve (MV) motion in a patient with mitral stenosis. The diastolic slope of valve motion is steeper in *B*. (Reproduced, with permission, from Kleid J, Schiller NB: *Echocardiography Case Studies*. Medical Examination Publishing Co., 1974.)

The peak velocity of blood flow in the jet of blood passing through the valve bears a relationship to the peak pressure difference across the valve (Chapter 4). Measurement of the half-time of the fall in blood velocity in the jet at the start of diastole has been shown to provide an indirect measure of the pressure difference across the valve in patients with mitral stenosis. The value empirically expressed as $220 \div t_{1/2}$ where $t_{1/2}$ is the half-time, correlates well with hemodynamic measurements of the mitral valve gradient.

2. Invasive techniques–

a. Cardiac catheterization–Cardiac catheterization is almost always indicated before surgery, and studies should be repeated before a second operation is performed. It is rarely needed for diagnosis because the classification of patients into the categories of mitral stenosis, mixed mitral stenosis and incompetence, and mitral incompetence is not based on cardiac catheterization findings. The left atrial ("wedge") pressure, the left ventricular pressure, and the cardiac output are needed for full assessment of the severity of mitral stenosis. Measurements of pulmonary arterial pressure, the left atrial (wedge) pressure, and the cardiac output are necessary to calculate pulmonary vascular resistance, which is an important variable in mitral stenosis. In most laboratories, the wedge pressure is considered to be an acceptable substitute for left atrial pressure. In some centers, however, direct left atrial pressure measurement by transseptal catheterization is preferred. In patients with distorted cardiac anatomy due to marked left atrial enlargement, kyphoscoliosis, unsuspected left atrial thrombus, or left atrial tumor, transseptal catheterization is less successful and more dangerous because of the likelihood of cardiac perforation and systemic embolization. It is not always possible to pass a catheter across the mitral valve in patients with mitral stenosis, even though the left atrium can be entered. On the other hand, left ventricular retrograde catheterization from the aorta is normally easy. For these reasons and because left ventricular angiography is now almost routinely performed, simultaneous measurements of wedge pressure and left ventricular pressure are widely used in patients with mitral stenosis.

(1) Hemodynamic measurement of severity– There is no entirely satisfactory method for measuring the hemodynamic severity of mitral stenosis, even during cardiac catheterization. The calculation of mitral valve area by means of the hydraulic formula introduced by Gorlin and Gorlin is the best available method (see p 74). The 3 variables—cardiac output, length of diastole, and pressure difference across the valve— are included in the calculation. Mitral diastolic blood flow is only equal to cardiac output when there is no mitral incompetence, and the presence of significant mitral incompetence is the principal cause of error in applying the formula. When mitral incompetence is not taken into account, mitral diastolic flow is underestimated, giving a falsely low value in the measurement of valve area. Simpler alternative measurements of "gradient," ie, pressure difference across the valve, have been suggested. End-diastolic gradient, mean gradient, and the difference between mean wedge pressure and end-diastolic pressure have been advocated. Although these may give rough indications of the degree of stenosis in patients whose heart rates are in the normal range, they can never be as accurate as calculations that include the length of diastole. The patient's symptoms are best assessed by the level of the wedge pressure. In general, mild symptoms occur with resting wedge pressures below 20 mm Hg, moderate symptoms with wedge pressures between 20 and 30 mm Hg, and severe symptoms with resting wedge pressures over 30 mm Hg.

(2) Technique for patients with pulmonary hypertension–In patients who have marked increases in pulmonary vascular resistance, wedge pressure measurement is critical and may occasionally prove difficult because the high pulmonary arterial pressure is associated with rapid tapering of the vessels. If a satisfactory wedge pressure tracing cannot be recorded using a conventional cardiac catheter, a Swan-Ganz balloon-tipped catheter should be passed into a peripheral branch of the pulmonary artery and the balloon inflated to obtain an indirect measure of left atrial pressure.

(3) Risks in severely ill patients–Patients with mitral stenosis and markedly raised pulmonary vascular resistance are often severely ill when they undergo cardiac catheterization. Although measurement of simultaneous wedge and left ventricular pressures and cardiac output is important, the patient may be so ill that a limited study is all that is warranted. Such patients tolerate angiography poorly, particularly when large volumes of contrast material are injected rapidly into the pulmonary arteries.

(4) Relationship between clinical and hemodynamic findings–The results of cardiac catheterization in patients with mitral stenosis are often surprising because the hemodynamic severity differs from what might be expected based on the clinical features of the case. In some patients with severe symptoms, the hemodynamic data are unimpressive; in other patients, the wedge pressure is markedly raised even when symptoms are relatively mild. Discrepancies between hemodynamic data and symptoms are even more common after surgical treatment, and heart rate and rhythm must always be considered in interpreting the results of cardiac catheterization in patients with mitral stenosis. Errors in calibrating strain gauges, collecting expired gas for the determination of oxygen consumption, and collecting and analyzing blood samples may provide false information. An unduly anxious or excited patient, failure to achieve a steady state, or even simple computational errors may give a false impression of the severity of the lesion.

(5) Indications for cardiac catheterization–It has become almost routine to obtain baseline hemodynamic data before performing any surgery. Since mitral valve replacement is a more serious operation than valvotomy, most cardiologists believe that complete left and right heart catheterization should always be done before the patient undergoes mitral valve replacement.

(6) Exercise during cardiac catheterization– Patients with mitral stenosis must sometimes exercise during cardiac catheterization, because if the wedge pressure is only slightly raised, the pressure difference across the mitral valve may be too small to be measured accurately, and the calculation of mitral valve area may be unduly influenced by small pressure differences, especially when the heart rate is slow. When the patient exercises and increases the heart rate and cardiac output, it is possible to accentuate the hemodynamic findings and confirm or disprove resting values. As a rule, only mild exercise or the simple maneuver of raising the legs will cause a significant increase in wedge pressure in patients with mitral stenosis. Accurate pressure measurements and cardiac output determinations during steady-state exercise at significant work loads are difficult to obtain.

(7) Overall results– The results of cardiac catheterization in patients with mitral stenosis show considerable variation from case to case. However, the average values give some indication of the levels of pressure and flow. The data in Table 12–2 show the fall in cardiac output and the rise in pulmonary arterial systolic and diastolic pressures associated with raised pulmonary vascular resistance. Mean right atrial pressure is also raised in patients with high resistance.

b. Left ventricular angiography is now an important component of the overall study of patients with mitral stenosis. It is primarily used to evaluate left ventricular function and to determine the presence or absence of mitral incompetence. The multiple ectopic beats that so frequently follow the left ventricular injection of contrast material often cause mitral incompetence, even in patients with normal mitral valves. In patients with mitral stenosis, the small rigid orifice of the mitral valve may permit a small localized jet of contrast material to flow back into the left atrium. This finding does not invalidate the diagnosis of predominant mitral stenosis, however. It is important to assess the size of the left ventricle, measure its systolic and diastolic dimensions, and compare the measurements with the equivalent dimensions of the left atrium and the systemic cardiac output before concluding that significant mitral incompetence is present. Spurious mitral incompetence occurring after left ventricular injections of contrast material is useful in the diagnosis of left atrial myxoma because the contrast material that enters the atrium may outline the tumor and confirm the diagnosis. Injection of contrast material into the pulmonary artery can also be used for this purpose.

c. Coronary angiography– In many centers, coronary angiography is performed almost as a routine in patients with mitral valve disease who are over age 40. The yield from such investigations is low when there is no clinical evidence of coronary disease. In our opinion, coronary arteriography is only indicated if cardiac pain or electrocardiographic evidence of myocardial ischemia is present.

Differential Diagnosis

Left atrial myxoma (see Chapter 21) is the most important disorder in the differential diagnosis of mitral stenosis with or without raised pulmonary vascular resistance. The radiologic picture shown in Fig 12–8 closely resembles that of mitral stenosis, and left atrial appendage enlargement is seen. Episodic symptoms,

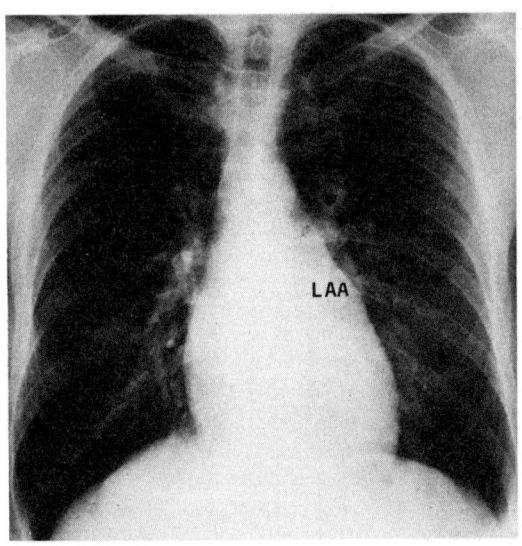

Figure 12–8. Chest x-ray in a 40-year-old man with left atrial myxoma. The left atrial appendage (LAA) is prominent.

Table 12–2. Cardiac catheterization data in patients with mitral stenosis.

	Pulmonary Vascular Resistance (mm Hg/L/min)	Indirect Left Atrial (Wedge) Pressure (mm Hg)	Cardiac Output (L/min)	Pulmonary Arterial Pressure (mm Hg)		Mean Right Atrial Pressure (mm Hg)
				Systolic	Diastolic	
Low resistance (< 4.0)	1.9 ± 1.0	26 ± 4	4.5 ± 1.1	47 ± 12	23 ± 6	7 ± 4
Intermediate resistance (4.0–7.5)	5.3 ± 1.0	29 ± 7	3.6 ± 1.1	71 ± 20	32 ± 8	8 ± 4
High resistance (> 7.5)	12.2 ± 5.0	31 ± 5	2.8 ± 0.7	94 ± 19	43 ± 8	13 ± 5

variable heart murmurs, fever, systemic embolism, a raised sedimentation rate, and hyperglobulinemia suggest the possibility of myxoma. The lesion is 100 times less common than mitral stenosis and 100 times more common than the rare congenital lesion cor triatriatum, in which the left atrium is divided into an upper and a lower chamber by an incomplete transverse septum. Cor triatriatum may also simulate mitral stenosis. Echocardiography and angiocardiography with injection of dye into the left ventricle or pulmonary artery are helpful in diagnosis.

In patients with raised pulmonary vascular resistance, pulmonary hypertension due to any other cause such as Eisenmenger's syndrome, idiopathic or thromboembolic pulmonary hypertension, or atrial septal defect with acquired pulmonary hypertension must be ruled out. Because mitral stenosis with pulmonary hypertension is amenable to surgery and patients with pulmonary hypertension due to other causes do not withstand exploratory thoracotomy well, it is essential to make the correct diagnosis.

Course & Complications

The course of mitral stenosis is long, lasting 20 years or more in many instances. The natural history of the lesion can be altered by surgical treatment, and an almost normal life expectancy may be possible with optimal treatment. If the stenosis is moderate or severe, mitral valvotomy will almost certainly be required before age 40 for the relief of dyspnea unless the level of activity is seriously curtailed by the patient. Restenosis of the valve may necessitate a second valvotomy, and mitral valve replacement is likely to be required. Coexistent left ventricular myocardial disease plays a smaller part in the course of mitral stenosis than in any other valvular lesion.

The course of mitral stenosis is, however, often different in tropical, subtropical, and developing countries. Pure mitral stenosis, with minimal myocardial involvement, is less frequent, and the latent period before symptoms develop is short. Associated pulmonary hypertension is particularly prevalent on the Indian subcontinent. Cardiac enlargement due to rheumatic myocardial damage is the rule, and the classic form of the disease, in which the patient is in sinus rhythm and the left atrium is the only chamber enlarged, is seldom seen. Atrial fibrillation occurs at an early age, and the response to surgical treatment is less than satisfactory.

A. Atrial Fibrillation: Atrial fibrillation occurs so frequently in the course of mitral stenosis that it hardly qualifies as a complication. The importance of both the effect of atrial fibrillation on the natural history of the lesion and its time of onset cannot be stressed too strongly. The circumstances precipitating atrial fibrillation and its clinical effects provide important diagnostic and prognostic information about the lesion. It is important to determine whether the onset of atrial fibrillation aggravated existing symptoms or heralded their appearance. If the onset of atrial fibrillation escapes notice in a patient with mitral stenosis, either the lesion is extremely mild or increased pulmonary vascular resistance is present. In the latter situation, the patient has presumably been so disabled that the additional stress of the arrhythmia goes unnoticed. The earlier atrial fibrillation occurs, the worse the prognosis because of the implication that rheumatic carditis must have damaged the atrial muscle. Conversely, if atrial fibrillation has not developed by age 50 in a patient with mitral stenosis, the stenosis is almost invariably mild. It is therefore imperative to determine the circumstances surrounding the onset of atrial fibrillation and to assess the patient's tolerance of the arrhythmia.

B. Bronchitis: The congested lungs of patients with mitral disease are prone to bronchitis. This is seen more frequently in patients with mitral stenosis, because pulmonary congestion is generally more severe than in other types of mitral valve disease.

C. Pulmonary Infarction: Pulmonary embolism and pulmonary infarction are common, especially in mitral stenosis with raised pulmonary vascular resistance. The lungs with their double arterial blood supply normally are not subject to infarction unless they are congested, and mitral stenosis is one of the commonest conditions in which pulmonary embolism is followed by pulmonary infarction. It is not always possible to determine the origin of the thrombus, and although emboli from the veins of the pelvis and legs are common, the possibility of thrombosis in situ should not be ruled out.

Treatment

A. Medical Treatment:

1. Penicillin prophylaxis to prevent recurrence of rheumatic fever–Prophylactic penicillin therapy to prevent recurrence of rheumatic carditis should be considered in all young patients with mitral stenosis. The younger the patient, the stronger the indication for treatment. The upper age limit for the initiation and cessation of prophylactic penicillin therapy is not clearly defined. Most physicians do not start prophylactic therapy if the patient is older than age 30 or if there has been no evidence of activity in the previous 5 years; treatment is seldom continued past age 40. The dosage schedules are given in Chapter 17 (p 536).

2. Prevention of infective endocarditis–Treatment to prevent infective endocarditis should always be recommended, especially if the valvular lesion is mild.

3. Restoration of sinus rhythm by DC countershock–Restoration of sinus rhythm in patients with atrial arrhythmia is rarely indicated before surgery in mitral stenosis. A patient with atrial fibrillation and symptoms severe enough to warrant restoration of sinus rhythm would almost certainly benefit from surgery.

B. Surgical Treatment:

1. Mitral valvotomy–Surgery in mitral valve disease is seldom if ever curative. However, it is the treatment of choice. Mitral valvotomy is indicated in any patient with mitral stenosis who has significant symptoms and a mitral valve area of about 1 cm² or less. The operation, which is now usually performed under direct vision during cardiopulmonary bypass, is palliative; its benefits do not last indefinitely. Open mitral valvotomy improves the surgeon's ability to treat left atrial thrombus, and mitral incompetence is less likely to result. This operation also enhances the possibility of mobilizing subvalvular structures such as fused papillary muscles and matted chordae tendineae. The decision whether to proceed with mitral valvotomy or to replace the mitral valve ultimately rests with the surgeon and is often made during the operation. In some cases, during the actual valvotomy, the surgeon encounters problems that make valve replacement essential and lead to a change in plans. Mitral valvotomy is not dangerous in patients with mitral stenosis and low pulmonary vascular resistance. The mortality rate is less than 2%, and in most centers patients with class II symptoms are readily selected for operation. The principal cause of morbidity and mortality is embolism. Occasionally, massive cerebral embolism occurs with disastrous results. Mitral stenosis often occurs with little or no rheumatic myocardial involvement, and in such cases the mechanical effects of obstruction to mitral flow predominate, so that the results of surgery are good. In patients with more evidence of myocardial disease, in older patients, in those with atrial fibrillation, and in those with enlarged hearts, the benefits of valvotomy are less dramatic. However, there is almost always some temporary benefit from surgery. There is often a discrepancy between improvement in the patient's symptoms, which is striking, and the objective evidence of benefit, which is often lacking.

2. Mitral valve replacement–Mitral valve replacement is seldom indicated as an initial operation in patients with mitral stenosis. If the patient is a woman of childbearing age, the use of long-term anticoagulation therapy, which is usually necessary after mitral valve replacement, is a distinct disadvantage. In patients with raised pulmonary vascular resistance, valve replacement may occasionally be indicated as an initial operation, especially in older patients with calcified valves. Valve replacement is generally performed only when mitral valvotomy has failed to control the patient's symptoms.

A second or even a third mitral valvotomy is not infrequently performed when stenosis recurs or when the first operation has not relieved the obstruction. Raised pulmonary vascular resistance does not contraindicate mitral valvotomy, and satisfactory reversal of pulmonary vascular disease following mitral valvotomy can be achieved.

3. Mortality rate in patients with pulmonary hypertension–The mortality rate of surgery in patients with raised pulmonary vascular resistance is roughly related to the level of resistance. In patients with severe right heart failure, the mortality rate is 10–15%. Late deaths in heart failure (10%) and survivors with persistent irreversible pulmonary vascular disease as shown in Fig 12–9A and B bring the percentage of cases with unsatisfactory results to about 50%. This figure reflects the fact that many patients seek treatment at a late stage of the disease.

Prognosis

The prognosis for patients with mitral stenosis is good now that mitral valve surgery is readily available. Although the lesion cannot be cured and myocar-

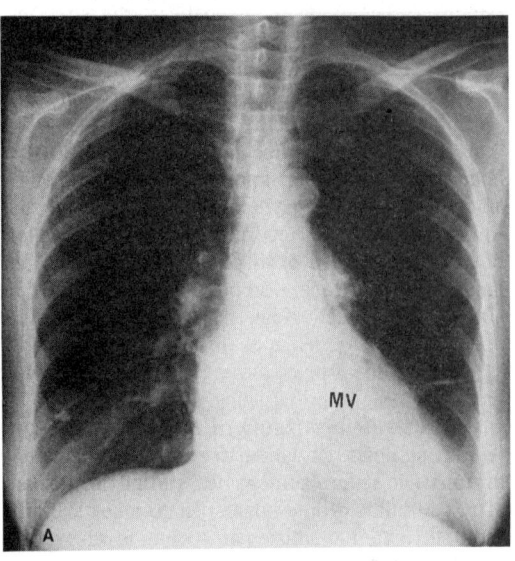
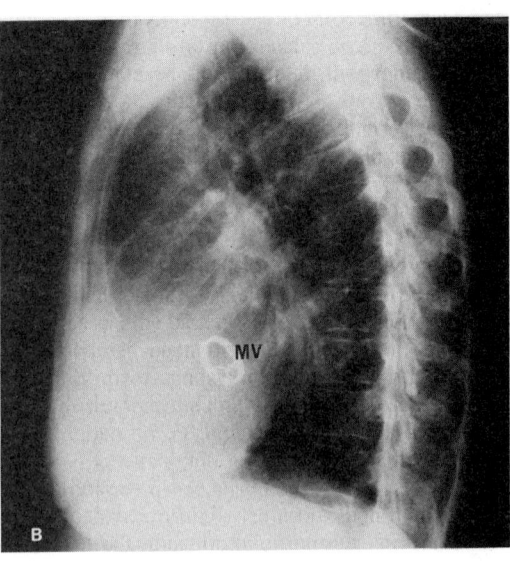

Figure 12–9. Postoperative chest x-rays of the 60-year-old woman whose preoperative x-ray is shown in Fig 12–5. Cardiac enlargement persisted after operation. The Björk-Shiley prosthetic valve (MV) is seen more clearly on the lateral view. *A,* posteroanterior view; *B,* lateral view.

dial involvement due to rheumatic carditis is not affected by surgery, relief of dyspnea and prevention of attacks of pulmonary edema are ensured. Most patients with mitral stenosis who have had mitral valvotomy will develop symptoms again some time later, probably with the onset of atrial fibrillation in early middle age. The benefits of mitral valvotomy in patients with mitral stenosis vary and tend to be best in those who develop severe stenosis at an early age and who have no evidence of myocardial disease. Age is an important factor; if the indications for mitral valvotomy are strong and if the operation is on a young adult, the relief may last for 10–15 years, but if operation is not indicated in early adult life and is not performed until the patient is 50, the relief is likely to be short-lived. Results are better in patients who are in sinus rhythm, which probably reflects the influence of age on prognosis. It is clear that age-related degenerative changes both in the valve itself and in the atrial and ventricular myocardium play an important role and that coexisting rheumatic and degenerative heart disease are seen more frequently now that surgical treatment is widely available.

Raised pulmonary vascular resistance worsens the prognosis of mitral stenosis. If developing pulmonary hypertension is diagnosed early and treatment is not delayed, the prognosis is better. In older patients, however, and in patients who do not receive early treatment, the prognosis is significantly worse. Relief of mitral stenosis reverses the course of pulmonary vascular disease; the speed of reversal depends on 2 factors: (1) how thoroughly the mitral stenosis has been eliminated and (2) how long the original pulmonary changes have been present. Improvement may continue for up to 2 years after operation.

Long-Term Results in Operated Cases

As experience has accumulated, it has become clear that mitral valvotomy is a palliative operation and that most patients ultimately require mitral valve replacement. The long-term results of mitral valve replacement are now becoming better defined as more data are available to determine the 10- to 20-year results. The 10-year survival rate after mitral valve replacement is about 50% irrespective of the type of valve used. Anticoagulation is required for all prosthetic valves and also for tissue valves if there is atrial fibrillation. Valve failure is around 10–15% over a 10-year period. No artificial valve has normal hemodynamic function, and some pressure difference is always found across the valve.

Embolism is an important complication that persists over the years and is responsible for both disability and death. It occurs at a rate of more than 5% per year, but only about half of emboli cause serious problems.

MIXED MITRAL STENOSIS & INCOMPETENCE

In some cases the rheumatic involvement of the mitral valve leads to dilation and stretching of the valve tissue and subsequent scarring and retraction in addition to narrowing. In this case, stenosis is present in addition to significant leakage through the valve. After severe mitral stenosis has been treated surgically, the stenosis is less severe, but the valve is still abnormal. With time, degenerative changes, fibrosis, and calcification stiffen and immobilize the valve and produce a mixture of stenosis and incompetence. The cardinal features of this lesion (Fig 12–10) include obstruction and leakage at the mitral valve, left atrial enlargement, and left ventricular enlargement (not hypertrophy). Variable features that may alter these findings are the severity of obstruction, the amount of regurgitation, and the severity of rheumatic myocardial damage.

Patients with mixed mitral stenosis and incompetence run a more constant clinical course than might be expected in view of the numerous possible combinations of severity of the components. Fig 12–11 illustrates the hemodynamic reasons for the constant clinical course. The blood that leaks back across the mitral valve during systole must flow forward during diastole, augmenting the normal forward stroke volume. Mitral incompetence thus increases mitral diastolic blood flow. The clinical severity of mitral valve disease is determined by left atrial pressure, which in turn depends on the length of ventricular diastole, the size and function of the left atrium, and mitral diastolic blood flow. The extra blood flow resulting from systolic mitral incompetence raises left atrial pressure and makes any mitral stenosis appear more severe. For these reasons, the clinical severity of mixed mitral stenosis and incompetence depends on the sum of the incompetence and the stenosis and tends to remain constant. If there is more stenosis than incompetence, there is a smaller amount of systolic backflow and a smaller diastolic forward flow across the valve. If there is more incompetence than stenosis, there is a larger systolic backflow and a larger diastolic forward flow. Thus, the symptoms in patients with mixed mitral lesions tend to vary less than might be expected. In contrast, the physical signs—which depend mainly on the volume of blood passing through the mitral valve during both systole and diastole—tend to depend on the severity of incompetence, and there is wide variation in the lengths and intensities of the systolic and diastolic mitral murmurs and in the degree of left ventricular volume overload.

Mixed mitral stenosis and incompetence, as a naturally occurring lesion, is commoner in subtropical and tropical countries than in the USA. The more widespread involvement of the myocardium, related to impaired nutrition, more frequent recurrences of streptococcal infections, and lack of penicillin prophylaxis may be responsible, together with the overcrowded housing resulting from larger families.

Mitral valve seen from left atrium

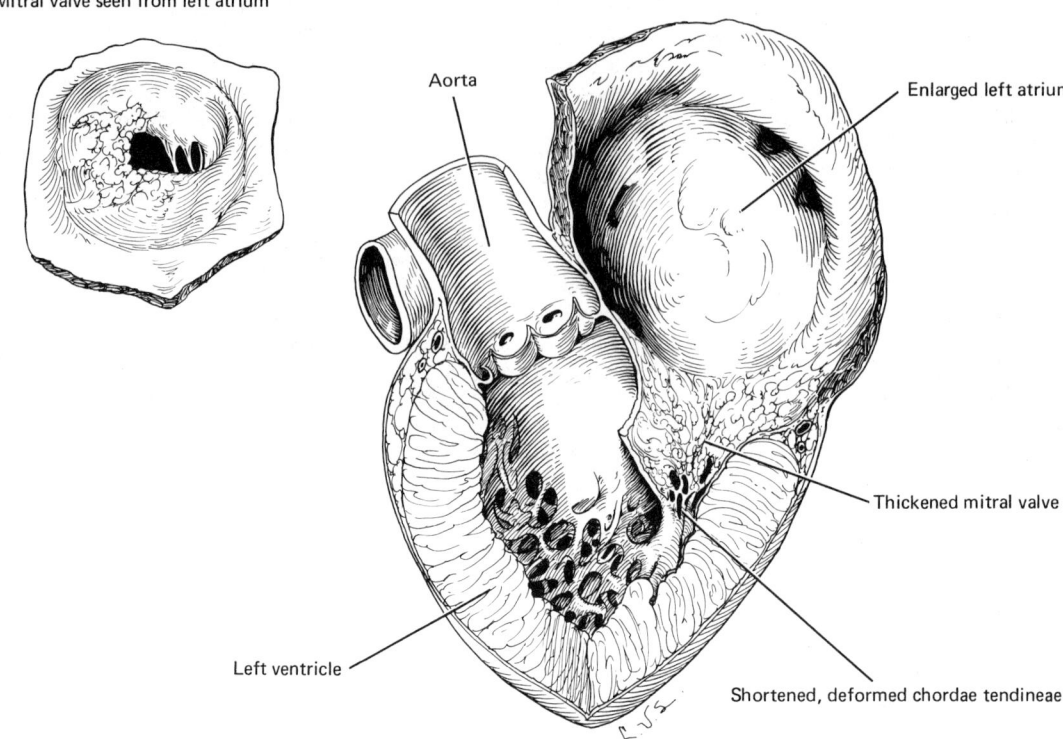

Drawing of left heart in left anterior oblique view showing anatomic features of mixed mitral stenosis and incompetence.

Cardinal features: *Obstruction and leakage at the mitral valve; left atrial enlargement; left ventricular enlargement (not hypertrophy).*

Variable factors: *Severity of obstruction; amount of leakage; severity of rheumatic myocardial damage.*

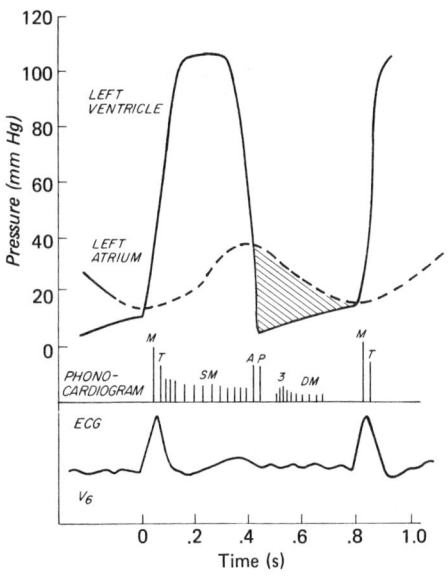

Diagram showing auscultatory and hemodynamic features of mixed mitral stenosis and incompetence. (Abbreviations are explained in Fig 11–1.)

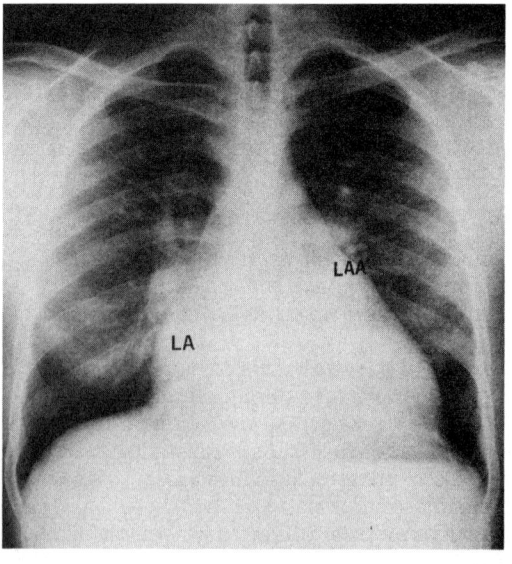

Chest x-ray showing left atrial (LA), left atrial appendage (LAA), and left ventricular enlargement in mixed mitral stenosis and incompetence.

Figure 12–10. Mitral stenosis and incompetence. Structures enlarged: left atrium, left ventricle.

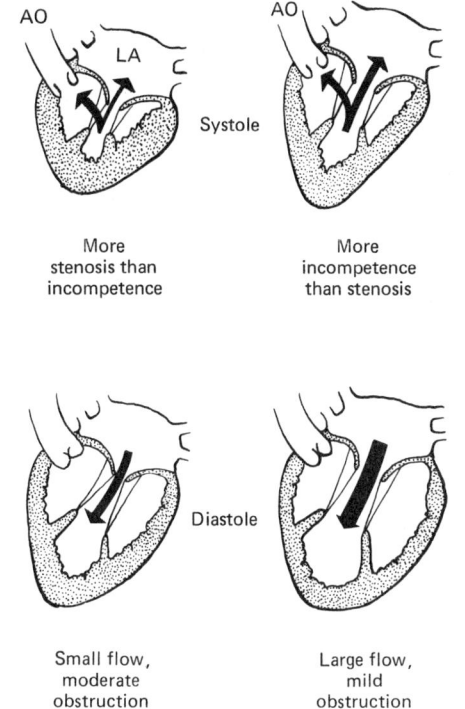

Figure 12-11. Diagram showing hemodynamic interaction between stenosis and incompetence in mixed mitral valve lesions. AO, aorta; LA, left atrium.

Clinical Findings

A. Symptoms:

1. Dyspnea–Dyspnea is the commonest presenting symptom in patients with mixed mitral stenosis and incompetence. It seldom occurs while the patient is in sinus rhythm. The patient often presents with an acute episode of dyspnea associated with the development of atrial fibrillation. This onset commonly heralds the approach of other symptoms, and the patient, who may have been living a relatively normal life, becomes acutely ill with severe dyspnea and perhaps pulmonary edema. Atrial fibrillation is sometimes triggered by an intercurrent infection such as influenza or pneumonia, and a systemic or pulmonary embolism may occur simultaneously. This clinical picture is so common that it is important to consider the possibility of mitral stenosis and incompetence in any patient who suddenly becomes short of breath, especially if the heart rate is rapid and atrial fibrillation is present. The physical signs can be difficult to interpret in the acute stage when the heart rate is rapid. Episodic dyspnea may be present when there is paroxysmal atrial arrhythmia. In such circumstances it is important to see the patient during an attack.

2. Palpitations–Palpitations are common in patients with mixed mitral stenosis and incompetence. Palpitations are generally due to atrial arrhythmia; if the heart rate is rapid, dyspnea is likely to occur.

3. Systemic embolism–The first symptom of mixed mitral stenosis and incompetence may be due to acute systemic embolism. Sudden pain and coldness in the leg, sudden paralysis, acute loin pain due to renal infarction, flank pain due to infarction of the spleen, and infarction of the bowel due to mesenteric artery emboli sometimes occur. Embolism usually occurs in patients with atrial fibrillation, particularly when the rhythm changes, but it may happen when the patient is in sinus rhythm.

4. Pressure from a large left atrium–Symptoms due to pressure from a greatly enlarged left atrium on surrounding structures are occasionally seen. Thus, cough, hoarseness, and recurrent lung infection involving the left lower lobe may occur.

B. Signs:

The signs in patients with mixed mitral stenosis and incompetence depend on the degree of incompetence. When incompetence is the predominant lesion, the left ventricular systolic ejection rate is more rapid than normal, and the peripheral pulse resembles a miniature "water-hammer" pulse. In patients with mixed mitral stenosis and incompetence it is not always easy to assess the relative importance of the stenosis, the incompetence, or the overall severity of the lesion. Many of the patients with this lesion have had mitral stenosis, and the mitral incompetence has resulted from either valvotomy or calcification and fixation of the deformed valve as well as degenerative, age-related changes and increased wear and tear.

The systemic venous pressure is not often raised unless there is associated tricuspid valve disease. Because pulmonary hypertension is seldom severe, the pulse is usually normal and the rhythm irregular in patients with atrial fibrillation. The heart is usually enlarged, with a hyperdynamic left ventricular impulse. The first sound may be loud and there may be an opening snap, especially if the patient has had a previous valvotomy for mitral stenosis. A third heart sound may also be heard, sometimes replacing the snap rather than accompanying it. Depending on the volume of mitral diastolic blood flow, there is a pansystolic mitral murmur transmitted to the axilla and a diastolic mitral murmur of variable length (Fig 12–12). In patients with moderate mitral incompetence, the murmur may last until the end of diastole at rapid heart rates (more than 100/min). The murmur is never accentuated during atrial systole, because even if the patient is in sinus rhythm, the mitral stenosis is not sufficient to limit atrial emptying, and the force of contraction of the distended left atrium is reduced. In patients with atrial fibrillation, the length of the mitral diastolic murmur depends on the RR interval of the preceding beat. A long diastolic pause allows time for equilibration between left atrial and left ventricular pressures. With long pauses, the murmur disappears toward the end of diastole. It is thus important to ascertain the length of the diastolic murmur during the longest pauses. In mixed mitral stenosis and incompetence, the murmur is less than full length at a normal heart rate of 70/min.

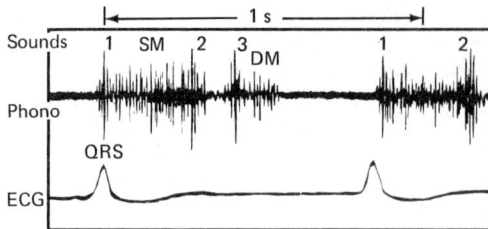

Figure 12-12. Phonocardiogram from a patient with mixed mitral stenosis and incompetence in atrial fibrillation. A pansystolic murmur (SM) and third heart sound (3) are followed by a short diastolic murmur (DM) at a slow heart rate. (Courtesy of Roche Laboratories Division of Hoffman-La Roche, Inc.)

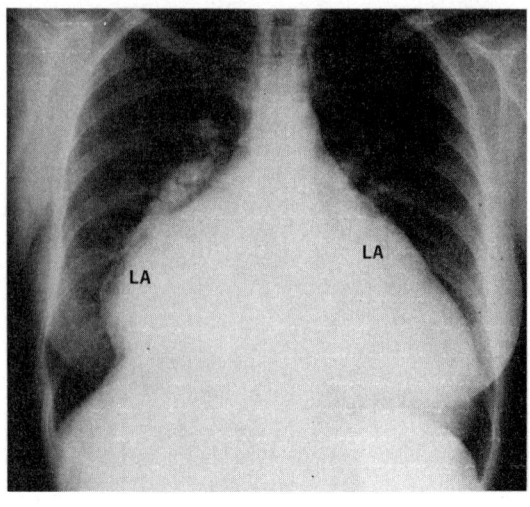

Figure 12-13. Chest x-ray of a 42-year-old woman with giant left atrium. The left atrium (LA) forms the left and right heart borders on the posteroanterior view.

Pulmonary congestion in mixed mitral valve disease is less marked than in mitral stenosis. Although pulmonary edema may occur at the onset of atrial fibrillation, control of the heart rate by digitalis usually leads to rapid improvement, and the symptom seldom recurs. Similarly, an increase in pulmonary vascular resistance seldom occurs and is not often severe in mixed mitral valve disease, presumably because left atrial pressure is lower than in pure stenosis. The most important factors to consider in mixed mitral valve disease are heart rate and heart rhythm. The whole clinical picture is greatly dependent on these factors, and the effects of changes in heart rate on the patient's condition offer the best means of assessing the severity of the lesion.

C. Electrocardiographic Findings: The electrocardiographic findings in patients with mixed mitral stenosis and incompetence are not of diagnostic value. A broad, notched, posteriorly oriented P wave (P mitrale) is seen if the patient is in sinus rhythm. Atrial fibrillation is usually present, whereas right ventricular hypertrophy is rarely seen.

Left ventricular hypertrophy on the ECG is common but not invariable, even when mitral incompetence is more prominent than stenosis. The hypertrophy is more commonly due to systemic hypertension, aortic valve disease, or rheumatic myocardial disease than to the valve lesion.

D. X-Ray Findings: Left ventricular enlargement is seen in patients with mixed mitral stenosis and incompetence, and it is roughly proportionate to the severity of the lesion. Left atrial enlargement is seen as a double density on the right border of the heart (Fig 12-10).

Left atrial enlargement tends to be greatest in patients with mixed mitral stenosis and incompetence. In patients with giant left atrium, shown in Fig 12-13, in which the chamber assumes enormous proportions with a volume of one liter or more, mixed mitral lesions are almost always present. The left atrium forms both the right and left borders of the heart and the picture can be mistaken for that of pericardial effusion (see Chapter 18).

Enlargement of the left atrial appendage, seen on the left border of the heart, is almost invariably present.

E. Special Investigations:

1. Noninvasive techniques–Because the mitral valve shows up so well on echocardiography, this form of investigation is particularly helpful in assessing the lesion. Echocardiography can determine the degree of stenosis, effects of incompetence, and the sizes of the left atrium and ventricle.

2. Invasive techniques–

a. Cardiac catheterization–Right and left heart catheterization are required before surgery in all patients with mixed mitral stenosis and incompetence. Simultaneous measurements of wedge pressure, left ventricular pressure, and cardiac output are essential. The patient is frequently in atrial fibrillation, and the effects of variation in the length of diastole from beat to beat can be clearly seen in Fig 12-14. The height and configuration of wedge pressure tracings depend on the severity of the lesion, the heart rate, and the compliance of the left atrium. Equalization of the pressures in the left atrium and left ventricle usually occurs by mid diastole at slow heart rates (less than 60/min). With faster heart rates (shorter diastolic intervals), wedge pressure rises, and an end-diastolic pressure difference usually occurs. The time course of the fall in left atrial pressure following the v wave is roughly exponential, and its time constant depends on the product of the resistance to flow across the mitral valve and the compliance of the left atrium. Thus, either mitral stenosis or a capacious left atrium may slow the rate of left atrial emptying and ventricular filling. The amount of left ventricular blood leaking back into the atrium cannot be accurately measured in mixed mitral lesions, with the result that mitral valve area cannot be accurately calculated. However, it is possible to calculate a lower limit, arbitrarily

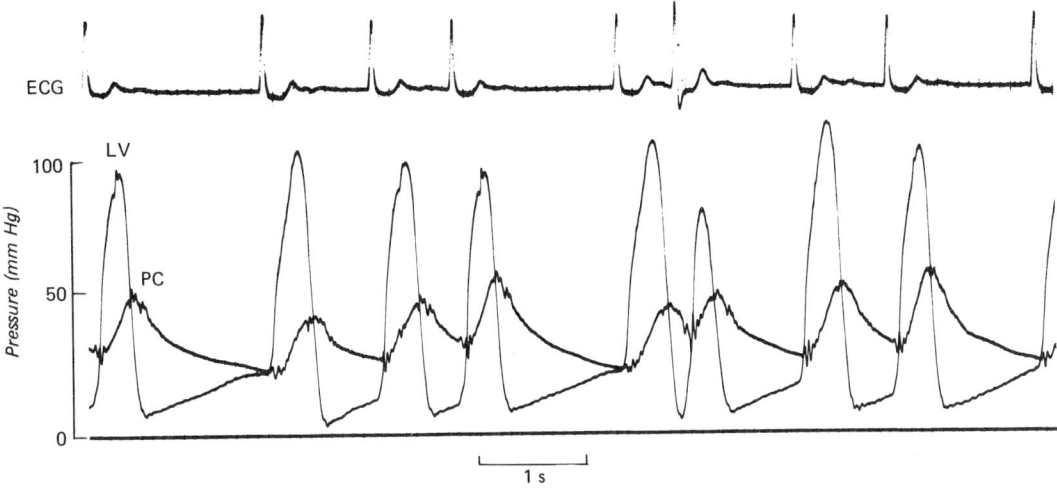

Figure 12-14. Wedge (PC) and left ventricular (LV) tracings from a patient with mixed mitral stenosis and incompetence in atrial fibrillation. The wedge pressure rises and the end-diastolic gradient increases when the heart rate increases. Lower wedge pressures are seen after a longer pause occurs between beats, and the end-diastolic gradient disappears.

assume there is no incompetence, and estimate that the valve area is greater than a certain value. The left ventricular end-diastolic pressure is ordinarily normal in patients with mixed mitral valve disease, and pulmonary congestion results from relative mitral stenosis rather than left ventricular failure. A raised end-diastolic left ventricular pressure in a patient with mixed mitral valve disease suggests that independent left ventricular myocardial disease is present and requires further investigation. Unrecognized rheumatic myocardial damage, systemic hypertension, uncontrolled atrial fibrillation, aortic valve disease, and coronary disease should be considered as possible causes.

b. Left ventricular angiography–Left ventricular angiography is needed in all patients. It provides the only means of measuring the amount of mitral incompetence. If the left ventricular stroke volume is subtracted from the forward stroke volume (calculated by means of the Fick principle), the difference is the volume of blood flowing back across the mitral valve per beat. This somewhat indirect measurement is not always accurate, but it is the best available. Left ventricular angiography also gives an indication of left ventricular function, which may be impaired because of either rheumatic myocardial damage or coronary artery disease.

Differential Diagnosis

A. Atrial Septal Defect: In atrial septal defect, atrial fibrillation, cardiac enlargement, and systolic and diastolic murmurs occur, and in the middle-aged patient an erroneous history of rheumatic fever in childhood is sometimes present. With these findings, the incorrect diagnosis of rheumatic heart disease is easily made. Radiologic examination is most useful because in atrial septal defect the chest x-ray shows a large pulmonary artery, a small aorta, a big heart, a big right atrium, and a left atrium that is usually unimpressive. The ECG almost invariably shows an incomplete or complete right bundle branch block with an rsR' pattern in lead V_1. This finding should always raise the suspicion that an atrial defect exists. Cardiac catheterization is ordinarily required to establish the diagnosis with certainty. The 2 lesions—mitral valve disease and atrial septal defect—may rarely coexist in Lutembacher's syndrome. In this condition, raised venous pressure, hepatomegaly, and peripheral edema are common, and the presence of right heart failure in a patient with mixed mitral stenosis and incompetence should always suggest an associated atrial septal defect.

B. Hypertrophic Cardiomyopathy: Patients with hypertrophic cardiomyopathy (who tend to be confused with those with mixed mitral valve disease) have lesions of the left ventricular inflow tract, with or without outflow obstruction. This lesion is rare, but when it is present mitral systolic and diastolic murmurs and mitral incompetence are seen. Significant left ventricular hypertrophy is always seen on the ECG. Echocardiography shows narrowing of the left ventricular outflow tract and systolic anterior motion of the aortic cusp of the mitral valve.

Course & Complications

A. Atrial Fibrillation: As in pure mitral stenosis, atrial fibrillation is such a frequent occurrence that it hardly qualifies as a complication. The age at which it occurs depends to some extent on the severity of the lesion and on the rheumatic myocardial damage. In patients with severe, recurrent attacks of rheumatic carditis, atrial fibrillation may occur even in adolescence. In the Western world, the onset is usually delayed until about age 40. In other countries, the onset of atrial fibrillation occurs much earlier, reflecting the higher incidence of rheumatic myocardial damage and recurrent episodes of rheumatic fever. The onset of atrial fibrillation often heralds the onset of dyspnea.

B. Rheumatic Myocarditis: Acute rheumatic myocarditis is an important complication of valve disease. It is common in patients with mixed mitral stenosis and incompetence and is so difficult to diagnose that it is usually only in retrospect that it can be identified. The standard major and minor criteria for rheumatic fever activity are seldom present. The early onset of atrial fibrillation, disproportionate cardiac enlargement, disproportionate tachycardia, and left ventricular hypertrophy or left bundle branch block on the ECG all point to rheumatic myocardial damage. On cardiac catheterization, low cardiac output, high left ventricular end-diastolic pressure, and diminished left ventricular ejection fraction indicate an important myocardial factor, which is generally assumed to be active rheumatic carditis in patients under age 40. Since histologic evidence of rheumatic activity in the form of Aschoff's nodes can be found in the left atrial appendage in virtually all patients undergoing operation, even the histologic criteria for the diagnosis of active rheumatic carditis are of doubtful value in identifying patients with clinically important rheumatic myocarditis. Patients with severe myocardial damage have a worse prognosis following surgery than patients with pure mechanical lesions, but management is not altered significantly by the finding.

The severe myocardial damage so commonly seen in patients with mixed mitral valve disease in tropical countries may be due to several factors. In addition to frequent recurrences of rheumatic fever, malnutrition, anemia due to hookworm infestation, and other tropical diseases may play a part. Left ventricular failure tends to occur as a result of myocardial damage and raises the left atrial pressure to levels sufficient to cause an increase in pulmonary vascular resistance, which further worsens the prognosis.

C. Coronary Artery Disease: In older patients, atherosclerotic coronary arterial disease may influence the clinical picture with a myocardial factor that alters prognosis.

D. Systemic Embolism: Systemic embolization is a frequent and important complication. Embolism is detected in about 20% of cases, but the true incidence is almost certainly higher when asymptomatic cases are included. Cerebral, femoral, renal, intestinal, and coronary emboli comprise most of the clinically recognized cases. Left atrial thrombi form because of stasis and account for most emboli in mixed valvular disease. The emboli resulting from left atrial thrombus clear more readily than those associated with endocarditis. Embolism is more common in patients with atrial fibrillation and is more likely to occur when heart rhythm changes, either at the onset of atrial fibrillation or at the restoration of sinus rhythm.

E. Infective Endocarditis: Endocarditis is a serious complication in patients with mixed mitral stenosis and incompetence. It occurs more frequently than in mitral stenosis, but not as often as in mitral incompetence. The patient is almost invariably in sinus rhythm at the time of onset (see Chapter 16).

F. Pulmonary Vascular Disease: The development of a raised pulmonary vascular resistance is much less common than in mitral stenosis, because the left atrial pressure is usually lower. In patients with severe myocardial involvement, left ventricular failure may contribute significantly to the increase in left atrial pressure and lead to the development of important pulmonary hypertension.

Treatment

A. Medical Treatment:

1. Prophylactic penicillin–Since rheumatic myocarditis is so commonly associated with mixed mitral stenosis and incompetence, prophylactic penicillin treatment to prevent recurrence of rheumatic fever is essential. The younger the patient, the more important the treatment. Penicillin prophylaxis should be continued up to about age 40 and is seldom started in patients over age 30 (see Chapter 17).

2. Prevention of endocarditis–Antibiotic therapy to prevent infective endocarditis should always be recommended, especially if the lesion is mild. It should be administered before the patient undergoes major dental work or minor surgical procedures (see Chapter 16).

3. Restoration of sinus rhythm by DC conversion–Restoration of sinus rhythm before surgery is sometimes indicated. If the patient develops atrial fibrillation with a rapid heart rate during an intercurrent infection or in relation to some other special stress, the mitral valve lesion may be too mild to warrant surgical treatment. In this case, restoration of sinus rhythm by DC countershock (as described in Chapter 7) may be effective in maintaining sinus rhythm for several years. In general, however, the results of cardioversion are poor, not because the patient fails to obtain relief but because atrial fibrillation soon recurs. The addition of propranolol for the control of heart rate may be useful in some patients. The deleterious effects of the drug on myocardial function may be outweighed by the benefits of a reduced heart rate, but, in general, medical treatment provides only temporary relief.

4. Anticoagulant therapy–Anticoagulant therapy is often advised in patients with atrial fibrillation who are not treated surgically. Unfortunately, it does not always prevent embolism, and if embolism occurs in a patient who has been given anticoagulants in full doses, hemorrhage into the area of infarction may be disastrous.

B. Surgical Treatment: Mitral valve replacement is the only operation indicated for the treatment of mixed mitral stenosis and incompetence. Starr-Edwards valves have generally proved to be the most satisfactory. Annuloplasty, valvuloplasty, and other conservative reconstructive operations on the mitral valve have not proved successful. Mitral valvotomy is contraindicated because significant mitral stenosis is not present by definition. Since mixed mitral stenosis and incompetence is a mechanically less severe lesion than mitral stenosis, the results of surgery are less dramatic. By the time the question of surgery arises, patients are older, there is a greater likelihood of associated myocardial disease, and atrial fibrillation has almost inevitably occurred. Since mitral valve replacement is a more serious operation than valvotomy, surgery is generally undertaken with much greater caution than in mitral stenosis. It is important to observe the response to medical treatment in patients presenting with dyspnea at the onset of atrial fibrillation. It may be possible to postpone mitral valve replacement for several years if the arrhythmia has been precipitated by some intercurrent illness; if the heart rate was extremely rapid at the onset but has slowed significantly with digitalis therapy; and if the patient can lead a quiet life. The decision to replace the mitral valve in patients with mixed mitral stenosis and incompetence is always a serious one because the mortality rate of the operation is about 10% and improvement is seldom dramatic. On the other hand, if the operation will ultimately be necessary, it may be advantageous to do it before increasing age, degenerative changes, and coronary artery disease increase the mortality rate.

1. Influence of myocardial disease on surgery–A frequent problem confronting the physician who treats patients with mixed mitral stenosis and incompetence is to determine the relative severity of the mechanical and the myocardial elements of the lesion. Many patients who have had previous mitral valvotomy are left with either mild mitral stenosis or mixed stenosis and incompetence. The patient may have symptoms, but on cardiac catheterization the lesion does not seem to be significant enough to warrant the drastic step of mitral valve replacement. The dilemma is one of choosing between temporizing measures such as cardioversion on the one hand and valve replacement on the other. It is generally helpful to compare the original catheterization data with the more recent studies to try to decide whether the patient's status is the same as that which prompted the original surgery.

2. Restoration of sinus rhythm after surgery–Restoration of sinus rhythm by DC countershock should always be considered after surgery in patients who are not in sinus rhythm. It is not indicated in patients with giant left atrium or other lesions with marked cardiac enlargement, however. Quinidine should always be used in an attempt to prevent recurrence of atrial fibrillation.

3. Digitalization and heart rate–The immediate treatment of a patient with mixed mitral stenosis and incompetence and atrial fibrillation often consists of controlling the heart rate with digitalis because patients so commonly present with this arrhythmia. The diagnosis by auscultation of mixed mitral stenosis and incompetence can be difficult at this stage, since murmurs are more difficult to hear when the heart rate is rapid and cardiac output is low. The physician must assume that any patient presenting with rapid atrial fibrillation, dyspnea, and pulmonary congestion has mitral disease until it is proved otherwise, and full digitalization is indicated. Prophylactic digitalis may be indicated for patients in sinus rhythm in whom atrial fibrillation is expected. There is some evidence that the heart rate may be slower when atrial fibrillation occurs, but lack of certain knowledge of the blood level of digitalis complicates the emergency management of an acutely ill patient. The control of heart rate is often a serious problem, and the easier it is to achieve such control, the easier it is to manage the patient. Mitral valve replacement seldom makes the heart rate easier to control, and the anticipation that surgery will help in difficult cases should not be used as an indication for operation. Propranolol has proved valuable in some cases. A search for precipitating factors such as intercurrent chest infection, a febrile illness, anemia, or thyrotoxicosis is always indicated.

Prognosis

The prognosis in mixed mitral stenosis and incompetence is not greatly influenced by surgery, because there is usually an important myocardial factor influencing the overall clinical picture. Rheumatic myocardial disease is more likely to be present in mixed valvular disease, and the severe mechanical lesions seen in pure mitral stenosis do not occur. If a patient with mixed mitral stenosis and incompetence experiences significant dyspnea before age 30, the prognosis is poor because rheumatic myocarditis is almost certainly present. If myocardial function is good and the heart is not overly large, the patient can usually live a relatively normal sedentary life, and the heart rate can be controlled by digitalis. Systemic embolization is always a hazard but usually causes morbidity rather than death. Patients with extreme cardiac enlargement can nonetheless live strikingly long lives and are relatively uninfluenced by surgical treatment. Such patients develop a chronic low output state and, although seriously incapacitated by fatigue and dyspnea, manage to live a sedentary existence for 10–15 years after the lesion has become too far advanced for surgery.

Long-Term Results in Operated Cases

The late results of mitral valve replacement are worse in mixed mitral valve disease than in mitral stenosis. The amount of myocardial involvement is generally greater, and the heart is larger. In addition, there is not as severe pulmonary hypertension, and consequently less room for improvement because of regression of pulmonary vascular disease.

MITRAL INCOMPETENCE

Mitral incompetence differs from other forms of mitral valve disease in that it occurs as both an acute and a chronic lesion. The chronic lesions are further subdivided into hemodynamically insignificant and significant lesions. The hemodynamically insignificant form is present in those patients with the "click-murmur" syndrome described by Barlow, sometimes referred to as the floppy valve syndrome or mitral valve prolapse, but these terms are unsatisfactory because prolapse and "floppy valves" may cause acute mitral incompetence and imply a pathologic process that cannot be determined at the bedside.

Causes of Mitral Incompetence

The causes of mitral incompetence are diverse and are different for acute and chronic lesions.

A. Rheumatic Fever: A history of rheumatic fever is present in about 10% of cases; taking into account that rheumatic fever is subclinical in about 50% of cases, this figure suggests that a rheumatic cause is present in about 20% of patients with mitral incompetence. The lesion may be of any degree of hemodynamic severity.

B. Degenerative Changes: Degenerative changes in the mitral valve figure prominently in the development of mitral incompetence, and the effects of abnormal wear and tear on a slightly abnormal valve may be important in the aggravation of mitral incompetence. Stretching, tearing of the chordae tendineae, atrophy of valve tissue, and myxomatous degeneration are commonly found at operation in both acute and chronic cases. It is not clear whether the degenerative changes are superimposed on congenital or mild rheumatic lesions or whether they occur in previously normal valves. However, it is striking that a history of a previous murmur is present in half of patients with acute mitral incompetence. This suggests that degenerative changes occur more readily in abnormal valves and that patients with the click-murmur syndrome may develop acute mitral incompetence.

C. Infective Endocarditis: Infective endocarditis plays a particularly important role in the clinical course of mitral incompetence. It is both a causative factor and a complication. A valve that is the site of a minor, hemodynamically insignificant lesion seems to be especially prone to endocarditis, with the subsequent exacerbation of mitral incompetence in patients with click-murmur syndrome. Endocarditis is also a direct cause of mitral incompetence when highly invasive organisms become established in the bloodstream and lodge on a normal mitral valve. The resulting mitral incompetence is of varying degrees of severity; rarely, repeated attacks of infective endocarditis may be the sole cause of chronic mitral incompetence.

D. Ischemic Heart Disease: Ischemic heart disease may be important in the development of mitral incompetence. Posteroinferior myocardial infarctions may cause ischemia or even rupture of the papillary muscle supporting the valve. Acute rupture is usually fatal, but less severe degrees of ischemia may lead to ruptured chordae tendineae or produce acute mitral incompetence in the course of myocardial infarction. After myocardial infarction, temporary interference with the function of the mitral valve sufficient to cause a murmur of mitral incompetence commonly occurs. It is difficult to decide whether such lesions are hemodynamically significant.

E. Congenital Heart Disease: Clefts in the mitral and tricuspid valves are part of atrioventricular canal lesions. They are also part of the lesion in endocardial cushion defects, which are seen in association with ostium primum atrial septal defects. Isolated mitral incompetence seen in association with Marfan's syndrome, Ehlers-Danlos syndrome, or osteogenesis imperfecta is congenital in origin, and it may be that the click-murmur syndrome seen in young women is often congenital in origin. There seems to be an association between abnormalities of the coronary circulation and mitral incompetence, and some cases of click-murmur syndrome have been found to have abnormalities of the coronary circulation that may be responsible for the tendency toward ventricular arrhythmia in this condition. Another rare cause of mitral incompetence is coronary arteriovenous fistula.

F. Mitral Valve Ring Calcification: Calcification of the mitral valve ring is a rare cause of mitral incompetence. It occurs in elderly women and produces a pathognomonic radiologic picture (see p 394). The condition is associated with conduction defects and is not necessarily benign.

G. Traumatic Heart Disease: Steering wheel chest injuries in automobile accidents and other forms of direct trauma to the thorax, or even the effort of attempting to lift a heavy object, may apparently cause acute disruption of the mitral valve, usually by rupture of the chordae tendineae. The patient may have forgotten the episode of trauma and must be questioned directly about accidents while the history is being taken.

1. HEMODYNAMICALLY INSIGNIFICANT MITRAL INCOMPETENCE: CLICK-MURMUR SYNDROME (Mitral Valve Prolapse)

The cardinal features of hemodynamically insignificant mitral incompetence (Fig 12–15) include normal heart size and normal hemodynamics. A late systolic murmur with or without a late systolic click is present. The ECG and chest x-ray are usually normal, but ST and T wave changes suggestive of myocardial ischemia are not infrequently seen, and the chest x-ray may show evidence of skeletal abnormalities, with pectus excavatum, straight thoracic spine, or scoliosis.

Click-murmur syndrome is extremely common and has been recognized more frequently since the development of echocardiography. If echocardiographic rather than clinical criteria are used as the basis of

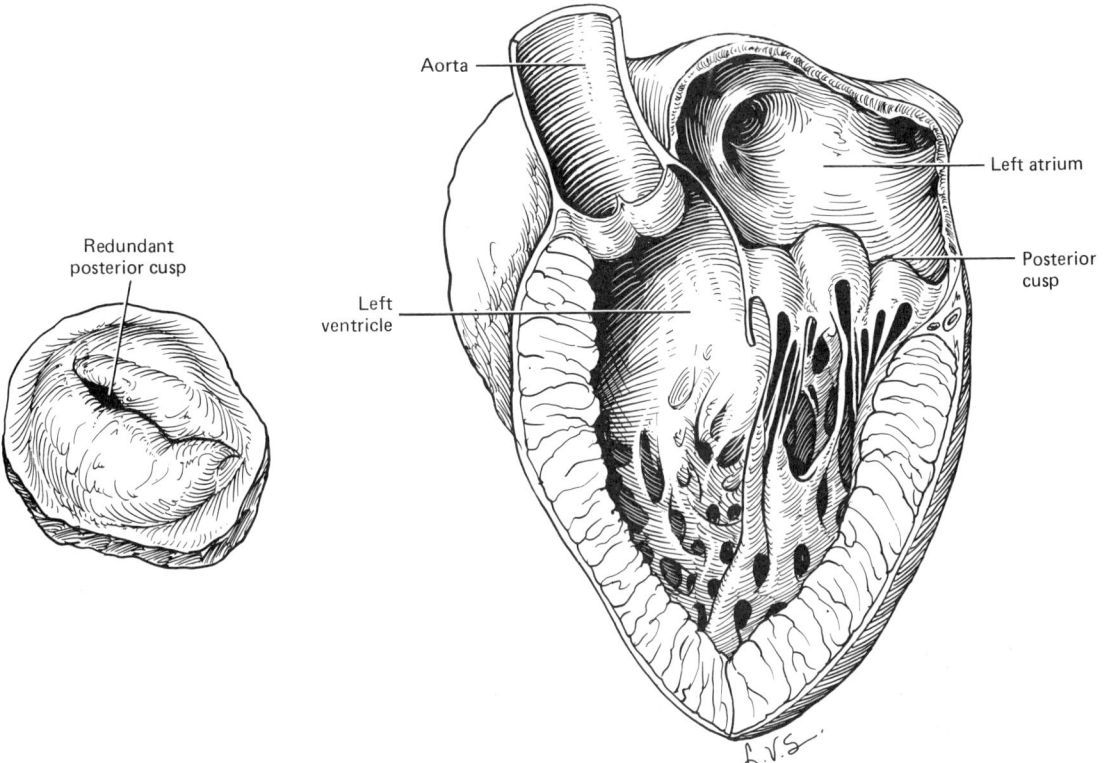

Drawing of left heart in left anterior oblique view showing anatomic features of hemodynamically insignificant mitral incompetence.

Cardinal features: *Normal heart size; redundant valve tissue.* **Variable factors:** *Clicks and murmurs.*

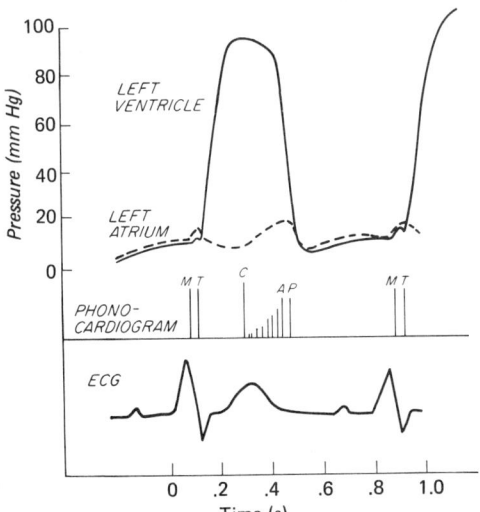

Diagram showing auscultatory and hemodynamic features of insignificant mitral incompetence. C, click. (Other abbreviations are explained in Fig 11–1.)

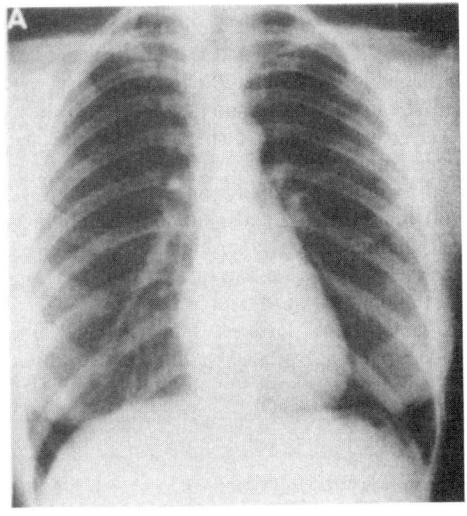

Chest x-ray in posteroanterior view of patient with click-murmur syndrome. (Reproduced, with permission, from Bontempo CP et al: Radiographic appearance of thorax in systolic click–late systolic murmur syndrome. *Am J Cardiol* 1975;**36**:27.)

Figure 12–15. Hemodynamically insignificant mitral incompetence (click-murmur syndrome). Structures enlarged: none.

diagnosis, about 5% of a normal population and up to 15% of young normal females would be found to have this lesion (Savage, 1983). Clinical examination of normal subjects with this echocardiographic abnormality reveals that while about 10% (0.5% of the normal population) have a click and 7% have a systolic murmur, the fully developed "click-murmur syndrome" is present in less than 2% (ie, 0.1% of the normal population). In spite of the fact that clinical evidence of abnormality is rare in subjects with echocardiographic evidence of prolapse, the "click-murmur" syndrome is the commonest form of valvular abnormality found in Western countries.

Click-murmur syndrome is associated with the same causes as the other forms of mitral incompetence and occurs at all ages. The click and murmur may be present in infancy or may develop at any age. The incidence is highest in women in the third and fourth decades. As with other forms of mitral disease, it is logical to base the diagnostic classification on physical findings. Echocardiography to confirm the presence of mitral valve prolapse—the commonest "cause" of the lesion—is always indicated. There is no doubt that the classic physical findings can occur without mitral valve prolapse, eg, after mitral valvotomy, and also that mitral valve prolapse can occur without the physical findings in "silent" cases or with the physical signs of significant mitral incompetence.

Late systolic mitral incompetence associated with posterior displacement of the posterior cusp of the mitral valve may be due to congenital abnormality of the valve tissue (floppy valve or billowing posterior leaflet). The redundant valve tissue bulges back into the left atrium, causing incompetence late in ventricular systole, and it is this mechanism that is thought to cause the click or murmur. In later life, degenerative myxomatous changes occur in the valve, which tends to stretch, and these changes cause similar redundancy of valvular tissue. Rheumatic disease and infective endocarditis can also cause a minor late systolic mitral valve leak. Mitral incompetence is most closely related to the presence of the late systolic murmur, and a click can be present without mitral incompetence.

The hemodynamic status as evidenced by the murmur is variable, and posture, exercise, and other mechanisms that alter systemic vascular resistance may influence the murmur. All the pathologic processes that cause click-murmur syndrome can progress either acutely or slowly to produce hemodynamically significant mitral incompetence. Thus, mitral valve prolapse, myxomatous degeneration, and floppy valves are seen in patients in whom mitral incompetence is far from minor. The proportion of cases with progressive lesions is not yet clearly established.

Clinical Findings

A. Symptoms: Most patients are entirely symptom-free, and the condition is found accidentally on routine physical examination. In some cases, atypical chest pain is present, and palpitations, fatigue, and dyspnea unrelated to exertion also occur. Exercise tolerance is almost always normal. Symptoms are more common in patients who know they have the lesion, and it seems clear that cardiac neurosis (see Chapter 21) readily develops when the presence of this lesion is brought to the attention of the patient. A family history of the lesion is occasionally found, and there may be a familial history of sudden death.

B. Signs: The only abnormalities are usually auscultatory in nature. The characteristic sign is a late systolic murmur, as shown in Fig 12–16. It is often preceded by one or more midsystolic clicks. The murmur increases in intensity up to the second heart sound, making it difficult to time and often leading to an incorrect diagnosis of diastolic murmur. It may become pansystolic with exercise or when the patient stands up. It often has a honking quality and may on occasion be loud enough to be heard without a stethoscope. It is not uncommonly the only abnormal finding, and

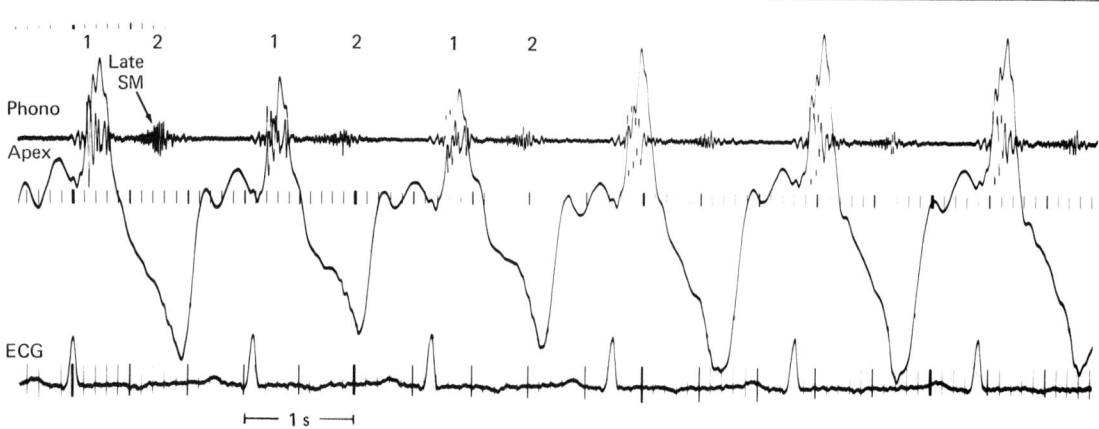

Figure 12–16. Phonocardiogram, apexcardiogram, and ECG from a patient with hemodynamically insignificant mitral incompetence. The late systolic accentuation of the murmur (late SM) can be seen.

its timing is its most consistent feature. In some cases a click is heard without a murmur. In such patients, mitral valve prolapse without mitral incompetence is thought to be present.

C. Electrocardiographic Findings: The ECG is usually normal. An abnormal P wave (P mitrale) may be seen, and in some cases there are nonspecific ST and T wave changes in the inferior leads that suggest the possibility of myocardial ischemia. An example is shown in Fig 12–17. Atrial and ventricular premature beats are often seen in long-term recordings, and atrial and ventricular tachyarrhythmias occasionally occur. The infrequent complication of sudden death is attributed to arrhythmia.

D. Chest X-Ray: The cardiac silhouette is ordinarily normal. Minor left atrial enlargement is sometimes seen. The thoracic cage is not infrequently abnormal, with pectus excavatum, straight thoracic spine, or scoliosis.

E. Special Investigations:

1. Noninvasive techniques–Echocardiography has been primarily responsible for the great increase in the frequency of diagnosis in the last 10 years. Even in patients with a click alone, echocardiographic tracings are abnormal. Echocardiography appears to be a particularly sensitive means of detecting minor degrees of mitral valve prolapse in apparently normal subjects. In addition to the movements of the valve itself, the size of the left atrium and ventricle can also be determined. A negative echocardiogram does not exclude the diagnosis, and reliance on echocardiographic findings alone, in the absence of a click or murmur (or both), may result in overdiagnosis of the lesion that may do more harm than good.

2. Invasive techniques–Since the diagnosis of chronic hemodynamically insignificant mitral incompetence is based on clinical findings and since no specific treatment is indicated, cardiac catheterization is not needed to establish the diagnosis. However, if cardiac catheterization is performed, the findings are not striking. Pressures on the right side of the heart, including the wedge pressure, are normal, and although mitral incompetence can be demonstrated by left ventricular angiography, cardiac chambers are normal in size. The anatomic features of the prolapsing mitral valve can be seen on the angiogram, but this investigation is not necessary for diagnosis. Mitral incompetence may appear more severe on superficial examination of the angiogram than it actually is after left ventricular stroke volume and forward stroke volume are measured.

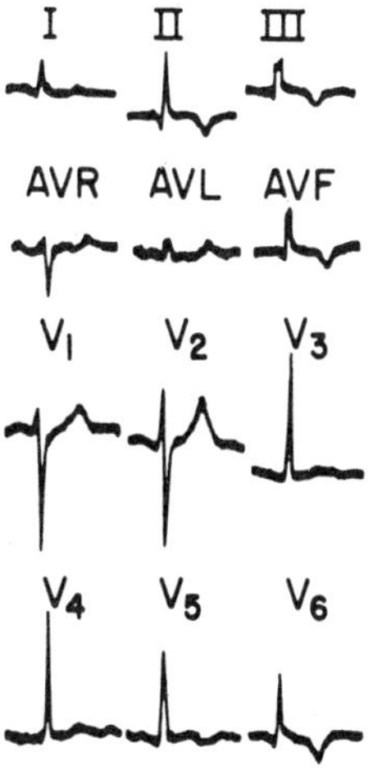

Differential Diagnosis

The physical signs of click-murmur syndrome are sufficiently specific to make the diagnosis of hemodynamically insignificant mitral incompetence reasonably certain. The underlying pathology and the cause are more difficult to determine, however, and the significance of the lesion is always open to question. The presence of associated coronary artery disease may have to be ruled out by angiography in some cases.

Course & Complications

Most patients with click-murmur syndrome live a completely normal life. The lesion is seen in elderly persons known to have had a murmur for years. The complications that occur are thus dramatic and important, but fortunately rare.

A. Infective Endocarditis: Infective endocarditis is an important complication of click-murmur syndrome. Since the hemodynamic status of the patient is virtually normal, the potential for acute valvular disruption with severe exacerbation of mitral incompetence is great. Maintaining a high index of suspicion, performing early blood culture studies, and avoiding blind treatment of intercurrent infections with antibiotics are important in minimizing the risks of endocarditis. Intravenous drug abuse is particularly dangerous. The patient is almost invariably in sinus rhythm at the onset of endocarditis (see also Chapter 16).

B. Acute Disruption of the Mitral Valve: Acute mitral incompetence can develop either spontaneously or as the result of trauma in patients with click-murmur syndrome. Rupture of the chordae tendineae or stretching of a myxomatously degenerated valve is thought to be responsible for mitral valve disruption in those cases in which endocarditis is absent. The number of patients who have this complication is not yet clearly defined.

C. Coronary Artery Disease: The role of coronary artery disease in producing or exacerbating the effects of click-murmur syndrome is not clear. Hemodynamically insignificant mitral incompetence occurs in patients with coronary artery disease, especially

Figure 12–17. Schematic representation of an electrocardiographic pattern seen in patients with the prolapsing mitral valve leaflet syndrome. (Reproduced, with permission, from O'Rourke RA et al: Prolapsing mitral valve syndrome. *West J Med* 1975;**122**:217.)

those with minor degrees of papillary muscle dysfunction. Click-murmur syndrome occurs often enough in patients in late middle age that chance associations with coronary disease must be quite frequent.

D. Ventricular Arrhythmias and Sudden Death: Patients with click-murmur syndrome show an increased tendency to develop ventricular arrhythmias, and there is undoubtedly an increased incidence of sudden death associated with this lesion. The patient whose echocardiogram is shown in Fig 12–18 subsequently died suddenly, and since no obvious cause was found at autopsy, arrhythmia was felt to be the responsible mechanism. The incidence of sudden death is not known, but even an occurrence rate of 0.1% per year is important because the condition is so common.

E. Cerebral Ischemic Events: An association has been noted between click-murmur syndrome and transient ischemic attacks in patients under the age of 45. The most likely explanation is thought to be embolization resulting from small pieces of thrombotic material formed in association with stasis around the abnormal mitral valve. A statistically significant relationship has been found between the echocardiographic finding of mitral valve prolapse and angiographic and clinical evidence of transient ischemia or partial stroke. The association was significant in patients under age 45 but not in older persons.

Treatment

Although antibiotic prophylaxis for the prevention of infective endocarditis is mandatory (see Chapter 16), click-murmur syndrome is generally so benign that no other specific treatment is needed. The patient should be followed and monitored for the development of complications. The possibility of sudden death from arrhythmia is always present, but fortunately this is rare, as no form of treatment has been shown to affect the development of this complication. Quinidine or propranolol should be given if premature beats are shown to be frequent (see Chapter 15). Patients with click-murmur syndrome in general do not lead happier lives when they are aware of the possibility of sudden death. The physician must exercise extreme care to ensure that patients with hemodynamically insignificant mitral incompetence do not become cardiac invalids. The physician should make a clear mental distinction between the patient who presents with no complaints and whose lesion is therefore discovered on routine or incidental examination and the patient who has consulted a physician because of some specific symptom thought to be related to cardiac disease.

Prognosis

The prognosis of hemodynamically insignificant mitral incompetence is not yet clear. The results of 20-year follow-up studies of patients with a late systolic murmur as the only finding indicate that infective endocarditis and acute disruption of the mitral valve due to rupture of the chordae tendineae are not infrequent sequelae. This finding correlates well with the information obtained from patients with significant mitral incompetence. A long history of a heart murmur is found in 3 types of patients with mitral incompetence: those with infective endocarditis, those with acute mitral valve disruption, and those with chronic hemodynamically significant mitral incompetence. It seems that many of these patients have had hemodynamically insignificant lesions that have subsequently become more severe. As in rheumatic mitral valve disease, it is clear to physicians who are now treating more patients in older age groups that age-related degenerative changes figure more prominently in the development of sequelae than was first thought. The mitral valve is a common site for degenerative changes of a calcific, myxomatous, or mechanical nature.

2. HEMODYNAMICALLY SIGNIFICANT MITRAL INCOMPETENCE

The cardinal features of hemodynamically significant mitral incompetence (Fig 12–19) include left ventricular enlargement (hypertrophy in acute lesions), systolic backflow into the left atrium, and left atrial enlargement. The variable features that influence atrial and ventricular enlargement are the severity of the leak and the acuteness or chronicity of the process.

Pathophysiology

A. Acute Lesions: In acute mitral incompetence, the degree of pulmonary congestion is much greater

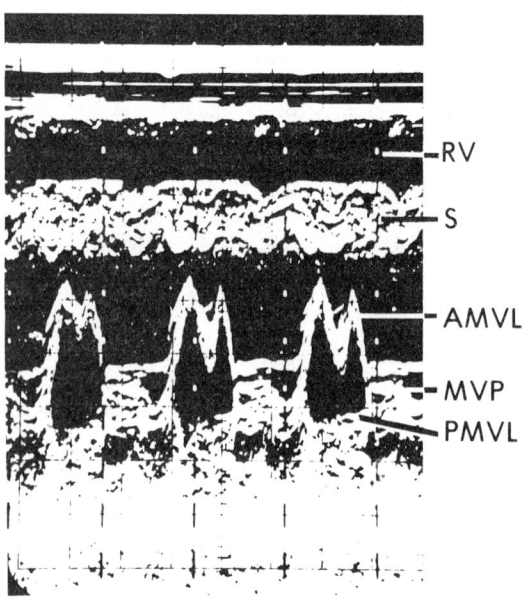

Figure 12–18. Echocardiogram showing mitral click-murmur syndrome in a patient who subsequently died suddenly. RV, right ventricle; S, septum; AMVL, anterior, and PMVL, posterior mitral valve leaflets; MVP, mitral valve prolapse. (Courtesy of NB Schiller.)

Incompetent mitral valve seen from the atrial surface

Drawing of left heart in left lateral view showing anatomic features of mitral incompetence.

Cardinal features: *Systolic backflow into left atrium; left atrial enlargement; left ventricular enlargement (hypertrophy in acute lesions).*

Variable factors: *Severity of leak; acuteness or chronicity; etiology; severity of associated left ventricular disease.*

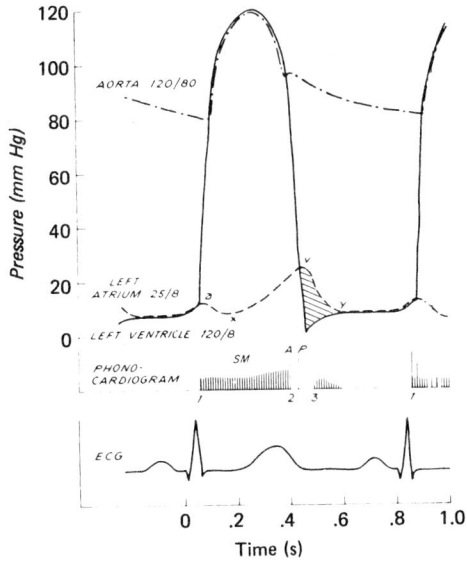

Diagram showing auscultatory and hemodynamic features of mitral incompetence. 3, third sound. (Other abbreviations are explained in Fig 11–1.)

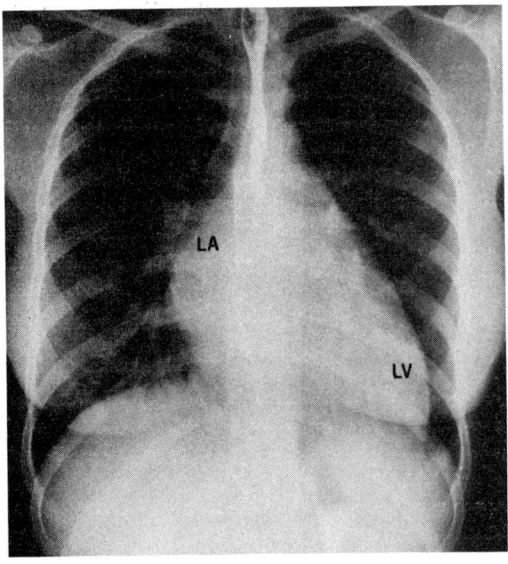

Chest x-ray of a patient with mitral incompetence showing left atrial (LA) and left ventricular (LV) enlargement.

Figure 12–19. Hemodynamically significant mitral incompetence. Structures enlarged: left atrium and left ventricle.

than in chronic lesions. A large proportion of the force of left ventricular contraction is expended in pumping blood back across the incompetent valve into a noncompliant atrium of normal size. The volume of blood flowing forward through the aortic valve falls, reducing arterial pressure and causing reflex tachycardia and peripheral vasoconstriction, which aggravate the lesion. Pulmonary venous pressure rises, and pulmonary congestion and edema occur acutely. If the acute mitral incompetence is severe, the patient cannot survive without surgical treatment. With time, pulmonary vascular resistance rises, and right heart failure ultimately develops if the patient does not die in pulmonary edema. In less severe cases, the hemodynamic picture gradually changes, and the left atrium dilates and becomes more compliant. The left ventricle enlarges, and as left atrial pressure falls, the resistance against which the left ventricle pumps decreases. In this way the left ventricular pressure load of acute mitral incompetence gradually changes to the volume load of chronic mitral incompetence. In the acute, severe stage of mitral incompetence, left ventricular hypertrophy occurs, and it is possible that part of the left ventricular hypertrophy sometimes seen on the ECG in chronic mitral incompetence may be due to a previous acute lesion.

1. Hemodynamic effects–The hemodynamic picture in acute mitral incompetence is shown in Fig 12–20. The findings are unique because there is pulmonary congestion with raised left atrial pressure but no left ventricular failure and no mitral stenosis. The systolic left atrial pressure is markedly raised owing to the late v wave, but the wedge pressure falls to normal levels by the end of diastole, and there is no appreciable end-diastolic pressure difference across the mitral valve. However, the average left atrial pressure is high enough to cause pulmonary edema, especially when diastole is shortened by tachycardia. Thus, the patient with acute mitral incompetence suffers from "relative" mitral stenosis and not from left ventricular failure in the initial stages.

2. Associated left ventricular disease–The hemodynamic changes mentioned above are seen in pure mechanical lesions, but the clinical picture is different in patients whose mitral incompetence is due to left ventricular disease.

The unique hemodynamic state of the patient with acute mitral incompetence is particularly susceptible to changes in systemic arterial resistance. The left ventricle pumps against 2 impedances in parallel during systole—aortic impedance and the impedance of the left atrium seen through the mitral valve. The magnitude of each impedance determines the overall load. If aortic impedance is reduced by vasodilator therapy, aortic flow will increase and mitral incompetence will decrease, lowering left atrial pressure and relieving any tendency toward pulmonary edema. This principle forms the basis for the successful use of nitroprusside and nitroglycerin in the treatment of acute mitral incompetence. If the patient survives, the acute lesions come to look more and more like those of chronic mitral incompetence, and after about a year, mitral incompetence that had an acute onset is usually indistinguishable from the chronic form of the lesion.

B. Chronic Lesions: Chronic mitral incompetence is the best tolerated of all the major valvular lesions.

1. Hemodynamic effects–Chronic mitral incompetence causes less hemodynamic stress than any other left-sided lesion. The left atrium bears the brunt of the load and in chronic cases dilates and becomes more compliant than normal. The mean left atrial pressure in chronic cases is thus usually less than 20 mm Hg, and left ventricular ejection against the low

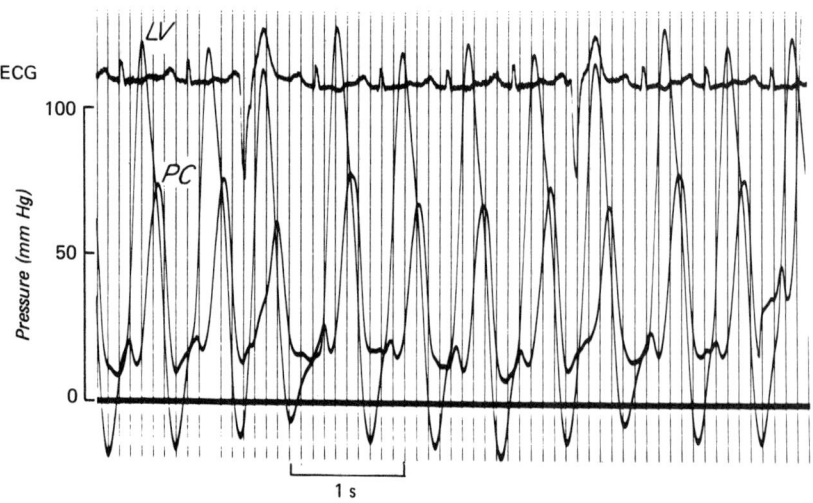

Figure 12–20. Pressure tracings in a patient with acute severe mitral incompetence showing large (70 mm Hg) v wave in wedge (PC) tracing and nearly normal left ventricular (LV) diastolic pressure.

atrial pressure results in a pure volume overload on the left ventricle. Left ventricular stroke volume is increased, but left ventricular hypertrophy does not necessarily follow. Associated left ventricular disease due to hypertension, coronary artery disease, or even possibly normal aging processes plays an important part in aggravating the hemodynamic effects of mitral incompetence. A raised systemic vascular resistance increases the leak through the mitral valve and compromises the left ventricular output. A low output causes tachycardia and peripheral vasoconstriction, which further aggravate the lesion. Thus, age-related degenerative changes in left ventricular function may be the precipitating cause of symptoms. Left atrial dilatation secondary to mitral incompetence usually leads to atrial fibrillation in middle age, but since there is no obstruction to mitral diastolic flow, patients with mitral incompetence withstand this arrhythmia better than do patients with any degree of mitral stenosis. The commonly held view is that chronic mitral incompetence of moderate or severe degree results in left ventricular hypertrophy on the ECG and leads to left ventricular failure. In our experience, this is incorrect. Undoubtedly, some patients with mitral incompetence have both of these features. It is equally clear, however, that some patients with severe lesions do not, and if the hemodynamic load were responsible for these findings, left ventricular hypertrophy and left heart failure would be the inevitable result in severe cases, as seen in patients with aortic valve incompetence or stenosis.

2. Associated left ventricular disease– Mitral incompetence also occurs as a secondary lesion in patients with left ventricular dilatation due to hypertensive heart disease or cardiomyopathy. It is also seen temporarily during the course of myocardial infarction. If these "functional" forms are included in the category of mitral incompetence, it becomes the commonest of all valvular lesions. It seems reasonable, however, to discount these temporary lesions and concentrate instead on those cases in which actual valve disease is present.

Clinical Findings

A. Symptoms:

1. Acute lesions–Dyspnea is the principal presenting symptom in patients with acute mitral incompetence. The onset may be acute (eg, when a cusp perforates or tears) or subacute (eg, when the mitral valve gradually shrinks and retracts after treatment of endocarditis). Dyspnea may progress to acute pulmonary edema with acute circulatory collapse, shock, and frothy pink, blood-tinged sputum. The patient may be ill at the time of onset, with a high fever and septicemia. Episodic attacks of dyspnea may occur and are associated with minor increases in cardiac output in response to the exertion of meals, washing, bowel movements, or even the excitement of visitors. Left atrial pressure is markedly dependent on the peripheral resistance in this lesion, and any increase in arterial pressure may provoke an attack of dyspnea.

2. Chronic lesions–In hemodynamically significant lesions, dyspnea is the principal presenting symptom. It is not usually as severe as in mitral stenosis, and the effects of an increase in heart rate are less prominent. The onset of atrial fibrillation is generally well tolerated and does not provoke the acute symptoms seen in patients who have mitral stenosis. Palpitations are more common than in other forms of mitral disease; atrial fibrillation is the commonest cause.

B. Signs: The physical signs are depicted in Fig 12–19. The first heart sound is usually buried in the pansystolic murmur, but there is never an opening snap. The presence of an opening snap indicates that significant rheumatic mitral stenosis is present. There is almost invariably a loud third heart sound associated with the rapid phase of left ventricular filling. It is a dull, low-pitched, thudding sound occurring about 0.10–0.18 second after the second sound (Fig 12–21). Some observers may consider it long enough to be called a diastolic murmur. Differences of opinion may arise about whether any degree of mitral stenosis is present. The characteristic murmur is a loud, high-pitched, pansystolic apical murmur transmitted to the axilla. It is louder on expiration and decreases when systemic vascular resistance decreases acutely, as occurs with amyl nitrite inhalation.

Signs of right heart failure and raised pulmonary vascular resistance are rare except in patients with severe acute mitral incompetence resulting from acute disruption of the valve. The presence of right-sided failure with increased venous pressure in a patient with mitral incompetence should suggest the possibility of associated organic tricuspid valve disease.

In patients with severe mitral incompetence, the cardiac impulse is hyperdynamic. The pulse is jerky and has been called a "small water-hammer pulse" because it resembles the pulse of aortic incompetence and has a rapid upstroke. The size of the heart varies with the severity and acuteness of the lesion. Chronic severe lesions show large overactive hearts because of increased systolic and diastolic flows across the incompetent valve. A prominent substernal impulse

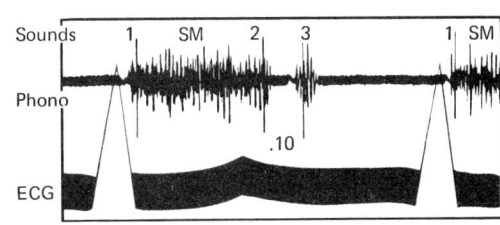

Figure 12–21. Phonocardiogram in a patient with hemodynamically significant mitral incompetence. The pansystolic murmur (SM) lasts until the second heart sound (2). The third heart sound (3) occurs 0.10 second after S_2 and lasts for about 0.05 second. Atrial fibrillation is present. (Courtesy of Roche Laboratories Division of Hoffman-La Roche, Inc.)

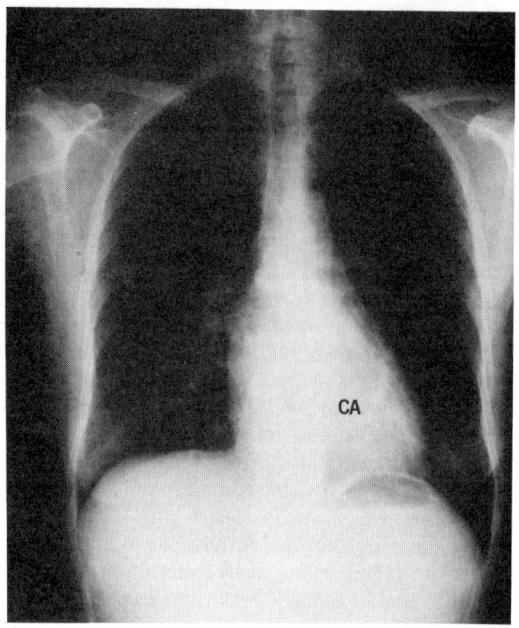

Figure 12–22. Chest x-ray of a 69-year-old woman with progressive mitral incompetence showing calcification (CA) of the mitral valve ring.

is sometimes seen as a result of the wide amplitude of the left atrial pressure pulse, and this impulse is often confused with right ventricular overactivity. In acute or less severe lesions, the heart is small, but it is still hyperdynamic.

C. Electrocardiographic Findings: Electrocardiographic evidence of left ventricular hypertrophy is more likely to occur in patients with acute rather than chronic lesions. The ventricle pumps into a small noncompliant left atrium and generates systolic pressures of up to 80 mm Hg in the atrium. This is a greater load than occurs in chronic mitral incompetence, and some evidence of left ventricular hypertrophy may be found. The electrocardiographic changes are not usually severe, and in most cases only high voltage is found. An incomplete right bundle branch block pattern (rsR' in lead V_1) is seen in about 5% of patients with mitral incompetence. Left bundle branch block is less common and is evidence of left ventricular disease. In patients in whom acute mitral incompetence is not treated in the early stages, right ventricular hypertrophy may ultimately develop owing to raised pulmonary vascular resistance. Atrial arrhythmias almost inevitably develop with time in patients with mitral incompetence. Although atrial premature beats, atrial tachycardia, and atrial flutter are occasionally seen, atrial fibrillation is much more common. Atrial arrhythmia may be paroxysmal at first and become chronic later. The onset of atrial fibrillation is more closely related to the patient's age than to any other variable in mitral incompetence. It is least common in acute mitral incompetence. The absence of atrial fibrillation in a symptomatic patient is also important. Significant symptoms in the presence of sinus rhythm suggest acute mitral incompetence.

D. X-Ray Findings: In patients with acute mitral incompetence, the heart is often of normal size at the outset, and marked pulmonary congestion and edema may be the only visible signs. Starting within a week or 2, however, the left atrium and ventricle enlarge and reach the proportions seen in chronic cases by the end of a year if the patient survives.

In hemodynamically significant chronic lesions, the left ventricle and left atrium are enlarged in proportion to the severity of the lesion (Fig 12–19).

The principal form of mitral incompetence in which cardiac fluoroscopy is valuable is mitral ring calcification. In this lesion, which is virtually confined to elderly women, the radiologic picture is striking (Fig 12–22). The entire calcified mitral ring can be seen moving up and down with the heartbeat, and the lesion can be distinguished from calcification of other sites in the chest.

E. Special Investigations:

1. Noninvasive techniques–Mitral incompetence can be diagnosed echographically (Fig 12–23), especially in acute disruption of the mitral valve. In addition to the valve itself, the size of the relevant heart chambers (left atrium and left ventricle) can be measured in the planes that are accessible to echographic investigation. Enlargement in one plane gen-

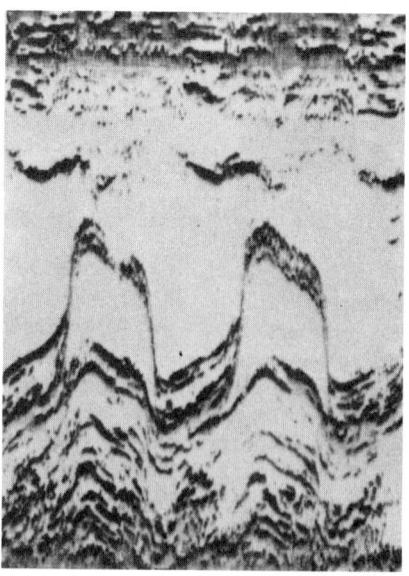

Figure 12–23. An echocardiogram from a patient with severe mitral regurgitation secondary to rheumatic heart disease. There is no abnormal systolic motion, but because the leaflets are thickened, they are moving (abnormally) parallel to each other in diastole. (Reproduced, with permission, from Fortuin NJ: Echocardiography. *Hosp Pract* [Nov] 1975;**10**:78.)

erally correlates with enlargement in other planes, and by concentrating on echographic views that show the mitral valve in a consistent manner, the physician can obtain reproducible tracings that can be used to follow changes in chamber size. Echocardiography is particularly useful in detecting and following the progress of annular calcification of the mitral valve.

2. Invasive techniques–

a. Acute mitral incompetence–Right and left heart catheterization are required in virtually all patients with acute disruption of the mitral valve in order to differentiate the mechanical effects of the lesion from those of associated myocardial disease. The hallmark of acute severe mitral incompetence is a wide pulse pressure in the wedge or left atrial tracing. The giant v wave, averaging over 50 mm Hg with values as high as 80 mm Hg in some cases, is quite characteristic. The v wave can usually also be seen in the pulmonary arterial pressure tracing as a second systolic peak which may equal that due to right ventricular contraction (Fig 12–24). The level of the diastolic left atrial pressure is also important as a clue to the state of the myocardium. In lesions that are mainly mechanical, the left ventricular and left atrial diastolic pressures are both about 15 mm Hg, indicating that there is no left ventricular failure. The mean left atrial pressure in a group of 20 patients with this lesion was 28 mm Hg, indicating that pulmonary congestion was moderately severe. Considerable emphasis should be placed on the measurement of left atrial pulse pressure in such cases, since it provides a simple means of assessing left ventricular function. A wide atrial pulse pressure with a high systolic and a low diastolic pressure indicates a powerfully contracting left ventricle with a low filling pressure. Conversely, a low systolic pressure with a high diastolic pressure indicates a poorly contracting left ventricle with a high filling pressure. Left ventricular angiography is an essential part of the study, because it shows the magnitude of mitral incompetence and demonstrates the hyperdynamic state found in pure mechanical lesions, as opposed to the sluggish ventricular contraction with mitral incompetence occurring in lesions that have poor left ventricular function. In patients who have cardiac pain and any suggestion of prior infarction, coronary angiography is indicated. In about 15% of cases, especially in younger patients, the raised left atrial pressure resulting from acute disruption of the mitral valve may cause a marked increase in pulmonary vascular resistance. If the patient survives the acute stage of the lesion or if the acute incompetence is less severe, circulatory adaptations occur. The left atrium and ventricle become more compliant, and left atrial pressure falls. The hemodynamic picture then comes to resemble that of chronic mitral incompetence, and raised pulmonary vascular resistance may persist.

b. Chronic mitral incompetence–In symptomatic patients with hemodynamically significant mitral incompetence, cardiac catheterization is indicated to determine the severity of the lesion before considering surgery. Left atrial pressure is usually only moderately raised, with a v wave of up to 30 mm Hg. The size of the left atrium is an important determinant of the hemodynamic findings, and in patients with a large atrium, the pressures are not usually impressive.

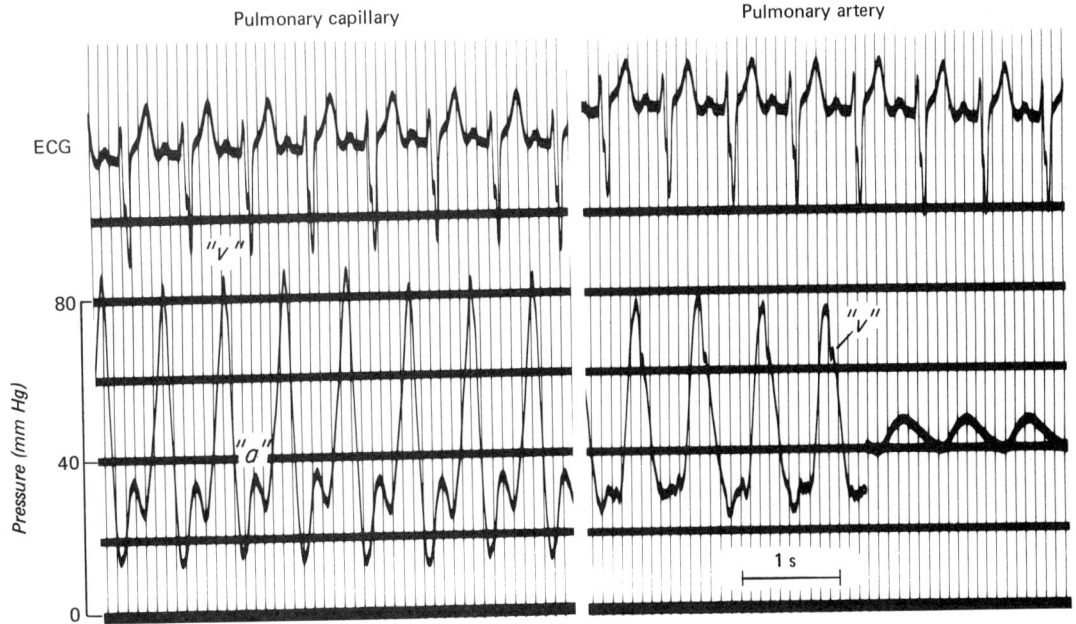

Figure 12–24. Pulmonary capillary (wedge) and pulmonary artery pressure tracings in a patient with acute mitral incompetence. The giant v wave seen in the wedge tracing is also visible in the pulmonary arterial pressure tracing.

The end-diastolic left ventricular pressure is of considerable importance. If it is raised, hypertension, active or inactive rheumatic myocarditis, or coronary disease should be suspected. The cardiac output may be abnormally low in patients with chronic mitral incompetence, especially in older persons, and the hemodynamic findings in patients with severe lesions may be unimpressive if this is the case. It is important to remember these factors when assessing the need for surgery, since valve replacement in patients with wedge pressures of less than 20 mm Hg may have surprisingly good results. Assessment of left ventricular function by left ventricular angiography is essential in any patient with mitral incompetence. Measurements of left ventricular ejection fraction and left ventricular wall motion should be obtained. The more obvious the mechanical lesion is on angiography, the higher the chances the patient will benefit from surgery.

Differential Diagnosis

Mitral incompetence must be distinguished from hypertrophic cardiomyopathy. There is a long pansystolic murmur in both conditions, and although the murmur in mitral incompetence is usually higher-pitched, has a timing that is not of the ejection type, and is transmitted to the axilla rather than centrally, the 2 lesions can be confused on diagnosis. Both show a third heart sound and a prominent left ventricle.

Ventricular septal defect is another condition that can be confused with mitral incompetence both in acute and chronic lesions. Again, the auscultatory findings are similar, with an overactive left ventricle, a pansystolic murmur, and third heart sound. Endocardial cushion defects with an associated ostium primum atrial defect and mitral incompetence are also difficult to differentiate from pure mitral incompetence, and cardiac catheterization is almost invariably needed to confirm the diagnosis. In the case of acute lesions, especially in patients who have suffered a recent myocardial infarction, the distinction between acquired ventricular septal defect due to rupture of the ventricular septum and acute mitral incompetence due to papillary muscle involvement can be extremely difficult.

Course & Complications

The course of mitral incompetence is not yet fully understood. Acute exacerbations, not severe enough to cause pulmonary edema, may be an important cause of progression. It is difficult to decide, in a patient seen with a moderately severe lesion, whether gradual progression or a moderately severe exacerbation was responsible for the worsening of the clinical picture.

A. Systemic Embolism: Systemic embolization is an important complication. It is more common in mixed mitral stenosis and incompetence, but it also occurs in pure mitral incompetence, where it is more frequently due to infective endocarditis. Embolism is detected in about 20% of cases and almost certainly occurs more frequently without causing symptoms. Cerebral, femoral, renal, intestinal, and coronary emboli comprise most of the clinically recognized cases. Left atrial thrombi do not occur as frequently in mitral incompetence as in mitral stenosis because there is less stasis. The emboli resulting from left atrial thrombus clear more readily than those associated with endocarditis. Embolism is more common in patients with atrial fibrillation and is more likely to occur when the rhythm changes, either when atrial fibrillation begins or when sinus rhythm is restored.

B. Infective Endocarditis: Infective endocarditis is an important complication of mitral valvular disease in general and occurs most frequently in patients with mitral incompetence (20%). The patient is almost invariably in sinus rhythm at the onset of this complication (see also Chapter 16).

C. Rheumatic Myocarditis: See above under Mixed Stenosis and Incompetence for discussion of rheumatic myocarditis as a complication.

D. Coronary Artery Disease: In older patients, atherosclerotic coronary arterial disease may influence the clinical picture with a myocardial factor that alters prognosis. This is especially true of those patients with mitral incompetence, whose lesions are frequently degenerative in origin. Coronary arterial disease, hypertension, and atherosclerosis are almost invariably present in elderly patients with mitral incompetence, and distinguishing between the mechanical and myocardial components of the lesion in a given patient often presents an insoluble problem.

E. Pulmonary Vascular Disease: Pulmonary hypertension, with a raised pulmonary vascular resistance, is uncommon except in acute mitral incompetence. The levels of left atrial pressure resulting from chronic mitral incompetence alone are virtually never high enough to cause this complication. In patients with associated left ventricular disease, however, left atrial pressure may occasionally reach levels that result in pulmonary hypertension and right heart failure.

Treatment

A. Medical Treatment: See above under Mitral Stenosis for a discussion of medical measures used in the treatment of mitral incompetence.

B. Surgical Treatment:

1. Valvuloplasty in acute mitral incompetence—Acute mitral incompetence is the major disorder that can be treated satisfactorily with mitral valvuloplasty. In cases in which the chordae tendineae supporting the posterior (mural) cusp of the mitral valve are torn, wedge resection of the affected part of the cusp gives excellent results. This operation, which is not indicated in lesions involving the anterior cusp, has the advantage of not requiring long-term anticoagulant therapy. The only comparable palliative operation for mitral incompetence is the suturing of the cleft in the mitral valve in a patient with an endocardial cushion defect. This procedure is undertaken in young persons, for whom a prosthetic valve and a lifetime of anticoagulation are the only other alternative until the long-term effectiveness of heterograft valves is established.

2. Mitral valve replacement in mitral incompetence—Mitral valve replacement is the treatment of choice in almost all cases of mitral incompetence. In acute lesions it may be difficult to decide when to operate. In patients with infective endocarditis or acute myocardial infarction, surgery should be delayed, if possible, until the acute lesion is completely healed. The hemodynamic load of acute mitral incompetence is generally not as severe as that of acute aortic incompetence, and it is usually possible to delay, particularly if systemic vasodilator therapy (afterload reduction) is employed. In most acute cases, surgery will be needed eventually, and there is some justification for operating before left atrial dilatation and atrial fibrillation have occurred. These changes ordinarily take from several months to a year to develop following an acute episode, and the optimal time for operation is 6 weeks to 3 months after the episode. The timing of surgery is most critical in patients suffering from endocarditis following intravenous drug abuse or endocarditis caused by drug-resistant organisms. No satisfactory regimen has yet been established for the management of such cases, and the long-term results are poor whether valve replacement is performed early or late in the course of the disease. Patients with known associated left ventricular disease also present problems in management. In patients with a narrow left atrial pulse pressure, left ventricular diastolic pressure over 25 mm Hg, and a reduced left ventricular ejection fraction (less than 40%), surgery is not indicated, but in borderline cases, especially those with previous myocardial infarction, the decision to withhold surgery can be extremely difficult. Studies during cardiac catheterization in which afterload reduction is carried out, ie, in which systemic arterial resistance is acutely lowered by vasodilator drugs such as intravenous nitroprusside or hydralazine, may be helpful. If cardiac output rises by 1 liter or more per minute and the left atrial pressure falls by 5–10 mm Hg, the outlook for surgery may be more encouraging.

3. Timing of surgery—In acute mitral incompetence the problem facing the cardiologist is no longer one of diagnosis because the clinical features distinguishing acute lesions are becoming widely recognized. Instead, the problem now is to decide when to operate on patients with endocarditis and how to determine the relative proportions of mechanical load and myocardial damage in patients with ischemic heart disease.

Prognosis

A. Acute Mitral Incompetence: In patients with mitral incompetence the prognosis depends more on the cause of the valvular lesion than on its severity and acuteness. The prognosis in acute mitral incompetence is good with surgery provided that myocardial infarction or uncontrollable infective endocarditis is not the basic cause. Early diagnosis and operation performed as soon as any associated lesions have healed improve the prognosis by preventing the changes of chronic mitral incompetence.

B. Chronic Mitral Incompetence: Chronic mitral incompetence carries a good prognosis once the lesion has stabilized. The load on the left ventricle is a pure "flow" load, and left ventricular hypertrophy is by no means inevitable. Atrial fibrillation is well tolerated, and provided that systemic hypertension or coronary artery disease does not develop, valve replacement can often be put off until age 50 or later. Age-related degenerative changes in the valve and in the heart as a whole are the most important causes of progression necessitating mitral valve replacement.

Long-Term Results in Operated Cases

A. Acute Mitral Incompetence: The late results of operation in acute mitral incompetence are better than in other forms of mitral valve disease. In some cases, valve replacement can be avoided and anticoagulation therapy is not needed. Postoperative atrial fibrillation is less frequent, and rheumatic myocardial damage is not necessarily present. Consequently, left ventricular function is better and the incidence of embolism is lower.

B. Chronic Mitral Incompetence: The results of mitral valve replacement in patients with chronic mitral incompetence resemble those in mixed mitral valve disease. The operation is palliative rather than curative, and some residual and usually progressive damage is present.

REFERENCES

General

Barnes CG, Finlay HVL: Cor triatriatum. *Br Heart J* 1952;**14**:283.

Besterman EMM: The use of phenylephrine to aid auscultation of early rheumatic diastolic murmurs. *Br Med J* 1951;**2**:205.

Braunwald E et al: Effects of mitral valve replacement on the pulmonary vascular dynamics of patients with pulmonary hypertension. *N Engl J Med* 1965;**273**:509.

Brickman RD et al: Cor triatriatum. *J Thorac Cardiovasc Surg* 1970;**60**:523.

Denbow CE, Pluth JR, Giuliani ER: The role of echocardiography in the selection of mitral valve prosthesis. *Mayo Clin Proc* 1980;**99**:586.

Fowler NO, Van der Bel-Kahn JM: Operations on the mitral valve: A time for weighing the issues. *Am J Cardiol* 1980;**46**:159.

Goodwin JF: Diagnosis of left atrial myxoma. *Lancet* 1963;**1**:464.

Law W et al: Radionuclide regurgitant index: Value and limitations. *Am J Cardiol* 1981;**47**:292.

McIntosh CL, Michaelis LL, Morrow AG: Atrio-ventricular valve replacement with the Hancock porcine xenograft: A five-year clinical experience. *Surgery* 1975;**78**:768.

Pridie RB, Oakley CM: Echocardiographic evaluation of the mitral valve. *Prog Cardiovasc Dis* 1978;**21**:92.

Rapaport E et al: Natural history of aortic and mitral valve disease. *Am J Cardiol* 1975;**35**:221.

Reichek N, Shelburne JC, Perloff JK: Clinical aspects of rheumatic valvular disease. *Prog Cardiovasc Dis* 1973;**15**:491.

Roberts WC, Perloff JK: Mitral valvular disease: A clinicopathologic survey of the conditions causing the mitral valve to function abnormally. *Ann Intern Med* 1972;**77**:939.

Sandrasagra FA, Oliver WA, English TAH: Myxoma of the mitral valve. *Br Heart J* 1979;**42**:221.

Schuler G et al: Temporal response of left ventricular performance in mitral valve surgery. *Circulation* 1979;**59**:1218.

Sherrid MV, Clark RD, Cohn K: Echocardiographic analysis of left atrial size before and after operation in mitral valve disease. *Am J Cardiol* 1979;**43**:171.

Wooley CF et al: Tricuspid stenosis: Atrial systolic murmur, tricuspid opening snap and right atrial pressure pulse. *Am J Med* 1985;**78**:375.

Mitral Stenosis

Bower BD et al: Two cases of congenital mitral stenosis treated by valvotomy. *Arch Dis Child* 1953;**28**:91.

Cowdery CD et al: New vectorcardiographic criteria for diagnosing right ventricular hypertrophy in mitral stenosis: Comparison with electrocardiographic criteria. *Circulation* 1980;**62**:5.

Dalby AJ et al: Preoperative factors affecting the outcome of isolated mitral valve replacement. *Am J Cardiol* 1981;**47**:826.

Gross RI et al: Long-term results of open radical mitral commissurotomy: Ten year follow-up study of 202 patients. *Am J Cardiol* 1981;**47**:821.

Heger JJ et al: Long-term changes in mitral valve area after successful mitral commissurotomy. *Circulation* 1979;**59**:443.

Lundstrom NR: Echocardiography in the diagnosis of congenital mitral stenosis and in evaluation of the results of mitral valvotomy. *Circulation* 1972;**46**:44.

Marshall R, McIlroy MB, Christie RV: The work of breathing in mitral stenosis. *Clin Sci* 1954;**13**:137.

McCall BW, Price JL: Movement of mitral valve cusps in relation to first heart sound and opening snap in patients with mitral stenosis. *Br Heart J* 1967;**29**:417.

Rowe JC et al: The course of mitral stenosis without surgery: Ten- and twenty-year perspectives. *Ann Intern Med* 1960;**52**:741.

Selzer A, Cohn KE: Natural history of mitral stenosis: A review. *Circulation* 1972;**45**:878.

Thuillez C et al: Pulsed Doppler echocardiographic study of mitral stenosis. *Circulation* 1980;**61**:381.

Wells BG: Prediction of mitral pressure gradient from heart sounds. *Br Med J* 1957;**1**:551.

Wood P: An appreciation of mitral stenosis. (2 parts.) *Br Med J* 1954;**16**:1051, 1113.

Wood P et al: The effect of acetylcholine on pulmonary vascular resistance and left atrial pressure in mitral stenosis. *Br Heart J* 1957;**19**:279.

Click-Murmur Syndrome (Mitral Valve Prolapse)

Allen H, Harris A, Leatham A: Significance and prognosis of an isolated late systolic murmur: A 9 to 22 year follow-up. *Br Heart J* 1974;**36**:525.

Barlow JB, Pocock WA: Mitral valve prolapse, the specific billowing mitral leaflet syndrome, or an insignificant non-ejection systolic click. (Editorial.) *Am Heart J* 1979;**97**:277.

Barlow JB et al: Late systolic murmur and non-ejection ("mid-late") systolic clicks. *Br Heart J* 1968;**30**:203.

Barnett HJM et al: Further evidence relating mitral-valve prolapse to cerebral ischemic events. *N Engl J Med* 1980;**302**:139.

Becker AE, DeWit APM: Mitral valve apparatus: A spectrum of normality relevant to mitral valve prolapse. *Br Heart J* 1979;**42**:680.

Bisset GS III et al: Clinical spectrum and long-term follow-up of isolated mitral valve prolapse in 119 children. *Circulation* 1980;**62**:423.

Bontempo CP et al: Radiographic appearance of the thorax in systolic click–late systolic murmur syndrome. *Am J Cardiol* 1975;**36**:27.

Brown OR et al: Aortic root dilatation and mitral valve prolapse in Marfan's syndrome: An echocardiographic study. *Circulation* 1975;**52**:651.

Chesler E et al: The myxomatous mitral valve and sudden death. *Circulation* 1983;**67**:632.

Cohen MV, Shah PK, Spindola-Franco H: Angiographic-echocardiographic correlation in mitral valve prolapse. *Am Heart J* 1979;**97**:43.

Criley JM et al: Prolapse of the mitral valve: Clinical and cine-angiocardiographic findings. *Br Heart J* 1966;**28**:488.

Davies MJ, Moore BP, Braimbridge MW: The floppy mitral valve: Study of incidence, pathology, and complications in surgical, necropsy and forensic material. *Br Heart J* 1978;**40**:468.

Gottidiener JS, Sherber HS, Harvey WP: Mid-systolic click and mitral valve prolapse following mitral commissurotomy. *Am J Med* 1978;**64**:295.

Hancock EW, Cohn K: The syndrome associated with mid-systolic click and late systolic murmur. *Am J Med* 1966;**41**:183.

Hickey AJ, MacMahon SW, Wilcken DEL: Mitral valve prolapse and bacterial endocarditis: When is antibiotic prophylaxis necessary? *Am Heart J* 1985;**109**:131.

Jeresaty RM: *Mitral Valve Prolapse*. Raven Press, 1978.

Jeresaty RM: Mitral valve prolapse: An update. *JAMA* 1985;**254**:793.

Jeresaty RM: Mitral valve prolapse-click syndrome. *Prog Cardiovasc Dis* 1973;**15**:623.

Koch FH, Hancock EW: Ten year follow-up of forty patients with midsystolic click/late systolic murmur syndrome. (Abstract.) *Am J Cardiol* 1976;**37**:149.

Leatham A, Brigden W: Mild mitral regurgitation and the mitral prolapse fiasco. *Am Heart J* 1980;**99**:659.

Malcolm AD et al: Clinical features and investigative findings in presence of mitral leaflet prolapse: Study of 85 consecutive patients. *Br Heart J* 1976;**38**:244.

Markiewicz W et al: Mitral valve prolapse in one hundred presumably healthy young females. *Circulation* 1976;**53**:464.

Mason JW et al: Cardiac biopsy evidence for a cardiomyopathy associated with symptomatic mitral valve prolapse. *Am J Cardiol* 1978;**42**:557.

Mills P et al: Long-term prognosis of mitral valve prolapse. *N Engl J Med* 1977;**297**:13.

Olsen EGJ, Al-Rufaie HK: The floppy mitral valve: Study on pathogenesis. *Br Heart J* 1980;**44**:674.

O'Rourke RA et al: Prolapsing mitral valve leaflet syndrome. *West J Med* 1975;**122**:217.

Pocock WA et al: Sudden death in primary mitral valve prolapse. *Am Heart J* 1984;**107**:378.

Popp RL et al: Echocardiographic abnormalities in the mitral valve prolapse syndrome. *Circulation* 1974;**49**:428.

Reid JVO: Mid-systolic clicks. *S Afr Med J* 1961;**35**:353.

Rizzon P et al: Familial syndrome of midsystolic click and late systolic murmur. *Br Heart J* 1973;**35**:245.

Salomon J, Shah PM, Heinle RA: Thoracic skeletal abnormalities in idiopathic mitral valve prolapse. *Am J Cardiol* 1975;**36**:32.

Savage DD et al: Mitral valve prolapse in the general population. 1. Epidemiologic features: The Framingham Study. 2. Clinical features: The Framingham Study. 3. Dysrhythmias: The Framingham Study. *Am Heart J* 1983;**106**:571, 577, 582.

Shappell SD et al: Sudden death and the familial occurrence of mid-systolic click, late systolic murmur syndrome. *Circulation* 1973;**48**:1128.

Smith ER et al: Angiographic diagnosis of mitral valve prolapse: Correlation with echocardiography. *Am J Cardiol* 1977;**40**:165.

Wigle ED et al: Mitral valve prolapse. *Annu Rev Med* 1976;**27**:165.

Winkle RA et al: Life-threatening arrhythmias in the mitral valve prolapse syndrome. *Am J Med* 1976;**60**:961.

Mitral Incompetence

Abbasi AD et al: Detection and estimation of the degree of mitral regurgitation by range-gated pulsed Doppler echocardiography. *Circulation* 1980;**61**:143.

Austen WG et al: Ruptured papillary muscle. *Circulation* 1965;**32**:597.

Braunwald E: Mitral regurgitation: Physiologic, clinical and surgical considerations. *N Engl J Med* 1969;**281**:425.

Brigden W, Leatham A: Mitral incompetence. *Br Heart J* 1953;**15**:55.

Chatterjee K et al: Beneficial effects of vasodilator agents in severe mitral regurgitation due to dysfunction of subvalvular apparatus. *Circulation* 1973;**48**:684.

Child JS et al: M mode and cross-sectional echocardiographic features of flail posterior mitral leaflets. *Am J Cardiol* 1979;**44**:1383.

Davis RH et al: Myxomatous degeneration of the mitral valve. *Am J Cardiol* 1971;**28**:449.

D'Cruz IA et al: Clinical manifestations of mitral annulus calcification, with emphasis on its echocardiographic features. *Am Heart J* 1977;**94**:367.

Ellis LB, Ramirez A: The clinical course of patients with severe "rheumatic" mitral insufficiency. *Am Heart J* 1969;**78**:406.

Fowler NO, Van der Bel-Kahn JM: Indications for surgical replacement of the mitral valve: With particular reference to common and uncommon causes of mitral regurgitation. *Am J Cardiol* 1979;**44**:148.

Freed C, Schiller NB: Echocardiographic findings in Marfan's syndrome. *West J Med* 1977;**126**:87.

Fulkerson PK et al: Calcification of the mitral annulus: Etiology, clinical associations, complications and therapy. *Am J Med* 1979;**66**:967.

Goodman DJ et al: Effect of nitroprusside on left ventricular dynamics in mitral regurgitation. *Circulation* 1974; **50**:1025.

Greenberg BH et al: Beneficial effects of hydralazine in severe mitral regurgitation. *Circulation* 1978;**58**:273.

Kirklin JW: Replacement of the mitral valve for mitral incompetence. *Surgery* 1972;**72**:827.

Littler WA, Epstein EJ, Coulshed N: Acute mitral regurgitation resulting from ruptured or elongated chordae tendineae. *Q J Med* 1973;**42**:87.

Mehta J et al: Acute haemodynamic effect of oral prazosin in severe mitral regurgitation. *Br Heart J* 1980;**43**:556.

Mintz GS et al: Two dimensional echocardiographic evaluation of patients with mitral insufficiency. *Am J Cardiol* 1979;**44**:670.

Nestico PF et al: Mitral annular calcification: Clinical, pathophysiology, and echocardiographic review. *Am Heart J* 1984;**107**:989.

Oliveira DBG et al: Chordal rupture. 2. Comparison between repair and replacement. *Br Heart J* 1983;**50**:318.

Phillips HR et al: Mitral valve replacement for isolated mitral regurgitation: Analysis of clinical course and late postoperative left ventricular ejection fraction. *Am J Cardiol* 1981;**48**:647.

Pocock WA, Barlow JB: Etiology and electrocardiographic features of the billowing posterior mitral leaflet syndrome. *Am J Med* 1971;**51**:731.

Saltissi S et al: Assessment of prognostic factors in patients undergoing surgery for non-rheumatic mitral regurgitation. *Br Heart J* 1980;**44**:369.

Sanders CA et al: Etiology and differential diagnosis of acute mitral regurgitation. *Prog Cardiovasc Dis* 1971;**14**:129.

Wigle ED, Auger P: Sudden, severe mitral insufficiency. *Can Med Assoc J* 1967;**96**:1493.

Wynn A: Gross calcification of the mitral valve. *Br Heart J* 1953;**15**:214.

13 Aortic Valve Disease; Combined Valve Disease

Aortic valve disease is the next most common form of valvular heart disease after mitral disease and accounts for about 35% of patients with significant valvular lesions.

Classification

Aortic valve disease has been classified in this text into 3 main categories: (1) hemodynamically insignificant aortic valve disease, (2) hemodynamically significant predominant aortic stenosis, and (3) hemodynamically significant predominant aortic incompetence.

An indirectly recorded brachial arterial diastolic blood pressure of 70 mm Hg or more is used as an arbitrary measurement below which hemodynamically significant aortic incompetence is said to be present. This cutoff point is naturally not entirely satisfactory, but it represents the best single figure on which to base a classification.

Interaction of Stenosis & Incompetence

Aortic stenosis and aortic incompetence load the left ventricle in different ways. In the purest forms of stenosis, the extra left ventricular work is performed almost entirely against increased pressure, with no increase in flow. In pure incompetence there is an almost pure flow load with an increase in stroke volume, because the ventricle must eject both its normal stroke volume and the blood that returns as backflow through the valve during diastole. Falling between these 2 extremes is a spectrum of lesions in which the ventricular load consists partly of increased volume and partly of increased flow. Severe stenosis and severe incompetence cannot coexist; therefore, in mixed lesions neither component is severe. If incompetence is greater than stenosis, the stroke volume is larger, and the pressure difference between the left ventricle and the aorta is exaggerated because of the large flow. If stenosis is more severe than incompetence, the narrower orifice permits less backflow during diastole, but the pressure difference during systole is large because the stenosis is relatively severe. Since the left ventricle tolerates pressure loads less easily than volume loads, stenotic lesions are more important than incompetent ones. Therefore, all cases with significant stenosis are included in one group (predominant aortic stenosis), and predominantly incompetent lesions form another.

Subvalvular & Supravalvular Aortic Stenosis

Among patients with predominant aortic stenosis is a small group (1% of cases) who do not have disease affecting the valves but rather congenital supravalvular or subvalvular lesions. Supravalvular aortic stenosis usually results from congenital hypoplasia of the ascending aorta, whereas subvalvular stenosis is due to the presence of a fibrous ring or shelf of tissue immediately below the valve. Supravalvular stenosis occurs in a familial form in physically underdeveloped children with characteristic elfin facies and prominent ears. Surgical relief of the aortic obstruction is often difficult because of the diffuse hypoplasia of the aorta.

Subvalvular stenosis is also congenital and is due to ring lesions that are amenable to surgical relief, in contrast to those of supravalvular stenosis. The clinical picture resembles that of predominant aortic stenosis, and the valve often leaks, perhaps because the subvalvular ring interferes with normal valve closure. The condition is diagnosed by angiography. The obstructing ring is often so close to the aortic valve that withdrawal pressure tracings may fail to detect the lesion. In hypertrophic obstructive cardiomyopathy, the obstruction lies lower in the ventricle, and the clinical picture is different (see Chapter 17, p 539).

Acute & Chronic Aortic Incompetence

Aortic incompetence, like mitral incompetence, occurs in both acute and chronic forms. Acute lesions are almost always due to the effects of infective endocarditis but may rarely occur when acute aortic dissection involves the aortic root or the aorta is torn as a result of trauma. The acute load on the left ventricle causes a clinical picture that is different from that seen in chronic lesions.

Causes of Aortic Valve Lesions

It is difficult to determine both the cause and severity of aortic valve lesions. There is often a discrepancy between the patient's symptoms and the hemodynamic severity of the lesions, and the cause often remains in doubt, even after autopsy. Both aortic stenosis and aortic incompetence may run long clinical courses lasting 20–30 years, and the physician is often confronted with patients who have hemodynamically significant lesions and yet no symptoms. Just as frequently, the patient has symptoms that are out of proportion to the hemodynamic findings. Because aortic valve lesions can run such a long clinical course, factors responsible for the progressive deterioration of the patient's clinical state are not always clear. Long-term changes may be due to valvular calcification or myocardial fibrosis, but an acute exacerbation often cannot be explained.

As in mitral valve disease, rheumatic fever is an important cause of aortic valvular lesions. A history of previous rheumatic fever is present in 10% of patients with predominant stenosis and in 15% of those with predominant incompetence. Since congenital aortic valve lesions are relatively common, some patients who have been diagnosed as having had rheumatic fever in childhood actually have congenital aortic valve lesions. Seventy-five percent of patients with predominant aortic stenosis who have a past history of rheumatic fever are women, whereas 75% of those with pure incompetence who have a past history of rheumatic fever are men. This agrees with the finding in mitral valve disease that stenosis occurs more commonly in females and incompetence in males. Aortic valve disease is more prevalent in males by a factor of 3:1 in predominant stenosis and 3:2 in predominant incompetence. These proportions vary in different series for the reason that causes vary in different geographic areas.

HEMODYNAMICALLY INSIGNIFICANT LESIONS

The cardinal features of hemodynamically insignificant aortic lesions (Fig 13–1) include normal heart size and hemodynamics and a systolic ejection murmur. The variable features are a systolic ejection click and a short aortic diastolic murmur. Auscultatory physical signs arising from the aortic valve are usually the sole abnormality. These lesions constitute 10% of cases seen in university hospital practice but make up a much larger percentage in private practice. These cases probably represent a presymptomatic phase of aortic valve disease that if followed long enough would be seen to develop into either aortic stenosis or aortic incompetence. The most important complication in such cases is infective endocarditis, with associated development or exacerbation of aortic incompetence. These lesions are seen in patients of all ages. Congenital (bicuspid valve), rheumatic, and atherosclerotic causes account for two-thirds of cases; no causative factor is identified in the others.

Clinical Features

More than half of cases are entirely asymptomatic. In the others, palpitations, fatigue, dizziness, and noncardiac dyspnea occur but without evidence of heart failure. Symptoms are more common in patients who are aware that they have a heart murmur. The pulse and blood pressure are normal; a collapsing pulse or a slow-rising pulse is, by definition, absent. The heart is not enlarged on clinical or x-ray examination, and no evidence of ventricular hypertrophy is detectable. (If any of these signs are present, the lesion is no longer hemodynamically insignificant.) There is always a systolic murmur at the base of the heart, preceded by an ejection click in one-third of cases and followed by a faint aortic diastolic murmur in one-third. Slight aortic dilatation is occasionally seen, but valvular calcification is not necessarily present.

Cardiac catheterization is not indicated for diagnosis, but if it is performed, intracardiac pressures are normal, and there is no significant pressure difference between the left ventricle and the aorta.

The role of the deposition of calcium in these slightly abnormal valves is difficult to determine, but it seems likely that valvular calcification immobilizes and narrows the valve, causing stenosis that gradually progresses but does not significantly load the left ventricle until the valve is narrowed to about one-fourth its normal area ($5.0 \text{ cm}^2 \rightarrow 1.25 \text{ cm}^2$).

The other important development in such cases is infective endocarditis. Patients with hemodynamically insignificant aortic lesions are particularly prone to this complication, and the valve is likely to become acutely and severely incompetent as a result. Thus, the prevention and early recognition of endocarditis are important aspects of the management of patients with this lesion. Antibiotic prophylactic therapy preceding major dental work or minor surgery and early blood culture during febrile illnesses are mandatory. Intravenous drug abuse is particularly likely to result in infective endocarditis because contaminated needles and syringes are often used, and the drugs are seldom sterile. When a rheumatic origin for the lesion is suspected, prophylactic penicillin treatment is warranted to prevent recurrences of rheumatic fever (see p 536).

PREDOMINANT AORTIC STENOSIS

The cardinal features of predominant aortic stenosis (Fig 13–2) are left ventricular hypertrophy and a systolic ejection murmur. The variable factors are the severity, which affects the hypertrophy; the site of the obstruction; the cause; and the presence or absence of valvular calcification.

Importance of Aortic Stenosis

Predominant aortic stenosis has an importance in clinical cardiology that is out of proportion to its frequency. Aortic stenosis is easily missed on clinical examination, especially if the patient is in severe left ventricular failure and the cardiac output is so low that the aortic systolic murmur that might point toward a diagnosis of aortic stenosis is virtually inaudible. Aortic stenosis is often suspected in patients in whom there is no significant obstruction to aortic flow. In these cases, it is the presence of an aortic systolic murmur, often associated with calcification of the aortic valve on fluoroscopy, that indicates possible aortic stenosis. Although echocardiography may be valuable in ruling out a diagnosis of aortic stenosis, left heart catheterization is needed to confirm that obstruction is severe. Approximately 10% of patients undergoing cardiac catheterization in a university hospital subsequently prove to have hemodynamically unimportant lesions despite a diagnosis of aortic stenosis before the procedure, but the risks of missing the correct diagnosis so far outweigh the dangers of cardiac catheterization that the study should be performed if there is the slightest doubt about the diagnosis.

402 / CHAPTER 13

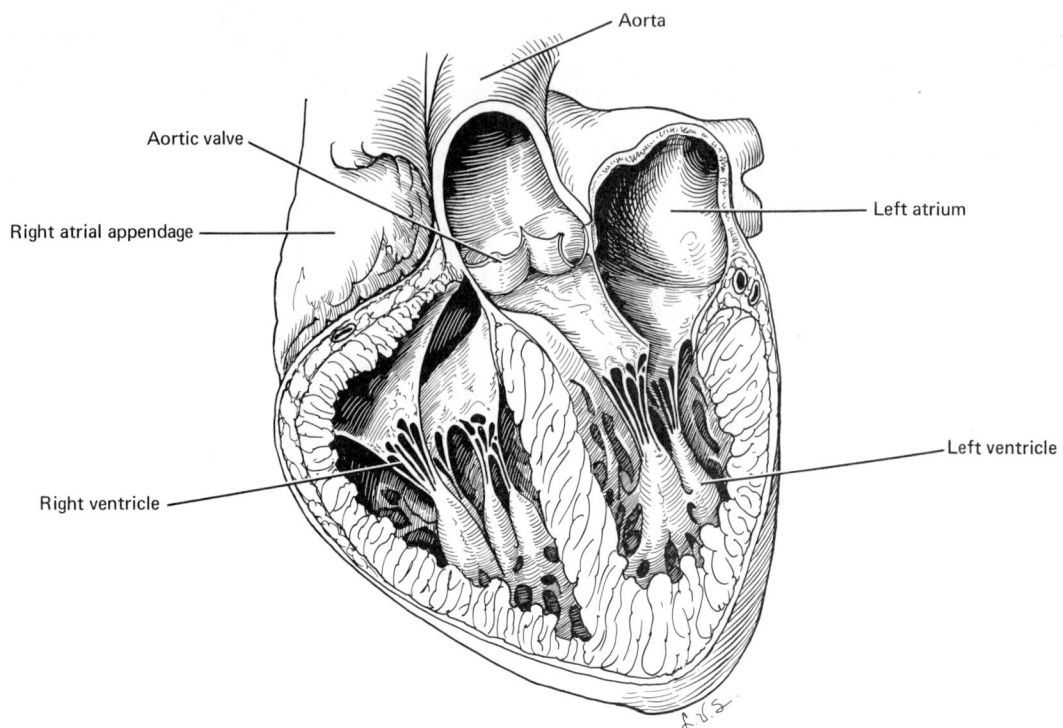

Drawing of left heart in left anterior oblique view showing anatomic features of hemodynamically insignificant aortic valve disease.

Cardinal features: *Normal heart size and hemodynamics; systolic ejection murmur.*

Variable factors: *Systolic ejection click; short aortic diastolic murmur.*

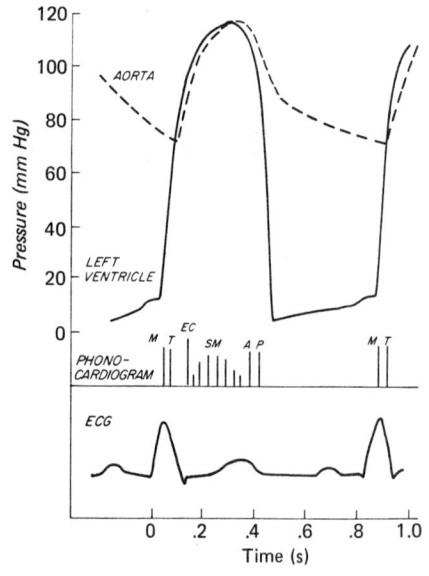

Diagram showing auscultatory and hemodynamic features of hemodynamically insignificant aortic valve disease. Note the absence of a gradient across the aortic valve. M, mitral; T, tricuspid; A, aortic; P, pulmonary valve; EC, ejection click; SM, systolic murmur.

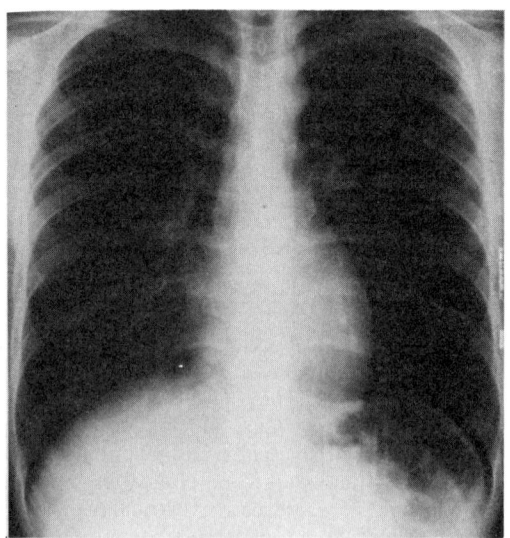

Chest x-ray showing normal heart size and shape.

Figure 13–1. Hemodynamically insignificant aortic valve disease. Structures enlarged: none.

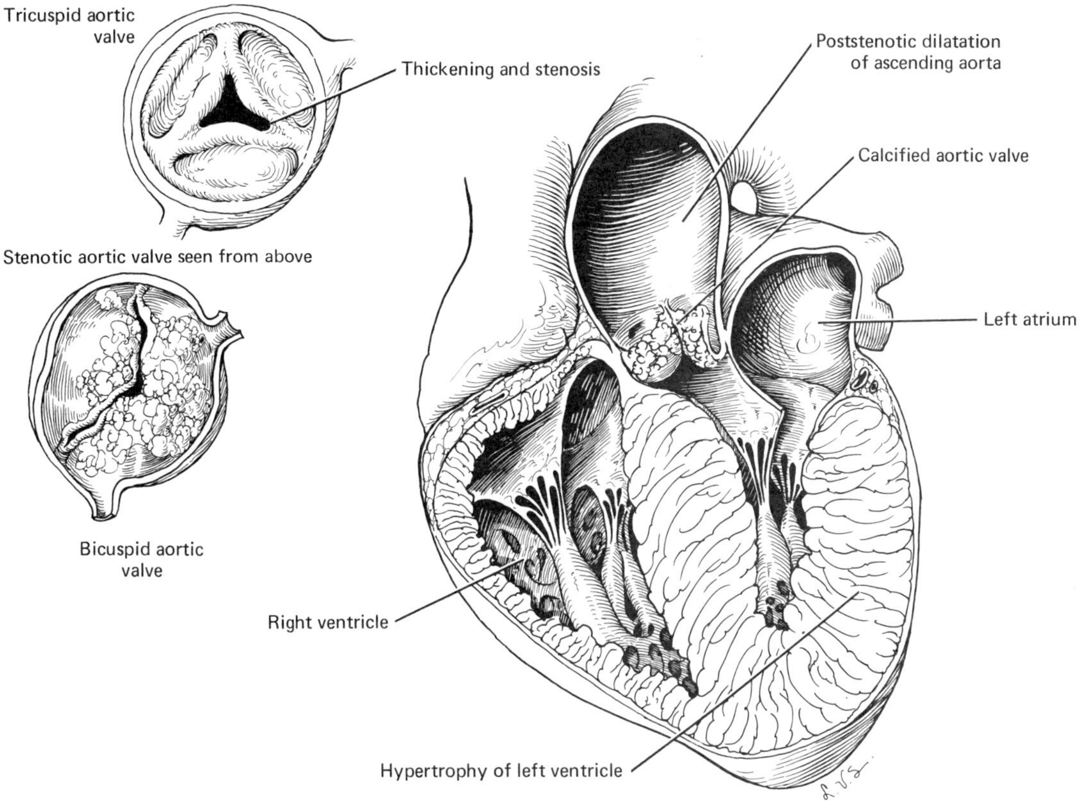

AORTIC VALVE DISEASE; COMBINED VALVE DISEASE / 403

Drawing of left heart in left anterior oblique view showing anatomic features of aortic stenosis.

Cardinal features: *Left ventricular hypertrophy; systolic ejection murmur.*

Variable factors: *Severity; site of obstruction; cause; valvular calcification.*

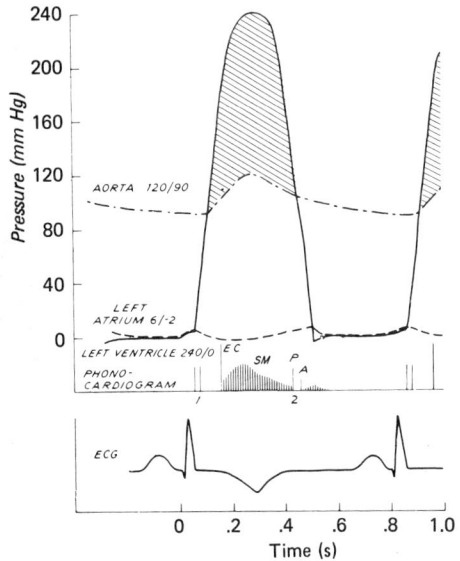

Diagram showing auscultatory and hemodynamic features of predominant aortic stenosis. (Abbreviations are explained in Fig 13–1.)

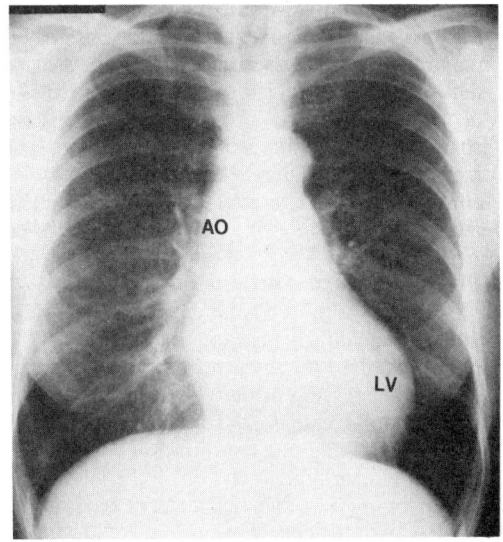

Chest x-ray of a patient with aortic stenosis showing left ventricular (LV) and aortic (AO) enlargement.

Figure 13–2. Aortic stenosis. Structures enlarged: left ventricle (thickened); poststenotic dilatation of the aorta.

Cause of Aortic Stenosis

The cause of aortic stenosis has been the subject of controversy for many years. In most cases (70%), there is no clinical clue to the cause. At autopsy the valve is usually so disorganized by calcification that it is difficult to count the number of cusps. Now that aortic valve replacement has become routine, the valve is available for study at an earlier stage of the disease, and it is easier to see if there are 2 or 3 cusps. Even so, separate cusps cannot be identified in some patients (15%). Since the normal aortic valve has 3 cusps, the finding of a bicuspid valve in 50% of patients indicates that the basic lesion is congenital in patients with predominant aortic stenosis who undergo surgery or die of the disease. Patients with bicuspid valves often have other congenital lesions, most commonly coarctation of the aorta. Some are known to have had a murmur since early infancy, but the majority (two-thirds) have had a murmur first heard only after age 20. This latter group generally does not have congenital aortic stenosis but rather a minor congenital valvular lesion that presents as hemodynamically insignificant aortic valve disease. The congenital abnormality apparently makes the valve more than normally susceptible to wear and tear.

Congenital aortic stenosis is rarely seen in adults and constitutes about 5% of cases. In such cases, a murmur has almost always been heard in infancy, and symptoms usually have developed in early adult life. Patients with predominant aortic stenosis tend to develop valvular calcification with increasing age, and after age 40, valvular calcification is present in virtually all cases, irrespective of the cause of the lesion.

In a small but increasing number of patients, atherosclerotic, age-related degenerative changes in a normal valve appear to be the sole cause of aortic stenosis. In this group, the valve is tricuspid, the patient is over age 60, and a murmur has not been present for more than 5 years. This group of patients constitutes about 15% of cases. There is some suggestion that aortic stenosis may develop rapidly in such patients and run a shorter course. Associated coronary artery disease is common in this group.

Progression of Aortic Stenosis

The role played by the deposition of calcium in the consequent progression of the disease seems unpredictable. Physicians must learn to recognize the signs of increasing severity of stenosis: progressive cardiac enlargement, decreasing peripheral pulse pressure, slowing of carotid upstroke, and increasing left ventricular hypertrophy on the ECG and echocardiograms. Aortic valve replacement is so much more successful in patients who have not yet developed left ventricular failure that early diagnosis and recognition of increasing severity are of the utmost importance. A special problem is the increased incidence of acquired aortic stenosis resulting from atherosclerosis in elderly persons. The disease can be extremely insidious and difficult to diagnose.

Clinical Findings

In all forms of aortic stenosis a fixed, disorganized, calcified, thickened, radiopaque mass of tissue replaces the normal flexible, thin, filmy valve structure. In congenital aortic stenosis the valve is often dome-shaped, and no cusps can be distinguished. Calcification is most closely related to age and occurs at the earliest in the late teens and 20s. The development of calcification is commonly associated with the development of an aortic systolic ejection murmur.

Aortic stenosis increases the work of the left ventricle. In cases of pure stenosis, hypertrophy first occurs at the expense of the left ventricular cavity, causing a decrease in ventricular compliance. The ventricle becomes more rounded, but overall heart size is not increased. If there is associated aortic incompetence, the left ventricle is larger, and in most cases heart size is increased by the time symptoms appear. The narrowing of the aortic valve produces turbulence, and the increased energy in the blood causes poststenotic dilatation of the aorta. The calcification of the aortic valve may spread to the valve ring and thence to the anterior (aortic) cusp of the mitral valve and the membranous part of the interventricular septum, where it may cause atrioventricular conduction defects. The coronary vessels are usually large and not atherosclerotic in younger patients with bicuspid valves, but calcific emboli may occur and cause coronary occlusion or other serious systemic embolism. Aortic stenosis developing de novo in elderly persons is more likely to be associated with coronary artery disease, and the combination carries a poor prognosis.

Blood is subject to extremely severe mechanical stress as it passes through the turbulent areas associated with a stenotic aortic valve. Damage to red cells in the form of excessive hemolysis may occur in patients with aortic stenosis, especially if the cells are abnormally fragile. This rare form of hemolytic anemia is also seen after aortic valve replacement.

A. Symptoms: Symptoms appear late in the course of aortic stenosis, and many patients with hemodynamically significant lesions have no complaints. The disease is not recognized in its earlier stages, usually because the patient does not seek medical advice. In some cases, the murmur has been present without any symptoms for so many years that the physician overlooks the possibility of aortic stenosis until it becomes severe.

The stage at which symptoms develop depends to some extent on the patient's activity level. In sedentary people the disease may be far advanced before the patient complains of symptoms. Half of patients with surgically significant aortic stenosis have had at least one episode of left ventricular failure before they undergo surgery for stenosis. In active persons, dyspnea on exertion occurs before overt left ventricular failure develops, but especially in sedentary people, an episode of paroxysmal nocturnal dyspnea may be the first symptom of disease.

That aortic stenosis runs a long presymptomatic course is evident from the finding that significant stenosis—as judged by the presence of a systolic murmur and left ventricular hypertrophy on the ECG—may be present for 20 years without causing any symptoms. The course of the disease after symptoms develop is rapid. Progressive left ventricular failure leads to death in 2–8 years if surgery is not performed. The symptoms in the later stages of aortic stenosis are some of the most difficult to manage in the entire spectrum of cardiac disease. Nightly attacks of paroxysmal dyspnea, with sweating, collapse, extreme restlessness, and intractable shortness of breath, cause severe distress. Morphine and potent diuretics are the drugs of choice in the medical management of such patients, but physicians who have had to treat patients at this stage of the disease tend to favor surgical treatment for all patients with significant aortic stenosis, regardless of age.

Dyspnea on exertion is the commonest presenting symptom (75% of cases) in predominant aortic stenosis. As in other forms of left ventricular overload, shortness of breath is quantitatively related to exertion and is often accompanied by a heavy, tight feeling in the chest that is discomfort rather than pain and is only perceived in association with dyspnea. This sensation may occasionally radiate to the arms and is often interpreted as angina pectoris. Dyspnea on effort ordinarily precedes the episodes of paroxysmal nocturnal dyspnea that herald the onset of left ventricular failure. Dizziness (10% of patients) and cardiac pain (10%) are the next most common presenting symptoms of aortic stenosis; syncope on unaccustomed effort is the other principal symptom. It occurs in about 5% of cases, usually early in the disease before the left ventricle has failed. In many patients it only occurs once, because the patient associates the syncope with overexertion and subsequently avoids lifting heavy objects, shoveling snow, running upstairs, or performing whatever activity precipitated the first attack. Loss of consciousness is usually preceded by dyspnea, which the patient disregards, perhaps because of the circumstances surrounding the overexertion. Recovery from the syncopal attack is rapid, and sudden death, which is common in aortic stenosis, seldom occurs on exertion. It is of great importance to obtain a clear history of the circumstances surrounding a syncopal episode in a patient suspected of having aortic stenosis. If syncope is provoked only by severe effort, stenosis is already severe. Syncope unrelated to excessive effort is more common than effort syncope in aortic stenosis (10%) but is not necessarily an indication that severe stenosis is present. Such syncope is often due to arrhythmia rather than an inadequate increase in cardiac output during stress. It is often confused with transient cerebral ischemic attacks due to atherosclerosis of the cerebral vessels in patients who have aortic systolic murmurs but no aortic stenosis.

It is important to distinguish 2 types of cardiac pain in aortic stenosis. The commonest form is a heavy substernal discomfort, described as a bursting, choking, constricting feeling that only comes when the patient is dyspneic. It may occur more readily after meals and radiate to the arms, but it never occurs without dyspnea. It differs from true angina of effort, in which the pain or discomfort is clearly the primary event and occurs before dyspnea. If both of these forms of cardiac distress are termed angina, then the commonest symptom of aortic stenosis is indeed angina. However, if the term angina is reserved for pain that is not associated with or preceded by dyspnea, then angina is the presenting symptom of only 10% of patients with aortic stenosis.

B. Signs: The arterial pulse in patients with predominant aortic stenosis is of small amplitude and is slow-rising because left ventricular ejection time through the narrowed aortic valve is prolonged. Such an arterial pulse is termed an anacrotic pulse, plateau pulse, or pulsus tardus, because the wave takes longer than normal to pass beneath the examiner's fingers. The examiner should feel the radial, brachial, femoral, and carotid pulses. The carotid pulse, being closest to the aortic valve, gives the most accurate information. The rise time is slowed and the time taken to reach peak pressure is increased in the central pulse in aortic stenosis. This sign is less reliable in older patients, in whom compliance of the arterial bed is reduced. In patients with mixed lesions in whom there is also aortic incompetence, the upstroke of the pulse is more rapid, and a double-peaked pulse (pulsus bisferiens) may be found (Fig 13–3). Pulsus bisferiens is more likely to be present in a more peripheral artery (eg, radial or brachial) and is not usually seen in the central aortic pulse. The presence of pulsus bisferiens is not of diagnostic significance.

Blood pressure is ordinarily low, with a narrow pulse pressure, and reflects the small stroke volume in aortic stenosis. However, it may be normal, especially in patients with mixed lesions. Systemic hypertension, although uncommon, does not rule out surgically significant aortic stenosis. An *a* wave may be seen in the jugular venous pulse if the ventricular septum bulges to the right and impairs right ventricular filling, or if severe pulmonary hypertension develops. The heart rate is usually regular, but about 10% of patients are in atrial fibrillation at the time of surgery. The incidence of atrial fibrillation in cases with a past history of rheumatic fever is no greater than in those with congenitally bicuspid aortic valves, but atrial fibrillation should always alert the physician to the possibility of coexisting associated mitral valve disease. The degree of left ventricular hypertrophy on physical examination—as shown by the prominence of the left ventricular heave—depends on the severity and purity of the stenosis. If the chest wall is thin, a left ventricular heave is readily seen and felt, but in many patients it is necessary to rely on the ECG for evidence of left ventricular hypertrophy. The degree of left ventricular enlargement on physical examination depends largely on the degree of aortic incompetence accompanying the aortic stenosis. The examining hand readily perceives the dynamic quality of the ventricular impulse, which primarily reflects left ventricular stroke volume. The degree of left ven-

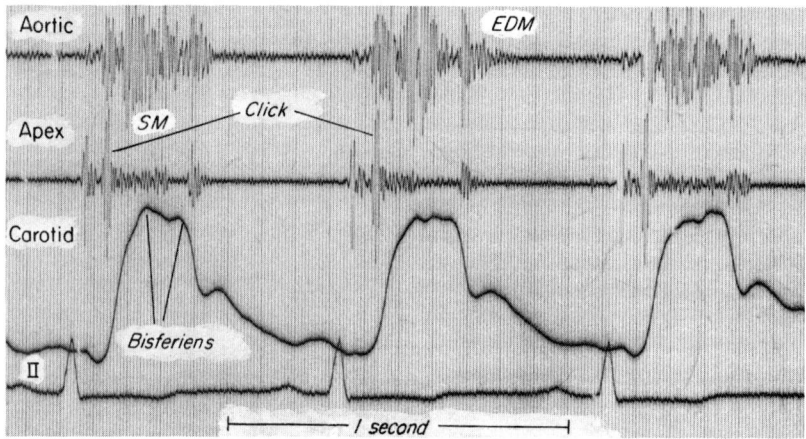

Figure 13–3. Phonocardiogram of a 36-year-old man with aortic stenosis and insufficiency. Note systolic ejection click, crescendo-decrescendo systolic murmur (SM), and short early aortic diastolic murmur (EDM). First sound faint at aortic area. Clinically, thought to be triple rhythm with presystolic gallop. The carotid pulse shows 2 peaks (bisferiens) whose relative heights vary.

tricular enlargement is better detected on the chest x-ray than on physical examination, especially when left ventricular failure has reduced the stroke volume.

Some degree of aortic incompetence is usually present. The greater the incompetence, the larger the heart. Predominant aortic stenosis varies from cases with no incompetence to those with an aortic leak sufficient to give a normal or slightly widened pulse pressure and a slightly hyperdynamic left ventricular impulse.

Depending on the anatomy of the valve, an aortic valve closure sound may or may not be present. If A_2 is audible, paradoxic (reversed) splitting of the second heart sound may be heard if severe stenosis or left bundle branch block is present (Fig 13–4). Third and fourth heart sounds are commonly heard. The characteristic murmur of aortic stenosis is harsh and chugging, and its timing is ejection in nature, starting after isovolumetric contraction has occurred, ie, 0.06 second or more after the first heart sound (Fig 13–2). It is usually associated with a systolic thrill at the base. It is preceded by an ejection click (Fig 13–3) only in mild cases, when the aortic valve is more flexible and ventricular ejection more rapid. The murmur may be heard at the base or the apex of the heart. It is often heard well in the neck, but this does not mean it is aortic in origin, since pulmonary systolic murmurs and bruits of carotid artery stenosis are also well heard there. The murmur starts after the first heart sound and stops before the second heart sound. It is louder after a long pause following an ectopic beat, and it varies with cardiac filling in atrial fibrillation. It may be audible only at the apex of the heart and can be easily missed if the patient is in severe left ventricular failure. A faint aortic diastolic murmur along the left sternal edge is usually present, but its loudness does not necessarily correspond to the severity of associated aortic incompetence, which is judged

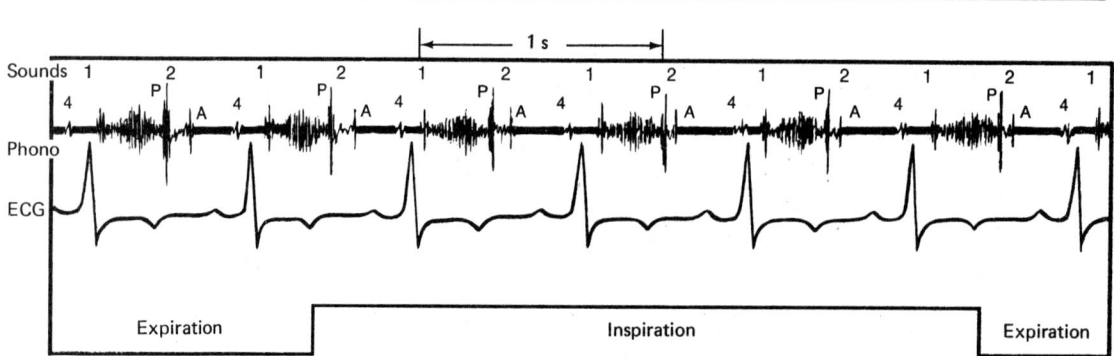

Figure 13–4. Phonocardiogram and ECG in aortic stenosis. The phonocardiogram shows ejection murmur, presystolic gallop (4), soft late A_2, and paradoxic splitting of the second heart sound (2). (Courtesy of Roche Laboratories Division of Hoffman-La Roche, Inc.)

instead by the character of the pulse, the size of the heart, and the dynamic qualities of the left ventricular impulse.

Rales at the bases of the lungs are heard in patients with left ventricular failure, and signs of right ventricular failure with raised jugular venous pressure, hepatomegaly, and peripheral edema are late manifestations of the disease. They are generally due to the development of a raised pulmonary vascular resistance (> 3.5 mm Hg/L/min), which occurs in about 10% of cases.

C. Electrocardiographic Findings: Electrocardiographic evidence of left ventricular hypertrophy is characteristically severe in predominant aortic stenosis. In about 10% of cases, left or—equally commonly—right bundle branch block or even complete block is found. Left bundle branch block interferes with the electrocardiographic recognition of left ventricular hypertrophy, but right bundle branch block does not. Significant aortic stenosis may be present in patients in whom the ECG shows little or no evidence of left ventricular hypertrophy (Fig 13–5). Moderately severe or gross evidence of left ventricular hypertrophy on the ECG is seen in about 75% of cases. Relatively slight changes occur in patients whose stenosis has developed more rapidly and in persons (most often women) who have refrained from physical exertion. Changes due to associated myocardial ischemia or myocardial infarction may be present, making electrocardiographic interpretation difficult.

D. X-Ray Findings: The chest x-ray shows a rounded shadow forming the left border of the heart; this represents the hypertrophied left ventricle. The overall heart shadow is enlarged in patients with left ventricular failure and in those with significant aortic incompetence, but not necessarily in those with early stenotic lesions in whom the left ventricle hypertrophies at the expense of the left ventricular cavity. The progression of the lesion over 10 years is shown in Fig 13–6A and B. Poststenotic dilatation confined to the origin of the ascending aorta is the rule. It is best seen on the left anterior oblique view (Fig 13–7). Calcification of the aortic valve, although often visible on the x-ray, should be sought at fluoroscopy. The characteristic dense shadow of the calcified aortic valve lies surprisingly low in the cardiac silhouette, moves up and down with the heartbeat, and lies more medially and less posteriorly than a calcified mitral valve. The presence of calcium in the aortic valve can readily be detected during cardiac catheterization when the catheter comes up against the aortic valve, or during angiocardiography. Signs of pulmonary congestion and slight left atrial enlargement are common, but prominence of the pulmonary artery is only seen in a few patients (5%) presenting late in the course of the disease.

E. Special Investigations:

1. Noninvasive techniques–Echocardiography is most helpful in excluding aortic stenosis by demonstrating that the aortic valve echo is normal. Unfortunately, this form of noninvasive investigation cannot determine the severity of aortic stenosis because it can only detect the thickening and lack of motion of the valve, as shown in Fig 13–8. Abnormalities of the aortic valve with calcification occurring in patients in whom there is no significant obstruction to left

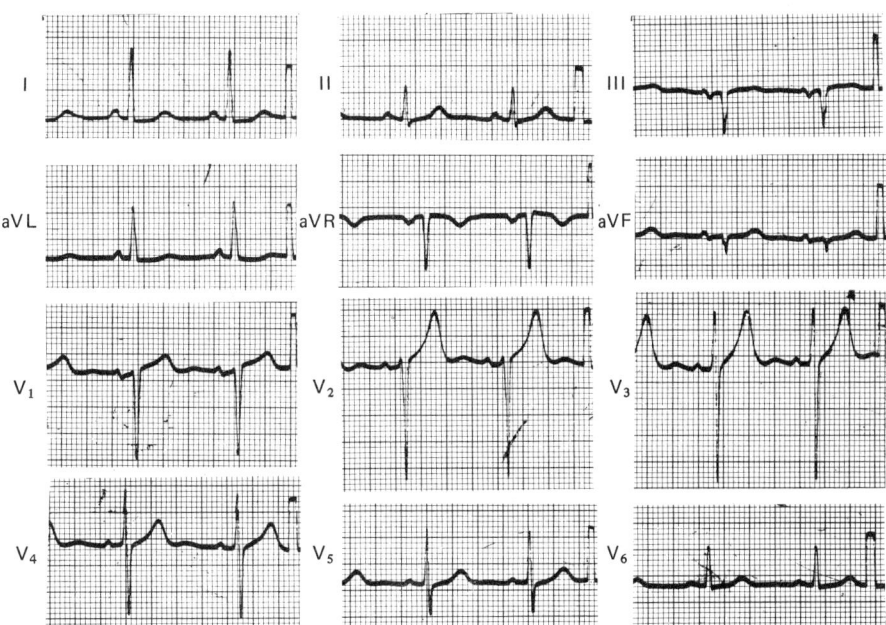

Figure 13–5. ECG of a 77-year-old woman with severe aortic stenosis. Left ventricular pressure 260/5 mm Hg; aortic pressure 130/67 mm Hg. There is little evidence on the ECG of left ventricular hypertrophy.

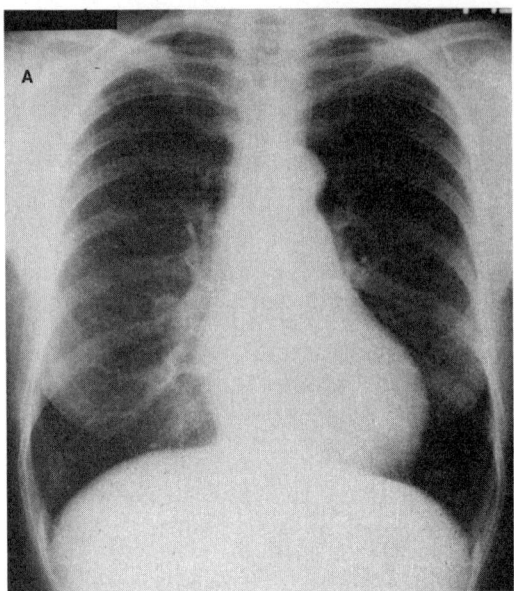
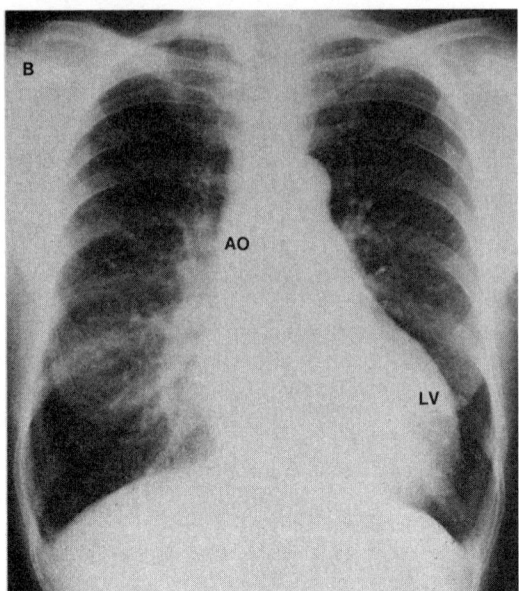

Figure 13-6. Serial chest x-rays of a patient with aortic stenosis taken 10 years apart. The left ventricle (LV) and aorta (AO) are prominent in both x-rays. The heart is larger and the right hilar vessels more prominent in the film shown at right, which was taken after the development of symptoms. Pressure tracings from this patient are shown in Fig 13-9.

ventricular outflow can give echocardiographic findings similar to those in patients with severe stenosis.

Doppler blood velocity measurements provide a better means of establishing severity. The peak velocity in the jet of blood passing through a stenotic valve depends on the severity of the obstruction. An indication of the pressure difference can be obtained by applying a simplified form of the Bernouilli equation

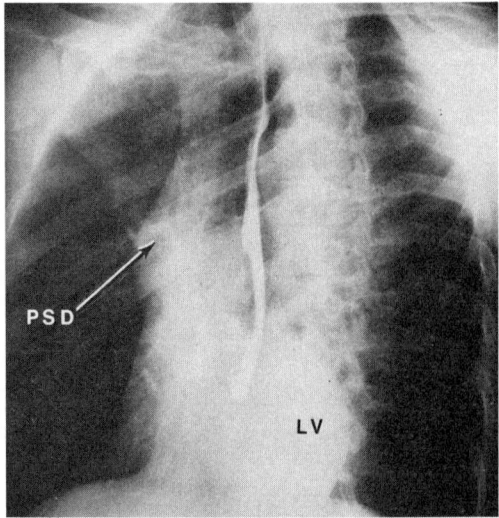

Figure 13-7. Chest x-ray showing poststenotic dilatation (PSD) of the aorta on left anterior oblique view in a patient with aortic stenosis. (LV, left ventricle.)

(see Chapter 4). The values for the pressure gradient across the aortic valve calculated from continuous wave Doppler measurements have been shown to correlate well with measurements made at cardiac catheterization.

2. Invasive techniques–

a. Right and left heart catheterization–The definitive study for the assessment of severity is always the measurement of the pressure difference between the left ventricle and the aorta, together with the systolic blood flow across the aortic valve; therefore, left heart catheterization is always indicated. Right heart catheterization may show a large right atrial a wave, raised pulmonary arterial pressure, and even moderately raised pulmonary vascular resistance in patients with severe lesions who are seen late in the course of the disease. In most cases, the right-sided pressures are normal, and the left atrial (wedge) pressure shows a large left atrial a wave due to increased force of left atrial contraction against a poorly compliant left ventricle. Left heart catheterization is most commonly performed using the retrograde aortic route.

Retrograde percutaneous femoral arterial catheterization is not always successful. Transseptal catheterization passing a catheter across the mitral valve into the left ventricle and simultaneous retrograde aortic catheterization are preferred in some centers, and this approach succeeds in about 85% of cases. It is important to measure left ventricular pressure, aortic pressure, and cardiac output simultaneously. An example of left ventricular and aortic pressure tracings in a patient with severe aortic stenosis is shown in Fig 13-9. Calculation of the valve area by the Gorlin

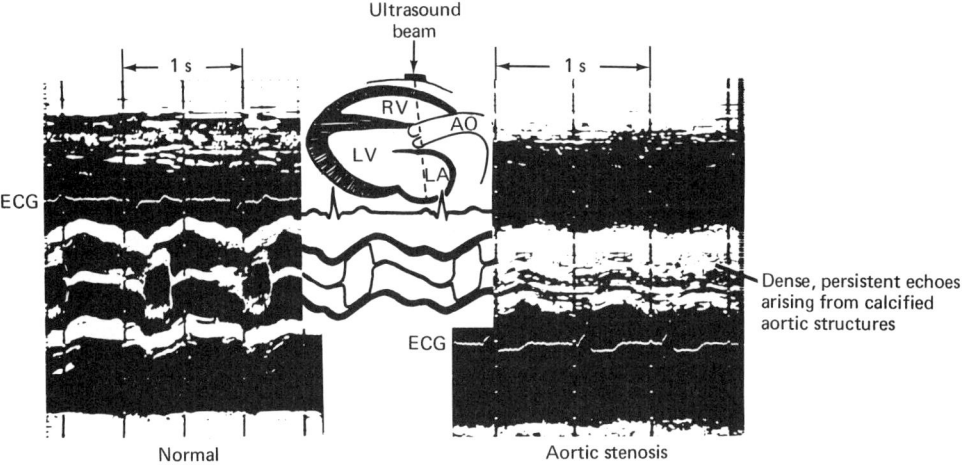

Figure 13–8. Comparison of echocardiograms of normal and stenotic aortic valves. RV, right ventricle; AO, aorta; LV, left ventricle; LA, left atrium. (Reproduced, with permission, from Kleid J, Schiller NB: *Echocardiography Case Studies.* Medical Examination Publishing Company, 1974.)

formula provides the most valuable index of severity. As in mitral disease, the presence of incompetence invalidates the measurement of valve area, but the Gorlin formula can provide a minimal value for valve area if it is assumed that incompetence is absent.

If it proves difficult to pass a catheter across the aortic valve, supravalvular angiography may be helpful in indicating the position of the aortic valve orifice, but the angiographic findings cannot be used as an indication of the severity of stenosis. In retrograde studies, the severity of aortic stenosis does not correlate directly with the ease with which a catheter can be passed across a stenotic valve. The degree of aortic dilatation and the position of the valve are more important factors in determining success of the procedure.

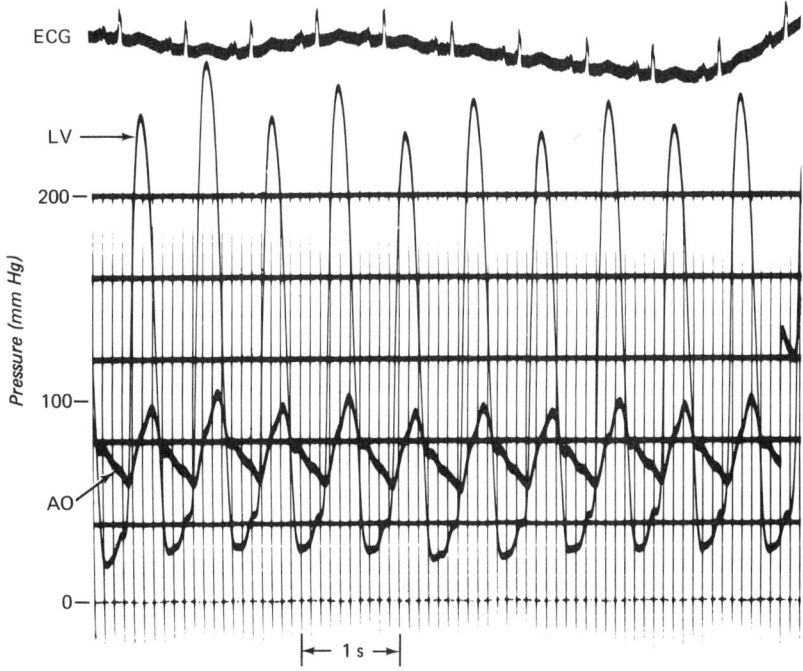

Figure 13–9. Simultaneous left ventricular (LV 270–240/40) and aortic (AO 100/60) pressure tracings in the patient whose chest x-rays are shown in Fig 13–6A and B. Pulsus alternans is present and is more prominent on the left ventricular tracing.

b. Left ventricular puncture–When retrograde aortic catheterization fails, direct left ventricular puncture via the apex of the heart is indicated. In some centers, transseptal catheterization may be tried before resorting to this procedure, but in most hospitals the last resort is left ventricular puncture. The procedure is performed with a 20-gauge lumbar puncture needle under fluoroscopic control, using 50–100 mg of intravenous meperidine as an analgesic. It is surprisingly well tolerated and usually painless. Satisfactory tracings are obtained in about 85% of cases, and since the left ventricle is almost invariably hypertrophied, the dangers of hemorrhage and tamponade are minimal. A small pneumothorax is the most frequent complication and occurs in about 10% of cases. The patient's status must be monitored for several hours after the procedure in order to detect any early evidence of complications.

c. Selective coronary angiography–Some cardiologists advocate coronary arteriography in all patients with aortic stenosis. If the surgeon plans to perfuse the coronary arteries, the investigation may indeed be indicated in order to confirm that the anatomy of the main branches of the coronary vessels is normal. In general, however, the state of the coronary vessels alters the prognosis of aortic stenosis but not the treatment or the decision to operate, which depend on the severity of the obstruction. Because coronary arteriography increases the morbidity and mortality rates of an already difficult investigation, it is not advised in patients with severe or moderately severe aortic stenosis. In cases in which the hemodynamic severity of the stenosis does not definitely warrant surgery, coronary angiography can help the cardiologist decide whether or not to operate. Coronary angiography is definitely indicated in those patients with prominent angina pectoris or in those who have suffered myocardial infarction. Increasing numbers of patients are being found to have both aortic stenosis and coronary artery disease. This probably reflects the increasing late development of aortic stenosis in older patients who already have coronary lesions. Now that aortocoronary bypass has come to be a commonplace operation with a low mortality rate, a larger number of patients are being treated by combined aortic valve replacement and aortocoronary bypass. There is still some difference of opinion about the indications for coronary bypass surgery in patients with aortic stenosis in whom coronary lesions are found at angiography. The results of replacing the aortic valve without carrying out bypass surgery have been shown to be similar, both in operative mortality rate and long-term survival, to those in which comparable coronary lesions were bypassed. In the authors' view, there should be a clear indication that coronary disease is a clinical problem before bypass surgery is undertaken. If a left main coronary lesion is present or the aortic valve disease is mild and angina is a dominant symptom, bypass surgery is indicated; but the value of "prophylactic" bypass surgery in patients with aortic valve disease is not yet established.

F. Hemodynamic Values: The means and standard deviations of measurements obtained during cardiac catheterization in patients with predominant aortic stenosis are shown in Table 13–1. In addition to the values for the entire group of patients, the results have been broken down into 2 subgroups: those with clear evidence of left ventricular failure and those without such evidence. This difference is not reflected in the duration of the history, the cardiac output, or the hemodynamic severity of the stenosis but is only manifested in the level of the wedge pressure.

Diagnosis

The most pressing problems in the diagnosis of aortic stenosis are (1) to detect when left ventricular failure will occur in the course of the disease, (2) to accurately assess the severity of stenosis, and (3) to decide whether to recommend surgery for asymptomatic and mildly symptomatic patients. The presence of left ventricular hypertrophy on the ECG or physical examination may raise the possibility of surgery but is not an absolute indication for further clinical investigation, since a patient with the disease can be asymptomatic for up to 20 years with moderate left ventricular hypertrophy.

On the other hand, the possibility that dyspnea, syncope, dizziness, or cardiac pain is due to aortic stenosis is a strong indication for left heart catheterization. Echocardiography can reduce the number of patients in whom cardiac catheterization is performed by showing that the aortic valve is thin and mobile, but it cannot be used to establish a diagnosis of aortic stenosis. The physician must maintain a strong index of suspicion and a sense of urgency in dealing with patients whose symptoms may be due to aortic stenosis, because delay is more dangerous in aortic stenosis than in any other cardiac lesion in adults.

Differential Diagnosis

A. Left Ventricular Failure: Aortic stenosis enters into the differential diagnosis of all patients with left

Table 13–1. Cardiac catheterization data, including length of history, in patients with predominant aortic stenosis.

	Mean Wedge Pressure (mm Hg)	Left Ventricular Systolic Pressure (mm Hg)	Aortic Systolic Pressure (mm Hg)	Aortic Diastolic Pressure (mm Hg)	Cardiac Output (L/min)	Length of History (Years)
Predominant aortic stenosis	20 ± 10	208 ± 40	132 ± 28	69 ± 13	4.7 ± 1.5	2.4 ± 2.0
Without left ventricular failure	13 ± 6	215 ± 40	138 ± 26	73 ± 14	4.8 ± 1.5	2.2 ± 1.8
With left ventricular failure	28 ± 9	202 ± 41	126 ± 29	85 ± 13	4.6 ± 1.5	2.6 ± 2.2

ventricular failure, especially when there is a basal systolic murmur and a history of syncope, dizziness, or conduction defect. The possibility of aortic stenosis must be considered in hypertension, cardiomyopathy, and even in coronary artery disease, especially when heart failure is severe. It is important to recognize the systolic murmur and rule out the possibility of aortic stenosis by all available means, including cardiac catheterization.

B. Hypertrophic Obstructive Cardiomyopathy: Aortic stenosis should not be confused with hypertrophic obstructive cardiomyopathy. In the latter condition (see Chapter 17, p 539), the pulse is jerky and the upstroke rapid and often bifid, in contrast to the slow-rising pulse of aortic stenosis. If there is associated aortic incompetence modifying the upstroke of the pulse in a patient with predominant aortic stenosis, there will almost certainly be an aortic diastolic murmur, which virtually rules out a diagnosis of obstructive cardiomyopathy. The murmur of hypertrophic cardiomyopathy is longer and harsher and usually heard best to the left of the sternum. The variation occurring in the murmur when diagnostic measures are used to influence the extent of outflow tract narrowing is helpful in establishing the diagnosis of obstructive cardiomyopathy. Echocardiography is particularly helpful in differential diagnosis because it shows systolic anterior motion of the mitral valve in hypertrophic cardiomyopathy and aortic valve thickening in aortic stenosis.

C. Other Lesions: The physical signs in mitral incompetence and ventricular septal defect are seldom confused with those of predominant aortic stenosis. In these disorders, the murmur is pansystolic, and the carotid upstroke is rapid. When the patient has both aortic stenosis and mitral incompetence, it is difficult to distinguish between them, and clinical assessment of the relative severity of the 2 lesions is usually impossible. In some cases there is a characteristic high-pitched "seagull cry" murmur (see p 423).

Coarctation of the aorta is another lesion that may occasionally coexist with aortic stenosis and be confused with it. The murmur of coarctation occurs later in systole and reaches its peak about the time of the second heart sound. There is characteristically a prominent carotid arterial pulsation as well as delay between the peaks of the brachial and femoral pulses, with hypertension in the arms (Chapter 11). Although coarctation of the aorta is commonly associated with bicuspid aortic valve, the coarctation is likely to cause problems long before the abnormal valve gives rise to difficulties that are associated with the development of aortic stenosis.

Complications

A. Sudden Death: Patients with predominant aortic stenosis are likely to die suddenly. The incidence of sudden death is unknown and is likely to be underestimated. Sudden death is clearly not confined to patients with severe stenosis, since it is one of the common causes of late death following aortic valve replacement. This finding suggests that residual myocardial damage may cause arrhythmias or that valve malfunction may occur acutely. The general consensus is that arrhythmia is responsible for most cases of sudden death in aortic stenosis. In aortic stenosis, the effects of a sudden fall in arterial pressure resulting from arrhythmia are probably greater than normal for both mechanical and reflex reasons. In terms of mechanics, cardiac output takes longer to return to normal after an arrhythmia has developed. In terms of reflexes, the central nervous system tends to receive contradictory information from the carotid and aortic baroreceptors on the one hand and the left ventricular stretch receptors (von Bezold receptors) on the other, because left ventricular pressure is high and aortic pressure is relatively low.

B. Left Ventricular Failure: Left ventricular failure is an almost inevitable consequence of aortic stenosis and occurs relatively late. It is the strongest possible indication for surgical treatment because it is consistently relieved by surgery. Medical measures for its control should be regarded as part of the preoperative preparation and not as a substitute for surgery.

C. Conduction Defects: Complete atrioventricular block occasionally complicates aortic stenosis, and its association with slow heart rates and large stroke volumes makes clinical assessment of the lesion difficult. The hemodynamic signs of aortic stenosis seem more severe when the heart rate is slow. The heart is larger, the systolic murmur and thrill are more impressive, and the pressure difference between the left ventricle and the aorta is greater. Usually, however, all that is necessary is a calculation of the aortic valve area by means of the Gorlin formula, since the heart rate does not influence the calculated valve area.

D. Infective Endocarditis: Infective endocarditis is an important but rare complication of aortic stenosis. It occurs in about 2% of cases and is less common than in mitral or aortic incompetence.

Treatment

A. Medical Treatment: It is important that the treatment for left ventricular failure in aortic stenosis not be restricted to medical means. Surgery is the first and not the last resort. Digitalis, diuretics, and salt restriction are effective in left ventricular failure caused by aortic stenosis, and they should be used preoperatively. Surgical treatment in severe aortic stenosis is a matter of some urgency.

B. Surgical Treatment:

1. Aortic valve replacement–Replacement of the aortic valve is required in all patients with moderate or severe stenosis (pressure difference 50 mm Hg or more or aortic valve area 0.8 cm^2 or less). Age is no bar to surgery, and the discomfort of intractable left ventricular failure should be avoided if at all possible. In young patients (under age 30), palliative open aortic valvotomy may be justified because the long-term hazards of valve replacement are not yet known. The physician should remember that after valvotomy a

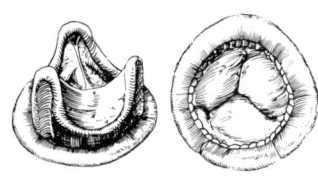

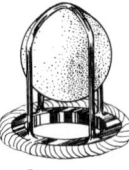 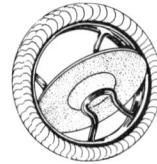

Caged ball   Tilting disk

Figure 13–10. Examples of artificial heart valves. (Reproduced, with permission, from Way LW [editor]: *Current Surgical Diagnosis & Treatment,* 7th ed. Lange, 1985.)

second operation to replace the aortic valve will almost certainly be necessary in a decade or two.

The choice of artificial valve rests with the surgeon. Homograft, heterograft, ball, flap, and disk valves have been used (Fig 13–10). The Starr-Edwards ball and cage valve has been used most frequently and has proved most successful. It is generally thought that homograft and heterograft tissue valves do not require postoperative anticoagulant therapy indefinitely, as opposed to all types of prosthetic valves, in which lifetime anticoagulation is needed. The mortality rate of aortic valve replacement depends on the stage of the disease at the time of surgery; the average is about 5%. The mortality rate is greatest in patients with marked left ventricular hypertrophy or severe heart failure.

2. Surgical treatment of nonvalvular lesions– Supravalvular aortic stenosis is more difficult to treat than valvular stenosis because the ascending aorta is often hypoplastic. Congenital subvalvular ring stenosis can be excised, bringing dramatic relief. Valve replacement is not needed.

3. Results of surgery–Like the mortality rate, the results of surgical treatment vary depending on when operation is performed and whether coronary artery disease or other valve lesions are present. If the left ventricle is markedly dilated as a result of long-standing left ventricular failure, results will be worse than in early cases with hearts of normal size. Ideally, patients should be closely followed and operation recommended at the first sign of significant symptoms. In practice, however, diagnosis is made late in the course of the disease in about half of cases, usually because the patient does not seek help, and sometimes because the correct diagnosis is missed.

Prognosis

Without surgery, the prognosis in aortic stenosis after the development of signs and symptoms of heart failure is poor. With treatment of heart failure, the patient may live for up to 8 years, but distressing episodes of recurrent left ventricular failure with pulmonary edema make the average survival time shorter.

Long-Term Results in Operated Cases

Aortic valve replacement for predominant aortic stenosis is the most satisfactory of all valve replacement operations. The degree of disability in the survivors is much less than in unoperated patients, and left ventricular failure is almost inevitably relieved. Approximately 70% of those who survive to leave hospital are still alive 5 years later, and after 10 years 50% are still living.

The results of valve replacement are better in patients in whom the operation is performed before severe left ventricular failure and marked left ventricular dilatation have occurred. In spite of this finding, operation is advised in all patients with significant aortic stenosis irrespective of the severity of left ventricular failure, because it is impossible to predict which patients will have an unsatisfactory result.

PREDOMINANT AORTIC INCOMPETENCE

The cardinal features of hemodynamically significant predominant aortic incompetence (Fig 13–11) include a large hypertrophied left ventricle, a large aorta, increased stroke volume, and wide pulse pressure. Variable factors include the severity of the process, the nature of the lesion (acute or chronic), and the cause.

Hemodynamically significant aortic incompetence creates an important extra load on the left ventricle. The blood that flows back across the aortic valve during diastole must be ejected during systole, and the consequent large stroke volume increases the work of the heart. The extra work is mainly "flow" work rather than "pressure" work, but peak systolic pressure tends to be raised and aortic diastolic pressure lowered because of rapid runoff of aortic blood into the peripheral arterial bed and back into the left ventricle. The arbitrary basis on which aortic incompetence is classified as hemodynamically significant here is the level of diastolic pressure. As stated on p 400, a value of less than 70 mm Hg constitutes the arbitrary dividing line, and patients with aortic incompetence and arterial diastolic pressures higher than that are considered to have hemodynamically insignificant aortic incompetence. Exceptions do exist, especially in patients with severe heart failure, in whom peripheral vasoconstriction has occurred and caused an increase in diastolic pressure.

Acute Lesions

Aortic incompetence occurs both as an acute lesion (20% of cases) and as a single chronic lesion (80% of cases). Acute aortic incompetence occurs when valve lesions develop either instantaneously—when a cusp perforates or tears—or over a few days or weeks—

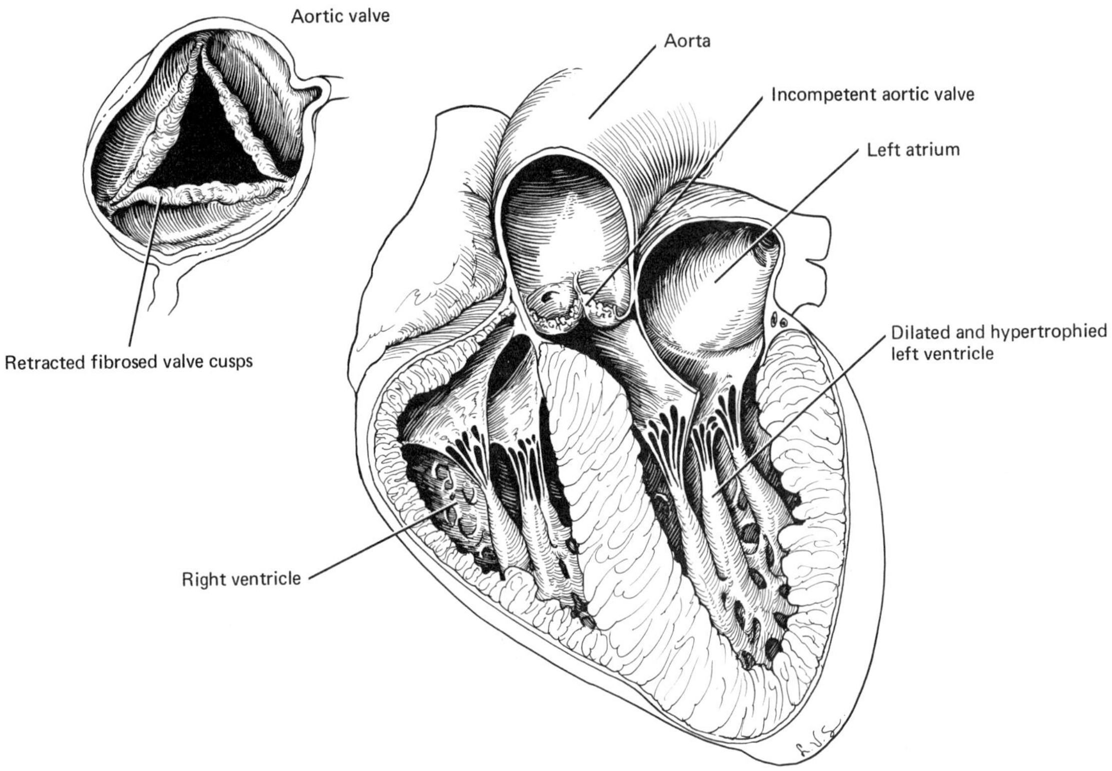

Drawing of left heart in left anterior oblique view showing anatomic features of aortic incompetence.

Cardinal features: Large hypertrophied left ventricle; large aorta; increased stroke volume; wide pulse pressure.

Variable factors: Severity; acuteness or chronicity; cause.

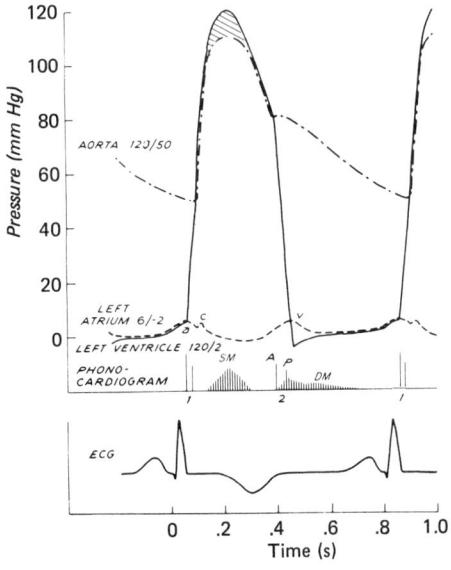

Diagram showing auscultatory and hemodynamic features of predominant aortic incompetence. DM, diastolic murmur. (Other abbreviations are explained in Fig 13–1.)

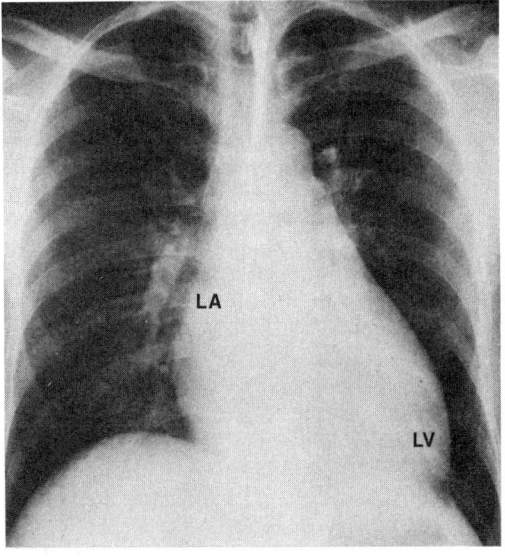

Chest x-ray of a patient with aortic incompetence and no signs of left heart failure. The long shadow of the enlarged left ventricle (LV) and slight left atrial (LA) enlargement can be seen.

Figure 13–11. Aortic incompetence. Structures enlarged: left ventricle, aorta.

when valve tissue is gradually eroded by infection, or when fibrosis, associated with healing of an infection, scars and contracts the valve. Acute aortic incompetence throws a more serious load on the left ventricle than acute mitral incompetence, and the chances that the patient's hemodynamic status will stabilize without surgical treatment are small. If the damage is less severe or less acute, the possibility for survival is better; and if the patient survives, the clinical picture in acute aortic incompetence by the end of about one year resembles that in chronic lesions.

Chronic Lesions

Chronic aortic incompetence results in marked peripheral vasodilatation, which is attributable in part to reflex baroreceptor effects. The wide aortic and carotid pulse pressures cause reflex vasodilation and relative bradycardia. With exercise, the cardiac output increases, there is peripheral vasodilatation of the muscular capillaries, and a further fall in systemic vascular resistance occurs. As a result, the proportion of the left ventricular stroke volume returning to the left ventricle during diastole falls, and the hemodynamic status becomes closer to that seen in normal subjects. In contrast, anything that increases the systemic vascular resistance, such as isometric exercise, exposure to cold, sympathetic nervous system stimulation, mental stress, or cardiac failure, tends to increase the volume of blood returning to the ventricle during diastole and makes the load on the heart more a "pressure" load and less a "flow" load.

Left Ventricular Hypertrophy & Dilatation

Aortic incompetence leads to left ventricular dilatation, which constitutes an important stimulus to hypertrophy of the left ventricular muscle. Hypertrophy involves an increase in the size of muscle cells and an increase in the connective tissue elements of the heart. In time, long-standing hypertrophy almost inevitably leads to myocardial fibrosis and becomes irreversible, so that heart muscle cells do not return to normal when the stimulus causing the hypertrophy is removed. With time, the left ventricle fails, probably as a result of myocardial fibrosis and age-related changes in ventricular muscle. This occurs relatively late in the course of chronic lesions. The development of ventricular failure is influenced by the severity of the incompetence and the state of myocardium, which in turn depend on the degree of atherosclerosis or the extent of rheumatic myocardial damage. It is also possible that the patient's activity level may play a part; earlier failure may develop in patients with more strenuous occupations. When it occurs, left ventricular failure is often acute and severe because reflex vasoconstriction takes the place of the normal vasodilatation seen in chronic lesions, and it further aggravates ventricular failure by increasing systemic vascular resistance and hence the amount of incompetence. The most striking clinical manifestations of left ventricular failure are an increase in arterial diastolic pressure and the change from vasodilatation to vasoconstriction that often accompanies failure and tends to obscure peripheral signs of aortic incompetence.

Causes of Aortic Incompetence

A. Acute Lesions: The most important cause of acute aortic incompetence is infective endocarditis. Patients who initially have normal aortic valves may contract infective endocarditis when they are debilitated because of immunosuppressive therapy, chronic illness, or intravenous drug abuse or when the infecting organism is highly invasive; in these cases, organisms of minimal pathogenicity may be the infective agent. Infective endocarditis also affects valves that are already diseased as a result of rheumatic or congenital involvement. The milder the original valve disease, the greater the potential for acute hemodynamic deterioration.

Another and rarer cause of acute aortic incompetence is aortic dissection. In this condition, a tear in the aortic intima extends to the neighborhood of the noncoronary cusp of the aortic valve and causes the valve lesion. Marfan's syndrome, aortic atherosclerosis with hypertension, and arteritis are the main causes of aortic dissection. Traumatic lesions may cause aortic incompetence, with either blunt trauma or penetrating wounds.

B. Chronic Lesions: Chronic aortic incompetence has several causes and occurs at all ages. It is more common in males by a factor of 3:2 and appears in our experience to be the commonest valvular lesion in black males. Rheumatic fever probably still accounts for the majority of cases. If it is assumed that rheumatic fever is subclinical in 50% of cases, a confirmed history of previous rheumatic fever in 25% of cases of chronic aortic incompetence indicates that about half of cases are rheumatic in origin.

Syphilis is a decreasingly common cause of aortic incompetence, but it is still found in 10% of cases. The average age of these patients is over 60 years, and associated atherosclerosis is almost always present.

Cases in which a congenital cause is confirmed account for about 10%, but this may be an underestimate. A congenital cause should be suspected when associated lesions such as ventricular septal defect, Fallot's tetralogy, patent ductus arteriosus, or coarctation of the aorta are seen; when noncardiac congenital lesions such as Marfan's syndrome are present; or when the murmur is heard in infancy.

Ankylosing spondylitis and Reiter's syndrome are rare causes of aortic incompetence (5% of cases) in which the atrioventricular conduction system may be involved. The characteristic hip or sacroiliac joint involvement of ankylosing spondylitis may precede or follow the valve lesion and is sometimes only detected on x-ray examination.

Hypertension and atherosclerosis are rarely (3% of cases) the cause of hemodynamically significant aortic incompetence. More commonly these conditions produce an aortic diastolic murmur, with only slight widening of the aortic pulse pressure and no lowering of the aortic diastolic pressure.

Clinical Findings

In rheumatic lesions, fibrosis and retraction of the valve cusps start early in the course of rheumatic infection and progress slowly over several years. Syphilis attacks the aortic valve secondarily, by extension of disease from the aorta. Endarteritis obliterans of the vasa vasorum of the aorta is the basic pathologic lesion of syphilitic aortitis, and aortic dilatation with swelling and thickening of the intima involves the root of the aorta and perhaps also the coronary ostia, leading to myocardial ischemia. In congenital lesions, the valve may be bicuspid. Alternatively, incompetence may be secondary to aortic dilatation, as in Marfan's syndrome, or to prolapse of unsupported valvular tissue, as in association with ventricular septal defects involving the membranous part of the interventricular septum. There is no associated myocarditis in congenital cases; as a result, muscle damage is less prominent. In ankylosing spondylitis and Reiter's syndrome, the pathologic lesion is again primarily in the aorta and in the connective tissues supporting the valve. In atherosclerotic lesions, too, it is aortic involvement that secondarily affects the valve, principally by means of dilatation.

A. Symptoms:

1. Acute lesions–Dyspnea is the commonest presenting cardiac symptom in acute lesions (50% of cases). Since infective endocarditis is by far the commonest cause, the patient usually is febrile and may be acutely ill with septicemia at the time that the aortic valve lesion develops. In other cases, the onset is slower and subacute: the aortic lesion appears or worsens as endocarditis heals, and the valve shrinks as it fibroses weeks or months after the endocarditis has responded to antibiotic therapy. In other patients, systemic embolism may be the presenting symptom, with a cerebrovascular accident, an acute coronary occlusion, or a cold, painful leg as the first sign of acute aortic incompetence. Acute aortic incompetence occurring in a person who is not ill with infective endocarditis suggests the possibility of acute aortic dissection involving the noncoronary cusp of the aortic valve. This uncommon lesion is not always painful. If either the left or right coronary artery is involved, the patient almost inevitably dies.

The dyspnea of acute aortic incompetence is often paroxysmal and associated with orthopnea and cough, with frothy pink sputum resulting from acute pulmonary edema. Chest pain may occur because of acute myocardial ischemia and peripheral circulatory collapse. Symptoms of shock, with anxiety, confusion, and mental obtundation, are occasionally seen.

2. Chronic lesions–

a. Symptoms unrelated to severity–There are 2 varieties of symptoms in chronic aortic incompetence, those due to the patient's awareness of increased force of the heartbeat and those due to left ventricular disease and heart failure. One-third of patients with hemodynamically significant aortic incompetence complain of palpitations, which on questioning turn out to be associated with sensations arising from forceful left ventricular contraction. The patient often notices the symptoms when lying in bed at night. These sensations sometimes provoke the symptoms of anxiety seen in cardiac neurosis, with stabbing inframammary pain, fatigue, and dyspnea with sighing respirations. The patient may have ventricular premature beats that further accentuate the symptoms. These symptoms usually occur in early adult life and can be present for 20 years or more without significant progression of the valvular lesion. More frequently (two-thirds of cases), the patient has no symptoms and is able to lead a surprisingly normal, active life in spite of a hemodynamically serious lesion. It is important to recognize certain symptoms as "functional" in patients with aortic incompetence and not interpret them as a necessary indication for surgery. Ventricular arrhythmia is probably the most important cause of symptoms at this stage, since it is thought that it may precede ventricular tachycardia or fibrillation, and these developments may account for the sudden death that is rarer in aortic incompetence than in stenosis but that nevertheless occurs. The presence of symptoms in a patient with aortic incompetence is always an indication for thorough investigation; but if the valvular lesion is well tolerated, the patient (especially if young) should usually simply be closely followed, and the physician should watch for the development of serious symptoms.

b. Symptoms of left ventricular failure–When aortic incompetence is the sole lesion, serious symptoms due to left ventricular failure occur late in the course of the disease. Dyspnea is by far the commonest symptom (75% of cases) and may be associated with a feeling of heaviness in the chest and substernal discomfort. If significant dyspnea occurs before age 30 and left ventricular failure is found, it is most likely that past or present rheumatic myocardial involvement is influencing the clinical picture. Left ventricular failure due solely to chronic aortic incompetence usually occurs after age 40, and patients who lead sedentary lives may not be aware of the insidious progression of pulmonary congestion because they have never exerted themselves sufficiently. In these patients, an acute episode of paroxysmal nocturnal dyspnea or frank pulmonary edema may be the presenting event. Chest pain is the next most common symptom in aortic incompetence. It is particularly common in patients with syphilitic lesions and in older persons with associated coronary arterial disease. Anginal pain may be present at rest or during exercise; in general, it is due to increased metabolic demands of the hypertrophied myocardium rather than to decreased supply resulting from obstructive atherosclerotic lesions in major coronary vessels. Syncope and dizziness are less common than in patients with predominantly stenotic lesions, and syncope during unaccustomed effort (the type seen in aortic stenosis) does not occur.

c. Development of left ventricular failure–The late symptoms in aortic incompetence carry a poor prognosis. This is in part due to reflex factors that cause a vicious circle. When cardiac output falls as the left ventricle fails, the normal peripheral vasodilatation seen in aortic incompetence is replaced by vasoconstriction. This peripheral vasoconstriction increases the work of the left ventricle, increases aortic incompetence, and aggravates left ventricular failure. The relatively high arterial diastolic pressure that results may mislead the physician into thinking that significant aortic incompetence is not present. Left ventricular failure is thus especially sudden in aortic incompetence and is often provoked by factors involving autonomic nervous system control of blood pressure and blood volume, such as excitement, excessive sodium intake, recumbency, overexertion, excessive mental stress, and violent dreams, all of which cause a rise in systemic arterial pressure. The patient's occupation may also influence the occurrence of left ventricular failure. Patients with strenuous jobs involving heavy manual labor may develop larger hearts corresponding to a given level of severity in the lesion and hence develop left ventricular failure earlier than patients who avoid excessive exertion. The role of mental stress may also be important in patients with this lesion, because it is increased systemic arterial pressure and increased peripheral resistance that tend to aggravate incompetence more than any increase in cardiac output.

d. Sweating–Patients with predominant aortic incompetence have a tendency to sweat more, a finding that is unexplained.

B. Signs: The rapid runoff of blood from the aorta during diastole dominates the physical signs of hemodynamically significant aortic incompetence. Prominent carotid pulsations in the neck, throbbing peripheral arteries, and a prominent left ventricular impulse that moves the whole left side of the chest produce easily visible evidence of the large left ventricular stroke volume and increased rate of systolic ejection seen in this lesion. These peripheral circulatory signs are seen in both acute and chronic lesions and are present in all patients except those in severe left ventricular failure. The rapid aortic runoff is due to increased blood flow back into the left ventricle and into the dilated peripheral arterial bed. It is important to remember that rapid runoff from the aorta into cardiac chambers or blood vessels other than the left ventricle is an equally potent cause of the peripheral signs ordinarily associated with aortic incompetence. Large patent ductus arteriosus, aortopulmonary window, rupture of an aneurysm of the aortic sinus (sinus of Valsalva) with consequent left-to-right shunt, or a major systemic arteriovenous fistula may produce similar physical signs.

Systemic arterial pressure is the most readily measured indication of the severity of the peripheral signs of rapid aortic runoff. There is a wide pulse pressure, with high systolic and low diastolic pressure. Arterial pressure measured indirectly with a blood pressure cuff is not always accurate, and a diastolic pressure reading of zero—ie, an audible sound over the artery with no cuff in position—is never correct although it is often seen in patients with aortic incompetence. The wide pulse pressure gives rise to the typical collapsing pulse in which the pulse wave rises rapidly to a peak and falls away quickly. Secondary physical signs due to rapid aortic runoff are numerous and usually have eponymic designations. Head movement in time with the heartbeat is called Musset's sign after the French poet Alfred de Musset, in whom it was noticed by his brother, who was a physician. Quincke's pulse denotes capillary pulsation in the extremities; Duroziez's sign refers to systolic and diastolic murmurs over the femoral artery; and Hill's sign denotes increased blood pressure in the legs above that measured in the arms. Corrigan's pulse refers to the collapsing pulse, which is also called a "water-hammer" pulse after a 19th century children's toy of that name. Pulsations in the digital and ulnar arteries are readily felt, and the hands and feet are warm and sweaty.

Pulsation can be seen in the second and third intercostal spaces to the right of the sternum when the aorta is dilated, especially in syphilitic lesions with or without associated aortic aneurysm. It is seen best from the side of the bed, with the examiner's eye at chest level.

In chronic aortic incompetence, the left ventricular impulse is heaving and hyperdynamic, and the apex beat is displaced downward and to the left. These physical signs depend largely on the size of the heart and are less obvious in acute aortic incompetence in which left ventricular hypertrophy has not yet developed. The characteristic physical sign on auscultation is a high-pitched, blowing diastolic murmur beginning immediately after the second sound at the start of diastole (Fig 13–11). It is called an "immediate" diastolic murmur to distinguish it from the "delayed" diastolic murmur of mitral stenosis, which does not start until left ventricular pressure has fallen below the level of left atrial pressure, ie, about 0.1 second after the start of diastole. The diastolic murmur of aortic incompetence lasts until backflow through the valve stops; the length of the murmur thus depends on the severity of the lesion and the compliance of the left ventricle. In severe cases, the murmur lasts throughout diastole and may be associated with a third heart sound (Fig 13–12).

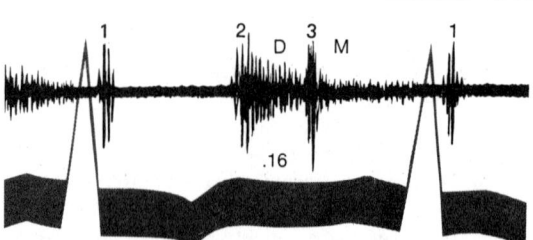

Figure 13–12. Phonocardiogram of a patient with aortic incompetence. A third sound is buried in the murmur (DM) that follows immediately after the second sound (2). (Courtesy of Roche Laboratories Division of Hoffman-La Roche, Inc.)

The inevitable increase in left ventricular stroke volume ordinarily causes a systolic murmur that is of no value in diagnosis or in the differentiation of aortic incompetence from predominant aortic stenosis. The site at which the immediate diastolic murmur of aortic incompetence is heard best depends on the degree of aortic dilatation. If the aorta is large, as in syphilitic lesions, the murmur is heard best to the right of the sternum. If the aorta is small, as in rheumatic lesions, the murmur is heard best to the left of the sternum. The murmur of aortic incompetence is sometimes only heard in the lower intercostal spaces (fourth or fifth) beside the sternum and is usually not heard well at the apex. When aortic incompetence is severe, an additional, separate apical diastolic murmur is heard. This murmur, which is called an Austin Flint murmur (Fig 13–13), is middiastolic or presystolic and is thought to be due to fluttering of the anterior, aortic cusp of the mitral valve as it is caught between the 2 streams of blood flowing into the ventricle during diastole, one from the aorta and the other from the left atrium. Atrial contraction can influence the pattern of flow in this region and cause presystolic accentuation of the murmur, which is only heard in patients with severe aortic incompetence. Thus, the differential diagnosis is not between mitral stenosis and aortic incompetence, but between aortic incompetence and aortic incompetence plus mitral stenosis.

Although murmurs of aortic incompetence are similar in both the acute and the chronic form, the physical signs due to the hemodynamic effects of aortic incompetence may be strikingly different in the 2 lesions. For example, left ventricular dilatation and hypertrophy and aortic dilatation are not seen at the onset of acute aortic incompetence, whereas peripheral circulatory collapse, sweating, marked tachycardia, and signs of shock, with tachypnea, basal rales, and other signs of acute severe incompetence are not seen in patients with chronic lesions, except in severe left ventricular failure. The aortic diastolic murmur and the pulse pressure are the 2 signs that should be monitored continuously in patients with infective endocarditis who are at risk of developing aortic incompetence.

C. Electrocardiographic Findings: Electrocardiographic evidence of left ventricular hypertrophy is always present in patients with chronic hemodynamically significant aortic incompetence unless left bundle branch block or complete atrioventricular block obscures the changes. The degree of left ventricular hypertrophy—as judged by the height of the R wave in the left-sided chest leads, the depth of the S wave in the right-sided leads, and the associated ST–T changes—is moderate or considerable in more than half of patients. In about 10% of patients, right or, more commonly, left bundle branch block or even complete atrioventricular block is present. Atrial fibrillation is less common than in any other isolated left-sided lesion (5% of patients), perhaps because left ventricular failure is seldom chronic, and unrec-

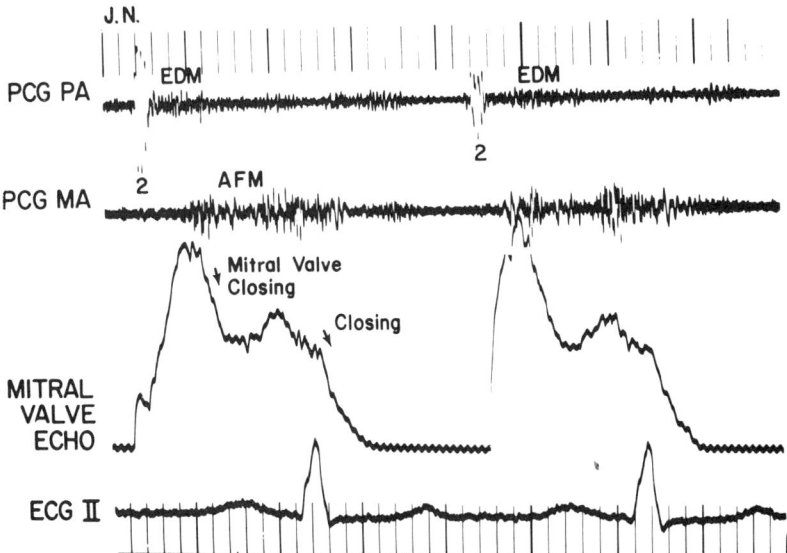

Figure 13–13. Phonocardiogram (PCG), echocardiogram, and ECG of a patient with a 2-component Austin Flint murmur (AFM). The murmur has its onset in mid diastole as the early diastolic aortic murmur (EDM) is diminishing, and it occurs while the mitral valve is closing. The second component of the murmur occurs coincidentally with atrial systole. At the time of this murmur, the mitral valve opens incompletely. The mitral valve echocardiogram shows the position of the anterior cusp. The rapid backward motion associated with mitral valve closure is interrupted by atrial systole. PA, pulmonary area; MA, mitral area. (Reproduced, with permission, from the American Heart Association, Inc., Fortuin NJ, Craige E: On the mechanism of Austin Flint murmur. *Circulation* 1972;**45**:558.)

ognized mitral valve disease occurs less frequently. In acute aortic incompetence, left ventricular hypertrophy may be absent when the patient is first seen and may develop over a period of months. In other patients in whom aortic incompetence is present before infective endocarditis develops, left ventricular hypertrophy may become progressively more severe. Age does not prevent its development.

D. X-Ray Findings: The cardiac silhouette in severe aortic incompetence shows evidence of both dilatation and hypertrophy of the left ventricle, as shown in Fig 13–11. The long wide curve of the left lateral wall of the heart on the posteroanterior view extends below the diaphragm; on the left anterior oblique view, the posterior sweep of the left ventricle overlies the dorsal spine and extends posterior to the inferior vena caval shadow. The physician must exercise care in interpreting x-ray evidence of left ventricular enlargement, since the left and right ventricles can on occasion be confused with one another. Electrocardiographic confirmation is always helpful and is required before the physician concludes that x-ray findings are due to the enlargement of a particular ventricle. Aortic dilatation, as shown in Fig 13–14, is an important finding in patients with nonrheumatic aortic incompetence. Although calcification of the aortic valve is rare ($< 10\%$ of cases), linear "eggshell" calcification of the ascending aorta (Fig 20–2) is diagnostic of aortitis and almost pathognomonic of a syphilitic lesion. Calcification of the arch and descending portions of the aorta is not important as a diagnostic sign and is commonly seen in older, atherosclerotic patients.

In acute aortic incompetence, left ventricular enlargement on the chest x-ray may be absent when the patient is first seen. If the patient survives, the left ventricle enlarges at about the same rate as the electrocardiographic changes of hypertrophy develop (3 weeks–6 months). X-ray evidence of pulmonary congestion with acute or subacute pulmonary edema is commonly seen in acute lesions. It is important to distinguish these changes from those seen in pulmonary infarction or pneumonia. The lesions are almost always bilateral but not always symmetric, and the characteristic "bat's wing" distribution of subacute pulmonary edema with shadows extending out from the roots of the lungs is often seen.

E. Special Investigations:

1. Noninvasive techniques–Echocardiography is valuable in detecting diastolic fluttering of the aortic leaflet of the mitral valve during diastole (Fig 13–15), but in general the finding is confirmatory rather than diagnostic. In severe, acute cases of aortic incompetence, the mitral valve closes early in diastole as the diastolic rush of blood from the aorta enters the ventricle. Although this echocardiographic sign has been used as an indication of severity, it is probably not always valid, because in patients with a slow heart rate and large stroke volume due to any cause, the mitral valve may drift into a closed position relatively early in diastole. The sign is useful, however, in following patients with endocarditis in whom aortic incompetence may be developing.

Doppler blood velocity measurements have been used to assess the severity of aortic incompetence. Ascending aortic blood flow is normally confined to systole, and diastolic flow is an indication of abnormal runoff via a low resistance pathway. In aortic incompetence, the flow takes place both forward, into the dilated peripheral bed; and backward, into the left ventricle. Semiquantitative estimates of the magnitude of backflow can be made using Doppler techniques to measure blood velocity in the ascending aorta. The results correlate well with other estimates of the regurgitant flow.

Radionuclear measurement of the left ventricular ejection fraction is proving valuable in following the course of patients with aortic incompetence. The technique can be applied during exercise, and the exercise does not have to be maximal to bring out the impairment in left ventricular function. The ease with which serial studies can be done makes this an attractive means of following patients.

2. Invasive techniques–

a. Cardiac catheterization–Cardiac catheterization and angiocardiography are mandatory in any patient in whom surgical treatment is contemplated. It is essential to demonstrate that the aortic valve is the site of the lesion and that it is the cause of the peripheral signs of rapid aortic runoff. In rare cases, especially in acute lesions, paravalvular lesions or rupture of an aortic sinus (sinus of Valsalva) aneurysm may not be suspected until the time of study.

Since left ventricular failure occurs so late in the course of aortic incompetence, most patients with chronic lesions show normal right heart pressures when they are first studied. In older patients with clinical

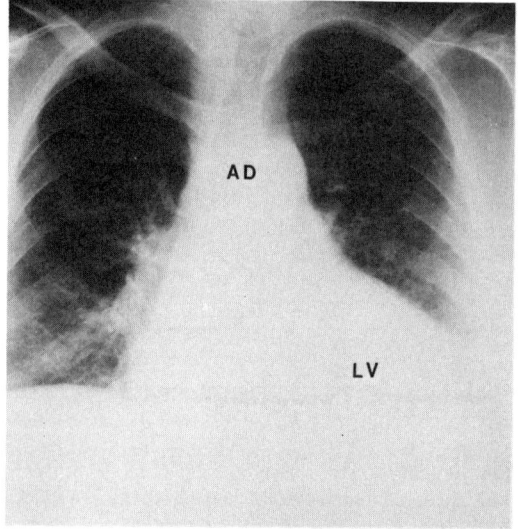

Figure 13–14. Chest x-ray of a patient with severe aortic incompetence and left heart failure. The large left ventricle (LV) and aortic dilatation (AD) are clearly seen.

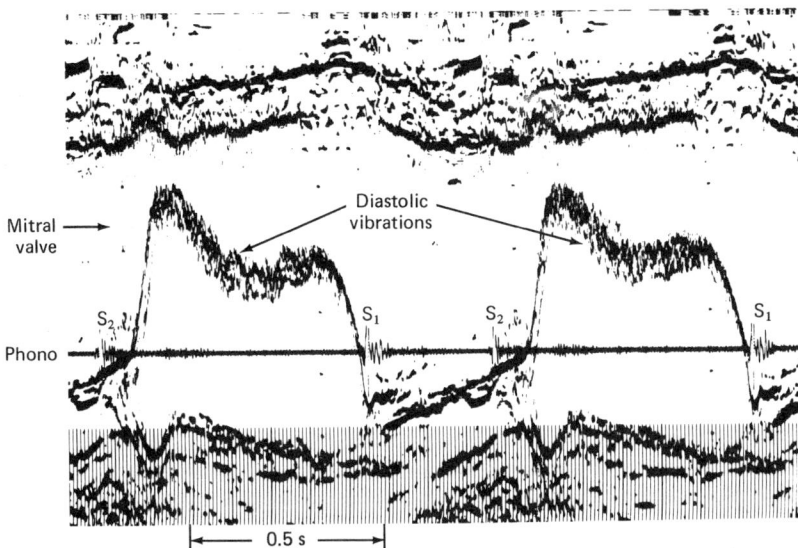

Figure 13–15. Echocardiogram showing diastolic vibration of mitral valve leaflet in a patient with aortic incompetence.

evidence of left heart failure, raised wedge and left ventricular diastolic pressures are found, although the cardiac output is usually normal or even slightly raised. The pressure levels are usually lower than expected, and pulmonary vascular resistance is rarely increased (< 10% of cases); the increase is at most moderate (3.5–7.5 mm Hg/L/min). In acute lesions, the hemodynamic findings are much more impressive, as shown in Table 13–2, and the wedge pressure and left ventricular diastolic pressure are often at a level at which pulmonary edema is likely to occur (> 35 mm Hg). The pressure in the left ventricle may rise rapidly during diastole to high levels, and a reversed gradient across the mitral valve may be seen in severe cases (Fig 13–16). The characteristic finding of a wide aortic pulse pressure is present in all patients except those

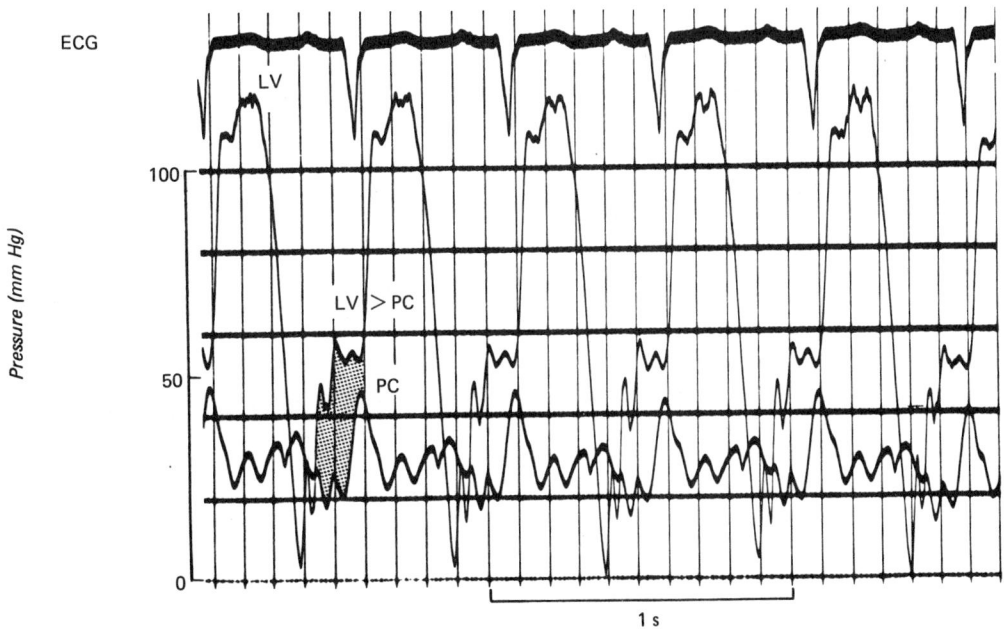

Figure 13–16. Left ventricular (LV) and wedge (PC, pulmonary capillary) pressure tracings in a patient with acute severe aortic incompetence. During the crosshatched period of diastole, the left ventricular pressure exceeds the pulmonary capillary pressure; this constitutes the reverse mitral gradient.

in severe left ventricular failure. The aortic pulse pressure is usually less than that in a peripheral artery, and that in turn is less than the indirectly recorded pulse pressure. As left ventricular failure develops, left ventricular diastolic pressure rises, establishing a lower limit to the aortic pressure of about 40 mm Hg. The level of left ventricular diastolic pressure varies with the compliance of the left ventricle. This is greater in large dilated ventricles in chronic lesions. The highest ventricular diastolic pressures are seen in patients with acute lesions and small hearts. In such patients, values of 60 mm Hg can occur, as seen in Fig 13–17.

b. Angiography–Supravalvular angiocardiography is important in assessing aortic incompetence. The speed with which the left ventricle opacifies is roughly proportionate to the severity of the leak. Angiocardiography establishes the valvular nature of the lesion and provides opacification of the left ventricle sufficient to assess left ventricular function without a catheter in the chamber. Angiography also makes it possible to detect or rule out associated mitral incompetence with greater certainty because ectopic beats (which often produce spurious mitral incompetence) occur less frequently, and positioning of the catheter to avoid interfering with the action of the mitral valve apparatus is not a problem. The end-diastolic volume of the left ventricle is increased in aortic incompetence, often with a normal end-diastolic pressure, indicating increased compliance of the ventricle. The total stroke volume is always greater than normal, and the ejection fraction is reasonably well maintained until left ventricular failure occurs. If the forward stroke volume is measured independently from the systemic cardiac output, it is possible to calculate the volume of blood flowing back across the aortic valve during diastole. This is usually expressed as a proportion of the total stroke volume. A value of 50% or more is found in patients with severe lesions and indicates that half the stroke volume returns to the ventricle during diastole. Coronary arteriography is frequently performed as a routine procedure in patients with aortic incompetence, but as in aortic stenosis, the state of the coronary arteries should not influence the decision to operate, which depends instead on the hemodynamic severity of the aortic valve lesion. As in aortic stenosis, it seems more logical to reserve coronary arteriography for those patients with a history of chest pain.

F. Hemodynamic Values: Hemodynamic data obtained at cardiac catheterization in a group of patients with aortic incompetence are shown in Table 13–2. Cardiac output is well maintained in both acute and chronic lesions. The pulse pressure is larger in chronic cases, although aortic diastolic pressure is reduced in both groups.

Differential Diagnosis

A. Pulmonary Incompetence: The murmur of aortic incompetence can be readily confused with the murmur of pulmonary incompetence in patients with

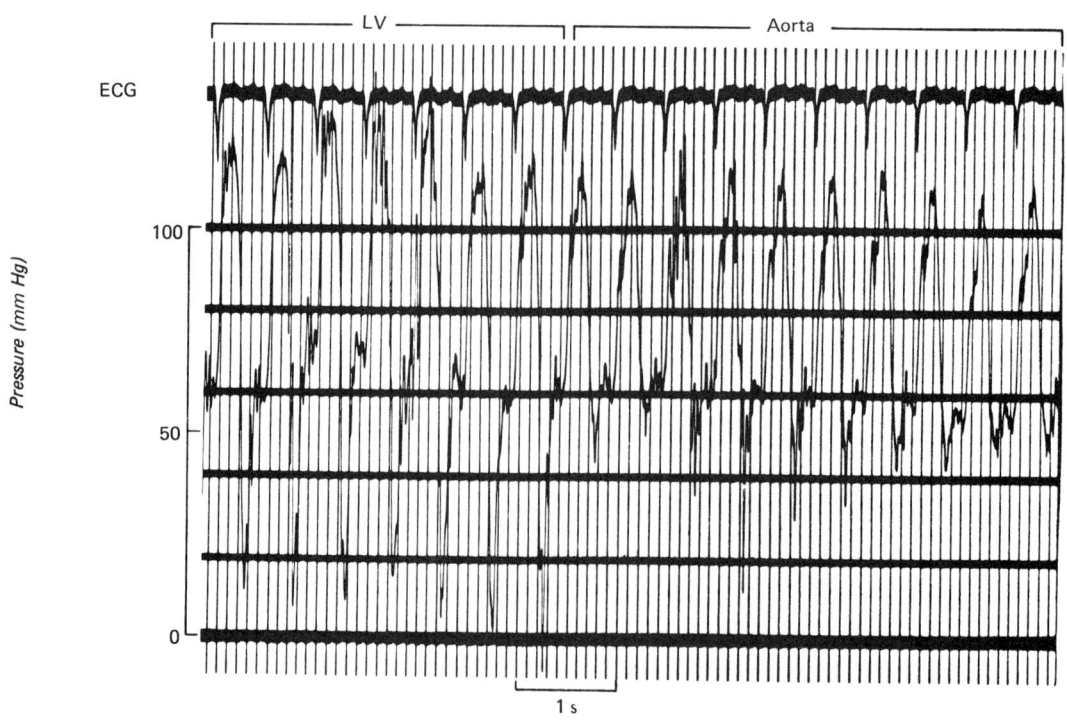

Figure 13–17. Withdrawal pressure tracing from left ventricle (LV) to aorta in a patient with acute severe aortic incompetence showing equalization of end-diastolic pressure at 60 mm Hg.

Table 13-2. Cardiac catheterization data in patients with hemodynamically significant predominant aortic incompetence.

	Mean Wedge Pressure (mm Hg)	Left Ventricular Systolic Pressure (mm Hg)	Aortic Systolic Pressure (mm Hg)	Aortic Diastolic Pressure (mm Hg)	Cardiac Output (L/min)
Pure aortic incompetence					
Chronic	18 ± 9	158 ± 31	157 ± 31	56 ± 12	5.1 ± 1.4
Acute	32 ± 10	134 ± 24	135 ± 24	54 ± 12	5.1 ± 1.7

severe pulmonary hypertension. Pulmonary incompetence rarely occurs in patients who do not have moderate or severe pulmonary hypertension. In patients with pulmonary hypertension, the hypertrophied right ventricle relaxes at about the same time as the left ventricle, causing the characteristic immediate, high-pitched diastolic murmur that is indistinguishable from that of aortic incompetence.

In patients with low pulmonary arterial pressure, the murmur of pulmonary incompetence is different and is therefore not likely to be confused with an aortic murmur. When pulmonary arterial pressure is low, the right ventricle relaxes more slowly and the murmur starts later and is not as high-pitched.

B. Sinus of Valsalva Aneurysm: Aneurysm of the sinus of Valsalva is a congenital abnormality that generally does not cause a problem until it ruptures, into either the right atrium or the right ventricle. Rupture produces a clinical picture that is readily confused with the development of acute aortic incompetence. Rupture may be spontaneous and occur acutely or subacutely; it also occurs in the course of infective endocarditis. The presenting symptom is usually dyspnea, with paroxysmal nocturnal dyspnea, and the most important physical sign is the development of a murmur that may be almost continuous and is usually both systolic and diastolic. There are signs of rapid runoff, with a collapsing pulse, and a wide pulse pressure resembling that seen in aortic incompetence.

C. Rapid Aortic Runoff in Other Conditions: Other disorders can cause the characteristic physical signs of rapid runoff of blood from the aorta into some low-pressure area or into other areas in the circulation. These disorders include patent ductus arteriosus, aortopulmonary window, systemic arteriovenous fistula, truncus arteriosus, and associated ventricular septal defect. Anemia without organic valvular disease occasionally causes aortic incompetence.

Course & Complications

A. Left Ventricular Failure: Left ventricular failure occurs late in the course of uncomplicated chronic aortic incompetence and should be thought of as part of the disease rather than a complication. The part played by myocardial fibrosis in causing left heart failure is difficult to determine. Myocardial hypertrophy results in an increase in connective tissue elements of the heart as well as an increase in the size of the individual muscle cells. The progress of myocardial fibrosis is probably influenced by inflammatory changes due to current or previous rheumatic myocarditis, which lead to left ventricular failure in younger patients. The diagnosis of active rheumatic myocardial disease is usually impossible except by retrospective analysis of the history.

Severe coronary arterial disease is not usually present in patients with hemodynamically significant aortic incompetence who present in a hospital, presumably because the 2 lesions together are not compatible with life and are mutually exclusive. In syphilitic aortic incompetence, coronary ostial stenosis is an important associated finding that may cause transient edema of the aortic intima, resulting in acute ostial obstruction and acute myocardial ischemia.

Left ventricular failure is difficult to predict in aortic incompetence, and the premonitory symptoms of increasing dyspnea with decreasing effort over several months or years are not always seen. The onset of left ventricular failure is more abrupt in aortic incompetence than in any other form of chronic left ventricular disease, probably because the change from marked peripheral vasodilatation to severe vasoconstriction associated with a falling cardiac output is so abrupt.

B. Infective Endocarditis: Infective endocarditis is the most important complication of aortic incompetence. Therapeutic advances, increased use of intravenous medication by physicians and patients, and the use of immunosuppressive drugs have since increased both the variety of organisms and the range of pathogenicity. Infective endocarditis is a greater hazard at the aortic valve than at any other site and is most dangerous when aortic incompetence is mild. Patients with mild lesions and those with no aortic valve disease at all are likely to suffer the most severe hemodynamic insults. Patients who have already developed significant aortic incompetence and whose cardiovascular systems have already adapted to the lesion are not exposed to comparable hemodynamic risks. The reason that endocarditis involving the aortic valve carries such a poor prognosis is that the valve is of crucial hemodynamic importance and is situated close to the main coronary vessels and conduction system. Ulcerative lesions of the cusps and the aortic root can cause acute, subacute, or chronic exacerbation of aortic incompetence, with or without perforation into adjacent cardiac chambers. (See Chapter 16 for details of treatment of infective endocarditis.)

C. Conduction Defects: Atrioventricular conduction defects are an occasional complication, especially in patients with ankylosing spondylitis or Reiter's syndrome. In patients with marked left ventricular hypertrophy and dilatation, left bundle branch block may occur, and all varieties of atrioventricular conduction delay are seen.

Treatment

Aortic valve replacement is the only effective treatment for aortic incompetence. However, this lesion is the one with the most problematic indications for surgery. Both the timing of surgery and the choice of prosthetic valve are still controversial. Since aortic valve replacement has become widely available, surgical treatment of chronic aortic incompetence has been instituted at progressively earlier stages of the disease. The chief difficulty is that if surgery is delayed until heart failure is obvious, the results of operation are poor because the large, hypertrophied, dilated, and often fibrotic heart does not recover normal function because irreversible myocardial fibrosis has irrevocably compromised left ventricular function.

The dilemma is that heart failure develops late in the course of the disease, and its onset cannot be predicted with sufficient accuracy to enable the surgeon to make a rational decision about surgical treatment. If the long-term durability of prosthetic valves were good and the surgical mortality rate were negligible, earlier valve replacement could be recommended. However, since the long-term (20-year) durability of prosthetic valves is not yet known and because as yet neither the mortality and morbidity rates of aortic valve replacement nor the long-term lack of complications associated with artificial valves or homografts is sufficiently low, prophylactic valve replacement is not warranted.

If surgery is performed, an additional difficulty lies in anchoring the valve securely. In aortic stenosis there is almost always a firm fibrous or calcific ring of tissue around the valve that holds surgical sutures securely, but in aortic incompetence, this ring is not present. Furthermore, there is often associated disease of the aortic wall that makes sutures more likely to tear out and necessitate a second open heart operation. Severe morbidity or even death may then result.

A 20-year-old asymptomatic patient with uncomplicated hemodynamically significant aortic incompetence can probably expect an average of about 20 years of life free from symptoms. Some more precise indications for surgery, such as massive cardiac enlargement, an arbitrary age (eg, 40 years), or the hemodynamic response to some stress such as salt loading or angiotensin infusion, might be more logical than the present situation in which some "excuse" is generally required before surgery is recommended in an asymptomatic patient. When significant dyspnea and left heart failure develop, surgery is mandatory. Medical treatment of left ventricular failure should only be a prelude to operation.

Exercise testing is less helpful than might be expected, because the patient with aortic incompetence generally tolerates exercise well. Signs of increasing left ventricular hypertrophy on the ECG and chest x-ray are not too helpful, since both have been documented 20–30 years before left ventricular failure occurred. Recent studies have suggested that radionuclide angiography, with measurement of the left ventricular ejection fraction during exercise, may be useful in detecting early evidence of left ventricular failure in patients with aortic incompetence. In addition, the degree of left ventricular emptying—as indicated by the end-systolic volume—has been shown to correlate with the level of left ventricular function.

Our recommendation is that patients with isolated hemodynamically significant aortic incompetence be followed at yearly intervals and observed for signs of deteriorating left ventricular function. If a patient shows an increasing heart size and progression of electrocardiographic changes indicative of left ventricular hypertrophy between ages 35 and 40, valve replacement is advisable, and this operation should be given serious consideration in any patient reaching age 40. The development of left ventricular failure in a patient under age 30 who has chronic aortic incompetence suggests the presence of associated myocardial damage—usually rheumatic carditis or unrecognized mitral valve disease. Although the results of surgery in such patients are not good, operation is still indicated in order to relieve the load on the left ventricle.

In patients with acute or acutely exacerbated lesions, surgery is almost always needed, and acute and progressive hemodynamic deterioration may force operation. Patients with infective endocarditis, especially those with acute fulminant lesions, should be treated at a center where emergency cardiac surgery is available, because the need for operation may arise at any time in the course of the disease. When endocarditis is present, surgery should be delayed if possible until the infection involving the valve has been controlled and sufficient healing has occurred to ensure that there is adequate tissue to hold the sutures securing the valve. Achieving such a result in actual practice is difficult. The course of infective endocarditis is so unpredictable and varies so widely with the type of causative organism, the prior state of the valve, and the general health of the patient that it is impossible to set up any rational guidelines for the management of patients with this lesion. Medical treatment alone is unlikely to stabilize the hemodynamic status of patients with aortic incompetence occurring de novo. In these patients, aortic valve replacement is almost inevitable, and the principal question is the timing of surgery.

Serious problems arise in patients who are addicted to heroin and in whom saprophytic organisms and fungi are often present. The reinfection rate is extremely high, and the prognosis is dismal. In our opinion, the most logical course to follow in the management of acute aortic incompetence with infective endocarditis is to wait and follow the patient as closely as possible and to use digitalis and diuretic therapy where indicated but withhold vasodilator therapy with nitroprusside infusion except for emergency use, ie, just to maintain the patient for the few hours needed to prepare for open heart surgery. There is little doubt that satisfactory results can be obtained in no more than 50% of patients. The patient must be closely followed for over one year because hemodynamic deterioration following infective endocarditis may occur late in the disease, when healing causes retraction and fibrosis of the damaged valvular tissue. Another complicating feature is toxic myocarditis accompanying endocarditis, but there is some disagreement about the existence and significance of this complication.

As it does in aortic stenosis, the choice of artificial valve rests with the surgeon. Homograft aortic valves have the advantage of not requiring long-term anticoagulation, but this factor must be balanced against their tendency to stiffen, calcify, and leak with time. The mortality rate of surgery depends on the clinical status of the patient and the experience of the surgeon and averages 2–5% in chronic cases.

The mortality rate is 2–3 times higher in second operations, mainly because the patient's clinical condition is almost inevitably worse. In patients with infective endocarditis, it is clearly advantageous to wait until the infection has been controlled, if possible. It has been shown, however, that it is possible to operate in the presence of infection without significantly compromising the results. Thus, the patient's hemodynamic state clearly takes precedence over management of the infection.

Prognosis

Aortic incompetence has a better prognosis than aortic stenosis, since the load on the ventricle is better tolerated, primarily because it is a "flow" load. In acute lesions, aortic incompetence carries a worse prognosis than mitral incompetence because there is an increased possibility of coronary arterial involvement; because a severe systemic infection is often present when the lesion develops; and because fistula formation and conduction defects are more likely to occur.

The prognosis of left ventricular failure in aortic incompetence is poor because it occurs at such a late stage in the disease. In milder lesions, the threat of endocarditis is the most important and least predictable factor in prognosis.

Long-Term Results in Operated Cases

The late results of valve replacement in patients with aortic incompetence are the least satisfactory of all valve replacement surgery. Most patients who come to surgery with chronic lesions at the stage of early left ventricular failure have large, fibrotic left ventricles which, though their function improves, never return to normal size or recover a normal ejection fraction. Patients with congenital lesions, in whom myocardial damage is less of a problem, fare better than patients with rheumatic lesions.

Patients with acute lesions almost all have infective endocarditis; in some of these patients, the valve may be dislodged because of ulcerative lesions in the area in which it is anchored. If stitches tear out from an area where inflammatory changes have weakened the tissues, the valve ring may become unseated and move with each heartbeat. This tends to tear out more sutures and is an urgent indication for reoperation.

MULTIPLE VALVE INVOLVEMENT

Combined Mitral & Aortic Valve Disease

Involvement of both aortic and mitral valves is almost pathognomonic of rheumatic heart disease, and patients with lesions of both valves have a higher incidence of a history of rheumatic infection in childhood (70%) than any other group of patients with valve disease. When both aortic and mitral valves are involved, the variability of the clinical picture greatly increases. The importance of the lesion at each valve can vary; the nature of each lesion (stenosis, incompetence, or mixture of the two) is diverse; and rheumatic myocardial involvement tends to play a more important part in the clinical course because the rheumatic infection is more severe and more often recurrent in these cases. It can be seen from the classification of mitral and aortic disease in this text that 20 or more subclassifications of different mixed valvular diseases can be described. It is beyond the scope of this text to do more than point out some of the more obvious relationships between aortic and mitral disease and to make a few general comments about the clinical picture. Combined mitral and aortic valve disease constitutes about 10% of cases of valvular disease. Such patients have hemodynamically significant disease of each valve. Predominant aortic and predominant mitral disease are about equal in frequency in combined lesions. Mitral stenosis decreases the apparent severity of aortic disease, particularly in aortic incompetence, and the combination of mitral stenosis and aortic incompetence is surprisingly well tolerated. After mitral stenosis has been relieved by valvotomy, aortic incompetence often appears to be more severe, and the presence on the ECG of left ventricular hypertrophy owing to aortic incompetence in a patient with predominant mitral stenosis is sufficient warning to warrant serious consideration of aortic valve replacement at the time of mitral valve surgery.

Mitral stenosis and aortic stenosis tend to mask one another, so that one or the other appears to be the dominant lesion clinically. The significance of the less dominant lesion is often underestimated.

When aortic valve disease is the major lesion, significant mitral incompetence is more serious than mitral stenosis. In either aortic stenosis or aortic incompetence, mitral incompetence is aggravated, and extreme cardiac enlargement and early heart failure are common.

Among the characteristic clinical pictures of combined valvular disease that should be mentioned is the combination of aortic stenosis with insignificant or mild mitral incompetence. This lesion gives rise to a characteristic high-pitched "seagull cry" murmur. In some cases, extension of aortic calcification into the aortic cusp of the mitral valve can be demonstrated, and this is one of the few combined aortic and mitral valve lesions that does not always have a rheumatic origin.

Clinical Course of Combined Lesions

Patients with combined mitral and aortic valve lesions tend to be symptomatic at an earlier age than patients with single valve lesions. The heart is usually larger, and atrial fibrillation tends to develop at an earlier age. The disease of each valve is less advanced in combined lesions because the valvular lesions are additive and because myocardial disease is so often present. Physical signs are more difficult to interpret in mixed lesions, and it is not always easy to distinguish the delayed diastolic or presystolic murmur of severe aortic incompetence (Austin Flint murmur) from the murmur of associated mitral stenosis. Similarly, an immediate basal diastolic murmur of pulmonary incompetence (Graham Steell murmur) in mitral stenosis with a raised pulmonary vascular resistance can be confused with the murmur of associated aortic incompetence. In patients with predominant aortic valve disease, the distinction between functional and organic mitral incompetence is often difficult. In the presence of left heart failure, a systolic murmur of mitral incompetence is often found, but it may be difficult to distinguish from the aortic systolic murmur; in mixed mitral stenosis and incompetence, the organic nature of the systolic murmur can be more readily recognized. In combined aortic and mitral valve disease, either valve lesion may become acutely worse in the course of infective endocarditis. The presence of a chronic lesion of one valve exaggerates the effects of an acute lesion of the other valve. Infective endocarditis and systemic embolism are as common in combined aortic and mitral valve disease as they are in aortic or mitral incompetence alone.

Double Valve Replacement

Surgical replacement of both valves, or aortic valve replacement with mitral valvotomy, generally leads to less satisfactory results than single valve replacement. This is probably because more extensive myocardial disease is present in patients with combined lesions. Simultaneous valve replacement is preferable to serial valve replacement, since the second cardiotomy is always more difficult than the first. The surgeon should have as much information as possible on which to base the decision whether to replace one valve or 2, and full preoperative hemodynamic studies are mandatory. Long-term survival after double valve replacement is not significantly shorter than after single valve replacement. This may be because valve lesions are additive, and double valve replacement is therefore usually undertaken at an earlier stage of development of each individual valve lesion.

The management of patients with combined aortic and mitral valve lesions always presents problems because the cases are naturally more complex and different, and sufficient experience of treatment regimens is generally lacking. Fortunately, the number of patients with combined mitral and aortic disease is decreasing in the Western world.

Combined Mitral & Tricuspid Valve Disease

Functional tricuspid incompetence has already been mentioned as a common complication of mitral stenosis with raised pulmonary vascular resistance (Chapter 12). In about 2% of patients with mitral valve disease, organic tricuspid valve disease is present and causes right heart failure. The mitral valve lesion is almost always mixed mitral stenosis and incompetence, and pulmonary vascular resistance is not greatly raised (average 2 mm Hg/L/min). Markedly raised systemic venous pressure (average 24 mm Hg) is the most striking clinical feature, and cardiac enlargement is usually massive, but not as great as in giant left atrium. Low cardiac output and atrial fibrillation are almost inevitable, and the lesions tend to run a chronic course in which valve replacement provides less benefit than in disease of the mitral valve alone. Isolated tricuspid valve disease without mitral valve involvement can theoretically occur, but for practical purposes it is rare enough to be of negligible importance.

Triple-Valve Disease

The remarks that have been made about double-valve disease are even more applicable to triple-valve disease, in which aortic, mitral, and tricuspid valves are involved. Since the lesions are additive and rheumatic myocarditis is almost inevitably present, the results of surgery are never as satisfactory as in disease affecting a single valve. All artificial valves currently available are functionally inferior to a normal valve. The presence of 3 such valves in series in the heart is likely to cause a significant load on the myocardium and tends to make the prognosis worse and decrease the degree of functional improvement that the patient experiences after surgery.

CARCINOID VALVULAR HEART DISEASE

Carcinoid tumors that arise from the chromaffin tissue in the gastrointestinal tract—usually in the ileum—produce vasoactive substances such as serotonin, bradykinin, and tryptophan. These vasoactive substances cause endothelial damage to the right side of the heart, resulting in fibrosis and thickening of the heart valves. Tricuspid incompetence and, less frequently, pulmonary stenosis are the end results of the damage, which also affects the endocardium of the right atrium and ventricle. The primary tumors can be small, and hepatic metastases are usually present in patients with cardiac involvement.

Clinical Findings

A. Symptoms: Patients with carcinoid syndrome complain of episodes of facial and upper trunk flushing in response to alcohol ingestion, eating, and emotional reactions. The release of vasoactive substances into the bloodstream is thought to be responsible. Abdominal pain, diarrhea, and renal and hepatic failure are also seen. Dyspnea is uncommon.

B. Signs: Hepatic enlargement and a peculiar violaceous color of the face and neck are often seen, and abdominal distention and ascites occur. The cardiac signs are not present in all cases. A systolic murmur of tricuspid incompetence is the commonest finding. It is louder on inspiration and often associated with *a* and *v* waves in the jugular venous pulse. A systolic ejection murmur due to pulmonary stenosis is less common, and diastolic murmurs are a late manifestation. Frank right heart failure with edema appears late in the disease and may be difficult to assess in the presence of severe hepatic involvement.

C. Electrocardiographic Findings: P wave abnormalities are usually all that are seen, and right ventricular hypertrophy is rare.

D. X-Ray Findings: Dilatation of the right heart occurs late in the disease.

E. Special Investigations: The diagnosis of carcinoid tumor is established by finding 5-hydroxyindoleacetic acid in the urine. It is a metabolic product of serotonin. A value of more than 25 ng/24 h is considered diagnostic and usually implies hepatic metastases. An amount exceeding 200 ng/24 h is usually found in patients with cardiac involvement. A variety of foods (bananas, apples) or drugs (phenothiazines) may cause false-positive reactions. Liver scans may reveal defects from metastases, and biopsy of the liver or the primary tumor shows the characteristic histologic findings.

Echocardiography may show dilatation of the right heart and abnormal motion of the ventricular septum. Cardiac catheterization is seldom indicated, because the cardiac involvement is usually not severe.

Differential Diagnosis

Isolated tricuspid incompetence is rare in rheumatic heart disease. Infective endocarditis involving the tricuspid valve and tumor involving the right atrium are the most important differential diagnostic problems.

Course & Complications

The tumor grows slowly in most cases, although it metastasizes early. The cardiac manifestations rarely cause serious problems but can progress to the stage at which valve replacement must be considered. Atrial fibrillation may occur in severe cases. In some patients the vasoactive substances are not inactivated in the lungs, and left-sided lesions have been reported.

Treatment

Resection of the primary tumor is the most helpful procedure. Chemotherapy with cytotoxic drugs (eg, cyclophosphamide) is used to treat hepatic metastases. Various serotonin antagonists (eg, methysergide) have been used to treat the flushing attacks, with generally disappointing results. Phenothiazines have been useful in some cases. Digitalis and diuretics are used for the treatment of right heart failure, and tricuspid or pulmonary valve replacement is seldom needed.

Prognosis

The disease is more slowly progressive than might be expected, and survival for 5–10 years after the initial symptoms develop is not uncommon. The cardiac involvement seldom influences the prognosis, which depends on the hepatic metastases.

IATROGENICALLY MODIFIED VALVULAR HEART DISEASE

1. MITRAL VALVOTOMY

Mitral commissurotomy is an important iatrogenic factor modifying the course of valvular heart disease. Even relatively ineffective closed mitral valvulotomy was—and still is—capable of influencing the clinical course of mitral stenosis. The operation is palliative rather than curative, and in 2–15 years after valvotomy the patient is likely to experience a recurrence of dyspnea. In some cases (about 20%), a second valvotomy is performed, but in most cases mitral valve replacement is necessary at the second operation. The clinical features of these patients with iatrogenically modified mitral stenosis warrant description.

Clinical Findings

A. Symptoms: In patients who have had a previous mitral valvotomy, symptoms are difficult to assess. Dyspnea is the commonest symptom, and, as in all patients with mitral valve disease, the relation between the onset of atrial fibrillation and the onset of dyspnea is of prime importance. A clinical picture resembling that of mixed mitral valve disease is common. Patients who have gained relief through mitral valvotomy are likely to experience a significant increase in dyspnea when atrial fibrillation occurs at about age 40. There is often a relationship between the length of the asymptomatic interval following valvotomy and the age of the patient. A woman who has had a mitral valvotomy in her 20s is likely to have 15 symptom-free years before atrial fibrillation develops, whereas a 35-year-old woman is likely to develop atrial fibrillation within about 5 years of operation.

B. Signs: The physical signs in iatrogenically modified cases usually reflect the preoperative findings. A loud opening snap and loud first heart sound are often present, and the timing of the opening snap reflects the preoperative and not the postoperative status of the patient. In such cases, the length of the diastolic murmur measured at the bedside becomes the best indicator of the severity of stenosis. A systolic murmur may appear after surgery, but, as is the case in patients who have not undergone operation, its significance is open to question, and other clinical evidence of mitral incompetence must always be sought.

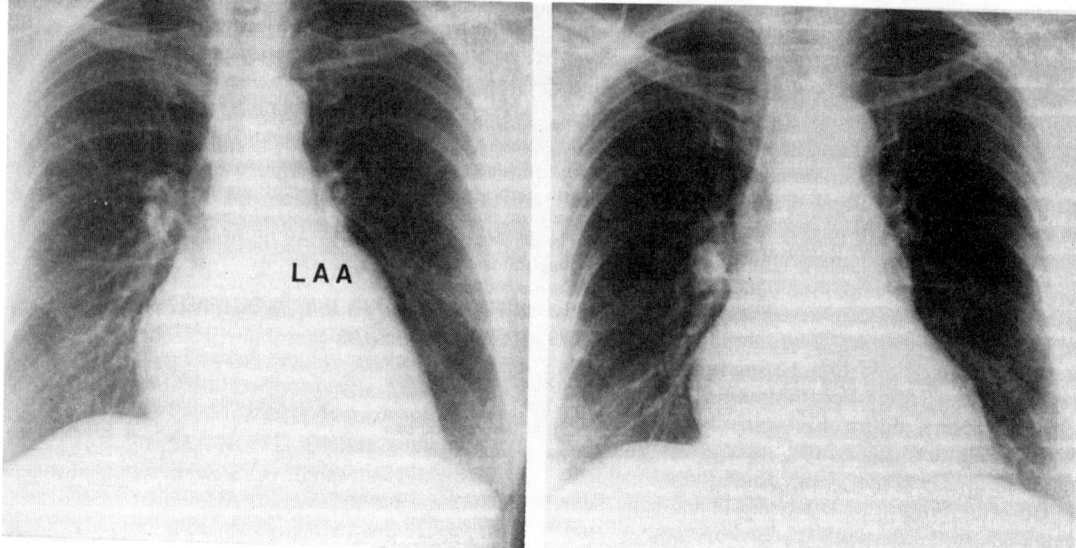

Figure 13–18. Preoperative and postoperative chest x-rays of a patient with mitral stenosis. The left atrial appendage (LAA) has been resected.

C. Electrocardiographic Findings: In a few cases, regression of the changes of right ventricular hypertrophy is seen, but in most patients the ECG shows little change from the preoperative tracing. Sooner or later, atrial fibrillation will almost certainly develop.

D. X-Ray Findings: The absence of the left atrial appendage as a bulge on the left heart border is a characteristic finding in patients who have undergone operation (Fig 13–18). If the pulmonary artery was enlarged before operation, it seldom returns to normal size, and the same is true of the left atrium. Changes in the degree of pulmonary congestion are perhaps the best indicators of the success of surgical treatment.

E. Special Investigations: Exercise testing and echocardiography are helpful noninvasive techniques used in screening patients to decide whether they should undergo catheterization again. However, echocardiographic findings tend to be influenced by the preoperative status of the valve. Cardiac catheterization, with measurement of the wedge pressure, left ventricular pressure, and cardiac output, constitutes the only acceptable objective evidence of the patient's postoperative status. It is thus highly advantageous to have a preoperative study available for comparison. The decision to perform a second operation is important, since the chances are high (80%) that valve replacement will be needed at that time.

Treatment

Almost all patients who have had mitral valvotomy ultimately require valve replacement. Temporizing with a second valvotomy is generally attempted when the valve is flexible and shows little or no calcification.

The principal problem posed by patients who have had a previous valvotomy is for the physician to decide when the patient's condition has deteriorated sufficiently to require further surgery. The subjective improvement after mitral valve surgery is so much more impressive than the objective evidence of improvement that the decision to operate again is often somewhat arbitrary.

A later form of iatrogenically modified mitral valve disease occurs after mitral valve replacement. Pulmonary vascular disease is sometimes irreversible, and when its development is arrested, cardiac function often continues to deteriorate as degenerative age-related changes occur. Patients with raised pulmonary vascular resistance often develop chronic severe right heart failure that responds poorly to treatment. In such cases, left ventricular failure may also be present, as shown by a rise in end-diastolic left ventricular pressure. Patients with such lesions are usually subjected to investigation in the hope of finding some surgically treatable lesion, but in practice they are usually exhibiting the long-term effects of rheumatic carditis.

2. PATIENTS WITH ARTIFICIAL VALVES

Patients who have had mitral or aortic valve replacement are becoming more common in everyday medical practice. By far the largest number of such patients have Starr-Edwards ball and cage prostheses. Other forms of plastic and metal valves, such as the Björk-Shiley disk valve, and homograft or heterograft (Hancock) tissue valves are also used.

The clinical picture in patients who have had valve

replacement varies greatly and depends on the type of valve used, the nature of the original lesion, the stage at which operation was performed, and the success of the operation. Few patients are free of symptoms; the problems encountered are most commonly related to thrombosis, embolism, valve dehiscence, leakage or obstruction of the valve, infective endocarditis, hemolysis, and hemorrhage from excessive anticoagulant therapy.

Clinical Findings

A. Symptoms: Many patients with artificial valves have residual shortness of breath on exertion. Most have at least a small pressure gradient across the valve at rest that becomes larger when the cardiac output and heart rate increase during exercise. The patient may also complain of the loud noise made by the artificial valve as it opens and closes with each heartbeat, but most patients become accustomed to the sensation within a few weeks after operation.

B. Signs: The physical signs arising from an artificial valve depend on the nature and type of valve used. Tissue valves do not give rise to the loud opening and closing clicks heard with metal and plastic prostheses. However, they do tend to leak with the passage of time as the tissue stiffens and calcifies. Thus, mitral systolic and aortic diastolic murmurs are not uncommon. The opening and closing clicks of plastic and metal valves are characteristic for each individual brand of valve. In general, there is a loud opening click at the start of systole and a loud closing click at the end of systole. The clicks are usually louder than the normal heart sounds and interfere with auscultation of natural valves. Systolic and diastolic murmurs are difficult to interpret in patients with artificial valves, and more importance should be given to changes in the auscultatory findings than to the findings themselves.

C. Electrocardiographic Findings: There are no characteristic electrocardiographic changes in patients with artificial heart valves. Postoperative electrocardiographic changes reflect surgical results.

D. X-Ray Findings: Artificial heart valves composed of metal are clearly seen on chest x-rays, and each has a characteristic shape. Even the plastic ball can usually be seen moving up and down with the heartbeat on cinefluoroscopy. The position of the artificial valve varies considerably from case to case, and a change in the position of the valve or in its movement during the cardiac cycle is important evidence of valvular dysfunction. Tissue valves may calcify with time and become visible on the chest x-ray.

E. Special Investigations:

1. Noninvasive techniques–Because plastic and metal valves reflect ultrasound well, they are readily detected by echocardiography. However, it is difficult to determine valve function by this means of study.

2. Invasive techniques–Cardiac catheterization and angiography are usually needed to decide whether prosthetic valve malfunction is severe enough to warrant reoperation. Most physicians carefully avoid passing a catheter through a prosthetic valve for fear of causing damage. When catheters have been inadvertently passed through artificial valves, little ill effect has been noticed. The most important information sought in studies of patients with artificial valves is the pressure difference across the valve and the flow through it. Angiography is commonly used to test for valvular incompetence.

Particular problems arise in the investigation of patients with combined mitral and aortic valve replacement. Retrograde catheterization of the left ventricle with passage of a catheter across the artificial aortic valve is not recommended. In addition to the possibility of damage to the valve, the fact that leakage of the valve may disturb the hemodynamic pattern contraindicates this approach. The only alternative is direct left ventricular puncture (see p 410). If angiography is essential, a 16-gauge multihole needle may be used, but the risk of complications is greater than when a 20-gauge needle is used.

Differential Diagnosis

The principal problem in differential diagnosis is distinguishing artificial valve malfunction from disease of another valve.

Long-Term Results & Complications

The long-term results of valve replacement depend to a considerable extent on the type of valve used—prosthetic versus homograft or xenograft. Data for Starr-Edwards ball and cage valves are now available for 20 years, while the commonest other prosthetic valve—the Björk-Shiley disk valve—has been in use for about 15 years. The several other types of prosthetic valves that have been introduced have either been abandoned or not used widely enough to generate adequate follow-up data. Data for tissue valves are also available for almost 20 years, but only in small numbers of patients with aortic homografts. The results with porcine xenografts (Hancock valves) now cover about 10 years and those for the Ionescu-Shiley valve made of glutaraldehyde-treated pericardial tissue a slightly shorter time.

A. Prosthetic Valves: The principal problem with prosthetic valves, as typified by the Starr-Edwards valve, has always been thromboembolism. Anticoagulation with coumarin anticoagulants is essential, and in spite of this therapy the incidence of thromboembolism is about 5% per patient year and about half of the emboli are serious—ie, cause a stroke, hematuria, or a painful cold limb. The incidence of embolism has tended to remain constant over the years of follow-up, and sudden cessation of anticoagulation is particularly likely to result in a "rebound" hypercoagulable state. The durability of the Starr-Edwards valve is well established now that problems related to ball variance have been dealt with. The Bjork-Shiley valve provides a slightly larger area for flow and appears to have approximately similar thrombogenic and durability characteristics.

Valve failure does occur with prosthetic valves,

which may stick either in the open or the closed position, especially when thrombus or pannus grows into the valve. This form of valve failure is more likely in the mitral than in the aortic position and can occur abruptly without warning. Both survival and maintenance of adequate valve function are more likely in the aortic than in the mitral position, probably because there is less stasis in the neighborhood of the aortic valve.

B. Tissue Valves: The principal advantage of a tissue valve is that anticoagulation is not required, except in patients in atrial fibrillation after mitral valve replacement and for the first few months after insertion. Thromboembolism still occurs, but less commonly than with prosthetic valves. Tissue valves are preferable, therefore, in young people or in those in whom anticoagulation is undesirable or difficult. The tendency for tissue valves to stiffen, calcify, leak, and cause obstruction to flow detracts from their overall durability. This tendency was most marked in formaldehyde-treated freeze-dried aortic homografts. While the results with glutaraldehyde-treated porcine xenograft (Hancock) valves were encouraging after 4 years of follow-up, longer-term studies have shown that late failure between 5 and 10 years is an important problem. One advantage of tissue valves is that their failure occurs relatively slowly, and an increase in symptoms, with changes in the physical signs and often calcification of the valve, makes it possible to recognize the problem and replace the valve.

C. Infective Endocarditis: Infective endocarditis involving an artificial valve is a rare but dangerous complication, occurring at a rate of about 1% per patient year with all types of valve (see Chapter 16). The later the infection occurs after surgery, the better the chance of cure with antibiotic therapy. Endocarditis involving tissue valves may be curable without replacing the valve, but if the infection occurs on a prosthetic valve, a second operation is almost inevitable. The mortality rate of endocarditis on an artificial valve approaches 50%, and since the complication is so serious, antibiotic coverage for major dental work and other minor surgical procedures is highly important.

D. Hemolysis: Hemolysis due to trauma to red cells is virtually confined to patients with prosthetic valves. It is seldom a serious problem but is more likely to occur after multiple valve replacement. Perivalvular leak is likely to aggravate hemolysis, which should be suspected in any patient with anemia. A raised serum LDH level is the most satisfactory indicator to follow.

E. Hemorrhage From Anticoagulant Therapy: Long-term anticoagulation with coumarin anticoagulant is not without its complications, especially in older patients. Hemorrhage, particularly from the gut, requires thorough investigation, looking for peptic ulceration, carcinoma of the colon, and other noncardiac lesions. Similarly, hematuria and hemoptysis and in fact hemorrhage from any site require full investigation before the conclusion that the anticoagulant therapy is responsible can be justified. It is inadvisable to stop anticoagulant therapy suddenly or completely, but reduction in the dose of anticoagulant, with close monitoring of the prothrombin level, is essential. Anticoagulant therapy may have to be stopped 3 or 4 days before noncardiac surgery and should be started again immediately after operation.

F. Thromboembolism: Thrombosis around the artificial valve, with consequent stenosis and systemic embolism, is the commonest complication of artificial valves. Anticoagulant therapy is needed in all types of valves except tissue valves, and hemorrhage due to excessive anticoagulation is also encountered. When thrombus forms around a prosthetic valve, it may disturb valve function and interfere with both the opening and the closing of the valve. Thus, both stenosis and incompetence can result from thrombus formation around an artificial valve. In some cases, especially early after operation, valve displacement due to tearing out of the sutures anchoring the valve leads to paravalvular leak. In other cases the valve mechanism itself may fail and cause leakage. Sudden death is still an important complication of valve replacement. The mechanism is not always clear, but escape of a worn ball from the cage mechanism has been reported. In other cases, the valve mechanism sticks shut.

Treatment

A second valve replacement is the only effective therapy for artificial valve malfunction. Both the patient and the physician are naturally reluctant to take this major step, and clear evidence of malfunction is required before a second artificial valve is inserted. In some cases, one of the natural valves proves to be the cause of the problem and needs replacement.

Prognosis

The long-term prognosis of patients with artificial valves is not yet established.

REFERENCES

General

Cosh JA, Lever JV: The aortic valve. *Cardiovasc Rev Rep* 1985;**6**:743.

Diebold B et al: Quantitative assessment of tricuspid regurgitation using pulsed Doppler echocardiography. *Br Heart J* 1983;**50**:443.

Jamieson WRE et al: Cardiac valve replacement in the elderly: A review of 320 consecutive cases. *Circulation* 1981;**64**(Suppl 2):177.

Kloster FE, Morris CD: Key references: Natural history of valvular heart disease. *Circulation* 1982;**65**:1283.

Krayenbuehl HP et al: Pre- and postoperative left ventricular contractile function in patients with aortic valve disease. *Br Heart J* 1979;**41**:204.

Krivokapich J, Child JS, Skorton DJ: Flail aortic valve leaflets: M-mode and two-dimensional echocardiographic manifestations. *Am Heart J* 1980;**99**:425.

Morrison GW et al: Incidence of coronary artery disease in patients with valvular heart disease. *Br Heart J* 1980;**44**:630.

Paton BC et al: Ruptured sinus of Valsalva. *Arch Surg* 1965;**90**:209.

Terdjman M et al: Aneurysms of sinus of Valsalva: Two-dimensional echocardiographic diagnosis and recognition of rupture into right heart cavities. *J Am Coll Cardiol* 1984;**3**:1227.

Thompson R, Ross I, Elmes R: Quantification of valvular regurgitation by cardiac gated pool imaging. *Br Heart J* 1981;**46**:629.

Wilson WR et al: Valve replacement in patients with aortic infective endocarditis. *Circulation* 1978;**58**:585.

Aortic Stenosis

Bacon APC, Matthews MB: Congenital bicuspid aortic valves and the aetiology of isolated aortic valvular stenosis. *Q J Med* 1959;**28**:545.

Campbell M: Calcific aortic stenosis and congenital bicuspid aortic valve. *Br Heart J* 1968;**30**:606.

Carabello BA et al: Hemodynamic determinants of prognosis of aortic valve replacement in critical aortic stenosis and advanced congestive heart failure. *Circulation* 1980;**62**:42.

Chizner MA, Pearle DL, deLeon AC Jr: The natural history of aortic stenosis in adults. *Am Heart J* 1980;**99**:419.

Davies CE, Steiner RE: Calcified aortic valve: Clinical and radiological features. *Br Heart J* 1949;**8**:733.

Denie J, Verheugt SP: Supravalvular aortic stenosis. *Circulation* 1958;**18**:902.

Emanuel RW et al: Congenitally bicuspid aortic valves: Clinicogenetic study of 41 families. *Br Heart J* 1978;**40**:1402.

Exadactylos N, Ugrue DD, Oakley CM: Prevalence of coronary artery disease in patients with isolated aortic valve stenosis. *Br Heart J* 1984;**51**:121.

Fenoglio JJ Jr et al: Congenital bicuspid aortic valve after age 20. *Am J Cardiol* 1977;**39**:164.

Gewitz MH et al: Role of echocardiography in aortic stenosis: Pre- and postoperative studies. *Am J Cardiol* 1979;**43**:67.

Henry WL et al: Evaluation of aortic valve replacement in patients with valvular aortic stenosis. *Circulation* 1980;**61**:814.

Johnson JR, Myers GS, Lees RS: Evaluation of aortic stenosis by spectral analysis of the murmur. *J Am Coll Cardiol* 1985;**6**:55.

Jones M, Barnhart GR, Morrow AG: Late results after operation for left ventricular outflow tract obstruction. *Am J Cardiol* 1982;**50**:569.

Leech G, Mills P, Leatham A: The diagnosis of a nonstenotic bicuspid aortic valve. *Br Heart J* 1978;**40**:941.

Mills P et al: The natural history of a non-stenotic bicuspid aortic valve. *Br Heart J* 1978;**40**:951.

Murphy ES et al: Severe aortic stenosis in patients 60 years of age and older: Left ventricular function and 10 year survival after valve replacement. *Circulation* 1981;**64**(Suppl 2):184.

Nair CK et al: Cardiac conduction defects in patients older than 60 years with aortic stenosis with and without mitral anular calcium. *Am J Cardiol* 1984;**53**:169.

Pansegrau DG et al: Supravalvular aortic stenosis in adults. *Am J Cardiol* 1973;**31**:535.

Perloff JK: Clinical recognition of aortic stenosis: The physical signs and differential diagnosis of the various forms of obstruction to left ventricular outflow. *Prog Cardiovasc Dis* 1968;**10**:323.

Presbitero P et al: Open aortic valvotomy for congenital aortic stenosis: Late results. *Br Heart J* 1982;**47**:26.

Reis RL et al: Congenital fixed subvalvular aortic stenosis. *Circulation* 1971;**43**(Suppl 1):11.

Roberts WC: The congenitally bicuspid valve: A study of 85 autopsy cases. *Am J Cardiol* 1970;**26**:72.

Smith N, McAnulty JH, Rahimtoola SH: Severe aortic stenosis with impaired left ventricular function and clinical heart failure: Results of valve replacement. *Circulation* 1978;**58**:255.

Thompson R et al: Evaluation of combined homograft replacement of aortic valve and coronary bypass grafting in patients with aortic stenosis. *Br Heart J* 1979;**42**:447.

Thompson R et al: Influence of preoperative left ventricular function on results of homograft replacement of the aortic valve for aortic stenosis. *Am J Cardiol* 1979;**43**:929.

Wagner S, Selzer A: Patterns of progression of aortic stenosis: A longitudinal hemodynamic study. *Circulation* 1982;**65**:709.

Wood P: Aortic stenosis. *Am J Cardiol* 1958;**1**:553.

Young JB et al: Diagnosis and quantification of aortic stenosis with pulsed Doppler echocardiography. *Am J Cardiol* 1980;**45**:987.

Aortic Incompetence

Abdulla AM et al: Limitations of echocardiography in the assessment of left ventricular size and function in aortic regurgitation. *Circulation* 1980;**61**:148.

Bonow RO et al: The natural history of asymptomatic patients with aortic regurgitation and normal left ventricular function. *Circulation* 1983;**68**:509.

Borer JS et al: Left ventricular function at rest and during exercise after aortic valve replacement in patients with aortic regurgitation. *Am J Cardiol* 1979;**44**:1297.

Borow KM et al: End-systolic volume as a predictor of postoperative left ventricular performance in volume overload from valvular regurgitation. *Am J Med* 1980;**68**:655.

Botvinick EH et al: Echocardiographic demonstration of early mitral valve closure in severe aortic insufficiency: Its clinical implications. *Circulation* 1975;**51**:836.

Bulkley B, Roberts WG: Ankylosing spondylitis and aortic regurgitation: Description of the characteristic cardiovascular lesion from study of eight necropsy patients. *Circulation* 1973;**48**:1014.

Carroll JD et al: Regression of myocardial hypertrophy: Electrocardiographic-echocardiographic correlations after aor-

tic valve replacement in patients with chronic aortic regurgitation. *Circulation* 1982;**65**:980.
Clark DG, McAnulty JH, Rahimtoola SH: Valve replacement in aortic insufficiency with left ventricular dysfunction. *Circulation* 1980;**61**:411.
Fioretti P et al: Postoperative regression of left ventricular dimensions in aortic insufficiency: A long-term echocardiographic study. *J Am Coll Cardiol* 1985;**5**:856.
Fleming PR: The mechanism of the pulsus bisferiens. *Br Heart J* 1957;**19**:519.
Fortuin NJ, Craige E: On the mechanism of the Austin Flint murmur. *Circulation* 1972;**45**:558.
Goldschlager N et al: The natural history of aortic regurgitation. *Am J Med* 1973;**54**:577.
Greves J et al: Preoperative criteria predictive of late survival following valve replacement for severe aortic regurgitation. *Am Heart J* 1981;**101**:300.
Griffin FM Jr, Jones G, Cobbs CG: Aortic insufficiency in bacterial endocarditis. *Ann Intern Med* 1972;**76**:23.
Henry WL et al: Observations on the optimum time for operative intervention for aortic regurgitation. 1. Evaluation of the results of aortic valve replacement in symptomatic patients. *Circulation* 1980;**61**:471.
Henry WL et al: Observations on the optimum time for operative intervention for aortic regurgitation. 2. Serial echocardiographic evaluation of asymptomatic patients. *Circulation* 1980;**61**:484.
Hockings BEF et al: Comparison of vasodilator drug prazosin with digoxin in aortic regurgitation. *Br Heart J* 1980;**43**:550.
Hunt D et al: Quantitative evaluation of cineaortography in the assessment of aortic regurgitation. *Am J Cardiol* 1973;**31**:696.
Huxley RL et al: Early detection of left ventricular dysfunction in chronic aortic regurgitation as assessed by contrast angiography, echocardiography, and rest and exercise scintigraphy. *Am J Cardiol* 1983;**51**:1542.
Jaffe HW: The laboratory diagnosis of syphilis: New concepts. *Ann Intern Med* 1975;**83**:846.
Massie BM et al: Ejection fraction response to supine exercise in asymptomatic aortic regurgitation: Relation to simultaneous hemodynamic measurements. *J Am Coll Cardiol* 1985;**5**:847.
Morganroth J et al: Acute severe aortic regurgitation: Pathophysiology, clinical recognition, and management. *Ann Intern Med* 1977;**87**:223.
Najafi H et al: Acute aortic regurgitation secondary to aortic dissection: Surgical management without valve replacement. *Ann Thorac Surg* 1972;**14**:474.
Paulus HE, Pearson CM, Pitts W Jr: Aortic insufficiency in five patients with Reiter's syndrome: A detailed clinical and pathologic study. *Am J Med* 1972;**53**:464.
Peter CA, Jones RH: Cardiac response to exercise in patients with chronic aortic regurgitation. *Am Heart J* 1982;**104**:85.
Roberts WC, Day PJ: Electrocardiographic observations in clinically isolated, pure, chronic, severe aortic regurgitation: Analysis of 30 necropsy patients aged 19 to 65 years. *Am J Cardiol* 1985;**55**:431.
Samuels DA et al: Valve replacement for aortic regurgitation: Long-term follow-up with factors influencing the results. *Circulation* 1979;**60**:647.
Schuler G et al: Serial noninvasive assessment of left ventricular hypertrophy and function after surgical correction of aortic regurgitation. *Am J Cardiol* 1979;**44**:585.
Spagnuolo M et al: Natural history of rheumatic aortic regurgitation: Criteria predictive of death, congestive heart failure, and angina in young patients. *Circulation* 1971;**44**:368.
Stone PH et al: Determinants of prognosis of patients with aortic regurgitation who undergo aortic valve replacement. *J Am Coll Cardiol* 1984;**3**:1118.
Turina J et al: Improved late survival in patients with chronic aortic regurgitation by earlier operation. *Circulation* 1984;**70(Suppl 1)**:147.
Urquhart J et al: Quantification of valve regurgitation by radionuclide angiography before and after valve replacement surgery. *Am J Cardiol* 1981;**47**:287.
Wigle ED, Labrosse CJ: Sudden, severe aortic insufficiency. *Circulation* 1965;**32**:708.
Wise JR et al: Urgent aortic-valve replacement for acute aortic regurgitation due to infective endocarditis. *Lancet* 1971;**2**:115.

Multiple Valve Disease

Gash AK et al: Left ventricular performance in patients with coexistent mitral stenosis and aortic insufficiency. *J Am Coll Cardiol* 1984;**3**:703.
Gersh BJ et al: Results of triple valve replacement in 91 patients: Perioperative mortality and long-term follow-up. *Circulation* 1985;**72**:130.

Carcinoid Valve Disease

Bean WB et al: The syndrome of carcinoid and acquired valve lesions of the right side of the heart. *Circulation* 1955;**12**:1.
Mengel CE: Carcinoid and the heart. *Mod Concepts Cardiovasc Dis* 1966;**35**:75.
Pernow B, Waldenstrom J: Paroxysmal flushing and other symptoms caused by 5-hydroxytryptamine and histamine in patients with malignant tumors. *Lancet* 1954;**2**:951.
Reid CL et al: Echocardiographic features of carcinoid heart disease. *Am Heart J* 1984;**107**:801.
Roberts WC, Sjoerdsma A: The cardiac disease associated with the carcinoid syndrome (carcinoid heart disease). *Am J Med* 1964;**36**:5.
Trell E et al: Carcinoid heart disease: Clinicopathologic findings and follow-up in 11 cases. *Am J Med* 1973;**54**:433.
Ureles AL: Diagnosis and treatment of malignant carcinoid syndrome. *JAMA* 1974;**229**:1346.

Artificial Valves

Alam M, Goldstein S: Echocardiographic features of a stenotic porcine aortic valve. *Am Heart J* 1980;**100**:517.
Barratt-Boyes BG: Homograft aortic valve replacement in aortic incompetence and stenosis. *Thorax* 1964;**19**:131.
Barratt-Boyes BG et al: Homograft valves. *Med J Aust* 1972;**2(Suppl 1)**:38.
Baxley WA, Soto B: Hemodynamic evaluation of patients with combined mitral and aortic prostheses. *Am J Cardiol* 1980;**45**:42.
Bonow RO et al: Aortic valve replacement without myocardial revascularization in patients with combined aortic valvular and coronary artery disease. *Circulation* 1981;**63**:243.
Cohn LH et al: Five to eight-year follow-up of patients undergoing porcine heart-valve replacement. *N Engl J Med* 1981;**304**:258.
Copans H et al: Thrombosed Björk-Shiley mitral prostheses. *Circulation* 1980;**61**:169.
Cunha CLP et al: Echophonocardiographic findings in patients with prosthetic heart valve malfunction. *Mayo Clin Proc* 1980;**55**:231.
Effron MK, Popp RL: Two dimensional echocardiographic assessment of bioprosthetic valve dysfunction and infec-

tive endocarditis. *J Am Coll Cardiol* 1983;**2**:597.

Eyster E, Mayer K, McKenzie S: Traumatic hemolysis with iron deficiency anemia in patients with aortic valve lesions. *Ann Intern Med* 1968;**68**:995.

Forman R, Firth BG, Barnard MS: Prognostic significance of preoperative left ventricular ejection fraction and valve lesion in patients with aortic valve replacement. *Am J Cardiol* 1980;**45**:1120.

Hirshfeld JW et al: Indices predicting long-term survival after valve replacement in patients with aortic regurgitation and patients with aortic stenosis. *Circulation* 1974;**50**:1190.

Ivert TSA et al: Prosthetic valve endocarditis. *Circulation* 1984;**69**:223.

Kotler MN et al: Noninvasive evaluation of normal and abnormal prosthetic valve function. *J Am Coll Cardiol* 1983;**2**:151.

Kouchoukos NT, Karp RB: Fundamentals of clinical cardiology: Management of the postoperative cardiovascular surgical patient. *Am Heart J* 1976;**92**:4.

Lakier JB et al: Porcine xenograft valves: Long-term (60–80 month) follow-up. *Circulation* 1980;**62**:513.

Lytle BW et al: Replacement of aortic valve combined with myocardial revascularization: Determinants of early and late risk for 500 patients, 1967–1981. *Circulation* 1983;**68**:1149.

McClung JA et al: Prosthetic heart valves: A review. *Prog Cardiovasc Dis* 1983;**26**:237.

McGoon MD et al: Aortic and mitral valve incompetence: Long-term follow-up (10 to 19 years) of patients treated with the Starr-Edwards prosthesis. *Circulation* 1984;**3**:930.

Mehlman DJ: A guide to the radiographic identification of prosthetic heart valves: An addendum. *Circulation* 1984;**69**:102.

Mikell FL et al: Two-dimensional echocardiographic demonstration of left atrial thrombi in patients with prosthetic mitral valves. *Circulation* 1979;**60**:1183.

Morton MJ et al: Risks and benefits of postoperative cardiac catheterization in patients with ball valve prostheses. *Am J Cardiol* 1977;**40**:870.

Ott DA et al: Ionescu-Shiley pericardial xenograft valve: Hemodynamic evaluation and early clinical follow-up of 326 patients. *Cardiovasc Dis* 1980;**7**:137.

Pacifico AD, Karp RB, Kirklin JW: Homografts for replacement of the aortic valve. *Circulation* 1972;**45(Suppl 1)**:36.

Penta A et al: Patient status 10 or more years after "fresh" homograft replacement of the aortic valve. *Circulation* 1984;**70(Suppl 1)**:182.

Quireshi SA et al: Late results of mitral valve replacement using unstented antibiotic sterilised aortic homografts. *Br Heart J* 1983;**50**:564.

Reis RL et al: The flexible stent: A new concept in the fabrication of tissue heart valve prostheses. *J Thorac Cardiovasc Surg* 1971;**62**:683.

Richardson JV et al: Combined aortic valve replacement and myocardial revascularization: Results in 220 patients. *Circulation* 1979;**59**:75.

Santinga JT et al: Factors relating to late sudden death in patients having aortic valve replacement. *Ann Thorac Surg* 1980;**29**:249.

Sayed HM et al: Haemolytic anemia of mechanical origin after open heart surgery. *Thorax* 1961;**16**:356.

Somerville J et al: Long-term results of pulmonary autograft for aortic valve replacement. *Br Heart J* 1979;**42**:533.

Watanakunakorn C: Prosthetic valve infective endocarditis. *Prog Cardiovasc Dis* 1979;**22**:180.

Weinstein L: Infected prosthetic valves: A diagnostic and therapeutic dilemma. *N Engl J Med* 1972;**286**:1108.

Yacoub MH, Keeling DH: Chronic haemolysis following insertion of Ball valve prosthesis. *Br Heart J* 1968;**30**:676.

14 Conduction Defects

ELECTROPHYSIOLOGY

Our understanding of disorders of the formation (initiation) and conduction (transmission) of the electrical impulse of the heart is based on the descriptions of electrophysiologic events in Chapter 1. The contents of this chapter and of Chapter 15 (Cardiac Arrhythmias) describe disturbances in the electrical activity of the heart manifested by electrocardiographic changes and by symptoms and signs of heart disease.

Electrical Properties of Cardiac Cells

The understanding of disorders of conduction and cardiac rhythm requires knowledge of the inherent properties of cardiac tissue—automaticity, excitability and refractoriness, conductivity, and the capacity for reentry.

The sinoatrial node is a small group of cells situated at the junction of the superior vena cava and the right atrium that initiates the cardiac impulse and results in normal sinus rhythm. Spread of the impulse as it passes through the heart is represented on the ECG as the P wave, QRS complex, ST segment, and T wave. Normally, the heart rate is determined by the rate of diastolic depolarization of the sinus node cells, as shown by the degree of the phase 4 slope (see Figs 1–17 to 1–19). The sinoatrial node is under the influence of the autonomic nervous system; stimulation of the vagus nerve, either spontaneously, by reflex, or by drugs, slows the heart rate, decreasing the slope of phase 4. Sympathetic cardiac stimulation by drugs or via the central nervous system directly or reflexly increases the heart rate and increases the slope of phase 4.

A. Automaticity: All cardiac cells possess the capacity to beat spontaneously. Certain cells of the specialized conduction system are able to initiate an action potential that sequentially activates the entire heart; this capability is known as automaticity. Automaticity is most marked in the sinoatrial nodal cells, as shown by the steepest phase 4 slope of any of the specialized cardiac cells, and these cells normally serve as the pacemaker of the heart. The more distal the cell from the sinoatrial node, the more gradual the slope of phase 4 (ie, the slope is more gradual in cells at the atrioventricular junction and most gradual in cells in the Purkinje fibers). If any of the more proximal pacemaker cells fail, a more distal latent cell may become the pacemaker, preventing cardiac standstill and producing **escape rhythms.** The rate of automatic discharge is slower in the more distal pacemakers. Cells in the junctional tissues near the atrioventricular node in the bundle of His or in the Purkinje system commonly take over when the sinoatrial node pacemakers fail for any reason.

Automaticity in any cardiac cell may be increased by disease, drugs, or overactivity of the sympathetic nervous system, and latent cells may assume the role of pacemaker when not needed. When secondary pacemakers take over because of failure of the primary pacemakers, they are like junior officers taking command of the ship when the captain collapses. When subsidiary pacemakers take over because of increased automaticity, they are like mutineers, because the primary pacemakers are still functioning. Although increased automaticity does occur, the role of latent pacemakers is basically to provide a backup mechanism in the event that the more proximal cells fail to "fire."

B. Excitability and Refractoriness: The ability of a cell to respond to a stimulus and initiate an action potential is called excitability. The term also denotes the ability of a cell to respond to a propagated impulse from a neighboring cell. The action potential itself serves as a stimulus to excite neighboring cells, and in this way, in a sequential and orderly manner, the heart is depolarized.

Refractoriness is the property by which cardiac cells fail to respond to an oncoming stimulus because repolarization is incomplete and the voltage of the interior of the cell has not become sufficiently negative to initiate or propagate an action potential. It is related to excitability in that the cell is totally unexcitable when the voltage is less negative than threshold and no stimulus, no matter how strong, can evoke a propagated response. This is the absolute refractory period. As the voltage of the cell becomes more negative at the end of phase 3, the resting membrane potential may not have reached its normal value of -90 mV but may be sufficiently negative that a powerful stimulus can evoke a response even though it may not be sufficiently strong to be fully propagated and may depolarize only a few neighboring cells. Shortly after this relative refractory period and before the normal resting maximum diastolic pressure potential has been reached, there is a short "supernormal" phase corresponding to the downstroke of the T wave, during which time a smaller than usual current can induce a propagated response. The supernormal, or vulnerable, phase is responsible for the so-called R on T phenomenon, in which a ventricular premature beat falling on the descending limb of the T wave may induce repetitive ventricular ectopic discharges, including ventricular fibrillation.

The refractory period varies in different parts of the heart, being shortest in the atrium and longest in the Purkinje system and in the atrioventricular node.

This variability of recovery of excitability, or refractoriness, is exaggerated in portions of the ventricle or conduction system in diseases such as ischemic heart disease. Altered, uneven recovery of excitability in ischemic cells may be responsible for the frequency of ventricular arrhythmias in coronary heart disease. Recovery of refractoriness, excitability, and conduction velocity varies from one cell to another and from one tissue region to another. This variability affects repolarization, heart rate, and duration of the action potential and can thus initiate reentry arrhythmias (Han, 1971). Drugs rather than disease may exaggerate these changes; digitalis, for example, shortens the action potential, whereas quinidine prolongs it. Hypokalemia lengthens and hyperkalemia shortens the action potential.

C. Conductivity: Conduction of an electrical impulse from one cell to another is a fundamental property of cardiac tissue and results from the spread of electrical activity from one specialized cell to another and finally to myocardial cells. The velocity of conduction varies in different tissues of the heart and is 100 times more rapid in the Purkinje system than in the atrioventricular node. It is about 20–30 mm/s in the atrioventricular node, 3000–5000 mm/s in the Purkinje system, and about 500–600 mm/s in the ventricle. Slow conduction through the atrioventricular node prolongs the absolute refractory period in nodal cells and prevents rapid atrial impulses from activating the ventricles at the same rapid rate as the atria. In normal adults, this prevents them from beating so rapidly that they cannot maintain a normal cardiac output. Infants do not have the same conduction delay in the atrioventricular node and can have atrial arrhythmias with ventricular rates as high as 300/min.

Velocity of conduction. The velocity of conduction is related to the magnitude of the resting membrane potential when the action potential begins. The velocity is slower and there is a decreased rate of rise of phase 0 when the resting membrane potential is less negative. The velocity of the conduction is also related to the heart rate. Decrease in the slope and amplitude of phase 4 depolarization increases the time between successive action potentials and the velocity of conduction in the subsequent beat. When the velocity of conduction is slowed sufficiently as a result of decreased maximum resting membrane potential, conduction may be sufficiently impaired so that it decreases as the depolarization wave spreads distally, with the result that the impulse may not be propagated throughout the entire conduction system. The ability of the excitation wave to propagate may progressively deteriorate. The term **decremental conduction** refers to the progressive decrease in conduction that results from alterations in the characteristics of the action potential owing to cellular abnormalities in the conduction pathway until ultimately a propagated impulse cannot be sustained. Decremental conduction may leave in its wake cells that have been incompletely repolarized and therefore have become refractory to an oncoming antegrade stimulus. It may not be obvious on the ECG and is one form of **concealed conduction,** which may also result when premature beats partially penetrate but do not pass through the atrioventricular node to the remainder of the conduction system. Such failure to conduct completely is called concealed conduction regardless of whether the spread is antegrade from the atria or retrograde from the ventricles. Decreased conduction may cause conduction delay or block anywhere along the normal pathway. Failure or delay in conduction may not be uniform, ie, it may be more manifest in one fiber than in a neighboring one and may be important in setting up a reentry circuit, causing premature beats or tachycardia. Failure of conduction is usually due to disease such as fibrosis, ischemia, hypoxia, acidosis, or drugs or hyperkalemia, any of which decreases the maximum resting membrane potential or shortens repolarization, allowing the resting membrane potential during diastole to be closer to the threshold potential. This decreases the velocity of the upstroke of phase 0 of depolarization, which determines the velocity of conduction.

D. Reentry: Reentry is not a property of cardiac cells per se but is thought to be the mechanism by which arrhythmias can develop in any portion of the heart through disturbances in the fundamental properties noted above. An automatic cell, by increasing the slope of phase 4 depolarization and increasing its automaticity, can become the pacemaker of the heart, producing either a premature beat or tachycardia. Similarly, through operation of a reentry mechanism, a premature beat can be propagated by a circuitous route through an area of the heart and permit continuous repetitive depolarization and tachycardia.

Fig 14–1 shows in schematic fashion a reentrant pathway and how it can be modified.

1. Requirements for reentry–Normally, the cardiac impulse propagates evenly through the distal conducting system to the ventricles, with equal velocity in each of the closely related cardiac fibers (for purposes of illustration called "limbs" of a terminal Purkinje fiber bundle, as illustrated in Fig 14–1). Use of the term limb is not meant to imply that every area of the Purkinje system has only 2 fibers. Reentry requires that one portion of the myocardial fiber in a bundle of fibers be blocked in one direction (usually antegrade) because that limb is partially depolarized and cannot conduct properly (unidirectional block). Reentry also requires that antegrade activation through the other limb of the distal Purkinje fiber be slowed but spread in the normal direction to the ventricle. It then returns to the point of origin in a retrograde manner and activates the initially blocked limb or fiber. The impulse proceeds slowly in retrograde fashion through the segment that had antegrade block until it reaches the proximal conducting fiber, which by this time has recovered its excitability and is no longer refractory as a result of excitation; this allows a retrograde impulse from the originally blocked segment to reenter the normal segment or limb, setting up a reentry circuit which may then become repetitive.

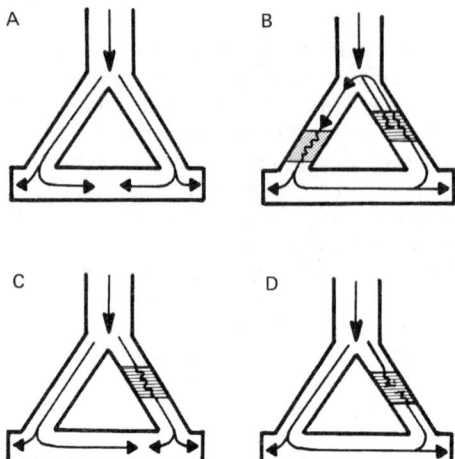

Figure 14-1. Schematic diagram of reentrant pathway and means for its modification. **A:** Normal propagation through the distal conducting system to the ventricle. Conduction proceeds with equal velocity through both limbs of a terminal Purkinje fiber bundle and then activates the myocardium. **B:** Shaded area on right indicates diseased tissue, including partially depolarized Purkinje fibers. Antegrade activation through the site is blocked. Activation is slowed (shaded area on left) but proceeds normally through the other limb to the myocardium and then activates the depressed segment (which is no longer refractory) in a retrograde direction. This impulse succeeds in propagating slowly through the depressed segment and reenters the proximal conducting system. **C:** If physiologic changes occur or appropriate pharmacologic agents are administered (see text), conduction may improve through the depressed segment and result in reestablishment of antegrade activation and abolition of reentry. **D:** If changes occur (or are induced) that result in block of retrograde activation as well as antegrade activation, then bidirectional conduction block occurs. This condition, too, would suppress a reentrant arrhythmia. (Modified and reproduced, with permission, from Rosen MR et al: Electrophysiology and pharmacology of cardiac arrhythmias. 5. Cardiac antiarrhythmic effects of lidocaine. Am Heart J 1975;**89**:526.)

Reentry requires, then, both impaired conduction (in one limb) and unidirectional block (in the other). Decremental conduction (as discussed above) may slow conduction in one fiber or produce antegrade unidirectional block in another fiber and so foster reentry. Parts C and D of Fig 14–1 show how the reentry rhythm can be terminated, either by improving conduction in the depressed segment and thus allowing the initial impulse to spread equally through both limbs of the fibers, or by increasing the retrograde block in the blocked segment so that the original impulse cannot be conducted to the proximal site.

A new stimulus, either from an atrial premature beat or from retrograde excitation of the atria by ventricular premature beats, is the usual mechanism for initiating paroxysmal atrial tachycardia, with the reentry circuit involving the atrioventricular node. A repetitive reentry circuit can be interrupted by drugs such as digitalis or verapamil if the reentry circuit involves the atrioventricular node. These drugs increase atrioventricular block, prolonging conduction in the atrioventricular node and making it refractory to any new impulse that reaches the atrioventricular node as part of the reentry circuit. Return, or echo, beats find the atrioventricular node unexcitable, so that it cannot continue to propagate the reentry circuit impulse.

2. Occurrence and causes of reentry–A reentry circuit can occur anywhere in the heart. In paroxysmal atrial tachycardia it usually includes the atrioventricular node. Atrial flutter is thought to result from a reentry pathway in the atria. In the ventricle it may occur in a diseased portion of the tissue. If there is an "excitable gap" between the head and tail of the reentry pathway (circus movement), there may be a continuous excitation wave that sets up a paroxysm of arrhythmia. Unidirectional block in one segment may be induced by ischemia, hypoxia, acidosis, potassium leak from necrotic cells, or (experimentally) by cooling. As a result of the relative automaticity of one group of cells, currents may be set up that stimulate neighboring cells and may lead to a propagated paroxysmal arrhythmia either via the reentry mechanism or via a direct ectopic rhythm (automaticity). Pathologic states such as ischemia do not affect all fibers uniformly, and irregular distribution of ischemia, with resulting irregular return of cells to their maximum resting diastolic potential and with varying conduction velocity, may lead to arrhythmias. Ventricular arrhythmias may be due to propagation from an ectopic site that has assumed greater automaticity because of early recovery of excitability; in other cases, reentry may be the mechanism. Recovery of excitability and altered refractory periods are common, especially in the border zone between necrotic and surviving cells that behave as chronically ischemic cells. This may explain the high incidence of arrhythmias after healed myocardial infarction and why unexpected ventricular fibrillation and sudden death may occur.

SPECIFIC TYPES OF CONDUCTION DEFECTS

BRADYCARDIA

Clinical Findings

A. Symptoms and Signs: The assessment of sinus bradycardia is difficult, since the definition itself is by no means uniform. Many authorities state that any regular sinus rate less than 60/min constitutes sinus bradycardia. Others use lower figures, such as 55 or 50/min. The age of the patient plays a role because slower heart rates (< 55/min) are more prevalent in healthy young individuals, especially athletes; are usually attributed to high vagal tone; are rarely associated with symptoms; and require no special investigative studies or treatment. Equivalent slow rates or more marked bradycardia (< 45/min) may produce symptoms in older individuals because with the development of coronary artery disease and impaired left ventricular function, stroke volume may not be able to increase to compensate for the slow heart rate and there may be a fall in cardiac output. Sinus bradycardia at any age is fairly common unless one defines it as a rate less than 40/min.

The sinus node is controlled by both cholinergic and adrenergic autonomic nervous impulses from any part of the body. Noncardiac causes of sinus bradycardia involving this system must be evaluated in light of the function of the sinus node as the common end pathway for many efferent impulses from the central nervous system.

Pathologically, there may be various infiltrative and inflammatory changes in the tissue framework of the sinoatrial node as well as lesions involving the sinus node artery (James, 1977).

The clinical significance of sinus bradycardia or sinus node or atrial dysfunction depends on whether atrioventricular junctional escape pacemakers or His bundle escape pacemakers take over the rhythm of the heart at rates that are only slightly slower than the normal sinus rate. If there is concomitant involvement of both sinoatrial and atrioventricular nodal areas, so that bundle branch or ventricular pacemakers are required, the prognosis for life is worse because these lower pacemakers are slower and less reliable, and artificial pacemakers are often indicated. The role of drugs—especially beta-adrenergic blocking agents, opiates, tranquilizers, and phenothiazines—must always be considered in sinus bradycardia. The decreased phase 4 depolarization slope that occurs in hypothyroidism and other metabolic disturbances should also be considered in the analysis of sinus bradycardia.

B. Myocardial Infarction and Bradycardia: The artery to the sinus node arises in most people from the right coronary artery, but in about one-third of individuals it arises from a branch of the left circumflex artery; sinus bradycardia, therefore, is usually found in patients with acute inferior myocardial infarction resulting from occlusion of the right coronary artery. Bradycardia is often transient or reversible, owing to ischemia of the sinus node and increased vagal tone, and can be reversed with time or with atropine. The slow heart rate is significant for 2 reasons: (1) By decreasing cardiac output, bradycardia may interfere with coronary perfusion and thus extend the infarction; and (2) a slow ventricular rate with variable conduction delay and repolarization may allow ectopic impulses to take over the rhythm of the heart in the ischemic or damaged ventricular muscle supplied by the right coronary artery.

C. His Bundle Recordings: His bundle recordings (Fig 14–2) have shown that the PR interval includes the spread of the impulse from the sinoatrial node through the atria and the bundle of His as well as the

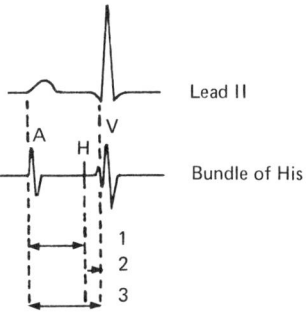

Figure 14–2. Diagrammatic illustration of His bundle recordings with normal atrioventricular conduction. (1), AH interval, approximately 120 ms, which is the time from beginning of atrial depolarization to the beginning of the bundle of His spike. (2), HV interval, approximately 50 ms (upper limits of normal are 55–60 ms), which represents the time from the bundle of His spike to the beginning of ventricular depolarization. (3), AV time, which is the PR interval. (Reproduced, with permission, from Goldman MJ: *Principles of Clinical Electrocardiography*, 12th ed. Lange, 1986.)

first part of its 2 main branches. The current from the His bundle is of sufficiently small magnitude that the surface ECG does not pick up its individual potentials. It can be recorded by an electrode catheter placed across the tricuspid valve near the His bundle and can be seen to occur during the PR interval of the surface ECG. The activity and timing of the conduction system between the sinoatrial node and the ventricles can then be determined. His bundle recordings have enhanced our understanding of the pathophysiology of atrioventricular conduction defects, especially the diagnostic, prognostic, and therapeutic significance of pacemaker activity above, in, and below the atrioventricular node.

Electrophysiologic methods of determining sinus node activity, such as sinus node recovery time, are useful but have significant limitations. The recovery time can be determined by noting the recovery time for a sinus beat when rapid atrial pacing is stopped. Sinus node recovery time is variable in the same patient at different times, and there is a considerable overlap between normal and abnormal patients (Table 14–1).

Differential Diagnosis

Because there is evidence that sinus bradycardia may not be as benign as once thought and because varying degrees of sinus node and atrial dysfunction as well as atrioventricular conduction defects may develop over a period of years, a 12- to 24-hour Holter monitor electrocardiographic recording should be obtained on older patients (over age 50) with otherwise unexplained rates less than 50/min at rest to rule out transient unrecognized atrial arrhythmias or conduction defects. Ambulatory monitoring is more strongly indicated if the rate is slower, if there is concomitant evidence of intraventricular conduction

Table 14–1. Clinical test for evaluation of sinus node function.*
($SNRT_c$, sinus node recovery time corrected; SNRT, observed sinus node recovery time; BCL, basic cycle length; IHR, intrinsic heart rate; SACT, sinoatrial conduction time.)

Test	Criteria of Abnormal Response	Comments
Atropine (0.04 mg/kg IV)	<50% increase in sinus rate	Relatively easy, safe test; helpful only if positive.
Isoproterenol (3 μg/min IV)	<25% increase in sinus rate	Helpful if positive; may be dangerous in ventricular arrhythmia and ischemic heart disease.
Sinus node recovery time (SNRT)	$SNRT_c$ > 450 ms $SNRT_c$ = SNRT − BCL or SNRT > 140% BCL	Highly specific, moderately sensitive; invasive procedure.
Sinoatrial conduction time (SACT)	SACT > 120 ms	Moderately specific, highly sensitive; invasive procedure.
Ambulatory electrocardiographic monitoring	Sinus bradycardia, sinus arrest, sinoatrial block, bradytachyarrhythmias	Excellent test; can correlate symptoms with arrhythmias.
Treadmill testing	<90% of predicted maximum heart rate for age and sex; development of exercise-induced sinus bradycardia	Difficult to assess in the elderly and debilitated patient.
Intrinsic heart rate	>10% decrease in age-predicted rate; IHR = 117.2 beats/min (0.53 × age)	Wide experience unavailable.

*Reproduced, with permission, from Talano JV et al: Sinus node dysfunction: An overview with emphasis on autonomic and pharmacologic consideration. Am J Med 1978;**64**:773.

defects such as right or left bundle branch block or bifascicular block (usually right bundle branch block and left anterior hemiblock), or if the patient complains of dizziness. (See section on atrioventricular conduction defects, below.) If the patient is young, with no symptoms and only modest bradycardia (eg, < 50/min), and has normal exercise tolerance, further investigation is not indicated, but the patient should be seen once a year and told to report any unusual symptoms such as near-syncope or dizziness or awareness of cardiac arrhythmias. If dizziness, palpitations, or syncope occurs, a 24-hour electrocardiographic monitor should be employed to determine the presence or absence of tachy- or bradyarrhythmias (Table 14–2).

Treatment

See Bradycardia-Tachycardia Syndrome.

TACHYCARDIA

Sinus tachycardia (> 100 beats/min) can occur in any condition that increases the slope of phase 4 depolarization of the sinus node cells, which therefore reach "threshold" sooner and thus result in rapid heart rates. This occurs in exercise, anemia, fever, emotional stress, thyrotoxicosis, following administration of adrenergic drugs such as epinephrine, or following any stimuli that increase adrenergic activity, which increases the release of norepinephrine. Beta-adrenergic blocking agents slow the heart rate at rest and during exercise by interfering with the adrenergic activity in the sinus node. Cholinergic or vagal stimuli slow the sinus rate; the effects can be reversed by atropine.

Table 14–2. Holter monitoring findings in 95 patients with dizziness or syncope.*†

Clinical Findings	Number of Patients
No abnormalities detected	22
Findings definitely correlating with symptoms	**46**
Paroxysmal atrial fibrillation	6
Paroxysmal atrial flutter	1
Paroxysmal atrial tachycardia	11
Ventricular tachycardia	10
Sinus bradycardia	3
Sinoatrial block or standstill	5
Atrioventricular block, second-degree	4
Atrioventricular block, third-degree	3
Defective pacemaker	5
Findings possibly related to symptoms	**42**
Frequent premature atrial contractions	11‡
Frequent premature ventricular contractions	31§
Findings not related to symptoms	**17**
Sinus tachycardia (≥ 120 beats/min)	8
Sinus bradycardia (≤ 50 beats/min)	1
Intermittent bundle branch block	3
Atrioventricular block, first-degree	5

*Reproduced, with permission, from Van Durme JP: Tachyarrhythmias and transient cerebral ischemic attacks. Am Heart J 1975;**89**:538.
†Patients who presented different types of arrhythmia or conduction defect were listed under each separate item.
‡Five patients developed paroxysmal atrial tachycardia; 2 patients developed atrial fibrillation.
§Ten patients developed ventricular tachycardia.

When sinus tachycardia occurs in acute myocardial infarction, it increases the work of the heart and may extend the size of the myocardial infarction. If the patient has an obstructive lesion such as mitral stenosis, tachycardia decreases the duration of ventricular filling and causes an increase in the pulmonary artery wedge pressure that induces pulmonary venous congestion and dyspnea.

BRADYCARDIA-TACHYCARDIA SYNDROME
(Sick Sinus Syndrome)

The bradycardia-tachycardia syndrome, consisting of alternating bradycardia due to sinus arrest, sinus bradycardia, or sinoatrial exit block combined with tachycardia from paroxysmal atrial or junctional arrhythmias, may produce symptoms referable to either slow or fast heart rates (Short, 1954). It is being reported with increasing frequency as its importance becomes recognized. The term sick sinus syndrome is offered by Ferrer (1974; 1981) because the symptoms due to the slow rate result from failure of impulse formation in the sinoatrial node or its conduction to the atrioventricular node, causing dizziness, syncope, and bradycardia. The term bradycardia-tachycardia syndrome is preferred by others because patients characteristically have paroxysmal atrial or junctional tachyarrhythmias in addition to the slow heart rates; this is because the pathologic process, usually fibrosis, is not confined to the sinoatrial node but may involve parts of the atrium, the atrioventricular node, the bundle of His, and the His-Purkinje system. Recent pathologic investigations have shown that the process is much more common than was once thought. The mechanism of bradycardia-tachycardia syndrome can therefore be sinus bradycardia, sinus node arrest, sinoatrial conduction defect, or disease of the atrioventricular node, with escape mechanisms in junctional pacemakers and resulting in the development of atrial arrhythmias.

In addition to the pathologic finding of nonspecific fibrotic degenerative disease of the conduction system, the bradycardiac syndromes may be associated with the more common diseases such as coronary disease, hypertension, aortic and mitral valve disease, and primary cardiomyopathy, but these conditions may be only incidental.

Clinical Findings

A. Symptoms and Signs: Characteristic findings of bradycardia-tachycardia syndrome are intermittent symptoms referable to a slow heart rate or to rapid supraventricular arrhythmia (paroxysmal atrial or junctional tachycardia, atrial flutter, or atrial fibrillation).

In some patients, the fast and slow rates may alternate. On one occasion the patient may have paroxysmal arrhythmia with palpitations and impaired cerebral, coronary, and extremity flow from rapid ventricular rates, and on another occasion, the slow heart rate caused by dysfunction of the sinus node or transmission from the sinoatrial to the atrioventricular node may result in inadequate perfusion of the brain, with dizziness, impaired cerebral function, and either presyncope or syncope. Impairment of coronary flow may result in angina pectoris or symptoms of cardiac failure or general weakness. In patients who present with paroxysmal atrial arrhythmias, the disorder of the sinus node or sinoatrial conduction dysfunction may only be recognized by the presence of sinus bradycardia between attacks or by noting that when the tachycardia is terminated (either with drugs or with cardioversion), the sinoatrial node shows a period of standstill and slow return to normal function. Five to 10% of cases of cardiovascular syncope were found by Easley (1971) to occur in this manner. A history of syncope that immediately follows the cessation of tachycardia suggests the diagnosis.

In a prospective study (Rokseth, 1974), sinoatrial or sinus node disease occurred in about one-third of all clinical conduction defects. Many patients were seen by a neurologist because the symptoms were vague and misinterpreted. Sixty percent of patients had atrial arrhythmias, and the incidence was higher if long-term ambulatory monitoring of the ECG was used. It is estimated that over a 5- to 10-year period, about half of patients with sinoatrial dysfunction will have symptoms suggesting Stokes-Adams attacks (Ferrer, 1974).

Sinus bradycardia, especially in older individuals, should be looked on with suspicion and not dismissed as a sensitive carotid sinus or "vagotonia." Patients with marked sinus bradycardia or with symptoms that could be related to a slow heart rate should have ambulatory monitoring of the ECG for 12–24 hours or more (Table 14–3). Episodes of short or long paroxysmal atrial tachycardia, atrial fibrillation, or atrial flutter may not have been suspected on the basis of the clinical history. His bundle recordings of atrial and His bundle depolarizations may show a variety

Table 14–3. Incidence of sinus abnormalities and atrioventricular block in patient population.*

	Number of Cases†	Percentage of Total Cases
Sinus		
Bradycardia	129	7.7
Tachycardia	429	25.6
Pause, arrest, or sinoatrial block	63	3.8
Atrioventricular block		
First-degree	32	1.9
Second-degree	39	2.3
Third-degree (complete)	10	0.6

*Reproduced, with permission, from Bleifer SB et al: Diagnosis of occult arrhythmias by Holter electrocardiography. *Prog Cardiovasc Dis* 1974;**16**:569.
†These are not mutually exclusive, since a patient may demonstrate more than one abnormality.

of conduction disturbances between the sinoatrial node and other parts of the specialized conduction system (not solely the atrioventricular node) in a reentry circuit, as is usual in paroxysmal atrial tachycardia.

Although most patients with bradycardia-tachycardia syndrome are older (usually at least in the seventh decade), the disease may occur in young people, and the possibility of degenerative disease of the sinoatrial node and the atria should not be dismissed on the basis of age. Patients who develop angina pectoris should be investigated for possible episodic bradycardia or tachycardia.

B. Electrophysiologic and Special Studies, Including His Bundle Studies: Electrophysiologic methods of determining sinus node activity, such as sinus node recovery time, are useful but have significant limitations. The recovery time can be determined by noting the recovery time for a sinus beat when rapid atrial pacing is stopped. Sinus node recovery time is variable in the same patient at different times, and there is a considerable overlap between normal and abnormal patients (Table 14–1).

In addition to continuous monitoring of the ECG over a period of hours, either while the patient is ambulatory or in the coronary care unit, other studies may be helpful in making the diagnosis. The response of the sinus rate to exercise or atropine, His bundle recordings, atrial pacing, atrial extrastimulus testing, and overdrive suppression of the sinus node may reveal dysfunction of the sinoatrial node or its connections to the atrioventricular node. Examples of such dysfunction are delayed recovery of the sinus node following rapid atrial pacing (sinoatrial node recovery time) and prolonged sinoatrial conduction time after atrial extrastimulus testing with progressively increasing prematurity. These studies are still investigational, and their role in diagnosis is uncertain. If the prolonged pauses during atrial pacing studies reproduce the spontaneous symptoms of the patient, the role of bradycardia can be considered established, and placement of a right atrial pacemaker may relieve the symptoms. The atrial arrhythmias are often due to chance reexcitation of already repolarized fibers; differences in the rate of repolarization result from variable refractory periods that are prevalent when the heart rate is slow. Han (1966) has shown that vagal stimulation decreases the refractory period unevenly in different parts of the atrium, which might lead to reentry atrial arrhythmias.

If the patient with sinus bradycardia is asymptomatic and yet has both bifascicular block and a prolonged PR interval on the ECG, suggesting trifascicular block, the hazard of complete atrioventricular block is sufficient to make one follow the patient closely and proceed with His bundle and other specialized studies if symptoms appear.

C. Precautions Before Undertaking Special Investigations in Chronic Sinoatrial Disease: Before resorting to invasive techniques such as atrial pacing and His bundle recordings, one should (as indicated earlier) rule out paroxysmal arrhythmias, drug effects, hypothyroidism, anemia due to blood loss or hematologic disorders, postural hypotension, transient ischemic attacks, what in early days was called swooning (vasovagal attacks), and the vague dizziness and confusion of cerebrovascular disease without focal neurologic signs. The differential diagnosis of nonspecific dizziness and weakness in elderly people includes many noncardiac conditions. This problem is discussed in more detail in Chapter 2. Twenty-four-hour monitoring of the ECG is indicated in all such patients to exclude a tachy- or bradyarrhythmia that is amenable to treatment. The variety of abnormalities detected is illustrated in Table 14–2. Myocardial ischemia induced by effort may be associated with hypotension and cerebral symptoms. Electrocardiographic monitoring may identify these patients. The specialized studies discussed below require equipment that is available only in larger centers. Simple noninvasive tests (eg, exercise tests or 24-hour monitoring of the ECG) (see pp 93 and 94) should be performed in symptomatic patients before they are referred to a major center for invasive studies.

D. Atropine Test: Atropine sulfate, 0.5 mg intravenously, usually increases the heart rate in normal individuals to over 100/min. In a group of patients with bradycardia-tachycardia syndrome, Rosen (1971) found that no patient developed a heart rate greater than 90/min after administration of 1 mg of atropine intravenously. The electrophysiologic effects of atropine have been summarized by Schweitzer (1980).

Although atropine can be used as a test of the ability of the sinoatrial node to increase its rate of discharge, there are occasions when atropine produces tachycardia and may induce angina pectoris or an arrhythmia, especially in the presence of coronary heart disease. Small doses (eg, 0.25 or 0.5 mg intravenously) should be given first, therefore, and the effect on heart rate noted before larger doses are used. Slow heart rates with varying rates of recovery of excitability in different parts of the atrium can lead to reentry atrial premature beats and perhaps atrial tachycardia or fibrillation.

Differential Diagnosis

Differential diagnosis includes all conditions causing bradycardia and atrial tachyarrhythmias. In addition, because the symptoms are often vague and nonspecific, one must consider psychophysiologic reactions, transient ischemic attacks due to cerebrovascular disease, vasovagal fainting, and all conditions in which elderly individuals may have transient cerebral symptoms other than sinus, sinoatrial, or atrioventricular conduction disturbances. Cerebral symptoms are nonspecific when due to conduction defects and may result from abnormalities anywhere in the transmission system from the sinus node to the Purkinje system. Special studies are needed to identify the site of delay in conduction.

If vague symptoms suggesting cerebral or cardiac ischemia appear with exercise and the sinus rate is slow (usually < 45/min), one should exercise the patient to determine if the atrial rate can be increased appropriately. If the cardiac rate does not increase following moderate exercise to more than 110/min or if symptoms suggest decreased perfusion of the brain or heart, one can conclude that bradycardia is responsible for the symptoms and proceed to evaluate the effect of atropine.

Treatment

A. Drug Treatment: If the patient is asymptomatic but the atrial rate fails to increase with exercise, and the rate is nonetheless still not slow enough to warrant a ventricular pacemaker, one may try to increase the atrial rate with atropine, sublingual isoproterenol, or ephedrine combined with a mild sedative. If, in addition to a slow heart rate that fails to respond adequately to exercise and to atropine, the patient has symptoms of cerebral insufficiency suggesting sinoatrial syncope, a demand right ventricular pacemaker should be considered.

The physician should make certain that the symptoms and slow heart rate are not due to use of phenothiazines, quinidine, or beta-adrenergic blocking drugs given to prevent atrial arrhythmias. Digitalis given in large doses to prevent or treat paroxysmal atrial fibrillation may cause or prolong the period of sinus arrest. Withdrawal of these medications is an important first step before use of a pacemaker is considered.

B. Pacemaker Implantation: The most effective method of therapy in symptomatic patients is insertion of a demand transvenous pacemaker in the right ventricle to maintain an adequate heart rate and prevent syncopal attacks. The physician can then use antiarrhythmic drugs to prevent atrial tachyarrhythmias without being concerned about their cardiac depressant effects. With the improvement in cardiac function that follows restoration of a normal heart rate by the introduction of a demand pacemaker, the atrial arrhythmias may not recur. Sinus node dysfunction with bradycardia-tachycardia syndrome is the indication for implantation of about one-third of all demand pacemakers for cardiac syncope.

Before use of a pacemaker is considered, it must be established that the symptoms are caused by a conduction defect, either sinus node abnormality or alternating bradycardia and tachycardia. The presence of sinus bradycardia alone, while requiring careful follow-up, is not an indication for pacemaker therapy. Patients with vague symptoms such as dizziness, fatigue, or even syncope do not require a pacemaker unless it is established that the symptoms are due to a conduction defect. Sudden death is rare in sinus node disease, in contrast to atrioventricular block, and pacemaker therapy is used for relief of symptoms. The indications for pacemaker insertion are controversial, and many physicians believe it is performed too frequently in sinus node disease.

Although patients with sinoatrial disease are an average of 10 years younger than those with atrioventricular conduction disease and generally have a more benign prognosis than those with atrioventricular block, major Stokes-Adams attacks may occur. A pacemaker should be inserted when it has been established that presyncope or syncope is due to sinoatrial disease.

The slow progression of bradycardia-tachycardia syndrome to complete atrioventricular block makes it difficult sometimes to decide whether to be conservative or aggressive in treatment. In general, as long as the patient is asymptomatic or has not developed bi- or trifascicular block, nothing is necessary except to carefully note the response to noninvasive procedures such as exercise, posture, Valsalva's maneuver, squatting, or atropine. If the cause has been identified as coronary heart disease, if the progress of the disease seems rapid, or if the patient develops symptoms due to both bradycardia and tachycardia, then definitive pacemaker and antiarrhythmic therapy should be initiated. Before a permanent transvenous pacemaker is introduced—especially if there is doubt about the relationship between the cerebral symptoms and bradycardia—a temporary pacemaker should be tried, and the effect of increased heart rate on the cerebral symptoms should be noted.

Pacemakers are not innocuous (see Chapter 7, p 127) and should be used only on adequate indications, but it is just as wrong not to use pacemakers when they are clearly indicated as to recommend their introduction unnecessarily. The results of transvenous pacing in patients with bradycardia-tachycardia syndrome have been uniformly good with respect to relief of symptoms from slow heart rates, but additional drugs are often necessary to control the paroxysmal arrhythmia.

Prognosis

Because the most common pathologic process is fibrosis of the conduction system, which is usually slowly progressive, the physician should follow the patient even if there are no symptoms, in order to note the development of any symptoms, arrhythmias, or atrioventricular conduction defects that may presage the development of Stokes-Adams attacks. Atypical symptoms may not be interpreted correctly, and sinoatrial disease may be found only if special studies such as 24-hour monitoring of the ECG are periodically undertaken. Unexplained cerebral symptoms are most important to note in patients with bradycardia. Unexplained atrial fibrillation, especially when associated with bradycardia occurring between paroxysmal attacks, should also alert the physician to the possibility of the condition and its long-term guarded prognosis.

ATRIOVENTRICULAR CONDUCTION DEFECTS

Atrioventricular conduction defects may occur anywhere from the atrioventricular node to both bundle branches. His bundle recordings have demonstrated single and multiple blocks, which may be localized in the atrioventricular node, the bundle of His, or anywhere in the conduction system distal to the bundle of His. Atrioventricular defects may be acute and transient, reversible, or chronic. Examples of acute defects are those associated with acute myocardial ischemia or infarction (discussed in detail below because of its importance) and those associated with acute myocarditis, rheumatic fever, heart block following surgery, drug toxicity, and hyperkalemia (discussed in other chapters). See Table 14–4.

Chronic atrioventricular defects may be intermittent or permanent and are usually due to structural defects in the conduction system that occur during the course of chronic disease. The most common causes of chronic defects are coronary heart disease, dilated cardiomyopathy, fibrosis of the conduction system (Lev's disease or Lenegre's disease), and myocardial infiltrative diseases (Table 14–4). In coronary heart disease, the conduction defect may be acute, as in acute myocardial ischemia or infarction, or chronic, as in chronic coronary heart disease following myocardial infarction.

Atrioventricular defects, whether acute or chronic, are important because they may lead to advanced heart block, syncope, or Stokes-Adams attacks (see p 446) with ventricular standstill or ventricular fibrillation. Insertion of a pacemaker may be required if advanced or complete heart block occurs.

Atrioventricular conduction defects vary from partial (first-degree) block to second-degree block to complete (third-degree) block (Figs 14–3 to 14–6). Partial atrioventricular block consists of prolongation of the PR interval to 0.21 second or more at normal heart rates and represents a delay in conduction of the cardiac impulse from the sinoatrial node to the ventricles, recognized only on ECG. In second-degree block, not every sinus impulse reaches the ventricles, with the result that failure of ventricular contraction occurs and is apparent by the absence (dropping) of a beat. Failure of conduction on the part of the ventricles allows the conduction system to recover, so that a subsequent beat is transmitted to the ventricles. The basic definition and classification of second-degree block were proposed by Mobitz (1924) (Mobitz type 1 and Mobitz type 2; see below) and have been clarified by His bundle recordings and electrical stimulation of the heart. In complete (third-degree) atrioventricular block, the lesion is in the atrioventricular node or distal to the His bundle. It is often part of a generalized pathologic process (Table 14–4) and associated with bilateral bundle branch block, but it may occur without any conduction defect in either the right or left bundle branches.

Table 14–4. Causes of atrioventricular block.

1. Degenerative disease of conduction system (Lev's disease, Lenegre's disease).
2. Myocardial infarction or ischemia without infarction.
3. Dilated cardiomyopathy.
4. Drug toxicity due to digitalis, quinidine, phenothiazines, tricyclic antidepressants.
5. Valvular heart disease (especially aortic stenosis and aortic insufficiency).
6. Connective tissue and myocardial disorders (eg, sarcoidosis, scleroderma, amyloidosis, systemic lupus erythematosus, thyroid disease).
7. Surgical heart block.
8. Hyperkalemia and following use of antiarrhythmic drugs.
9. Cardiac tumors (usually secondary but sometimes primary).
10. Chagas' disease of the heart; rarely, syphilitic gumma.
11. Congenital.

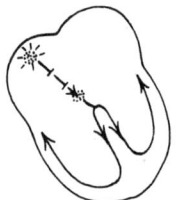
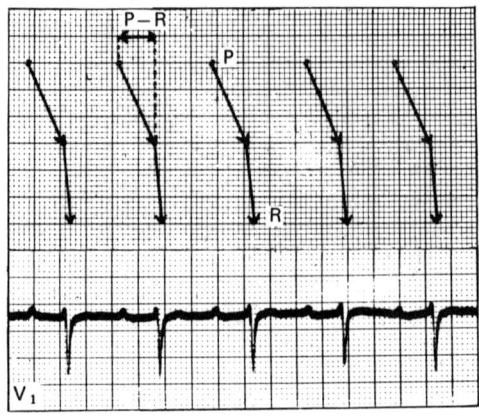

Figure 14–3. First-degree atrioventricular block. The PR interval is prolonged to 0.28 second. (Reproduced, with permission, from Goldman MJ: *Principles of Clinical Electrocardiography*, 12th ed. Lange, 1986.)

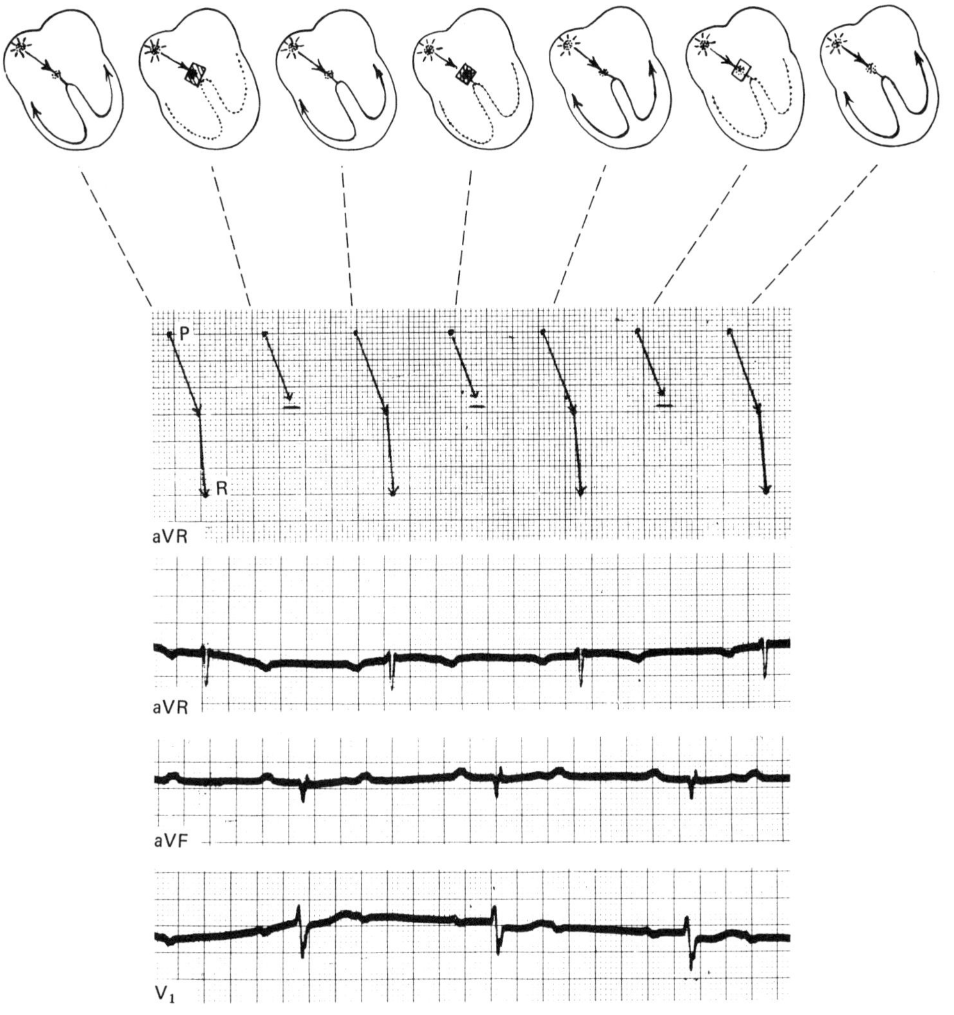

Figure 14–4. 2:1 atrioventricular block. The atrial rhythm is regular at a rate of 82/min. Every other atrial beat produces ventricular stimulation. (Reproduced, with permission, from Goldman MJ: *Principles of Clinical Electrocardiography*, 12th ed. Lange, 1986.)

Figure 14–5. Second-degree atrioventricular block of Wenckebach type. The atrial rhythm is regular. In lead II, the first PR interval = 0.18 second, the second = 0.28 second, and the third = 0.36 second. The fourth atrial beat fails to activate the ventricle. (Reproduced, with permission, from Goldman MJ: *Principles of Clinical Electrocardiography*, 12th ed. Lange, 1986.)

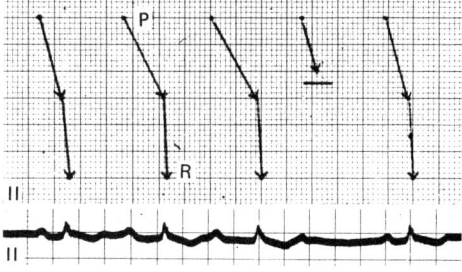

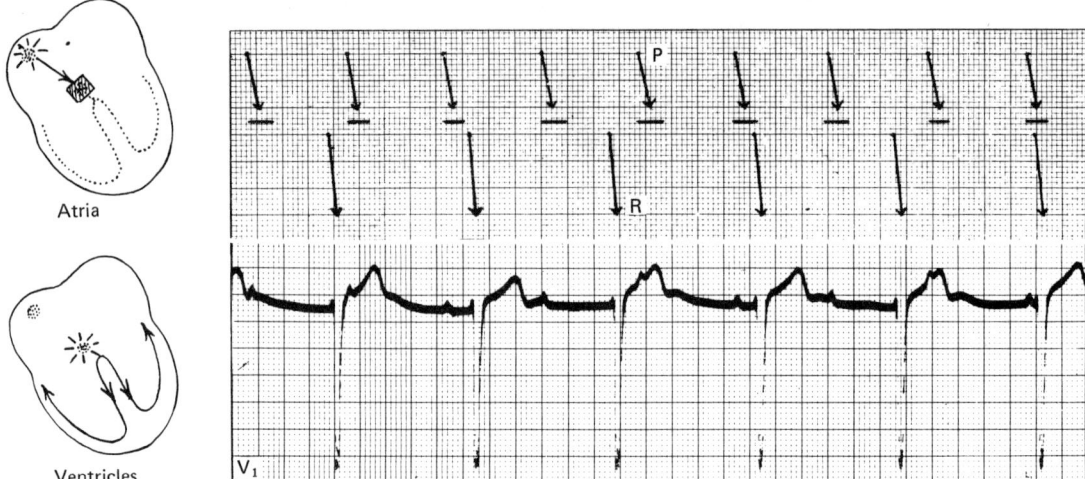

Figure 14–6. Diagram of complete atrioventricular block. The atria are activated by impulses arising normally in the sinoatrial node. In this example, the atrial rate = 72/min. The atrial impulses do not activate the ventricles. A second cardiac pacemaker is located near the atrioventricular node and stimulates the ventricles. The ventricular rate = 54/min. The atrial and ventricular rhythms are independent of each other. (Reproduced, with permission, from Goldman MJ: *Principles of Clinical Electrocardiography,* 12th ed. Lange, 1986.)

1. ACUTE ATRIOVENTRICULAR CONDUCTION DEFECTS

Myocardial Infarction & Acute Conduction Defects*

Continuous electrocardiographic monitoring of patients in coronary care units has shown that atrioventricular conduction defects are common in acute myocardial infarction. Overall, complete atrioventricular block occurs in 6–10% of cases, depending on the sample of patients, and is associated with a high mortality rate not necessarily as a result of the heart block itself. Atrioventricular block, especially in the presence of anterior myocardial infarction, implies a large infarct with considerable myocardial damage in the area of the septum and consequent cardiac failure or cardiogenic shock.

A. Inferior Infarcts: When atrioventricular conduction defects occur in inferior infarction, the damage to the conduction tissue is usually reversible and transient. It is due to temporary ischemia or edema of the atrioventricular node caused by occlusion of the atrioventricular nodal artery—a branch of the right coronary artery—and is characterized by progression through all degrees of atrioventricular block to complete atrioventricular block, though Stokes-Adams attacks are uncommon. The QRS complex is almost always normal in width. With complete atrioventricular block, there is a junctional pacemaker, resulting in a heart rate greater than 50/min. His bundle recordings indicate that the atrioventricular block is usually in the atrioventricular node and rarely involves the bundle of His or its branches, and the prognosis is correspondingly better than when the block is infranodal. Artificial cardiac pacemakers are less often required than in anterior infarction and in many centers are not used at all unless the patient has episodes of syncope, especially if the junctional pacemaker is satisfactory (> 50 beats per minute). The conduction defect usually lasts for a few days—rarely as long as a week—and the prognosis is good for the acute episode. The frequency of transient complete atrioventricular block in inferior infarctions is at least twice that in anterior infarctions.

B. Anterior Infarcts: In anterior myocardial infarction with conduction defects, there is usually widespread necrosis of the septum involving the bundle of His and its branches, usually preceded by the sudden onset of unifascicular or bifascicular block—most often right bundle branch block or left anterior hemiblock (see p 451). The sequential change to and from bundle branch block to left anterior hemiblock (fascicular block) and complete atrioventricular block as well as various arrhythmias may be rapid and take place over minutes to an hour. His bundle recordings show that the conduction defect is below the atrioventricular node, the QRS duration is usually widened, the interval between the bundle of His spike and the beginning of the QRS complex (the HV interval) is prolonged, the heart rate is usually fewer than 40 beats/min, and the escape pacemaker is in the bundle branches or lower in the Purkinje system. Stokes-Adams attacks and sudden death are an ever-present danger. For this reason, the development of conduction defect in a patient with anterior myocardial infarction usually indicates severe stenosis of the left anterior descending artery or the left main coronary artery and is much more serious than is the case in inferior

---

*See also Chapter 8, pp 167– 168.

infarctions. Insertion of a prophylactic demand ventricular pacemaker is indicated when certain manifestations of ventricular conduction defect such as bilateral bundle branch block or type II second-degree (Mobitz type II) atrioventricular block develop during the course of acute anterior infarction, because complete atrioventricular block and Stokes-Adams attacks may appear rapidly. The mortality rate is high when atrioventricular conduction defects develop for the first time in anterior infarction, because the necrosis is extensive and left ventricular function is severely impaired, with decreased cardiac output, raised left ventricular filling pressure, decreased ejection fraction, and a low stroke work index. There may be ventricular hypokinesia and even an abrupt development of ventricular aneurysm, septal perforation, or mitral insufficiency. The mortality rate is high even if a pacemaker is introduced, because cardiac function is sufficiently impaired by the widespread necrosis so that even if Stokes-Adams attacks are prevented, the patient may die of "pump failure," cardiogenic shock, or ventricular fibrillation. If the patient survives the episode of complete atrioventricular block with Stokes-Adams attacks in anterior infarction, it may be wise to replace the temporary ventricular pacemaker with a permanent one because there are some (though few) data that indicate that these patients have a high incidence of sudden death within the next 1–2 years if they are not paced.

2. CHRONIC ATRIOVENTRICULAR CONDUCTION DEFECTS

Clinical Findings

A. Partial (First-Degree) Atrioventricular Block: Clinically, patients with partial atrioventricular block alone are usually asymptomatic, and the diagnosis is made on routine electrocardiography. It may be suspected clinically if there is a very soft first heart sound, because of the inverse relationship between the PR interval and the loudness of the first sound. With long PR intervals, the mitral valve leaflets have become nearly apposed prior to ventricular systole; when they finally close completely with ventricular systole, closure of the valve is associated with minimal sound. Conversely, a loud first heart sound indicates that the mitral valve leaflets were wide apart just before ventricular systole, making first-degree atrioventricular block unlikely. This is correlated with a normal or short PR interval.

Although there is conduction delay between the atria and the ventricles in partial atrioventricular block, each atrial impulse is transmitted regularly to the ventricles. Conduction is delayed following an early premature beat, and partial atrioventricular block may be seen only in one or 2 beats following the long pause after an early premature beat. The refractory periods of the atrioventricular node and of the ventricular myocardium are inversely proportionate to the preceding cycle length. Partial atrioventricular block that occurs unexpectedly in one or 2 beats should suggest an atrial premature beat (often nonconducted) or a His bundle premature beat that may not be easily visible on the ECG; this has been termed **concealed conduction** by Langendorf (1948) and refers to incomplete penetration of the atrioventricular node by the atrial premature beats, which are not discernible on the routine ECG but which can be seen in His bundle recordings. The next sinus beat finds the atrioventricular node partially refractory, which results in prolongation of the PR interval. An abrupt, transient prolonged PR interval may thus justify the inference that conduction has been delayed by an event such as an atrial premature beat that is not visible by conventional means. The finding has no more significance than the atrial premature beat itself.

1. His bundle recordings–The PR interval has been shown by His bundle recordings to divide into the AH interval (65–145 ms), representing the spread of the impulse from the low atrial region to the bundle of His, and the HV interval (35–55 ms), representing the spread of the impulse from the bundle of His to the beginning of the QRS complex. Electrophysiologic studies have shown that when the prolongation of the PR interval is due to prolongation of the AH interval, the disease process is in the atrioventricular node; when the HV interval is prolonged, the pathologic processes are distal to the His bundle. The AH interval is prolonged by drugs such as digitalis and by acute myocarditis, thyrotoxicosis, acute inferior infarction, and rapid atrial pacing. In general, a prolonged AH interval (proximal block) is of better prognostic significance than a prolonged HV interval (distal block). When the AH interval is normal but the HV interval is prolonged (especially to more than 70 ms), the conduction delay is distal to the His bundle or its branches. This infranodal delay is more serious because it indicates disease of the ventricular conduction system, with more chronic myocardial disease, and an adverse clinical course that may lead to sudden death. However, deaths (including sudden deaths) are usually the result of underlying cardiac disease and infrequently due to the development of heart block and Stokes-Adams attacks (Dhingra, 1981). The incidence of sudden death was no different in patients with a prolonged HV interval who were not paced from that in those who were (Morady, 1984; McAnulty, 1984). Pacemakers are not advised unless the HV interval exceeds 80–100 ms, and even this is controversial. Neurologic symptoms due to paroxysmal complete atrioventricular block require a pacemaker.

2. Trifascicular block with prolonged PR and HV intervals and bundle branch block–This consists of an HV interval greater than 70 ms in the presence of left or right bundle branch block. If symptoms related to atrioventricular block develop, a permanent pacemaker should be inserted to relieve symptoms; this has not been shown to prolong life, however (Morady, 1984; Scheinman, 1982). Patients with prolonged HV intervals are more apt to have a greater

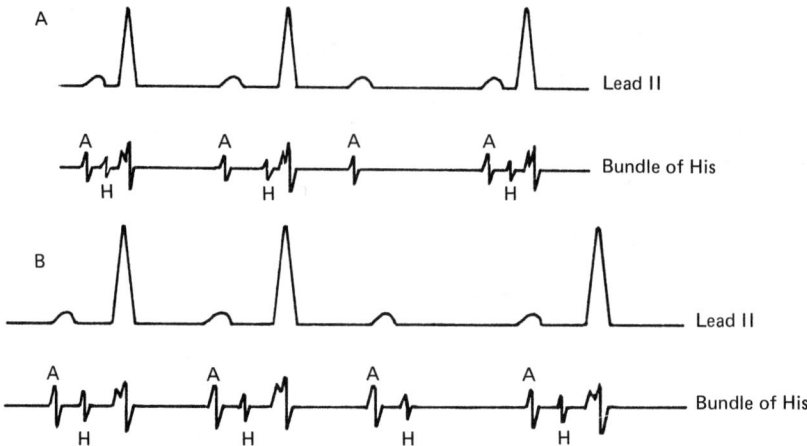

Figure 14–7. Diagrammatic illustrations of bundle of His recordings in second-degree atrioventricular block. **A:** Mobitz type I (Wenckebach) block: The first complex has a normal PR interval with normal AH and HV intervals. The second complex has a prolonged PR interval owing to lengthening of the AH interval. The third P wave is not conducted and is not followed by a bundle of His spike. This indicates that the site of the block is proximal to the His bundle in the atrioventricular node. **B:** Mobitz type II block: The first 2 beats are sinus-conducted, with a prolonged PR interval due to lengthening of the HV interval. The third P wave is not conducted and is followed by a His spike. This indicates that the block is distal to the His bundle. The PR interval is constant for the conducted beats, and the QRS interval is prolonged. (Reproduced, with permission, from Goldman MJ: *Principles of Clinical Electrocardiography*, 12th ed. Lange, 1986.)

incidence of coronary disease, ventricular arrhythmias, and cardiac failure; the high mortality rate is usually due to these causes. If the atrioventricular block is associated with a prolonged AH interval only, one can conclude that although heart disease is present, the risk of complete atrioventricular block is minimal.

B. Second-Degree Atrioventricular Block: In second-degree atrioventricular conduction delay, not every sinus impulse reaches the ventricles, with the result that failure of ventricular contraction occurs and is apparent on auscultation at the bedside by the absence (dropping) of the beat. The failure of conduction on the part of the ventricles allows the conduction system to recover, so that a subsequent beat is transmitted to the ventricles (Figs 14–5 and 14–7).

Second-degree atrioventricular block may be of 2 forms: partial progressive atrioventricular block, in which the PR interval progressively increases, culminating in a dropped beat (Wenckebach or Mobitz type I); or 2:1 block, in which every other beat is not conducted but the PR interval is not progressively prolonged in the beat prior to the dropped beat (usually Mobitz type II as commonly defined) (Fig 14–8). The classification of Mobitz type I and Mobitz type II is only partially helpful, because some patients dem-

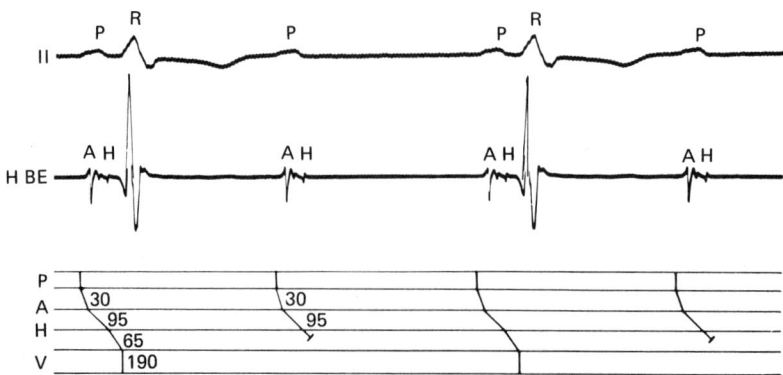

Figure 14–8. Second-degree atrioventricular block (Mobitz type II). Every other atrial impulse is blocked. The QRS is wide (0.12 second). The block occurs below the His bundle owing to a sudden decrement in conduction below the His bundle. HBE, His bundle electrogram. (Reproduced, with permission, from Dreifus LS et al: Atrioventricular block. *Am J Cardiol* 1971;28:371.)

onstrate both type I and type II in the same lead and because the site of the block in 2:1 block cannot be predicted with complete reliability. Although in most patients with 2:1 block the block is distal to the bundle of His, it may be in the atrioventricular node. The width of the QRS complex in the conducted beats is helpful in locating the block—narrow if the block is in the atrioventricular node and wide if below it. Multiple blocks may also be present.

Clinical correlation has shown that Mobitz type I, or partial progressive atrioventricular block, is usually due to conduction delay in the atrioventricular node and associated with a QRS complex of normal width and a heart rate of more than 50 beats/min; it rarely produces Stokes-Adams attacks. This is in contrast to Mobitz type II, which has been shown by His bundle recordings to be due in most cases to conduction delay within or distal to the bundle of His but definitely distal to the atrioventricular node; this form is usually associated with a wide QRS complex, is more apt to progress to complete atrioventricular block with Stokes-Adams attacks, and is associated with a prolonged HV interval in about half of cases. It seems paradoxic that 2:1 atrioventricular block may be associated with a normal HV interval in the conducted beat, but this occurs because of variable conduction delay in different parts of the system. A similar situation obtains in complete atrioventricular block without a phase of partial or complete atrioventricular block. A balanced discussion of second-degree atrioventricular block is that of Zipes (1979).

1. Wenckebach pauses–In partial progressive atrioventricular block (Wenckebach type), the increment in the PR interval between the first and second conducted beats is usually greater than in subsequent conducted beats, with the PR intervals becoming longer and the RR shorter with each beat. The pauses may vary, so that the rhythm can be 2:1, 4:3, 5:4, etc. Although in Mobitz type II the second-degree block is usually associated with a 2:1 rhythm, there may be other intervals such as 3:1 or 4:1. As implied above, His bundle recordings are needed in 2:1 block to see whether the HV interval is prolonged and whether the block is proximal or distal to the His bundle.

2. Dropped beats–Dropped beats must be differentiated from premature beats by noting that there is no heart sound at the apex. Premature beats, even when quite premature, can usually be heard (unless they are blocked supraventricular premature beats) faintly at the apex although not necessarily felt at the wrist. Patients are usually unaware of the dropped beat, and the diagnosis is often made incidentally from a routine ECG or during continuous monitoring of the ECG.

3. His bundle recordings–The division of the PR interval into the AH interval and the HV interval (see p 443) by His bundle recordings has led to an attempt to classify second-degree atrioventricular block by the duration of the HV interval (nodal if the HV interval is normal; infranodal if it is prolonged). But measurement of the HV interval is imprecise, and the interval may be either normal or abnormal, with either a normal or abnormal PR interval or with evidence of infranodal ventricular conduction defect such as left or right bundle branch block or hemiblock (see below).

C. Complete (Third-Degree) Atrioventricular Block: Block usually progresses from first- to second- to third-degree (Fig 14–9), but complete block may occur without preceding partial block, or the PR interval may be normal immediately after a period of complete block. Runs of ventricular tachycardia or fibrillation may interrupt complete atrioventricular block, may be precipitated by exercise, and may be the mechanism for a Stokes-Adams attack (Fig 14–10). The site of the complete atrioventricular block is often suggested by the width of the QRS complex and the ventricular rate. The former is usually normal, and the escape pacemaker has a rate of more than 50/min in atrioventricular nodal complete block (Narula, 1971).

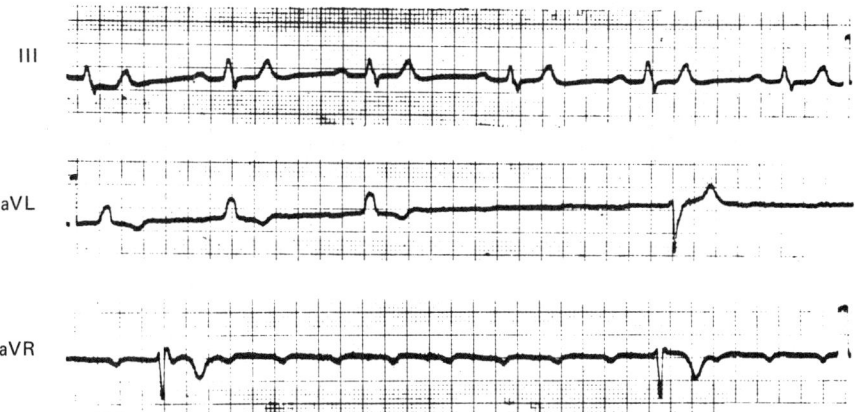

Figure 14–9. Transition from 2:1 atrioventricular block to complete block with ventricular escape following a period of ventricular standstill in a 53-year-old man.

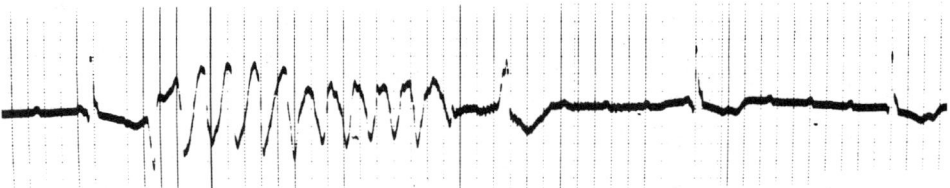

Figure 14–10. Complete atrioventricular block with run of ventricular tachycardia in a 55-year-old woman with atrial flutter.

The QRS complex is usually widened and the heart rate slower when the block is distal to the His bundle. Because of the block, there is dissociation between the atrial and ventricular contractions, but atrioventricular dissociation is not synonymous with atrioventricular block. Atrioventricular dissociation is always present in complete atrioventricular block but may also be present in its absence, as in nonparoxysmal junctional tachycardia or ventricular tachycardia. In these situations, the junctional or ventricular pacemaker rate is faster than the sinus rate and does not permit the latter to activate the ventricles.

1. "Escape" pacemakers–In complete atrioventricular block, survival of the patient depends upon activation of pacemakers distal to the block, which are called "escape" pacemakers. When the block is in the atrioventricular node, the pacemaker may be in the bundle of His, which has an inherently faster rate of spontaneous phase 4 depolarization than do pacemakers lower in the Purkinje system. When the atrioventricular block is distal to the bundle of His, the "escape" pacemaker may be in one of the bundle branches or in the ventricles. These are less reliable and may fail temporarily, leading to cessation of ventricular activity, with Stokes-Adams attacks.

2. Stokes-Adams attacks–Stokes-Adams attacks are manifested by cerebral symptoms due to cerebral ischemia from ventricular asystole in complete atrioventricular block or ventricular conduction defects. Ventricular asystole may follow a period of ventricular fibrillation; therefore, a patient seen late may be thought to have primary ventricular asystole when in fact it was preceded by ventricular fibrillation. In almost all cases of cardiac arrest observed at onset, the mechanism is ventricular fibrillation followed by asystole. The latter obviously can occur de novo. The cerebral symptoms reflect a continuum from momentary transient giddiness to loss of consciousness, convulsions, and sudden death, depending upon the duration of interruption of the cardiac output. The momentary lapse of consciousness resembles a petit mal episode and may last only a few seconds. The attacks are abrupt and unpredictable, can occur without warning many times a day or at intervals of days to years, are variable in severity (duration of syncope), and occur in recumbency as well as in the erect position. The patient falls to the ground without warning and becomes pale and pulseless but rapidly recovers when the ventricles resume beating. There is usually a postischemic flush, and the reactive hyperemia is often so obvious that both the patient and witnesses can describe it. As soon as the ventricles resume beating, the patient feels well and can resume activity. This is in sharp contrast to epilepsy or vasovagal fainting, in which the patient has premonitory symptoms and feels weak and nauseated both before and after. Absence of premonitory symptoms, pallor during and hyperemia after the attack, and rapid recovery are characteristic of Stokes-Adams attacks.

3. Symptoms other than syncope–Depending upon the heart rate and the underlying condition of the ventricle, the patient may be totally asymptomatic despite the presence of complete atrioventricular block or may complain of fatigue and weakness because a normal cardiac output cannot be maintained at the slow rate, especially with physical activity. Any manifestations of cardiac failure or cerebral symptoms due to impaired cerebral perfusion may then develop. A ventricular rate of more than 40/min is usually necessary for the patient to be free of symptoms. There may be episodes of transient dizziness rather than typical Stokes-Adams attacks if the duration of ventricular standstill is short. If ventricular fibrillation occurs, defibrillation is necessary. Asystole lasting 2–3 minutes is usually fatal if not treated.

4. Signs–The physical signs of complete atrioventricular block are due to the slow ventricular rate, the long period of variable diastolic ventricular filling, the large stroke volume resulting from the slow heart rate, and the presence of independent atrial and ventricular contractions. The slow ventricular rate increases only slightly (approximately 5 beats/min) with exercise or following a sympathomimetic drug and is associated with a wide pulse pressure and raised systolic pressure. The large stroke volume produces a variable pulmonary systolic ejection murmur and third heart sound. The most important signs are those related to independent atrial and ventricular contractions with evidence of atrioventricular dissociation. Depending upon the timing of the contractions of the atrium and ventricles, the first sound varies in intensity, so that there may be intermittent loud first sounds as well as atrial sounds. There may be intermittent **"cannon" *a* waves** when the right atrium contracts against a closed tricuspid valve.

5. His bundle recordings–Patients with slow ventricular rates and symptoms should have continuous (Holter) monitoring of the ECG to determine if the episodes of near-syncope or syncope are associated with the development of complete atrioventricular block. Dizziness is a common symptom in older people, and it must be definitely established that the symptom is due to complete block before inserting a pacemaker. Even with other evidence of conduction delay in the bundle branches with bilateral bundle branch block or a prolonged HV interval by His bundle recording, dizziness and weakness may be due to other arrhythmias, postural hypotension, anemia, diffuse cerebral arteriosclerosis, or general debility and not to complete block. This is especially important in patients with bilateral bundle branch block with or without a prolonged PR interval who have syncope or near syncope. His bundle recordings have shown that whether or not the PR interval or HV interval is prolonged, one cannot automatically assume that episodes of syncope or near syncope are due to intermittent complete atrioventricular block. The longer the HV interval, the more likely that episodic syncope is due to the development of complete atrioventricular block, but this is not invariable.

Treatment

A. Partial (First-Degree) Atrioventricular Block: Treatment involves serial observation with ECGs if the conduction defect is chronic. Attempts should be made to eliminate the cause if block is due to use of digitalis or other antiarrhythmic agents, beta-blocking agents, quinidine, or procainamide; to hyperkalemia; or to myocarditis. A decrease in the PR interval following exercise is an encouraging sign, indicating that the conduction defect is benign and in the atrioventricular node. If the patient is symptomatic, with episodic dizziness or syncope suggesting intermittent Stokes-Adams attacks, 24-hour continuous Holter monitoring is indicated to determine if symptoms are due to complete atrioventricular block or another cause (eg, ventricular arrhythmias) not related to bradyarrhythmia. His bundle recordings should should be reserved for symptomatic patients with atrioventricular block, in order to determine if the block is distal to the His bundle.

Patients with first-degree atrioventricular block who have cerebral symptoms proved to be due to bradyarrhythmia are generally advised to undergo insertion of a pacemaker, especially if Holter monitoring reveals episodes of more advanced block. If symptomatic patients are shown by His bundle recordings to have a prolonged AH interval and a normal HV interval, the conduction defect is atrioventricular nodal or supranodal, and the risk of development of complete atrioventricular block is minimal even in the presence of known heart disease. Insertion of a pacemaker in patients with a prolonged HV interval is indicated only if the interval exceeds 80–100 ms, if the patient has neurologic symptoms, or if episodes of syncope are known to be due to high-grade atrioventricular block. Insertion is not indicated in asymptomatic individuals with an HV interval shorter than 80 ms.

B. Second-Degree Atrioventricular Block: If second-degree block is in the atrioventricular node (Mobitz type I), even with inferior myocardial infarction, clinical observation is usually sufficient because progression to complete atrioventricular block and Stokes-Adams attacks is uncommon. It is still not clear if a temporary demand pacemaker should be introduced in patients with inferior myocardial infarction with complete atrioventricular block. Although the likelihood of Stokes-Adams attacks is less than in complete atrioventricular block distal to the atrioventricular node, it is still significant, and we believe it is wise in inferior infarction to insert a pacemaker when the patient develops complete atrioventricular block, especially if early or if symptoms develop that suggest Stokes-Adams attacks. In chronic Mobitz type II atrioventricular block, careful observation with serial ECGs is usually sufficient unless the patient has symptoms suggesting episodic syncope or its equivalent or unless the block develops acutely in the setting of acute anterior infarction with the acute development of bifascicular block, in which case a temporary demand pacemaker is immediately indicated. The decision on what course of action to take will depend upon the age of the patient and the degree of associated atherosclerosis. It is important to determine whether the bifascicular block preceded the acute infarction, because in this instance the prognosis is better and a pacemaker need not be inserted, as would be the case if the bifascicular block developed after the acute infarction.

C. Complete (Third-Degree) Atrioventricular Block: Drugs are rarely used today in complete atrioventricular block because of the almost universal availability of pacemakers. During the interval between recognition of a Stokes-Adams attack and introduction of a temporary or permanent pacemaker, it is wise for the patient to be in the hospital with continuous electrocardiographic monitoring and an intravenous infusion of isoproterenol available.

The treatment of asymptomatic complete atrioventricular block discovered accidentally is a matter of some dispute. The prognosis is worse when a pacemaker is not used, because patients with complete block, especially if over age 60, may develop Stokes-Adams attacks, ventricular arrhythmias, or cardiac or cerebral perfusion abnormalities.

In the past, it was thought that congenital complete atrioventricular block had a favorable prognosis if patients were asymptomatic. However, in long-term follow-up, 35 patients, most less than age 20 years when first seen, developed symptoms presumably due to atrioventricular block, and two-thirds required pacemaker insertion. Symptoms were often absent for many years. The prognosis was worse in patients who developed symptoms in infancy, but most patients required pacemakers before age 50 (Reid, 1982).

If the patient has had a single unequivocal Stokes-Adams attack, a demand pacemaker should be introduced because recurrent attacks are the rule, and any individual episode may be fatal. When atrioventricular block is varying from 2:1 to complete, a demand pacemaker should be inserted because during the transition there may be ventricular asystole with Stokes-Adams attacks and the patient is at greater risk of ventricular fibrillation. Dramatic improvement in cardiac failure, relief of cerebral symptoms and of syncope or near-syncope, and improved survival result from the use of pacemakers in patients with permanent or intermittent complete atrioventricular block. The pacemaker should be set at 70–80 beats/min; the new programmable pacemakers permit variation of rate, depending upon the response of the patient.

The effect of a temporary pacemaker should always be determined before permanent insertion. Even though it may not be established that dizziness or near-syncope is due to complete atrioventricular block, this diagnosis is strongly suspected if a patient has partial or 2:1 atrioventricular block. If the symptoms are thought to be due to complete atrioventricular block that has not been documented, a temporary ventricular pacemaker should relieve the symptoms and clarify the diagnosis. If the patient has documented complete atrioventricular block with Stokes-Adams attacks, a temporary pacemaker is not required and a permanent pacemaker should be inserted promptly. The mortality rate in a group of patients paced for atrioventricular block compared to that expected in the population at large was 1.7 to 1 in one study (Ginks, 1979). The mortality rate was higher in the first year of pacing than subsequently. The most important factor influencing prognosis was a history of myocardial infarction. Late sudden death occurred in one-fourth of patients.

D. Proper Functioning of Pacemakers: (See Chapter 7.) After being provided with a pacemaker, the patient should be closely observed to confirm its proper functioning, especially during the first month. Recurrence of symptoms suggests that positioning of the electrode catheter has been faulty or that the catheter has moved, and Holter monitoring should be employed to correlate symptoms with the possibility of such faulty pacing. The rate of the pacemaker and its functioning should be checked periodically—weekly for the first month, monthly for 1–2 years, and then more frequently as battery failure is anticipated. The patient or a family member should be taught to count the pulse rate, learn the significance of changes in rate, and immediately report such changes to the physician. Details of the newer types and modes of demand and atrioventricular synchronous pacing are described by Harthorne (1981).

E. Unexplained Syncope: Electrophysiologic studies in patients with unexplained syncope have shown that about one-third have ventricular arrhythmias, a smaller percentage conduction defects, and approximately half an unknown cause. Appropriate therapy can be instituted in one-fourth to one-third of these patients, and about half have no further episodes of syncope even in the absence of definitive treatment (Hess, 1982).

VENTRICULAR CONDUCTION DEFECTS & BUNDLE BRANCH BLOCK

Bundle branch block is an electrocardiographic finding, usually an unexpected one. It is uncommon before age 60 and increases in frequency with age. Most patients with bundle branch block have associated cardiovascular disease or develop it within a few years; approximately 20% have no obvious abnormality of the heart. Bundle branch block is diagnosed when the QRS complex exceeds 0.12 second, with late delay in the right precordial leads in right bundle branch block and in the left ventricular leads in left bundle branch block, combined with depressed ST and asymmetrically inverted T waves opposite to the direction of the QRS delay in the leads with late delay in the QRS complex (rsR' complexes). The block may be intermittent (Fig 14–11) or may develop over a period of years.

The concept of bundle branch block, whether right or left, implies that the branch is in fact blocked, whereas anatomically and functionally there is merely a delay in conduction in the bundle branches. The term "conduction delay" rather than "block" is therefore preferable, and the degree of the delay can be expressed as minor, incomplete, or complete.

Left Bundle Branch Block

Left bundle branch block is most frequently found in individuals with clinical evidence of heart disease. In the absence of other evidence of heart disease, it can be associated with many years of normal life. When left bundle branch block occurs for the first time and is known not to have been present before, the chances of developing clinical cardiac disease and of sudden death are greater. Latent coronary disease may be the cause (Rabkin, 1980; Fisch, 1980; Schneider, 1979).

The left bundle is not a discrete entity, as is the right bundle, and the division into left anterior and right posterior divisions is purely arbitrary. When left bundle branch block occurs in the presence of anterior myocardial infarction, the prognosis is better and the incidence of complete atrioventricular block lower than when right bundle branch block is present in association with acute myocardial infarction. Left bundle branch block obscures the electrocardiographic diagnosis of acute myocardial infarction (Fig 14–12); radioisotopic methods (see Chapter 8) may be useful in diagnosis under these circumstances.

Myocardial ischemia can also be masked by a pacemaker rhythm and may become apparent when the pacemaker is turned off (Fig 14–13). Care must be taken to exclude nonspecific T wave changes.

Right Bundle Branch Block

Right bundle branch block, especially incomplete block, occurs in many normal individuals. If one includes as showing right ventricular conduction defects those ECGs with an r' in the right precordial leads, the percentage in the general population may be as

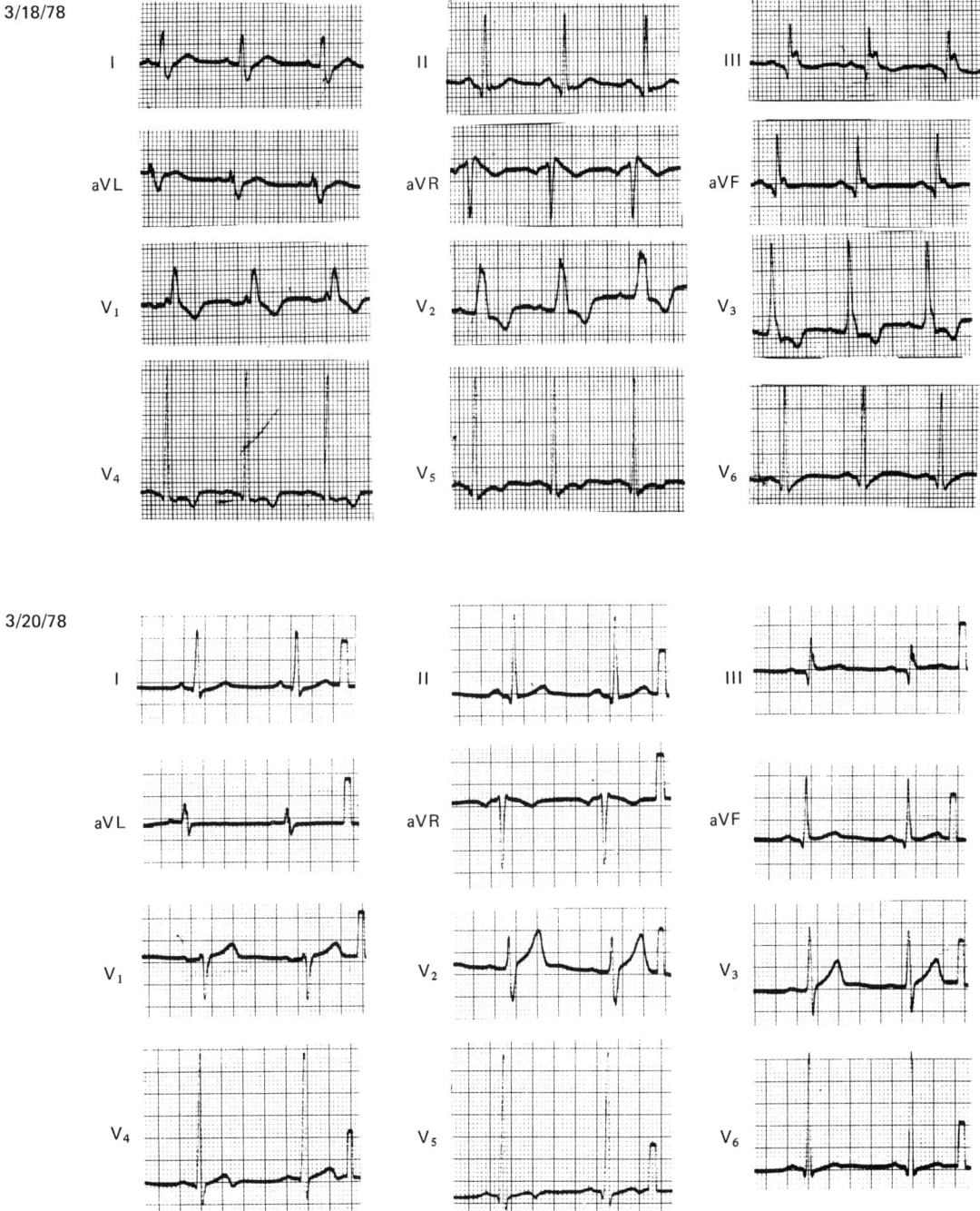

Figure 14–11. Intermittent right bundle branch block (top tracing) in a 63-year-old man with postoperative esophagitis. Two days later, conduction was normal (bottom tracing).

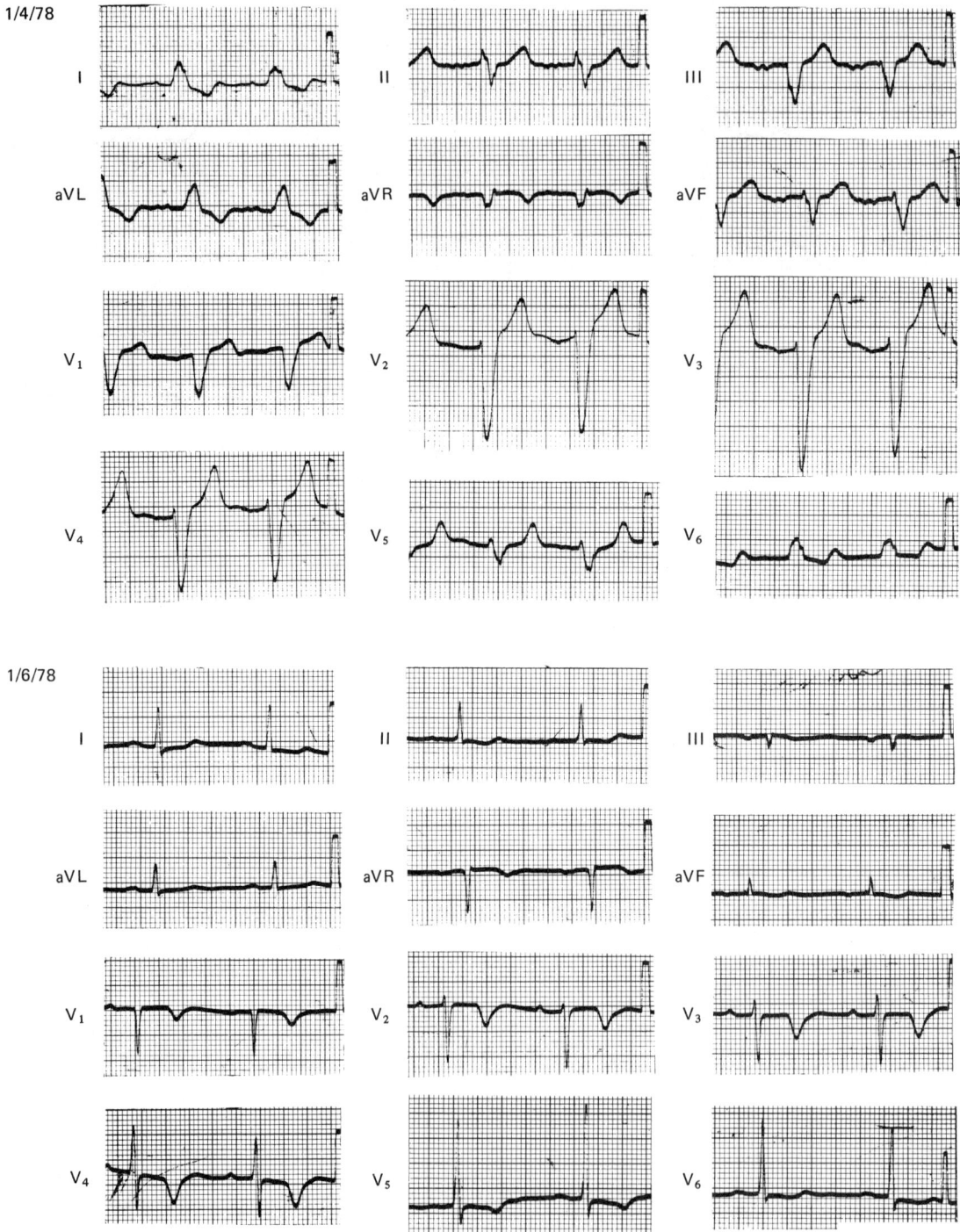

Figure 14–12. Intermittent left bundle branch block (top tracing) in an 80-year-old man following gastric bleeding. Second tracing 2 days later (bottom tracing) reveals apparent acute myocardial ischemia, but repolarization changes after left bundle branch block occur in the absence of any known heart disease.

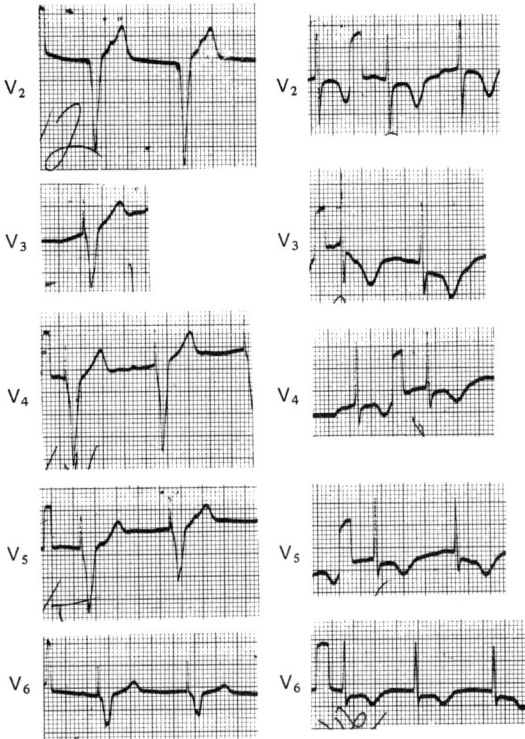

Figure 14–13. ECG on the left shows pacemaker precordial leads (rate 73/min), with upright T waves obscuring myocardial ischemia in an 84-year-old man. ECG on the right shows inverted T waves probably due to myocardial ischemia in leads V_{2-6} when demand pacemaker is "turned off" by a slightly faster heart rate of 87/min. Inverted T waves may also occur in the absence of ischemia.

high as 10%. When a right or left bundle branch block occurs in the presence of associated cardiac disease, its significance depends on the nature of the cardiac disease, associated defects in the fascicles of the left bundle, a prolonged PR interval, and symptoms suggesting intermittent, more advanced heart block. Bundle branch block may be intermittent (Figs 14–11) or may progress over a period of years. Transient right bundle branch block (complete or incomplete) may follow the development of acute right ventricular dilatation in acute pulmonary embolism. Pulmonary hypertension develops transiently, causing right ventricular dilatation and an electrocardiographic pattern of right ventricular conduction defect.

Right bundle branch block is more common in acute myocardial infarction than is left bundle branch block and may be rapidly followed by complete atrioventricular block, especially if the patient has associated left anterior hemiblock. The right bundle is supplied anatomically by the first septal perforator branch of the left anterior descending artery. Right bundle branch block, therefore, is common when necrosis of the proximal portion of the septum occurs as a result of occlusion of the proximal left anterior descending artery. In chronic right just as in chronic left bundle branch block, His bundle recordings have shown that HV prolongation, indicating extension of the conduction defect to the more distal branches of the right and left bundles, is present in many instances of left bundle branch block (less so in right bundle branch block), whether the PR interval is normal or prolonged.

Isolated right bundle branch block has been subdivided into proximal block and distal block, with different prognoses. Patients with distal delay have episodes of syncope or near-syncope, which are rare in proximal block. The distinction can be made by noting whether the delay in pulmonary valve opening is mainly between mitral and tricuspid valve closure (proximal block) or between tricuspid valve closure and pulmonary valve opening (distal block) (Dancy, 1982).

Examination over a period of months or years or monitoring of the ECG for 24 hours in patients with either right or left bundle branch block will often reveal paroxysmal atrioventricular block, indicating that the ventricular conduction defects precede and may be the earliest precursors of complete atrioventricular block. Twenty-four-hour monitoring and careful clinical observation are indicated in patients with isolated bundle branch block who have symptoms suggesting bradyarrhythmia.

Bilateral Bundle Branch Block

In bilateral bundle branch block (right bundle branch block and left anterior hemiblock, right bundle branch block and left posterior hemiblock, or right or left bundle branch block with prolonged PR interval or alternating right and left bundle branch block), the heart presumably depends on the remaining fascicle for conduction of the atrial impulse to the ventricle (Fisch, 1980). The incidence of complete atrioventricular block is probably about 1% per year in unselected asymptomatic patients found or known to have bifascicular block (Fig 14–14).

The presence of an atrioventricular conduction defect, whether it be a prolonged HV interval or second-degree block, does not necessarily mean that Stokes-Adams attacks are likely or that a pacemaker is necessary. *Further prospective studies and clinical judgment are required before pacemaker implantation can be justified solely on the basis of the ECG or His bundle findings in the absence of symptoms shown to be due to bradyarrhythmias.*

Unifascicular & Bifascicular Block

The main left bundle branch of the bundle of His usually divides into 2 main branches, the left anterior superior and the left posterior fascicles. Anatomically, the division is often much more complex, but for clinical purposes it is sufficient to assume only the 2 divisions. Left anterior hemiblock is diagnosed when the frontal plane QRS axis is to the left and superior, between −45 and −90 degrees in association with right bundle branch block. There is an *r* wave and a

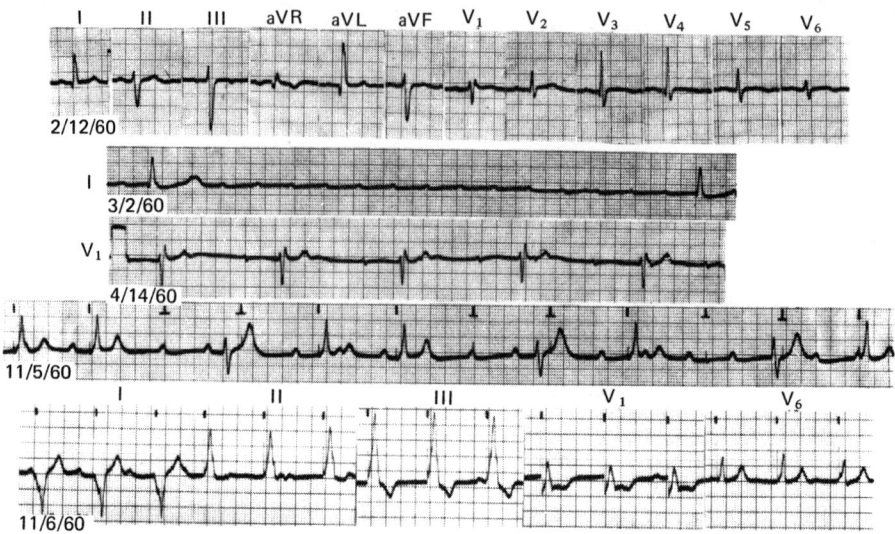

Figure 14–14. Five successive ECGs of a 58-year-old man suffering from Stokes-Adams attacks. First tracing, February 12, 1960. Regular sinus rhythm 66/min, practically normal PR interval measuring 0.20 second, atypical right bundle branch block with QRS axis –60 degrees and left anterior hemiblock (bifascicular block), T axis +20 degrees, QRS duration = 0.12 second, rSr' pattern in V_1 (r' delay = 0.08 second), qr or QR pattern in aVR and aVL; measured in aVL, the left ventricular activation time would be delayed to 0.09 second. The third tracing, recorded on April 14, 1960, showed a complete atrioventricular block (76/36), with a right ventricular delay (identical in pattern as when in sinus rhythm); a ventricular pause of 7 seconds is seen in the record of March 2. The last 2 tracings, recorded after electrical stimulation, showed one an intermittent and the other a regular response. (Reproduced, with permission, from Lenegre J: Etiology and pathology of bilateral bundle branch block in relation to complete heart block. *Prog Cardiovasc Dis* 1964;**6**:409.)

prominent S wave in leads II and III. There are also q waves in leads I and aVL. The differentiation from an old inferior myocardial infarction is not always easy. Left posterior hemiblock is diagnosed when there is right axis deviation greater than 120 degrees, provided that right ventricular hypertrophy or old lateral myocardial infarction (both of which may cause right axis deviation) can be excluded.

Left anterior hemiblock is much more common than left posterior hemiblock. Although the incidence of chronic asymptomatic left anterior hemiblock increases with age, it is not a sensitive indicator of clinical cardiac disease (Corne, 1978). The prevalence of left anterior hemiblock in 16,000 life insurance applicants was only 2.5%.

The causes of bifascicular block are chiefly those of ventricular conduction defects anywhere: hypertensive or coronary heart disease, fibrosis of the conduction system, and primary myocardial disease. Bifascicular block is more common in men. The average age of patients when first seen is about 60 years. Coronary disease, arrhythmias on Holter monitoring, and congestive heart failure are more common when the HV interval is prolonged (Dhingra, 1981).

In bifascicular block with right bundle branch block and left anterior or left posterior hemiblock, it is assumed that 2 of the 3 fascicles that are extensions from the bundle of His are involved, and survival depends on adequate functioning of the remaining third fascicle. Careful follow-up (including ambulatory ECG monitoring) is sufficient in asymptomatic bifascicular block unless the patient develops cerebral symptoms thought (or found by Holter monitoring) to be due to atrioventricular block. If the symptoms strongly suggest Stokes-Adams attacks and the diagnosis is documented by continuous monitoring of the ECG, a prophylactic right ventricular pacemaker is recommended (Scheinman, 1982).

Although patients with bifascicular block may die suddenly, only 5% in one study had developed documented complete atrioventricular block over a period of years. Many patients with bifascicular block have a history of angina, bundle branch block, or ventricular arrhythmias, and sudden death can occur without complete atrioventricular block. Although sudden death is a major cause of death in these patients, most deaths are due to ventricular arrhythmias or cardiac failure and not to atrioventricular block. Prophylactic pacing is therefore not recommended unless patients with dizziness or syncope have documented bradyarrhythmias associated with their symptoms. In these chronically ill patients, dizziness and syncope may be due to many causes, including drugs, conduction defects, bleeding, postural hypotension, paroxysmal arrhythmias, aortic stenosis, cardiomyopathy, and vasovagal fainting, among others. Table 14–5 tabulates the causes of syncope in patients with chronic bifascicular block and demonstrates the rarity with which atrioventric-

Table 14–5. Causes of syncope in 30 of 186 patients with chronic bifascicular block.*
RBBB, right bundle branch block; LAH, left anterior hemiblock; LPH, left posterior hemiblock; LBBB, left bundle branch block.

Cause	RBBB and LAH (124)†	RBBB and LPH (24)†	LBBB (38)†
Second- or third-degree atrioventricular block	3	1	1
Sinoatrial block	–	1	–
Orthostatic hypotension	2	–	–
Seizure disorders	3	–	–
Gastrointestinal bleeding	–	–	1
Ventricular arrhythmia	5	1	3
Unknown	8	–	1
Total	21	3	6

*Reproduced, with permission, from Dhingra RC et al: Evaluation and management of conduction disease. *Cardiovasc Med* 1978;**3**:493.
†Number of patients in subgroup.

ular or sinoatrial block occurs in these patients. Table 14–6 sets forth the criteria for permanent pacemaker therapy in patients with conduction defects.

Because of the hazard of abrupt onset of complete atrioventricular block and syncope, a conservative course of action is *not* advised in acute anterior myocardial infarction, in which a pacemaker should be promptly introduced when left anterior hemiblock with right bundle branch block (bifascicular block) develops.

Bifascicular block with right bundle branch block and left posterior hemiblock is often overdiagnosed because right axis deviation exceeding 110 degrees can be found in normal thin individuals or those with right ventricular hypertrophy. A marked superior axis, even to the right, can occur with some varieties of anterolateral myocardial infarction. Left posterior hemiblock is an uncommon condition.

Indications for His Bundle Studies

These are still in the process of being evaluated, but a list of definitive indications by one experienced physician is as follows: (1) Cardiac arrhythmias with difficulties in management; (2) Wolff-Parkinson-White syndrome; (3) patients with sinus node dysfunction, to evaluate the site of pacemaker insertion (whether atrial or ventricular); (4) patients with calcific aortic stenosis who have syncope; (5) patients who have abnormal ECGs and are scheduled for major cardiac surgery; and (6) symptomatic patients with atrioventricular block or bundle branch block, to confirm or exclude atrioventricular conduction defects as the underlying mechanism for syncope (Narula, 1977). Many cardiologists would not agree on some of these indications, especially (4) and (5). Transient complete heart block occurred only once in 52 operating procedures in patients with chronic bundle branch block and left axis deviation who required noncardiac surgery (Pastore, 1978).

Intermittent or Rate-Dependent Conduction Defects

Conduction defects are not static, and electrocardiographic abnormalities may be present on one occasion and absent at other times (Fig 14–14). Atrioventricular block, bundle branch block, and bifascicular block may vary with the heart rate and be either bradycardia- or tachycardia-dependent.

Table 14–6. Criteria for permanent pacemaker therapy in patients with conduction disease.*

	Without Acute Myocardial Infarction		During Acute Myocardial Infarction	
	Bifascicular Block	Second- or Third-Degree Atrioventricular Block	Bifascicular Block	Second- or Third-Degree Atrioventricular Block
Pacemaker	Symptomatic patients with documented bradyarrhythmia. Recurrent syncope due to unknown cause. Repetitive atrioventricular block distal to His bundle on pacing in symptomatic patients.	Symptomatic patients with block at any site. Asymptomatic patients with block in or distal to His bundle.	With prolonged HV interval.	Type II second-degree block. Third-degree atrioventricular block with wide QRS rhythm.
Pacemaker not needed	Asymptomatic patients with or without PR prolongation.	Asymptomatic patients with block proximal to His bundle.		
Controversial	Symptomatic patients with prolonged HV interval and without documented bradyarrhythmia.		Without prolonged HV interval.	Type I second- or third-degree atrioventricular block with narrow QRS. Transient third-degree atrioventricular block.

*Reproduced, with permission, from Dhingra RC et al: Evaluation and management of conduction disease. *Cardiovasc Med* 1978; **3**:493.

VENTRICULAR PREEXCITATION
(Accelerated Conduction Syndrome; Wolff-Parkinson-White Syndrome)

Ventricular preexcitation is usually congenital and can be defined as preexcitation (premature excitation) of the ventricles resulting from accessory or anomalous bypass pathways between the atria and the ventricle, either bypassing the atrioventricular node or being conducted through the atrioventricular node in an accelerated fashion through special pathways.

Preexcitation may occur by a number of accessory pathways (Fig 14–15). In addition to the normal spread of activation from the atria to the ventricles via the atrioventricular node, early activation of the ventricle occurs along a complex system of accessory pathways, as shown by epicardial mapping and surgical interruption of the pathways (Gallagher, *Circulation* 1978). The lateral accessory pathway (bundle of Kent) enters a portion of the ventricular myocardium from the atrium. Mahaim fibers may pass from the bundle of His to the ventricular myocardium, and pathways may spread from the internodal atrial tracks to the ventricular myocardium, bypassing the upper part of the atrioventricular node via the James fibers. The precise anatomy of the bypass track can only be determined by epicardial mapping. The orientation of the delta wave gives a clue to the location of the accessory pathways, which may be anterior, posterior, septal, lateral, or a combination of these sites (Fig 14–15).

Preexcitation may be constant or intermittent, the latter often brought on by a change in atrial rate. Because the ventricle is activated both via the accessory pathway and through the normal atrioventricular nodal pathway, fusion ventricular beats may occur. The syndrome occurs in 0.5–2% of the population,

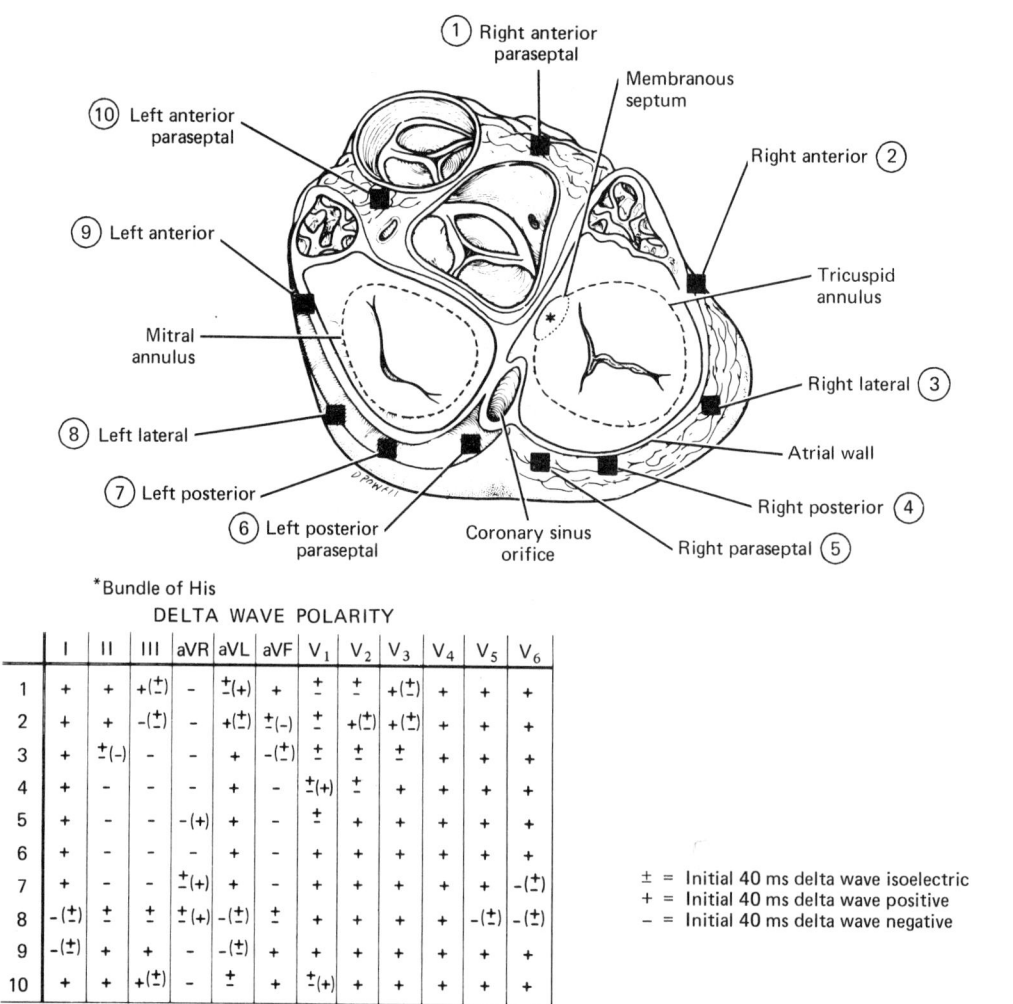

Figure 14–15. Polarity of the delta wave in different leads in various types of preexcitation. (Reproduced, with permission, from Gallagher JJ et al: The preexcitation syndromes. *Prog Cardiovasc Dis* 1978;**20**:285.)

Table 14–7. Effect of drugs in Wolff-Parkinson-White syndrome.*

Drug	Duration of Effective Refractory Period					Shortest RR Interval Between 2 Preexcited Beats During Atrial Fibrillation
	Atrium	Atrio-ventricular Node	His-Purkinje	Ventricle	Accessory Pathway	
Digitalis	±	+	0	±	−	−
Quinidine	+	−	+	+	+	+
Procainamide	+	−	+	+	+	+
Lidocaine	±	±	−	+	+	+
Disopyramide	+	−	±	+	+	?
Amiodarone	+	+	+	+	+	+
Ajmaline (IV)†	+	0	+	+	+	+
Propranolol	0	+	0	0	0	0
Phenytoin	±	−	−	±	±	?
Verapamil	±	+	0	±	±	?

*Modified and reproduced, with permission, from Gallagher JJ et al: The preexcitation syndromes. *Prog Cardiovasc Dis* 1978; 20:285.
†Investigational; +, prolonged; −, shortened; 0, no change; ±, variable; ?, unknown.

and paroxysmal atrial arrhythmias occur in half of affected individuals. Tables 14–7 and 14–8 summarize the effect of drugs and the results of surgery in 83 patients.

1. LOWN-GANONG-LEVINE SYNDROME

The Lown-Ganong-Levine syndrome (Lown, 1952) is a "forme fruste" of Wolff-Parkinson-White syndrome, characterized on the ECG by a short PR interval and normal QRS interval without a delta wave. It is thought to represent a variety of short-circuiting of the upper part of the atrioventricular node (via James fibers) and is also associated with increased frequency of paroxysmal atrial arrhythmias. The arrhythmias observed in Lown-Ganong-Levine syndrome include mostly atrial and ventricular premature beats; however, paroxysmal supraventricular tachycardia as well as ventricular tachycardia may occur (Benditt, 1978; Monahan, 1975). Concealed accessory pathways for retrograde conduction occur in some patients with paroxysmal tachycardia, and individual electrophysiologic evaluation is necessary (see p 457). A fast intranodal pathway in the typical dual atrioventricular nodal pathway that occurs normally may be the mechanism for the reentrant paroxysmal tachycardia in Lown-Ganong-Levine syndrome (Josephson, 1977). Aberrancy occurs because the ventricular complex resulting from the atrial premature beat occurs during the relative refractory period of the preceding depolarization before repolarization is complete. Ven-

Table 14–8. Summary of Wolff-Parkinson-White syndrome surgery, 1968–1977.*

Results	First 40 Patients	Last 43 Patients	Comment
Cure	21	37	No preexcitation, no antiarrhythmic drug, no arrhythmia
Preexcitation syndrome modified			
Preexcitation persists; no antiarrhythmic drugs required	2	1	No arrhythmias; preexcitation in 2 due to second AP distinct from one operated on
Preexcitation persists; antiarrhythmic drugs required	6	3	Arrhythmia easily managed on drugs in contrast to preoperative state
AP intact; His bundle ablated (pacemaker); no antiarrhythmic drugs required	3	2	No arrhythmia
AP intact; His bundle ablated (pacemaker); antiarrhythmic drugs required	2	0	Arrhythmia controlled
No change in preexcitation or arrhythmia control	3	0	One death 4 years postoperatively due to persistent arrhythmia
Surgical deaths	3	0	Cardiomyopathy in 2; persistent arrhythmia in ?Wolff-Parkinson-White syndrome in one
Asymptomatic or markedly improved	34/37	43/43	

*Reproduced, with permission, from Gallagher JJ et al: The preexcitation syndromes. *Prog Cardiovasc Dis* 1978;20:285.
AP, accessory pathway.

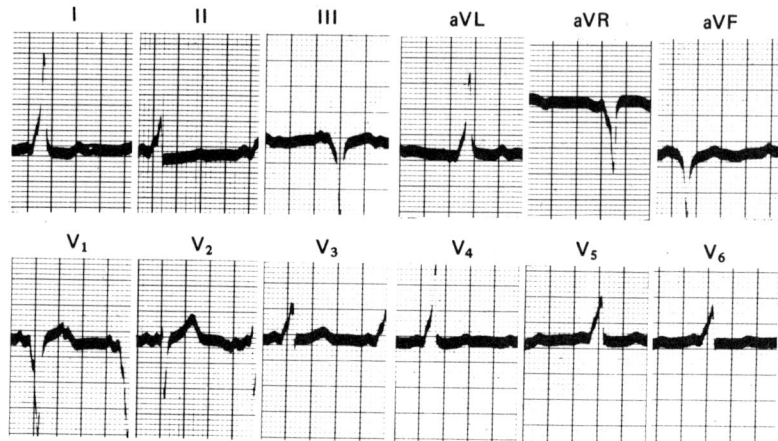

Figure 14–16. Wolff-Parkinson-White syndrome in a 26-year-old woman. The superior orientation of the delta vector (type B) produces QS complexes in aVF that simulate inferior infarction. Note the short PR and the slurred initial upstroke of the QRS (the delta wave) producing a wide QRS complex in leads I, aVL, V_5, and V_6.

tricular depolarization following the atrial premature beat begins, therefore, at a less negative maximum resting potential and alters phase 0 of the action potential.

We know of no attempts at surgical correction. This may be because a dual pathway in the atrioventricular node rather than an accessory bypass track may be responsible for the preexcitation.

2. WOLFF-PARKINSON-WHITE SYNDROME

Preexcitation due to Wolff-Parkinson-White syndrome (Wolff, 1930) has been classified according to the location of the accessory bypass, but the classification is incomplete because a variety of subtypes have recently been discovered by electrophysiologic study. Conventionally, type A preexcitation is from the left accessory bypass, producing an electrocardiographic pattern in V_1 resembling right ventricular hypertrophy or right bundle branch block. Type B preexcitation results from early activation via the right lateral accessory pathway, producing an electrocardiographic change similar to that of left bundle branch block (Figs 14–16 and 14–17). Subgroups can be identified by special electrophysiologic techniques that by epicardial mapping may identify patients who may be helped by ablation of the accessory or anomalous pathways.

The electrocardiographic classification originally proposed by Rosenbaum (1945) has been extended by the work of Gallagher (*Prog Cardiovasc Dis* 1978), with special reference to the polarity of the delta wave, resulting in probable identification of 10 different anatomic locations of accessory pathways (Fig 14–15).

The spatial orientation of the delta vector in patients

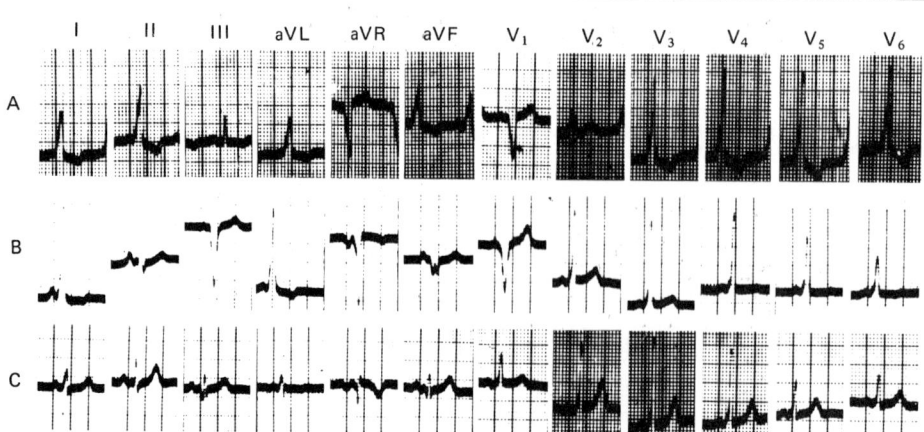

Figure 14–17. Three examples of Wolff-Parkinson-White syndrome. *A:* Woman age 17. *B:* Man age 39. *C:* Woman age 57.

with Wolff-Parkinson-White syndrome gives some indication of the location of the accessory pathway, but electrophysiologic studies are required for precise localization. Some pathways are difficult to identify, but some can be inferred. The polarity of the delta wave in various types of epicardial preexcitation is illustrated in Fig 14–15. Epicardial mapping to determine the site of the accessory pathways should be performed only if the patient has disabling atrial arrhythmias and cardiac surgery is contemplated. On the other hand, His bundle recordings with programmed electrical stimulation are desirable in almost all cases of Wolff-Parkinson-White syndrome to determine the refractory period of the accessory pathway. If the refractory period is short, drugs such as digitalis, which shorten it further, are hazardous, especially if the patient has atrial fibrillation (Table 14–7).

The effective refractory period of the accessory pathway ranges from 200 ms to as long as 900 ms, with most of the periods between 200 and 400 ms (Gallagher, 1976). This wide range must be appreciated, as must the significance of the short refractory periods, which may result in rapid ventricular responses to atrial fibrillation.

Clinical Findings

A. Symptoms and Signs: The diagnosis is made electrocardiographically, even in patients who do not have a history of paroxysmal arrhythmia. During the arrhythmia it may be difficult to see the characteristic pattern, especially if there is a rapid atrial rate. The typical findings include a short PR interval, a wide QRS complex, and a slurred delta wave at the onset of the QRS, representing ventricular preexcitation via the bypass through the accessory pathway. The total PR interval plus the QRS interval is essentially normal (Fig 14–17). The delta wave is usually short—about 0.05 second—and the PR interval in rare cases may be essentially normal. About half of patients have no symptoms; the remainder have episodes of paroxysmal atrial arrhythmia which in some cases may only be noted by 12- to 24-hour Holter monitoring. Palpitations due to arrhythmia are the presenting symptom in many patients; they may last a few seconds and produce trivial or no concern or may last hours and be disabling. It was once thought that death was rare during an attack of arrhythmia. This opinion has been modified, possibly because of the very rapid ventricular rates that may occur if the patient has atrial fibrillation and because of the adverse effect of digitalis in such circumstances, with occasional deterioration to ventricular fibrillation and death. Digitalis increases conduction through the accessory pathway and does not slow the ventricular rate.

Approximately one-third of patients with Wolff-Parkinson-White syndrome develop atrial fibrillation at some time. The duration of the refractory period of the accessory pathway is of considerable therapeutic importance in these patients; if it shortens at rapid atrial rates, the frequent impulses from the atrium in atrial fibrillation may spread directly to the ventricle via the accessory pathway, causing rapid ventricular rates and collapse. Ventricular fibrillation may follow. Patients in whom the accessory pathway has a short refractory period usually have a rapid ventricular response if atrial fibrillation occurs. If the ventricular rate cannot be determined during an attack of atrial fibrillation, atrial fibrillation should be induced experimentally by rapid atrial stimulation to determine the ventricular rate. If the rate is rapid, indicating direct transmission of rapid atrial impulses to the ventricle via the accessory pathway, drugs such as digitalis that shorten the effective refractory period of the accessory pathway should not be used (see p 459).

The mechanism of the atrial arrhythmia is that of reentry, in which impulses from the atria usually pass through the normal atrioventricular conduction system to the ventricle and then return in retrograde fashion to the atria via the anomalous pathway (Fig 14–18). When the atria, the atrioventricular junction, and the atrioventricular node are no longer refractory, the retrograde impulse may reexcite portions of the specialized normal atrioventricular pathway that conduct to the ventricles and so set up a self-perpetuating circuit and normalize the QRS. Recent electrophysiologic studies have shown that the circuit is antegrade through the normal atrioventricular pathway and retrograde through the anomalous bypass pathway because the refractory period of the latter is usually (not always) shorter. Rarely, the reverse pathway may be the mechanism of the reentry tachycardia. The impulse is retrograde via the atrioventricular node and antegrade through the accessory pathway (Fig 14–18), and the pattern thus simulates ventricular tachycardia because of the aberrant QRS complexes.

B. His Bundle and Intracardiac Recordings: His bundle recordings and epicardial mapping have further delineated the mechanisms of Wolff-Parkinson-White syndrome.

The relationship of the His bundle spike to the delta wave is a function of the HV interval. The HQ or the HV interval is less than normal (usually 30–50 ms) when Wolff-Parkinson-White syndrome is present. When conduction from the atrioventricular node is prolonged, the H spike may either follow the delta wave or be "lost" in the QRS complex because excitation of the ventricles precedes that of the His bundle, presumably by bypass tracks.

Wellens (1974) found an almost linear relationship between the shortest RR interval (the most rapid ventricular response) during atrial fibrillation and the effective refractory period of the accessory pathway. When the effective refractory period was 200 ms, the RR interval was 200 ms. When the effective refractory period was 300 ms, the shortest RR interval during atrial fibrillation was 300 ms. This was true not only in a series of 16 patients but also in each patient in the series in whom consecutive RR intervals were measured. The duration of the refractory period following administration of various antiarrhythmic agents was determined by Wellens (1975) (see also Table

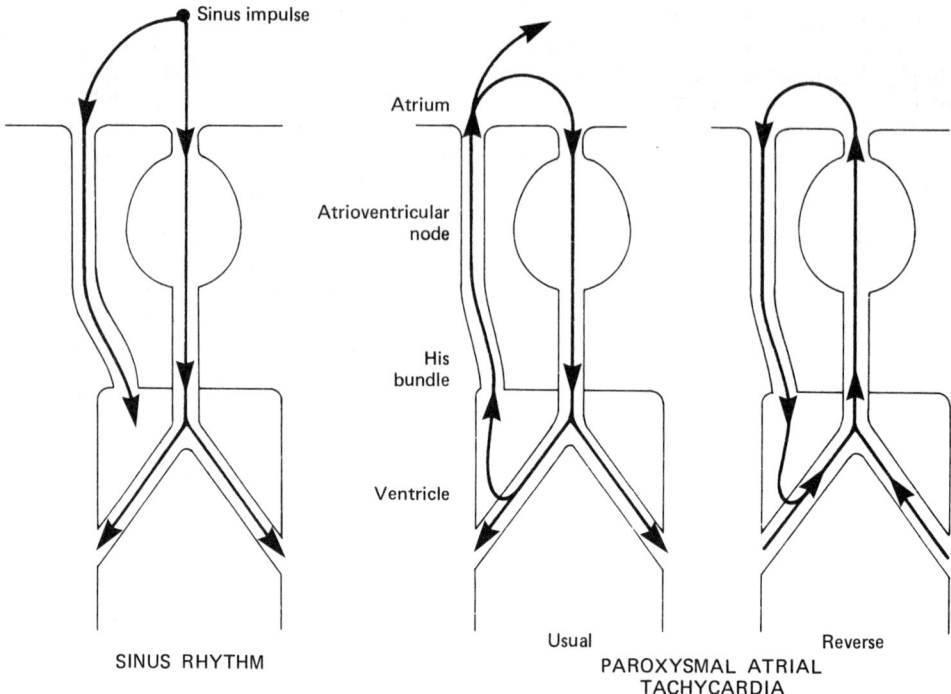

Figure 14-18. Diagram of the normal conduction system and the accessory atrioventricular connection showing the conduction sequence during sinus rhythm in the left-hand panel and during tachycardia in the 2 right-hand panels. (Arrows show the direction of the reverse of the conduction sequence during tachycardia if the impulse spreads from the atrium via the bypass accessory pathway and returns through the atrioventricular node in retrograde fashion.) (Modified and reproduced, with permission, from Spurrell RAJ, Krikler DM, Sowton E: Problems concerning assessment of anatomical site of accessory pathway in Wolff-Parkinson-White syndrome. *Br Heart J* 1975;**37**:127.)

14-7 and p 459). All of the common antiarrhythmic agents either increased the refractory period of the accessory pathway or had no effect—with the exception of digitalis, which decreased it. Procainamide and quinidine increased the HV interval, but digitalis, phenytoin, atropine, propranolol, lidocaine, and verapamil had no effect. The drugs had contrasting effects on the refractory period of the atrioventricular node. Digitalis, propranolol, and verapamil prolonged it; quinidine had a variable effect, decreasing it in some and increasing it in others; and atropine decreased the refractory period of the atrioventricular node, as did lidocaine. Procainamide may increase the refractory period of the accessory pathways from 275 to 400 ms and is therefore a safe drug to use in Wolff-Parkinson-White syndrome.

C. Epicardial Mapping: Epicardial mapping reveals the basis of the ECG in Wolff-Parkinson-White syndrome and identifies the accessory pathways by noting the activation of the ventricles that coincides with the delta wave. Fig 14-19 shows this graphically. At 2 the delta wave coincides with the antegrade activation of the right ventricle at the time of the delta wave. The latter part of the QRS is a fusion wave that results from activation of the ventricle from both the accessory pathway and the normal pathway. When the ventricle is activated early but the QRS complex is normal in duration, the connection between the atria and the His bundle is by way of the James fibers, bypassing the upper part of the atrioventricular node. This is probably the mechanism of the Lown-Ganong-Levine syndrome.

The technique of epicardial mapping is described in detail by Boineau (1975). The timing of the arrival of the excitation wave in various parts of the ventricle defines the site of the accessory pathway and is best predicted by the delta vectors, as in Fig 14-15.

The technique of electrophysiologic epicardial mapping has been further described by Gallagher (*Circulation* 1978). Details of the procedure are given, and the authors describe their efforts to define both the atrial and ventricular insertions of the accessory pathways by both retrograde and antegrade mapping. Epicardial mapping is a highly technical procedure requiring skilled personnel, but it can provide data on antegrade and retrograde preexcitation. It should not be undertaken without careful preoperative electrophysiologic study. The technique has limited application because of the difficult technical procedures involved.

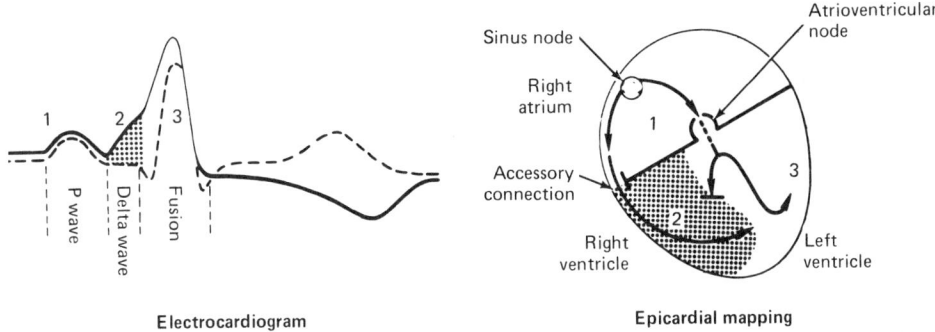

Figure 14-19. Basis of the ECG in Wolff-Parkinson-White syndrome. (Reproduced, with permission, from Boineau JP et al: Epicardial mapping in Wolff-Parkinson-White syndrome. *Arch Intern Med* 1975;**135**:422.)

Treatment

Asymptomatic patients in whom the condition is discovered by chance during a routine ECG should be informed of the nature and significance of the syndrome. Electrophysiologic investigation of paroxysmal arrhythmias is indicated in patients whose attacks of tachycardia are severe and not readily prevented or treated or if the arrhythmia is paroxysmal atrial fibrillation. The most important purpose of these special investigations is to determine the effective refractory period of the accessory pathway, the RR interval during induced atrial fibrillation, and the effect of pharmacologic agents on it, not only to be certain that the drug selected does not decrease the refractory period of the accessory pathway but also to determine which of several drugs effectively terminates the reentry circuit. The effects of various drugs on the refractory period of the accessory pathway, the atrioventricular node, and the HV interval of atrioventricular conduction have already been discussed. Amiodarone prolongs the effective refractory period of both the atrium and the ventricle, preventing the initiation of reentry tachycardia as well as prolonging the refractory period of the accessory pathway.

A. Hazard of Digitalis When Atrial Fibrillation Occurs in Wolff-Parkinson-White Syndrome: If the atrial arrhythmia is fibrillation, digitalis should *not* be used, because it increases the block in the atrioventricular node while decreasing the refractory period of the anomalous pathway, permitting favored passage of the cardiac impulse via the accessory pathway. The rapid atrial impulses may then be transmitted without the protective blocking action of the atrioventricular node directly to the ventricle, and rapid ventricular rates of atrial fibrillation, ventricular tachycardia, or even ventricular fibrillation may ensue. Patients with RR intervals of 220 ms or less during spontaneous atrial fibrillation may develop ventricular fibrillation following administration of digitalis. Digitalis could be directly related to the onset of ventricular fibrillation in slightly less than half of patients who had atrial fibrillation with a short refractory period of the accessory pathway (Sellers, *Circulation* 1977;**56**:260; Campbell, 1977). Sudden death in patients with Wolff-Parkinson-White syndrome may be due to rapid conduction across an accessory pathway with a short refractory period. The cycle length of the anomalous pathway is not shortened by digitalis in all patients; the ventricular rate during spontaneous or induced atrial fibrillation may be a more direct measure of the likelihood of ventricular fibrillation if digitalis is given.

The frequency of atrial fibrillation becomes greater with age; it is uncommon in children. Digitalis should be avoided, although some authors suggest that it may be given safely in patients in whom elective induction of atrial fibrillation has demonstrated that the accessory pathway has a long refractory period and in whom, therefore, the risk of developing ventricular fibrillation is low. Drugs that prolong the refractory period of the accessory pathway (procainamide, quinidine) are preferable and safer (Table 14-7).

B. Management of Paroxysmal Atrial Arrhythmia in Wolff-Parkinson-White Syndrome: Patients who have episodes of paroxysmal atrial arrhythmia require a different approach; some authorities believe it wise in all patients to determine the refractory period of both the normal and the anomalous pathways to the ventricle so as to avoid drugs that decrease the refractory period of the anomalous pathway. Most cases of paroxysmal atrial tachycardia can be treated in the usual fashion, ie, with interruption of the reentry circuit. This can be achieved by increasing the block in the atrioventricular node by maneuvers such as carotid sinus massage or with drugs that stimulate the vagus nerve—or with digitalis if the rhythm is paroxysmal atrial tachycardia and not atrial fibrillation. Drugs that *increase* the block in the anomalous pathway—procainamide and quinidine—are the most effective. Propranolol has little effect on the anomalous pathway but a selective blocking effect on the atrioventricular node. About 20% of patients who have paroxysmal atrial tachycardia in the absence of obvious evidence of Wolff-Parkinson-White syndrome on the ECG have a retrograde accessory pathway, so-called **concealed Wolff-Parkinson-White syndrome** (see p 471). Determination of the refractoriness of the accessory pathway may have to be considered in older people with paroxysmal atrial tachycardia, because those with a short refractory period should not be given digitalis. There are no clear diagnostic criteria on the surface ECG by which those with a concealed accessory atrioventricular pathway can be identified. It may be helpful if paroxysmal atrial tachycardia occurs without an antecedent atrial premature beat, especially if paroxysmal atrial tachycardia occurs after shortening of the preceding cycle length (Sung, 1977).

Some of the new investigational drugs (eg, lorcainide and encainide) and amiodarone have suppressed arrhythmias in patients with preexcitation who did not respond to conventional drugs. These newer drugs increase the refractoriness of the accessory pathway (Reid, 1977; Zipes, 1977; Prystowsky, 1984).

1. Atrial pacing–Atrial pacing has been used therapeutically with the hope that a random beat might by chance excite a portion of the reentry pathway, making it refractory to the oncoming circuit wave. There is a risk that atrial pacing may increase the ventricular rate.

2. Emergency treatment–DC shock (cardioversion) or intravenous procainamide should be considered in emergency situations. It is unwise to use beta blockers and verapamil, because although they do not decrease the refractory period of the accessory pathway per se, they decrease it *relative* to that of the atrioventricular node (see pp 458 and 459). The refractory period of the atrioventricular node is prolonged by propranolol and verapamil. If the attacks of atrial arrhythmia are frequent and difficult to control, major efforts to prevent the arrhythmia are indicated (drugs, atrial pacing, and surgery).

3. Prevention of atrial arrhythmias in the preexcitation syndromes–Drugs that prevent the reentry phenomena by slowing conduction in the atrioventricular node or increasing the refractory period of the atrioventricular node may be helpful, as in paroxysmal atrial tachycardia in the absence of Wolff-Parkinson-White syndrome. Quinidine and procainamide are valuable, and *if one is certain that the arrhythmia is not atrial fibrillation,* digitalis may prevent the attacks. Drugs used in combination rather than one alone may sometimes be more effective in preventing atrial arrhythmias. Side effects may prevent one drug from being used to maximum effect, eg, bradycardia complicating propranolol therapy. A ventricular pacemaker may be inserted and may be activated externally in the hope that a chance premature beat may interrupt the reentry cycle.

4. Operative treatment–Surgical interruption of the aberrant pathway is being performed with increasing frequency, preceded by careful electrophysiologic studies and epicardial mapping at the time of surgery to determine the area of earliest ventricular excitation. When the anomalous pathway is clearly mapped, resection may interrupt the pathway and prevent both the delta wave and the subsequent arrhythmias. The procedure should not be undertaken lightly, because the sequence of ventricular activation varies in different patients (Holmes, 1982).

Cryosurgical ablation of the accessory atrioventricular connections is a technique now being used in some centers. If found to be consistently beneficial, this will be a useful addition to surgical treatment, because thoracotomy alone rather than cardiopulmonary bypass is sufficient, decreasing operating time by several hours. The site of preexcitation can be abolished by local application of the cryoprobe at $-60\ °C$. Evidence of preexcitation and arrhythmias disappeared in these patients (Gallagher, 1976).

5. Catheter ablation of His bundle–A new technique used in relatively few cases of recurrent atrial tachycardia is catheter ablation of the His bundle with electric shock. A catheter is placed in the region of the His bundle, and a shock of about 300 J is given when the largest His spike is noted. Preliminary results indicate that partial or complete atrioventricular block may occur, decreasing or preventing episodes of supraventricular tachycardia. A ventricular pacemaker is required in these patients to prevent Stokes-Adams attacks. Catheter ablation of the His bundle has been used only in refractory cases with frequent attacks of tachycardia causing severe hemodynamic deterioration that are unresponsive to conventional drugs. Amiodarone should be tried first because of its powerful electrophysiologic effect on the sinoatrial and atrioventricular nodes (Scheinman, 1983; Gallagher, 1982).

IDIOPATHIC LONG QT SYNDROME

Idiopathic long QT syndrome is an uncommon condition first described in deaf siblings, although deafness is not always present. The syndrome is characterized by recurrent syncope, a long QT interval (usually 0.5–0.7 s), ventricular arrhythmias (torsade de pointes), and sudden and unexpected death. Patients with the disease demonstrate neural degeneration of the conduction system. The syndrome may be acquired, resulting from electrolyte imbalance, neurologic disorders, or toxicity to cardiac drugs (eg, quinidine or amiodarone) or psychotropic drugs. The role of these various causes in producing sudden death is unclear (Milne, 1982).

The sympathetic nervous system (especially the left stellate ganglion) and autonomic imbalance play a role in the pathogenesis of the syndrome. Acute arrhythmic episodes are treated by local anesthetic block of the left stellate ganglion, and recurrent episodes are treated by resection of this ganglion as well as of the first 3 or 4 thoracic ganglia. Before resection of the left stellate ganglion is considered, patients should be treated with propranolol or other beta-adrenergic blocking drugs or with phenytoin, which has proved beneficial in some patients.

The role of prolongation of the QT interval by antiarrhythmic agents is being investigated. One of the newer such agents, encainide, greatly increases the QT interval yet is effective in treating ventricular tachyarrhythmias without producing syncope. Quinidine prolongs the QT interval and, in the cases in which syncope has been reported, has been associated with ventricular fibrillation and not with asystole. Prolongation of the QT interval from drugs and procedures must be distinguished from the specific syndrome known as the idiopathic long QT syndrome.

REFERENCES

Electrophysiology

Castellanos A Jr, Castillo CA, Agha AS: Symposium on electrophysiological correlates of clinical arrhythmias. 3. Contribution of His bundle recordings to the understanding of clinical arrhythmias. *Am J Cardiol* 1971;**28**:499.

Denes P et al: The effects of cycle length on cardiac refractory periods in man. *Circulation* 1974;**49**:32.

Fisch C: Concealed conduction. *Cardiol Clin* 1983;**1**:63.

Fozzard HA: Cardiac muscle: Excitability and passive electrical properties. *Prog Cardiovasc Dis* 1977;**19**:343.

Fozzard HA, DasGupta DS: Electrophysiology and the electrocardiogam. *Mod Concepts Cardiovasc Dis* 1975;**44**:29.

Han J: The concepts of re-entrant activity responsible for ectopic rhythm. *Am J Cardiol* 1971;**28**:253.

Hoffman BF, Cranefield PF: *The Electrophysiology of the Heart.* McGraw-Hill, 1960.

James TN et al: De subitaneis mortibus. 30. Observations on the pathophysiology of long QT syndromes with special reference to the neuropathology of the heart. *Circulation* 1978;**57**:1221.

Josephson ME, Seides SF: *Clinical Cardiac Electrophysiology: Techniques and Interpretations.* Lea & Febiger, 1979.

Langendorf R: Concealed A–V conduction: The effect of blocked impulses on the formation and conduction of subsequent impulses. *Am Heart J* 1948;**35**:542.

Lewis T: *The Mechanism and Graphic Registration of the Heart Beat,* 3rd ed. Shaw & Sons, 1925.

Massing GK, James TN: Anatomical configuration of the His bundle and bundle branches in the human heart. *Circulation* 1976;**53**:609.

Moe GK, Mendez C: The physiologic basis of reciprocal rhythm. *Prog Cardiovasc Dis* 1966;**8**:461.

Monahan JP, Denes P, Rosen KM: Portable electrocardiographic monitoring: Performance in patients with short P-R intervals without delta waves. *Arch Intern Med* 1975;**135**:1188.

Narula OS (editor): *His Bundle Electrocardiography and Clinical Electrophysiology.* Davis, 1975.

Parsonnet V et al: Optimal resources for implantable cardiac pacemakers. (Pacemaker Study Group.) *Circulation* 1983;**68**:226A.

Scheinman MM, Morady F: Invasive cardiac electrophysiologic testing: The current state of the art. (Editorial.) *Circulation* 1983;**67**:1169.

Singer DM, Lazzara R, Hoffman B: Interrelationships between automaticity and conduction in Purkinje fibers. *Circ Res* 1967;**21**:537.

Watanabe Y, Dreifus LS: Factors controlling impulse transmission with special reference to A–V conduction. *Am Heart J* 1975;**89**:790.

Wellens HJJ: Contribution of cardiac pacing to our understanding of the Wolff-Parkinson-White syndrome. *Br Heart J* 1975;**37**:231.

Zipes DP et al: Role of the slow current in cardiac electrophysiology. *Circulation* 1975;**51**:761.

Pathology & Causes

Davies MJ: *Pathology of Conducting Tissue of the Heart.* Appleton-Century-Crofts, 1971.

Demoulin J, Kulbertus HE: Histopathological correlates of sinoatrial disease. *Br Heart J* 1978;**40**:1384.

Evans R, Shaw DB: Pathological studies in sinoatrial disorder (sick sinus syndrome). *Br Heart J* 1977;**39**:778.

Fraser GR, Froggatt P, James TN: Congenital deafness associated with electrocardiographic abnormalities, fainting attacks and sudden death: A recessive syndrome. *Q J Med* 1964;**33**:361.

Frink RJ, James TN: Normal blood supply to the human His bundle and proximal bundle branches. *Circulation* 1973;**47**:8.

Hudson REB: Surgical pathology of the conducting system of the heart. *Br Heart J* 1967;**29**:646.

James TN: Cardiac innervation: Anatomic and pharmacologic relations. *Bull NY Acad Med* 1967;**43**:1041.

James TN: The connecting pathways between the sinus node and the A–V node and between the right and left atrium in the human heart. *Am Heart J* 1963;**66**:498.

James TN et al: De subitaneis mortibus. 30. Observations on the pathophysiology of the long QT syndromes with special reference to the neuropathology of the heart. *Circulation* 1978;**57**:1221.

Lenegre J: Etiology and pathology of bilateral bundle branch block in relation to complete heart block. *Prog Cardiovasc Dis* 1964;**6**:409.

Lev M: The pathology of atrioventricular block. *Cardiovasc Clin* 1972;**4**:159.

Mackenzie J: *Diseases of the Heart.* Oxford, 1908.

Moss AJ, Schwartz PJ: Sudden death and the idiopathic long Q–T syndrome. *Am J Med* 1979;**66**:6.

Schwartz PJ, Periti M, Malliani A: The long Q–T syndrome. *Am Heart J* 1975;**89**:378.

Titus JL: Cardiac arrhythmias. 1. Anatomy of the conduction system. *Circulation* 1973;**47**:170.

Bradycardiac Syndromes

Alpert MA, Flaker GC: Arrhythmias associated with sinus node dysfunction: Pathogenesis, recognition, and management. *JAMA* 1983;**250**:2160.

Bleifer SB et al: Diagnosis of occult arrhythmias by Holter electrocardiography. *Prog Cardiovasc Dis* 1974;**16**:569.

DeSanctis RW: Diagnosis and therapeutic uses of atrial pacing. *Circulation* 1971;**43**:748.

Easley RM Jr, Goldstein S: Sino-atrial syncope. *Am J Med* 1971;**50**:166.

Eraut D, Shaw DB: Sinus bradycardia. *Br Heart J* 1971;**33**:742.

Ferrer MI: *The Sick Sinus Syndrome.* Futura, 1974.

Ferrer MI: Sick sinus syndrome. *J Cardiovasc Med* 1981;**6**:743.

Gillette PC: Recent advances in mechanisms, evaluation, and pacemaker treatment of chronic bradydysrhythmias in children. *Am Heart J* 1982;**102**:920.

Han J et al: Temporal dispersion of recovery of excitability in atrium and ventricle as a function of heart rate. *Am Heart J* 1966;**71**:481.

James TN: The sinus node. *Am J Cardiol* 1977;**40**:965.

Kang PS et al: Role of autonomic regulatory mechanisms in sinoatrial conduction and sinus node automaticity in sick sinus syndrome. *Circulation* 1981;**64**:832.

Kirk JE, Kvorning SA: Sinus bradycardia: A clinical study of 515 consecutive cases. *Acta Med Scand [Suppl]* 1952;**266**:625.

Lloyd-Mostyn RH, Kidner PH, Oram S: Sinus-atrial disorder including the brady-tachycardia syndrome. *Q J Med* 1973;**42**:41.

Margolis JR et al: Digitalis and the sick sinus syndrome. *Circulation* 1975;**52**:162.

Mazuz M, Friedman HS: Significance of prolonged electrocardiographic pauses in sinoatrial disease: Sick sinus syndrome. *Am J Cardiol* 1983;**52**:485.

Moss AJ, Davis RJ: Brady-tachy syndrome. *Prog Cardiovasc Dis* 1974;**16**:439.

Narula OS: Sick sinus syndrome. (2 parts.) *Primary Cardiol* (Jan) 1978;**4**:27 and (Feb) 1978;**4**:12.

Phibbs B et al: Indications for pacing in the treatment of bradyarrhythmias: Report of an independent study group. *JAMA* 1984;**252**:1307.

Rokseth R, Hatle L: Prospective study on the occurrence and management of chronic sinoatrial disease, with follow-up. *Br Heart J* 1974;**36**:582.

Rosen KM et al: Cardiac conduction in patients with symptomatic sinus node disease. *Circulation* 1971;**43**:836.

Schweitzer P, Mark H: The effect of atropine on cardiac arrhythmias and conduction. Part 1. *Am Heart J* 1980;**100**:119.

Shaw DB, Kekwick CA: Potential candidates for pacemakers: Survey of heart block and sinoatrial disorder (sick sinus syndrome). *Br Heart J* 1978;**40**:99.

Short DS: The syndrome of alternating bradycardia and tachycardia. *Br Heart J* 1954;**16**:208.

Strauss HC et al: Electrophysiologic evaluation of sinus node function in patients with sinus node dysfunction. *Circulation* 1976;**53**:763.

Swiryn S, McDonough T, Hueter DC: Sinus node function and dysfunction. *Med Clin North Am* 1984;**68**:935.

Talano JV et al: Sinus node dysfunction: An overview with emphasis on autonomic and pharmacologic consideration. *Am J Med* 1978;**64**:773.

Van Durme JP: Tachyarrhythmias and transient cerebral ischemic attacks. *Am Heart J* 1975;**89**:538.

Wohl AJ et al: Prognosis of patients permanently paced for sick sinus syndrome. *Arch Intern Med* 1976;**136**:406.

Atrioventricular Conduction Defects

Barold SS, Coumel P: Mechanisms of atrioventricular junctional tachycardia: Role of reentry and concealed accessory bypass tracts. *Am J Cardiol* 1977;**39**:97.

Campbell M, Suzman SS: Congenital complete heart-block. *Am Heart J* 1934;**9**:304.

Childers R: Concealed conduction. *Med Clin North Am* 1976;**60**:149.

Dhingra RC et al: Significance of the HV interval in 517 patients with chronic bifascicular block. *Circulation* 1981;**64**:1265.

Dollery CT, Paterson JW, Conolly ME: Clinical pharmacology of beta-receptor blocking drugs. *Clin Pharmacol* 1969;**10**:765.

Erlanger J: On the physiology of heart block in mammals, with especial reference to the causation of Stokes-Adams disease. *J Exp Med* 1906;**8**:8.

Gilchrist AR: Clinical aspects of high grade heart block. *Scott Med J* 1958;**3**:53.

Ginks W, Leatham A, Siddons H: Prognosis of patients paced for chronic atrioventricular block. *Br Heart J* 1979;**41**:633.

Guidelines for permanent cardiac pacemaker implantation, May 1984. *J Am Coll Cardiol* 1984;**4**:434.

Harthorne JW: Indications for pacemaker insertion: Types and modes of pacing. *Prog Cardiovasc Dis* 1981;**23**:393.

Hess DS, Morady F, Scheinman MM: Electrophysiologic testing in the evaluation of patients with syncope of undetermined origin. *Am J Cardiol* 1982;**50**:1309.

Hinkle LE Jr, Carver ST, Stevens M: The frequency of asymptomatic disturbances of cardiac rhythm and conduction in middle-aged men. *Am J Cardiol* 1969;**24**:629.

Johansson BW: Longevity in complete heart block. *Ann NY Acad Sci* 1969;**167**:1031.

Kapoor WN et al: A prospective evaluation and follow-up of patients with syncope. *N Engl J Med* 1983;**309**:197.

Kastor JA: Atrioventricular block. (2 parts.) *N Engl J Med* 1975;**292**:462, 572.

Lagergren H et al: Three hundred and five cases of permanent intravenous pacemaker treatment for Adams-Stokes syndrome. *Surgery* 1966;**59**:494.

Landegren J, Biörck G: The clinical assessment and treatment of complete heart block and Adams-Stokes attacks. *Medicine* 1963;**42**:171.

Langendorf R: Concealed A–V conduction: The effect of blocked impulses on the formation and conduction of subsequent impulses. *Am Heart J* 1948;**35**:542.

Langendorf R, Cohen H, Gozo EG Jr: Observations on second degree atrioventricular block, including new criteria for the differential diagnosis between type I and type II block. *Am J Cardiol* 1972;**29**:111.

Lewis JK: Stokes-Adams disease: An account of important historical discoveries. *Arch Intern Med* 1958;**101**:130.

Lie KI et al: Mechanism and significance of widened QRS complexes during complete atrioventricular block in acute inferior myocardial infarction. *Am J Cardiol* 1974;**33**:833.

Lown B, Kosowsky BD: Artificial cardiac pacemakers. (3 parts.) *N Engl J Med* 1970;**283**:907, 971, 1023.

Luceri RM et al: The arrhythmias of dual-chamber cardiac pacemakers and their management. *Ann Intern Med* 1983;**99**:354.

Marriott HJL, Menendez MM: A–V dissociation revisited. *Prog Cardiovasc Dis* 1966;**8**:522.

McAnulty JH, Rahimtoola SH: Bundle branch block. *Prog Cardiovasc Dis* 1984;**26**:333.

Mobitz W: Uber die unrollständige störung der erregungsüberleitung zwischen vorhoff und kammer des menschlichen herzens. *Z Gesamte Exp Med* 1924;**41**:180.

Moore EN, Knoebel SB, Spear JF: Concealed conduction. *Am J Cardiol* 1971;**28**:406.

Morady F, Peters RW, Scheinman MM: Bradyarrhythmias and bundle branch block. Chap 7, pp 135–151, in: *Cardiac Emergencies.* Scheinman MM (editor). Saunders, 1984.

Mullins CB, Atkins JM: Prognoses and management of ventricular conduction blocks in acute myocardial infarction. *Mod Concepts Cardiovasc Dis* 1976;**45**:129.

Nakamura FF, Nadas AS: Complete heart block in infants and children. *N Engl J Med* 1964;**270**:1261.

Narula OS: Pacing and the His bundle electrogram. 3. The significance of H–V interval prolongation. *Medtronic News* 1977;**7**:3.

Narula OS, Gann D, Samet P: Prognostic value of H–V intervals. Pages 437–449 in: *His Bundle Electrocardiography and Clinical Electrophysiology*. Narula OS (editor). Davis, 1975.

Narula OS et al: Atrioventricular block: Localization and classification by His bundle recordings. *Am J Med* 1971;**50**:146.

O'Rourke RA: The Stokes-Adams syndrome. 1. Definition and etiology. *West J Med* 1972;**117**:96.

Penton GB, Miller H, Levine SA: Some clinical features of complete heart block. *Circulation* 1956;**13**:801.

Phibbs B, Marriott HJL: Complications of permanent transvenous pacing. *N Engl J Med* 1985;**312**:1428.

Puech P: Atrioventricular block: The value of intracardiac recordings. Page 81 in: *Cardiac Arrhythmias: The Modern Electrophysiological Approach*. Krikler DM, Goodwin JF (editors). Saunders, 1975.

Reid JM, Coleman EN, Doig W: Complete congenital heart block. *Br Heart J* 1982;**48**:236.

Rosen KM et al: Chronic heart block in adults. *Arch Intern Med* 1973;**131**:663.

Rowe JC, White PD: Complete heart block: A follow-up study. *Ann Intern Med* 1958;**49**:260.

Rowland E, Evans T, Krikler D: Effect of nifedipine on atrioventricular conduction as compared with verapamil: Intracardiac electrophysiological study. *Br Heart J* 1979;**42**:124.

Scarpelli FM, Rudolph AM: The hemodynamics of congenital complete heart block. *Prog Cardiovasc Dis* 1964;**6**:327.

Scheinman MM et al: Value of the H–Q interval in patients with bundle branch block and the role of prophylactic permanent pacing. *Am J Cardiol* 1982;**50**:1316.

Vohra J et al: The effect of toxic and therapeutic doses of tricyclic antidepressant drugs on intracardiac conduction. *Eur J Cardiol* (Oct) 1975;**3**:219.

Watanabe Y, Dreifus LS: Factors controlling impulse transmission with special reference to A–V conduction. *Am Heart J* 1975;**89**:790.

Wenckebach KF: Zur analyse des unregelmässigen pulses. *Z Klin Med* 1899;**36**:181.

Zipes DP: Second-degree atrioventricular block. *Circulation* 1979;**60**:465.

Ventricular Conduction Defects & Bundle Branch Block

Bigger JT Jr et al: Ventricular arrhythmias in ischemic heart disease: Mechanism, prevalence, significance, and management. *Prog Cardiovasc Dis* 1977;**19**:255.

Brohet CR et al: Vectorcardiographic diagnosis of right ventricular hypertrophy in the presence of right bundle branch block in young subjects. *Am J Cardiol* 1978;**42**:602.

Brooks N, Leech G, Leatham A: Complete right bundle-branch block: Echophonocardiographic study of first heart sound and right ventricular contraction times. *Br Heart J* 1979;**41**:637.

Castellanos A Jr, Lemberg L: Diagnosis of isolated and combined block in the bundle branches and the divisions of the left branch. *Circulation* 1971;**43**:971.

Cohen HC et al: Tachycardia and bradycardia-dependent bundle branch block alternans: Clinical observation. *Circulation* 1977;**55**:242.

Corne RA, Beamish RE, Rollwagen RL: Significance of left anterior hemiblock. *Br Heart J* 1978;**40**:552.

Dancy M, Leech G, Leatham A: Significance of complete right bundle-branch block when an isolated finding. *Br Heart J* 1982;**48**:217.

Demoulin JC, Kulbertus HE: Histopathologic correlates of left posterior fascicular block. *Am J Cardiol* 1979;**44**:1083.

Dhingra RC et al: Significance of the HV interval in 517 patients with chronic bifascicular block. *Circulation* 1981;**64**:1265.

Fisch GR, Zipes DP, Fisch C: Bundle branch block and sudden death. *Prog Cardiovasc Dis* 1980;**23**:187.

Fleg JL, Das DN, Lakatta EG: Right bundle branch block: Long-term prognosis in apparently healthy men. *J Am Coll Cardiol* 1983;**3**:887.

Havelda CJ et al: The pathologic correlates of the electrocardiogram: Complete left bundle branch block. *Circulation* 1982;**65**:445.

Hindman MC et al: The clinical significance of bundle branch block complicating acute myocardial infarction. (2 parts.) *Circulation* 1978;**58**:679, 689.

Kunkel F, Rowland M, Scheinman MM: The electrophysiologic effects of lidocaine in patients with intraventricular conduction defects. *Circulation* 1974;**49**:894.

Lancaster MC, Schechter E, Massing GK: Acquired complete right bundle branch block without overt cardiac disease. *Am J Cardiol* 1972;**30**:32.

Lenegre J: Bilateral bundle branch block. *Cardiologia* 1966;**48**:134.

Lie KI et al: Factors influencing prognosis of bundle branch block complicating acute antero-septal infarction: The value of His bundle recordings. *Circulation* 1974;**50**:935.

Luy G, Bahl OP, Massie E: Intermittent left bundle branch block. *Am Heart J* 1973;**85**:332.

McAnulty JH, Rahimtoola SH: Bundle branch block. *Prog Cardiovasc Dis* 1984;**26**:333.

Narula OS: Pacing and the His bundle electrogram. 3. The significance of H–V interval prolongation. *Medtronic News* 1977;**7**:3.

Narula OS, Samet P: Right bundle branch block with normal, left or right axis deviation: Analysis by His bundle recordings. *Am J Med* 1971;**41**:432.

Norris RM, Mercer CJ, Croxson MS: Conduction disturbances due to anteroseptal myocardial infarction and their treatment by endocardial pacing. *Am Heart J* 1972;**84**:560.

Pastore JO et al: The risk of advanced heart block in surgical patients with right bundle branch block and left axis deviation. *Circulation* 1978;**57**:677.

Rabkin SW, Mathewson FAL, Tate RB: Natural history of left bundle-branch block. *Br Heart J* 1980;**43**:164.

Rosenbaum MB et al: The differential electrocardiographic manifestations of hemiblocks, bilateral bundle branch block and trifascicular blocks. Pages 145–182 in: *Advances in Electrocardiography*. Schlant RC, Hurst JW (editors). Grune & Stratton, 1972.

Rotman M, Triebwasser JH: A clinical and follow-up study of right and left bundle branch block. *Circulation* 1975;**51**:477.

Sandler IA, Marriott H: The differential morphology of anomalous ventricular complexes of RBBB type in lead V_1: Ventricular ectopy versus aberration. *Circulation* 1965;**31**:551.

Scheinman MM, Morady F: Invasive cardiac electrophysiologic testing: The current state of the art. (Editorial.) *Circulation* 1983;**67**:1169.

Schneider JV et al: Newly acquired left bundle-branch block: The Framingham Study. *Ann Intern Med* 1979;**90**:303.

Sung RJ et al: Clinical and electrophysiologic observations in patients with concealed accessory atrioventricular bypass tracts. *Am J Cardiol* 1977;**40**:839.

Talbot S et al: QRS waveforms in right and left bundle-branch aberration. *Br Heart J* 1980;**44**:184.

Trevino AS, Beller BM: Conduction disturbances of the left bundle branch system and their relationship to complete heart block. (2 parts.) *Am J Med* 1971;**51**:362, 374.

Warner RA et al: Improved electrocardiographic criteria for the diagnosis of left anterior hemiblock. *Am J Cardiol* 1983;**51**:723.

Ventricular Preexcitation Syndromes

Becker AE et al: The anatomic substrates of Wolff-Parkinson-White Syndrome: A clinicopathologic correlation in seven patients. *Circulation* 1978;**57**:870.

Benditt DG et al: Characteristics of atrioventricular conduction and the spectrum of arrhythmias in Lown-Ganong-Levine syndrome. *Circulation* 1978;**57**:454.

Benson DW et al: Localization of the site of ventricular preexcitation with body surface maps in patients with Wolff-Parkinson-White syndrome. *Circulation* 1982;**65**:1259.

Boineau JP: Mapping: Cardiac activation and repolarization. *Circulation* 1981;**64**:208.

Boineau JP et al: Epicardial mapping in Wolff-Parkinson-White syndrome. *Arch Intern Med* 1975;**135**:422.

Campbell RW et al: Atrial fibrillation in the preexcitation syndrome. *Am J Cardiol* 1977;**40**:514.

Caracta AR et al: Electrophysiologic studies in the syndrome of short PR interval, normal QRS complex. *Am J Cardiol* 1973;**31**:245.

Dreifus LS, Haiat R, Watanabe Y: Ventricular fibrillation: A possible mechanism of sudden death in patients with Wolff-Parkinson-White syndrome. *Circulation* 1971;**43**:520.

Dreifus LS et al: Sinus bradycardia and atrial fibrillation associated with the Wolff-Parkinson-White syndrome. *Am J Cardiol* 1976;**38**:149.

Durrer D et al: The role of premature beats in the initiation and the termination of supraventricular tachycardia in the Wolff-Parkinson-White syndrome. *Circulation* 1967;**36**:644.

Flensted-Jensen E: Wolff-Parkinson-White syndrome: A long term follow-up of 47 cases. *Acta Med Scand* 1969;**186**:65.

Gallagher JJ et al: Epicardial mapping in the Wolff-Parkinson-White syndrome. *Circulation* 1978;**57**:854.

Gallagher JJ et al: The preexcitation syndromes. *Prog Cardiovasc Dis* 1978;**20**:285.

Gallagher JJ et al: Techniques of intraoperative electrophysiologic mapping. *Am J Cardiol* 1982;**49**:221.

Gallagher JJ et al: The Wolff-Parkinson-White syndrome and the preexcitation dysrhythmias: Medical and surgical management. *Med Clin North Am* 1976;**60**:101.

Gillette PC, Garson A, Kugler JD: Wolff-Parkinson-White syndrome in children: Electrophysiologic and pharmacologic characteristics. *Circulation* 1979;**60**:1487.

Harper RW et al: Effects of verapamil on the electrophysiologic properties of the accessory pathway in patients with the Wolff-Parkinson-White syndrome. *Am J Cardiol* 1982;**50**:1323.

Holmes DR et al: The Wolff-Parkinson-White syndrome: A surgical approach. *Mayo Clin Proc* 1982;**57**:345.

Josephson ME, Kastor JA: Supraventricular tachycardia in Lown-Ganong-Levine syndrome: Atrionodal versus intranodal reentry. *Am J Cardiol* 1977;**40**:521.

Kerr CR et al: Electrophysiologic effects of disopyramide phosphate in patients with Wolff-Parkinson-White syndrome. *Circulation* 1982;**65**:869.

Lown B, Ganong WF, Levine SA: The syndrome of short P-R interval, normal QRS complex, and paroxysmal rapid heart action. *Circulation* 1952;**5**:693.

Mandel WJ, Danzig R, Hayakawa H: Lown-Ganong-Levine syndrome: A study using His bundle electrograms. *Circulation* 1971;**44**:696.

Monahan JP, Denes P, Rosen KM: Portable electrocardiographic monitoring: Performance in patients with short P-R intervals without delta waves. *Arch Intern Med* 1975;**135**:1188.

Morady F et al: Electrophysiologic testing in the management of patients with the Wolff-Parkinson-White syndrome and atrial fibrillation. *Am J Cardiol* 1983;**51**:1623.

Prystowsky EN et al: Clinical efficacy and electrophysiologic effects of encainide in patients with Wolff-Parkinson-White syndrome. *Circulation* 1984;**69**:278.

Reid PR, Greene HL, Varghese PJ: Suppression of refractory arrhythmias by aprindine in patients with the Wolff-Parkinson-White syndrome. *Br Heart J* 1977;**39**:1353.

Rosenbaum FF et al: The potential variations of the thorax and the esophagus in anomalous atrioventricular excitation (Wolff-Parkinson-White syndrome). *Am Heart J* 1945;**29**:281.

Rosenbaum MB et al: Control of tachyarrhythmias associated with Wolff-Parkinson-White syndrome by amiodarone hydrochloride. *Am J Cardiol* 1974;**34**:215.

Scheinman MM, Morady F: Invasive cardiac electrophysiologic testing: The current state of the art. (Editorial.) *Circulation* 1983;**67**:1169.

Sellers TD, Bashore TM, Gallagher JJ: Digitalis in the preexcitation syndrome: Analysis during atrial fibrillation. *Circulation* 1977;**56**:260.

Sellers TD Jr et al: Effects of procainamide and quinidine sulfate in the Wolff-Parkinson-White syndrome. *Circulation* 1977;**55**:15.

Strasberg B et al: Treadmill exercise testing in the Wolff-Parkinson-White syndrome. *Am J Cardiol* 1980;**45**:742.

Sung RJ et al: Clinical and electrophysiologic observations in patients with concealed accessory atrioventricular bypass tracts. *Am J Cardiol* 1977;**40**:839.

Tonkin AM, Gallagher JJ, Wallace AG: Tachyarrhythmias in Wolff-Parkinson-White syndrome: Treatment and prevention. *JAMA* 1976;**235**:947.

Tonkin AM et al: Refractory periods of the accessory pathway in the Wolff-Parkinson-White syndrome. *Circulation* 1975;**52**:563.

Wallace AG et al: Ventricular excitation in the Wolff-Parkinson-White syndrome. Pages 613–630 in: *The Conduction System of the Heart*. Wellens HJJ, Lie KI, Janse MJ (editors). HE Stenfert Kroese BV, 1976.

Wellens HJJ: Effect of drugs on Wolff-Parkinson-White syndrome. Page 367 in: *His Bundle Electrocardiography*. Narula O (editor). Davis, 1975.

Wellens HJJ: The electrophysiologic properties of the accessory pathway in the Wolff-Parkinson-White syndrome. Pages 567–587 in: *The Conduction System of the Heart*. Wellens HJJ, Lie KI, Janse MJ (editors). HE Stenfert Kroese BV, 1976.

Wellens HJJ: Wolff-Parkinson-White syndrome. 1. Diagnosis, arrhythmias, and identification of the high-risk patient.

2. Treatment. *Mod Concepts Cardiovasc Dis* 1983; **52:**53, 57.

Wellens HJJ, Durrer D: Wolff-Parkinson-White syndrome and atrial fibrillation: Relation between refractory period of accessory pathway and ventricular rate during atrial fibrillation. *Am J Cardiol* 1974;**34:**777.

Wolff L, Parkinson J, White PD: Bundle branch block with short P–R interval in healthy young people prone to paroxysmal tachycardia. *Am Heart J* 1930;**5:**685.

Zipes DP et al: Aprindine for treatment of supraventricular arrhythmias. *Am J Cardiol* 1977;**40:**586.

Idiopathic Long QT Syndrome

Crampton R: Preeminence of the left stellate ganglion in the long Q–T syndrome: *Circulation* 1979;**59:**769.

DeSilvey DL, Moss AJ: Primidone in the treatment of the long QT syndrome: QT shortening and ventricular arrhythmia suppression. *Ann Intern Med* 1980;**93:**53.

Gallagher JJ et al: Catheter technique for closed-chest ablation of the atrioventricular conduction system: A therapeutic alternative for the treatment of refractory supraventricular tachycardia. *N Engl J Med* 1982;**306:**194.

Gallagher JJ et al: Techniques of intraoperative electrophysiologic mapping. *Am J Cardiol* 1982;**49:**221.

Jackman WM et al: Ventricular tachyarrhythmias in the long QT syndromes. *Med Clin North Am* 1984;**68:**1079.

James TN et al: De subitaneis mortibus. 30. Observations on the pathophysiology of the long QT syndromes with special reference to the neuropathology of the heart. *Circulation* 1978;**57:**1221.

Kay GN et al: Torsade de pointes: The long-short initiating sequence and other clinical features: Observations in 32 patients. *J Am Coll Cardiol* 1983;**2:**806.

Milne JR et al: The long QT syndrome: Effects of drugs and left stellate ganglion block. *Am Heart J* 1982;**104:**194.

Moss AF et al: The long QT syndrome: A prospective international study. *Circulation* 1985;**71:**17.

Moss AJ, Schwartz PJ: Sudden death and the idiopathic long Q–T syndrome. *Am J Med* 1979;**66:**6.

Pryor R: The long Q–T syndrome. *Primary Cardiol* (Feb) 1981;**7:**52.

Rubin SA et al: Usefulness of Valsalva manoeuvre and cold pressor test for evaluation of arrhythmias in long QT syndrome. *Br Heart J* 1979;**42:**490.

Surawicz B, Knoebel SB: Long QT: Good, bad or indifferent? *J Am Coll Cardiol* 1984;**4:**398.

15 Cardiac Arrhythmias

Cardiac arrhythmias can occur in a wide variety of circumstances in patients with no evidence of heart disease or in those with heart disease due to any cause. For purposes of description, we have divided disturbances of rhythm into (1) supraventricular (atrial or junctional) arrhythmias and (2) ventricular arrhythmias. The electrophysiologic principles applicable to the study of cardiac arrhythmias are included with the discussion of that subject in Chapter 14.

The usual history of cardiac arrhythmia is of a sudden onset of palpitations that the patient may describe as regular or irregular, although it may not always be possible to characterize them one way or the other. It may help if the physician taps out various rhythms and rates and asks, "Is it like this? Or like this?" etc. The patient may not complain of palpitations but rather of the consequences of the arrhythmia, such as weakness, chest pain, dizziness, dyspnea, and confusion. Some patients have no symptoms with arrhythmia.

If the arrhythmia occurs in an older patient with coronary heart disease, severe symptoms of near-syncope, chest pain, palpitations, dyspnea, and disturbed left ventricular function with low cardiac output may develop.

In arrhythmias of longer duration, there may be progressive deterioration of cardiac function, with impaired perfusion of vital organs from decreased cardiac output. The patient may then develop symptoms resulting from inadequate perfusion of the brain, heart, kidneys, skin, and extremities. The fact that the patient tolerates the arrhythmia at the outset does not guarantee that circulatory embarrassment will not develop with time. This is especially true in patients in the coronary care unit, in whom cardiac failure may develop gradually.

Palpitations may be due to increased forcefulness of the heartbeat as well as to arrhythmia or due to one or the other at different times (see p 38). Continuous ambulatory electrocardiographic monitoring to determine the rhythm is often necessary. Some arrhythmias last seconds or minutes, while others, such as atrial fibrillation, last hours or days or indefinitely.

The diagnosis may be simple after a routine ECG, or it may be complex, requiring extensive studies with carotid sinus massage, Valsalva's maneuver, rapid atrial pacing, His bundle studies with intracardiac recording and stimulation, and, in selected cases, echocardiography, coronary arteriography, and left ventricular cineangiograms. It may be necessary to determine the relationship of the QRS complex and the P wave to the His bundle deflection, the effect of posture and drugs, and the adequacy of the baroreceptor reflexes in order to identify the type of arrhythmia and determine whether it is ventricular or supraventricular. The examiner should obtain a history of previous episodes, an indication of the patient's tolerance for them, their frequency and duration, the extent of circulatory impairment, and the response to treatment, if any.

It is important to estimate the severity of the arrhythmia (ie, the impact on left ventricular function, blood pressure, cerebral and coronary perfusion, and renal function). The importance of the heart rate, duration of the arrhythmia, and the presence of underlying heart disease must be emphasized. The arrhythmia may be trivial or urgent, depending on the cause, the effect on the circulation, and the age of the patient.

The consequences of a cardiac arrhythmia depend upon its effect on cardiac hemodynamics; on cerebral, coronary, and renal perfusion; on blood pressure, left ventricular function, and cardiac rate (rapid or slow); on the duration of the arrhythmia; and on the presence or absence of underlying heart disease. If the arrhythmia occurs in a young person with no underlying heart disease and the increase in ventricular rate is only modest (<160/min), hemodynamic function is rarely impaired, and perfusion of vital organs (brain, heart, and kidneys) and extremities is adequate.

Whether the disturbance in rhythm is regular or irregular has an important influence on the patient's tolerance; an irregular rhythm such as atrial fibrillation is less well tolerated than paroxysmal atrial tachycardia at a similar rate. Incomplete ventricular filling in the absence of atrial systole can significantly reduce cardiac output in a cardiac arrhythmia.

SUPRAVENTRICULAR (ATRIAL OR JUNCTIONAL) ARRHYTHMIAS

SUPRAVENTRICULAR PREMATURE BEATS (Atrial Extrasystoles)

Premature beats are important only if they interfere with hemodynamic function of the left ventricle, impair cardiac output, and decrease perfusion to vital organs, or if they are precursors of more serious arrhythmias. Supraventricular premature beats are rarely important in this sense.

Supraventricular premature beats are more apt to occur if there is atrial or conduction system disease such as left atrial enlargement in mitral stenosis. Beats occurring in these conditions may presage the development of atrial fibrillation. When atrial fibrillation is converted to sinus rhythm, reappearance of atrial premature beats often indicates that atrial fibrillation will soon recur.

In community prospective studies, supraventricular beats are not related to sudden death, as are ventricular premature beats in coronary disease.

Clinical Findings

A. Symptoms: Atrial premature beats are conducted in antegrade or retrograde manner; they commonly depolarize the sinus node, and therefore there may be a pause following the premature beat that is longer or shorter than the pause between 2 normally conducted sinus beats. With the exception of hypertrophic cardiomyopathy, in which the stroke output following a pause is usually weaker than normal, the ventricular beat following the pause is usually stronger, and the patient may have a variety of symptoms referable to awareness of the strength of this beat. When supraventricular beats are frequent or occur in runs, such beats may decrease the cardiac output and impair perfusion to the essential organs, causing mental confusion, dyspnea, angina, palpitations, or weakness.

Supraventricular premature beats are common in healthy individuals and increase in frequency with age. They are not by themselves an indication of cardiac disease, and antiarrhythmic drug therapy is not indicated (Hinkle, 1969).

B. Signs: Supraventricular premature beats, like ventricular premature beats, may be recognized at the bedside when an extra beat is detected that disturbs the dominant rhythm. The origin of the extra beat, whether supraventricular or ventricular, is difficult to distinguish on auscultation. If the premature beat retrogradely penetrates the sinus node and discharges it, the next normal sinus beat is delayed, but the pause is not "compensatory" and the basic rhythm is altered. Unless the premature beats occur near the junction of the atria and the atrioventricular node (junctional premature beats), cannon waves do not occur (see Chapter 3). They may occur if the atria contract when the tricuspid valve is closed, since both atria and ventricles contract within a short interval.

The pause that follows the premature beat may allow the physician to diagnose the underlying cardiac condition, and it is useful to listen carefully to the postpause beat. In aortic stenosis, for example, the murmur may be louder as a result of the more forceful ventricular contraction following the pause. However, this is not the case in mitral incompetence. The long pause with increased left ventricular volume may produce or increase left ventricular outflow obstruction in hypertrophic cardiomyopathy (see Chapter 17, p 539), and the first sound may be diminished in the postpause beat. When long pauses are felt in the radial or carotid arteries, the possibility of a "dropped" beat due to atrioventricular block must be considered. Early premature beats can be heard (unless they are nonconducted atrial premature beats), whereas "dropped" beats cannot.

1. Electrocardiography–Supraventricular premature beats are best recognized on the ECG, especially after careful inspection of a long strip (Fig 15–1). The usual pattern is that of P waves having a contour different from that of regular sinus P waves. These P waves are premature and may be associated with an aberrant QRS complex that usually has a right bundle branch block configuration. They may be nonconducted if they occur early and may be missed unless careful inspection of the T wave preceding a pause shows that it is slurred or notched or otherwise different from other T waves in the lead, thus indicating that a premature P wave is buried in the T wave complex.

The ectopic (premature) P wave has been called P′ and should be carefully sought if the RR interval or the dominant rhythm is disturbed or if the PR interval in the succeeding beat is prolonged because of concealed conduction in the atrioventricular node. Search for P′ complexes may often explain unsuspected bradycardia by demonstrating ectopic P waves. When atrial premature beats occur in bigeminy, ie, in every other beat, the patient may be thought to have 2:1 block or sinus bradycardia when in fact the rhythm is that of atrial premature beats, which are clinically less significant.

2. Concealed atrial premature beats–Occasionally, the premature beat or P′ beat may be isoelectric to the lead examined and thus not obvious and only suspected or recognized by its effects on the subsequent PR interval or by the pause that follows the so-called concealed premature beat. Atrial premature beats may be "concealed" when they partially penetrate the atrioventricular node and do not spread to the ventricles, but they nonetheless influence the refractory period of the atrioventricular node and so alter the succeeding PR interval. Supraventricular beats may not be recognized despite careful inspection but may be found and proved by His bundle recording that reveals a premature atrial or His bundle spike. If the presence of a premature beat that is not obvious on the ordinary ECG is strongly suspected, the ECG can be recorded at double standardization, or different leads that tend to exaggerate the size of the P′ wave may be employed.

Other means of amplifying the size of the supraventricular depolarizations include the bipolar Lewis lead (see also p 473) (right arm electrode in the second intercostal space to the right of the sternum 2 interspaces above lead V_1 and left arm electrode in the fourth intercostal space to the right of the sternum, the normal position for lead V_1, and both recorded on lead I), esophageal leads (electrode directly posterior to the left atrium), and right atrial electrode catheters that display large P′ as well as P waves. The P′ or ectopic atrial depolarization usually has a polarity different from the normal sinus P wave and may be inverted in leads II, III, and aVF and upright in aVR. These are low atrial or junctional.

3. Initiation of paroxysmal tachycardia–If the atrial premature beats occur at a critical time after the

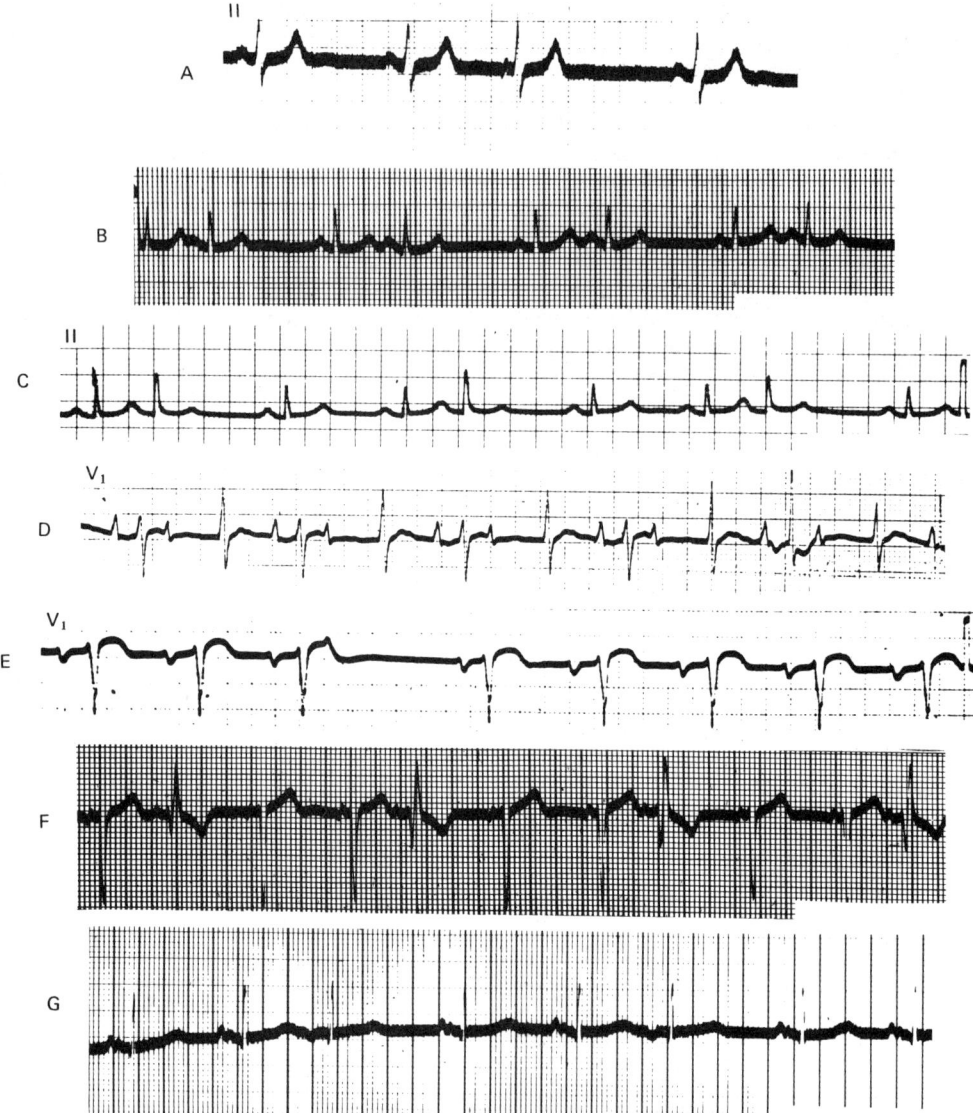

Figure 15–1. Atrial premature beats. **A:** Atrial premature beats, lead II. **B:** Atrial bigeminal rhythm, lead II. **C:** Atrial premature beats with slight aberrant conduction and subtle changes when P is superimposed on T waves, lead II. **D:** Normal sinus rhythm with atrial bigeminy that represents either nonconducted premature beats followed by junctional escape beats with aberrant intraventricular conduction or atrial premature beats with prolonged PR interval, lead V_1. **E:** Nonconducted atrial premature beat after third QRS complex, lead V_1. **F:** Atrial premature beats with aberrant conduction of right bundle branch block pattern, lead V_1. **G:** Atrial or junctional premature beats, lead II.

previous QRS complex (so-called **critical coupling interval**) and if conduction delay through a portion of the conduction system, usually the atrioventricular node, is present, a reentry circuit may be established, and the premature atrial beat may initiate supraventricular tachycardia. Programmed electrical stimulation has shown that atrial premature beats with a progressively shorter coupling interval combined with delay in conduction through the atrioventricular node are the causal mechanism in most cases of supraventricular tachycardia, although such tachycardias may be due to increased automaticity, such as occurs in coronary disease or following digitalis.

Treatment

Atrial premature beats rarely require drug treatment, unless they are frequent, multiform, chaotic, or associated with hemodynamic changes.

SUPRAVENTRICULAR TACHYCARDIA

With supraventricular tachycardia, there is a rapid regular rhythm (varying in rate from 150 to 250/min) in which the QRS complex is normal in appearance and similar to that seen in sinus rhythm. The tachycardia may be episodic paroxysmal reentry (reciprocating) supraventricular atrial tachycardia or "near-incessant" paroxysmal junctional reciprocating tachycardia (PJRT), often associated with retrograde posterior atrial septal accessory pathways. Tachycardia may also be nonparoxysmal supraventricular (junctional) tachycardia due to increased automaticity of the junctional cells (see p 472) and is reversed when the underlying condition is treated or subsides. Junctional rhythm due to the fault of the sinus pacemaker has a slow rate (60–80/min) and is not a tachycardia.

If ectopic P waves or P' waves are seen distorting the T waves or occurring prior to the QRS complexes with a 1:1 conduction and a normal PR interval, then atrial tachycardia is present (Fig 15–2). If the P' wave immediately precedes or is coincident with the QRS complex, then a junctional or His bundle rhythm is present, as shown by His bundle recordings. Often, however, no P' can be seen, and the site of origin of the ectopic focus cannot be identified other than to say that it is above the ventricles. If the QRS complex is distorted and wide (aberrant conduction), the rapid regular rhythm may be confused with ventricular tachycardia, and a number of clinical features have been described to help in the differentiation. A bizarre, aberrant QRS complex in a rapid ventricular rhythm does not establish the site of origin as ventricular; a narrow QRS complex does not automatically mean that the site of origin is in the atria, because it may be in the bundle of His. When the origin of the P' is inferior, indicating a low origin spreading superiorly, it favors atrial flutter; the reverse is true of atrial tachycardia.

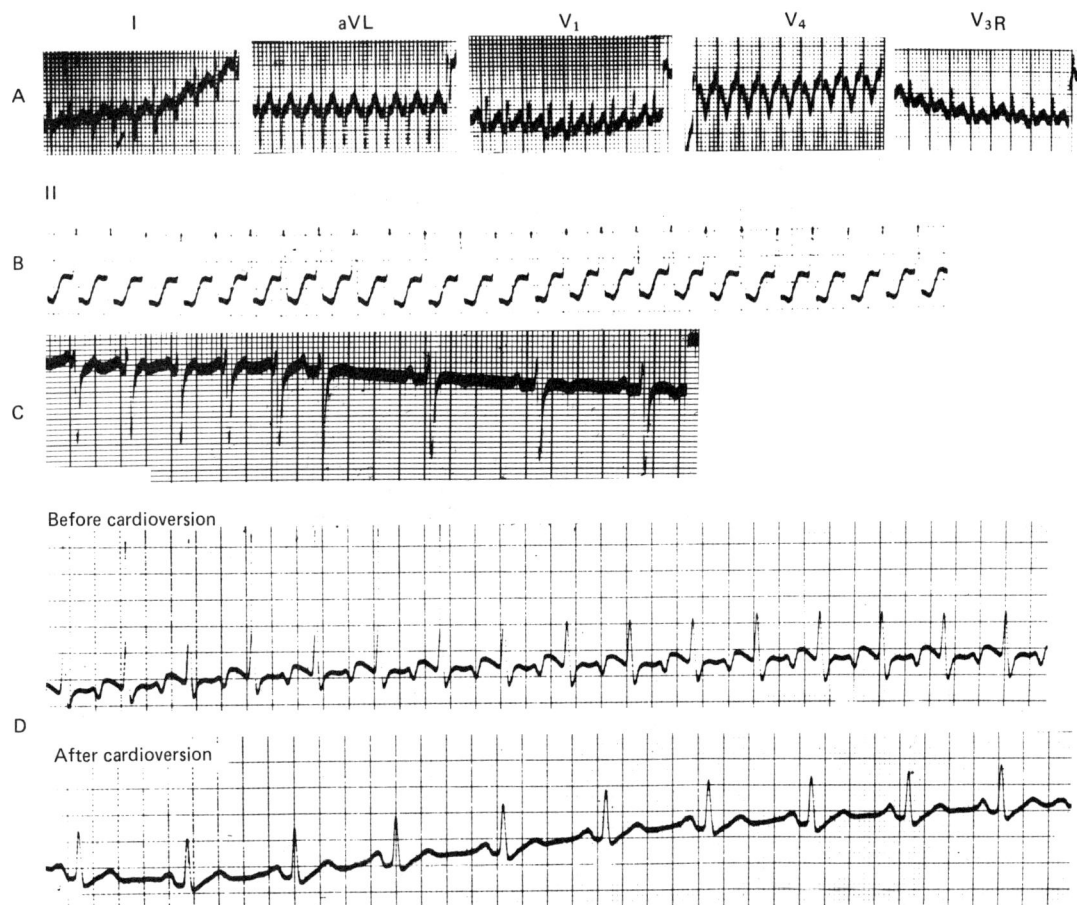

Figure 15–2. Supraventricular tachycardia. **A:** Supraventricular tachycardia in 3-week-old girl with a heart rate of 300/min. **B:** Probable myocardial ischemia during supraventricular tachycardia at a rate of 220/min. **C:** Supraventricular tachycardia with spontaneous subsidence in a 57-year-old woman. **D:** Paroxysmal atrial tachycardia with 1:1 conduction. Change in height of R waves indicates altered ventricular conduction converted by cardioversion in a 36-year-old woman to 2:1 conduction.

The mechanism of paroxysmal supraventricular tachycardia is reentry in about 75% of cases. The remainder of cases are due to increased automaticity or, in a small percentage of cases, to triggered activity as a result of increased afterpotentials (see Reentry, Chapter 14).

Supraventricular tachycardia is due to the same causes as premature beats. It often occurs in individuals with no evident heart disease. It may result from disease of the atria or bundle of His, as in atrial septal defect, mitral stenosis, or coronary disease involving the artery to the sinoatrial or atrioventricular node. The latter is usually confined to acute myocardial infarction, and paroxysmal supraventricular tachycardia is infrequent in patients with chronic coronary heart disease. Tobacco, coffee, stimulant drugs, and, most importantly, alcohol have been invoked as causal factors.

1. PAROXYSMAL SUPRAVENTRICULAR (ATRIAL) TACHYCARDIA

Paroxysmal supraventricular tachycardia results in a sudden increase in heart rate to 150–250/min, although rates of 300/min have been observed in infants, probably because atrioventricular conduction is accelerated in infants and the refractory period of the atrioventricular node is shorter. Young adults may have ventricular rates of 300/min for short periods at the onset that may result in syncope.

Many normal individuals have rapid heart rates with paroxysmal atrial tachycardia but do not develop "ischemic" ST segments during the attack or after it, or if they do, the ST changes may last only minutes to hours. Since patients rarely die during an attack, pathologic confirmation is not available. Some patients who develop "ischemic" ST segments during paroxysmal atrial tachycardia but who do not have angina on effort when they are in sinus rhythm may over a period of a few years develop angina pectoris, suggesting that subclinical coronary disease was unmasked by the rapid rate of the paroxysmal atrial tachycardia. The amount of ischemia or cellular damage that results from rapid rates with paroxysmal atrial tachycardia must be small, because few of these patients develop serum enzyme abnormalities or clinical manifestations suggesting subendocardial infarction. Nevertheless, it is common to find ischemic ST segment changes during paroxysmal atrial tachycardia in patients who have no symptoms and who do not have angina pectoris between attacks.

Clinical Findings

A. Symptoms: Palpitations may be the only symptom, but if there is underlying heart disease, the patient may complain of weakness, dizziness, anginal pain, or dyspnea. Central nervous system disturbances, when they occur, are usually diffuse in nature and not focal, as they are apt to be in cerebral ischemic attacks due to internal carotid artery disease. Angina pectoris may appear with the onset of tachycardia even if the patient has had no history of angina. The patient may be unaware of the rapid heart rate and complain only of angina. It is important to consider the onset of arrhythmias as a cause of the angina pectoris that appears at rest or during the night and is unrelated to exercise. The presence of underlying coronary disease is suggested not only by the appearance of angina during tachycardia but also by the appearance of typical ischemic ST segments on the ECG during the attack of rapid heart action. Infants may develop heart failure, especially if the heart rate exceeds 300/min; this is often the presenting manifestation of supraventricular tachycardia.

B. Signs:

1. Urine–In paroxysmal atrial tachycardia, the patient may pass a large quantity of urine within a few minutes of onset, a phenomenon that is thought to be due to stimulation of atrial natriuretic factors induced by volume changes in the atria.

2. Degree of atrioventricular conduction– Conduction is almost always 1:1, and there is no clinical evidence of atrial and ventricular asynchrony, so there is nothing abnormal to be heard at the bedside other than the rapid heart rate. The first sound does not vary in intensity, and no cannon waves can be seen in the jugular venous pulse. The major exception occurs when the atrial tachycardia is due to digitalis toxicity, in which instance, because digitalis also decreases conduction through the atrioventricular node, 2:1 block is frequent and may be overlooked when the atrial rate is about 150/min and the ventricular rate about 75/min. As the ventricular rate is normal, the patient has no palpitations or other symptoms, and were it not for the evidence on the ECG of rapid atrial rates with 2:1 ventricular response, digitalis toxicity could be overlooked. Fig 15–3 shows ECGs in coronary heart disease before and after treatment. Although digitalis is the usual cause of atrial tachycardia with 2:1 conduction, there are well-documented instances in which the patient with this disorder has not received digitalis; the physician is thus not warranted in diagnosing digitalis toxicity on the basis of the arrhythmia alone.

Digitalis toxicity is less commonly manifested by atrial tachycardia with 1:1 conduction or by varying degrees of atrioventricular block with or without atrial tachycardia or atrial fibrillation. Digitalis may not only cause atrial tachycardia with 2:1 conduction but may also produce partial progressive atrioventricular block with Wenckebach phenomenon, as shown in Fig 15–3C.

3. Jugular venous pulse–It is helpful to study the jugular venous pulse carefully in these instances; rapid *a* waves at twice the rate of the ventricular response may lead to the correct diagnosis. The same is true in atrial flutter (see below), when the conduction from the atria to the ventricles is 4:1 and the ventricular rate at 75/min does not make one suspect that the atria are beating at a more rapid rate. The ECG can usually define the atrial rate unless the atrial waves are isoelectric.

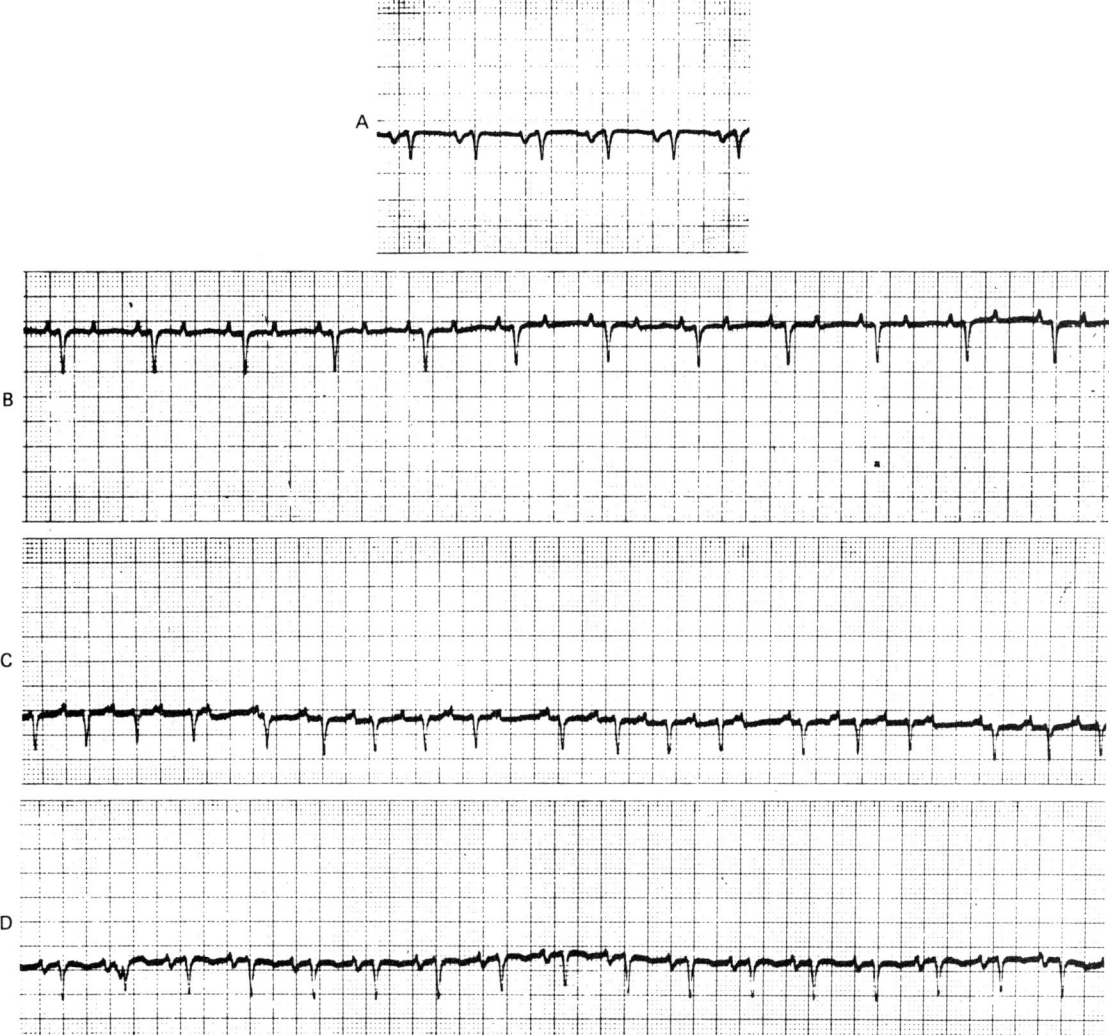

Figure 15–3. Atrial tachycardia before, during, and after treatment in a man age 52 weighing 60 kg, with coronary heart disease. *A:* 5:00 PM 7/22/55. Coronary heart disease before treatment with digoxin and a mercurial diuretic (Mercuhydrin, 2 mL intramuscularly). Note sinus rhythm. *B:* Atrial tachycardia with an atrial rate of 150/min and a ventricular rate of 75/min with 2:1 block after digoxin, 2.5 mg, and Mercuhydrin, 1 mL intramuscularly in 24 hours, with weight loss of 3.6 kg not recognized. On second day, a further dose of 1 mg digoxin and 1 mL Mercuhydrin was given, with weight loss of 5.9 kg in 48 hours. *C:* 9:00 PM 7/25/55, 4 hours after administration of 11 meq potassium orally. Atrial tachycardia (rate 125/min) with Wenckebach phenomenon is now present. *D:* 11:45 PM 7/25/55, 1 hour and 45 minutes after a second dose of 11 meq potassium. Sinus tachycardia is now present. (All strips are lead V_1.)

4. Concealed Wolff-Parkinson-White syndrome–As many as 20% of patients with supraventricular tachycardia may have concealed Wolff-Parkinson-White syndrome, primarily with a retrograde anomalous pathway (Pritchett, 1978). In childhood these patients may have had a definite delta wave that disappeared in later life; electrophysiologic studies demonstrate the anomalous pathway. The differentiation of Wolff-Parkinson-White syndrome from ordinary supraventricular tachycardia is difficult without special studies. In centers that do frequent electrophysiologic examination of such patients, surgical ablation of the anomalous pathway has been recommended if the arrhythmia cannot be prevented by drugs.

Hemodynamic Studies

Hemodynamic studies in paroxysmal atrial tachycardia may in some cases show not only a marked increase in heart rate but also prolongation of the PR interval, fall in arterial pressure, decrease in the cardiac index, and increase in the pulmonary artery diastolic pressure and right atrial pressure (Goldreyer, 1976).

Differential Diagnosis

Atrial flutter is an atrial arrhythmia thought to be due to a circus movement, arising low in the atria, with atrial rates varying from 150 to 350/min; at the lower range, it may be difficult to distinguish from atrial tachycardia, just as atrial tachycardia with a rapid atrial rate may be difficult to distinguish from atrial flutter. One must then rely upon probabilities. In the usual case of supraventricular tachycardia, the atrial rate is less than 200/min, and in most cases of atrial flutter, the atrial rates are approximately 300/min. Atrial or supraventricular tachycardia usually occurs in younger individuals, often those with no heart disease or with heart disease that obviously involves the atria; it can then be inferred that the rapid supraventricular rhythm is more likely to be supraventricular tachycardia than atrial flutter. In contrast, atrial flutter, like atrial fibrillation, is more apt to occur in older individuals with obvious heart disease such as coronary heart disease or mitral stenosis. A conduction delay from atria to ventricles of 4:1—or variable conduction such as alternating 2:1, 3:1, 4:1—occurs in atrial flutter but is uncommon in supraventricular tachycardia.

Treatment

For treatment, see p 475.

2. NONPAROXYSMAL SUPRAVENTRICULAR (JUNCTIONAL) TACHYCARDIA

When sinoatrial nodal function is depressed, as during digitalis therapy, in acute myocardial infarction, or often after open heart surgery, supraventricular tachycardia with a rate usually less than 130/min may occur, either because the secondary junctional pacemakers "escape" as a result of depressed sinus node function or because the automaticity of the junctional tissues is enhanced by metabolic abnormalities secondary to hypoxia, ischemia, and associated digitalis therapy.

This condition is called nonparoxysmal junctional tachycardia and is usually associated with a narrow QRS complex. The junctional pacemaker may activate the atria retrogradely or may beat independently of the atria and result in atrioventricular dissociation. Knoebel (1974) believes that most of these tachycardias are due to increase in automaticity of the junctional tissues and are not passive escape rhythms, because the ventricular rate is often faster than in passive rhythms (usually <60/min) and because atrioventricular dissociation occurs, indicating that both sinus and junctional pacemakers are intact.

When the mechanism is not "escape" but enhanced automaticity, it is postulated that the released metabolites or potassium from the ischemic and hypoxic myocardial cells may increase the slope of phase 4 diastolic depolarization of the action potential of the involved cells, leading to increased automaticity of the junctional tissues.

Atrioventricular Dissociation

In some instances, both the sinus node and the junctional area "fire" independently, and atrioventricular dissociation occurs. This can be recognized on the ECG by noting intermittent capture of the ventricles by a sinus impulse that fortuitously reaches the ventricle when it has recovered excitability following depolarization from the junctional beat. Pick (1957) described nonparoxysmal junctional tachycardia and noted that the ventricular rate was slower than with ordinary supraventricular tachycardia. In contrast to the sudden onset and sudden offset that characterize supraventricular tachycardia, nonparoxysmal junctional tachycardia has a gradual onset and offset and is often seen transiently in the first few days after acute myocardial infarction. Although the QRS interval is often normal, it may be wide and slurred if there is aberrant conduction to the ventricles.

Clinical Findings

A. Symptoms: The symptoms in nonparoxysmal junctional tachycardia depend upon the ventricular rate and hemodynamic effects. Symptoms may be absent because the ventricular rate is usually between 80 and 120/min, or there may be palpitations, dyspnea, or fatigue. The diagnosis is often not suspected clinically but made from the echocardiographic abnormalities and the clinical setting.

B. Signs: The signs are similar to those of paroxysmal atrial tachycardia, but there may be signs of atrioventricular dissociation (see above).

Differential Diagnosis

Nonparoxysmal junctional tachycardia with aberrancy must be differentiated from accelerated idioventricular rhythm during acute myocardial infarction, but this is often not possible with conventional ECGs. This latter condition usually has more abnormal ventricular complexes, but His bundle recordings may be necessary if a clear diagnosis is felt to be clinically required. The ventricular origin is also more obvious when the clinical situation abruptly worsens or when the signs of ventricular tachycardia (see Clinical Differentiation, below) can be elicited. If fusion beats of gradual onset and offset occur preceding and following the run of tachycardia, the rhythm is ventricular in origin.

In sinus tachycardia, the rate is rapid, essentially regular at short intervals, and almost always less than 180/min. It may be slightly irregular and vary with simple maneuvers such as posture, mild exercise, respiration, breath-holding, or carotid sinus pressure. The regularity of the heart rate in paroxysmal atrial tachycardia may differentiate this rhythm from sinus tachycardia, in which the heart rate may be rapid and apparently regular but can be altered by posture, respiration, or slight exercise. If the heart rate is counted for a full minute, especially after changes in position and other maneuvers mentioned in the preceding sentence, it will be shown to be slightly irregular and variable in sinus tachycardia. In paroxysmal atrial tachycardia, however, the heart rate is not influenced by these procedures unless the attack is terminated abruptly.

Sinus tachycardia results from a number of factors, eg, fever, infection, anemia, anxiety, leukemia, thyrotoxicosis, or connective tissue disorders.

A. Differentiation of Ventricular and Supraventricular Rhythms on the ECG: The differentiation between ventricular tachycardia and supraventricular tachycardia with aberrant conduction is often difficult (Fig 15–4). It is easy if the QRS complex is narrow and preceded by P waves; the difficulty arises when one cannot see P waves and the QRS complexes are wide. The key to the differentiation is identification of the P waves and their relationship to the ventricular complex. In ventricular tachycardia, atrioventricular dissociation occurs, although in rare cases there may be retrograde conduction to the atria, with retrograde 1:1 conduction and one P wave for every QRS complex. Usually, however, the ventricles are beating at a faster rate than the atria in ventricular tachycardia, whereas they are both the same in paroxysmal atrial tachycardia. Careful inspection of the T waves and QRS complexes for the possible presence of "buried" P waves is important in determining the atrial rate and in deciding if there are 2 independent pacemakers. Multiple conventional or Lewis leads, esophageal leads, right atrial electrode catheter electrograms, or His bundle recordings may be required to amplify the P waves or to relate them to the QRS complexes (Figs 15–5 and 15–6).

When the QRS complex is wide, the differentiation between ventricular tachycardia and supraventricular tachycardia with aberrant conduction is more difficult. Supraventricular tachycardia is inferred when the pattern in lead V_1 is that of right bundle branch block with an rSr′ or rsR′ pattern because of a prolonged refractory period in the right bundle or when the QRS configuration in the first few beats of tachycardia is similar to the pattern of premature beats that may have been present previously. These criteria are only probable and not absolute indications of supraventricular tachycardia. Although the odds favor supraventricular tachycardia on the basis of what has been said, the rSR′ pattern in lead V_1 could still represent junctional tachycardia with aberrancy and not paroxysmal atrial tachycardia. Ventricular tachycardia is the more likely diagnosis if the QRS pattern is of the left bundle branch type or has a QR pattern in lead V_1. If the patient has had ventricular premature beats on a previous ECG that are similar in configuration to the QRS complexes of the current tachycardia, ventricular tachycardia is the more probable diagnosis.

B. Differentiation From Ventricular Tachycardia: The differentiation of ventricular tachycardia from supraventricular tachycardia with aberrant conduction is often difficult in patients with a QRS duration of 0.12 second or more. Utilizing His bundle recordings to establish the site of origin of the tachycardia, Wellens (1985) found that the following changes favored (but did not establish) a ventricular origin: (1) QRS duration exceeding 0.14 second; (2) left axis deviation; (3) atrioventricular dissociation; (4) capture or fusion beats (infrequent); (5) monophasic (R) or biphasic (qR, QR, or RS) complexes in V_1; and (6) a qR or QS complex in lead V_6. The diagnosis of a supraventricular origin was favored by the following: (1) a triphasic QRS complex, especially if there was initial negativity in leads I and V_6; (2) ventricular rates exceeding 170/min; (3) QRS duration greater than 0.12 second but less than or equal to 0.14 second; and (4) the presence of preexcitation syndrome.

With wide QRS complexes, the diagnosis of ventricular tachycardia can also be made on the basis of the following criteria: (1) The QRS complexes during the tachycardia are 120 ms or greater in duration and totally different from the complexes during supraventricular rhythm. (2) Atrioventricular dissociation or ventriculoatrial block is present. (3) Intermittent fusion and normal capture beats occur. (4) Atrial pacing to rates in excess of the tachycardia does not produce aberration. (5) No His bundle potential precedes ventricular activation during the tachycardia. A His bundle potential precedes each QRS complex with a normal HV interval when sinus rhythm is restored (Puech, 1970; Waxman, 1977).

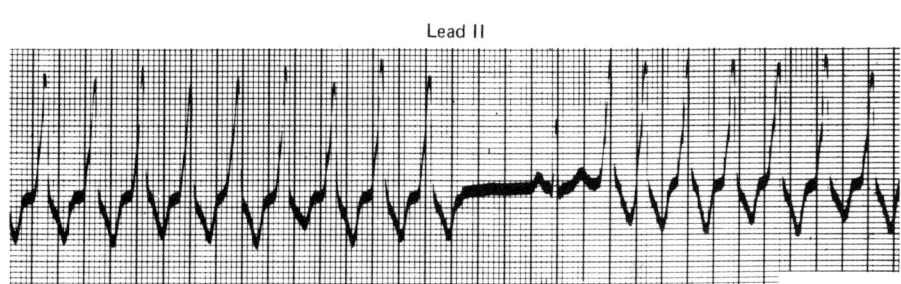

Figure 15–4. Tachycardia (ventricular or junctional) interrupted by single normal beat in a 43-year-old man.

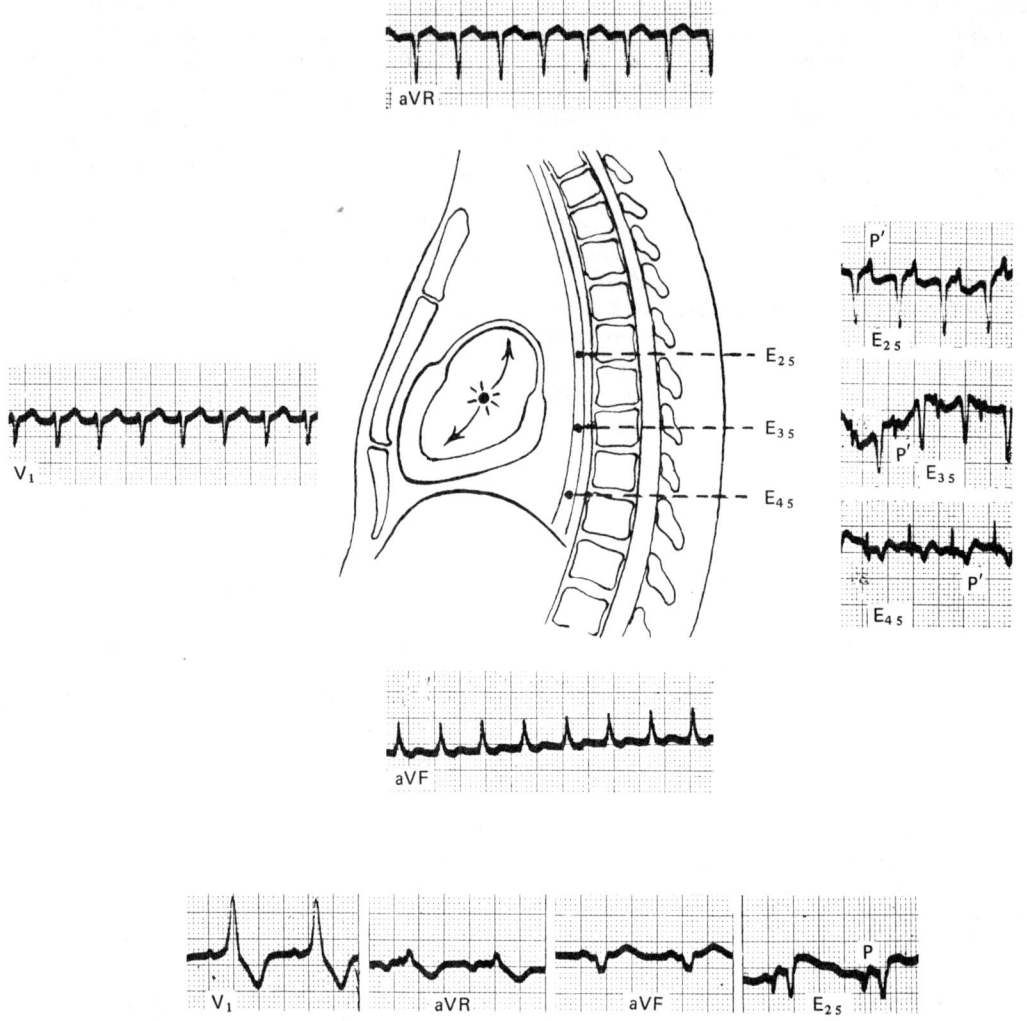

Figure 15–5. Supraventricular paroxysmal atrial or junctional tachycardia, diagnosed with the aid of esophageal leads that amplify the P waves. The bottom strip was taken after reversion to sinus rhythm and demonstrates a typical Wolff-Parkinson-White syndrome conduction (type A). (Reproduced, with permission, from Goldman MJ: *Principles of Clinical Electrocardiography*, 12th ed. Lange, 1986.)

C. Clinical Differentiation: Clinical bedside evaluation may provide evidence of atrial and ventricular asynchrony, eg, varying intensity of the first heart sound and cannon waves in the jugular venous pulse. Cannon waves are large abrupt *a* waves in the jugular venous pulse ("venous Corrigan waves") occurring as the atria contract when the tricuspid valve is closed (see p 48).

D. Value of Underlying Condition in Differentiation: The age of the patient and the setting in which the tachycardia occurs are helpful in diagnosis. Ventricular tachycardia is more likely if the patient has acute myocardial infarction, coronary heart disease, or other disease of the left ventricle, such as hypertrophic cardiomyopathy, aortic stenosis, or hypertensive disease. As noted previously, if the patient is young and free of heart disease and the precipitating factor was an acute emotional event, supraventricular tachycardia is the more likely diagnosis. It must be emphasized again, however, that none of these criteria are absolute and all indicate only the probable site of origin of the tachycardia. About 5–10% of patients with ventricular tachycardia have no known or obvious heart disease, whereas supraventricular tachycardia may occur in patients with known heart disease even if the patient is young. If it is essential to make the differentiation in order to determine therapy, His bundle recordings are helpful by demonstrating the presence of a His bundle spike preceding the QRS complex, in which case the tachycardia is supraventricular. His bundle recordings with intracardiac stimulation by programmed, critically timed supraventricular pre-

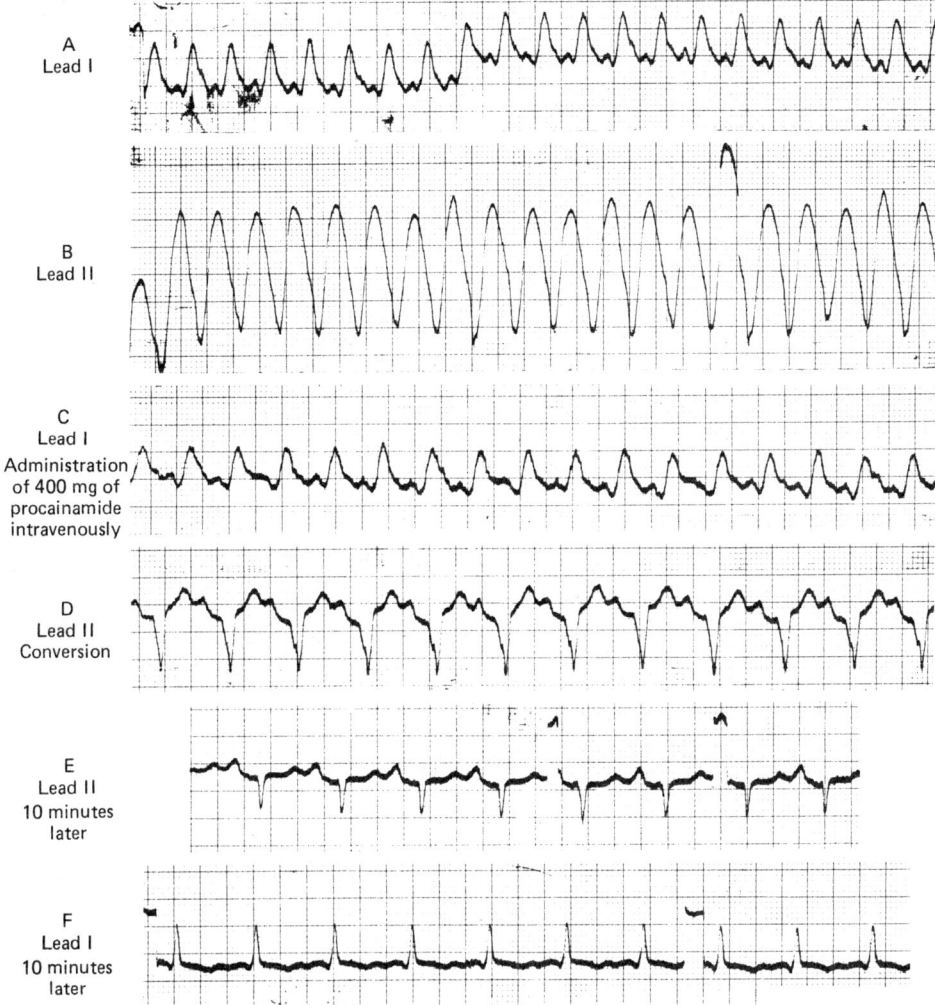

Figure 15-6. Paroxysmal supraventricular tachycardia 7 days after aortoiliac thromboendarterectomy. Sudden tachycardia after bowel movement. *A* and *B:* Before treatment. The pattern resembles ventricular tachycardia because of the wide QRS complexes, but a P wave is seen before each QRS complex in *A,* indicating that the rhythm is atrial tachycardia with aberrant conduction. *C:* Ventricular slowing following administration of 400 mg of procainamide intravenously (2 hours after 1 g quinidine gluconate intramuscularly over a 4-hour period with a quinidine blood level of 3.1 mg/mL). *D:* Sinus rhythm with intraventricular block at time of conversion. *E* and *F:* 10 minutes later, showing normal intraventricular conduction.

---

mature beats may establish the supraventricular origin of a tachycardia of unknown cause, but such procedures are indicated only if therapy is ineffective and the prognosis doubtful. In troublesome cases, treatment should be directed toward the more serious condition, ventricular tachycardia; lidocaine with or without DC electric shock is helpful in both supraventricular and ventricular tachycardia.

Treatment

In the treatment of supraventricular tachycardia, drugs should be given orally unless serious cardiovascular deterioration indicates the need for rapid reversion to sinus rhythm. It is most important for the physician to estimate the degree of urgency. This estimate is made in part by observing how the patient is handling the rapid rate and whether the tachycardia is producing dyspnea, angina, faintness, confusion, hypotension, or oliguria. The history of previous attacks is most helpful in determining not only their usual duration but also the degree of disability produced. The duration of the attack when the patient is first seen is of importance, because if arrhythmia has been present for hours or days and the patient is still asymptomatic, the urgency is not great unless the patient's age and the presence of underlying heart disease such as mitral stenosis or coronary heart disease suggest that problems may arise if the attack continues. Therapeutic decisions are also influenced by ineffective treatment that the patient may already have received or by a history of therapeutic agents that have or have not succeeded in stopping previous attacks. If the patient is in a coronary care unit, a Swan-Ganz catheter may be inserted to allow bedside hemodynamic observations of pulmonary capillary wedge pressure, pulmonary artery pressure, and cardiac output, as in patients with acute myocardial infarction. If the patient is hypotensive, raising the arterial pressure with pressor agents may stop the attack or allow other therapeutic agents to become effective, and this form of treatment is often the most valuable immediate measure.

A. Underlying Condition: Treatment of underlying metabolic abnormalities such as hypoxia, ischemia, alkalosis, acidosis, or anemia is of first importance. Treatment of ventilatory problems is more important than the use of cardiac drugs in postoperative patients or in patients with chronic lung disease.

B. Sedation: If the ventricular rate is not over 150–180/min in a patient who has no or minimal heart disease with good left ventricular function and who is tolerating the tachycardia without symptoms other than palpitation—and especially if the attack was precipitated by an acute emotional event—sedation may be the initial and only treatment for the first few hours. Seconal, 0.1–0.2 g orally; diazepam (Valium), 5–10 mg orally; or flurazepam (Dalmane), 30 mg orally, may relax the patient and induce sleep, and the tachycardia may abruptly stop.

C. Stimulation of Vagus Nerve: If sedation fails or if the patient has dyspnea, severe palpitations, cerebral symptoms, polyuria, fall in blood pressure, or angina, maneuvers should be tried to increase atrioventricular block by stimulating the vagus nerve to increase the refractory period of the atrioventricular node and delay atrioventricular nodal transmission of the impulse.

Noninvasive methods of stimulating the vagus may be used first, eg, carotid sinus massage, Valsalva's maneuver (Fig 15–7), breath-holding, squatting, or placing the face in ice water for a few seconds (Waxman, 1980). As with all methods of increasing vagal stimulation, patients may have a few ventricular premature beats or a short run of them at the time of conversion, and, rarely, ventricular fibrillation may develop. For this reason, resuscitative equipment should be immediately available. Gentle unilateral carotid sinus massage should be performed for up to 10 seconds (with the patient's head comfortably supported by a pillow), first on one side and then the other but not on both sides together or continuously. ***Caution:*** Do not use carotid sinus stimulation if the patient has carotid bruits or a history of transient cerebral ischemic attacks. Pressure on the eyeball should be avoided because of the risk of retinal detachment. Inducing vomiting is an unpleasant measure but may be effective.

D. Drug Treatment:

1. Decrease of atrioventricular conduction–If vagal stimulation fails, drugs can be used that directly decrease atrioventricular conduction.

a. Calcium entry–blocking drugs–These drugs are the treatment of choice in paroxysmal atrial tachycardia. Verapamil has the greatest inhibiting effect on the atrioventricular node, nifedipine the least, and diltiazem is intermediate. Verapamil (Isoptin), 5–10 mg, or diltiazem (Cardizem), 150–300 ug/kg, can be given intravenously over 3–5 minutes; nifedipine is likely to be ineffective (Sung, 1980; Sakurai, 1983; Svinarich, 1984). Verapamil may be combined with propranolol unless the patient has left ventricular failure. The data are inadequate to determine the value of verapamil combined with digitalis. Bradycardia and hypotension may occur with verapamil, and caution must be used before giving it to patients already receiving digitalis or beta-adrenergic blocking drugs. The combination may produce various bradycardia syndromes, including sinus arrest.

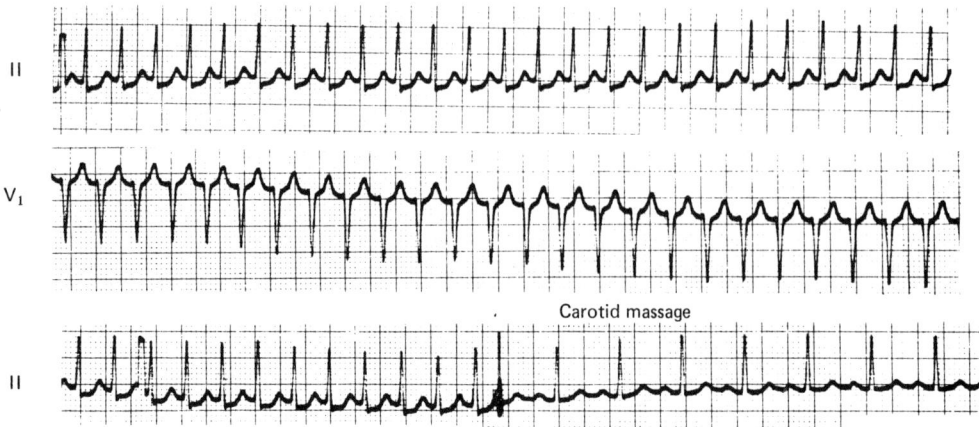

Figure 15–7. Carotid massage abruptly terminates paroxysmal atrial tachycardia in a 54-year-old man with carcinoma of the neck. ST ischemic depression is seen just prior to cessation of the attack.

b. Other drugs–Edrophonium (Tensilon), 5–10 mg intravenously, is usually given by bolus injection. A bolus of 10 mg converted 9 (17%) of 51 patients with paroxysmal atrial tachycardia within 15 minutes; 34 (67%) responded within 35 minutes. An infusion of 0.75–1 mg/min converted almost all within 1 hour (Reddy, 1978). Such vagal stimulation may induce gastrointestinal symptoms such as abdominal cramps, nausea, and vomiting. In older patients, it is wise to begin with a smaller dose, repeating it at 5- to 10-minute intervals, until a dose of 10 mg has been given. Other agents include propranolol, 0.5–1 mg intravenously every 5 minutes, up to a total of 1–5 mg; other beta-adrenergic drugs; and digitalis (digoxin), 0.75–1 mg intravenously. Patients should be monitored closely, and hypotension should be avoided. Caution should be used if the patient has evidence of impaired cardiac function, because cardiac failure may result. Fig 15–8 shows an example of supraventricular tachycardia promptly abolished by means of intravenous lanatoside C therapy. As with vagal stimulation, intravenous digitalis may cause ventricular premature beats at the time of conversion of supraventricular tachycardia to sinus rhythm. These premature beats may be due to digitalis toxicity but this is doubtful, since the beats are similar to those occurring after carotid sinus massage or placing the face in ice water; furthermore, the ST segment is normal 5 minutes later, without premature beats.

If these drugs fail, one of the noninvasive methods of stimulating the vagus (such as carotid sinus massage) should be used during the time of drug action to produce additive vagal stimulation. If the tachycardia persists, therapeutic agents that reflexly increase vagal stimulation can be used, including such pressor drugs as phenylephrine, 2–4 mg subcutaneously or 0.1–0.2 mg intravenously, which raise blood pressure and stimulate the baroreceptor reflexes. Caution should be used; one should begin with small doses to avoid excess hypertension.

Among the newer drugs, one of the most powerful in treating severe cases of supraventricular tachycardia unresponsive to conventional therapy is amiodarone, given in a dosage of 5 mg/kg over a 15-minute period, followed by an infusion of 600 mg over a 12- to 24-hour period. Side effects are frequent when the drug is used chronically (see p 490) in dosages of 300–600 mg/d (Morady, 1982).

2. Decrease of automaticity–(See Tables 15–5 and 15–6 and p 487.) Drugs that decrease excitability and automaticity may occasionally be helpful in an acute paroxysm of tachycardia. Give quinidine sulfate, 0.2–0.4 g orally every 4 hours; procainamide, 100 mg/5 min intravenously to a total of 1 g; or phenytoin or lidocaine, 50–100 mg of either drug intravenously followed by an infusion of 1–2 mg/min. Quinidine is most effective in atrial arrhythmias but may produce hypotension and ventricular arrhythmias. Propranolol, 20–40 mg 2–4 times daily orally or in small doses (0.1–2 mg) intravenously, may be used to increase atrioventricular block. Its mechanism of action is to block beta-adrenergic receptors, increase atrioventricular nodal transmission time, and block the reentry circuit. Begin with 0.1 mg intravenously every 1–5 minutes until the desired effect is achieved or early toxic manifestations force abandonment of this therapy.

Electrophysiologic testing of the effect of various drugs may be helpful, as in ventricular tachycardia (see below).

E. Cardioversion: In many cases of supraventricular tachycardia, if the conventional drugs are ineffective, cardioversion is the treatment of choice. However, if the patient has digitalis toxicity, car-

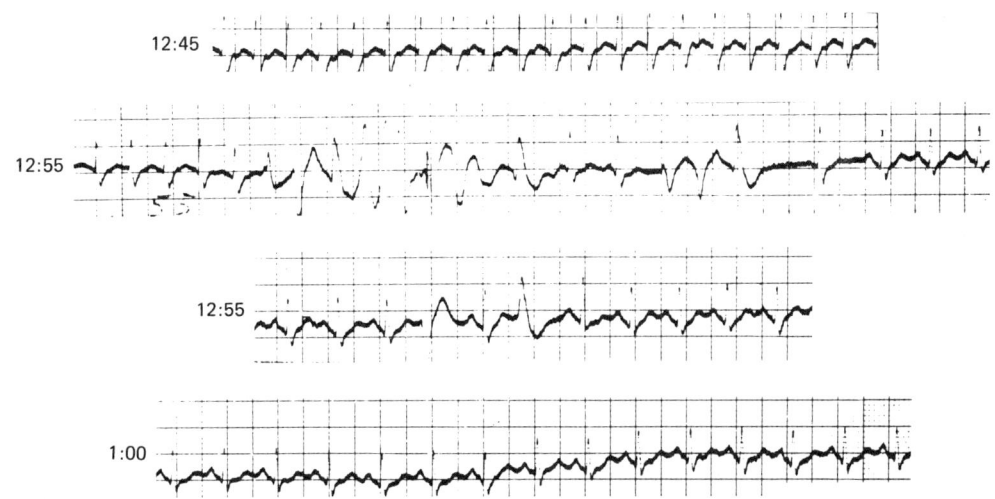

Figure 15–8. Supraventricular tachycardia promptly abolished with intravenous lanatoside C therapy at 12:45 in a 59-year-old man. Note the ventricular premature beats lasting 3 seconds at the time of reversion to sinus rhythm.

dioversion should be avoided or used in small increments of current beginning with 5–10 J, since it can produce serious ventricular arrhythmias. Amiodarone may also be tried (Morady, 1982). Catheter ablation of the His bundle and implanted pacemakers are to be considered only when patients fail to respond to intensive medical treatment and have recurrent attacks with severe hemodynamic consequences (Scheinman, 1982).

F. Rapid Atrial Pacing: If there is digitalis toxicity, if supraventricular tachycardia occurs following cardiac surgery, or if the patient fails to revert to sinus rhythm with vigorous pharmacologic therapy, rapid atrial pacing to produce overdrive suppression of the ectopic focus may be the treatment of choice (Waldo, 1981; Wiener, 1980). Pacing of the atrium at heart rates above that of the ectopic tachycardia may terminate the tachycardia during pacing or immediately after pacing is stopped or may induce atrioventricular block, effectively slowing the ventricular rate. Discontinuing the atrial pacing causes transient depression of both the ectopic tachycardia and the sinus node; the latter recovers first, restoring sinus rhythm. Atrial pacing not only restores sinus rhythm by this "overdrive suppression," but it may interrupt the reentry circuit of the paroxysmal atrial tachycardia by depolarizing the atrium so that the reentry pathway is refractory to an oncoming pulse. Occasionally, atrial pacing may induce atrial fibrillation, which may then spontaneously revert to sinus rhythm.

G. Paroxysmal Atrial Tachycardia With Block: As indicated previously, paroxysmal atrial tachycardia with block is usually (not always) due to digitalis toxicity. It is wise to stop digitalis and diuretics to minimize potassium loss and, if the situation is not urgent, allow tachycardia with block to gradually disappear over 1–3 days. If the serum potassium is less than 3 meq/L, potassium chloride may be given in a dosage of 40–100 meq orally; or, if the need is urgent or deemed possibly so, the potassium can be given intravenously in a dosage of 10–20 meq/h. Cardioversion should be avoided in the presence of digitalis toxicity because of the risk of inducing ventricular arrhythmias.

H. Junctional Rhythms With Atrioventricular Dissociation: This rhythm is usually due to increased automaticity (most commonly from digitalis toxicity), acute inferior myocardial infarction, acute myocarditis, or following cardiac surgery. Treatment is the same as for paroxysmal atrial tachycardia with block. Digitalis and diuretics should be stopped, and if the serum potassium is low, potassium may be given intravenously at a rate of 10–20 meq/L/h. If the abnormal rhythm is due to acute myocardial infarction, treatment should be directed at the acute infarction and should consist of rest, oxygen, and other therapy monitored by frequent determination of hemodynamic indices, noting the response of the patient (see Chapter 8). In the "near-incessant" variety or "permanent" form of paroxysmal junctional reciprocating tachycardia, amiodarone or aprindine may abolish the arrhythmia, but conventional drugs are usually ineffective. If unresponsive to all drugs, the arrhythmia has been abolished by surgical ablation of the retrograde accessory pathway, which is usually near the coronary sinus in the posterior atrial septum (Guarnieri, 1984).

I. Arrhythmias During Cardiac Catheterization: The irritation of the right atrium or the right ventricle may induce atrial or ventricular premature beats. The catheter should be removed from the involved chamber until the premature beats disappear, and the procedure can then be continued.

J. Prevention of Recurrences:

1. Drug treatment–Recurrences of supraventricular tachycardia can be prevented by long-term administration of digitalis, beta-adrenergic blocking agents, verapamil (Sakurai, 1983), or amiodarone (see p 477). Margolis (1980) has advocated episodic rather than chronic antiarrhythmic therapy, following determination of the combination of drugs and procedures that terminate an individual attack. A useful review of supraventricular tachycardia is that of Bigger (1980).

2. Implantation of pacemakers–Externally activated pacemakers designed to interrupt the reentry circuit have been used successfully. More recently, implanted automatic atrial pacemakers, activated by rapid atrial tachycardia, have been used in resistant, recurrent cases associated with considerable hemodynamic deterioration during tachycardia (Spurrell, 1982). The results seem promising, but more experience is required.

3. Cryotherapy–Disabling episodes of paroxysmal tachycardia that cannot be controlled by antiarrhythmic therapy have occasionally been treated by cold ablation of the atrioventricular node, which is usually involved in the reentry circuit. Patients should first have an electrophysiologic study to define the reentry pathway and exclude accessory connections. When it is established that the atrioventricular node is involved in the reentry circuit and temporary cooling produces atrioventricular block, cryotherapy at -60 to $-65\,°C$ may destroy the atrioventricular node and prevent recurrent arrhythmias (Scheinman, 1983). This procedure is rarely necessary, especially with the availability of drugs such as verapamil or amiodarone, and should be considered only after electrophysiologic studies by experienced physicians.

4. Catheter ablation of His bundle–A new procedure used in disabling recurrent attacks is electrical ablation via catheter to damage or destroy the His bundle, producing partial or complete atrioventricular block with beneficial clinical effects (Scheinman, 1982; Josephson, 1984). This technique should only be used in desperate cases by experienced individuals. A catheter is placed across the tricuspid valve near the bundle of His, and a current of about 300 J is then given to damage the area and prevent rapid atrial impulses from reaching the ventricle. A ventricular pacemaker must be simultaneously inserted if this technique is used. Further data are awaited.

ATRIAL FIBRILLATION & ATRIAL FLUTTER
(See Fig 15–9.)

Atrial Fibrillation

Atrial fibrillation is the most common atrial arrhythmia in older people. It can be paroxysmal or established, as is true of atrial flutter (see p 480). Paroxysmal attacks usually last hours or days rather than seconds or minutes and almost never longer than 2 or 3 weeks. If the rhythm persists after this period, atrial fibrillation is said to be established, or chronic; this is in contrast to supraventricular tachycardia, which rarely lasts days or weeks and usually lasts minutes or hours. Paroxysmal atrial fibrillation may occur without known heart disease or other obvious reason but most commonly occurs after pulmonary or cardiac surgery or in older individuals with mitral stenosis, atrial septal defect, myocarditis, thyrotoxicosis, or constrictive pericarditis. It is most common in older people with left atrial enlargement due to any cause. It may be precipitated by an acute emotional event even if the patient has underlying cardiac disease such as mitral stenosis. It is not especially common in chronic coronary heart disease and is infrequent in acute myocardial infarction, although continuous monitoring has shown that it may occur. It is common when hypoxia and infection occur in chronic lung disease with cor pulmonale.

Following pulmonary embolism or surgery—perhaps as a result of hypoxia from inadequate ventilation or pericardial injury—as many as one-third of patients may develop paroxysmal atrial fibrillation. Transient atrial fibrillation is also common following cardiac surgery, especially mitral valve surgery. Even if the rhythm reverts to sinus rhythm preoperatively, it often recurs after surgery. It is common during the course of untreated thyrotoxicosis and usually disappears spontaneously when the thyrotoxicosis is treated. It may be precipitated by cardiac catheterization in patients with mitral stenosis or atrial septal defect. Atrial fibrillation may occur after infective endocarditis is established in aortic or mitral valvular heart disease but is uncommon in acute endocarditis occurring in drug users with tricuspid or aortic valve lesions.

Atrial fibrillation is rare in pure aortic valve disease in the absence of heart failure, and its presence should prompt the physician to think of associated mitral valve disease, even if the typical murmurs are not readily heard.

A prospective Framingham study found that in the absence of known heart disease, the incidence of chronic atrial fibrillation increased with age but still developed infrequently (2% over a period of 20 years). Cardiovascular disease was usually associated with the arrhythmia or developed shortly after the arrhythmia occurred (Kannel, 1982). Isolated or "lone" atrial fibrillation is usually asymptomatic but may result in systemic emboli, although less frequently than in mitral valve disease. Ten percent of the patients in the Framingham study had strokes, some of which may have been due to cerebral emboli.

A. Clinical Course: The onset of atrial fibrillation may provoke dyspnea in the patient with mitral stenosis and may also produce cardiac failure in the patient with atrial septal defect, when the rapid ventricular rate prevents atrial emptying and left ventricular filling. In mitral stenosis (see Chapter 12), left atrial pressure may rise quickly, producing pulmonary venous congestion, severe dyspnea, and acute pulmonary edema. The atrial transport function of atrial systole may be required to preserve adequate left ventricular filling in patients with low cardiac reserve;

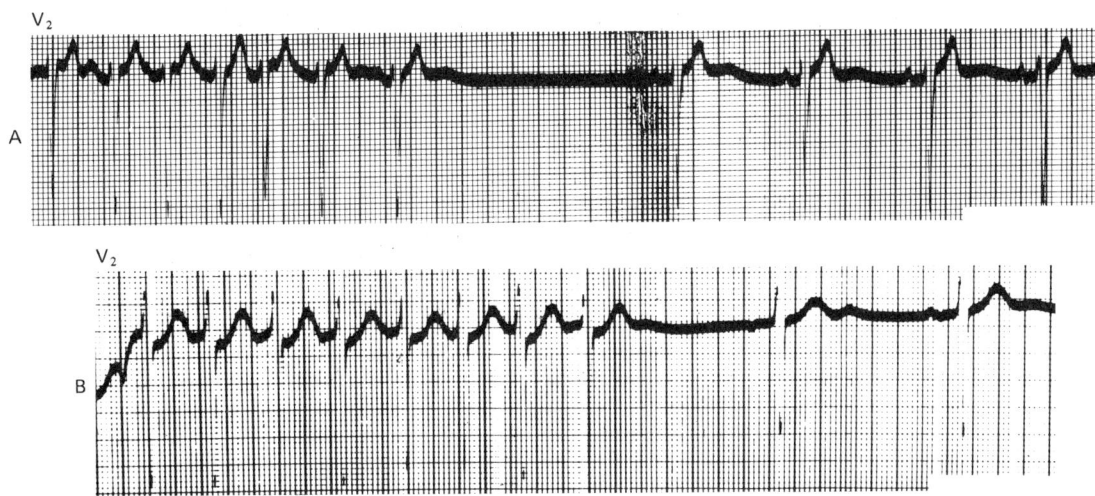

Figure 15–9. Spontaneous changes in atrial arrhythmia. **A:** Spontaneous conversion of atrial fibrillation with rapid irregular ventricular response to sinus rhythm in a 71-year-old woman. **B:** Spontaneous subsidence of supraventricular tachycardia, followed by junctional escape prior to sinus rhythm in a 62-year-old woman.

the onset of atrial fibrillation may produce severe left ventricular failure in these patients. Some individuals merely have palpitations; a few may have no symptoms whatever, and the atrial fibrillation in these cases is discovered accidentally.

B. Chronic Atrial Fibrillation: In chronic atrial fibrillation—especially if the ventricular rate is controlled with digitalis—the patient may be asymptomatic and may be unaware of the atrial fibrillation or its irregularity except when exercising. Some patients describe what they think are paroxysmal episodes of atrial fibrillation when in fact they have chronic fibrillation but are aware of the rapid, irregular ventricular rate only with exercise or emotion.

C. Risk of Systemic Emboli: In addition to the possibility that pulmonary venous congestion and decreased cardiac output may occur when atrial fibrillation supervenes in mitral valve disease, patients with chronic atrial fibrillation have the added risk of systemic emboli, which are uncommon in patients with supraventricular tachycardia. Systemic embolism may be the initial clinical manifestation of mitral stenosis, eg, cerebral embolization with hemiplegia, and a major embolus to an extremity may require surgery. The likelihood that an embolism will develop is greatest in the year following onset of atrial fibrillation, but the course is unpredictable and patients may develop major emboli after they have had atrial fibrillation for several years. Systemic emboli are less common in nonrheumatic types of heart disease and occur rarely in thyrotoxicosis.

D. Atrial Rate and Ventricular Response: The atrial rate in atrial fibrillation is approximately 450–600/min, and the ventricular response is almost always irregular because of variable "concealed" conduction in the atrioventricular node. Without treatment, the ventricular rate usually varies between 130 and 160/min, but it may be less than 100/min. The so-called F (fibrillation) waves seen on the ECG reflecting the circus movements thought to be the cause of atrial fibrillation, with multiple wave fronts simultaneously exciting the atria, may be obvious on the ECG or may be fine and difficult to see. The differentiation of so-called coarse and fine atrial fibrillation is rarely of clinical importance. When the ventricular rate is rapid and only slightly irregular, the presence of obvious F waves is helpful in diagnosis. When the ventricular rate is rapid or when it is slow as a result of digitalis therapy, the irregularity may not be gross or obvious unless the ventricular rate is timed carefully.

If the ventricular rate is rapid, atrial fibrillation with aberrant conduction may be confused with ventricular tachycardia. The presence of a right bundle branch block pattern in lead V_1 is helpful, as noted previously in the differential diagnosis of tachycardia, and favors aberrancy of interventricular conduction.

E. Pulse Deficit: Before digitalis is given, there is a substantial difference between the ventricular rate as determined at the apex of the heart and that felt at the radial pulse—the so-called pulse deficit. This occurs because the more rapid beats may not result in a sufficient stroke output to cause a pulse wave to reach the wrist. Following digitalis therapy, when the ventricular rate is slowed, each beat has a more forceful output and the pulse deficit diminishes.

Atrial Flutter

Atrial flutter is similar to atrial fibrillation in its age distribution and causative factors, but it is less common than atrial fibrillation in mitral valve disease and atrial septal defect. It may be paroxysmal or established, as in atrial fibrillation, but the atrial rate is slower, usually 260–350/min, and the ventricles usually respond to every other atrial excitation wave, so that the pattern is a 2:1 atrioventricular conduction with an atrial rate of about 300/min and a regular ventricular rate of 150/min. In some patients, atrioventricular conduction may be variable and show alternating 2:1, 3:1, or 4:1 conduction with an irregular ventricular rate, simulating atrial fibrillation. Atrioventricular conduction is less predictable than in atrial fibrillation, and patients may have abrupt changes from 4:1 to 2:1 with postural changes or excitement or while eating. They may have a ventricular rate of 75/min when recumbent and 150/min when sitting. They may then have an abrupt onset of palpitations and symptoms without a change in the basic atrial flutter, reflecting only a change in the ventricular response to the flutter.

For these reasons, atrial flutter is a more unstable and troublesome rhythm than atrial fibrillation. The abrupt jumps in ventricular rate with minor activities may produce pulmonary venous congestion if the patient has underlying cardiac disease such as severe mitral stenosis. This is in contrast to atrial fibrillation, in which there is a more gradual and smaller increase in ventricular response following trivial activity. Atrial flutter and atrial fibrillation may occur in the same patient on different occasions, as may atrial tachycardia.

Treatment

A. Atrial Fibrillation: The principal aim of therapy, whether the patient has acute or chronic atrial fibrillation, is to slow the ventricular rate by increasing atrioventricular block with digitalis. A secondary consideration is restoration of sinus rhythm, and a third important therapeutic aim is to prevent recurrences.

1. Digitalis–(See Table 15–5 and Chapter 10 for details of dosage.) When restoration of sinus rhythm is not urgent, because severe symptoms of dyspnea, angina, palpitations, confusion, or hypotension are absent, digitalis—with or without the addition of a beta-adrenergic blocking drug or a calcium entry–blocking drug such as verapamil—is the treatment of choice and can be used orally or parenterally, depending upon the urgency of the need to slow the ventricular rate by increasing the atrioventricular block. Verapamil may replace both digitalis and beta-blocking drugs as agents to slow the ventricular rate in atrial fibrillation. Once the ventricular rate is controlled, the decision to attempt restoration of sinus rhythm can be undertaken in nonurgent circumstances. Digitalis alone is often relatively ineffective in slowing the ventricular rate in acute atrial fibrillation or in chronic atrial fibrillation in the setting of severe cardiovascular disease. In these cases there is little relation between the "therapeutic" serum digoxin levels (0.8–2 ng/mL) and the ventricular rate (Goldman, 1975). The addition of verapamil may slow the ventricular rate, especially with exercise, and may be of considerable benefit.

2. Quinidine–Almost all patients with atrial fibrillation who are treated with quinidine go through a transitional phase of atrial flutter prior to the development of sinus rhythm, because quinidine slows the atrial rate. It has a vagolytic action that improves atrioventricular conduction, leading to a more rapid ventricular rate as the atrial rate slows. Digitalis is therefore given before quinidine to prevent a rapid ventricular rate. In these instances, the atrial rate varies from 150 to 300/min and may be irregular.

3. Other drugs–If quinidine is ineffective, the following drugs may be used, alone or in combination: procainamide, 250–500 mg 2 or 3 times a day; disopyramide (in the absence of cardiac failure), 0.8–1.2 g/d; propranolol, 10–60 mg 2 or 3 times a day (or its equivalent); verapamil, 40–80 mg 3 or 4 times a day. Amiodarone is probably the most effective of the newer drugs for the prevention of recurrent atrial fibrillation, especially in the presence of Wolff-Parkinson-White syndrome, and can be used in doses of 300–600 mg/d. Side effects are frequent, however (see Table 15–7). Verapamil may not be effective and may be harmful. In chronic atrial fibrillation or in paroxysmal fibrillation when the ventricular rate cannot be controlled with digitalis (especially during exercise), beta blockers (propranolol, 10–20 mg orally 4 times daily and increased as needed, or metoprolol, 50–100 mg twice daily) can be added with benefit to slow the ventricular rate during exercise. They should be used with caution if the patient has a history of asthma or left ventricular failure, atrioventricular conduction defects, or bradycardia. Propranolol can be added to quinidine in an effort to prevent recurrences, and there are some data to suggest that the combination is more effective than quinidine alone. If quinidine alone or in combination with propranolol is not tolerated, procainamide, 250–500 mg orally 3 or times a day alone or combined with quinidine, is sometimes effective but should be used cautiously.

4. Cardioversion–Restoration of sinus rhythm is usually performed by electric shock cardioversion. If an electric defibrillator is not available, quinidine can be used. When quinidine is given to patients receiving digoxin, the mean serum digoxin almost doubles, and some patients develop symptoms of digitalis toxicity (Leahey, 1980). Fig 15–10 shows the relationship between the daily dose of quinidine, peak serum quinidine concentrations, and myocardial toxicity. As the dose of quinidine is increased, there is an average progressive increase in serum quinidine concentration, but there are many departures from the average. Serum levels of 8–10 μg/mL may be achieved

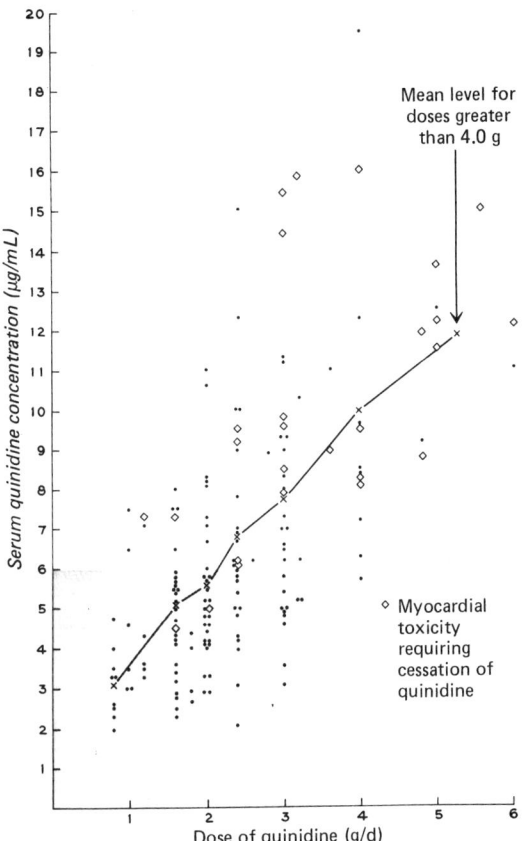

Figure 15–10. Relationship between daily dose, peak serum quinidine concentration, and myocardial toxicity. (Reproduced, with permission, from the American Heart Association, Inc., Sokolow M, Ball RE: Factors influencing conversion of chronic atrial fibrillation with special reference to serum quinidine concentration. *Circulation* 1956;**14**:568.)

with doses of 2–2.5 g/d in some patients, whereas serum concentrations below 7 μg/mL can be obtained in others with 3 g quinidine per day. Myocardial toxicity is more closely related to the serum concentration than to the dose and progressively increases as the serum concentration rises (Fig 15–10). If quinidine is used to restore sinus rhythm because countershock is not available, it can be started at a dose of 0.2 g every 2 hours for 5 doses on day 1, with serum levels obtained 2 hours after the last dose. The individual dose can be increased by 0.1 g daily, but it is unwise to increase the dose beyond 3 g/d unless serum concentrations of the drug can be determined and the patient can be seen before each dose. It should be reemphasized that cardioversion is the treatment of choice in attempted conversion of chronic atrial fibrillation and that quinidine is used only if cardioversion is not possible.

Countershock should be used with caution in the presence of digitalis toxicity. If large doses of digitalis have been required to slow the ventricular rate, it is wise to stop digitalis for 1 or more days and to attempt cardioversion with small stimuli such as 5 J, increasing the strength of the shock as necessary. Because atrial fibrillation recurs so often, quinidine is usually begun 2 days before cardioversion to build up an adequate blood level of the drug in order to prevent recurrence of the arrhythmia. When quinidine (0.3 g 4 times daily) is given, about 20% of patients revert to sinus rhythm, and countershock is not necessary. This dose of quinidine may produce a blood quinidine concentration of 2–4 μg/mL, which may be sufficient to restore sinus rhythm. It is also a level that is usually adequate to prevent recurrences.

If digitalis or verapamil cannot be used (usually because of preexcitation syndromes; see Chapter 14) or are ineffective in the treatment of acute paroxysmal atrial fibrillation, other drugs may sometimes convert the arrhythmia to sinus rhythm. Give procainamide, 50 mg/min intravenously up to a total dose of 1–1.5 g, or in more critical situations, amiodarone (see above and Ventricular Tachycardia).

5. Anticoagulation prior to cardioversion–A controversial area with respect to cardioversion is the necessity for anticoagulation prior to conversion to sinus rhythm. The incidence of systemic emboli following restoration of sinus rhythm without anticoagulation is small—about 0.5%—although some authors have reported rates as high as 2–3%. If the patient has had recent systemic emboli or has a large left atrium, anticoagulant therapy with a coumarin drug for several weeks prior to countershock is desirable, although many physicians do not use anticoagulants prior to cardioversion.

6. Rapid atrial pacing–If atrial fibrillation or flutter with rapid ventricular rates cannot be controlled by conventional pharmacologic therapy, especially following open heart surgery, continuous rapid atrial pacing at rates of 450/min can be initiated. Pacing increases the atrioventricular block, slowing the ventricular rate. If atrial flutter is the arrhythmia, atrial pacing may induce atrial fibrillation with a slower ventricular rate; digitalis may then increase the atrioventricular block and further slow the ventricular rate (Waldo, 1981). The use of rapid atrial pacing for paroxysmal atrial tachycardia is discussed on p 478. As with paroxysmal atrial tachycardia, atrial flutter may abruptly stop when rapid atrial pacing is discontinued.

7. Prevention of recurrences–Because the recurrence rate following cardioversion is high, especially in patients who have long-standing atrial fibrillation or considerable enlargement of the heart or whose arrhythmias developed following cardiac surgery, it becomes a matter of judgment whether to control the ventricular rate with digitalis and leave the patient in chronic atrial fibrillation or to attempt to restore normal sinus rhythm with cardioversion. Quinidine is effective in preventing frequent recurrent attacks of paroxysmal atrial fibrillation of relatively short duration (usually hours to days), the dose and frequency of administration being gradually increased until the attacks no longer occur or are less frequent.

Fig 15–11 depicts the serum quinidine concentration measured at 2:00 PM in patients given 0.4 g 4 times a day. Although the mean value is 4.7 ± 1.9 μg/mL, the serum concentration ranges from 2 to 11 μg/mL, indicating differences in absorption, distribution, and metabolism of the drug. Myocardial toxicity may occur with increasing doses of quinidine and is manifested by the presence of ventricular arrhythmias—usually ventricular premature beats but occasionally ventricular tachycardia or even ventricular fibrillation. Ventricular fibrillation occurs infrequently when quinidine is given with the patient in a stable state with no other drug therapy, but the likelihood of fibrillation is enhanced when patients are receiving increasing doses of digitalis with or without diuretic therapy and resultant hypokalemia. When both quinidine and digitalis are given under these circumstances—especially if diuretics are also used—it is an open question whether the ventricular fibrillation is due to digitalis or quinidine. Prolongation of the QT interval is common and represents the electrophysiologic action of quinidine delaying repolarization. Intraventricular block or bundle branch block that develops after quinidine is due to a marked conduction defect. When the QRS duration exceeds 30–50% of the control value, it is wise to stop quinidine.

If quinidine is given at regular intervals (eg, 4 times daily), a blood level plateau is reached in 48–72

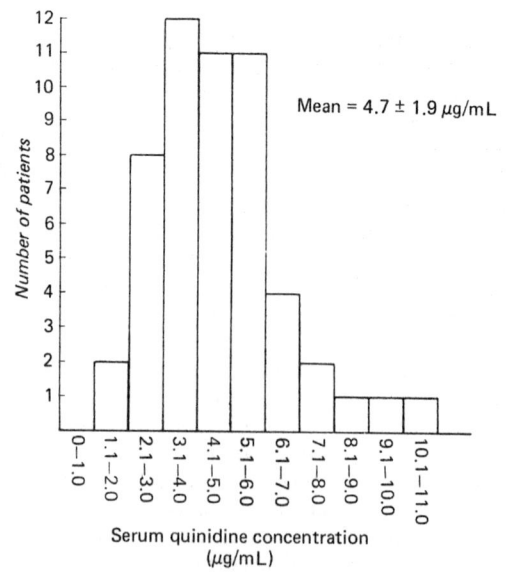

Figure 15–11. Distribution of 2:00 PM serum quinidine levels, dose of 0.4 g 4 times daily for at least 3 days (53 patients). (Reproduced, with permission, from the American Heart Association, Inc., Sokolow M, Ball RE: Factors influencing conversion of chronic atrial fibrillation with special reference to serum quinidine concentration. *Circulation* 1956;**14**:568.)

hours. A larger dose or administration at shorter intervals is required to achieve higher, more effective blood levels (Table 15–1).

A rare complication of quinidine therapy is thrombocytopenia, resulting from the affinity of quinidine and its antibody for a receptor on the surface of platelets, provoking their immunologic destruction. The process is usually reversible when quinidine is stopped (Christie, 1982).

Not only is the recurrence rate of atrial fibrillation high after cardioversion in patients with large hearts and a long history of atrial fibrillation, but the drug that is most effective in preventing recurrences is quinidine, which is unpleasant for some patients to take because of its side effects: diarrhea, nausea, and tinnitus. The same symptoms occur when quinidine is used to convert atrial fibrillation to sinus rhythm, and various medications can be used to counteract the symptoms, but this is unwise in patients receiving chronic quinidine therapy. In patients whose atrial fibrillation has lasted less than 6 months and whose hearts and left atria are normal in size or only slightly enlarged, cardioversion should be tried at least once, combined with an effort to prevent recurrences with oral quinidine therapy, 0.2–0.3 g 4 times daily, or long-acting quinidine preparations that require only twice-daily dosage. Under these circumstances, about half the patients remain in sinus rhythm for a year or more and are much more comfortable than when they were in atrial fibrillation, primarily because of relief of disproportionate tachycardia with mild exercise. Patients who have been repeatedly converted to sinus rhythm almost always indicate that their cardiac function is much better when they are in sinus rhythm. Quinidine decreases the recurrence rate of atrial fibrillation after restoration of sinus rhythm. In a multicenter study from Stockholm, approximately 50% of patients were still in sinus rhythm a year after treatment of atrial fibrillation or flutter when they received quinidine, whereas only 25% of the control group remained in sinus rhythm (Södermark, 1975).

Long-acting quinidine is superior to short-acting quinidine in maintaining sinus rhythm after DC cardioversion. After 18 months, 65% of patients remained in sinus rhythm while receiving long-acting quinidine and 30% while receiving short-acting quinidine of comparable dosage (Normand, 1976). In the whole series, sinus rhythm was maintained for 18 months in 50% of patients, which is consistent with the results of the Stockholm study.

8. Mitral stenosis or coronary disease—In patients with minimal or moderate mitral valve or coronary artery disease, control of atrial fibrillation or flutter is often decisive in determining whether symptoms of dyspnea or angina are due to the arrhythmia or to the anatomic defect. If the former, drug therapy and not surgery is the treatment of choice. Hemodynamic study with cardiac catheterization is often necessary to determine the magnitude of the structural defect. Cardiac catheterization should be delayed until the ventricular rate is controlled and the patient is in a steady state. The severity of mitral stenosis, for example, can be overestimated if cardiac catheterization is done when the ventricular rate is rapid, in which instance the pulmonary capillary wedge pressure may be high and evidence of pulmonary venous congestion present. The various formulas for determining the valve areas are theoretically not influenced by rapid ventricular rates, but this is often not the case.

B. Atrial Flutter: Paroxysmal atrial flutter responds to cardioversion in about 95% of cases, and this is the treatment of choice in almost all cases. Patients should not be allowed to remain in chronic atrial flutter because of the instability of the rhythm, as noted above. Quinidine by mouth is a relatively ineffective method of treatment of chronic atrial flutter and should be used only to prevent recurrences. If the patient has a history of paroxysms lasting hours that are not prevented by quinidine or quinidine plus propranolol, digitalis can be used to increase the atrioventricular block and slow the ventricular rate. Systemic emboli are much less frequent than in atrial fibrillation, because atrial systole is made stronger by the slower atrial rate and more uniform atrial contractions, decreasing the likelihood of atrial thrombus formation. As in chronic

Table 15–1. Effects of quinidine on 2 patients with coronary heart disease, paroxysmal atrial fibrillation, and paroxysmal atrial flutter.

	Dose of Quinidine	Average Midday Blood Level	Comment
Male, age 57 years Coronary heart disease. Paroxysmal atrial fibrillation 2–4 times per month for 12 years.	None	0	4 attacks in 6 weeks
	0.2 g 3 times daily	0.5 µg/mL	3 attacks in 6 weeks
	0.4 g 3 times daily	2.9 µg/mL	8 attacks in 24 weeks
	0.4 g 4 times daily	3.2 µg/mL	3 attacks in 6 weeks
	0.4 g 4 times daily (Enseals)	1.5 µg/mL	2 attacks in 1 week
	0.6 g 3 times daily	4.5 µg/mL	2 attacks in 6 weeks
	0.5 g 4 times daily	5.2 µg/mL	No attacks in 6 months
Male, age 54 years Coronary heart disease. Paroxysmal atrial flutter 2–4 times per week for 4 years.	0.2 g 5 times daily	1.3 µg/mL	No effect
	0.4 g 4 times daily	1.9 µg/mL	Slight decrease in attacks
	0.4 g 5 times daily	2.7 µg/mL	1 attack in 9 weeks
	0.4 g 5 times daily	3.7 µg/mL	1 attack in 6 weeks
	Quinidine stopped	0	Many attacks within 48–72 hours
	0.6 g 4 times daily	4.6 µg/mL	No attacks for 3 months

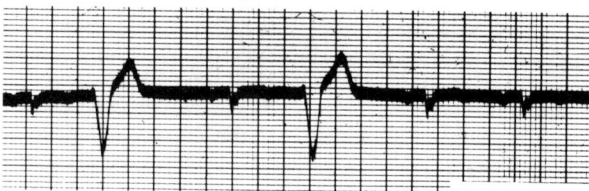

Figure 15–12. Ventricular premature beats with bigeminy in a 48-year-old man not receiving digitalis.

atrial fibrillation, it is wise to begin quinidine therapy 1–2 days prior to cardioversion if the patient has recurrent episodes of atrial flutter and to realize that an increased ventricular rate may result. The usefulness of digitalis to prevent recurrences should not be overlooked, because it may increase the atrioventricular block. Digitalis is always worth a trial, because if it is successful, the patient can be maintained on a single daily dose, which is tolerated much better than multiple doses of quinidine.

VENTRICULAR ARRHYTHMIAS

VENTRICULAR PREMATURE BEATS (Extrasystoles)

Ventricular premature beats are the most common of all arrhythmias (Figs 15–12 and 15–13). In the absence of heart disease, they are usually not of great clinical significance, but in patients with coronary heart disease, they represent a constant danger of ventricular tachycardia or fibrillation and sudden death.

Many epidemiologic studies of the incidence and prognostic significance of ventricular premature beats have been performed in recent years in the hope of identifying and perhaps treating a high-risk group liable to sudden death. Whereas in the past a single ECG was used to determine the presence of ventricular premature beats, more recent epidemiologic studies have used 6-, 12-, or 24-hour ambulatory monitoring of the ECG or continuous ECGs during graded exercise to evaluate the type and frequency of ventricular premature beats in population groups. It has been shown, for example, that multihour ambulatory monitoring reveals at least 10 times as many premature beats, as well as complex arrhythmias, as does a single routine ECG. Ventricular premature beats may cause concern in as many as one-third of patients convalescing from acute myocardial infarction.

Lown (1977) has devised a grading system for ventricular premature beats (Table 15–2). Since sudden deaths are most apt to occur in people with known coronary disease—especially with ventricular premature beats—efforts have been made to identify those who have frequent or complex premature beats spontaneously or after exercise that might warrant long-term antiarrhythmic therapy, especially if the angiographically identified disease is severe. However,

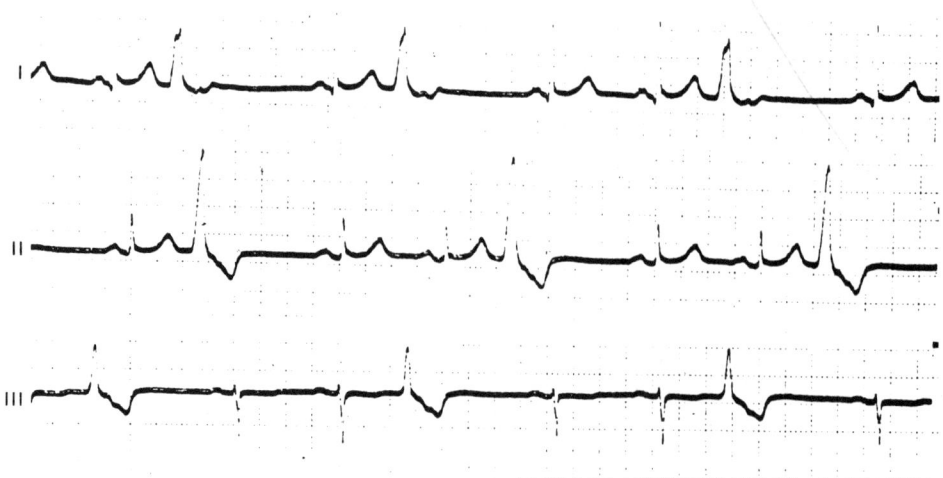

Figure 15–13. Sinus rhythm with frequent unifocal premature ventricular beats occurring in bigeminy (every other beat) and trigeminy (every third beat). The basic ventricular rate is 75/min.

Table 15-2. A grading system for ventricular premature beats.*†

Grade	Characteristics of Beat
0	No ventricular beats
1A	Occasional, isolated ventricular premature beats (less than 30/h): Less than 1/min
1B	Occasional, isolated ventricular premature beats (less than 30/h): More than 1/min
2	Frequent ventricular premature beats (more than 30/h)
3	Multiform ventricular premature beats
4A	Repetitive ventricular premature beats: Couplets
4B	Repetitive ventricular premature beats: Salvos
5	Early ventricular premature beats (ie, abutting or interrupting the T wave)

*Reproduced, with permission, from Lown B, Graboys TB: Sudden death: An ancient problem newly perceived. *Cardiovasc Med* 1977;2:219.
†This grading system is applied to a 24-hour monitoring period and indicates the number of hours within that period that a patient has ventricular premature beats of a particular grade.

premature beats are capricious and variable in coronary disease, and, just as in normal subjects, they may be present on one occasion and absent on another. In a large study of over 1000 patients who had had a myocardial infarction in the previous year, patients with complex ventricular beats noted in a 1-hour recording showed a 3-fold incidence of sudden death in 3 years, as compared to patients who had only single or no arrhythmias during the recording. See Fig 15-14 (Ruberman, 1977). Later follow-up indicates that the effects persist over a 5-year period.

Premature beats are also common in asymptomatic patients with coronary disease (Table 15-3). Even in

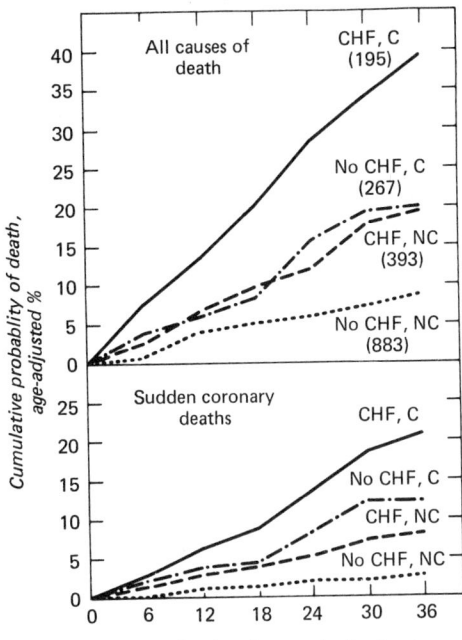

Figure 15-14. Mortality rates over 3 years after baseline monitoring in relation to the presence of complex (C) ventricular premature beats or their absence (NC) and congestive heart failure (CHF). (Reproduced, with permission, from Ruberman W et al: Ventricular premature beats and mortality after myocardial infarction. *N Engl J Med* 1977; 297:750.)

Table 15-3. Incidence of various ventricular arrhythmias in patient population.*

Arrhythmias	Number of Cases	Percent of Total Cases
Premature beats (unifocal)		
< 6/min†	523	31.3
6-12/min†	90	5.4
> 12/min†	70	4.2
Premature beats (multifocal)		
< 6/min†	206	12.3
6-12/min†	81	4.8
> 12/min†	69	4.1
Paired premature ventricular contractions	169	10.1
R wave encroaching on the T wave	72	4.3
Tachycardia	69	4.1
Fibrillation	0	0

*Reproduced, with permission, from Bleifer SB et al: Diagnosis of occult arrhythmias by Holter electrocardiography. *Prog Cardiovasc Dis* 1974;16:569.
†In *any* 1-minute period.

the coronary care unit, it has been shown that conventional monitoring of the ECG has limitations, and many arrhythmias are missed with ordinary monitoring techniques. The number of diagnostic errors resulting from such unreliable estimates of the frequency of ventricular arrhythmias and their response to treatment has led to greater reliance on computer detection and analysis of ventricular arrhythmias in the coronary care unit. The frequency of ventricular arrhythmias, including multiform and complex varieties as well as ventricular tachycardia, has been underestimated.

Seventy percent of subjects who had frequent complex ventricular premature beats discovered accidentally on Holter monitoring had no significant coronary disease when angiograms were subsequently performed. Most patients with ventricular premature beats in the absence of known coronary disease or symptoms do not, in fact, have coronary disease. On the other hand, 30% of such patients do.

Ventricular premature beats are said to occur during public speaking in 70% of patients with coronary disease but in only 10% of normal subjects (Lown, 1978). The risk of sudden death increases if there are more than 10 ventricular premature beats per 1000 complexes (Hinkle, 1969).

Role of Central Nervous System

The role of the central nervous system in ventricular premature beats is particularly important because excitement, anxiety, or fear increases autonomic adrenergic stimuli to the heart and may induce increased automaticity in the Purkinje fibers, leading to premature beats. Ventricular premature beats are common in patients on the day or so preceding elective surgery and disappear spontaneously in the postoperative period after successful surgery. Premature beats may be frequent during the day, but less frequent or even absent during sleep. Alcohol, tobacco, and coffee are important causes. Premature beats may come and go and are apt to occur during periods of emotional stress, even if the source of stress is not clearly defined. In rare cases, ventricular fibrillation may occur.

Significance of Ventricular Premature Beats

The greatest hazards of ventricular premature beats—in contrast to atrial premature beats—are ventricular tachycardia and ventricular fibrillation. Any tachycardia, atrial or ventricular, may have adverse hemodynamic effects if sufficiently rapid. Ventricular tachycardia, because it is more apt to occur in a setting of organic heart disease—particularly coronary heart disease or cardiomyopathy—is feared because of the likelihood of abrupt hemodynamic worsening or of ventricular fibrillation and sudden death.

Ventricular premature beats are common in older people with no heart disease. They increase in frequency with age, and the patients are often asymptomatic; but, as with atrial premature beats, the premature beat may produce symptoms referable to the postpause forceful beat that produces a thump, a sense of skipping or of emptiness in the chest, or a twinge of local pain. The premature beats may be the first sign of coronary heart disease, especially when they occur following exercise, but by themselves they are not a reliable sign of coronary disease. They are apt to occur in patients with slow heart rates because the long diastolic pause slows the subsequent velocity of conduction, increases the likelihood of variable refractory periods among cells, and favors the development of both reentry and automatic ectopic foci. In coronary disease, there may be scattered areas of ischemia or fibrosis, with different rates of recovery of excitability in neighboring fibers. This nonuniform recovery of excitability during the relative refractory period may induce chaotic propagation of the cardiac impulse and lead to ventricular fibrillation. This may occur with ventricular premature beats or with supraventricular premature beats with aberrant conduction. Aberrantly conducted beats also increase the likelihood of ventricular fibrillation, especially if the premature beats are closely coupled (Yoon, 1975). Prematurity and variable responsiveness are conditions within segments of the cardiac muscle of the ventricle that lead to reentry rhythms. If there is persistent ischemia, hypoxia, ventricular aneurysm, or left ventricular dilatation, phase 4 of the action potential may have an increased slope, with resultant increased automaticity. Ventricular premature beats may then be due to increased automatic ectopic firing rather than to reentry. Patients whose premature beats occur when the heart rate is slow are often benefited by increasing the rate, as with exercise, but when the rate slows following exercise, the premature beats may reappear. It is generally thought that premature beats are more significant when they occur only during or following exercise, but this requires further validation by prognostic studies. Multiform (grade 3) beats occurring during inducement of unifocal ventricular premature beats are associated with left ventricular wall motion abnormality, prior myocardial infarction, and a decreased ejection fraction. The first was the most important factor in distinguishing multiformity from nonmultiformity (Booth, 1982). Premature beats occurring during acute myocardial infarction are discussed in Chapter 8.

Clinical Findings

A. Symptoms: Patients may be asymptomatic or may complain of a forceful heartbeat that follows the extrasystolic pause. In contrast to atrial premature beats, when there is a normal sequence of conduction via the atrioventricular node through to the ventricles, ventricular premature beats by retrograde activation depolarize the atrioventricular node and interrupt the normal regular rhythm.

B. Signs:

1. Cannon waves–(See Chapter 3.) Right atrial systole may find the tricuspid valve closed because of recent intermittent ectopic ventricular systoles and produce, irregularly, a cannon wave in the neck as atrial systole forces blood back into the jugular vein. Cannon waves are presystolic, are of relatively large amplitude, and have a rapid ascent and descent that have suggested the term "venous Corrigan waves." The ventricular premature contractions occur irregularly; the sinus P wave and the ectopic QRS complexes may occur relatively simultaneously, usually with the P wave following the QRS complex, so that atrial contraction finds the tricuspid valve closed. Occasionally, there may be 1:1 synchronous retrograde conduction to the sinus node with ventricular premature beats, and cannon waves do not occur, as is true also if the patient has atrial fibrillation or atrial flutter with an insignificant or absent atrial systole.

2. Asynchrony of atria and ventricles–The first heart sound may vary in intensity because of the asynchronous contraction of the atria and the ventricles. The pause that follows the premature beat is usually "compensatory" because the basic rhythm is not altered. The premature beat, although it may have retrograde atrioventricular conduction, infrequently depolarizes the sinus node. For this reason, the pause following a ventricular premature beat is "prolonged," making up for the prematurity of the ectopic beat and keeping the basic sinus rhythm constant. This is in contrast to the usual atrial premature beat, in which the atrial ectopic beat depolarizes the sinus node, resetting its rate so that the pause is not "compensatory." The basic rate of sinus rhythm is not altered with ventricular premature beats. If the ventricular premature beats are frequent or occur in irregular runs, the cardiac rhythm may be so irregular that it may be confused with atrial fibrillation. Cannon waves in the neck (see above) may be helpful in the differentiation, as may the recognition of a "quick" premature beat before each pause.

3. Hemodynamic changes–Hemodynamic changes occur infrequently unless the ventricular premature beats are frequent or occur in runs, so that they decrease the cardiac output. When they are frequent and impair cardiac output, coronary perfusion may be reduced, and patients may have angina pectoris as a result of the premature beats.

4. Occurrence during anesthesia and surgery–Ventricular premature beats are common during anesthesia and are more apt to be noted in patients whose ECGs are being continuously monitored. They are related to hypoxia, hypotension, ischemia, and alterations in acid-base balance and are usually improved by careful attention to ventilation and arterial pressure. They may occur during intubation, especially if this is traumatic and ventilation is inadequate. Postoperatively, ventricular premature beats may also result from disturbances in ventilation or factors listed previously. Blood gas tensions should be monitored, so that possible causes such as acidosis, alkalosis, hypercapnia, or hypoxia will not be missed, especially in patients who have had pulmonary or cardiac surgery. Hypokalemia resulting from chronic diuretic or corticosteroid therapy combined with excessive digitalis therapy may be the cause of ventricular premature beats during or after surgery.

5. Beats induced by ambulation or graded exercise–Various studies have shown that ambulatory monitoring and graded treadmill exercise may complement each other in identifying the presence of ventricular premature beats, neither procedure being clearly superior. At least 6 hours are required for ambulatory monitoring. In some patients, exercise is more effective in inducing ectopic beats than ambulation; in others, the opposite is true. Ventricular premature beats should be counted and noted as being unifocal, multiform, occurring in pairs or runs, appearing early on the T wave (during the "vulnerable" period), or occurring in short runs of ventricular tachycardia or ventricular fibrillation.

In community epidemiologic studies, some middle-aged men with no history of angina or other evidence of coronary heart disease and no risk factors develop ventricular premature beats following graded exercise on a treadmill or cycle ergometer. These men have an incidence of sudden death similar to those who do not develop premature beats with exercise. To further complicate the task of clinical assessment, antiarrhythmic therapy in patients with coronary heart disease during convalescence from acute myocardial infarction is of only limited benefit and does not eliminate the arrhythmia in many cases, and the side effects of drug therapy may be significant. Further prospective studies are necessary to determine the prognostic significance of simple and complex ventricular premature beats that occur during ambulatory monitoring and following exercise and the benefits of various antiarrhythmic regimens, including newer drugs not yet approved by the FDA.

Treatment

In treating ventricular premature beats it is not necessary to abolish all such beats but only the complex ones. The main objective is to prevent ventricular tachycardia, ventricular fibrillation, and sudden death. Most ambulatory noncoronary patients with only occasional ventricular premature beats require no treatment other than reassurance and elimination of the precipitating cause if it is known to be alcohol, tobacco, anxiety, or digitalis therapy.

If the patient has chronic pulmonary disease or is recovering from anesthesia, improvement in ventilation should precede the use of drug therapy. The possible role of cardiac catheters, displacement of a central venous pressure line into the right ventricle, or insertion of pacemakers as causes of arrhythmias should be considered.

Discontinuation of any drugs that may be respon-

Table 15–4. Effectiveness of drugs against specific cardiac arrhythmias.*†‡

	Q	PA	P	PH	L
Supraventricular					
Atrial premature depolarizations	4	4	2	2	1
Paroxysmal atrial tachycardia	3	3	3	2	1
Atrial flutter	2	2	2§	1	1
Atrial fibrillation					
Conversion	4	4	2§	1	1
Maintenance	4	4	1	1	1
Atrioventricular junctional tachycardia and premature contractions	3	3	1	1	1
Ventricular					
Ventricular premature depolarizations	3	4	2	4	4
Ventricular tachycardia	2	4	2	4	4
Digitalis-induced arrhythmias					
Supraventricular	2	2	3	4	4
Ventricular	2**	2**	3**	4	4

*Reproduced, with permission, from Hoffman BF, Bigger JT Jr: Antiarrhythmic drugs. Chapter 40 in: *Drill's Pharmacology in Medicine*, 4th ed. DiPalma JR (editor). McGraw-Hill, 1971.
†Abbreviations: Q, quinidine; PA, procainamide; P, propranolol; PH, phenytoin; L, lidocaine.
‡Scale of relative effectiveness: 1, poor; 2, fair; 3, good; 4, excellent.
§Propranolol is very effective in reducing the ventricular response in atrial flutter and atrial fibrillation but does not convert these arrhythmias to sinus rhythm.
**All these drugs may be effective in treating digitalis-induced ventricular arrhythmias; however, significant undesirable effects have been encountered with each of them.

sible for the premature beats is part of treatment. Often overlooked as possible causes are aminophylline and similar drugs used in chronic obstructive lung disease and the so-called psychotropic drugs, particularly the phenothiazines and tricyclic antidepressants. Thioridazine (Mellaril) is particularly important in this respect.

A. Reassurance and Sedation: If premature beats are discovered during routine examination or because of a complaint of a "skipped" beat or palpitations, reassurance and mild sedation are often sufficient. Sedation and relief of anxiety are important therapeutic measures and must never be overlooked. Fatal cardiac arrhythmias have been attributed to central sympathetic influences on cardiac rhythm. Diazepam, 2.5–5 mg 2–4 times daily, may be very effective but must be used cautiously by ambulatory patients because it may cause undesirable oversedation.

B. Antiarrhythmic Drugs: (Tables 15–4 to 15–9.) If premature beats are frequent (> 5/min), multiform, or of the potentially dangerous variety with early R on T phenomenon (premature beats occurring on the downstroke of the T wave during the supernormal phase of excitability), if ambulatory monitoring demonstrates or exercise induces short runs of ventricular tachycardia, and especially if the patient has coronary heart disease with severe symptoms induced by the

Table 15–5. Guide for rapid administration of antiarrhythmic drugs.* See Table 15–7 for newer agents.

Drug	Dose	Therapeutic Plasma Level (μg/mL)	Side Effects	Comments
Lidocaine	100-mg bolus IV over several minutes followed by 2–4 mg/min constant infusion	1.4–6	Focal seizures; grand mal seizures; respiratory arrest; dizziness; heart block (usually associated with preexisting abnormal His-Purkinje conduction); sinoatrial arrest.	Significant reduction in dose in patients with heart failure; moderate reduction in dose in patients with hepatic disease; no oral form available; no significant myocardial depression; toxicity usually seen at high plasma levels; toxicity at low plasma levels may be caused by metabolites.
Digoxin	0.75–1 mg followed by 0.25 mg IV every 2–4 hours	0.8–2 (ng/mL)	Nausea; vomiting; ventricular arrhythmias; conduction defects; atrioventricular dissociation.	Exercise caution if patient is receiving digitalis; then use in smallest doses. Exercise caution in elderly patients and in those with impaired renal function or acute myocardial infarction.
Propranolol	0.1–1 mg/min IV up to 10 mg	40–85 (ng/mL)	Hypotension; bradycardia; prolonged atrioventricular conduction and heart block; myocardial depression; bronchospasm.	Extreme caution and decreased dose in the presence of heart failure; many of the side effects reversed by large doses of isoproterenol.
Procainamide	100 mg slowly (< 50 mg/min) IV every 5 minutes (or more often in life-threatening situations) up to 1000 mg. (May also give 1 g IM.)	4–8	Hypotension; prolonged atrioventricular and His-Purkinje conduction.	Myocardial toxicity usually only at high plasma levels or after rapid administration.
Phenytoin	50–100 mg IV slowly (< 50 mg/min) every 5 minutes up to 1000 mg. Additional 500 mg on following day.	10–18	Hypotension; 1:1 conduction in atrial flutter; respiratory arrest; idioventricular rhythm; ventricular fibrillation; asystole; nystagmus.	Administration IM provides erratic blood levels; toxicity usually seen only after rapid administration.
Quinidine	6–10 mg/kg of quinidine gluconate IV slowly over 22–45 minutes or orally 200–400 mg every 2 hours for 5 doses. (May also be given IM.)	2.3–5 (in double extraction assay; higher if protein precipitation assay used).	Hypotension; prolonged His-Purkinje conduction; ventricular arrhythmias.	Generally given parenterally only in emergencies and is hazardous unless close supervision by an experienced physician is maintained. IM use is preferred. Doubles serum digoxin levels when given along with digoxin and may cause digitalis toxicity.

*Modified and reproduced, with permission, from Winkle RA, Glantz SA, Harrison DC: Pharmacologic therapy of ventricular arrhythmias. *Am J Cardiol* 1975;36:629.

Table 15-6. Guide for long-term oral administration of antiarrhythmic drugs.* See Table 15-7 for newer agents.

Drug	Usual Total Daily Dose	Frequency of Administration	Therapeutic Plasma Level (µg/mL)	Slow Phase Half-Life (hours)	Side Effects	Comments
Propranolol	80–320 mg	Every 6 hours	Uncertain	3–4.6	Myocardial depression; prolonged atrioventricular conduction and heart block; bradycardia; bronchospasm; nausea; vomiting; fatigue; depression; peripheral vascular insufficiency; hyperglycemia; alopecia.	Active metabolites may play a role in clinical effect. Dose chosen empirically. Should be tapered slowly in patients with angina. Caution needed in patients with cardiac function dependent on sympathetic tone.
Procainamide	3–6 g	Every 3–6 hours	4–8	3–4	Nausea; vomiting; agranulocytosis; lupuslike syndrome; myocardial depression; prolonged atrioventricular and His-Purkinje conduction.	Toxic myocardial effect, usually only at toxic plasma levels. Half-life markedly prolonged in renal failure or alkaline urine. Oral absorption erratic after acute myocardial infarction.
Phenytoin	300–400 mg	Once daily	10–18	22	Nystagmus; ataxia; lethargy; nausea; vertigo; rashes; pseudolymphoma; megaloblastic anemia; peripheral neuropathy; hyperglycemia; seizures.	Half-life higher at higher doses. Rate of metabolism affected by many drugs. Clinically significant decrease in plasma binding in azotemia and hypoproteinemia.
Quinidine	1–2.4 g	Every 6 hours	3–5	7	Hypotension; anorexia; nausea and vomiting; diarrhea; tinnitus; vertigo; prolonged His-Purkinje conduction; rash; fever; thrombocytopenia; hepatic dysfunction; hemolytic anemia; ventricular arrhythmias.	Minor gastrointestinal side effects controlled with symptomatic therapy. Clinically significant decrease in plasma binding in hypoproteinemia and hepatic disease. Myocardial toxicity usually only at toxic plasma levels. Protein precipitation drug assay measures inactive metabolites. Accumulation of metabolites in renal disease. Doubles serum digoxin levels when given along with digoxin and may cause digitalis toxicity.
Digoxin	0.125–0.25 mg	Once daily	0.8–2 (ng/mL)	36	Nausea; vomiting; ventricular arrhythmias; conduction defects; atrioventricular dissociation.	Decrease dose when early toxic symptoms or signs appear in order to prevent more serious ones. May require larger daily doses. Use with caution in older patients and in those with impaired renal function and Wolff-Parkinson-White syndrome.

*Modified and reproduced, with permission, from Winkle RA, Glantz SA, Harrison DC: Pharmacologic therapy of ventricular arrhythmias. *Am J Cardiol* 1975;**36**:629.

premature beats, an attempt should be made to suppress them with quinidine, propranolol, or procainamide, alone or in combination.

1. Quinidine–Quinidine is effective but may be unpleasant to take over a prolonged period because of side effects of nausea, diarrhea, and tinnitus. Quinidine cardiotoxicity may also result, causing ventricular tachycardia or fibrillation and ventricular conduction defects.

2. Procainamide–Procainamide, 250–500 mg orally every 4–6 hours, is effective for acute tachycardia, but when given over a period of many months for therapy of premature beats, it is likely to cause a lupuslike connective tissue disorder with arthritis and LE cells in the blood (Fig 15–15). The major metabolite of procainamide, acetylprocainamide, is effective and is less likely to cause the development of antinuclear antibodies, but side effects are prominent (Lahita, 1979).

3. Phenytoin–Phenytoin, 300 mg/d orally, is relatively ineffective as an antiarrhythmic agent in ventricular premature beats unless they are induced by digitalis toxicity, but it can be tried if other agents are ineffective.

Table 15-7. Clinical characteristics of newer antiarrhythmic agents.*

Drug	Dose - Intravenous	Dose - Oral	Effective Serum or Plasma Concentration (μg/mL)	Elimination Half-Life (h)	Absorption	Metabolism Secretion Route	Side Effects	Onset of Action - Intravenous (min)	Onset of Action - Oral (h)
Amiodarone†	5–10 mg/kg.	Maintenance: 200–800 mg.	...	...	Fair	...	Ophthalmologic, endocrine, neurologic, dermatologic, cardiovascular.	5–10	4–6
Disopyramide†	2 mg/kg over 15 min; then 2 mg/kg over 1 hour.	Loading: 300 mg. Maintenance: 150 mg every 6 hours.	2–8	5–8	Good	Renal 50%, probably hepatic 50%	Anticholinergic, cardiovascular.	<5	½–3
Encainide‡	0.6–0.9 mg/kg over 15 min.	25–100 mg every 6–12 hours.	0.48	1.9–3.8	...	...	Prolongation of PR, HV, and QRS.	15	1½
Ethmozin	Loading: 1–3 mg/kg.§	Maintenance: 75–150 mg every 6 hours.**	0.5–1	5–10**	Good§	Probably hepatic§	Neurologic, gastrointestinal, cardiovascular.	<5§	2§
Mexiletine	Loading: 1200 mg/12 hours. Maintenance: 250–500 mg/12 hours.	Loading: 400–600 mg. Maintenance: 200–300 mg every 8 hours.	0.5–2	10–26	Good	Probably hepatic	Neurologic, gastrointestinal, cardiovascular.	<5	1–2
Tocainide†	0.5–0.75 mg/kg/min for 15 min.	Loading: 400–600 mg. Maintenance: 400–800 mg every 8 hours.	3.5–10	10–17	Good	Renal 40%, probably hepatic 60%	Neurologic, gastrointestinal, cardiovascular.	5–10	1½
Verapamil†	0.075–0.15 mg/kg.	Maintenance: 80–120 mg every 8 hours or every 6 hours.	...	3–7	Good	Hepatic	Neurologic, gastrointestinal, cardiovascular.	<5	1–2

*Modified and reproduced, with permission, from Zipes DP, Troup PJ: New antiarrhythmic agents: Amiodarone, aprindine, disopyramide, ethmozin, mexiletine, tocainide, verapamil. *Am J Cardiol* 1978;41:1005.
†Amiodarone, disopyramide, tocainide, and verapamil are the only drugs that have been approved by the FDA.
‡Roden (1980), Sami (1979).
§Animal data.
**According to studies in progress, maintenance doses may be in the range of 250 mg every 8 hours and provide a slightly longer half-life.

Table 15-8. Management of arrhythmias in acute myocardial infarction.*

Arrhythmia	First Choice	Second Choice	Comments
Atrial premature complexes	Observation only, if few beats	Quinidine Digitalis	Atrial premature complexes are frequently forerunners of atrial fibrillation or flutter. *Caution:* Avoid excessive dosage of digitalis because of increased susceptibility to arrhythmia in acute myocardial infarction.
Paroxysmal atrial tachycardia	Digitalis	Precordial DC shock	An uncommon complication of acute infarction. Avoid excessive digitalis.
Atrial fibrillation	Digitalis	Precordial DC shock	Arrhythmia tends to recur, hence first aim of treatment is control of ventricular rate. If patient tolerates arrhythmia poorly or needs "atrial kick" or if stroke volume is low, immediate DC conversion may be necessary. Eventual spontaneous reversion is the rule.
Atrial flutter	Digitalis	Precordial DC shock	Comments above on atrial fibrillation are applicable to flutter. Some authorities recommend immediate DC shock in all instances of atrial flutter or fibrillation.
Paroxysmal junctional tachycardia	Digitalis	Precordial DC shock	See atrial tachycardia. If rate is only moderately increased and associated with atrioventricular dissociation, consider digitalis toxicity as causative.
Ventricular premature complexes	Lidocaine	Quinidine Procainamide Phenytoin Overdriving with pacemaker	Decision to treat depends on setting. More than 5 ventricular premature complexes per minute, occurrence in salvos, or R on T phenomena (closely coupled) demand immediate and adequate treatment. Once ventricular premature complexes are initially suppressed with lidocaine, a plan for long-term therapy with longer-acting agent should be considered.
Ventricular tachycardia	Precordial DC shock	Lidocaine Quinidine Procainamide Phenytoin Overdriving with pacemaker	Forerunner of ventricular fibrillation. Best combination is immediate precordial shock followed by long-term administration of suppressive drugs.
Ventricular fibrillation	Precordial DC shock	Closed-chest cardiac massage Intubation and ventilatory support	When cardiac arrest occurs in the coronary care unit, precordial shock should be administered immediately. If unsuccessful, it may be necessary to resort to cardiopulmonary resuscitation. The longer fibrillation persists, the less likely is survival.

*Reproduced, with permission, from Killip T: Management of arrhythmias in acute myocardial infarction. *Hosp Pract* (April) 1972; 7:131; and from Braunwald E (editor): *The Myocardium: Failure and Infarction.* Hospital Practice Publishing Co, 1974.

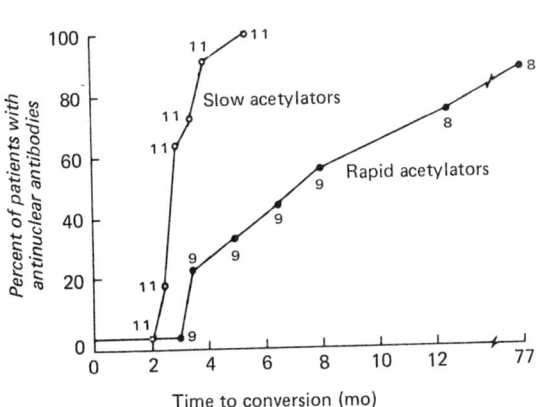

Figure 15-15. Development of procainamide-induced antinuclear antibody in slow acetylators (open circles) and rapid acetylators (closed circles) with time. The number of patients followed is listed at each point. (Reproduced, with permission, from Woosley RL et al: Effect of acetylator phenotype on the rate at which procainamide induces antinuclear antibodies and the lupus syndrome. *N Engl J Med* 1978;**298**:11257.)

4. Propranolol–Propranolol, 80–320 mg/d orally in 3–4 doses, is helpful in controlling ventricular premature beats but may further slow the ventricular rate and in some instances may increase their frequency, especially if they become more frequent with slow heart rates.

5. Digitalis–Digitalis has been helpful in the treatment of ventricular premature beats resulting from heart failure, provided no digitalis has previously been given. Recent observations suggest that digitalis may also be valuable in the treatment of ventricular premature beats in the absence of heart failure (Lown, *N Engl J Med* 1977). Treatment of heart failure may improve coronary perfusion and decrease the nonhomogeneous excitability of ventricular fibers that may cause variable refractory periods and be responsible for reentry premature beats. Premature beats may disappear following treatment of heart failure.

6. New investigational antiarrhythmic agents–A variety of new antiarrhythmic agents, none of which have been approved by the FDA except for amiodarone, disopyramide, tocainide, and verapamil, are listed in Table 15-7. Investigational drugs not included in Table 15-7 that are receiving increasing therapeutic trial include (1) flecainide (Bigger, 1984), 100–300 mg

Table 15-9. Cardiac drugs of use in the coronary care unit in management of arrhythmias.*

Drug	Dosage	Indications	Comments
Atropine	0.5–1 mg IV	Bradycardia due to sinus slowing; atrioventricular dissociation	May be repeated 2–3 times. Urinary retention common. May rarely cause atropine psychosis or acute glaucoma. Excess dosage may cause sinus tachycardia.
Lidocaine	60–100 mg IV	Ventricular premature complexes	Effective in 3–5 minutes. May be repeated 3 times. Duration of action variable, usually 20–40 minutes. Bolus should be followed by steady infusion at 2–4 mg/min to maintain desired effect.
Quinidine	0.2–0.4 g every 6 hours orally	Long-term suppression of ventricular arrhythmia	Aim is to achieve adequate blood level (3–6 mg/L) for effective suppression. May depress ventricular function, lower blood pressure, or widen QRS. Usually reserved for long-term suppression of ventricular arrhythmias after initial treatment with lidocaine. The problem is to give adequate dosage without causing toxicity. "Usual" dosage is often too small and does not achieve therapeutic blood levels, but higher dosage may depress myocardial function. Idiosyncrasy to quinidine is well known. Procainamide may cause fever, leukopenia, or lupus erythematosus.
Procainamide	2–4 g daily in divided doses every 3–6 hours		
Isoproterenol	1 mg in 500 mL 5% dextrose as a continuously regulated infusion	Bradycardia; sinus slowing; atrioventricular block; asystole	Provides short-term support until pacemaker or other definitive therapy is instituted. May induce ventricular arrhythmia. Markedly increases myocardial oxygen demand. Probably contraindicated in cardiogenic shock.
Propranolol	0.5 mg IV every 2 minutes; total dosage no more than 5 mg. 80–320 mg/d orally in divided doses.	Recurrent atrial fibrillation or flutter with rapid ventricular rate	Use with great caution. May induce profound atrioventricular block or asystole. Reserve for special situations only.
Digoxin	0.5 mg IV, followed by 0.25 mg in 6 hours, then 0.125 mg at 12 and at 18 hours. Maintenance dose 0.125–0.375 mg daily, orally or IV.	Congestive failure; supraventricular arrhythmias	Use cautiously in acute myocardial infarction because of apparent reduced toxic threshold. Excreted by kidneys; therefore, reduce dose when blood urea nitrogen is elevated. Avoid hypokalemia.

*Reproduced, with permission, from Killip T: Management of arrhythmias in acute myocardial infarction. *Hosp Pract* (April) 1972; 7:131; and from Braunwald E (editor): *The Myocardium: Failure and Infarction.* Hospital Practice Publishing Co, 1974.

orally twice a day or 2 mg/kg intravenously (the half-life is about 20 hours, and side effects, which occur in one-third to one-half of cases, usually involve the gastrointestinal system or central nervous system); (2) lorcainide, 100–200 mg orally twice a day or 2 mg/kg intravenously over a 10-minute period (side effects are similar to those of flecainide [Somberg, 1984], except that insomnia is more prominent); (3) propafenone, intravenous loading dose of 2 mg/kg over a 10-minute period, followed by an infusion of 2 mg/min to suppress ventricular tachycardia. Oral doses of 300–900 mg/d in 3 divided doses may also be given (Shen, 1984; Connolly, 1983). Zipes (1978) and Kupersmith (1985) present a comprehensive review of the newer antiarrhythmic drugs (Table 15–7). Detailed analysis of the newer drugs are listed in the references. Most of them are 75–80% effective in suppressing ventricular premature beats or in preventing ventricular tachycardia, but side effects are substantial.

Disopyramide is still used sparingly. It may be an alternative to lidocaine for ventricular arrhythmias in the coronary care unit when given by intravenous infusion in doses of 2–4 mg/kg followed by 250–400 mg orally every 6 hours. It has anticholinergic activity, and many patients develop dry mouth and urinary hesitancy. The most important side effect of disopyramide is the development of cardiac failure that occurs in about half of patients with a history of cardiac failure. The drug has significant negative inotropic action; the development of cardiac failure may be delayed, or failure may appear within 48 hours. Cardiac failure is uncommon in patients with no history of cardiac failure. The management of arrhythmias in general and of those associated with acute myocardial infarction is shown in Tables 15–8 and 15–9.

C. Digitalis Toxicity: The chance that ventricular premature beats due to excessive digitalis will induce ventricular fibrillation increases with more severe heart disease or if there is associated hypokalemia. When digitalis is taken for suicidal purposes by individuals with normal hearts, ventricular arrhythmias are relatively uncommon. When ventricular premature beats are absent before treatment and appear after treatment, digitalis toxicity should be considered.

D. Autonomic Discharge Due to Central Nervous System Activity: Treatment of autonomic impulses caused by emotional stress or central nervous system stimulants may prevent ventricular fibrillation in patients with frequent ventricular premature beats. If there is no contraindication and patients appear to be hyperkinetic and excitable (suggesting that autonomic activity may be playing a role), propranolol, 80–320 mg/d orally in divided doses, metoprolol, 50–200 mg/d orally in divided doses, or other beta-blocking drugs may be given a trial. Stimulants such as alcohol, tobacco, and coffee should be used in moderation or should be avoided if their relationship to ventricular arrhythmias can be documented.

E. Coronary Arterial Disease: Goldschlager (1973) found that ventricular premature beats occurred in only 11% of patients with insignificant coronary disease but were 3 times as common after exercise when there was prior myocardial infarction, an abnormal contractile pattern, and 2- or 3-vessel disease. This worker believes that ventricular premature beats in the presence of coronary disease imply an adverse prognosis, presumably because of the likelihood of more severe anatomic disease when premature beats were present. Exercise-induced ventricular premature beats therefore identify a high-risk group of patients with coronary heart disease in whom therapy of the premature beats should be attempted.

F. Resection of Ventricular Aneurysm: (See ¶D, p 499.) Ventricular premature beats and ventricular tachycardia may be precursors of ventricular fibrillation in patients with ventricular aneurysms following acute myocardial infarction. Identification and resection of the aneurysm in patients with cardiac failure and resistant arrhythmias may sometimes (not always) be followed by disappearance of ventricular arrhythmias and may therefore prevent sudden death. Cardiac failure is often strikingly benefited (Chapter 8).

G. Prevention of Ventricular Fibrillation: The prevention of ventricular fibrillation is an important goal in the treatment of ventricular premature beats, but there is no unanimity of opinion on how to distinguish the 50% of patients whose premature beats are unimportant prognostically from the other half, in whom ventricular fibrillation or hemodynamic effects are produced. It seems established, however, that in coronary disease, hypertrophic cardiomyopathy, idiopathic dilated cardiomyopathy, mitral valve prolapse, and aortic valve disease, as well as in connective tissue disorders, frequent complex arrhythmias, those that occur in short runs, those that occur early on the T wave, or those that are associated with longer bursts of ventricular tachycardia predispose to sudden death. Every effort should be made to suppress these premature beats, with careful attention to precipitating factors; ventilation; central nervous system autonomic influences; and iatrogenic factors such as cardiac catheters or pacemakers, sedation, and antiarrhythmic drugs. Graded exercise and long-term monitoring should be used to count the various types of ventricular premature beats as an aid in deciding whether or not to give treatment. Monitoring should be continued during the recovery period after exercise because most premature beats occur during this period. Monitoring should be repeated some months following recovery from a myocardial infarction because the incidence of subsequent sudden death is at least tripled when there are many ventricular premature beats as compared to when there are none.

VENTRICULAR TACHYCARDIA

Ventricular tachycardia (Figs 15–16 and 15–17) is a rapid, essentially regular (may be slightly irregular) tachycardia of abrupt onset with an average ventricular rate of 150–200/min. Because this is similar to the rate of supraventricular tachycardia, the rate is not helpful in differential diagnosis. Ventricular tachycardia may occur during complete atrioventricular block and may cause Stokes-Adams attacks. Depending upon the underlying state of the heart and the rapidity and duration of the tachycardia, the patient may develop hemodynamic abnormalities fostered by the decreased ventricular filling and low cardiac output caused by the rapid rate and the lack of an appropriately timed atrial contraction. Patients may develop any of the clinical manifestations noted in the discussion of the hemodynamic significance and impact of arrhythmias in general, with dyspnea, angina, hypotension, oliguria, and syncope. If the ventricular rate is not too rapid (< 160/min), patients may have only mild symptoms of weakness or dizziness. When the more severe symptoms occur in the setting of acute myocardial infarction, ventricular fibrillation is likely, and the tachycardia should be treated immediately with intravenous lidocaine, 50–100 mg, followed by an infusion of 1–2 mg/min, for 1–3 days. If the tachycardia is not terminated promptly by this means or by a trial of procainamide, 100 mg intravenously every 5 minutes up to a total of 1 g, external countershock should be employed. Some patients with ventricular tachycardia during acute myocardial infarction complain only of weakness and dizziness. The frequency with which ventricular tachycardia degenerates into ventricular fibrillation is not known, but in monitored cases in coronary care units, ventricular tachycardia usually precedes ventricular fibrillation, although the latter may occur unexpectedly and de novo early in the course of myocardial infarction.

Diagnosis

By definition, ventricular tachycardia is present when 3 or more ventricular premature beats occur consecutively. Although this definition overestimates the frequency of ventricular tachycardia, which is hemodynamically important, it does not minimize the potential of this arrhythmia to precipitate ventricular fibrillation. Paroxysms of ventricular tachycardia may occur in the same record with single premature beats.

Ventricular tachycardia is most common in the presence of acute myocardial infarction, usually in the first 1–3 hours, when by continuous monitoring it may be found in as many as 40% of cases. The incidence falls precipitously with the passage of hours, and in only 5% is the onset after the first day. Patients

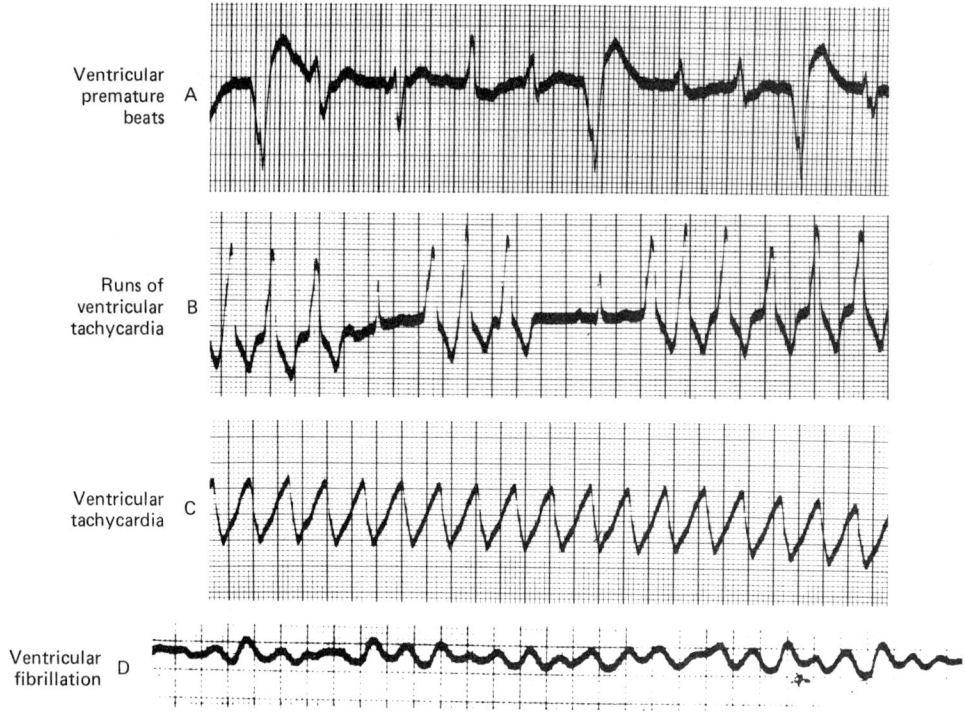

Figure 15–16. Ventricular arrhythmias. **A:** Ventricular premature beats, lead II. **B:** Runs of ventricular tachycardia, lead II. **C:** Ventricular tachycardia, lead V_1. **D:** Ventricular fibrillation, lead II.

who have ventricular tachycardia early in the course of acute myocardial infarction do not necessarily have recurrences later in the disease or following convalescence, even after exercise. Ventricular tachycardia and ventricular fibrillation occurring early (in the first few minutes or hours) in acute myocardial infarction are thought to be due to myocardial ischemia resulting in reentry or to automatic ectopic ventricular discharge. Patients with large infarcts and cardiac failure are more apt to have ventricular tachycardia and ventricular fibrillation. The former may occur in the setting of sinus bradycardia with inferior myocardial infarction and is less likely to occur when the ventricular rate is increased by administration of small doses of atropine. Large doses of atropine (1 mg or more intravenously) may induce ventricular arrhythmias because of the induced sinus tachycardia and the variable recovery of excitability in different portions of the infarcted heart. Ventricular tachycardia early in the course of acute myocardial infarction must be differentiated from nonparoxysmal junctional tachycardia with aberrant conduction. In the latter the rate is usually slower (70–120/min), and a careful search for P waves may indicate its supraventricular origin. Accelerated idioventricular rhythm (Fig 15–18) looks the same, but there is atrioventricular dissociation and often capture or fusion beats at the onset and termination of the run of the idioventricular rhythm.

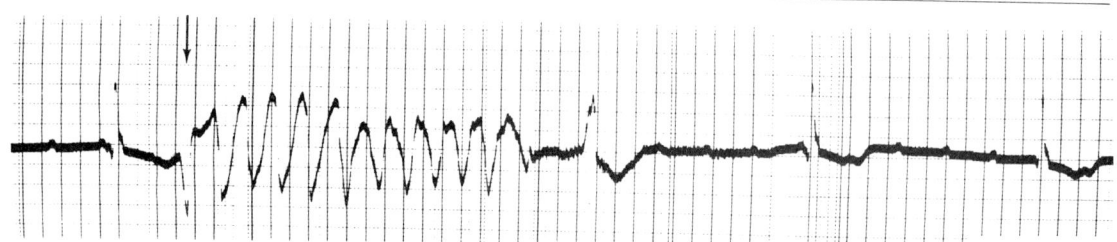

Figure 15–17. Complete atrioventricular block with a run of ventricular tachycardia (arrow) initiated by a ventricular premature beat occurring at the end of the T wave (R on T phenomenon).

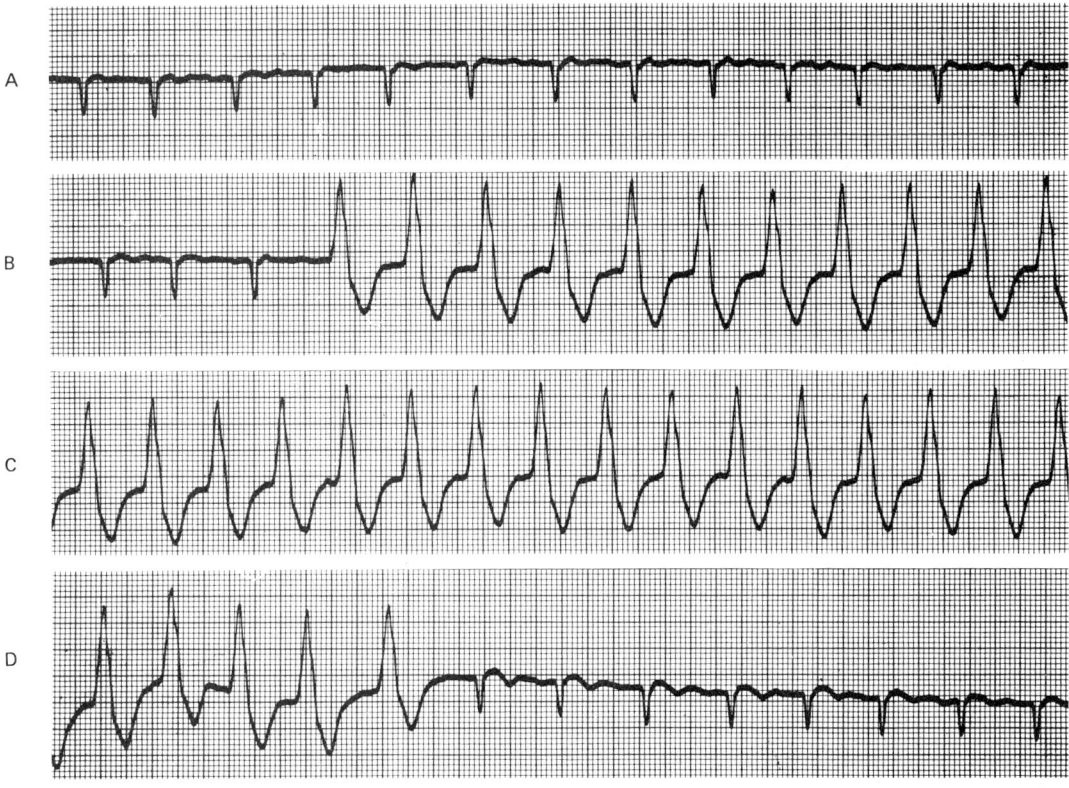

Figure 15–18. Accelerated idioventricular rhythm. Continuous recording of lead V$_1$ in a patient with acute myocardial infarction. **A:** Atrial fibrillation with irregular ventricular response, rate = 100. **B–C:** Appearance of idioventricular rhythm, which initially has a rate of 100 and then increases to 120. **D:** Spontaneous reversion. (Reproduced, with permission, from Goldman MJ: *Principles of Clinical Electrocardiography*, 12th ed. Lange, 1986.)

Clinical Findings
(Fig 15–19)

Ventricular tachycardia should be strongly suspected when an abrupt tachycardia with syncope or near-syncope occurs in an older patient with coronary heart disease, especially if the patient had ventricular premature beats before the tachycardia and the QRS complexes are wide and bizarre, with QR or QS complexes in lead V$_1$, or if the complexes are similar to those seen in the ventricular premature beats present on a prior occasion. The T wave is usually large and in the direction opposite to that of the complex. Prolongation of the QRS complex and atrioventricular dissociation are not absolute criteria to establish the ventricular origin of a tachycardia. (See Tables 15–10 and 15–11.)

A. Asynchrony of Atrial and Ventricular Contractions:
The most important clinical feature of ventricular tachycardia is asynchrony of atrial and ventricular contractions, with the atria beating at a slower rate. This is not an absolute criterion because independence of atrial and ventricular activity is occasionally due to junctional atrioventricular rhythms with retrograde atrioventricular block causing atrioventricular dissociation. Further, it must be remembered that retrograde activation of the atria may occur in ventricular tachycardia with a one-to-one conduction, so that asynchronous atrial and ventricular activity do not occur.

On auscultation, because of the wide QRS complexes and atrioventricular dissociation, there is wide splitting of the first and second heart sounds, beat-to-beat variation in arterial pressure and systolic murmurs, changing intensity of the first heart sound depending upon the relation of the P wave to the QRS complex, and intermittent, large cannon *a* waves in the jugular venous pulse. When the atria contract with the tricuspid valve closed, large cannon waves appear in the jugular venous pulse unless the patient has atrial fibrillation or flutter or 1:1 retrograde conduction to the atria. When the relationship between atrial and ventricular contraction is such that the mitral and tricuspid valves are wide open at the onset of ventricular systole, they close with a snap and the first heart sound is louder. When the atria and the ventricle contract close together, the mitral valve leaflets are relatively closed and the first sound is soft. The systolic blood pressure varies from beat to beat depending upon the sequence of the atrial and ventricular contraction and the contribution of atrial systole to ventricular filling.

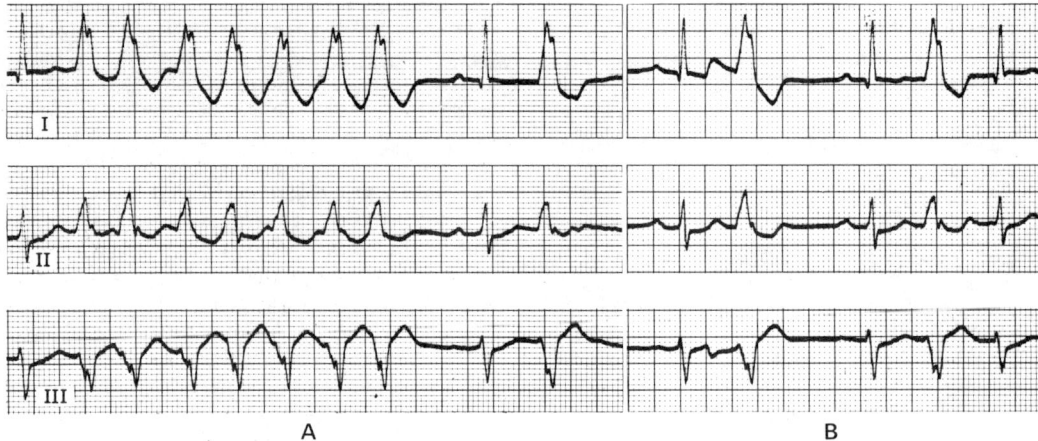

Figure 15–19. Ventricular tachycardia and ventricular premature beats. **A:** Following one sinus beat, there are 7 consecutive ventricular premature beats, indicating ventricular tachycardia. The ventricular rate is 150, and the rhythm is irregular. **B:** The above is followed by sinus rhythm with ventricular bigeminy. The configuration of the ventricular ectopic beats is identical to that of the tachycardia. This indicates that both are arising from the same ventricular focus. (Reproduced, with permission, from Goldman MJ: *Principles of Clinical Electrocardiography*, 12th ed. Lange, 1986.)

If ventricular excitation is transmitted backward to the atrium or sinus node, the result is 1:1 ventriculoatrial conduction with no variation in the intensity of the first heart sound and no cannon waves in the jugular venous pulse.

B. Capture and Fusion Beats and Supraventricular Tachycardia With Aberrant Conduction: The appearance of "capture" beats with normal QRS duration between the abnormal ventricular beats suggests ventricular tachycardia and indicates that a supraventricular impulse conducted across the atrioventricular node has "captured" the ventricles, a sign of the presence of atrioventricular dissociation rather than atrioventricular block.

Supraventricular tachycardia can only be diagnosed with confidence when P waves are found with the same frequency as the QRS complexes unless ventricular tachycardia with retrograde atrioventricular conduction is present, with one-to-one atrial and ventricular activity. The P waves may precede or be buried in the QRS complex or may be retrograde when atrioventricular junctional tachycardia is present. If the P waves cannot be definitely distinguished, one should explore the right precordial leads, obtain a Lewis lead (see p 467), and do esophageal or right atrial electrograms (Fig 15–5).

Fusion beats (Dressler beats) are those in which an impulse from the sinus node fortuitously "captures" an independent ventricular beat to produce a QRS complex that is a fusion of both atrial and ventricular depolarizations. Carotid sinus pressure or edrophonium may impair atrioventricular conduction and allow P waves to be seen in supraventricular tachycardia with aberration. Ventricular capture beats can sometimes be elicited by accelerating the sinoatrial nodal discharge, slowing the ventricular rate, blocking ventriculoatrial conduction without affecting the atrioventricular conduction, and by intracavitary stimulation (Puech, 1975).

It bears reemphasis that rapid (> 250/min) tachycardia with wide, slightly irregular QRS complexes should suggest atrial fibrillation with Wolff-Parkin-

Table 15–10. Some mechanisms causing widening of the QRS complex in supraventricular rhythms (after Puech, 1970).

---

1. Preexisting bundle branch block.
2. Aberrant ventricular conduction (functional bundle branch block).
    a. Short coupling interval with long preceding cycle.
    b. Different rates of recovery of excitability in the ventricular conduction system.
3. Drug-induced intraventricular conduction delay.
4. Ectopic activity of supranodal origin, with conduction through an accessory pathway in Wolff-Parkinson-White syndrome.
5. Other more complex mechanisms.

Table 15–11. Criteria of Puech (1970) and Waxman (1977) for the diagnosis of ventricular tachycardia.

QRS complexes exceeding 0.12 second not associated with preexisting bundle branch block.

Atrioventricular dissociation or ventriculoatrial block present.

Irregular fusion and normal capture beats.

Normalization of the QRS complexes by a ventricular capture during a tachycardia with a wide QRS complex.

Failure to produce aberration by rapid atrial pacing at a rate greater than the underlying tachycardia.

Absence of a His bundle potential preceding ventricular activation during the tachycardia, whereas during sinus rhythm such a potential precedes the QRS complex.

son-White conduction and lead to a search for slurred initial delta waves.

C. Electrocardiography: Review of long strips of the ECG in different leads with double sensitivity and a careful search for P waves may show independent atrial beats at a rate slower than the ventricular tachycardia. These are often not seen or may be buried in the QRS complex. The absence of P waves on a routine ECG does not exclude ventricular tachycardia. Furthermore, in junctional or ventricular tachycardia there may be retrograde activation of the atria that prevents independent sinus beats. Onset of tachycardia with an ectopic P wave is strong evidence of supraventricular tachycardia with aberrant conduction.

D. His Bundle Recordings: His bundle recordings may establish the diagnosis by noting the relationship of the His spike and the P wave to the QRS complexes. In supraventricular arrhythmia, the P wave and the His spike precede the QRS complex, whereas in ventricular tachycardia the QRS complex with retrograde conduction precedes the His potential.

E. Comparison of Previous Premature Beats and Tachycardia: The diagnosis can be clarified in retrospect if, after cessation of tachycardia, ventricular premature beats can be seen that have a configuration similar to that seen during tachycardia. As mentioned in the discussion of supraventricular arrhythmias, if the initial or first few QRS complexes of tachycardia are normal in configuration and later ones become bizarre, this favors a supraventricular over a ventricular origin. Monitoring of the ECG during graded exercise may produce short bursts of ventricular tachycardia as well as ventricular premature beats and clarify the nature of the preceding tachycardia.

F. Accelerated Idioventricular Rhythms: Accelerated idioventricular rhythms (Fig 15–18) may "escape" when there is suppression of higher pacemakers due to sinoatrial and atrioventricular block but may also represent "slow" ventricular tachycardia due to reentry or increased automaticity due to ischemia. Norris (1974), in his experience with 61 patients with accelerated idioventricular tachycardia in acute myocardial infarction, noted that the attacks of tachycardia consisted of paroxysms of relatively short duration which were relatively slow (< 100/min), often beginning with sinus bradycardia or sinoatrial block, and therefore were probably escape rhythms because the sinus node was depressed. The first beat almost always occurs after a long diastolic pause; the initial and final beats of a paroxysm may have a normal, nonpremature P wave and a QRS configuration combining sinus and ventricular origin (fusion beats). The incidence of ventricular fibrillation is only about one-fourth that of patients with ectopic (nonescape) ventricular tachycardia with a more rapid rate. Atrioventricular dissociation occurs in most patients with accelerated idioventricular rhythms because although the ventricular rhythm is usually "escape" in nature, the sinus node still discharges at a slower rate.

Accelerated idioventricular rhythms must be differentiated from idioventricular rhythm that occurs in complete atrioventricular block with ventricular rates less than 40/min. Not only is the ventricular rate slower, but evidence of complete atrioventricular block is found on the ECG and in the clinical features noted in the discussion above. In congenital atrioventricular block when the ventricular rate is faster (approximately 60–70/min), the differentiation may be more difficult, but it still depends upon the presence of complete block. Atrioventricular dissociation, such as occurs in accelerated idioventricular rhythm, also has independent atrial and ventricular pacemakers, but atrioventricular block is not present. Atrioventricular dissociation is always present in complete atrioventricular block but may occur in its absence when the atria and ventricles depolarize independently.

G. Torsade de Pointes: Torsade de pointes is an atypical variety of ventricular tachycardia that has received renewed attention recently. The QRS complex of the tachycardia varies in polarity and twists around the isoelectric line in irregular bursts. It is particularly found in patients who have a long QT interval, in those using drugs such as quinidine, in acute myocardial ischemia, in hypokalemia, or spontaneously in those with congenital QT syndrome. The changing configuration of the QRS complex is thought to be an ominous sign of imminent ventricular fibrillation when the QRS widens in response to antiarrhythmic drugs, and the drug should be stopped. However, some effective drugs prolong the QT interval without producing torsade de pointes. Bradycardia in association with atypical ventricular tachycardia is a warning sign. Cardiac pacing or cardioversion has been recommended as the most effective treatment. Prolongation of the QT_C interval is usually substantial, with a mean of 0.59 second (Kay, 1983). Coronary disease was the most common condition in Kay's series of 32 patients; he also emphasized the long-short initiating sequence of torsade.

Treatment*

In the relatively asymptomatic patient with coronary disease whose premature beats are frequent or occur in short runs of tachycardia, treatment can be started with procainamide, 250–500 mg orally every 4–6 hours, or quinidine, 0.2–0.4 g orally 4 times daily, or lidocaine, 50–100 mg as an intravenous bolus. If the runs are prolonged or the patient is symptomatic, lidocaine, 50–100 mg intravenously, or procainamide, 100 mg/5 min intravenously up to a total of 1 g, can be given as an emergency measure while the patient is being prepared for external countershock. Fig 15–20 shows the effects of intramuscular quinidine gluconate. If 50–100 mg of intravenous lidocaine does not terminate the arrhythmia, a second injection can be given in 2–5 minutes with the hope of achieving blood levels of 1.5–4 $\mu g/mL$. If this is ineffective or if the patient has important clinical symptoms, cardioversion preceded by intravenous anesthesia,

---
*The details of dosage and other information about antiarrhythmic drugs are presented in Tables 15–4 to 15–9.

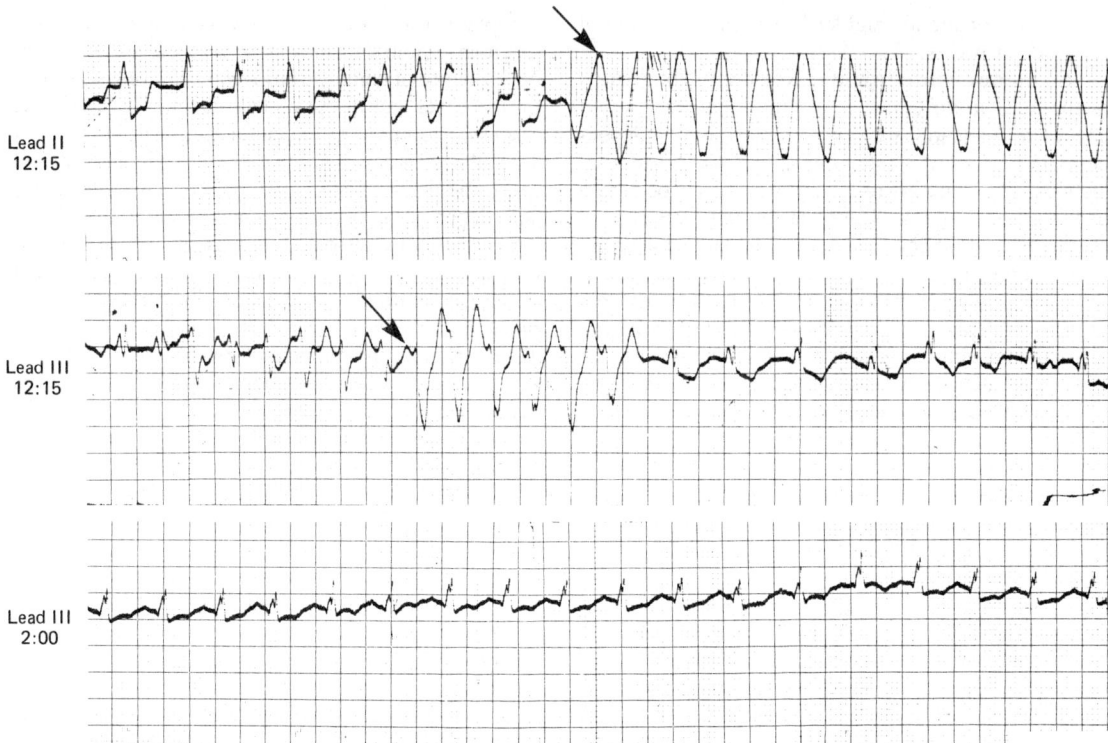

Figure 15–20. Woman age 30 years with myocarditis and runs of ventricular tachycardia (arrows) at 12:15 PM. Quinidine gluconate (0.8 g) given intramuscularly at 12:30 PM. Sinus rhythm without premature beats noted at 2:00 PM. Blood quinidine level at this time was 4.8 μg/mL.

---

usually diazepam, 5–15 mg, should be accomplished promptly; almost all patients revert to sinus rhythm, often with low-energy currents. A thump over the chest should be tried prior to electric external countershock; it may be successful in restoring sinus rhythm. Most instruments for defibrillation deliver 10 J as the lowest dose. If this amount of energy is insufficient, repetitive and larger amounts of energy—up to 400 J—should be given as soon as possible to convert the arrhythmia to sinus rhythm. In patients with recurrent attacks, hypoxia and metabolic or electrolyte factors should all be corrected, since they may be predisposing factors. Bedside hemodynamic monitoring with appropriate treatment may also help improve the function of the left ventricle and eliminate factors that predispose to ventricular tachycardia. Management of these hemodynamic abnormalities revealed by hemodynamic monitoring is discussed in detail in the chapter on coronary heart disease (see Chapter 8).

The clinical pharmacokinetics and present status of some of the currently approved agents and some newer agents not approved by the FDA are summarized by Winkle (1975), Harrison (1977), and Zipes (1978).

A. Sedation: It is important to treat anxiety in patients in the coronary care unit. Drugs such as diazepam, 5–10 mg orally as needed, or other tranquilizers should be given to decrease anxiety. Propranolol, 80–160 mg/d orally in divided doses, metoprolol, 50–200 mg/d orally in divided doses, or other beta-blocking drugs are occasionally effective early in the course of acute myocardial infarction to counteract the effects of autonomic discharge; later, this drug may be dangerous because it may increase the likelihood of left ventricular failure.

B. Emergency Cardioversion and Prevention of Recurrences: Direct current countershock should be employed promptly if the ventricular tachycardia is life-threatening, after which pharmacologic therapy should be employed to prevent recurrence. Following cardioversion, the patient should be given prophylactic intravenous infusions of lidocaine, 1–4 mg/min, which, if ineffective, should be supplemented with quinidine, 0.2–0.6 g orally 3–4 times daily, or procainamide, 250–500 mg orally every 4 hours. One should avoid large doses of lidocaine over long periods because the patient may develop central nervous symptoms, with dizziness, blurred vision, and excitement. Lidocaine blood levels are linearly dose-related and can be very helpful in avoiding toxicity. Lidocaine is metabolized in part by the liver, and smaller doses should be used in the presence of impaired liver function. If doses greater than 3–4 mg/min in an infusion must be exceeded or continued, one should consider combining lower doses of lidocaine with drugs such as quinidine and procainamide.

C. Overdrive Suppression by Rapid Pacing: If drugs and attention to precipitating factors are unsuccessful in preventing ventricular tachycardia, overdrive suppression of the ectopic focus by pacing may help prevent attacks (Fig 15–21). One should attempt to stop the initial attack and then use pacing at a rate somewhat faster than the ordinary sinus rate to prevent subsequent attacks. Overdrive suppression is ordinarily useful only temporarily, although long-term pacing has been used with success. Electrophysiologic study should be performed before permanent insertion of a long-term pacing unit. One must be certain that the tachycardia can be terminated by rapid pacing, and one must exclude Wolff-Parkinson-White syndrome to avoid ventricular fibrillation.

D. Resection of Ventricular Aneurysm and Ischemic Zone of Increased Excitability: If episodes of ventricular tachycardia occur frequently (some patients have 75–100 attacks over a period of days or weeks), the possibility of ventricular aneurysm should be considered. Two-dimensional echocardiography, radionuclide angiography, and cardiac catheterization with left ventricular angiography should be considered in order to establish the presence of a localized expansile pulsation of the left ventricle that might be treated surgically. Recurrent ventricular tachycardia unrelieved by other measures may be prevented in some cases by resection of the ventricular aneurysm, and cardiac failure may be reversed (see Chapter 8).

Before resection of an aneurysm for complex ventricular tachycardia that recurs despite good medical therapy, electrophysiologic studies should be employed to define the focus of origin of the arrhythmia. The initial electrical activity of the focus usually occurs in the border between the edge of the aneurysm and the neighboring viable myocardium. At surgery, intraoperative mapping should also be performed, and encircling endocardial resection (which includes the area of earliest electrical activity in the border zone) should be combined with resection of the ventricular aneurysm. When this localized endocardial area was resected in patients with recurrent ventricular tachycardia, the arrhythmia could no longer be induced by electrical stimulation, and the disabling ventricular tachycardia and complex ventricular premature beats were usually abolished (Josephson, 1980). Electrophysiologic studies, including electrical stimulation and mapping at the time of surgery, require experienced specialists in the field and cooperation between cardiologists and surgeons.

E. Recurrent Ventricular Tachycardia:

1. Drug treatment–When patients with recurrent ventricular tachycardia do not respond to intensive antiarrhythmic therapy given in the usual trial and error method, electrophysiologic studies should be considered. Programmed electrical stimulation in the electrophysiology laboratory in patients with spontaneous episodes of tachycardia allows the physician to initiate and terminate ventricular tachycardia by critically timed atrial or ventricular stimuli. Individual antiarrhythmic drugs can then be given to determine whether or not they prevent induction of tachycardia. Drugs found to be effective in preventing ventricular tachycardia in the laboratory have been found to be effective in preventing spontaneous occurrences of the arrhythmia. The induced and spontaneous arrhythmias are said to be identical in about 80–90% of patients. The method allows a more rational and rapid selection of the most potent antiarrhythmic agent (Vandepol, 1980). Wellens (1985) emphasized that these stimulation studies were primarily of value when clinically documented sustained ventricular tachycardia could be induced. Chronic oral therapy with the same drug proves to be effective in most patients. In some instances, especially with amiodarone, the drug may be effective clinically even though ventricular tachycardia can still be induced in the laboratory while the patient is receiving the drug.

2. Surgical or catheter ablation of site–As with surgical ablation of the accessory pathway or catheter interruption of the His bundle in atrial arrhythmias, identification of the location of the focus for recurrent ventricular tachycardia (by electrophysiologic drug testing) has led to surgical or electrical ablation with promising results (Horowitz, 1980, 1981; Scheinman, 1983). Techniques of catheter mapping (Josephson, *Am J Cardiol* 1982; 1984) and intraoperative mapping (Gallagher, 1982) have been well described. More experience is needed to determine the long-term effectiveness and safety of the procedure.

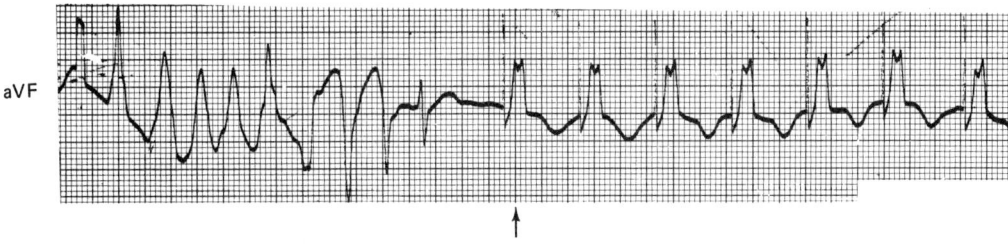

Figure 15–21. Short runs of ventricular tachycardia abolished (arrow) by artificial transvenous pacemaker in a 43-year-old man following the replacement of a mitral valve.

3. Implantation of pacemakers—Automatic surgically implanted pacemakers have been used successfully with increasing frequency. The pacemaker automatically monitors cardiac electrical activity and discharges defibrillatory pulses when ventricular tachycardia or ventricular fibrillation occurs (Mirowski, 1985; Reid, 1983). Potential problems and long-term results of the method remain to be determined (see p 502).

VENTRICULAR FIBRILLATION

Ventricular fibrillation (shown in Fig 15–22) is the most feared arrhythmia because of its relationship to sudden cardiac death.

Uncoordinated cardiac impulses spread rapidly across the ventricle from multiple areas of reentry and through pathways that vary in size and direction. As a result, there is failure of the normal sequential contraction of the heart. A heart in ventricular fibrillation is seen as a mass of multiple small twitches. The pressure within the ventricle does not rise, and the peripheral tissues are not perfused, because there is no effective cardiac output. In effect, the heart is in a state equivalent to cardiac arrest. The random reentry pathways of the excitatory wave result in perpetuation of the dysrhythmia. Spontaneous episodes of ventricular fibrillation may terminate without therapy. If the ventricular fibrillation persists for more than a few minutes, perfusion of the heart and brain essentially stops, and even if the patient is subsequently resuscitated, irreversible brain damage may have occurred. As a result, efforts aimed at recognizing the high-risk patient susceptible to ventricular fibrillation have been employed to alert everyone concerned to the need for immediate treatment should the arrhythmia occur. As indicated in the sections on ventricular tachycardia and ventricular premature beats, most instances of ventricular fibrillation are preceded by less severe varieties of ventricular arrhythmia, but some patients, particularly those in the early minutes or hours of acute myocardial infarction, may have ventricular fibrillation without warning arrhythmias. Furthermore, in patients who have fortuitously developed an acute myocardial infarction while being monitored, the immediate phase of the infarction was not associated with ventricular arrhythmias which developed later, within minutes to an hour. The frequency of ventricular arrhythmias—especially ventricular fibrillation—while well established in coronary heart disease (see Chapter 8), is a matter of dispute in prolapsed mitral valve syndrome.

On physical examination, the patient with ventricular fibrillation is usually unconscious, pulseless, with obvious poor perfusion and cold skin, and apparently dead.

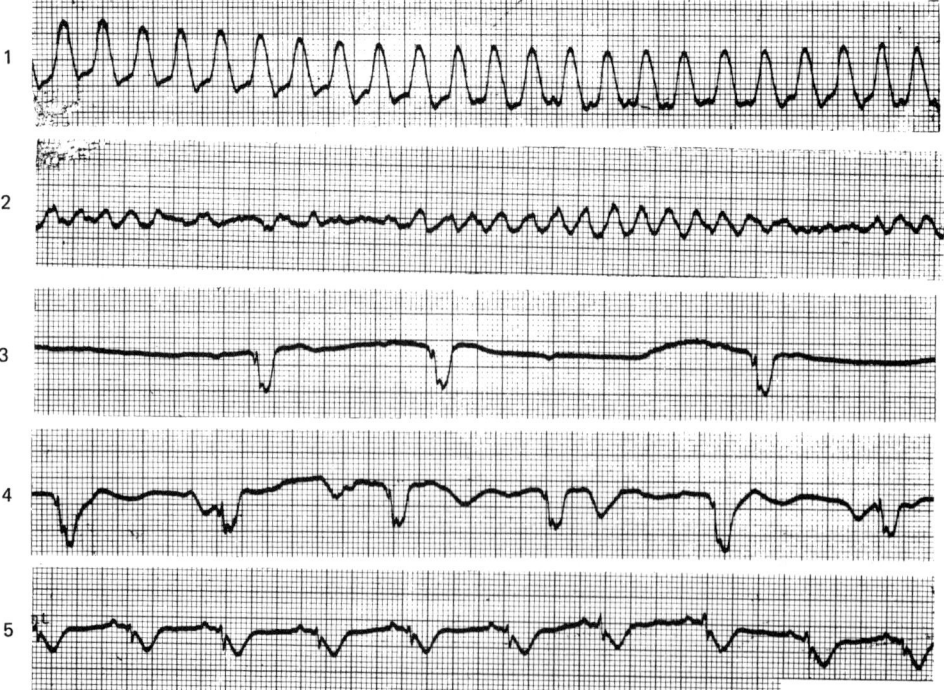

Figure 15–22. Sequential changes after cardiac arrest in a 55-year-old woman with unstable angina: Strip 1 shows ventricular tachycardia. Strip 2 shows ventricular fibrillation. Strip 3 shows idioventricular rhythm after defibrillation. Strip 4 shows ventricular premature beats. Strip 5 shows sinus rhythm. (Courtesy of K Gershengorn.)

Background of Patients Who Develop Ventricular Fibrillation

Most patients who develop ventricular fibrillation have known coronary heart disease or a history of hypertension, hypercholesterolemia, ventricular premature beats, or some other evidence of heart disease. Since approximately 60% of all coronary deaths are sudden and since most sudden deaths occur in patients with known coronary disease, identification of coronary patients at greatest risk of cardiac arrest and preventive treatment must take precedence over treatment of cardiac arrest itself if one hopes to decrease the mortality rate from sudden cardiac death.

Although many patients have seen their physician within the month preceding the ventricular fibrillation—and about one-fifth on the day of the arrest because of chest pain, dyspnea, or palpitations—most patients collapse instantaneously and therefore cannot be saved by a mobile team but only by a trained person who witnesses the episode and can immediately institute restorative measures. The American Heart Association makes available a film for the purpose of encouraging citizens, especially relatives or coworkers of patients who have once been defibrillated or have known coronary heart disease, to take special courses in resuscitation. Cobb (1975) has analyzed the types of activities immediately preceding ventricular fibrillation and notes that only about one-sixth have had unusual physical or mental stress. About one-third of cases occur during sleep, and the great majority of cases of ventricular fibrillation occur during ordinary activities at work or at home.

In some communities paramedical teams can reach a stricken individual within 5 minutes. Experience with out-of-hospital onset of ventricular fibrillation has shown that only about one-fourth of patients will have unequivocal evidence of acute myocardial infarction by electrocardiographic criteria—perhaps half if one includes enzyme changes. Sixty to 70% of patients are resuscitated, and about 30% of resuscitated victims leave the hospital alive (see also Table 15–12). The resuscitation efforts are therefore clearly worthwhile. Some prehospital cardiac arrests are found by mobile teams to be due to asystole rather than ventricular fibrillation, but it is not known whether or not the asystole followed a period of ventricular fibrillation. These patients rarely survive hospitalization.

Many patients who develop ventricular fibrillation have unwitnessed episodes that may be instantaneous or last only minutes, and death occurs before medical help can be obtained. In many communities, efforts are under way to train lay persons to perform resuscitative measures, with the hope that external cardiac massage and artificial respiration will be instituted pending the arrival of a trained ambulance or fire department rescue team.

Treatment

A. Emergency Treatment: Treatment consists of *immediate* emergency resuscitative measures (see Chapter 7) to restore the circulation by external cardiac massage combined with mouth-to-mouth breathing. Chest compression is applied by means of a sharp downward thrust over the lower sternum at a rate of approximately 80/min, combined with 2 or 3 quick breaths with the nose closed and the neck extended, and quick breaths are continued at a rate of 18/min until help arrives. If 2 people are available, the inflations and the chest compression should be continued without interruption until help arrives. The patient must be intubated and defibrillated at the earliest possible moment (DeSilva, 1980; Crampton, 1980).

In the coronary care unit, with electrocardiographic monitoring, resuscitation should be accomplished within 30 seconds after the onset of fibrillation. Specially trained nurses in the coronary care unit should defibrillate the patient if a doctor is unavailable. Defibrillation is accomplished with 400 J, repeated if necessary. Lack of tissue perfusion causes anaerobic metabolic acidosis, and it is necessary to give sodium bicarbonate, 44 meq intravenously every 5–10 minutes, for the duration of arrest. The accumulation of pyruvic and lactic acids and hypercapnia from absent ventilation lead to a low pH, which in turn may induce further arrhythmias and interfere with defibrillation by electric countershock. Arterial pH should be monitored when resuscitation is achieved so that excessive bicarbonate is not given to produce alkalosis.

In the coronary care unit, defibrillation is almost always successful, at least initially, but fibrillation may be recurrent, usually within the first day or so,

Table 15–12. Hospital follow-up data on surviving patients who had defibrillation.*

	Hospital Deaths (Percent)	Discharged Survivors (Percent)	Totals Prehospital Ventricular Fibrillation (Percent)
Acute myocardial infarction	37	31	35
Ischemia without infarction	34	29	32
No acute electrocardiographic change	10	26	17
Complete left bundle branch block†	19	14	17
Complete right bundle branch block	24	7	17
Repeat ventricular fibrillation	50	24	40
Congestive heart failure	69	53	63
Cardiogenic shock	39	5	25
Severe pulmonary complications‡	41	44	42
Severe neurologic deficit	95	12	61
Partial neurologic deficit	5	28	15
No neurologic deficit	...	60	25

*Reproduced, with permission, from Liberthson RR et al: Prehospital ventricular defibrillation: Prognosis and follow-up course. *N Engl J Med* 1974;291:317.
†Possibly masking an acute myocardial change.
‡Aspiration pneumonia or flail chest.

and antiarrhythmic therapy such as lidocaine, 1–4 mg/min by infusion, should be started promptly after the patient is resuscitated.

B. Bypass Coronary Surgery: Because of the extensive coronary disease found on coronary arteriography in most patients recovered from ventricular fibrillation, bypass surgery has been recommended to prevent recurrence. The data are limited, but it is not established that bypass surgery can prevent recurrent attacks of ventricular fibrillation.

C. Prophylactic Drugs to Prevent Recurrences: The same can be said for antiarrhythmic drugs such as quinidine, procainamide, and phenytoin (especially in digitalis toxicity). A number of studies have shown that these drugs may decrease the number of simple or complex ventricular premature beats seen on 24-hour monitoring, but the side effects are significant and there is as yet only minimal evidence that they will in fact prevent sudden cardiac death even though the number of ventricular premature beats seems to be decreased (Jelinek, 1974). Table 15–7 summarizes the clinical characteristics of some of these newer agents. The most promising appear to be amiodarone, flecainide, and encainide. Further clinical data are awaited. The unpredictability of the ventricular fibrillation is an especially devastating aspect of this fatal arrhythmia, and efforts are being made to preselect a high-risk group from the coronary heart disease population in which various forms of therapy can be prospectively tested.

Beta-adrenergic blocking agents are the only drugs that have decreased the incidence of sudden death when used prophylactically. Almost all beta-adrenergic blocking drugs tried have reduced the incidence of sudden death and cardiac death when used on a long-term basis following myocardial infarction. The value of beta-blocking drugs emphasizes the role of adrenergic central nervous system stimuli in causing ventricular arrhythmias. Decreasing these adrenergic stimuli with drugs such as tranquilizers, diazepam, or beta-adrenergic blocking drugs may prove to be more valuable than using purely antiarrhythmic drugs such as quinidine and procainamide.

D. Resection of Ventricular Aneurysm: One group of patients who might benefit from cardiac surgery are those who, following an acute myocardial infarction, develop a ventricular aneurysm with refractory ventricular arrhythmias that might degenerate into ventricular fibrillation, possibly because of persistence of a rim of viable but ischemic tissue on the edge of the aneurysm or because of the presence of cardiac failure. Resection of the aneurysm and the endocardial border zone of earliest activation (see p 499) may be successful in eliminating the ventricular arrhythmia even if bypass surgery has not been performed. Large, flabby ventricles with dyskinesia or akinesia but without a well-marked or demarcated aneurysm should not be treated by resection of the poorly contracting segments.

E. Implanted Automatic Pacemakers: Implanted automatic pacemakers may sense ventricular fibrillation and spontaneously fire a defibrillatory impulse. This dramatic new approach is encouraging in the several hundred cases in which it has been attempted, and further data are awaited with considerable interest (Mirowski, 1985; Reid, 1983).

F. Control of Risk Factors: Control of risk factors that increase the likelihood of clinical coronary events, especially control of hypertension and hyperlipidemia and cessation of smoking, have been shown to decrease the incidence of sudden death in patients with known coronary heart disease with or without ventricular fibrillation. See the discussion of myocardial infarction on p 163. Patients who have had ventricular fibrillation and have been resuscitated should be strongly advised to stop smoking. It is of considerable interest that overt diabetes is uncommon in this group of patients; however, diabetes should be treated if present.

Holter monitoring at intervals following recovery from acute myocardial infarction or from an episode of ventricular fibrillation may identify some individuals in whom spontaneous cardiac pain occurs coincidentally with the development of complex ventricular arrhythmias. This group may benefit from intensive antiarrhythmic or beta-adrenergic blocking therapy.

Prognosis
(Table 15–13)

Although about one-half to two-thirds of patients with ventricular fibrillation outside the hospital are satisfactorily defibrillated, most of these patients die in the hospital. However, 30% are discharged alive, often with only mild evidence of cardiac failure or pulmonary complications. Subsequent coronary arteriography almost always shows extensive coronary disease, and approximately half have left ventricular wall motion abnormalities. Severe neurologic deficits are uncommon in patients who are promptly defibrillated. Impaired memory is described by Cobb (1975) as the most common late neurologic sequela. The high

Table 15–13. Breakdown of the patient population showing the follow-up data on 301 subjects with prehospital ventricular fibrillation.*

	Patients Alive	Deaths
Monitored prehospital ventricular fibrillation patients	301	
		102
Defibrillation attempted	199	
		98
Sent to hospital	101	
		59
Discharged from hospital	42	

*Reproduced, with permission, from Liberthson RR et al: Prehospital ventricular defibrillation: Prognosis and follow-up course. *N Engl J Med* 1974;**291**:317.

incidence of recurrence of fibrillation within the months following release from the hospital indicates that chronic myocardial ischemia is still present. The incidence of recurrence of ventricular fibrillation is greater among persons who show no evidence of myocardial infarction than among those who do.

Without treatment, the patient with acute myocardial infarction who develops ventricular fibrillation almost always dies. Prospective follow-up of patients who have been resuscitated is unfavorable, with a 30% 1-year mortality rate and a 50% 3-year mortality rate. Most of the recurrences of "sudden cardiac death" occur within the first few months, and patients and their families should be instructed regarding resuscitation and the need to get professional help immediately if another attack occurs during this vulnerable period (Schaffer, 1975).

REFERENCES

Pathophysiology & Mechanisms

Adgey AAJ et al: Incidence, significance and management of early bradyarrhythmia complicating acute myocardial infarction. *Lancet* 1968;**2**:1097.

Anderson R et al: Relation between metabolic acidosis and cardiac dysrhythmias in acute myocardial infarction. *Br Heart J* 1968;**30**:493.

Arnsdorf MF: Membrane factors in arrhythmogenesis: Concepts and definitions. *Prog Cardiovasc Dis* 1977;**19**:413.

Ayres SM, Grace WJ: Inappropriate ventilation and hypoxemia as causes of cardiac arrhythmias. *Am J Med* 1969;**46**:495.

Califf RM et al: Relationships among ventricular arrhythmias, coronary artery disease, and angiographic and electrocardiographic indicators of myocardial fibrosis. *Circulation* 1978;**57**:725.

Chan AQ, Pick A: Re-entrant arrhythmias and concealed conduction. *Am Heart J* 1979;**97**:644.

Commerford PJ, Lloyd EA: Arrhythmias in patients with drug toxicity, electrolyte, and endocrine disturbances. *Med Clin North Am* 1984;**68**:1051.

Conolly ME, Kersting F, Dollery CT: The clinical pharmacology of beta-adrenoreceptor-blocking drugs. *Prog Cardiovasc Dis* 1976;**19**:203.

Dimarco JP, Garan H, Ruskin JN: Complications in patients undergoing cardiac electrophysiologic procedures. *Ann Intern Med* 1982;**97**:490.

Ferrer MI: The sick sinus syndrome. *Hosp Pract* (Nov) 1980;**15**:79.

Fisch C (editor): Symposium on electrophysiological correlates of clinical arrhythmias. (3 parts.) *Am J Cardiol* 1971;**28**:243, 371, 499.

Fowler NO et al: Electrocardiographic changes and cardiac arrhythmias in patients receiving psychotropic drugs. *Am J Cardiol* 1976;**37**:223.

Gallagher JJ, Damato AN, Lau SH: Electrophysiologic studies during accelerated idioventricular rhythms. *Circulation* 1971;**44**:671.

Goldreyer BN, Kastor JA, Kershbaum KL: The hemodynamic effects of induced supraventricular tachycardia in man. *Circulation* 1976;**54**:783.

Han J: Mechanisms of ventricular arrhythmias associated with myocardial infarction. *Am J Cardiol* 1969;**24**:800.

Han J et al: Incidence of ectopic beats as a function of basic rate in the ventricle. *Am Heart J* 1966;**72**:632.

Hinkle LE Jr, Carver ST, Stevens M: The frequency of asymptomatic disturbances of cardiac rhythm and conduction in middle-aged men. *Am J Cardiol* 1969;**24**:629.

Hoffman BF, Rosen MR, Wit AL: Electrophysiology and pharmacology of cardiac arrhythmias. 3. The causes and treatment of cardiac arrhythmias. (Part A.) *Am Heart J* 1975;**89**:115.

Horowitz LN, Josephson ME, Harken AH: Epicardial and endocardial activation during sustained ventricular tachycardia in man. *Circulation* 1980;**61**:1227.

Josephson ME et al: Comparison of endocardial catheter mapping with intraoperative mapping of ventricular tachycardia. *Circulation* 1980;**61**:395.

Katz LN, Pick A: *Clinical Electrocardiography*. Part 1: *The Arrhythmias*. Lea & Febiger, 1956.

Kinoshita S: Mechanisms of ventricular parasystole. *Circulation* 1978;**58**:715.

Langendorf R, Pick A, Winternitz M: Mechanisms of intermittent ventricular bigeminy. 1. Appearance of ectopic beats dependent upon length of the ventricular cycle, the "rule of bigeminy." *Circulation* 1955;**11**:422.

Lewis T: *Clinical Disorders of the Heartbeat*. Shaw & Sons, 1912.

Lown B, Verrier RL, Rabinowitz SH: Neural and psychologic mechanisms and the problem of sudden cardiac death. *Am J Cardiol* 1977;**39**:890.

Malliani A, Schwartz PJ, Zanchetti A: Neural mechanisms in life-threatening arrhythmias. *Am Heart J* 1980;**100**:705.

Michelson EL et al: Fixed coupling: Different mechanisms revealed by exercise-induced changes in cycle length. *Circulation* 1978;**58**:1002.

Myerburg RJ: Electrocardiographic analysis of cardiac arrhythmias. *Hosp Pract* (June) 1980;**15**:51.

Ochs HR et al: Single and multiple dose pharmacokinetics of oral quinidine sulfate and gluconate. *Am J Cardiol* 1978;**41**:770.

Podrid PJ, Schoeneberger A, Lown B: Congestive heart failure caused by oral disopyramide. *N Engl J Med* 1980; **302**:614.

Rodstein M, Wolloch L, Gubner RS: Mortality study of the significance of extra-systoles in an insured population. *Circulation* 1971;**44**:617.

Romero CA Jr: Holter monitoring in the diagnosis and management of cardiac rhythm disturbances. *Med Clin North Am* 1976;**60**:299.

Rosen MR, Hoffman BF, Wit AL: Electrophysiology and pharmacology of cardiac arrhythmias. 5. Cardiac antiarrhythmic effects of lidocaine. *Am Heart J* 1975;**89**:526.

Samet P: Hemodynamic sequelae of cardiac arrhythmias. *Circulation* 1973;**47**:399.

Scherf D, Schott A: Pages 381–441 in: *Extrasystoles and Allied Arrhythmias*. Grune & Stratton, 1953.

Schroeder JS: Ambulatory electrocardiographic monitoring: Technique and clinical indications. *JAMA* 1976;**236**:494.

Schwartz PJ et al (editors): *Neural Mechanisms in Cardiac*

Arrhythmias. Vol 2 in: *Perspectives in Cardiovascular Research.* Raven Press, 1979.

Stemple DR et al: Electrophysiological effects of edrophonium in the innervated and the transplanted denervated human heart. *Br Heart J* 1978;**60:**644.

Talbot S: Fixed and variable coupling of ventricular extrasystoles. *Cardiology* 1973;**58:**117.

Vaughan Williams EM: Classification of antiarrhythmic drugs. Pages 449–472 in: *Symposium on Cardiac Arrhythmias.* Sandoe E, Flensted-Jensen E, Olesen KH (editors). AB Astra, 1970.

Vera Z, Mason DT: Reentry versus automaticity: Role in tachyarrhythmia genesis and antiarrhythmic therapy. *Am Heart J* 1981;**101:**329.

Watanabe Y, Dreifus LS: *Cardiac Arrhythmias: Electrophysiologic Basis for Clinical Interpretation.* Grune & Stratton, 1977.

Wellens HJJ, Bär FWHM, Lie KI: The value of the electrocardiogram in the differential diagnosis of a tachycardia with a widened QRS complex. *Am J Med* 1978;**64:**27.

Wellens HJJ, Brugada P, Stevenson WG: Programmed electrical stimulation of the heart in patients with life-threatening ventricular arrhythmias: What is the significance of induced arrhythmias and what is the correct stimulation protocol? *Circulation* 1985;**72:**1.

Wellens HJJ, Durrer DR, Lie KI: Observations on mechanisms of ventricular tachycardia in man. *Circulation* 1976;**54:**237.

WHO/ISC Task Force: Definition of terms related to cardiac rhythm. *Am Heart J* 1978;**95:**796.

Wit AL, Hoffman BF, Rosen MR: Electrophysiology and pharmacology of cardiac arrhythmias. 9. Cardiac electrophysiologic effects of beta adrenergic receptor stimulation and blockade. (3 parts.) *Am Heart J* 1975;**90:**521, 665, 795.

Wit AL, Rosen MR, Hoffman BF: Electrophysiology and pharmacology of cardiac arrhythmias. 2. Relationship of normal and abnormal electrical activity of cardiac fibers to the genesis of arrhythmias. B. Reentry, Section II. *Am Heart J* 1974;**88:**798.

Wit AL, Rosen MR, Hoffman BF: Electrophysiology and pharmacology of cardiac arrhythmias. 8. Cardiac effects of diphenylhydantoin. *Am Heart J* 1975;**90:**265.

Supraventricular (Atrial or Junctional) Arrhythmias

Barold SS, Coumel P: Mechanisms of atrioventricular junctional tachycardia: Role of reentry and concealed accessory bypass tracts. *Am J Cardiol* 1977;**39:**97.

Betriu A et al: Beneficial effect of intravenous diltiazem in the acute management of paroxysmal supraventricular tachyarrhythmias. *Circulation* 1983;**67:**88.

Gillette PC: The mechanisms of supraventricular tachycardia in children. *Circulation* 1976;**54:**133.

Goel BG, Han J: Atrial ectopic activity associated with sinus bradycardia. *Circulation* 1970;**42:**853.

Goldreyer BN: Mechanisms of supraventricular tachycardias. *Annu Rev Med* 1975;**26:**219.

Goldreyer BN, Kastor JA, Kershbaum KL: The hemodynamic effects of induced supraventricular tachycardia in man. *Circulation* 1976;**54:**783.

Hinkle LE Jr, Carver ST, Stevens M: The frequency of asymptomatic disturbances of cardiac rhythm and conduction in middle-aged men. *Am J Cardiol* 1969;**24:**629.

Josephson ME, Horowitz LN, Kastor JA: Paroxysmal supraventricular tachycardia in patients with mitral valve prolapse. *Circulation* 1978;**57:**111.

Josephson ME, Kastor JA: Supraventricular tachycardia in Lown-Ganong-Levine syndrome: Atrionodal versus intranodal reentry. *Am J Cardiol* 1977; **40:**521.

Knoebel SB, Fisch C: Accelerated junctional escape: A clinical and electrocardiographic study. *Circulation* 1974; **50:**151.

Mauritson DR et al: Oral verapamil for paroxysmal supraventricular tachycardia: A long-term, double-blind randomized trial. *Ann Intern Med* 1982;**96:**409.

Morady F, Scheinman MM: Paroxysmal supraventricular tachycardia. 1. Diagnosis. *Mod Concepts Cardiovasc Dis* 1982;**51:**107.

Narula OS, Narula JT: Junctional pacemakers in man: Response to overdrive suppression with and without parasympathetic blockade. *Circulation* 1978;**57:**880.

Parkinson J, Papp C: Repetitive paroxysmal tachycardia. *Br Heart J* 1947;**9:**241.

Pick A, Dominguez P: Nonparoxysmal A-V nodal tachycardia. *Circulation* 1957;**16:**1022.

Pick A, Langendorf R: Recent advances in the differential diagnosis of AV junctional arrhythmia. *Am Heart J* 1968;**76:**553.

Prinzmetal M et al: *The Auricular Arrhythmias.* Thomas, 1952.

Pritchett ELC et al: Supraventricular tachycardia dependent upon accessory pathways in the absence of ventricular preexcitation. *Am J Med* 1978;**64:**214.

Puech P et al: The diagnosis of supraventricular arrhythmias and the differentiation between supraventricular tachycardia with aberrant conduction and ventricular tachycardias. Page 199 in: *Symposium on Cardiac Arrhythmias.* Sandoe E, Flensted-Jensen E, Olesen KH (editors). AB Astra, 1970.

Ross DL et al: Curative surgery for atrioventricular junctional ("AV nodal") reentrant tachycardia. *J Am Coll Cardiol* 1985;**6:**1383.

Scheinman MM, Morady F: Invasive cardiac electrophysiologic testing: The current state of the art. (Editorial.) *Circulation* 1983;**67:**1169.

Shine KI, Kastor JA, Yurchak PM: Multifocal atrial tachycardia: Clinical and electrocardiographic features in 32 patients. *N Engl J Med* 1968;**279:**344.

Waxman MB, Wald RW: Termination of ventricular tachycardia by an increase in cardiac vagal drive. *Circulation* 1977;**56:**385.

Waxman MB et al: Effects of respiration and posture on paroxysmal supraventricular tachycardia. *Circulation* 1980; **62:**1011.

Wellens HJJ, Brugada P, Stevenson WG: Programmed electrical stimulation of the heart in patients with life-threatening ventricular arrhythmias: What is the significance of induced arrhythmias and what is the correct stimulation protocol? *Circulation* 1985;**72:**1.

Wolff L: Clinical aspects of paroxysmal rapid heart action. *N Engl J Med* 1942;**226:**740.

Zipes DP, Fisch C: ECG analysis No. 10: Supraventricular arrhythmias with abnormal QRS complex. *Arch Intern Med* 1972;**130:**781.

Treatment of Supraventricular Arrhythmias

Abdollah H et al: Clinical efficacy and electrophysiologic effects of intravenous and oral encainide in patients with accessory atrioventricular pathways and supraventricular arrhythmias. *Am J Cardiol* 1984;**54:**544.

Bigger JT Jr: Supraventricular tachycardia. *Hosp Pract* (Aug) 1980;**15**:45.

Brugada P, Wellens HJJ: Effects of intravenous and oral disopyramide on paroxysmal atrioventricular nodal tachycardia. *Am J Cardiol* 1984;**53**:88.

Brugada P et al: Suppression of incessant supraventricular tachycardia by intravenous and oral encainide. *J Am Coll Cardiol* 1984;**4**:1255.

Camm J, Ward D, Spurrell R: Response of atrial flutter to overdrive atrial pacing and intravenous disopyramide phosphate, singly and in combination. *Br Heart J* 1980;**44**:240.

Camm J et al: Cryothermal mapping and cryoablation in the treatment of refractory cardiac arrhythmias. *Circulation* 1980;**62**:67.

Chang M et al: Nadolol and supraventricular tachycardia: An electrophysiologic study. *J Am Coll Cardiol* 1983;**2**:894.

DeSilva RA et al: Cardioversion and defibrillation. *Am Heart J* 1980;**100**:881.

Guarnieri T et al: The nonpharmacologic management of the permanent form of junctional reciprocating tachycardia. *Circulation* 1984;**69**:269.

Josephson ME: Catheter ablation of arrhythmias. *Ann Intern Med* 1984;**101**:234.

Josephson ME et al: The effects of carotid sinus pressure in re-entry paroxysmal supraventricular tachycardia. *Am Heart J* 1974;**88**:694.

Klein GJ et al: Cryosurgical ablation of the atrioventricular node–His bundle: Long-term follow-up and properties of the junctional pacemaker. *Circulation* 1980;**61**:8.

Klein HO, Hoffman BF: Cessation of paroxysmal supraventricular tachycardias by parasympathomimetic interventions. *Ann Intern Med* 1974;**81**:48.

Lown B, Levine SA: The carotid sinus: Clinical value of its stimulation. *Circulation* 1961;**23**:766.

Margolis B, DeSilva RA, Lown B: Episodic drug treatment in the management of paroxysmal arrhythmias. *Am J Cardiol* 1980;**45**:621.

Michaelson SP, Wolfson S: Treatment of supraventricular arrhythmias with propranolol. *Cardiovasc Med* 1976;**1**:213.

Morady F, Scheinman MM: Paroxysmal supraventricular tachycardia. 2. Treatment. *Mod Concepts Cardiovasc Dis* 1982;**51**:113.

Moss AJ, Aledort LM: Use of edrophonium (Tensilon) in the evaluation of supraventricular tachycardias. *Am J Cardiol* 1966;**17**:58.

Narula OS, Narula JT: Junctional pacemakers in man: Response to overdrive suppression with and without parasympathetic blockade. *Circulation* 1978;**57**:880.

Ochs HR et al: Intravenous quinidine: Pharmacokinetic properties and effects on left ventricular performance in humans. *Am Heart J* 1980;**99**:468.

Reddy CVR, Gould L: The efficacy of Tensilon (edrophonium) infusion in the treatment of atrial tachycardia. (Abstract.) *Clin Res* 1978;**26**:263A.

Rosen KM: Junctional tachycardia: Mechanisms, diagnosis, differential diagnosis, and management. *Circulation* 1973;**47**:654.

Sakurai M et al: Acute and chronic effects of verapamil in patients with paroxysmal supraventricular tachycardia. *Am Heart J* 1983;**105**:619.

Scheinman MM, Morady F: Invasive cardiac electrophysiologic testing: The current state of the art. (Editorial.) *Circulation* 1983;**67**:1169.

Scheinman MM et al: Catheter-induced ablation of the atrioventricular function to control refractory supraventricular arrhythmias. *JAMA* 1982;**248**:851.

Spurrell RJ et al: Implantable automatic scanning pacemaker for termination of supraventricular tachycardia. *Am J Cardiol* 1982;**49**:753.

Sung RJ, Elser B, McAllister RG Jr: Intravenous verapamil for termination of re-entrant supraventricular tachycardia: Intracardiac studies correlated with plasma verapamil concentration. *Ann Intern Med* 1980;**93**:682.

Svinarich JT, Sung RJ: The role of verapamil in the treatment and prophylaxis of supraventricular tachycardia. *Cardiovasc Rev Rep* 1984;**5**:1220.

Talano JV, Tommaso C: Slow channel calcium antagonists in the treatment of supraventricular tachycardia. *Prog Cardiovasc Dis* 1982;**25**:141.

Waldo AL et al: Temporary cardiac pacing: Applications and techniques in the treatment of cardiac arrhythmias. *Prog Cardiovasc Dis* 1981;**23**:451.

Waxman MB et al: Vagal techniques for termination of paroxysmal supraventricular tachycardia. *Am J Cardiol* 1980;**46**:655.

Weisberger AS, Feil H: Lanatoside C in the treatment of persistent paroxysmal auricular tachycardia. *Am J Cardiol* 1947;**34**:871.

Wellens HJJ: *Electrical Stimulation of the Heart in the Study and Treatment of Tachycardias.* University Park Press, 1971.

Wiener I: Pacing techniques in the treatment of tachycardias. *Ann Intern Med* 1980;**93**:326.

Wu D et al: Effects of procainamide on atrioventricular nodal re-entrant paroxysmal tachycardia. *Circulation* 1978;**57**:1171.

Zipes DP: A consideration of antiarrhythmic therapy. (Editorial.) *Circulation* 1985;**72**:949.

Atrial Fibrillation & Atrial Flutter

Bedford DE: The course and treatment of auricular flutter. *Q J Med* 1927;**21**:21.

Bloomfield AL: A bibliography of internal medicine: Auricular fibrillation. *Arch Intern Med* 1958;**102**:302.

Campbell M: Paroxysmal auricular fibrillation: A record of 200 cases. *Q J Med* 1930;**23**:67.

Campbell RWF et al: Atrial fibrillation in the preexcitation syndrome. *Am J Cardiol* 1977;**40**:514.

Christie DJ, Aster RH: Drug-antibody-platelet interaction in quinine- and quinidine-induced thrombocytopenia. *J Clin Invest* 1982;**70**:989.

Cramer G: Early and late results of conversion of atrial fibrillation with quinidine: A clinical and hemodynamic study. *Acta Med Scand [Suppl]* 1968;**490**:1.

Goldman S et al: Inefficacy of "therapeutic" serum levels of digoxin in controlling the ventricular rate in atrial fibrillation. *Am J Cardiol* 1975;**35**:651.

Gouaux JL, Ashman R: Auricular fibrillation with aberration simulating ventricular paroxysmal tachycardia. *Am Heart J* 1947;**34**:366.

Hillestad L et al: Quinidine in maintenance of sinus rhythm after electroconversion of chronic atrial fibrillation. *Br Heart J* 1971;**33**:518.

Hinton RC et al: Influence of etiology of atrial fibrillation on incidence of systemic embolism. *Am J Cardiol* 1977;**40**:509.

Kannel WB et al: Epidemiologic features of chronic atrial fibrillation. *N Engl J Med* 1982;**306**:1018.

Kastor JA: Digitalis intoxication in patients with atrial fibrillation. *Circulation* 1973;**47**:888.

Khalsa A, Edvardsson N, Olsson SB: Effects of metoprolol on heart rate in patients with digitalis treated chronic atrial fibrillation. *Clin Cardiol* 1978;**1**:91.

Kleiger R, Lown B: Cardioversion and digitalis. 2. Clinical studies. *Circulation* 1966;**33**:878.

Klein HO, Kaplinsky E: Verapamil and digoxin: Their respective effects on atrial fibrillation and their interaction. *Am J Cardiol* 1982;**50**:894.

Klein HO et al: The beneficial effects of verapamil in chronic atrial fibrillation. *Arch Intern Med* 1979;**139**:747.

Lahita R et al: Antibodies to nuclear antigens in patients treated with procainamide or acetylprocainamide. *N Engl J Med* 1979;**301**:1382.

Langendorf R, Pick A, Katz LN: Ventricular response in atrial fibrillation: Role of concealed conduction in the A–V junction. *Circulation* 1965;**32**:69.

Leahey EB Jr et al: The effect of quinidine and other oral antiarrhythmic drugs on serum digoxin: A prospective study. *Ann Intern Med* 1980;**92**:605.

Lown B: Electrical reversion of cardiac arrhythmias. *Br Heart J* 1967;**29**:469.

Mancini JGB, Goldberger AL: Cardioversion of atrial fibrillation: Consideration of embolization, anticoagulation, prophylactic pacemaker, and long-term success. *Am Heart J* 1982;**104**:617.

Miles WM et al: Evaluation of the patient with wide QRS tachycardia. *Med Clin North Am* 1984;**68**:1015.

Morady F et al: Electrophysiologic testing in the management of patients with the Wolff-Parkinson-White syndrome and atrial fibrillation. *Am J Cardiol* 1983;**51**:1623.

Normand JP et al: Comparative efficacy of short-acting and long-acting quinidine for maintenance of sinus rhythm after electrical conversion of atrial fibrillation. *Br Heart J* 1976;**38**:381.

Parkinson J, Campbell M: Paroxysmal auricular fibrillation: A record of 200 patients. *Q J Med* 1930;**24**:67.

Södermark T et al: Effect of quinidine on maintaining sinus rhythm after conversion of atrial fibrillation or flutter: A multicentre study from Stockholm. *Br Heart J* 1975;**37**:486.

Sokolow M: Some quantitative aspects of treatment with quinidine. *Ann Intern Med* 1956;**45**:582.

Sokolow M, Ball RE: Factors influencing conversion of chronic atrial fibrillation with special reference to serum quinidine concentration. *Circulation* 1956;**14**:568.

Sokolow M, Edgar AL: Blood quinidine concentration as a guide in the treatment of cardiac arrhythmias. *Circulation* 1950;**1**:576.

Waldo AL et al: Temporary cardiac pacing: Applications and techniques in the treatment of cardiac arrhythmias. *Prog Cardiovasc Dis* 1981;**23**:451.

Wetherbee DG, Brown MG, Holzman D: Ventricular rate response following exercise during auricular fibrillation and after conversion to normal sinus rhythm. *Am J Med Sci* 1952;**223**:667.

Zipes DP, Prystowsky EN, Heger JJ: Amiodarone: Electrophysiologic actions, pharmacokinetics and clinical effects. *J Am Coll Cardiol* 1984;**3**:1059.

Ventricular Arrhythmias

Armbrust CA Jr, Levine SA: Paroxysmal ventricular tachycardia: Study of 207 cases. *Circulation* 1950;**1**:28.

Bär FW et al: Differential diagnosis of tachycardia with narrow QRS complex (shorter than 0.12 second). *Am J Cardiol* 1984;**54**:555.

Benditt DG, Pritchett EL, Gallagher JJ: Spectrum of regular tachycardias with wide QRS complexes in patients with accessory atrioventricular pathways. *Am J Cardiol* 1978;**42**:828.

Bigger JT Jr et al: Ventricular arrhythmias in ischemic heart disease: Mechanism, prevalence, significance, and management. *Prog Cardiovasc Dis* 1977;**19**:255.

Booth D, Popio KA, Gettes LS: Multiformity of induced unifocal ventricular premature beats in human subjects: Electrocardiographic and angiographic correlations. *Am J Cardiol* 1982;**49**:1643.

Boudoulas H et al: Malignant premature ventricular beats in ambulatory patients. *Ann Intern Med* 1979;**91**:723.

Brodsky M et al: Arrhythmias documented by 24 hour continuous electrocardiographic monitoring in 50 male medical students without apparent heart disease. *Am J Cardiol* 1977;**39**:390.

Charlap S, Frishman WH: Calcium channel blockade: Effects of verapamil on arrhythmias. *J Cardiovasc Med* 1982;**7**:674.

Dressler W, Roesler H: The occurrence in paroxysmal ventricular tachycardia of ventricular complexes transitional in shape to sinoauricular beats. *Am Heart J* 1952;**44**:485.

Fisher JD: Role of electrophysiologic testing in the diagnosis and treatment of patients with known and suspected bradycardias and tachycardias. *Prog Cardiovasc Dis* 1981;**24**:25.

Greene HL, Reid PR, Schaeffer AH: The repetitive ventricular response in man: A predictor of sudden death. *N Engl J Med* 1978;**299**:729.

Harrison DC (editor): Proceedings of the symposium on cardiac arrhythmias: A decade of progress—1980. *Am Heart J* 1980;**100**:977. [Entire issue.]

Hinkle LE Jr, Carver ST, Stevens M: The frequency of asymptomatic disturbances of cardiac rhythm and conduction in middle-aged men. *Am J Cardiol* 1969;**24**:629.

Horowitz LN et al: Recurrent sustained ventricular tachycardia. 3. Role of the electrophysiologic study in selection of antiarrhythmic regimens. *Circulation* 1978;**58**:986.

Kay GN et al: Torsade de pointes: The long-short initiating sequence and other clinical features: Observations in 32 patients. *J Am Coll Cardiol* 1983;**2**:806.

Kennedy HL et al: Coronary artery status of apparently healthy subjects with frequent and complex ventricular ectopy. *Ann Intern Med* 1980;**92**:179.

Killip T: Management of arrhythmias in acute myocardial infarction. *Hosp Pract* (April) 1972;**7**:131.

Kluger J et al: The clinical pharmacology and antiarrhythmic efficacy of acetylprocainamide in patients with arrhythmias. *Am J Cardiol* 1980;**45**:1250.

Lahita R et al: Antibodies to nuclear antigens in patients treated with procainamide or acetylprocainamide. *N Engl J Med* 1979;**301**:1382.

Lown B, DeSilva RA, Lenson R: Roles of psychologic stress and autonomic nervous system changes in provocation of ventricular premature complexes. *Am J Cardiol* 1978;**41**:979.

Lown B, Temte JV, Arter WJ: Ventricular tachyarrhythmias: Clinical aspects. *Circulation* 1973;**47**:1364.

Lown B et al: Effect of a digitalis drug on ventricular premature beats. *N Engl J Med* 1977;**296**:301.

Marriott HJL: Differential diagnosis of supraventricular and ventricular tachycardia. *Geriatrics* 1970;**25**:91.

Moss AJ et al: Ventricular ectopic beats and their relation to sudden and nonsudden cardiac death after myocardial infarction. *Circulation* 1979;**60**:998.

Norris RM, Mercer CJ: Significance of idioventricular rhythms in acute myocardial infarction. *Prog Cardiovasc Dis* 1974;**16**:455.

Pedersen DH et al: Ventricular tachycardia and ventricular fibrillation in a young population. *Circulation* 1979;**60**:988.

Pick A, Langendorf R: *Interpretation of Complex Arrhythmias.* Lea & Febiger, 1979.

Reynolds EW, Vander Ark CR: Quinidine syncope and the delayed repolarization syndromes. *Mod Concepts Cardiovasc Dis* 1976;**45**:117.

Roden DM et al: Total suppression of ventricular arrhythmias by encainide: Pharmacokinetic and electrocardiographic characteristics. *N Engl J Med* 1980;**302**:877.

Rodstein M, Wolloch L, Gubner RS: Mortality study of the significance of extra-systoles in an insured population. *Circulation* 1971;**44**:617.

Ruberman W et al: Ventricular premature beats and mortality after myocardial infarction. *N Engl J Med* 1977;**297**:750.

Ryan M, Lown B, Horn H: Comparison of ventricular ectopic activity during 24-hour monitoring and exercise testing in patients with coronary heart disease. *N Engl J Med* 1975;**292**:224.

Rydén L et al: Prophylaxis of ventricular tachyarrhythmias with intravenous and oral tocainide in patients with and recovering from acute myocardial infarction. *Am Heart J* 1980;**100**:1006.

Sami M et al: Clinical electrophysiologic effects of encainide, a newly developed antiarrhythmic agent. *Am J Cardiol* 1979;**44**:526.

Schamroth L: Ventricular extrasystoles, ventricular tachycardia, and ventricular fibrillation: Clinical-electrocardiographic considerations. *Prog Cardiovasc Dis* 1980;**23**:13.

Swerdlow CD et al: Safety and efficacy of intravenous quinidine. *Am J Med* 1983;**75**:36.

Van Durme JP: Tachyarrhythmias and transient cerebral ischemic attacks. *Am Heart J* 1975;**89**:538.

Vlay SC, Reid PR: Ventricular ectopy: Etiology, evaluation, and therapy. *Am Heart J* 1982;**73**:899.

Waxman MB, Wald RW: Termination of ventricular tachycardia by an increase in cardiac vagal drive. *Circulation* 1977;**56**:385.

Wellens HJJ, Fritz WHM, Lie KI: The value of the electrocardiogram in the differential diagnosis of a tachycardia with a widened QRS complex. *Am J Med* 1978;**64**:27.

Wigle ED et al: Mitral valve prolapse. *Annu Rev Med* 1976;**27**:165.

Winkle RA, Glantz SA, Harrison DC: Pharmacologic therapy of ventricular arrhythmias. *Am J Cardiol* 1975;**36**:629.

Woosley RL et al: Effect of acetylator phenotype on the rate at which procainamide induces antinuclear antibodies and the lupus syndrome. *N Engl J Med* 1978;**298**:1157.

Yoon MS, Han J, Fabregas RA: Effect of ventricular aberrancy on fibrillation threshold. *Am Heart J* 1975;**89**:599.

Young MD et al: Treatment of ventricular arrhythmias with oral tocainide. *Am Heart J* 1980;**100**:1041.

Zipes DP (editor): Symposium on new aspects of antiarrhythmic therapy. *Am J Cardiol* 1978;**41**:975.

Treatment of Ventricular Arrhythmias

Anderson JL, Mason JW: Successful treatment by overdrive pacing of recurrent quinidine syncope due to ventricular tachycardia. *Am J Med* 1978;**64**:715.

Anderson JL et al: Antiarrhythmic drugs: Clinical pharmacology and therapeutic uses. *Drugs* 1978;**15**:271.

Antman EM et al: Calcium channel blocking agents in the treatment of cardiovascular disorders. 1. Basic and clinical electrophysiologic effects. *Ann Intern Med* 1980;**93**:875.

Bigger JT (guest editor): Symposium on flecainide acetate. *Am J Cardiol* 1984;**53**:1B. [Entire issue.]

Carey EL et al: Encainide and its metabolites: Comparative effects in man on ventricular arrhythmia and electrocardiographic intervals. *J Clin Invest* 1984;**73**:539.

Conard GJ, Ober RE: Metabolism of flecainide. *Am J Cardiol* 1984;**53**:41B.

Connolly SJ et al: Clinical pharmacology of probafenone. *Circulation* 1983;**68**:589.

Data JL, Wilkinson GR, Nies AS: Interaction of quinidine with anticonvulsant drugs. *N Engl J Med* 1978;**294**:699.

Fisher JD et al: Role of implantable pacemakers in control of recurrent ventricular tachycardia. *Am J Cardiol* 1982;**49**:194.

Gallagher JJ: Surgical treatment of arrhythmias: Current status and future directions. *Am J Cardiol* 1978;**41**:1035.

Gallagher JJ et al: Cryoablation of drug-resistant ventricular tachycardia in a patient with a variant of scleroderma. *Circulation* 1978;**57**:190.

Gallagher JJ et al: Techniques of intraoperative electrophysiologic mapping. *Am J Cardiol* 1982;**49**:221.

Garson A et al: Amiodarone treatment of critical arrhythmias in children and young adults. *J Am Coll Cardiol* 1984;**4**:749.

Goldschlager N, Cake D, Cohn K: Exercise-induced ventricular arrhythmias in patients with coronary artery disease: Their relation to angiographic findings. *Am J Cardiol* 1973;**31**:434.

Graboys TB et al: Long-term survival of patients with malignant ventricular arrhythmia treated with antiarrhythmic drugs. *Am J Cardiol* 1982;**50**:437.

Greenblatt DJ, Koch-Weser J: Drug therapy: Clinical pharmacokinetics. (2 parts.) *N Engl J Med* 1975;**293**:702, 964.

Guiraudon G et al: Encircling endocardial ventriculotomy: A new surgical treatment for life-threatening ventricular tachycardias resistant to medical treatment following myocardial infarction. *Ann Thorac Surg* 1978;**26**:438.

Harrison DC, Fitzgerald JW, Winkle RA: Contribution of ambulatory electrocardiographic monitoring to antiarrhythmic management. *Am J Cardiol* 1978;**41**:996.

Harrison DC, Meffin PJ, Winkle RA: Clinical pharmacokinetics of antiarrhythmic drugs. *Prog Cardiovasc Dis* 1977;**20**:217.

Hartzler GO: Treatment of recurrent ventricular tachycardia by patient-activated radiofrequency ventricular stimulation. *Mayo Clin Proc* 1979;**54**:75.

Helfant RH et al: The clinical use of DPH (Dilantin) in the treatment and prevention of cardiac arrhythmias. *Am Heart J* 1969;**77**:315.

Henningsen NC et al: Effects of long-term treatment with procaine amide: A prospective study with special regard to ANF and SLE in fast and slow acetylators. *Acta Med Scand* 1975;**198**:475.

Hess DS, Morady F, Scheinman MM: Electrophysiologic testing in the evaluation of patients with syncope of undetermined origin. *Am J Cardiol* 1982;**50**:1309.

Hoffman BF, Bigger JT Jr: Antiarrhythmic drugs. Pages 842–852 in: *Drill's Pharmacology in Medicine,* 4th ed. DiPalma JR (editor). McGraw-Hill, 1971.

Horowitz LN, Josephson ME, Kastor JA: Intracardiac electrophysiologic studies as a method for the optimization of drug therapy in chronic ventricular arrhythmia. *Prog Cardiovasc Dis* (Sept–Oct) 1980;**23**:81.

Horowitz LN et al: Surgical treatment of ventricular arrhythmias in coronary artery disease. *Ann Intern Med* 1981;**95**:88.

Horowitz LN et al: Ventricular resection guided by epicardial and endocardial mapping for treatment of recurrent ventricular tachycardia. *N Engl J Med* 1980;**302**:589.

Jelinek MV, Lohrbauer L, Lown B: Antiarrhythmic drug therapy for sporadic ventricular ectopic arrhythmias. *Circulation* 1974;**49**:659.

Josephson ME: Catheter ablation of arrhythmias. *Ann Intern Med* 1984;**101**:234.

Josephson ME, Horowitz LN: Recurrent ventricular tachycardia: An electrophysiologic approach. *Hosp Pract* (Sept) 1980;**15**:55.

Josephson ME et al: Role of catheter mapping in the preoperative evaluation of ventricular tachycardia. *Am J Cardiol* 1982;**49**:207.

Kay GN et al: Torsade de pointes: The long-short initiating sequence and other clinical features: Observations in 32 patients. *J Am Coll Cardiol* 1983;**2**:806.

Keefe DL, Somberg JC: New therapy focus: Tocainide. *Cardiovasc Rev Rep* 1984;**5**:1014.

Kimball JT, Killip T: Aggressive treatment of arrhythmias in acute myocardial infarction: Procedures and results. *Prog Cardiovasc Dis* 1968;**10**:483.

Kleinman S et al: Positive direct antiglobulin tests and immune hemolytic anemia in patients receiving procainamide. *N Engl J Med* 1984;**311**:809.

Koch-Weser J, Klein SW: Procainamide dosage schedules, plasma concentrations, and clinical effects. *JAMA* 1971;**215**:145.

Kupersmith J, Reder RF, Slater W: New antiarrhythmic drugs. *Cardiovasc Rev Rep* 1985;**6**:35.

Lahita R et al: Antibodies to nuclear antigens in patients treated with procainamide or acetylprocainamide. *N Engl J Med* 1979;**301**:1382.

Lerman BB et al: Disopyramide: Evaluation of electrophysiologic effects and clinical efficacy in patients with sustained ventricular tachycardia or ventricular fibrillation. *Am J Cardiol* 1983;**51**:759.

Lown B, Graboys TB: Management of patients with malignant ventricular arrhythmias. *Am J Cardiol* 1977;**39**:910.

Lown B et al: Effect of a digitalis drug on ventricular premature beats. *N Engl J Med* 1977;**296**:301.

Margolis B, DeSilva RA, Lown B: Episodic drug treatment in the management of paroxysmal arrhythmias. *Am J Cardiol* 1980;**45**:621.

Mason JW, Swerdlow CD, Mitchell LB: Efficacy of verapamil in chronic, recurrent ventricular tachycardia. *Am J Cardiol* 1983;**51**:1614.

Mason JW, Winkle RA: Accuracy of the ventricular tachycardia-induction study for predicting long-term efficacy and inefficacy of antiarrhythmic drugs. *N Engl J Med* 1980;**303**:1073.

Mead RH, Harrison DC: Therapy with investigational antiarrhythmic drugs. *Med Clin North Am* 1984;**68**:1321.

Mirowski M: The automatic implantable cardioverter-defibrillator: An overview. *J Am Coll Cardiol* 1985;**6**:461.

Mirowski M et al: Termination of malignant ventricular arrhythmias with an implanted automatic defibrillator in human beings. *N Engl J Med* 1980;**303**:322.

Morady F et al: Electrophysiologic testing in the management of survivors of out-of-hospital cardiac arrest. *Am J Cardiol* 1983;**51**:85.

Morady F et al: Intravenous amiodarone in the acute treatment of recurrent symptomatic ventricular tachycardia. *Am J Cardiol* 1983;**51**:156.

Morady F et al: Long-term efficacy and toxicity of high-dose amiodarone therapy for ventricular tachycardia or ventricular fibrillation. *Am J Cardiol* 1983;**52**:975.

Nademanee K, Singh BN: Advances in antiarrhythmic therapy: The role of newer antiarrhythmic drugs. *JAMA* 1982;**247**:217.

Nappi JM: Warfarin and phenytoin interaction. *Ann Intern Med* 1979;**90**:852.

Nestico PF, DePace NL, Morganroth J: Therapy with conventional antiarrhythmic drugs for ventricular arrhythmias. *Med Clin North Am* 1984;**68**:1295.

Opie LH: Drugs and the heart. 4. Antiarrhythmic agents. *Lancet* 1980;**1**:861.

Parsonnet V et al: Optimal resources for implantable cardiac pacemakers. (Pacemaker Study Group.) *Circulation* 1983;**68**:227A.

Podrid PJ, Ruskin J (editors): The role of oral mexiletine in the management of ventricular arrhythmias. (Symposium.) *Am Heart J* 1984;**107**:1053. [Entire issue.]

Podrid PJ et al: Ethmozin: A new antiarrhythmic drug for suppressing ventricular premature complexes. *Circulation* 1980;**61**:450.

Proceedings of the symposium on the role of oral mexiletine in the management of ventricular arrhythmias. November 13, 1983, at Anaheim, California. *Am Heart J* 1984;**107**:1053. [Entire issue.]

Prystowsky EN et al: Clinical efficacy and electrophysiologic effects of encainide in patients with Wolff-Parkinson-White syndrome. *Circulation* 1984;**69**:278.

Puech P: Ectopic ventricular rhythms: Ventricular tachycardia and His bundle recordings. Page 243 in: *His Bundle Electrocardiography and Clinical Electrophysiology*. Narula O (editor). David, 1975.

Reid PR et al: Clinical evaluation of the internal automatic cardioverter-defibrillator in survivors of sudden cardiac death. *Am J Cardiol* 1983;**51**:1608.

Roden DM et al: Antiarrhythmic efficacy, pharmacokinetics and safety of N-acetylprocainamide in human subjects: Comparison with procainamide. *Am J Cardiol* 1980;**46**:463.

Rotmensch HH et al: Steady-state serum amiodarone concentrations: Relationships with antiarrhythmic efficacy and toxicity. *Ann Intern Med* 1984;**101**:462.

Ruskin JN et al: Permanent radiofrequency ventricular pacing for management of drug-resistant ventricular tachycardia. *Am J Cardiol* 1980;**46**:317.

Schaeffer AH, Greene HL, Reid PR: Suppression of the repetitive ventricular response: An index of long-term antiarrhythmic effectiveness of aprindine for ventricular tachycardia in man. *Am J Cardiol* 1978;**42**:1007.

Scheinman MM, Morady F: Invasive cardiac electrophysiologic testing: The current state of the art. (Editorial.) *Circulation* 1983;**67**:1169.

Schoonmaker FW, Osteen RT, Greenfield JC Jr: Thioridazine (Mellaril)-induced ventricular tachycardia controlled with an artificial pacemaker. *Ann Intern Med* 1966;**65**:1076.

Shen EN et al: Electrophysiologic and hemodynamic effects of intravenous propafenone in patients with recurrent ventricular tachycardia. *J Am Coll Cardiol* 1984;**3**:1291.

Singh BN (moderator): Recent trends in the management of life-threatening ventricular arrhythmias. (Conference.) *West J Med* 1984;**141**:649.

Singh BN, Zipes DP (guest editors): The role of oral mexiletine in the management of ventricular arrhythmias. (Symposium.) *Am Heart J* 1984;**107**:1053. [Entire issue.]

Smith WM, Gallagher JJ: "Les torsades de pointes": An unusual ventricular arrhythmia. *Ann Intern Med* 1980;**93**:578.

Sokolow M, Perloff D: The clinical pharmacology and use

of quinidine in heart disease. *Prog Cardiovasc Dis* 1961; **3**:316.

Somberg JC (guest editor): Symposium on lorcainide: A new antiarrhythmic agent. *Am J Cardiol* 1984;**54**:1B. [Entire issue.]

Sung RJ et al: Electrophysiologic mechanism of exercise-induced sustained ventricular tachycardia. *Am J Cardiol* 1983;**51**:525.

Taylor J, Kosowsky B, Lown B: Complications of procainamide in a prospective antiarrhythmic study. *Circulation* 1971;**44**(Suppl 2):43.

Vandepol CJ et al: Incidence and clinical significance of induced ventricular tachycardia. *Am J Cardiol* 1980;**45**:725.

Velebit V et al: Aggravation and provocation of ventricular arrhythmias by antiarrhythmic drugs. *Circulation* 1982; **96**:337.

Waldo AL, Arciniegas JG, Klein H: Surgical treatment of life-threatening ventricular arrhythmias: The role of intraoperative mapping and consideration of the presently available surgical techniques. *Prog Cardiovasc Dis* 1981;**23**:247.

Wellens HJJ: Value and limitations of programmed electrical stimulation of the heart in the study and treatment of tachycardias. *Circulation* 1978;**57**:845.

Wellens HJJ, Brugada P, Stevenson WG: Programmed electrical stimulation of the heart in patients with life-threatening ventricular arrhythmias: What is the signficance of induced arrhythmias and what is the correct stimulation protocol? *Circulation* 1985;**72**:1.

Wellens HJJ, Durrer D: Effect of procainamide, quinidine, and ajmaline in Wolff-Parkinson-White syndrome. *Circulation* 1974;**50**:114.

Wellens HJJ et al: Medical treatment of ventricular tachycardia: Considerations in the selection of patients for surgical treatment. *Am J Cardiol* 1982;**49**:186.

Winkle RA: Ambulatory electrocardiography and the diagnosis, evaluation, and treatment of chronic ventricular arrhythmias. *Prog Cardiovasc Dis* 1980;**23**:99.

Winkle RA, Glantz SA, Harrison DC: Pharmacologic therapy of ventricular arrhythmias. *Am J Cardiol* 1975;**36**:629.

Winkle RA et al: Practical aspects of automatic cardioverter/defibrillator implantation. *Am Heart J* 1984;**108**:1335.

Woosley RL et al: Effects of acetylator phenotype on the rate at which procainamide induces antinuclear antibodies and the lupus syndrome. *N Engl J Med* 1978;**298**:1157.

Zipes DP: A consideration of antiarrhythmic therapy. (Editorial.) *Circulation* 1985;**72**:949.

Zipes DP (guest editor): Symposium on cardiac arrhythmias. (2 parts.) *Med Clin North Am* 1984;**68**:783, 1013. [Entire issues.]

Zipes DP, Troup PJ: New antiarrhythmic agents: Amiodarone, aprindine, disopyramide, ethmozin, mexiletine, tocainide, verapamil. *Am J Cardiol* 1978;**41**:1005.

Zoll PM, Linenthal AJ: Termination of refractory tachycardia by external countershock. *Circulation* 1962;**25**:596.

Ventricular Fibrillation & Sudden Death

Adgey AAJ et al: Management of ventricular fibrillation outside hospital. *Lancet* 1969;**1**:7607.

Chaudron JM et al: Attacks of ventricular fibrillation and unconsciousness in a patient with prolonged QT interval: A family study. *Am Heart J* 1976;**91**:783.

Cobb LA, Werner JA, Trobaugh GB: Sudden cardiac death. 1. A decade's experience with out-of-hospital resuscitation. *Mod Concepts Cardiovasc Dis* 1980;**49**:31.

Cobb LA et al: Resuscitation from out-of-hospital ventricular fibrillation: Four year follow-up. *Circulation* 1975;**52**(**Suppl 3**):223.

Crampton R: Accepted, controversial, and speculative aspects of ventricular fibrillation. *Prog Cardiovasc Dis* 1980; **23**:167.

DeSilva RA et al: Cardioversion and defibrillation. *Am Heart J* 1980;**100**:881.

Echt DS et al: Clinical experience, complications, and survival in 70 patients with the automatic implantable cardioverter/defibrillator. *Circulation* 1985;**71**:289.

Jelinek MV, Lohrbauer L, Lown B: Antiarrhythmic drug therapy for sporadic ventricular ectopic arrhythmias. *Circulation* 1974;**49**:659.

Koch FH, Hancock EW: Ten year follow-up of forty patients with the midsystolic click/late systolic murmur syndrome. *Am J Cardiol* 1976;**37**:149.

Koster RW, Wellens HJJ: Quinidine-induced ventricular flutter and fibrillation without digitalis therapy. *Am J Cardiol* 1976;**38**:519.

Lewis BH, Antman EM, Graboys TB: Detailed analysis of 24-hour ambulatory electrocardiographic recordings during ventricular fibrillation or torsade de pointes. *J Am Coll Cardiol* 1983;**2**:426.

Lie KI et al: Observations on patients with primary ventricular fibrillation complicating acute myocardial infarction. *Circulation* 1975;**52**:755.

Lown B, Verrier RL: Neural activity and ventricular fibrillation. *N Engl J Med* 1976;**294**:1165.

Lown B, Verrier RL, Rabinowitz SH: Neural and psychologic mechanisms and the problem of sudden cardiac death. *Am J Cardiol* 1977;**39**:890.

Mills P et al: Long-term prognosis of mitral-valve prolapse. *N Engl J Med* 1977;**297**:13.

Mirowski M et al: Mortality in patients with implanted automatic defibrillators. Part 1. *Ann Intern Med* 1983;**98**:585.

Myerburg RJ et al: Clinical, electrophysiologic and hemodynamic profile of patients resuscitated from prehospital cardiac arrest. *Am J Med* 1980;**68**:568.

Reid PR et al: Clinical evaluation of the internal automatic cardioverter-defibrillator in survivors of sudden cardiac death. *Am J Cardiol* 1983;**51**:1608.

Schaffer WA, Cobb LA: Recurrent ventricular fibrillation and modes of death in survivors of out-of-hospital ventricular fibrillation. *N Engl J Med* 1975;**293**:259.

Selzer A, Wray HW: Quinidine syncope: Paroxysmal ventricular fibrillation occurring during treatment of chronic atrial arrhythmias. *Circulation* 1964;**30**:17.

Swerdlow CD, Winkle RA, Mason JW: Determinants of survival in patients with ventricular tachyarrhythmias. *N Engl J Med* 1983;**308**:1486.

Yoon MS, Han J, Fabregas RA: Effects of ventricular aberrancy on fibrillation threshold. *Am Heart J* 1975;**89**:599.

Zoll PM: Resuscitation of the heart in ventricular standstill by external electrical stimulation. *N Engl J Med* 1952; **247**:768.

16 Infective Endocarditis

GENERAL CONSIDERATIONS

Infective endocarditis is infection of the endocardium, occurring on valve leaflets, congenital or acquired lesions, a prolapsed mitral valve, arteriovenous fistulas, walls of the heart cavities, or tissue surrounding prosthetic valves. The term "infective endocarditis" is now generally preferred to "bacterial endocarditis," because many different microorganisms other than bacteria (fungi, rickettsiae, viruses, animal parasites) can also cause the disease.

The infection may be acute or subacute (chronic), depending largely on the susceptibility of the host. Subacute disease usually occurs in patients with an underlying cardiac abnormality and has a less traumatic clinical course than acute disease. Acute infection usually occurs in persons with normal hearts following intravenous drug abuse or cardiovascular surgery due to acute development of heart disease. Rapid destruction of valves and a fulminant clinical course follow unless antibiotic therapy is quickly administered.

Infective endocarditis is often an insidious disease not diagnosed during life that tends to occur in patients already acutely or chronically ill from other causes. Early diagnosis and effective antibiotic therapy are vital not only for eradication of infection but also to prevent or minimize damage to heart valves, which becomes more severe the longer infection is uncontrolled. Changing patterns of disease have necessitated changes in treatment regimens.

Complexity of Management

Infective endocarditis is one of the most difficult of all cardiac diseases to manage. Not only is the diagnosis often difficult, but the choice of antibiotic, its route of administration, and the assessment of its effects cause problems. Effective drug treatment requires penetration of the vegetation in order to reach the bacteria in sufficient concentration to kill them. Surgical drainage in addition to antibiotics may be required for metastatic abscesses.

Close observation of the patient during therapy is essential because of the likelihood of development of acute heart failure due to acute valvular damage. Acute cardiac catastrophes, such as dislodgment of valve leaflets or prosthetic valves, perforation of valve cusps, rupture of aneurysms, or abscesses of the myocardium into other cardiac chambers with fistula formation—as well as the ever-present threat of serious systemic embolism—make the management of infective endocarditis a difficult and worrisome task. Since emergency cardiac surgery may become necessary at a few hours' notice, it is an advantage to treat the patient at a center where facilities and personnel for open heart surgery are available. The period during which the patient is at risk is long, because in some cases it is the fibrosis and shrinkage that occur with healing of the endocardial infection that cause or aggravate the valvular incompetence and are responsible for subacute heart failure.

A. Benefits and Complications of Antibiotic Therapy: Before penicillin became available, subacute infective endocarditis was uniformly fatal within months to about 2 years. Acute infective endocarditis was rare, because patients with overwhelming septicemic infections did not live long enough to develop clinical manifestations of cardiac involvement, although vegetations were often seen on the heart valves at autopsy. Penicillin usually eradicated the infection but did not prevent damage to heart valves. Patients with preexisting valvular disease—even minimal disease—were likely to have increased incompetence following treatment for subacute infection. Patients with acute infection were likely to suffer severe valvular incompetence following successful antibiotic therapy, leading to acute heart failure that was often fatal. Thus, prevention of valvular damage and surgical techniques for valvular repair have become almost as important as control of infection.

B. Differentiation of Acute From Subacute Infective Endocarditis: Although acute infective endocarditis is more fulminant and may be caused by organisms which in the past have produced subacute clinical pictures—and although the urgency is greater in the acute forms—the treatment of the 2 conditions is similar. The course of acute infective endocarditis is measured in days or weeks rather than months, as is the case in subacute infective endocarditis. *Staphylococcus aureus* rather than *Streptococcus viridans* is most apt to be the responsible organism, and valve destruction and perforation are more likely to occur quickly, leading to rapidly developing cardiac failure. Prompt treatment with specific anti-infective drugs is essential. Surgical treatment is more often required, because rapid destruction of valves may occur. The prognosis is better in subacute than in acute infective endocarditis, because valve destruction occurs more slowly. Acute infective endocarditis may be overlooked because it frequently occurs on a normal valve, whereas subacute infective endocarditis often occurs on previously damaged valves. Murmurs may be absent at the onset of acute infective endocarditis, but valve lesions may result in gross insufficiency of the involved valve even though the infection is controlled by antibiotic therapy.

PATHOGENESIS & PATHOLOGY

Hosts Likely to Develop Infective Endocarditis

Infective endocarditis most frequently occurs in patients who have undergone cardiac surgery, in those with prosthetic heart valves, in those receiving prolonged intravenous therapy, and in persons who are intravenous drug abusers. It also occurs in patients with atherosclerotic changes, in patients with immunosuppression due to drugs or disease (although endocarditis rarely develops due to immunosuppression alone), and in patients undergoing complex diagnostic or therapeutic procedures (eg, peritoneal dialysis, hemodialysis). The incidence of the disease is increasing owing to increased numbers of people in each of these groups.

A cooperative study of infective endocarditis by the American Heart Association in 1978 indicated that almost one-fourth of patients developed the infection following cardiovascular surgery, usually with insertion of a prosthetic valve or creation of a systemic to pulmonary artery shunt in congenital heart disease. One-fourth of these patients were 20 years of age, and most of this group were heroin addicts. There was no recognizable prior heart disease in a third of the patients. There were recurrent episodes in 10%. Three-fourths of the infected patients were alive 2 years following institution of antibiotic therapy (Kaplan, 1977).

The age distribution is bimodal, with younger individuals most apt to have acute infective endocarditis and older ones subacute endocarditis, probably because of the presence of unoperated rheumatic valvular disease in the older patients. Current data indicate that the median age at onset of the subacute cases is 45 years, that 25% of patients are over 60 years,

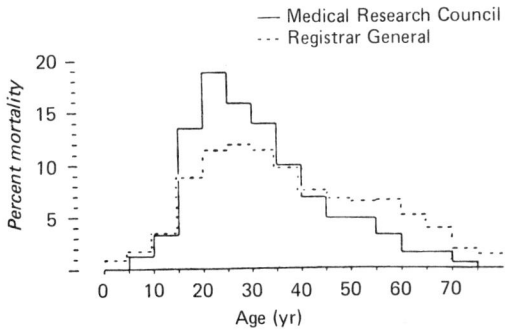

Figure 16–1. The age incidence in 408 cases in the Medical Research Council series, compared with the age incidence in 4531 deaths due to acute or subacute bacterial endocarditis derived from the Registrar General's Reviews 1940–1944. Ages are shown in groups of 5 years. *Note:* The age distribution has undergone a marked shift to the right (toward older patients) in the last 30 years. (Reproduced, with permission, from Cates JE, Christie RV: Subacute bacterial endocarditis. *Q J Med* [New Series] 1951;**20**:93.)

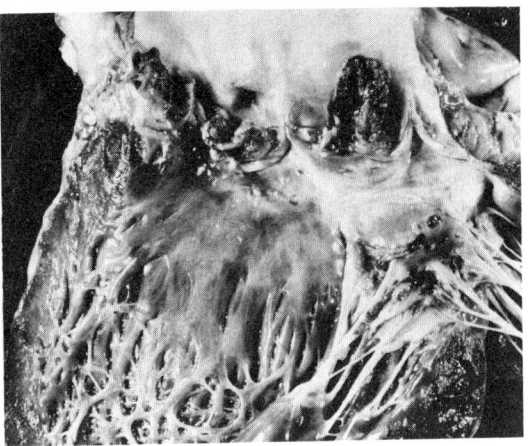

Figure 16–2. Rheumatic aortic valve in a 31-year-old male with *Streptococcus viridans* infection and subacute bacterial endocarditis. (Courtesy of O Rambo.)

and that only 7% are under 20 years of age (Mills, 1974).

Microorganisms Causing Infective Endocarditis

Microorganisms in the bloodstream may be deposited on damaged, roughened valves, such as congenital or rheumatic lesions; the organisms become enmeshed in deposits of fibrin and platelets on the endothelium of the valve to form irregular vegetations. Pathogens may invade the endothelium but are usually relatively superficial. A typical infected rheumatic aortic valve is seen in Fig 16–2. In patients who have died of infective endocarditis, host defenses with antibody formation, local attempts at repair, and local macrophage infiltration can be seen at autopsy but are not adequate to clear the infection.

Widespread, sometimes almost casual use of antibiotics has led to an increase in cases involving drug-resistant microorganisms rarely seen in the past. Fewer cases are now caused by pathogens highly susceptible to antibiotics. In the past, *Streptococcus viridans* and group D streptococci were responsible for 90–95% of cases of subacute infective endocarditis, but these organisms are now responsible for only about one-third of all cases of infective endocarditis. The relative frequency of infection with *Staphylococcus aureus*, *Staphylococcus epidermidis*, *Streptococcus faecalis* (enterococcus), gram-negative organisms both aerobic and anaerobic, and fungi is increasing. Each of these organisms may cause either acute or subacute endocarditis. Infections with certain organisms (eg, *Bacteroides*) are still infrequent, but all rare organisms must now be considered possible causative agents (Wilson, 1977). Subacute infection of chronically diseased rheumatic valves due to *S viridans* is less common now. Infection of calcified valves in elderly patients or in patients with prosthetic valves is seen more frequently.

Vegetations vary in size and may become quite large and friable in fungal infections. They may occur on the downstream side of the damaged valve, and small fragments may break off, causing embolization to the systemic circulation in left-sided mitral or aortic valve lesions and to the lungs in right-sided lesions, usually on the tricuspid valve. Embolism is responsible for many of the clinical features.

A precipitating cause of infection should always be sought. Dental procedures (extraction or deep scaling), recent instrumentation of the genitourinary tract, gynecologic procedures, or inflammatory gastrointestinal disease sometimes precedes the illness. In about half of subacute cases, no cause can be established; fewer cases of acute endocarditis are of unknown cause.

Involvement of Heart Valves

A. Normal Valves: Bacteria and fungi from intravenous injection of infective material (as in "mainline" heroin addicts), from indwelling venous catheters, from infection of arteriovenous shunts, or from bacteria that gain entry during renal dialysis may settle on normal valves. As the infective organisms become embedded in the fibrin-platelet matrix, further growth of organisms enlarges the vegetation and makes the organisms inaccessible to normal cellular host defenses. Massive bacteremia and infection may perforate the leaflets, cause progressive gross incompetence or destruction of the involved valves, and allow rapid development or worsening of cardiac failure.

The tricuspid valve is involved almost exclusively in intravenous drug users. The frequency of left- or right-sided lesions in such patients varies in different cities and institutions.

B. Diseased Valves: Endocarditis is more apt to occur in patients with mild to moderate valvular disease. Pulmonary stenosis, patent ductus arteriosus, ventricular septal defect, and bicuspid aortic valve are the most common congenital cardiac lesions in which endocarditis develops. Infective endocarditis is rare in atrial septal defect (especially in ostium secundum defects) and severe mitral stenosis and infrequent in patients with established atrial fibrillation.

CLINICAL FEATURES

1. SUBACUTE INFECTIVE ENDOCARDITIS

Diagnosis

The onset of endocarditis may be slow and insidious, and unless one searches for infections due to bacteria or fungi in every patient with fever and valvular lesions, the diagnosis can be missed for months. The presenting symptoms are nonspecific and are often attributed to a febrile illness (eg, "flu"), with fever, malaise, arthralgia, fatigue, and anemia. If short-term antibiotic treatment is given, the clinical picture is that of recurrent "flu."

The diagnostic features of endocarditis are given below. If the diagnosis is suspected, blood cultures must be obtained. The diagnosis may be difficult if antibiotics have been given earlier.

A. Fever: Fever is the most frequent presenting sign and may appear without apparent predisposing cause or may follow a surgical procedure. Prostatic and other urogenital operations in men and dilation and curettage of the uterus, abortion, and other gynecologic procedures in women are sometimes precursors of endocarditis. Weakness, malaise, and loss of weight without fever may occur in debilitated or elderly patients, especially if antibiotics have been given or sometimes because of renal failure secondary to endocarditis. The symptoms may be overlooked and the diagnosis made only at autopsy.

B. Emboli: The presenting symptom may be acute systemic embolism (especially to the brain, spleen, or kidney), which may occur at any time during the course of the disease. Emboli are usually small except in fungal or *Serratia* infections and usually produce microscopic hematuria or petechiae. Osler's nodes are painful erythematous nodules on the skin, chiefly of the hands and feet. These cutaneous manifestations are probably caused by minute emboli, or they might be due to an immune mechanism with vasculitis. Nontender nodules on the soles of the feet and the palms of the hands (Janeway's lesion) are probably a deposit of immune complexes with inflammation. Emboli to the systemic circulation are uncommon in right-sided endocarditis; the right-sided manifestations are recurrent pneumonia or pulmonary embolism.

1. Small emboli–In left-sided lesions, emboli to the skin may produce splinter hemorrhages in the nails of the fingers or toes (but these may occur in persons doing manual labor). Petechiae (usually on the conjunctiva or hard palate or around the neck and upper trunk) are more definite evidence of embolism. At first they are red and small, but over a period of days they become brown and gradually fade. Hemorrhagic areas with white centers may be seen in the fundi owing to emboli in the nerve fiber retinal layer (Roth spots). Emboli to the kidney may cause flank pain or hematuria.

2. Large emboli–Large emboli may involve (1) the cerebral arteries, causing hemiplegia, other central nervous system deficit, neurologic syndromes including headache, psychiatric symptoms, confusion, or sterile meningitis; (2) the coronary arteries, resulting in acute myocardial infarction; or (3) the vasa vasorum, leading to mycotic aneurysms. Mycotic aneurysms may appear anywhere, often in branches of the renal artery. Rupture is infrequent, and these lesions are often missed.

C. Septic Abscesses: If staphylococci are the infecting organisms in either acute or subacute cases, septic abscesses may develop, especially in the liver, heart, kidney, brain, and spleen. Septic abscesses may contribute to continued fever and require surgical incision even though the organisms on the endocardium of the valves have been eradicated.

D. Splenomegaly and Clubbed Fingers: These are usually late signs in untreated patients and, although they were common in the preantibiotic era, are much less common today (approximately 10% of cases). As in any systemic infection, splenomegaly may occur, although it is less frequent when antibiotic therapy is given early in the course of the disease.

E. Immune Complex Nephritis and Renal Emboli: Glomerulonephritis and renal failure frequently occur in infective endocarditis and were formerly thought to be embolic in origin. However, most renal lesions are due to the deposit of antigen-antibody complexes and complement on the glomerular basement membrane. The antigen in glomerular deposits corresponds to the organism found in blood cultures.

F. Anemia: Normocytic anemia is common, especially in long-standing infection, and probably accounts in part for the weakness and lassitude seen in patients with chronic infective endocarditis.

G. Cardiac Findings: Symptoms of heart disease such as dyspnea or palpitations develop late in subacute (in contrast to acute) infective endocarditis, and the cardiac origin of the illness may only be suspected if a valvular lesion or murmurs are present or if embolic manifestations appear. Left heart failure is the rule in subacute cases, because right-sided valvular lesions are infrequent, in contrast to acute endocarditis (see below).

In subacute infective endocarditis, a murmur is almost always present, indicating previous valve involvement of rheumatic or congenital origin. The valve involvement is usually mild, and patients may not know they have a cardiac lesion. Careful search for such a lesion is mandatory in suspicious cases, and subacute endocarditis is an important cause of fever of unknown origin in patients in whom cardiac disease is overlooked.

Disease has now been found to affect certain lesions that were not considered to be possible sites of infective endocarditis. These include prolapsed mitral valve (systolic click-murmur syndrome) and fibrosis and calcification of the mitral and aortic valves. Prolapse of the mitral valve can often be demonstrated by echocardiography (see Chapter 12) or angiography. Echocardiography may also be helpful in recognizing vegetations on the aortic valve, especially if they are large (> 5 mm), as in fungal infections (Fig 16–3). Echocardiography is less helpful when endocarditis involves the mitral valve.

Changing murmurs are rarely helpful in the diagnosis of subacute infective endocarditis, because the murmurs are often due in large part to anemia, tachycardia, or other hemodynamic variables. The abrupt appearance of a diastolic murmur, such as that of aortic insufficiency, is more helpful in diagnosis of acute infective endocarditis (see below).

Cardiac failure formerly was a late occurrence, as was the development of atrial fibrillation. Untreated patients often died of infection before cardiac failure could develop. In subacute cases, cardiac failure may not occur until months after bacteriologic cure, as

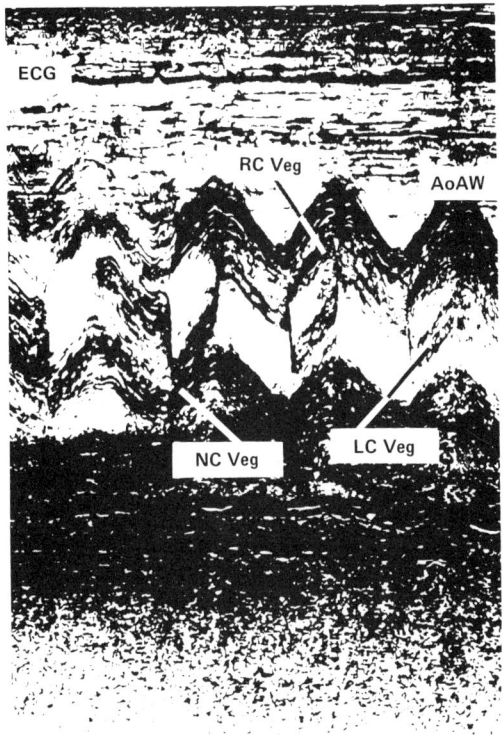

Figure 16–3. Echocardiogram shows dense posteriorly moving echoes indicating aortic valve vegetations in a patient with aortic valve endocarditis. NC, noncoronary cusp; LC, left coronary cusp; RC, right coronary cusp; AoAW, anterior aortic wall; Veg, vegetation. (Reproduced, with permission, from the American Heart Association, Inc., Hirschfeld DS, Schiller N: Localization of aortic valve vegetations by echocardiography. *Circulation* 1976;**53**:280.)

infection heals and valve lesions worsen (especially aortic valve lesions). Pericarditis is infrequent.

Laboratory Findings: Blood Cultures

In 80–90% of cases, definitive diagnosis is based on positive blood culture. Organisms are discharged into the circulation independently of the time of the fever.

Important principles regarding blood cultures for investigation of infective endocarditis are as follows:

(1) For subacute cases, 2 separate cultures should be obtained daily for 2–3 days. For acute cases, 2–3 cultures are obtained during the several hours of initial clinical workup.

(2) Both aerobic and anaerobic bacteria and fungi should be sought with appropriate techniques.

(3) The cultures must be incubated long enough (1–3 weeks) to allow slow-growing organisms to emerge, and appropriate subcultures must be performed. Venous blood is adequate.

(4) At least 2 cultures should yield the same organism to rule out contamination.

(5) Blood cultures must be obtained before anti-

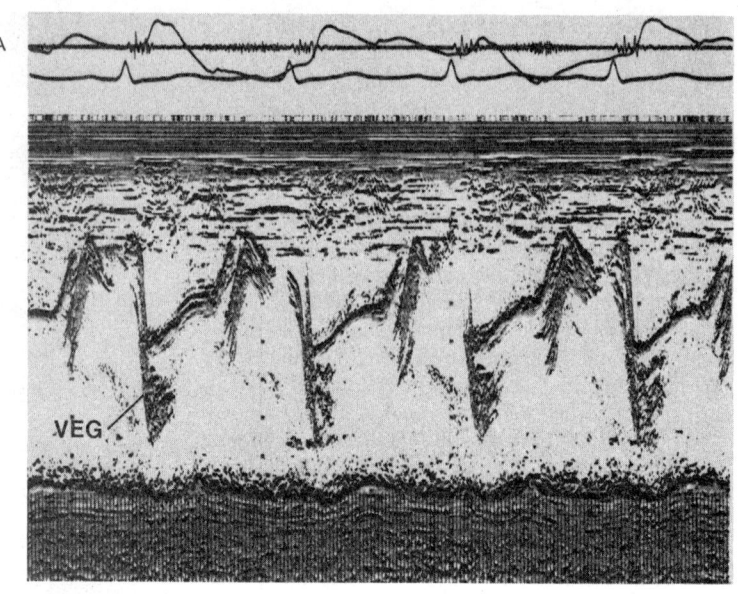
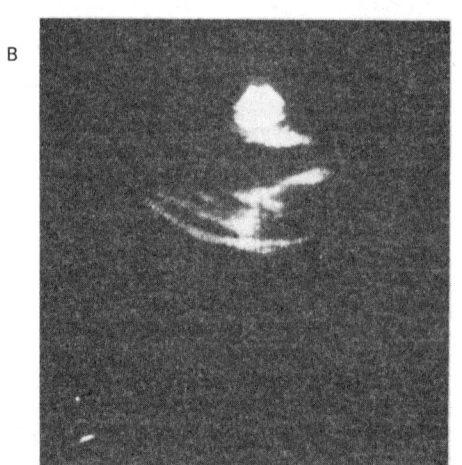
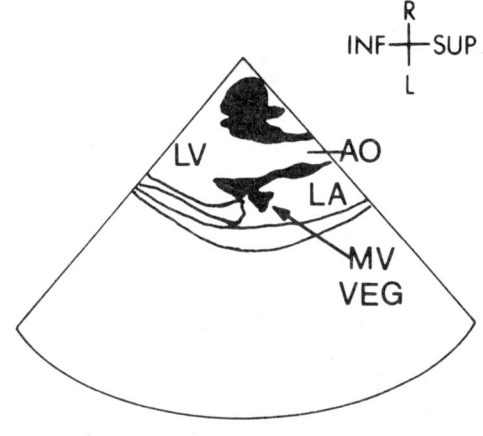
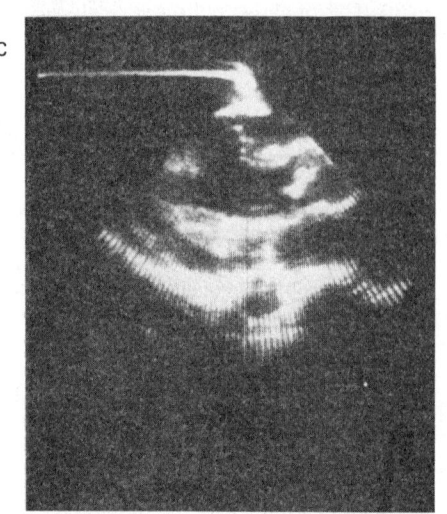
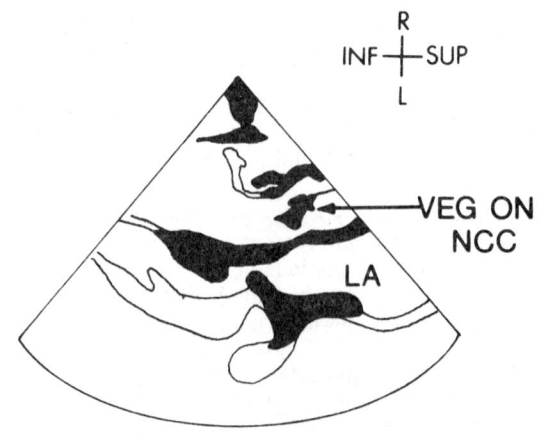

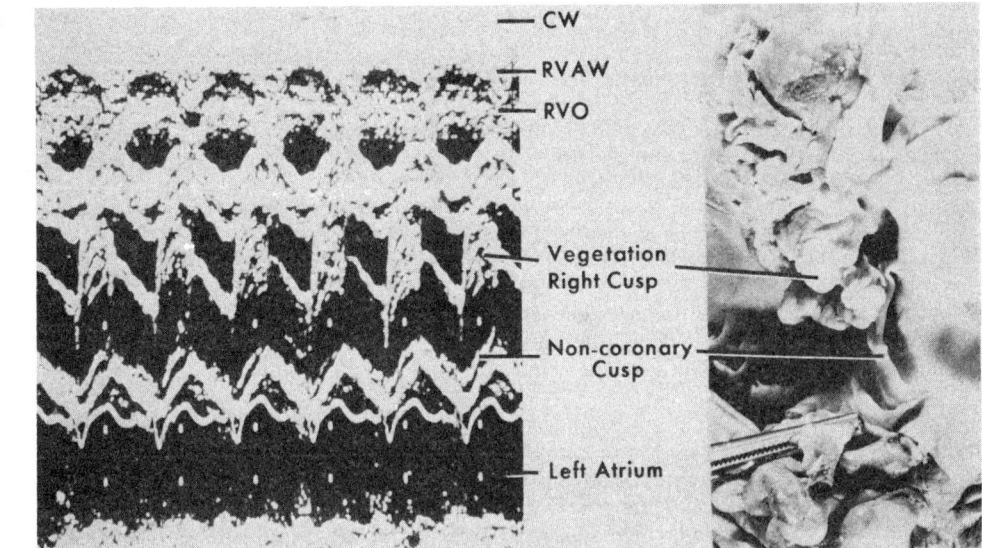

Figure 16–4 (at left and above). *A:* Dense echoes below the tricuspid valve in a patient with acute endocarditis of the tricuspid valve. M mode echocardiogram. VEG, vegetation. (Courtesy of NB Schiller.) *B:* Vegetation (VEG) on the mitral valve (MV). Real-time 2-dimensional echocardiogram. LV, left ventricle; AO, aorta; LA, left atrium. (Courtesy of NB Schiller and NH Silverman.) *C:* Vegetation (VEG) on the aortic valve. NCC, noncoronary cusp; LA, left atrium. Real-time 2-dimensional echocardiogram. (Courtesy of NB Schiller and NH Silverman.) *D:* Vegetation on the aortic valve shown with anatomic lesion at autopsy. M mode echocardiogram. CW, chest wall; RVAW, right ventricular anterior wall; RVO, right ventricular outflow tract. (Reproduced, with permission, from the American Heart Association, Inc., Hirschfeld DS, Schiller N: Localization of aortic valve vegetations by echocardiography. *Circulation* 1976;**53**:280.)

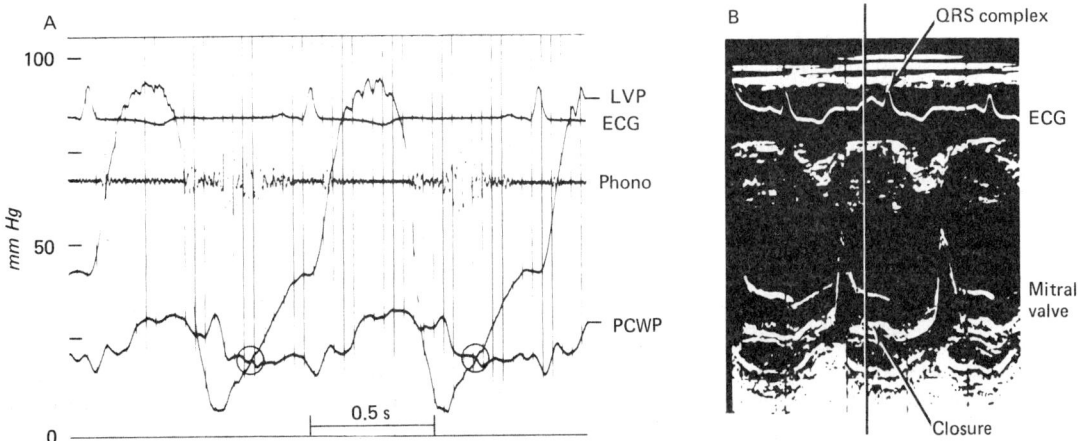

Figure 16–5. *A:* Early closure of the mitral valve. Simultaneous ECG, left ventricular pressure (LVP) and pulmonary capillary wedge pressure (PCWP), and phonocardiogram. Mitral valve closure (circled) occurs when LVP exceeds PCWP, clearly preceding electrocardiographic QRS complex. Phonocardiogram obtained at the cardiac apex demonstrates a middiastolic Austin Flint murmur. (Adapted and reproduced, with permission, from the American Heart Association, Inc., Botvinick EH et al: Echocardiographic demonstration of early mitral valve closure in severe aortic insufficiency: Its clinical implications. *Circulation* 1975;**51**:836.) *B:* Echocardiogram showing mitral valve closure (line) preceding the QRS complex. (Courtesy of NB Schiller.)

biotics are started. Alternatively, antimicrobials should be stopped for 3–7 days before blood is drawn for cultures.

(6) If cultures are positive, the sensitivity of the organism to various antibiotics, singly and in combination, should be determined as a guide to treatment (see below). Bactericidal effects are essential.

2. ACUTE INFECTIVE ENDOCARDITIS

This section emphasizes the differences between acute and subacute endocarditis, including the causative organisms, the involved valves, and the hemodynamic effects.

Diagnosis

The infection is apt to be more abrupt, with higher fever, chills, and the presence of septic abscesses, because the predominant organism is often *S aureus*. The symptoms of infection usually predominate, and organisms are more easily cultured and identified than in subacute cases. When the lesion is on the tricuspid valve, however (as is commonly the case), pulmonary complications of "pneumonia," pulmonary embolism, and pulmonary abscess are dominant. X-rays of the chest reveal pleural effusions and changing pulmonary infiltrates of variable size and shape that may recur. The major postmortem lesions in patients with *S aureus* endocarditis are listed in Table 16–1. There are geographic differences with respect to both the infecting organisms and the valves involved.

A. Emboli: In fungal endocarditis, emboli are more frequent and can be large and disabling. Cerebral embolism may produce hemiplegia, and the possibility of endocarditis must always be considered in patients who develop acute stroke. The lower frequency of systemic embolism in acute infective endocarditis is due to the frequency of right-sided lesions as well as to the rapid downhill course.

B. Cardiac Findings:

1. Changing murmurs and valve findings–The frequency with which acute infective endocarditis occurs on normal cardiac valves makes serial examination more important than in subacute endocarditis. The development of murmurs and evidence of valvular involvement may be noted if the patient is under close observation as the vegetations become larger. This is especially true of tricuspid insufficiency in heroin addicts. The progressive appearance and lengthening of a tricuspid systolic murmur can be noted and are made worse by inspiration as right atrial inflow increases with inspiration. A right-sided gallop rhythm may appear, as may the progressive development of a prominent *v* wave in the jugular venous pulse and enlargement of a tender, pulsating liver, with right-sided failure. Valvular vegetations can be demonstrated by echocardiography (Fig 16–4). When acute infective endocarditis involves the aortic valve, the diastolic murmur may be long and soft and the first sound may be soft because of early closure of

Table 16–1. Major postmortem lesions in 39 patients with *Staphylococcus aureus* endocarditis.*

Lesions	Patients Number	Percent
Myocardial abscesses	14	36
Purulent pericarditis	4	10
Pneumonia, lung abscesses, septic infarcts	19	49
Renal abscesses, septic infarcts, nephritis	22	56
Brain abscesses, septic emboli, or infarcts	11	28
With meningitis	6	
Without meningitis	5	
Meningitis	11	28
Without brain involvement	5	
With brain lesions	6	

*Reproduced, with permission, from Watanakunakorn C, Tan JS, Phair JP: Some salient features of *Staphylococcus aureus* endocarditis. *Am J Med* 1973;54:473.

the mitral valve (see below). The diastolic pressure may be maintained by reflex peripheral arteriolar vasoconstriction, and early mitral valve closure may be a sign of increasing aortic insufficiency. As the magnitude of the aortic regurgitant flow increases, there is a rapid early diastolic rise in left ventricular pressure and left atrial pressure before the onset of systole, causing a prominent Austin Flint diastolic murmur (see Chapter 13). If hemodynamic measurements are made, the crossover of left ventricular end-diastolic pressure and left atrial pressure precedes the Q wave of the ECG instead of slightly following it at the peak or downstroke of the R wave. Early closure of the mitral valve can be clearly demonstrated on echocardiography, when the anterior and posterior leaflets approximate each other well before the onset of the Q wave of the ECG with a normal PR interval (Fig 16–5). This ominous sign is a harbinger of severe left ventricular failure. The magnitude of the acute aortic insufficiency can also be shown by supra-aortic cineangiography, which shows the left ventricle fully opacified in a single beat of the regurgitant flow.

2. Cardiac failure–Cardiac failure is the most feared complication of acute infective endocarditis and may occur with startling rapidity in left-sided lesions, whether mitral or aortic. One cannot use the width of the pulse pressure, the loudness of the murmur, or the size of the left ventricle as a guide to the severity or imminence of left ventricular failure. The left ventricle is often only slightly enlarged, and the ECG may not reveal left ventricular hypertrophy in acute as compared to chronic aortic insufficiency because of the rapid development of aortic or mitral insufficiency (see Chapter 13). Symptoms of pulmonary edema and echocardiographic evidence of marked early closure of a mitral valve lead the physician to suspect perforation or destruction of the aortic valve and indicate the need for valve replacement. Vigorous medical treatment may be needed while the infection subsides so that the sutures will hold, but at times the situation is so urgent that a prosthetic valve must be inserted within days. Careful judgment is required to determine the timing of operation if cardiac failure worsens despite control of the infection.

3. Ventricular septum and muscle involvement–The infection on the aortic valve may spread to the ventricular septum, and abscesses may develop and rupture into the right heart or may interfere with conduction of the cardiac impulse and cause atrioventricular block with or without syncope. Septic abscesses can be suspected if there is sudden development of atrioventricular block or hemiblock. Mitral valve infections may cause septic abscesses of the papillary muscles or destruction of the mitral ring, resulting in flail mitral valves that require prompt surgical correction.

DIFFERENTIAL DIAGNOSIS

Infective endocarditis must be differentiated from all other causes of prolonged and obscure fever. The diagnosis is based on a positive blood culture in conjunction with the presence of a valve lesion and the absence of diagnostic signs or tests supporting an alternative diagnosis. Infection, neoplasm, and connective tissue disorders are the most common causes of fever of unknown origin (40%, 20%, and 20%, respectively), and these must be excluded.

The major difficulty in diagnosis occurs when blood cultures are negative, which means that reliance must be placed on associated diagnostic features. This emphasizes the importance of optimally obtained and examined blood cultures.

(1) Bacteremia may be due to pneumonia, septic thrombophlebitis, meningitis, cellulitis, or infected fistulas. There must be evidence of valve lesions as well as emboli before septicemia can be considered to have originated in the heart. Miliary tuberculosis must be kept in mind and serial chest x-rays obtained.

(2) Acute rheumatic fever occasionally is confusing, but only if blood cultures are negative. In acute rheumatic fever, the arthralgia or arthritis responds rapidly to salicylates, and there may be erythema marginatum, chorea, or previous beta-streptococcal infection which can be documented by increasing antistreptolysin O titers in the serum.

(3) Neoplasm can be diagnosed by appropriate measures or by biopsy of lymph nodes or bone marrow. If atrial myxoma is suspected, echocardiography and angiography can be diagnostic. (See Chapter 21 for discussion of atrial myxoma.)

(4) Connective tissue disorders must be suspected and diagnosed on the basis of skin or renal lesions, a positive LE cell preparation or antinuclear antibody test, renal biopsy, and negative blood cultures.

PREVENTION OF BACTERIAL ENDOCARDITIS

The American Heart Association has recommended chemoprophylaxis when bacteremia is likely, as with dental extraction or deep scaling, genitourinary instrumentation, and similar procedures (see below). Some dentists believe that prophylaxis is futile, because vigorous chewing may also produce transient bacteremia, and continuous prophylaxis to prevent infective endocarditis is ineffective or unreasonable.

Prevention of acute endocarditis involves prevention or early treatment of all causes of bacteremia; social and educational programs for control of "mainline" drug abuse; and early recognition of systemic infection in the compromised host.

Prevention of Bacterial Endocarditis

The following recommendations are taken from A Statement for Health Professionals by the Committee on Rheumatic Fever and Infective Endocarditis of the Council on Cardiovascular Disease in the Young and are published by permission of the American Heart Association, Inc (Shulman, 1984).*†

A. Standard Regimen: Oral penicillin for adults and children over 60 lb: penicillin V, 2 g 1 hour prior to the procedure and then 1 g 6 hours later. For children less than 60 lb: 1 g 1 hour prior to the procedure and then 500 mg 6 hours later.

For persons unable to take oral antibiotics, give 2 million units of aqueous penicillin G (50,000 units/kg for children) intravenously or intramuscularly 30–60 minutes prior to the procedure and 1 million units (25,000 units/kg for children) 6 hours later. Children's antibiotic doses should not exceed the maximum adult dose.

B. For Patients With Prosthetic Valves and Others With Highest Risk of Endocarditis: Ampicillin, 1–2 g (50 mg/kg for children), *plus* gentamicin 1.5 mg/kg (2 mg/kg for children), both intramuscularly or intravenously one-half hour prior to the procedure, followed by 1 g of oral penicillin V 6 hours later; or administer the parenteral regimen once 8 hours later.

C. Standard Regimen for Patients Allergic to Penicillin: Erythromycin, 1 g orally (20 mg/kg for children) 1 hour prior to the procedure, and then 500 mg (10 mg/kg for children) 6 hours later.

For patients unable to tolerate either penicillin or erythromycin, an oral cephalosporin (1 g 1 hour prior to the procedure plus 500 mg 6 hours later) may be useful, but complete data are lacking.

D. Regimen for High-Risk Patients Allergic to Penicillin: Vancomycin, 1 g (20 mg/kg for children) intravenously slowly over 1 hour starting 1 hour prior

---

*Pediatric doses: Ampicillin, 50 mg/kg/dose; gentamicin, 2 mg/kg/dose; amoxicillin, 50 mg/kg/dose; vancomycin, 20 mg/kg/dose. The intervals between doses are the same as for adults. Total doses should not exceed adult doses.

†Modified slightly from Shulman ST (chairman) et al: Prevention of bacterial endocarditis: A statement for health professionals by the Committee on Rheumatic Fever and Infective Endocarditis of the Council on Cardiovascular Disease in the Young. (Special report.) *Circulation* 1984;**70:**1123A.

to the procedure. A repeat dose is usually not necessary except in the case of delayed healing.

Antibiotic Regimens for Genitourinary & Gastrointestinal Tract Surgery & Instrumentation (Shulman, 1984)

A. Standard Regimen: Ampicillin, 2 g (50 mg/kg for children) intramuscularly or intravenously, plus gentamicin, 1.5 mg/kg intramuscularly or intravenously. Children may receive 2 mg/kg. The dose should be given one-half hour prior to the procedure and repeated 8 hours later.

B. For Patients Allergic to Penicillin: Vancomycin, 1 g for adults (20 mg/kg up to 1 g for children) given intravenously slowly over 1 hour, *plus* gentamicin, 1.5 mg/kg intramuscularly or intravenously (2 mg/kg for children) 1 hour prior to the procedure. These doses may be repeated once 8–12 hours later.

C. Oral Regimen for Minor or Repetitive Procedures in Low-Risk Patients: Amoxicillin, 3 g (50 mg/kg for children) orally 1 hour before the procedure and 1.5 g (25 mg/kg for children) 6 hours later. Modify the second dose in patients with compromised renal function.

TREATMENT OF INFECTIVE ENDOCARDITIS

General Principles

The cardinal principles of treatment of infective endocarditis are (1) to isolate the infecting organism by obtaining at least 2 positive blood cultures; (2) to determine susceptibility of the organism to various antibiotics, alone and in combination; (3) to choose antimicrobial therapy that is bactericidal and not merely bacteriostatic; and (4) to continue therapy long enough to totally eradicate the infection. If septic abscesses are present and do not respond to appropriate antibiotic therapy given long enough, surgical drainage is required if technically feasible. If severe valvular insufficiency develops, along with symptoms of progressive cardiac failure, surgical excision of the involved valve and insertion of a prosthesis must be undertaken with proper timing. The results are less good with tricuspid prostheses than with mitral or aortic ones.

A. Choice of Antibiotic: The choice of antibiotic is based on experience, the results of laboratory sensitivity tests, the status of renal function, and the presence or absence of allergic hypersensitivity to any particular antibiotic, eg, penicillin. Prior to the identification of the infecting organism, antibiotic therapy should be given intravenously in acutely ill patients, using a combination of antibiotics that appear most appropriate on the basis of experience and knowledge of the organisms usually responsible for acute endocarditis. (See also p 523 for discussion of the "best guess" approach.)

The least toxic but most effective antibiotics, such as the penicillins, are preferable; tetracyclines, erythromycins, lincomycins, and chloramphenicol generally cannot eradicate the infection even if the organism appears to be susceptible in vitro. Aminoglycosides are rarely single drugs of choice but occasionally participate in synergistic drug combinations that provide optimal bacterial action. The objective should be total eradication of the infection. One should choose a regimen shown by experience to result in the highest percentage of cures rather than one which may be more convenient to use or require a shorter course of therapy but has a lower percentage of cures. For example, an infection with *S viridans*, which usually is very sensitive to penicillin, might be cured with 2 weeks of oral therapy, but the likelihood of cure is much greater if one gives the drug parenterally for 3–4 weeks (Kaye, 1980).

Eradication of infection is almost always possible with one drug or a combination of drugs. Deaths are usually due to delayed or inadequate treatment, exotic organisms, septic abscesses, perforation of mycotic aneurysms, or destruction of valves, requiring surgery.

B. Steps in Management:

1. Obtain positive blood culture–For subacute endocarditis, it is best to try to withhold therapy until a positive blood culture is obtained, so that therapy can be specific. Any complications that occur within a few days before the report of the blood culture are apt to be embolic and probably will not be influenced by immediate therapy. Drugs can therefore be withheld unless the patient has acute endocarditis, in which case therapy is directed to the most common pathogens, *S aureus* and gram-negative organisms, until the reports of the blood culture permit change of therapy.

2. Parenteral therapy–The antimicrobial agent is best injected as a bolus over a 20-minute period (by Volutrol) into the tubing of a continuous intravenous infusion of 5% dextrose and water. Injections should be given every 4–6 hours to avoid deterioration of the antibiotic as well as irritation of the venous endothelium. Some drugs (eg, vancomycin) cause severe pain if given intramuscularly or if extravasation outside the vein occurs. Patients receiving therapy over a period of 4–6 weeks usually tolerate a slow intravenous drip of glucose and water and intermittent injection of a bolus of antibiotic. The patient can be ambulatory (in the hospital).

3. Duration of therapy–The duration of therapy has always been in some dispute. In general, infection with organisms such as sensitive *S viridans* can be cured in 3–4 weeks, whereas infections with *S aureus* require 5–6 weeks of therapy. The aim of treatment is to cure as many infections as possible, and it is advisable to err on the side of overtreating rather than risk the dangers of stopping too soon and allowing the infection to regain a foothold. Organisms that are more difficult to eradicate, such as *Candida* or *Pseudomonas*, may require early surgical excision of the involved valve because drug therapy alone is relatively ineffective.

4. Testing for bactericidal activity–When antimicrobial agents are used singly or in combination (Fig 16–6), it is wise to determine if bactericidal con-

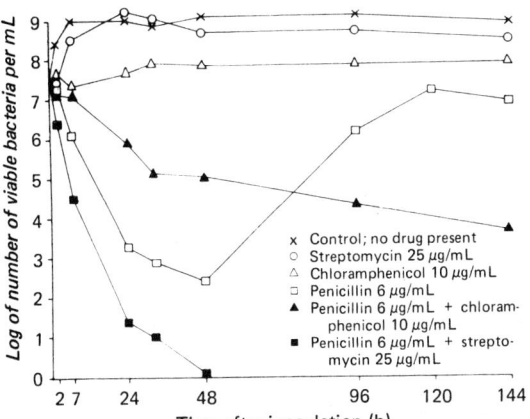

Figure 16-6. The effects of penicillin (6 μg/mL), chloramphenicol (10 μg/mL), and streptomycin (25 μg/mL), singly and in combination, on a strain of *Streptococcus faecalis* in vitro. The synergistic effect of combined therapy is obvious from the increased bactericidal effect of the combined penicillin and streptomycin (indicated by the dark squares). (Reproduced, with permission, from Jawetz E: Synergism and antagonism among antimicrobial drugs: A personal perspective. *West J Med* 1975;**123**:87.)

centrations have been achieved by determining the level of serum dilution that is bactericidal for the infecting organism 2 hours after the last dose of the antibiotic. It is believed that a dilution of at least 1:8 is desirable in order to assure a satisfactory result. Patients may continue to have occasional fever or embolic phenomena, yet the antibiotic program may be completely effective. Knowing that the serum dilution of 1:8 or higher is bactericidal for the organism gives the physician the confidence to continue the antibiotic regimen without changing drugs. Bacteriostatic drugs have not been successful in eradicating endocarditis. Once a course of treatment has been chosen on the basis of all the evidence, it should not be changed without a good reason.

Table 16–2 shows drug selections for various organisms and Table 16–3 their dosage when renal failure is present.

5. Observations during the course of treatment–If a satisfactory antimicrobial regimen has been selected, patients usually begin to feel well within a few days even though occasional fever or embolic phenomena may occur. A negative blood culture and serum bactericidal activity in adequate dilution (≥ 1:8) are important prognostic features. If the patient continues to have fever, especially with chills, after the start of a regimen that should be effective, the possibility of septic abscesses should be considered; radioactive isotope scans of the liver, kidney, and spleen may be helpful. Drug fever is another possibility.

a. Daily examination–The patient should be examined daily for the appearance of new murmurs, evidence of cardiac enlargement or cardiac failure, and evidence of embolic manifestations. The development of pain and friction rub in the left upper quadrant suggests an embolus to the spleen. Pain in the flank associated with hematuria suggests an embolus to the kidney. If aminoglycosides are used, hearing should be checked intermittently by audiometer. If the patient develops central nervous system symptoms with headache and somnolence, the possibility of brain abscess or mycotic aneurysm of a cerebral artery should be considered; if the symptoms are severe and progressive, cerebral angiography or CT scan should be performed with a view toward localizing an aneurysm whose rupture is imminent.

b. Check laboratory work–Renal function should be monitored frequently, because it may deteriorate either as a result of renal emboli or because of drug toxicity. The drug regimen should be adjusted to take account of renal failure (Table 16–3). Frequent blood counts should be performed to note the development of progressive anemia or a marked elevation of the white count that might suggest septic abscess. Frequent ECGs are desirable to detect intraventricular conduction defects or atrioventricular block suggesting abscess of the ventricular septum.

Course of the Disease

A. Valvular Changes:

1. Aortic insufficiency–If endocarditis involves the aortic valve, attention must be paid to signs suggesting worsening of aortic insufficiency. Frequent examination is required to measure diastolic blood pressure, to note the duration of the diastolic murmur, and to assess the possibility of early mitral valve closure and progressive enlargement of the heart or signs of left ventricular failure (eg, frank pulmonary edema or episodic dyspnea). Many of these patients are young adults with no previous valvular disease.

2. Mitral insufficiency–Progressive enlargement of the left atrium as shown by echocardiographic or radiologic examination, as well as progressive enlargement of the left ventricle, may signify serious dysfunction of the mitral valve (see Chapter 12).

3. Tricuspid insufficiency–In acute endocarditis involving the tricuspid valve, the patient should be examined daily for the appearance of signs of tricuspid insufficiency (see Diagnosis, above). (See also Fig 16–4A.)

B. Heart Failure: Progressive destruction of any of the valves associated with either left or right ventricular failure should force serious consideration of cardiac surgery, because many of these patients have perforation of the valve leaflets, septal abscess, or rupture of a mycotic aneurysm from the aortic sinus (sinus of Valsalva) into the right heart, and they can be helped by surgical repair. When heart failure occurs in a patient in whom the infection has not been controlled, a serious dilemma arises; surgery should be considered any time that an optimal anti-infectious program is under way and cardiac failure cannot be controlled medically.

Table 16–2. Anti-infective chemotherapeutic agents against suspected or proved causes of infective endocarditis.*

Suspected or Proved Etiologic Agent	Drug(s) of First Choice	Alternative Drug(s)
Gram-negative cocci		
Gonococcus	Penicillin,[1] ampicillin, tetracycline[2]	Spectinomycin, cefoxitin
Gram-positive cocci		
Pneumococcus *(Streptococcus pneumoniae)*	Penicillin[1]	Erythromycin,[3] cephalosporin[4]
Streptococcus, hemolytic groups A, B, C, G	Penicillin[1]	Erythromycin,[3] cephalosporin[4]
Streptococcus viridans	Penicillin[1] plus aminoglycoside (?)[5]	Cephalosporin,[4] vancomycin
Staphylococcus, nonpenicillinase-producing	Penicillin[1]	Cephalosporin,[4] vancomycin
Staphylococcus, penicillinase-producing	Penicillinase-resistant penicillin[6]	Vancomycin, cephalosporin[4]
Streptococcus faecalis (enterococcus)	Ampicillin plus aminoglycoside[5]	Vancomycin
Gram-negative rods		
Bacteroides (except *Bacteroides fragilis*)	Penicillin[1] or chloramphenicol	Clindamycin, cephalosporin[4]
Enterobacter	Aminoglycoside,[5] new cephalosporin[8]	Chloramphenicol
Escherichia coli sepsis	Aminoglycoside[5]	New cephalosporin,[8] ampicillin
Haemophilus (meningitis, respiratory infections)	Chloramphenicol plus ampicillin	New cephalosporin[8]
Klebsiella	New cephalosporin[8] or aminoglycoside[5]	Chloramphenicol
Proteus		
Proteus mirabilis	Ampicillin	New cephalosporin,[8] aminoglycoside[5]
Proteus vulgaris and other species	Aminoglycoside[5]	Chloramphenicol
Pseudomonas aeruginosa	Aminoglycoside[5] plus ticarcillin, piperacillin, or azlocillin	New cephalosporin,[8] polymyxin
Serratia, Providencia	Aminoglycoside[5]	TMP-SMX[7] plus polymyxin
Gram-positive rods		
Listeria	Ampicillin plus aminoglycoside[5]	Tetracycline[2]
Acid-fast rods		
Nocardia	Sulfonamide	Minocycline
Rickettsiae	Tetracycline[2]	Chloramphenicol

*Modified and reproduced, with permission, from Jawetz E: Anti-infective chemotherapeutic and antibiotic agents. Chapter 28 in: *Current Medical Diagnosis & Treatment 1986.* Krupp MA, Chatton MJ, Tierney LM Jr (editors). Lange, 1986.
[1] Penicillin G is preferred for parenteral injection; penicillin V for oral administration. Only highly sensitive microorganisms should be treated with oral penicillin.
[2] All tetracyclines have similar activity against microorganisms and comparable therapeutic activity and toxicity. Dosage is determined by the rates of absorption and excretion of different preparations.
[3] Erythromycin estolate is the best-absorbed oral form but carries greatest risk of hepatitis.
[4] Cefazolin, cephapirin, cephalothin, and cefoxitin are parenteral cephalosporins; cephalexin or cephradine the best oral forms.
[5] Aminoglycoside: Gentamicin, tobramycin, amikacin, netilmicin, selected by local pattern of susceptibility.
[6] Parenteral nafcillin or oxacillin. Oral dicloxacillin, cloxacillin, or oxacillin.
[7] TMP-SMX is a mixture of 1 part trimethoprim plus 5 parts sulfamethoxazole.
[8] New cephalosporins (1984–1985): Cefotaxime, moxalactam, cefoperazone, cefuroxime, ceftizoxime, etc.

Specific Antimicrobial Regimens*

A. Subacute Endocarditis Due to *Streptococcus viridans*: Viridans streptococci (usually originating in the oropharynx) are the infecting organism in more than 60% of spontaneously arising cases of typical slow-onset endocarditis. A majority of such organisms are susceptible to 0.1–1 unit/mL penicillin G in vitro. Penicillin G, 5–10 million units daily (in divided doses given as a bolus every 4 hours in an intravenous infusion of 5% dextrose in water), continued for 3–4 weeks, is generally curative. Enhanced bactericidal action is obtained if an aminoglycoside (eg, gentamicin, 3–5 mg/kg/d intramuscularly) is added during the first 10–14 days of treatment. More resistant organisms may require daily doses of penicillin G of 20–50 million units. Probenecid, 0.5 g 3 times daily orally, further enhances blood levels of penicillin by interfering with its tubular excretion.

*With the assistance of Dr Ernest Jawetz.

Because of the risk of new infection with local organisms, the catheter site must be cleaned carefully and changed every 2 days during prolonged intravenous infusions. To avoid phlebitis, the daily dose should be divided and given at the appropriate intervals by intermittent injection over a half-hour period in a continuous infusion of 5% glucose in water. The potassium content of potassium penicillin G (1.7 meq/million units) must be kept in mind if renal impairment is present.

B. Endocarditis Due to *Streptococcus faecalis*: This organism causes about 5–10% of cases of spontaneously occurring endocarditis and occasionally also follows abuse of intravenous drugs. Treatment is with penicillin plus an aminoglycoside. Penicillin G, 20–40 million units daily, or ampicillin, 6–12 g daily, is given in divided doses as bolus injections every 2–3 hours in an intravenous infusion of 5% dextrose in water. An aminoglycoside (kanamycin, 15 mg/kg/d; gentamicin, 5 mg/kg/d) selected by

Table 16-3. Half-life in serum and proposed dosage regimen for various antibiotics used in renal failure.*

	Principal Mode of Excretion or Detoxification	Approximate Half-Life in Serum		Proposed Dosage Regimen in Renal Failure		Significant Removal of Drug by Dialysis (H = Hemodialysis; P = Peritoneal Dialysis)
		Normal	Renal Failure†	Initial Dose‡	Give Half of Initial Dose at Interval of	
Penicillin G	Tubular secretion	0.5 h	6 h	4 g IV	8–12 h	H, P no
Ampicillin	Tubular secretion	1 h	8 h	6 g IV	8–12 h	H yes, P no
Carbenicillin, ticarcillin	Tubular secretion	1.5 h	16 h	3–4 g IV	12–18 h	H, P yes
Nafcillin	Liver 80%, kidney 20%	0.5 h	2 h	2 g IV	4–6 h	H, P no
Cephalothin	Tubular secretion	0.8 h	8 h	4 g IV	18 h	H, P yes
Cephalexin, cephradine	Tubular secretion and glomerular filtration	2 h	15 h	2 g orally	8–12 h	H, P yes
Cefazolin	Kidney	2 h	30 h	2 g IM, IV	24 h	H yes, P no
Cefoxitin, cefamandole	Tubular secretion and glomerular filtration	1–1.5 h	16–20 h	2 g IV	12–18 h	H, P yes
Cefotaxime, moxalactam	Tubular secretion and liver	1–2 h	20–30 h	2 g IV	24 h	H, P yes
Amikacin	Glomerular filtration	2.5 h	2–3 d	15 mg/kg IM	3 d	H, P yes
Tobramycin, gentamicin	Glomerular filtration	2.5 h	2–4 d	3 mg/kg IM	2–3 d	H, P yes§
Vancomycin	Glomerular filtration	6 h	6–9 d	1 g IV	5–8 d	H, P no
Tetracycline	Glomerular filtration	8 h	3 d	1 g orally or 0.5 g IV	3 d	H yes, P no
Chloramphenicol	Mainly liver	3 h	4 h	1 g orally or IV	8 h	H, P no
Erythromycin	Mainly liver	1.5 h	5 h	1 g orally or IV	8 h	H, P no
Clindamycin	Glomerular filtration and liver	2.5 h	4 h	600 mg IV or IM	8 h	H, P no

*Modified and reproduced, with permission, from Jawetz E: Anti-infective chemotherapeutic and antibiotic agents. Chapter 28 in: *Current Medical Diagnosis & Treatment 1986.* Krupp MA, Chatton MJ, Tierney LM Jr (editors). Lange, 1986.
†Considered here to be marked by creatinine clearance of 10 mL/min or less.
‡For a 60-kg adult with a serious systemic infection. The "initial dose" listed is administered as an intravenous infusion over a period of 1–8 hours, or as 2 intramuscular injections during an 8-hour period, or as 2–3 oral doses during the same period.
§Aminoglycosides are removed irregularly in peritoneal dialysis. Gentamicin is removed 60% in hemodialysis.

appropriate laboratory test for ribosomal susceptibility is injected intramuscularly 2–3 times daily in divided doses. The cell wall inhibitory drug (penicillin) enhances entry of the aminoglycoside and permits killing of enterococci. This treatment must be continued for 4–5 weeks. Cephalosporins cannot be substituted for penicillins in this regimen.

C. Endocarditis Due to Staphylococci (*Staphylococcus aureus, Staphylococcus epidermidis*): If the infecting staphylococci are *not* penicillinase producers, penicillin G, 10–20 million units in divided doses as an intravenous bolus, is the treatment of choice. If the staphylococci produce penicillinase, nafcillin, 8–12 g daily, given as a bolus every 2 hours in an intravenous infusion, is the first-choice alternative drug. In probable or established hypersensitivity to penicillin, the alternative drug is vancomycin, 2–3 g daily in divided doses every 4 hours intravenously. This treatment must usually be continued for 5–6 weeks, and a frequent careful check for metastatic lesions or abscesses must be conducted to avoid reseeding of cardiac lesions from such reservoirs of infectious organisms.

D. Endocarditis Due to Gram-Negative Bacteria: The susceptibility of these organisms to antimicrobial drugs varies so greatly that effective treatment must be based on laboratory tests. Aminoglycosides (gentamicin, 5–7 mg/kg/d; kanamycin, 15 mg/kg/d; amikacin, 15 mg/kg/d; or tobramycin, 5–7 mg/kg/d) are often combined with a cell wall–inhibitory drug (cephalothin, 6–12 g/d; cefazolin, 4 g/d; ampicillin, 6–12 g/d; ticarcillin 10–18 g/d; or cefotaxime or cefoperazone, 12 g/d) to enhance penetration by the aminoglycoside. (See Table 16–3 for methods of administration.) Laboratory guidance is essential not only for drug susceptibility tests but also for establishment of the presence of sufficient bactericidal activity in serum obtained during treatment. All aminoglycosides may not be equally effective in any given patient; if the clinical response and the laboratory tests warrant, one can, for example, switch from gentamicin to amikacin. The dosage of aminoglycosides must be adjusted if renal function is impaired as determined by serum creatinine levels and creatinine clearance. Suggested modifications in time-dose regimens for aminoglycosides and other nephrotoxic drugs are given in Table 16–3. Each of these drugs also is capable of causing eighth nerve damage, and the patient should be monitored daily for hearing loss and vestibular function. Auditory toxicity with either gentamicin or tobramycin occurred in about 10% of patients, whereas nephrotoxicity may be less after tobramycin (Smith, 1980).

E. Endocarditis Due to Fungi: These organisms

rarely arise spontaneously but are seen with increasing frequency in abusers of intravenous drugs, after cardiac surgery, or in immunosuppressed individuals. *Candida albicans, Candida parapsilosis,* and *Torulopsis glabrata* are among those encountered most commonly, but virtually any fungus, including *Aspergillus* and even *Histoplasma*, can be seen. *Candida* endocarditis is often associated with bulky, friable vegetations that tend to produce massive emboli in large arteries. *Candida* endocarditis has occurred early after the insertion of prosthetic valves, and the diagnosis may be based on the finding of pseudohyphae in emboli surgically removed from large vessels. It may take 1–3 weeks to grow these organisms in blood cultures.

The drugs most active against fungi are amphotericin B (0.4–0.8 mg/kg/d intravenously, and flucytosine, 150 mg/kg/d orally, alone or in combination). However, these drugs rarely eradicate fungal endocarditis. Early surgical excision of the involved valve tissue during antifungal therapy and the continuation of the latter for several weeks offer the best opportunity for cure.

Prosthetic Valve Endocarditis

Endocarditis on tissue surrounding a prosthetic valve occurs at a rate of about 1% per year and is one of the most serious postoperative complications of prosthetic valve surgery. Most cases have involved the aortic valve, but the mitral valve may be infected as well. Infection may occur early, within 2–8 weeks after operation, or late, as with any diseased valve. Early-onset infections are caused by organisms introduced at the time of surgery from such sources as an infected pump oxygenator, contaminated intravenous lines used during the procedure, or infected personnel. A postoperative wound infection, especially of the sternum, may be a source of infection of the prosthetic valve. Although only one-third of all infections of prosthetic valves occur early (within the first 2 months), the mortality rate is high (70–80%) in early-onset cases as compared to the more frequent late-onset endocarditis (often many months to a year or so after the valve was introduced); the overall mortality rate of all cases of prosthetic valve endocarditis approximates 50–60%. The causes of early death in Wilson's 1975 series were prosthetic valve dysfunction, infection, cardiac failure, and emboli.

Early-onset endocarditis of a prosthetic valve is usually due to *S epidermidis* or *S aureus;* gram-negative bacilli are the next most common cause. Late-onset endocarditis is usually due to streptococci *(S viridans* or *S faecalis)*, although staphylococci are also frequent (Table 16–4).

Late-onset endocarditis usually follows one of the common predisposing causes of endocarditis on a damaged valve and pathologically involves the neoendothelium that grows over cloth-covered valves.

On pathologic examination, all patients with prosthetic valve endocarditis have infection located behind the site of attachment of the prosthesis to the valve ring, with spread to the neighboring structures. Severe regurgitation through the involved valve follows the prosthetic detachment and may require urgent surgery.

A. Medical and Surgical Treatment: Medical treatment of prosthetic valve endocarditis is most disappointing, and it may be necessary to resect the valve, introduce a new one, and combine the procedure with effective antimicrobial therapy. The mortality rate is 50–60% even in properly treated patients. In *Candida* infections, large-artery embolism may be the signal for replacing the prosthetic valve.

The high mortality rate may be a function of delayed surgery, since delay allows destruction of the valve, progressive development of renal and cardiac failure, and development of emboli (especially cerebral) before the patient is operated on again. Early surgical replacement of the infected valve is required if the infection is not rapidly controlled by aggressive antibiotic therapy or if there is evidence of destruction of the involved valve, with progressive cardiac failure or valvular regurgitation.

B. Prevention: Preventing infection is obviously better than treating prosthetic valve endocarditis; efforts have been made to ensure adequate antibacterial prophylaxis when prosthetic valves are inserted. Since the most common bacteria that cause early-onset prosthetic valve endocarditis are *S aureus* and gram-negative organisms, vigorous therapy with combined drugs is recommended, eg, nafcillin, 8–12 g/d intravenously, and gentamicin, 3–5 mg/kg/d intramuscularly, in 3 equal doses for 3 or 4 postoperative days. The results with cephalothin have been poor, and the toxicity of amphotericin B makes its use to prevent the uncommon *Candida* infections unwise. Good studies to establish the most effective prophylactic regimen are not available, but vigorous prophylaxis against the most likely organisms is indicated.

For prophylaxis of late-onset endocarditis, antimi-

Table 16–4. Microbiology of prosthetic valve infective endocarditis.*

	Early Endocarditis† (%)	Late Endocarditis† (%)
Number of cases‡	146	140
Infecting organism		
Staphylococcus epidermidis	40 (27.4)	32 (22.9)
Staphylococcus aureus	28 (19.2)	16 (11.4)
Streptococci	11 (7.5)§	52 (37.1)§
Gram-negative bacilli	30 (20.5)	19 (13.6)
Fungi	14 (9.6)	6 (4.3)
Miscellaneous bacteria	15 (10.3)	7 (5.0)
Mixed organisms	8 (5.5)	8 (5.7)

*Reproduced, with permission, from Watanakunakorn C: Prosthetic valve infective endocarditis. *Prog Cardiovasc Dis* 1979; 22:181.
†Early endocarditis: occurring within 2 months of operation; late endocarditis: occurring 2 months or longer after operation.
‡From multiple references.
§$P < 0.001$ (χ^2 test with Yate's correction).

crobials are used as in patients with known rheumatic or congenital heart lesions (see p 517). The predisposing factors are similar, and *S viridans* is the most common organism.

Treatment of Subacute Endocarditis in Patients With Negative Blood Cultures

When the physician does not know which organism is causing the endocarditis, the "best guess" method is employed. A combination of penicillin, 20–40 million units, and tobramycin, 5–7 mg/kg/d intramuscularly, is given, because the most common organisms are *S viridans* and *S faecalis*. This combination may also be effective in *S epidermidis* endocarditis. If the patient fails to improve in 1–2 weeks, a trial of other bactericidal drugs is indicated, eg, vancomycin, 0.5 g every 4 hours intravenously. Because of its great frequency in autopsied cases, endocarditis must be assumed to be present in staphylococcal septicemia even if its clinical diagnosis is not certain.

Penicillin Hypersensitivity

For many forms of endocarditis, penicillins have the best record of cure. A history of allergic reaction to penicillin is notoriously unreliable. Only 5–10% of patients with such a history cannot be given penicillin in a situation where it is clearly the drug of choice. All penicillins are cross-reactive, and cephalosporins have a much less successful record than penicillins in the treatment of endocarditis. Therefore, in spite of a history of penicillin reaction—except one of anaphylaxis—it may be desirable to attempt penicillin treatment in cases of endocarditis where a penicillin-susceptible organism has been recovered.

The following steps are advisable:

(1) Skin tests with penicilloyl-polylysine, native penicillin (1–10 units), and penicillin degraded after prolonged storage in a refrigerator. Unless strongly positive reactions are observed within 1 hour, proceed with treatment.

(2) An available airway and a person skilled in its insertion and the use of resuscitation must be at the bedside (preferably in the intensive care unit) for 40–45 minutes. An intravenous infusion of 5% dextrose in water must be in place and running. A syringe with 5 mL of epinephrine 1:1000 must be available at the bedside. A test dose of 100 units of penicillin G is injected into the intravenous tubing with close observation for a possible immediate reaction. If none has occurred in 45 minutes, inject 50,000 units of penicillin G into the tubing and again observe for 40 minutes. Absence of a reaction permits beginning of regular penicillin dosage with the assurance that an immediate life-threatening anaphylactic reaction will not occur.

Delayed, serum sickness type reactions, with skin rashes, angioneurotic edema, fever, or arthritis, may develop in such individuals. Administration of corticosteroids or antihistamines can often suppress these reactions and permit completion of the planned treatment. In extremely penicillin-hypersensitive patients, vancomycin is the best drug.

Patient Follow-Up

The physician's responsibility does not end with completion of the course of therapy. The only proof of cure is persistence of good health, absence of relapse, and repeatedly negative blood cultures. The patient should be observed at weekly intervals and should keep a daily temperature record. Blood for culture should be taken once a week for one month. The patient should be examined carefully for evidence of embolic phenomena, splenomegaly, clubbed fingers, and microscopic hematuria. If after 2 months there are no clinical symptoms or signs and the blood cultures have been consistently negative, it is safe to consider that cure has been achieved. The patient is then seen every month for another 3 or 4 months. It is always advisable to keep the cultures of the organism, because in case of relapse or recurrence, a question will arise about whether the same organism is responsible.

Persistent & Resistant Infection or Development of Cardiac Failure

If effective antibiotic therapy fails to eradicate the infection and positive blood cultures persist or recur, or if adequate combinations of drugs are not bactericidal, one should change the antibiotics, as mentioned previously, and hope to find the combination that will eradicate the organism. This may be difficult in the case of gram-negative or unusual organisms, especially fungi, or if the patient has a prosthetic valve. Cardiac failure may develop late as a result of progressive damage with fibrosis of the valve, especially the aortic valve. The development of severe aortic insufficiency may be rapid, and surgical replacement with a prosthetic valve is essential. At times, the urgency of surgical replacement is such that patients must be operated on within hours of arrival at the hospital. A few such patients have been cured by antibiotic therapy combined with surgical removal of the infected valve. Cardiac failure may progressively worsen even though the infection is eradicated; the physician is then faced with a different situation—a destroyed valve producing cardiac failure—in which case the valve should be replaced because it is destroyed and not because it is infected.

PROGNOSIS

Antibiotic therapy has reduced the mortality rate of infective endocarditis from almost 100% in all untreated cases to about 20% in subacute cases and 20–50% in acute cases. This remarkable achievement is best appreciated by physicians who had to deal with endocarditis prior to the antibiotic era. The residual high mortality rate in acute staphylococcal infections is due to the destruction of valves and to occurrence of septic abscess that may be inaccessible to drainage. The prognosis in subacute infective endocarditis depends upon the time elapsed before diagnosis, the organism involved and its sensitivity to antibiotic agents, the presence of an artificial valve, and the delay in beginning effective treatment. In sensitive *S viridans* infections, for example, the mortality rate is about 10%. However, with more resistant *S viridans*, *S aureus*, or gram-negative organisms, the mortality rate increases to 30–40%.

The prognosis depends also upon the class of patient being reported. Deaths are more frequent in elderly debilitated patients, in whom fever may be absent or minimal in the subacute variety and in whom the diagnosis may be delayed or missed because of atypical features of the disease. In *S aureus* endocarditis, for example, there may be a 2- to 3-fold higher mortality rate in older patients as compared to younger ones; most of the unsuspected fatal cases have been in the age group over 70.

The significant residual mortality rate in acute and subacute endocarditis means that the physician should actively seek the diagnosis, obtain blood cultures whenever fever occurs in a patient with valvular disease, and look for septic abscesses that can be surgically drained. Cooperation between the infectious disease specialist and the cardiologist is necessary both to eradicate the infection and to recognize when the complications of valve destruction require surgical therapy.

The incidence of endocarditis following placement of an aortic homograft valve (frequently used in England, Australia, and some centers in the USA) was 2.6% in 539 patients in the experience of Barratt-Boyes of New Zealand (1972). Early endocarditis occurred in less than 1% and was almost universally fatal. The mortality rate was almost 50% in patients with late endocarditis associated with development of an aortic leak. This incidence of endocarditis is about the same as that following the insertion of Starr-Edwards prostheses.

Continuous prophylactic antibiotics are not required in patients with homograft valves, but "antibiotic cover" is recommended when dental or surgical procedures are required in patients with plastic valves.

If endocarditis presents with renal failure, the prognosis is good for return of renal function.

REFERENCES

Pathology

Anderson DJ, Bulkley BH, Hutchins GM: A clinicopathologic study of prosthetic valve endocarditis in 22 patients: Morphologic basis for diagnosis and therapy. *Am Heart J* 1977;**94**:325.

Cates JE, Christie RV: Subacute bacterial endocarditis: A review of 442 patients treated in 14 centres appointed by the Penicillin Trials Committee of the Medical Research Council. *Q J Med* 1951;**20**:93.

Ivert TSA et al: Prosthetic valve endocarditis. *Circulation* 1984;**69**:223.

Johnson CM, Rhodes KH: Pediatric endocarditis. *Mayo Clin Proc* 1982;**57**:86.

Kaplan EL et al: AHA Cooperative Study of the Occurrence of Infective Endocarditis. (Abstract.) *Circulation* 1977;**56(4–Part 2)**:III-39.

Mills J, Drew D: *Serratia marcescens* endocarditis: A regional illness associated with intravenous drug abuse. *Ann Intern Med* 1976;**84**:29.

Weinstein L, Schlesinger JJ: Pathoanatomic, pathophysiologic, and clinical correlations in endocarditis. (2 parts.) *N Engl J Med* 1974;**291**:832, 1122.

Wilkowske CJ: Enterococcal endocarditis. *Mayo Clin Proc* 1982;**57**:101.

Wilson WR, Washington JA II: Infective endocarditis: A changing spectrum? *Mayo Clin Proc* 1977;**52**:254.

Diagnosis

Alpert JS et al: Pathogenesis of Osler's nodes. *Ann Intern Med* 1976;**85**:471.

Bayliss R et al: The microbiology and pathogenesis of infective endocarditis. *Br Heart J* 1983;**50**:513.

Berger M et al: Two-dimensional echocardiographic findings in right-sided infective endocarditis. *Circulation* 1980;**61**:855.

Botvinick EH et al: Echocardiographic demonstration of early mitral valve closure in severe aortic insufficiency: Its clinical implications. *Circulation* 1975;**51**:836.

Chandraratna PAN, Aronow WS: Spectrum of echocardiographic findings in tricuspid valve endocarditis. *Br Heart J* 1979;**42**:528.

Cliff MM, Soulen RL, Finestone AJ: Mycotic aneurysms: A challenge and a clue. *Arch Intern Med* 1970;**126**:977.

Cohen PS, Maguire JH, Weinstein L: Infective endocarditis caused by gram-negative bacteria: A review of the literature, 1945–1977. *Prog Cardiovasc Dis* 1980;**22**:205.

Corrigall D et al: Mitral valve prolapse and infective endocarditis. *Am J Med* 1977;**63**:215.

Dreyer NP, Fields BN: Heroin-associated infective endocarditis: Report of 28 cases. *Ann Intern Med* 1973;**78**:699.

Durack DT, Kaplan EL, Bisno AL: Apparent failures of endocarditis prophylaxis: Analysis of 52 cases submitted to a national registry. *JAMA* 1983;**250**:2318.

Hall B, Dowling HF: Negative blood cultures in bacterial endocarditis: A decade's experience. *Med Clin North Am* 1966;**50**:159.

Hermans PE: The clinical manifestations of infective endocarditis. *Mayo Clin Proc* 1982;**57**:15.

Jacoby GA, Swartz MN: Current concepts: Fever of undetermined origin. *N Engl J Med* 1973;**289**:1407.

Johnson DH, Rosenthal A, Nadas AS: A forty-year review of bacterial endocarditis in infancy and childhood. *Circulation* 1975;**51**:581.

Kaplan EL et al: A collaborative study of infective endocarditis in the 1970's: Emphasis on infections in patients who have undergone cardiovascular surgery. *Circulation* 1979;**59**:327.

Kaye D (editor): *Infective Endocarditis.* University Park Press, 1976.

Mills J, Drew D: *Serratia marcescens* endocarditis: A regional illness associated with intravenous drug abuse. *Ann Intern Med* 1976;**84**:29.

Nastro IJ, Finegold SM: Endocarditis due to anaerobic gram-negative bacilli. *Am J Med* 1973;**54**:481.

Osler W: Chronic infectious endocarditis. *Q J Med* 1909;**2**:219.

Pesanti EL, Smith IM: Infective endocarditis with negative blood cultures: An analysis of 52 cases. *Am J Med* 1979;**66**:43.

Pringle TH et al: Clinical, echocardiographic, and operative findings in active infective endocarditis. *Br Heart J* 1982;**48**:529.

Pruitt AA et al: Neurologic complications of bacterial endocarditis. *Medicine* 1978;**57**:329.

Rubenson DS et al: The use of echocardiography in diagnosing culture-negative endocarditis. *Circulation* 1981; **64**:641.

Seelig MS et al: *Candida* endocarditis after cardiac surgery: Clues to earlier detection. *J Thorac Cardiovasc Surg* 1973;**65**:583.

Stafford A et al: Diagnostic shelf: Serial echocardiographic appearance of healing bacterial vegetations. *Am J Cardiol* 1979;**44**:754.

Tobin MJ et al: Q fever endocarditis. *Am J Med* 1982;**72**:396.

Turck WPG et al: Chronic Q fever. *Q J Med* 1976;**45**:193.

Washington JA II: The role of the microbiology laboratory in the diagnosis and antimicrobial treatment of infective endocarditis. *Mayo Clin Proc* 1982;**57**:22.

Watanakunakorn C: Prosthetic valve infective endocarditis. *Prog Cardiovasc Dis* 1979;**22**:181.

Welton DE et al: Recurrent infective endocarditis: Analysis of predisposing factors and clinical features. *Am J Med* 1979;**66**:932.

Welton DE et al: Value and safety of cardiac catheterization during active infective endocarditis. *Am J Cardiol* 1979;**44**:1306.

Wise JR Jr, Oakley CM, Goodwin JF: Acute aortic regurgitation in patients with infective endocarditis: The distinctive clinical features and the role of premature mitral valve closure. *J Maine Med Assoc* 1972;**63**:273.

Prevention

AHA Committee Report: Prevention of bacterial endocarditis. *Circulation* 1977;**56**:139A.

Kaplan EL et al: AHA Cooperative Study of the Occurrence of Infective Endocarditis. (Abstract.) *Circulation* 1977;**56**(4–Part 2):III-39.

Petersdorf RG: Antimicrobial prophylaxis of bacterial endocarditis: Prudent caution or bacterial overkill? *Am J Cardiol* 1978;**65**:220.

Shulman ST (chairman) et al: Prevention of bacterial endocarditis: A statement for health professionals by the Committee on Rheumatic Fever and Infective Endocarditis of the Council on Cardiovascular Disease in the Young. (Special report.) *Circulation* 1984;**70**:1123A.

Sipes JN, Thompson RL, Hook EW: Prophylaxis of infective endocarditis: A reevaluation. *Annu Rev Med* 1977; **28**:371.

Sugrue D et al: Antibiotic prophylaxis against infective endocarditis after normal delivery: Is it necessary? *Br Heart J* 1980;**44**:499.

Van Scoy RE: Prophylactic use of antimicrobial agents. *Mayo Clin Proc* 1977;**52**:701.

Treatment

Alsip SG et al: Indications for cardiac surgery in patients with active infective endocarditis. *Am J Med* 1985;**78**(**Suppl B**):138.

Appel GB, Neu HC: The nephrotoxicity of antimicrobial agents. (3 parts.) *N Engl J Med* 1977;**296**:633, 722, 784.

Barratt-Boyes BG et al: Homograft valves. *Med J Aust* 1972;**2**(**Suppl 1**):38.

Bennett JE: Flucytosine. *Ann Intern Med* 1977;**86**:319.

Bennett WM et al: Guidelines for drug therapy in renal failure. *Ann Intern Med* 1977;**86**:754.

Brandenburg RO et al: Infective endocarditis: A 25-year overview of diagnosis and therapy. *J Am Coll Cardiol* 1983;**1**:280.

Brewer NS: The aminoglycosides: Streptomycin, kanamycin, gentamicin, tobramycin, amikacin, neomycin. *Mayo Clin Proc* 1977;**52**:675.

Brooks GF, Barriere SL: Clinical use of the new beta-lactam antimicrobial drugs: Practical considerations for physicians, microbiology laboratories, pharmacists, and formulary committees. *Ann Intern Med* 1983;**98**:530.

Calderwood SB et al: Risk factors for the development of prosthetic valve endocarditis. *Circulation* 1985;**72**:31.

Delgado DG, Cobbs CG: Infections of prosthetic valves and intravascular devices. Chap 52, p 690, in: *Principles and Practice of Infectious Diseases*. Vol 1. Mandell GL, Douglas RG Jr, Bennett JE (editors). Wiley, 1979.

Galgiani JN et al: *Bacteroides fragilis* endocarditis, bacteremia and other infections treated with oral or intravenous metronidzole. *Am J Med* 1978;**65**:284.

Geraci JE et al: *Haemophilus* endocarditis: Report of 14 patients. *Mayo Clin Proc* 1977;**52**:209.

Green GR, Peters GA, Geraci JE: Treatment of bacterial endocarditis in patients with penicillin hypersensitivity. *Ann Intern Med* 1967;**67**:235.

Hermans PE: Antifungal agents used for deep-seated mycotic infections. *Mayo Clin Proc* 1977;**52**:687.

Hubbell G, Cheitlin MD, Rapaport E: Presentation, management, and follow-up evaluation of infective endocarditis in drug addicts. *Am Heart J* 1981;**102**:85.

Jawetz E: Anti-infective chemotherapeutic and antibiotic agents. Chapter 28 in: *Current Medical Diagnosis & Treatment 1986*. Krupp MA, Chatton MJ, Tierney LM Jr (editors). Lange, 1986.

Jawetz E: Synergism and antagonism among antimicrobial drugs: A personal perspective. *West J Med* 1975;**123**:87.

Jawetz E, Sonne M: Penicillin-streptomycin treatment of enterococcal endocarditis. *N Engl J Med* 1966;**274**:710.

Karchmer AW: Staphylococcal endocarditis: Laboratory and clinical basis for antibiotic therapy. *Am J Med* 1985;**78**(**Suppl 6B**):116.

Karchmer AW et al: Late prosthetic valve endocarditis: Clinical features influencing therapy. *Am J Med* 1978;**64**:199.

Kaye D: Antibiotic treatment of streptococcal endocarditis. *Am J Med* 1980;**69**:650.

Korzeniowski O, Sande MA: Combination antimicrobial therapy for *Staphylococcus aureus* endocarditis in patients addicted to parenteral drugs and in nonaddicts. *Ann Intern Med* 1982;**97**:496.

Kumin GD: Clinical nephrotoxicity of tobramycin and gentamicin: A prospective study. *JAMA* 1980;**244**:1808.

Lerner PI, Weinstein L: Infective endocarditis in the antibiotic era. (4 parts.) *N Engl J Med* 1966;**274**:159, 199, 323, 388.

Masur H, Johnson WD: Prosthetic valve endocarditis. *J Thorac Cardiovasc Surg* 1980;**80**:31.

Mayer KH, Schoenbaum SC: Evaluation and management of prosthetic valve endocarditis. *Prog Cardiovasc Dis* 1982;**25**:43.

McAnulty JH, Rahimtoola SH: Surgery for infective endocarditis. *JAMA* 1979;**242**:77.

Ostermiller WE Jr, Dye WS, Weinberg M: Fungal endocarditis following cardiovascular surgery. *J Thorac Cardiovasc Surg* 1971;**61**:670.

Pelletier LL Jr, Petersdorf RG: Infective endocarditis: A review of 125 cases from the University of Washington Hospitals, 1963–72. *Medicine* 1977;**56**:287.

Reisberg BE: Infective endocarditis in the narcotic addict. *Prog Cardiovasc Dis* 1979;**22**:193.

Sande MA, Scheld WM: Combination antibiotic therapy of bacterial endocarditis. *Ann Intern Med* 1980;**92**:390.

Smith CR et al: Double-blind comparison of the nephrotoxicity and auditory toxicity of gentamicin and tobramycin. *N Engl J Med* 1980;**302**:1106.

Sorrell TC et al: Vancomycin therapy for methicillin-resistant *Staphylococcus aureus*. *Ann Intern Med* 1982;**97**:344.

Stinson EB: Surgical treatment of infective endocarditis. *Prog Cardiovasc Dis* 1979;**22**:145.

Thompson RL, Wright AJ: Cephalosporin antibiotics. *Mayo Clin Proc* 1983;**58**:79.

Tumulty PA: Management of bacterial endocarditis. *Geriatrics* 1967;**22**:122.

Turck M: Alternative antibiotics for the penicillin-sensitive patient. *Hosp Pract* (Oct) 1981;**16**:77.

UCLA Conference (John Edwards, monitor): Severe candidal infections: Clinical perspective, immune defense mechanisms, and current concepts of therapy. *Ann Intern Med* 1978;**89**:91.

Varma MPS, Adgey AAJ, Connolly JF: Chronic Q fever endocarditis. *Br Heart J* 1980;**43**:695.

Watanakunakorn C: Prosthetic valve infective endocarditis. *Prog Cardiovasc Dis* 1979;**22**:181.

Westenfelder GO, Paterson PY: Life-threatening infection: Choice of alternate drugs when penicillin cannot be given. *JAMA* 1969;**210**:845.

Wilson WR, Geraci JE: Treatment of streptococcal infective endocarditis. *Am J Med* 1985;**78(Suppl 6B)**:128.

Wilson WR et al: Cardiac valve replacement in congestive heart failure due to infective endocarditis. *Mayo Clin Proc* 1979;**54**:223.

Wilson WR et al: Prosthetic valve endocarditis. *Ann Intern Med* 1975;**82**:751.

Working Party of the British Society for Antimicrobial Chemotherapy: The antibiotic prophylaxis of infective endocarditis. *Lancet* 1982;**2**:1323.

Wright AJ, Wilkowske CJ: The penicillins. *Mayo Clin Proc* 1983;**58**:21.

Myocardial Disease (Myocarditis & Cardiomyopathy) 17

This chapter discusses myocarditis, cardiomyopathy, and various disease and clinical states of which disease of the myocardium may be a manifestation. The common known causes of chronic myocardial disease (ischemic, hypertensive, valvular, congenital, as well as infective endocarditis and syphilis) are discussed in other chapters.

GENERAL CONSIDERATIONS

The myocardium is susceptible to diseases of various causes, not all of them known. The clinical manifestations vary from mild illness to cardiac failure and death. Myocarditis may be acute or chronic, and acute myocarditis may be benign or fulminant. The terms "chronic myocarditis" and "chronic cardiomyopathy" are often used interchangeably. The term "chronic idiopathic cardiomyopathy" includes disorders that have been called dilated cardiomyopathy, Fiedler's myocarditis, idiopathic myocarditis, primary myocardial disease, endocardial myofibrosis, Löffler's syndrome, and alcoholic cardiomyopathy. Myocarditis may be a primary disorder, or it may be secondary to systemic diseases such as connective tissue disorders.

The clinical diagnosis of myocardial disease is often one of exclusion. The physician must consider common diseases with unusual clinical features in the differential diagnosis. As hypertensive disease and rheumatic heart disease in adults become less common, cardiomyopathy and the acute myocarditides have come to form a larger percentage of cases of cardiac disease. Some forms of myocardial disease are inexplicably more common in tropical and subtropical areas than in temperate climates.

Myocarditis is often associated with pericarditis, especially in viral infections. The endocardium and the valves are less often involved except in acute rheumatic fever or endocardial fibrosis. Myocardial disease due to drug toxicity is becoming increasingly common with the use of many cardiotoxic drugs (eg, the phenothiazines, doxorubicin).

ETIOLOGY & CLASSIFICATION

A working classification of the myocardial disorders is given in Table 17–1. All classifications are arbitrary and none are completely satisfactory, because of the many unknown causes and overlapping among the cardiomyopathies. Many of the diseases are of unknown cause. In such cases the diagnosis must be inferred from the associated systemic features, as in secondary cardiomyopathy and primary viral myocarditis. Infiltrative diseases such as primary amyloidosis may be difficult to diagnose, but newer immunoelectrophoretic techniques and procedures such as endomyocardial, rectal, or gum biopsy may be helpful. In sarcoidosis, chest x-ray may reveal characteristic hilar adenopathy or pulmonary infiltration or, in advanced disease, right ventricular hypertrophy and cor pulmonale.

PATHOLOGY

The pathologic features of cardiomyopathy associated with systemic disease are rarely specific. They may be relatively minor and discovered only at autopsy. One should clearly distinguish myocarditis recognized only postmortem from clinically significant disease that produces cardiac symptoms and dysfunction.

Inflammatory changes often occur during viral infections and are often unassociated with cardiac symptoms. Varying degrees of myofibrillary hypertrophy, fibrosis, or inflammation involving the myocardial cells or conduction system may be found in any type of cardiomyopathy. Cardiac failure may be evident, including chronic passive congestion. Evidence of the primary systemic disease may be apparent in other organs.

The pathologic processes in cardiomyopathy and myocarditis may be focal or diffuse; may be a pathologic curiosity at autopsy; or may cause fatal cardiac failure, arrhythmias, or conduction defects.

Percutaneous transvenous endomyocardial biopsy is a simple, safe technique when performed by experienced personnel. Biopsy permits anatomic diagnosis of conditions such as acute myocarditis, drug toxicity, cardiac graft rejection, amyloidosis, sarcoidosis, hemochromatosis, and endomyocardial fibrosis (Fowles, 1982; Fenoglio, 1983). Biopsy is seldom useful in determining the prognosis, especially in dilated cardiomyopathy, but can be valuable in evaluating treatment.

Common Specific Pathologic Pictures

The following are common pathologic changes seen at autopsy with some examples of the underlying causes that may be responsible. Most cases of cardiomyopathy are of unknown cause. When the cause is known, the condition is not usually called simply cardiomyopathy but identified as, for example, hypertensive heart disease.

(1) Infiltration of the myocardium with inflammatory cells of a variety of types, disorganizing their

Table 17–1. Classification of diseases of the myocardium.

I. Acute or subacute myocarditis
  A. Infectious: Usually acute but may be subacute
      Viral (especially coxsackie, echo, or poliomyelitis)
      Mycotic (eg, histoplasmosis, toxoplasmosis, *Candida*)
      Parasitic (eg, schistosomiasis, trichinosis, trypanosomiasis [acute Chagas' disease])
      Rickettsial (eg, epidemic typhus, scrub typhus, Q fever)
      Bacterial (eg, pneumococcus, diphtheria)
  B. Acute rheumatic fever
II. Acute or subacute myocardial damage due to drugs:
      Antiarrhythmic agents (eg, digitalis)
      Antimony
      Corticosteroids
      Doxorubicin
      Emetine
      Hydralazine
      Methysergide
      Phenothiazines
      Phenytoin
      Procainamide
      Tricyclic antidepressants (eg, amitriptyline, imipramine)
III. Chronic cardiomyopathy
  A. Idiopathic, dilated, or primary congestive cardiomyopathy
  B. Hypertrophic cardiomyopathy
  C. Restrictive cardiomyopathy
IV. Cardiomyopathy associated with specific metabolic diseases:
      Thyrotoxicosis
      Myxedema
      Alcoholic cardiomyopathy
      Beriberi heart
      Nutritional cardiomyopathy
      Acromegaly
      Inherited metabolic disorders
V. Cardiomyopathy associated with recognized chronic diseases, usually of unknown cause:
  A. Connective tissue disorders:
      Systemic lupus erythematosus
      Scleroderma
      Rheumatoid arthritis
      Polyarteritis nodosa
  B. Sarcoidosis
  C. Hemochromatosis
  D. Amyloid disease
  E. Endomyocardial fibrosis
  F. Peripartum disease
  G. Sickle cell disease
  H. Chagas' disease
  I. Neurologic disorders (eg, Friedreich's ataxia)

structure; best seen by electron microscopy. (Acute myocarditis, connective tissue disorders.)

(2) Infiltration with infecting organisms. (Acute viral myocarditis, *Candida* infections, Chagas' disease.)

(3) Focal or diffuse fibrosis of any part of the myocardium or conduction system. (Scleroderma, sarcoidosis, endocardial fibrosis.) When the fibrosis affects the vascular bed of the lungs, pulmonary hypertension, cor pulmonale, and right heart failure may occur.

(4) Vasculitis in the walls of small arteries as well as perivascular and intestinal infiltration of cells with or without granuloma formation. (Systemic lupus erythematosus.)

(5) Injury to myocardial cells as a result of excessive deposition of various substances. (Immune complexes in lupus erythematosus, fibrils of light chain immunoglobulins in amyloid disease, glycogen in Gierke's disease, calcium in renal failure, iron in hemochromatosis, products of abnormal metabolism, invasive tumors.)

(6) Metabolic changes caused by biochemical substances produced by tumor. (Serotonin or bradykinins in carcinoid syndrome.) (See Chapter 13.)

(7) Direct injury of myocardial cells from drugs. (Doxorubicin, digitalis, sympathetic amines, alcohol, methysergide, and others.)

Pathology of Conduction System

In all cases of myocardial disease, the damage to cardiac muscle may include the conduction system, causing destruction of the sinoatrial or atrioventricular node or large portions of the Purkinje system. Stokes-Adams attacks, arrhythmias, and sudden death are common in such disorders as scleroderma, sarcoidosis, and Chagas' disease. Inflammatory or fibrotic lesions may interrupt the ventricular conduction system, so that patients may have symptoms of the conduction defect in the absence of cardiac enlargement or cardiac failure.

GENERAL PATHOPHYSIOLOGY

Myocarditis and cardiomyopathy cause clinical disease in several ways: (1) by impairing myocardial cell contractility and systolic function; (2) by restricting filling of the ventricles, owing to impaired diastolic function; (3) by decreasing or increasing cardiac output and cardiac work; (4) by inducing progressive myocardial dilatation and hypertrophy; (5) by inducing pericarditis or pericardial effusion; (6) by inducing ischemia of the myocardium; and (7) by causing endocardial thrombus formation, leading to embolization.

The resulting impairment of cardiac function usually consists of (1) low-output failure with decreased myocardial contractility and increased cardiac volume or (2) decreased diastolic function secondary to decreased compliance of the left ventricle, so that high filling pressure is required to maintain cardiac output (see below).

Occasionally, there may be increased cardiac output, as in thyrotoxicosis, severe anemia, or Paget's disease of bone. (See High-Output Failure, Chapter 10.) When impairment of left ventricular function is sufficiently great, the ejection fraction falls below 30%, and progressive cardiac failure usually ensues.

In restrictive cardiomyopathy, there is restricted

filling of both ventricles due to a fibrotic or infiltrative lesion; this leads to systemic congestive phenomena.

ACUTE MYOCARDITIS IN GENERAL

In acute myocarditis, there is an acute febrile illness, with fever, malaise, arthralgias, chest pain, dyspnea, syncope, and palpitations. The patient may have associated pericarditis.

Signs

A. Cardiac Signs: Tachycardia out of proportion to the degree of fever suggests myocarditis. The cardiac impulse may be displaced to the left. Palpation may disclose left ventricular heave. The blood pressure is usually normal. Auscultation may reveal equalization of the first and second sounds (**tictac rhythm**), and a "functional" systolic murmur due to cardiac dilatation may be present. There may be a gallop rhythm with S_3, and if definite cardiac failure is present, a raised pulmonary venous or jugular venous pressure may be seen. Various ventricular arrhythmias or atrioventricular conduction defects may be found.

Acute circulatory collapse, with hypotension, oliguria, and obtundation, may occur when myocardial damage is severe (eg, in severe infections). Emboli may form, and sudden death may occur.

B. Signs of Associated Disease: Signs of an underlying disease may be present in the lungs, skin, liver, kidneys, or elsewhere.

Electrocardiography

Nonspecific ST–T changes, often in the inferior leads, are the most common abnormalities. If the conduction system is involved, there may be conduction defects, including partial atrioventricular block. In a young person with acute viral infection, the development of ST–T abnormalities, partial atrioventricular block, and conduction defects suggests myocarditis; in an older person, ischemic cardiomyopathy must be excluded.

X-Ray Findings

The radiologic findings are also nonspecific. The heart may be enlarged and globular with signs of pericardial effusion. Pericardial effusion can be confirmed by the echocardiogram, which shows an echo-free zone between the epicardium of the left ventricle and the chest wall. (See Chapter 18.) With gross cardiac failure there may be pulmonary venous congestion, and with cor pulmonale there may be radiologic signs of pulmonary hypertension and right ventricular enlargement. If the patient has sarcoidosis, there may be hilar adenopathy and pulmonary infiltration. In lymphomatous and malignant disease, tumor in various parts of the body may be evident.

Noninvasive Tests

Echocardiography may demonstrate pericardial thickening, enlargement of specific chambers of the heart, wall motion abnormalities, and findings characteristic of other diseases.

Cardiac Catheterization

Cardiac catheterization is usually done to rule out surgically treatable lesions in congestive cardiomyopathy (see below) or to differentiate the latter from hypertrophic cardiomyopathy or constrictive pericarditis (see Chapter 18). It is rarely performed in acute myocarditis unless the diagnosis is in doubt. Catheterization and angiography in dilated cardiomyopathy will show a left ventricle of increased volume in diastole with poor pulsations; a decreased ejection fraction ($< 40\%$); normal coronary arteries; and symmetric, decreased wall motion without aneurysm or segmental contraction abnormalities.

The prognosis for survival is much less favorable when the ejection fraction is low—especially when it is less than 20%.

Prognosis

The cardiac failure of myocardial disease may differ from that due to ischemic cardiomyopathy or severe valvular disease depending upon the cause. In acute viral myocarditis or peripartum cardiomyopathy, for example, cardiac failure may be completely reversible over a period of 1–2 months. In viral myocarditis, it may be recurrent.

ACUTE MYOCARDITIS ASSOCIATED WITH SPECIFIC DISEASES

Acute myocarditis most commonly follows streptococcal infection leading to acute rheumatic fever or infection caused by type B coxsackievirus but may also be caused by infection due to type A coxsackievirus, echovirus, adenovirus; by other viral diseases such as poliomyelitis, varicella, mumps, and hepatitis; or by infection due to other organisms such as *Chlamydia trachomatis*. In one series, one-third of the patients with acute myocarditis developed IgM responses specific to type B coxsackievirus (El-Hagrassy, 1980). Most patients with myocarditis seen in infectious disease services in general hospitals are free of cardiac symptoms, and signs are discovered only by careful clinical examination (including ECG) (see p 531). The acute exanthems rarely cause cardiac failure or cardiac dysfunction.

Clinical Findings

A. Myocarditis Due to Type B Coxsackieviruses: Cardiac involvement occurs in 5–10% of coxsackievirus infections (Grist, 1974), and the histologic effects are shown in Figs 17–1 and 17–2. The disease may be mild or severe.

1. Symptoms and signs–Fig 17–3 shows the relative frequency of important clinical symptoms and signs in proved coxsackievirus heart disease, the most common cause of viral myocarditis. Types B3 and B5 are most commonly associated with myocarditis

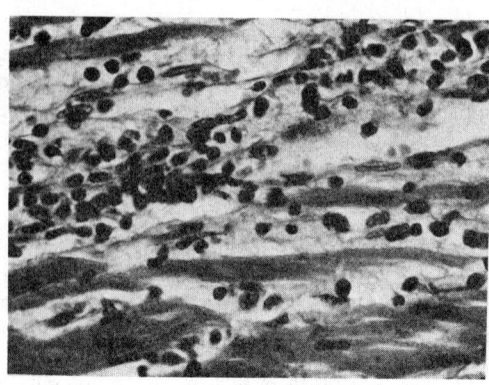

Figure 17–1. Focus of inflammatory cell infiltration in the myocardium in viral myocarditis. H&E stain. (Courtesy of O Rambo.)

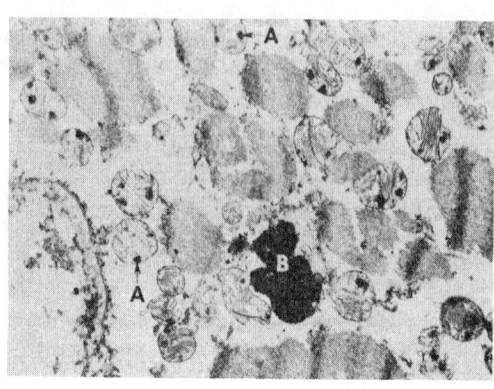

Figure 17–2. Electron micrograph of the myocardium in myocarditis due to type B4 coxsackievirus, showing fragmented myofibrils (B) and swollen mitochondria (A) and demonstrating the severity of the acute process. Original magnification of × 25,000 reduced by 36%. (Reproduced, with permission, from Rose HD: Recurrent illness following acute coxsackie B4 myocarditis. *Am J Med* 1973;**54**:544.)

in adults. Coxsackievirus myocarditis is usually suspected in adults on the basis of an acute febrile illness with lethargy, chest pain, dyspnea, enlargement of the heart, ventricular premature beats, ventricular tachycardia, and nonspecific ST–T changes. There may be obvious signs of cardiac failure in severe cases. Patients often have associated pericarditis; the presence of a pericardial rub in association with electrocardiographic abnormalities demonstrates pericardial involvement and distinguishes coxsackievirus infection with myocarditis from other influenzalike syndromes.

The illness usually lasts 1–4 weeks but may persist for months. Multiple recurrences may occur over a period of 1–2 years, but rarely is the condition severe, fulminant, or fatal. Patients are usually completely well months later, but chronic cardiac failure has continued over a period of 2–3 years in 5–10% of patients. Some observers believed that coxsackievirus myocarditis may be a cause of dilated cardiomyopathy

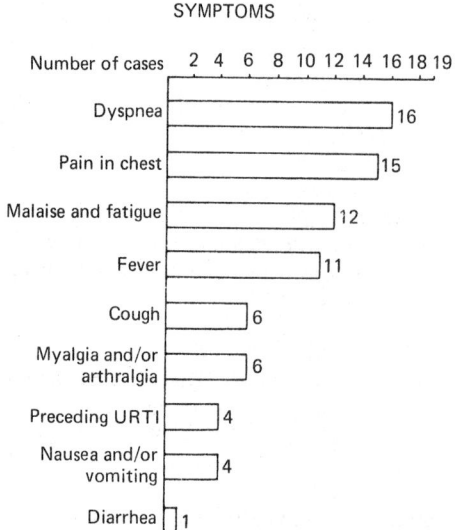

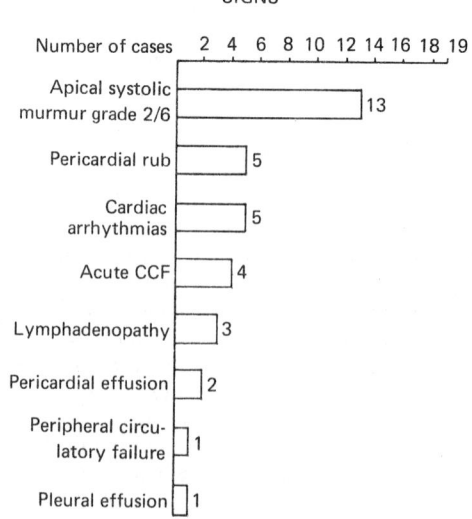

Figure 17–3. Clinical symptoms and signs in 19 proved cases of coxsackievirus heart disease. (Modified and reproduced, with permission, from Sainani GS, Dekate MP, Rao CP: Heart disease caused by coxsackievirus B infection. *Br Heart J* 1975;**37**:819.)

that occurs later in life. A relationship between coxsackievirus myocarditis and chronic constrictive pericarditis has also been proposed, but only a few well-documented examples of such patients have been reported.

2. Laboratory findings—The diagnosis is confirmed by virus isolation from throat washings or feces or by a 4-fold increase in neutralizing antibody in paired sera during the course of the disease.

3. X-ray findings—The chest film may demonstrate significant cardiac enlargement, often with pleural or pericardial effusion. If the latter is suspected, echocardiography can then establish its presence and magnitude (see Chapter 18).

4. Endomyocardial biopsy—Biopsy of the right ventricular endocardium occasionally establishes the specific diagnosis of the myocarditis. More commonly, the biopsy shows a nonspecific inflammatory infiltrate that establishes the diagnosis of myocarditis but not its cause. Serial biopsies may prove the value of treatment with corticosteroids or immunosuppressor drugs. Fig 17–4 shows the presence and disappearance of myocarditis following such therapy.

B. Myocarditis Due to Other Viruses: Myocarditis has been noted frequently, usually by electrocardiographic changes or some alteration of heart sounds, as an incidental feature of other viral diseases such as echovirus infection, mumps, varicella, poliomyelitis, infectious mononucleosis, measles, and hepatitis. Gallop rhythm, enlargement of the heart, or other signs of cardiac failure (see Chapter 10) may be present. Focal myocardial infiltration may be found on pathologic examination of the heart from patients with many types of viral infections who had no clinical evidence of heart disease during life.

C. Acute Myocarditis in Rickettsial Diseases:

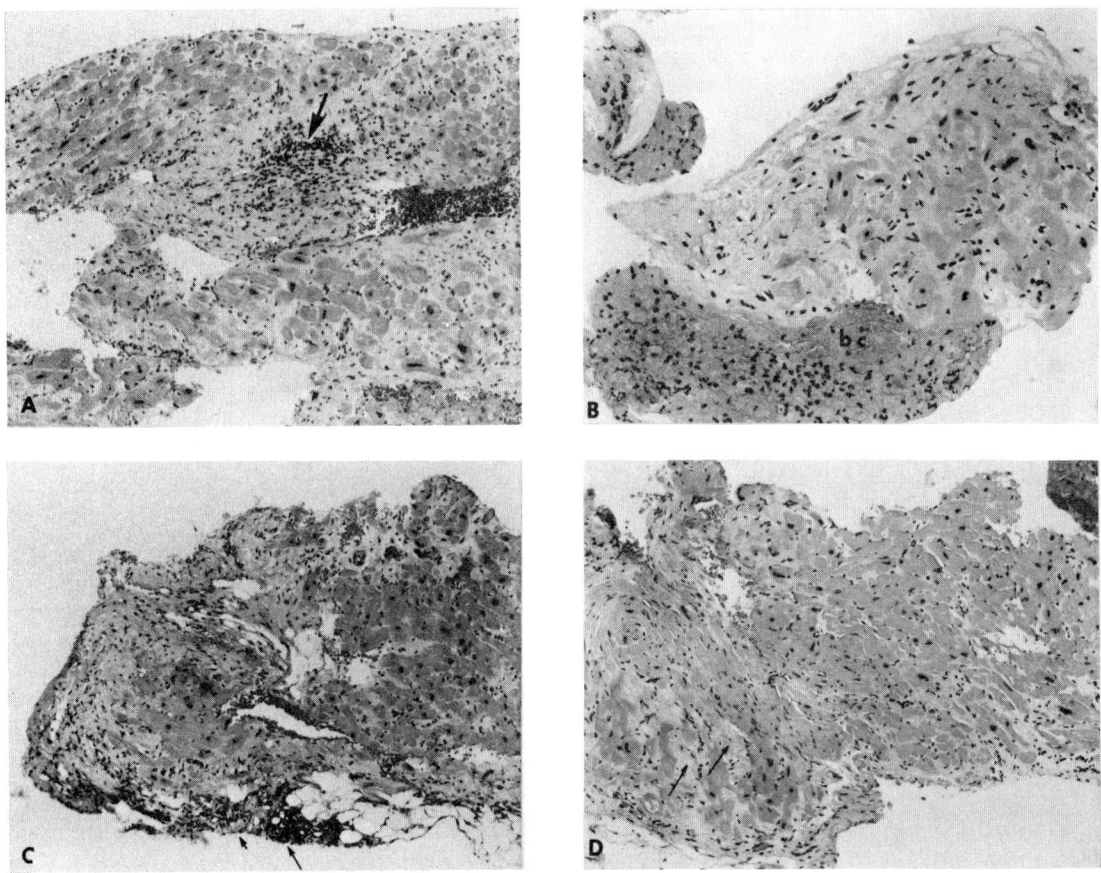

Figure 17–4. Endomyocardial biopsy specimens. *A,* obtained before immunosuppressive therapy, showing an obvious lymphocytic infiltrate (arrow) that was present in each biopsy specimen. (Hematoxylin-eosin × 120, reduced by 43%.) *B,* obtained after 4 months of immunosuppressive therapy; there is now complete absence of cell infiltrate. Blood clot (bc) is attached to the biopsy specimen. (Hematoxylin-eosin × 192, reduced by 43%.) *C,* after discontinuation of immunosuppressive therapy. There is a return of the lymphocytic infiltrate and, in addition, considerable pericardial infiltrate is present (arrows). (Hematoxylin-eosin × 120, reduced by 43%.) *D,* the final biopsy, taken 1 full year after initiation of immunosuppressive therapy, shows considerable fibrosis (arrows), but absence of cell infiltrate. (Hematoxylin-eosin × 120, reduced by 43%.) (Reproduced, with permission, from Mason JW, Billingham ME, Ricci DR: Treatment of acute inflammatory myocarditis assisted by endomyocardial biopsy. *Am J Cardiol* 1980;**45**:1037.)

In rickettsial diseases, infection may result in cardiac or circulatory failure in the second week of disease, but this is rarely a prominent feature. In typhus epidemics of 1915, cardiac failure was thought to be the cause of death in one-third of cases autopsied. In Q fever, there may be tachycardia out of proportion to the degree of fever, as well as dyspnea, fatigue, or chest pain suggesting myocardial involvement.

Rocky Mountain spotted fever may rarely cause myocarditis. Serologic confirmation can only be made late in the disease, and the diagnosis can be made earlier only on epidemiologic and clinical evidence.

Scrub typhus myocarditis in US military personnel during World War II was characterized by persistent fatigue, tachycardia, and electrocardiographic and radiologic evidence of cardiac involvement requiring prolonged convalescence even in otherwise healthy young men. Eventually, all patients recovered completely (Sokolow, 1945).

D. Acute Myocarditis in Trypanosomiasis: In Chagas' disease, the initial skin and eye lesions may be associated with acute myocarditis, but the dominant feature is late chronic cardiac failure or conduction defects. African trypanosomiasis can cause chronic pancarditis as well as valvulitis and lesions of the conduction system. The usual presenting symptoms are neurologic rather than cardiac, because meningoencephalitis is a frequent complication. The histologic pattern is similar to that of Chagas' disease, but myocarditis is less frequent in infections due to *Trypanosoma gambiense* than in those due to *Trypanosoma cruzi*. Cases of idiopathic hypertrophy occurring in African countries might be due to undiagnosed trypanosomiasis.

E. Diphtheritic Myocarditis: Diphtheria is rare in the USA as a result of widespread immunization with diphtheria toxoid, but it is a substantial health problem in some other countries. The disease occurs chiefly in children and is usually transmitted by nasopharyngeal secretions, but any underlying skin lesion may become infected. The diagnosis is made by bacteriologic examination of a grayish-green adherent membrane that may involve the nares, pharynx, larynx, bronchi, or skin. An exotoxin secreted by the bacilli causes the acute clinical disease.

Myocarditis occurs in 10–25% of cases, usually in the first few weeks, and is manifested by clinical features and by ST–T changes in the ECG. In more severe cases, acute circulatory or cardiac failure may occur, associated with various arrhythmias or conduction defects, especially ventricular tachycardia and atrioventricular block (Boyer, 1948).

Prevention by immunization in infancy with booster injections every 10 years is the most effective form of control.

Treatment consists of early intramuscular or intravenous injection of diphtheria antitoxin, combined with antibiotic treatment with penicillin, erythromycin, or ampicillin to eradicate the organism. Intensive care nursing may be necessary, especially if there is airway obstruction requiring tracheostomy or bronchoscopy. Bed rest and supportive care may be necessary for several weeks. Digitalis is rarely of value. Antitoxin is usually ineffective once myocarditis has occurred. Large doses of corticosteroids have been given in severe cases, but their therapeutic value has not been established.

The course of the disease varies from a mild illness to a fulminant, highly fatal process. In severe cases, with circulatory failure or atrioventricular block, the mortality rate approaches 60–70%, emphasizing the importance of preventive immunization and early treatment with antitoxin. Carrier states are relatively common and should be sought and treated with antibiotics after the patient has recovered. Permanent partial atrioventricular block may occur, but cardiac failure or complete heart block is rare in the years following the acute attack.

F. Acute Myocarditis in Trichinosis: Ingestion of *Trichinella spiralis* in inadequately cooked pork may cause disease leading to myocarditis. Disease is suspected in a patient with fever, periorbital edema, muscle pains, and eosinophilia who has eaten inadequately cooked meat. The larvae spread through the body, but focal inflammatory myocarditis and endocarditis with thrombosis are responsible for some deaths.

Myocarditis occurs 3–8 weeks after infection and is suspected on the basis of dyspnea, tachycardia, and electrocardiographic demonstration of ST–T changes, sinus tachycardia, and ventricular premature beats. Congestive failure occurs rarely. The diagnosis is strongly suspected on the basis of severe eosinophilia (often ≥ 50%) and splinter hemorrhages of the nails, and it is confirmed by serologic tests and skeletal muscle biopsy.

Treatment is supportive, with corticosteroid therapy added. The long-term prognosis of survivors is good, and chronic cardiac disease is rare.

Differential Diagnosis

Acute myocarditis due to infection with viruses (eg, coxsackievirus), protozoa (eg, trypanosomes), or bacteria (eg, pneumococci) must be distinguished from acute toxic myocarditis due to drugs or diphtheria and from myocarditis associated with acute rheumatic fever. Changes on the ECG in viral diseases may be due to acute circulatory failure from infection, metabolic abnormalities such as disturbances in acid-base balance, and hypoxia and not to myocarditis as such.

Nonviral myocarditis is recognized on the basis of manifestations of the underlying disease. The diagnosis of acute myocarditis in Chagas' disease is usually based on epidemiologic evidence as well as the presence of a chagoma at the site of entry of the parasites and recovery of trypanosomes in blood. The diagnosis should be considered in patients living in thatched huts providing the appropriate environment for triatomine bugs, which transmit the disease.

Acute rheumatic fever is associated with other major findings such as arthritis and a history of recent streptococcal infection; arthritis is relieved by salicylates, and recent streptococcal infection can be inferred from finding increasing titers of antistreptolysin (ASO) in the serum. Diphtheria causes a typical lesion in the throat but may infect the skin also (common in the Orient and Asia), and the organism can be identified from throat and skin cultures. In acute myocardial toxicity due to drugs, awareness of the use of drugs, their dosage, and the presence of the disease being treated with drugs helps differentiate myocardial toxicity from acute myocarditis. This may be difficult in patients with acute lupus erythematosus with fever, pericarditis, and vasculitis, and specific immunologic procedures may be required to make the differentiation.

Acute glomerulonephritis may present as acute cardiac failure, but the poststreptococcal state, hypertension, and urinary findings should simplify the diagnosis. Hemodynamic findings indicate that "cardiac failure" in acute nephritis is usually due to salt and water retention and not to cardiac failure per se. The cardiac index is often increased, averaging 5.4 L/min/m^2 at rest and 7.5 L/min/m^2 with exercise—in contrast to the low cardiac output in acute cardiac failure. The pulmonary capillary wedge pressure is slightly increased at rest but within the normal range after exercise (averaging 15 mm Hg at rest and 18 mm Hg after exercise) (Binak, 1975).

Treatment*

In the absence of effective specific antiviral therapy, treatment consists of general supportive care and management of cardiac failure, arrhythmias, or conduction defects if they occur. (See respective chapters.) The combination of prednisone and immunosuppressive drugs has been proved by endomyocardial biopsy to be valuable in some patients with acute myocarditis and cardiac failure (Mason, 1980). Clinical and experimental experience suggests that early exercise should be avoided to prevent multiplication of viruses and further impairment of cardiac function.

In nonviral acute myocarditis, treatment is directed toward the underlying cause if possible, as it is with diphtheria or pneumococcal infections. Some patients with *Candida* infections respond to amphotericin B or flucytosine, and patients receiving pyrimethamine and sulfonamide for toxoplasmosis show considerable clinical improvement. Most cases of disseminated toxoplasmosis with myocarditis result from infection in immunocompromised patients.

Prognosis

Follow-up of 14 of 19 patients with acute myocarditis due to type B coxsackievirus by Sainani (1975) revealed no deaths, but 3 patients had chronic heart failure.

RHEUMATIC FEVER

Rheumatic fever is a subacute or chronic systemic disease that may either be self-limiting or lead to slowly progressive valvular deformity. Rarely, it is acute and fulminant.

Rheumatic fever and its sequelae used to be the commonest cause of heart disease in people under 50 years of age in the USA, and as a cause of heart disease in people of all ages it ranked third behind hypertension and atherosclerotic coronary disease. The prevalence of rheumatic fever has decreased 5-fold or more in the last 50 years in the USA and Scandinavia but not in developing countries (Krause, 1979; Disciascio, 1980). The peak incidence occurs between ages 5 and 15; rheumatic fever is rare before age 4 or after age 50.

Etiology

Rheumatic fever occurs as a late sequela of infections with beta-hemolytic streptococci (eg, tonsillitis, nasopharyngitis, otitis media). Streptococcal antigens cross-react with antigens of human heart muscle, especially sarcolemma, and the resulting antigen-antibody response leads to rheumatic fever (Zabriskie, 1985). A genetic factor may be involved. Circulating immune complexes have been found in most adults with acute rheumatic fever, especially those positive for HLA-B5, and the concordance rate for occurrence of disease in identical twins is 5 times greater than in nonidentical twins (Disciascio, 1980). Nonsuppurative complications of streptococcal infections such as rheumatic fever should be differentiated from suppurative complications such as peritonsillar abscess, sinusitis, mastoiditis, and cervical adenitis.

Pathology

The acute phase of rheumatic fever may involve the endocardium, myocardium, pericardium, synovial joint linings, lungs, peritoneum, or pleura. The characteristic lesion is a perivascular granulomatous reaction and vasculitis (Aschoff nodule; Fig 17–5). The

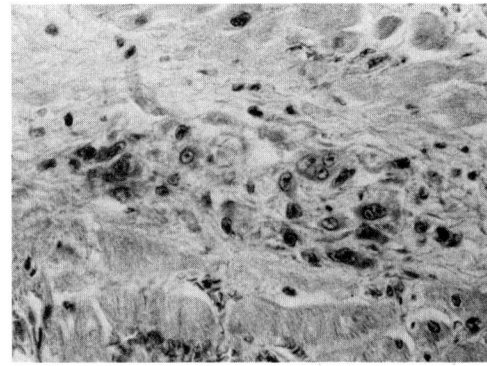

Figure 17–5. Typical multinucleated Aschoff nodule from the atrial appendage in a patient with rheumatic heart disease. Magnification × 100, H&E stain. (Courtesy of O Rambo.)

---

*Treatment of myocarditis associated with Chagas' disease is discussed on p 563.

mitral valve is attacked in 75–80% of cases, the aortic valve in 30%, and the tricuspid and pulmonary valves in less than 5%. Small pink granules appear on the surface of the edematous valves. Healing may be complete, or progressive scarring due to subacute or chronic inflammation may develop over months or years.

Diagnosis

The diagnosis is more readily made in epidemics of streptococcal infections such as occur in wartime, when the relationship of beta-hemolytic streptococcal infections and the subsequent nonsuppurative complications of rheumatic fever are more readily seen. Even mild cases can be recognized under these circumstances. When isolated cases of rheumatic fever occur, the diagnosis is often unsuspected and not made. This may explain the high percentage of patients with rheumatic heart disease who deny a previous history of rheumatic fever.

Children usually have more severe disease than adults and are therefore more easily diagnosed. The diagnosis may be difficult with minimal illness. The modified Jones criteria show major and minor criteria which are not absolute but should serve as guides. At least 2 major criteria are necessary for diagnosis.

Modified Jones Criteria

A. Major Criteria: The major criteria are peri-, myo-, or endocarditis, chorea, subcutaneous nodules, erythema marginatum, and polyarthritis.

B. Minor Criteria: The minor criteria are fever, malaise, abdominal pain (especially in children), arthralgias ("growing pains"), and laboratory findings of leukocytosis, raised sedimentation rate, and evidence of a preceding streptococcal infection (positive throat culture for group A *Streptococcus*, increased titer of antistreptolysin O). A history of rheumatic fever and the presence of rheumatic heart disease are also minor criteria.

Clinical Findings

A. Symptoms: The disease usually begins with fever or arthritis 2–3 weeks following infection due to beta-hemolytic streptococci.

1. Fever–The fever may be low-grade and intermittent, but in severe cases with pericarditis or myocarditis, it may be as high as 39 °C. It may last for weeks or months in conjunction with malaise, asthenia, weight loss, and anorexia, as with any chronic active disease.

2. Joint pains–"Growing pains" in joints, periarticular tissues, or muscle systems may be a symptom of rheumatic fever (polyarthralgia).

3. Arthritis–Arthritis with effusion is typically a migratory polyarthritis involving the large joints sequentially; as the inflammation in one involved joint subsides, another joint will become hot, red, swollen, and tender. Fever rises as each successive joint becomes inflamed. In adults, only a single or a small joint may be affected. The acute arthritis lasts 1–5 weeks and subsides without residual deformity. *Note:* Joint involvement is considered a major criterion only when definite effusion and signs of inflammation are present. This is in contrast to arthralgia, in which pain or stiffness is present without these objective signs. Prompt response of arthritis to therapeutic doses of salicylates is characteristic (but not diagnostic) of rheumatic fever.

4. Peri-, myo-, endocarditis ("carditis")–The symptoms of carditis in rheumatic fever are often slight and must be looked for specifically. The patient does not complain of dyspnea unless cardiac failure is present. Chest pain may be prominent, either made worse with breathing (pleuritis), related to posture if pericardial (see Chapter 18), or epigastric if there is peritoneal involvement. The interpretation of the symptoms is clarified by signs, an ECG, and x-ray findings (see below). The patient may complain of palpitations due to a rapid heart rate, but arrhythmias are uncommon.

5. Skin lesions and subcutaneous nodules–The patient may complain of skin lesions or subcutaneous nodules, but these are more frequently found on physical examination (see Signs, below).

6. Chorea–Chorea (Sydenham's) consists of purposeless jerky movements, continual and nonrepetitive, of the limbs, trunk, and facial muscles. Milder forms masquerade as undue restlessness as the patient attempts to convert uncontrolled movements into seemingly purposeful ones. Facial grimaces of infinite variety are common. These movements are made worse by emotional tension and disappear entirely during sleep. The episode lasts weeks or months.

Chorea may appear suddenly as an isolated entity or may develop in the course of overt rheumatic fever. Eventually, 50% of patients have other signs of rheumatic fever. Girls are more frequently affected, and occurrence in adults is rare.

B. Signs:

1. General appearance–The patient may seem well or may appear both acutely and chronically ill, with pallor, subdued affect, and general debility.

2. Arthritis–The joints may be normal on examination in patients with arthralgia and growing pains,

Table 17–2. Incidence of symptoms and signs of rheumatic fever in 1000 patients.*

Carditis	653
Chorea	518
Arthritis	410
Arthralgia	401
Epistaxis	274
Precordial pain	240
Pericardial rub	130
Abdominal pain	117
Subcutaneous nodules	88
Rash	71

*Reproduced, with permission, from the American Heart Association, Inc., Bland EF, Jones TD: Rheumatic fever and rheumatic heart disease: A 20-year report on 1000 patients followed since childhood. *Circulation* 1951;4:836.

or reddened and swollen in acute arthritis. Movement of the involved joint or even the weight of bedsheets over the joint is painful. There is marked disparity between the often slight effusion and faint blush over the affected joint and the magnitude of the pain. The arthritis may involve only one joint or may "migrate" to involve multiple joints as the patient is examined daily.

3. Carditis–Myocardial signs may be minimal or characterized by tachycardia that is out of proportion to the degree of fever and is increased by slight activity; by cardiac enlargement with the cardiac impulse displaced to the left; by pericardial friction rub with or without a raised jugular venous pressure, depending on the presence and amount of pericardial effusion; by painful engorgement of the liver (especially in cardiac failure in children); and by signs of left ventricular failure such as gallop rhythm or pulmonary rales. Cardiac murmurs are infrequent at onset, but gradually, a short, soft middiastolic murmur of mitral valve involvement **(Carey-Coombs murmur)**; a short early diastolic murmur of aortic valve involvement, or a soft pansystolic murmur of mitral incompetence may be heard. Short systolic murmurs are commonly due to fever or tachycardia. Tictac heart sounds may be present (see Acute Myocarditis).

4. Arrhythmias–Premature beats are uncommon; atrial fibrillation and ventricular tachycardia are rare.

5. Erythema marginatum (annulare)–This is frequently associated with skin nodules. The lesions begin as rapidly enlarging macules that assume the shape of rings or crescents with clear centers. They may be slightly raised and confluent. The rash may be transient or may persist for long periods.

6. Subcutaneous nodules–Subcutaneous nodules are commonest in children. They are usually small ($\leq$ 2 cm in diameter), firm, and nontender and are attached to fascia or tendon sheaths over bony prominences such as the elbows, the dorsal surfaces of the hands, the malleoli, the vertebral spines, and the occiput. They persist for days or weeks, are usually recurrent, and are clinically indistinguishable from the nodules of rheumatoid arthritis.

7. Recurrent spontaneous nosebleeds–Nosebleeds are frequent, but the cause is not clear.

C. Laboratory Findings: These are helpful in 3 ways:

1. As nonspecific evidence of inflammatory disease–The sedimentation rate and white count are almost always increased during active rheumatic fever except when chorea is the only clinical sign. Normochromic anemia, proteinuria, and microhematuria may appear without concomitant glomerulonephritis.

2. As evidence of antecedent beta-hemolytic streptococcal infection–A high or increasing antistreptolysin O titer indicates recent infection but does not mean that rheumatic fever is present. Throat culture is positive for beta-hemolytic streptococci in 50% of early cases of active rheumatic fever.

3. As strong evidence against the diagnosis–A low antistreptolysin O titer (< 100 Todd units) that does not rise on repeated tests tends to rule out rheumatic fever. A normal sedimentation rate is rare with rheumatic fever.

D. Electrocardiographic Findings: PR prolongation greater than 0.04 second above the patient's normal PR interval is the most significant abnormality; changing contour of P waves or inversion of T waves is less specific. Other characteristics are shown in Table 17–3.

E. X-Ray Findings: Chest x-ray may be normal or show cardiac enlargement. Pericardial effusion may develop (see Chapter 18).

F. Special Investigations: Echocardiograms are diagnostic if pericardial effusion develops but are of little value in early valvular involvement.

Differential Diagnosis

Rheumatic fever may be confused with the following: rheumatoid arthritis, osteomyelitis, chronic infections, traumatic joint disease, neurocirculatory asthenia or cardiac neurosis, infective endocarditis, pulmonary tuberculosis, chronic meningococcemia, meningitis, acute poliomyelitis, connective tissue diseases, serum sickness, drug sensitivity, leukemia, sickle cell anemia, inactive rheumatic heart disease, congenital heart disease, and "surgical abdomen."

Table 17–3. Electrocardiographic abnormalities in 700 cases of rheumatic fever.*

		No.	Percent
Total cases with abnormalities in the ECG		147	21
Of the 147 cases:			
1. Conduction defects		88	60
Partial atrioventricular block	83		
Complete atrioventricular block	3		
Intraventricular block	2		
2. T wave changes		52	35
Inversion of LV T waves†	17		
Diphasic LV T waves	11		
Flat LV T waves	24		
3. Abnormal rhythms		14	10
Shifting atrial pacemaker	7		
Junctional rhythm	4		
Junctional escape	2		
Atrial fibrillation	1		
4. Miscellaneous		12	8
Marked left axis deviation or right axis deviation	7		
Inversion P_2 and P_3	5		
Duration of atrioventricular block			
Of 76 cases:			
0–4 days		11	15
5–8 days		3	4
9–14 days		39	51
15–21 days		14	18
22–28 days		6	8
Over 3 months		3	4

*Modified and reproduced, with permission, from Sokolow M: Significance of electrocardiographic changes in rheumatic fever. *Am J Med* 1948;5:365.
†LV, left ventricular.

Complications

Congestive heart failure occurs in severe cases. Other complications include cardiac arrhythmias, pericarditis with large effusion, rheumatic pneumonitis, pulmonary embolism and infarction, cardiac invalidism, and early or late development of permanent heart valve deformity.

Prevention of Recurrent Rheumatic Fever

The principles of prevention are to avoid beta-hemolytic streptococcal infections if possible and to treat streptococcal infections promptly and intensively with appropriate antibiotics.

A. General Measures: Avoid contact with persons with suspected streptococcal infections.

B. Prevention of Infection: Two methods of prevention are now advocated.

1. Penicillin–The preferred method of prophylaxis is with benzathine penicillin G, 1.2 million units intramuscularly every 4 weeks. Oral penicillin (200,000–250,000 units daily before breakfast) may be used instead but is less reliable. Prophylaxis is advocated for children who have had one or more acute attacks and should be given at least until age 30. Adults should receive prophylaxis for about 5 years after an attack. Recurrences are rare in patients receiving prophylactic antibiotics.

2. Sulfonamides–If the patient is sensitive to penicillin, give sulfadiazine, 1 g orally daily throughout the year. *Caution:* Patients receiving sulfonamides should have periodic blood counts and urinalyses. If there is any tendency toward leukopenia or renal complications, the drug should be stopped immediately and a different drug (eg, erythromycin, 250 mg twice daily) substituted.

C. Treatment of Streptococcal Sore Throat: Prompt penicillin therapy (within 24 hours) of streptococcal infections will prevent most attacks of acute rheumatic fever.

Treatment

A. Medical Treatment:

1. Salicylates–The salicylates markedly reduce fever, relieve joint pain, and may reduce joint swelling. There is no evidence that they have any effect on the natural course of the disease. *Note:* The salicylates should be continued as long as necessary to relieve pain, swelling, or fever. If withdrawal results in recurrence of symptoms, treatment should be reinstituted immediately.

a. Sodium salicylate is the most widely used of this group of drugs. The maximum adult dose is 1 g orally every 4 hours to allay symptoms and fever; 4 g/d suffice in most adults. In an occasional patient, maximum doses may not be completely effective. There is no evidence that intravenous administration has any advantage over the oral route. Early untoward reactions to the salicylates include tinnitus, nausea and vomiting, and gastrointestinal bleeding. Salicylates may be used with antacids, after meals, or with milk to reduce gastric irritation. *Caution:* Do not use sodium salicylate or sodium bicarbonate in patients with acute rheumatic fever who have associated cardiac failure.

b. Aspirin may be substituted for sodium salicylate. A satisfactory daily dose for children is usually 15–25 mg/kg given in divided doses every 4 hours during the day for a week, with the dose then decreased by half. Adults initially may require 0.6–0.9 g every 4 hours during the day. Hyperpnea may occur with large doses. Other anti-inflammatory agents (eg, indomethacin) have not been used in large-scale studies.

2. Penicillin–Penicillin is given at the outset of disease to eradicate streptococcal infections.

3. Corticosteroids–A short course of corticosteroids usually causes rapid improvement in the acute manifestations of rheumatic fever and is indicated in severe cases. Give prednisone, 5–10 mg orally every 6 hours for 3 weeks, and then gradually withdraw over a period of 3 weeks. In severe cases, the dosage should be increased, if necessary, to levels adequate to control symptoms. There is, however, no evidence that either corticosteroids or salicylates prevent or reduce permanent myocardial damage.

B. General Measures: Bed rest should be enforced until all signs of active rheumatic fever have disappeared (ie, normal temperature with the patient at bed rest and without medications, normal sedimentation rate, normal resting pulse rate [< 100/min in adults], and normal heart function or fixation of abnormalities on ECG). Several months should elapse before return to full activity, unless the disease was very mild. Maintain good nutrition.

C. Treatment of Complications:

1. Congestive heart failure–Treat as for congestive heart failure due to other causes, with the following variations:

a. Digitalis is usually not as effective in congestive heart failure due to acute rheumatic fever as in other forms of congestive failure. It may accentuate myocardial irritability, producing arrhythmias, and should therefore be given with care.

b. Congestive failure and pericarditis may respond dramatically to corticosteroids, but the anti-inflammatory action may fail to modify subsequent valvular damage. When sodium-retaining drugs are employed, sodium intake is restricted and thiazide diuresis is used.

2. Pericarditis–Treat as for any acute nonpurulent pericarditis. The rheumatic effusion is sterile, and antibiotics are of no value. The general principles include relief of pain, by opiates if necessary, and removal of fluid by pericardiocentesis if tamponade develops. This, however, is rarely necessary. Corticosteroids and salicylates should be continued or started, as they aid resorption of fluid.

Prognosis

Initial episodes of rheumatic fever last months in children and weeks in adults. Twenty percent of children have recurrences within 5 years. Recurrences are uncommon after 5 years of well-being and rare after

Table 17–4. Fatalities in rheumatic fever in patients with special features.*

Onset (Number of Cases)	10 Years (Fatalities)	20 Years (Fatalities)
Greatly enlarged heart 70	56 (80%)	57 (81%)
Congestive failure 207	148 (71%)	152 (80%)
Pericarditis 130	73 (56 %)	77 (63%)
Nodules 88	34 (38%)	37 (43%)
Arthritis 410	91 (22%)	109 (27%)
Chorea 518	49 (9.4%)	63 (12%)

*Reproduced, with permission, from the American Heart Association, Inc., Bland EF, Jones TD: Rheumatic fever and rheumatic heart disease: A 20-year report on 1000 patients followed since childhood. *Circulation* 1951;4:836.

age 21. The immediate mortality rate is 1–2%. Persistent rheumatic activity with a greatly enlarged heart, heart failure, and pericarditis indicate a poor prognosis as shown in Table 17–4; 30% of children thus affected die within 10 years of the initial attack. Otherwise, the prognosis for life is good (more recent data on a comparable series are not available). Approximately one-third of young patients have detectable valvular damage after the initial episode, most commonly involving the mitral valve. After 10 years, two-thirds of surviving patients will have detectable valvular disease. In adults, residual heart damage occurs in less than 20% and is generally less severe (Engleman, 1954). Mitral incompetence is the commonest ultimate lesion, and aortic incompetence is much more common than in children. Twenty percent of patients who have chorea develop valvular deformity even after a long latent period of apparent well-being.

ACUTE MYOCARDIAL DAMAGE DUE TO DRUG TOXICITY

Acute myocardial damage is seen after the use of a variety of drugs, notably cytotoxic agents, emetine, digitalis, sympathomimetic drugs, arsenic, antimony, amphetamines, and tricyclic antidepressants. About one-fourth of patients (4 out of 15) receiving high-dose multiple chemotherapy may die of acute myopericardial failure during treatment as a result of endothelial injury, pericardial effusion, cardiac failure, and cardiac arrhythmias (Appelbaum, 1976).

Cytotoxic agents, eg, cyclophosphamide (Cytoxan) and doxorubicin (Adriamycin), may produce clinical as well as pathologic myocardial disease; the toxic effects are dose-related and more apt to occur when cytotoxic drugs are used in combination. As with any variety of acute myocardial disease or toxicity, the clinical presentation may be with arrhythmias or conduction defects rather than cardiac failure, or with postural hypotension or electrocardiographic T wave abnormalities. Patients receiving emetine (for amebiasis) or antimony (for schistosomiasis) may demonstrate electrocardiographic abnormalities without clinical symptoms or signs; it is then desirable to use alternative drugs or proceed with smaller dosages.

Cautious restriction of total dosage, using a weekly schedule (Torti, 1983), or continuous intravenous infusion of doxorubicin (Legha, 1982) may decrease toxicity (see above). Close clinical observation for early evidences of cardiac involvement is advised. Serial ECG, chest films, echocardiograms, and in selected cases, endomyocardial biopsy, may reveal early signs of myocardial toxicity. Decrease in the height of the R wave is an early sign of cardiac toxicity, and the risk:benefit ratio of continued therapy must be assessed. Cardiac enlargement and cardiac failure may develop slowly or rapidly.

Treatment

Withdraw cardiotoxic drugs and treat cardiac failure and arrhythmias as outlined in Chapters 10 and 15.

Prognosis

The prognosis is good if appropriate measures are taken before severe cardiac failure occurs, poor if the offending drug is continued after early cardiac toxicity is manifest. Mild to moderate cardiac failure subsides gradually after the cardiotoxic drug is stopped.

CHRONIC CARDIOMYOPATHIES

This is a miscellaneous group of diseases of unknown cause (not related to known causes such as coronary, hypertensive, valvular, or congenital heart

Table 17–5. Causes of death in 301 cases of rheumatic fever and heart disease among 1000 patients after 20 years.*

Rheumatic Heart Disease		
Rheumatic fever Congestive failure	231	(77%)
Subacute infective endocarditis	26	
Acute infective endocarditis	4	30 (10%)
Other causes:		
Cerebral embolism	3	
Sudden and unexpected	10	30 (10%)
Uncertain	8	
Unrelated disease or accident	9	
Possible Rheumatic Heart Disease		
Unrelated disease or accident	10	(3%)

*Modified and reproduced, with permission, from the American Heart Association, Inc., Bland EF, Jones TD: Rheumatic fever and rheumatic heart disease: A 20-year report on 1000 patients followed since childhood. *Circulation* 1951;4:836.

diseases), classified on the basis of clinical and hemodynamic features into 3 types: (1) congestive (dilated or primary) cardiomyopathy, with clinical features of cardiac enlargement, increased cardiac volume, and symptoms and signs of congestive failure with poor systolic pump function; (2) hypertrophic (obstructive) cardiomyopathy; and (3) restrictive cardiomyopathy, with infiltrative myocardial disease associated with endomyocardial fibrosis, amyloid disease, scleroderma, hemochromatosis, and other disorders that interfere with left ventricular filling and emptying (impaired diastolic function) (Goodwin, 1972).

The clinical division into these 3 types is imperfect because of overlap (eg, amyloid heart disease may be both restrictive and congestive). Conduction defects may be predominant in some cardiomyopathies (eg, Chagas' disease; sarcoid).

1. CONGESTIVE (DILATED OR PRIMARY) CARDIOMYOPATHY

Dilated cardiomyopathy is a nonspecific diagnosis; there are no clinical characteristics that differentiate it from other myocardial diseases leading to congestive failure. Possible causes are (1) excessive alcohol intake over a period of many years; (2) ischemic cardiomyopathy (see Chapter 8); (3) acute viral myocarditis (frequency is controversial); (4) diabetes mellitus affecting the small vessels of the heart, causing vasculitis, heart failure, and anginal pains similar to those of large-vessel coronary disease, but with the main coronary arteries often remaining normal; and (5) deficiencies of thiamine and other nutrients. Endomyocardial biopsy may be useful in establishing the underlying cause of cardiomyopathy in some patients (Parrillo, 1984).

As newer immunochemical techniques are applied to the investigation of congestive cardiomyopathy, specific etiology may become apparent.

Clinical Findings

A. Symptoms: The disease is suspected early in patients who have dyspnea, chest pain, or palpitations. Dyspnea may progress from dyspnea on exertion to orthopnea, paroxysmal nocturnal dyspnea, and pulmonary edema. When right heart failure supervenes, peripheral edema may be a prominent symptom.

The chest pain is nondescript and may be related to pulmonary congestion or, if pleuritic, to pulmonary embolism. Pericardial pain is rare.

Patients who complain of palpitations may have chronic atrial fibrillation or paroxysmal atrial or ventricular arrhythmias. Ventricular premature beats occur in about half of cases; ventricular tachycardia or fibrillation usually occurs late. Recognition of arrhythmias is increased if ambulatory monitoring or exercise electrocardiographic tests are used. Complex arrhythmias or conduction defects can be identified in at least one-third of symptomatic patients and may explain some cases of sudden death.

Dizziness or syncope may occur from bradyarrhythmia or ventricular conduction defects secondary to fibrosis.

Symptoms of pulmonary or systemic emboli may occur, sometimes dominating the clinical features.

B. Signs: The signs are those of cardiac hypertrophy or cardiac failure (see Chapter 10). The cardiac failure is usually left ventricular with pulmonary rales, left ventricular gallop rhythm, and left ventricular heave that is displaced downward and to the left. If the disease is more advanced, right ventricular enlargement and congestive heart failure are found with a raised venous pressure and pulsating neck veins and liver, an enlarged tender liver, and dependent edema of the legs or sacrum. Thirty to 40% of patients with cardiomyopathy have a history of hypertension, but hypertension is not usually present in patients presenting with cardiac failure.

Signs of pulmonary emboli (see Chapter 19) or systemic emboli (see Chapter 20) may be found.

C. Laboratory Findings: There are no specific laboratory findings unless the congestive cardiomyopathy is due to a specific disease such as myocardial ischemia.

D. Electrocardiographic Findings: Changes on the ECG include left ventricular hypertrophy (see Chapter 9), ventricular and atrial arrhythmias (see Chapter 15), conduction defects (see Chapter 14), and nonspecific ST–T abnormalities.

E. X-Ray Findings: There is cardiac enlargement, chiefly left ventricular, with a large cardiac volume and with pulmonary congestion but without disproportionate left atrial enlargement, calcified valves, or abnormalities of the aorta (see Chapter 10).

F. Echocardiography: Echocardiography is particularly helpful in excluding pericardial effusion (see Chapter 18), aortic stenosis (when murmur is not heard because of severely decreased cardiac output) (see Chapter 13), and mitral valve disease (see Chapter 12) and in estimating left ventricular volume and ejection fraction (see Chapter 10). Massive increases in diastolic volume or decreases in ejection fraction (<20%) are of bad prognostic import.

G. Hemodynamic Findings and Angiography: The findings are those of a large-volume heart with poor contractions and generalized hypokinesia, decreased ejection fraction (usually ≤ 30–40%), increased left ventricular filling pressure, and possibly increased right atrial and right ventricular pressure (see Chapter 10).

Differential Diagnosis

A. Ischemic Cardiomyopathy: Increased left ventricular volume with decreased ejection fraction and generalized hypokinesia are seen on angiography in both dilated and ischemic cardiomyopathy. The latter may also exhibit greatly increased cardiac volume, segmental defects in contraction rather than symmetric hypokinesia, and myocardial ischemia during exercise.

B. Other Disorders: Other forms of cardiac disease (eg, valvular heart disease), hypertension, and secondary cardiomyopathies are discussed elsewhere in this book.

Treatment

There are no specific measures for congestive cardiomyopathy. Treat cardiac failure as outlined in Chapter 10. Anticoagulant and antiarrhythmic treatment may be valuable in some cases.

With severe cardiac failure, the use of vasodilator or inotropic therapy should be considered if the usual therapeutic agents fail.

Prognosis

Without treatment, the prognosis for dilated cardiomyopathy is poor. Two-thirds of deaths occur within 2 years. The 5-year mortality rate is about 50%; roughly one-third to one-fourth of patients survive for 10 years (Fuster, 1981; Beahrs, 1983). Endomyocardial biopsies are of prognostic value; survival is twice as long if the biopsy is normal as when it shows abnormalities (Shirey, 1980). Prolonged bed rest and intensive treatment of cardiac failure may improve the prognosis.

2. HYPERTROPHIC (OBSTRUCTIVE) CARDIOMYOPATHY

Classification & Diagnosis

The term hypertrophic obstructive cardiomyopathy identifies the 2 main features of the entity, hypertrophy and obstruction. The latter is not always present. The terms **idiopathic hypertrophic subaortic stenosis** and **asymmetric left ventricular hypertrophy** have been proposed. The former term suggests that the disease involves the aorta rather than the ventricle and makes no provision for right-sided lesions. The latter is unsatisfactory both because asymmetry is not an inherent feature of the lesion and because asymmetric hypertrophy may affect either the septum or the ventricle.

The cardinal features of hypertrophic obstructive cardiomyopathy are illustrated in Fig 17–6. The considerable hypertrophy, involving predominantly the septum, leads to decreased compliance of the left ventricle, decreased left ventricular diastolic filling, and increased left ventricular filling pressure to maintain adequate flow; the last causes dyspnea and decreased exercise tolerance. The anterior leaflet of the mitral valve comes into apposition with the septal muscle, and narrowing of the outflow tract gives rise to the characteristic systolic murmur. The severity of the obstruction varies with the level of the peripheral resistance, the adequacy of the central blood volume, and the degree of ventricular emptying. In some cases, septal hypertrophy involves the right side of the heart in addition to or instead of the left, and a picture resembling that of infundibular pulmonary stenosis is then seen.

Cause

The cause is not known. Some cases are present at birth; HLA abnormalities and familial distribution have been reported. In other cases, the condition appears to develop later in life in a patient with a clear history of essential hypertension.

Age & Sex Incidence

The disease occurs with equal frequency in both sexes and is seen in all age groups. The possibility of associated skeletal muscle disease has been raised.

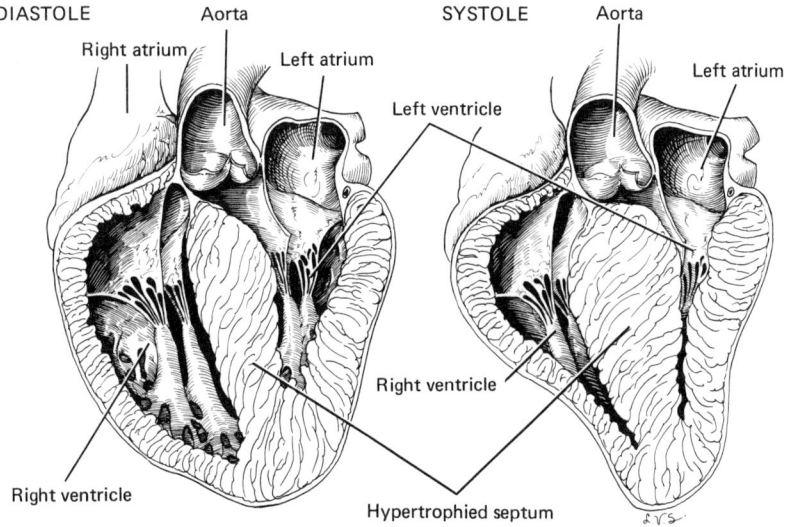

Cardinal features: *Left ventricular (especially septal) hypertrophy; systolic outflow obstruction; systolic anterior motion of mitral valve; excessive left ventricular emptying.*

Variable factors: *Severity; level of peripheral resistance; low resistance and low blood volume lead to obstruction.*

Figure 17–6. Hypertrophic obstructive cardiomyopathy (left lateral view). The cardinal features are displayed.

Criteria for Diagnosis

The criteria required for diagnosis are controversial but include left ventricular hypertrophy (predominantly in the septum), variable obstruction in the body of the left ventricle, decreased distensibility and impaired diastolic function and relaxation of the left ventricle, and a propensity to sudden death, especially after severe exertion. The best evidence of obstruction is a significant pressure difference between the body of the ventricle and the subvalvular area or aorta during left heart catheterization with a sidehole closed-tip catheter at left heart catheterization (Fig 17–7). Systolic anterior motion of the mitral valve on echocardiography is a sign of obstruction.

Evidence of hypertrophy can also be obtained in different ways (ECG, echocardiography, or angiography), but the results are often inconsistent. Emptying of the ventricle that is more complete than normal on angiocardiography is an important feature of the disease. Abnormalities in left ventricular diastolic function (impaired relaxation) have been described in most patients.

There are wide differences of opinion about the minimum abnormality required to establish the diagnosis. The dangers of creating cardiac neurosis by warning patients with minor or subclinical findings of the possibility of sudden death are obvious.

Clinical Findings

A. Symptoms:

1. History of heart murmur—The presence of a heart murmur is not an uncommon reason for referral to a cardiologist. A spurious history of rheumatic fever is sometimes given because the murmur was heard in childhood, perhaps in association with an episode of sore throat.

2. Dyspnea and chest pain—Dyspnea on exertion and chest pain are the commonest presenting symptoms. The pain is a dull, aching, substernal discomfort and radiates to the arm like angina pectoris. It is closely associated with dyspnea. Classic angina, in which there is pain without dyspnea, rapidly relieved by rest and nitroglycerin, is less common.

3. Other symptoms—Fatigue, dizziness, palpitations, and syncope are often reported. Sudden death occurs, especially in familial cases with marked septal hypertrophy, but the frequency of this outcome is not well documented, and it is not directly related to severity. Ventricular arrhythmias are common and may be responsible for symptoms or sudden death. Sudden death is more apt to occur in individuals under the age of 30 with a positive family history, and it even occurs in infants. The possibility of its occurrence cannot be predicted by symptoms, hemodynamic variables, or left ventricular septal thickness. The frequency of ventricular tachycardia with ambulatory ECG monitoring suggests at least one possible approach to prevention. Forty percent of cases of sudden death occur during or immediately after vigorous exercise (Maron, 1982). Progression of left ventricular hypertrophy is not prevented by treatment with propranolol (McKenna, 1982).

4. Factors influencing symptoms—The severity of symptoms varies with the state of the circulation. Anything that reduces peripheral resistance, such as a hot environment, pregnancy, standing up suddenly, exercise, or amyl nitrite inhalation, may induce or exaggerate outflow obstruction and bring on symptoms. Left ventricular failure occurs late and may follow the onset of atrial fibrillation. Congestive heart failure is uncommon.

B. Signs:

1. Pulse—The pulse has a bifid quality. The rapid initial upstroke is followed by a small tidal wave (Fig 17–8). The outflow obstruction develops after the start of systole, and the initial ejection of blood through an unobstructed outflow tract is responsible for the sharp rise in the pulse wave. As the obstruction develops during systole, it cuts down the rate of ejection and the pulse wave falls off, only to rise again later

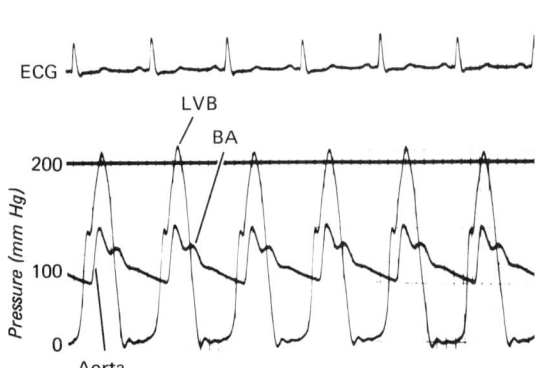

Figure 17–7. Simultaneous brachial arterial (BA) and left ventricular body (LVB) pressure tracings and ECG in a patient with hypertrophic obstructive cardiomyopathy.

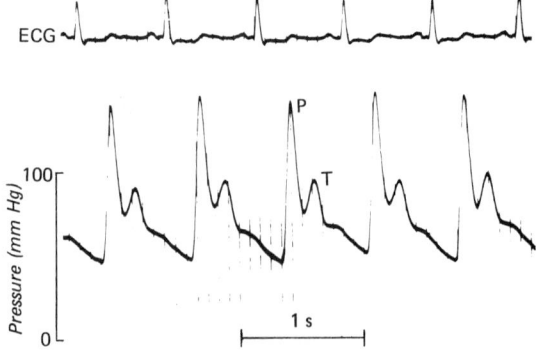

Figure 17–8. Bifid brachial arterial pulse in a patient with hypertrophic obstructive cardiomyopathy. The early percussion wave (P) is followed by a smaller tidal wave (T).

in systole. The characteristic carotid pulse can be helpful in elderly individuals whose systolic murmur may resemble aortic stenosis or mitral regurgitation.

2. Cardiac impulse—The same mechanism accounts for the findings on palpation at the apex of the heart in some cases, where a bifid impulse is felt during systole. The apical impulse may be bifid for another reason. The hypertrophied ventricle is less compliant than normal, and there is an abnormally forceful left atrial contraction. This produces a palpable presystolic impulse that gives a double apical impulse. When both of these factors are present, there is a triple cardiac impulse ("triple ripple") that is virtually pathognomonic of the condition (Fig 17–9).

3. Systolic murmur—There is almost invariably a harsh, long systolic murmur that peaks like other ejection murmurs in mid systole but starts early and may last for almost the whole of systole (Fig 17–9).

4. Other signs—Third and fourth heart sounds are commonly heard, but ejection clicks and aortic diastolic murmurs are rare. Mitral incompetence is often also present. The murmur may be best termed a **pansystolic ejection murmur**. Mitral diastolic murmurs may also occur. Left ventricular contraction may be prolonged, and paradox splitting of the second sound is sometimes present (Fig 17–10). Posture has a marked effect on the murmur, and sudden squatting often abolishes or lessens the intensity of the murmur, as it does the obstruction. The Valsalva maneuver (during the overshoot) increases the murmurs of mitral regurgitation and of obstruction to the outflow of the left ventricle by decreasing the size of the left ventricle as a result of the reduced venous return.

5. Effect of an ectopic beat—The peripheral arterial blood pressure is often smaller after a long diastolic pause following an ectopic beat (Brockenbrough's sign; Fig 17–11). The more forceful ventricular contraction (postectopic potentiation) increases the degree of outflow obstruction.

6. Effect of amyl nitrite—Amyl nitrite inhalation and isoproterenol induce or exaggerate the outflow obstruction murmur, whereas phenylephrine relieves obstruction (Fig 17–12). Such studies may help in determining the degree of associated mitral incompetence. Amyl nitrite also brings out the murmur of aortic stenosis, but this murmur is shorter and associated with a slowly rising pulse and should not lead to confusion.

C. Electrocardiographic Findings: Electrocardiographic evidence of left ventricular hypertrophy or left or (less often) right bundle branch block is almost always present, and the diagnosis is suspect if the ECG is normal. Arrhythmias are common, and Wolff-

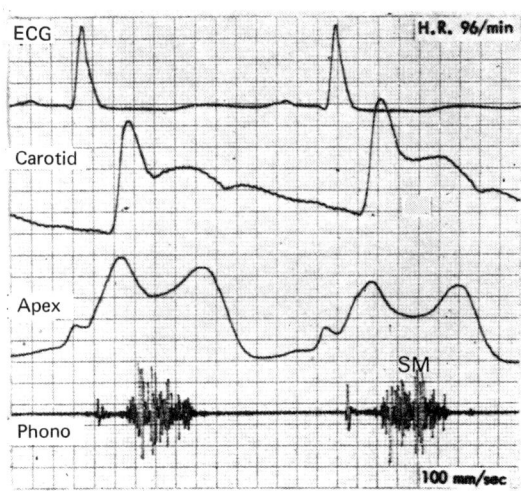

Figure 17–9. ECG, carotid pulse, apexcardiogram (Apex), and phonocardiogram (Phono) of a 36-year-old man with clinical and hemodynamic features of hypertrophic obstructive cardiomyopathy. Blood pressure was 120/50 mm Hg. Note the a wave and double humped apical impulse in the apexcardiogram, as well as the position of the systolic murmur (SM) late in systole. (Reproduced, with permission, from Burchell HB: Hypertrophic obstructive type of cardiomyopathy: Clinical syndrome. Pages 29–42 in: *Ciba Foundation Symposium: Cardiomyopathies.* Wolstenholme GEW, O'Connor M [editors]. Little, Brown, 1964.)

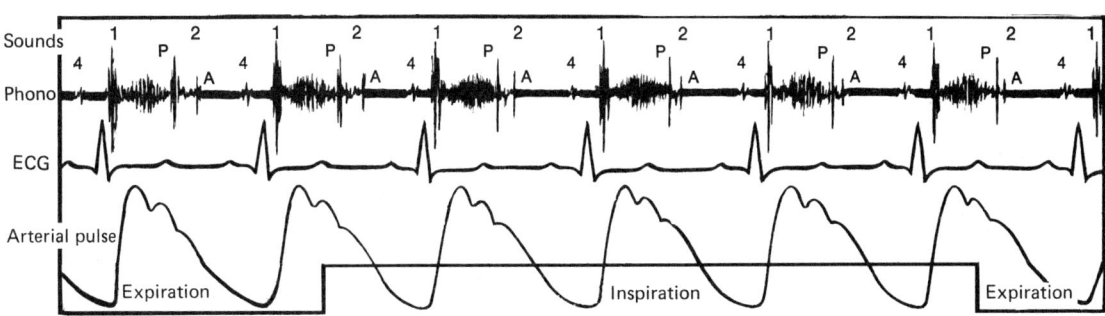

Figure 17–10. Phonocardiogram, ECG, and arterial pulse in hypertrophic obstructive cardiomyopathy. Phonocardiogram shows presystolic gallop, loud first sound, ejection murmur, and soft late A_2 with paradox splitting. (Courtesy of Roche Laboratories Division of Hoffman-La Roche, Inc.)

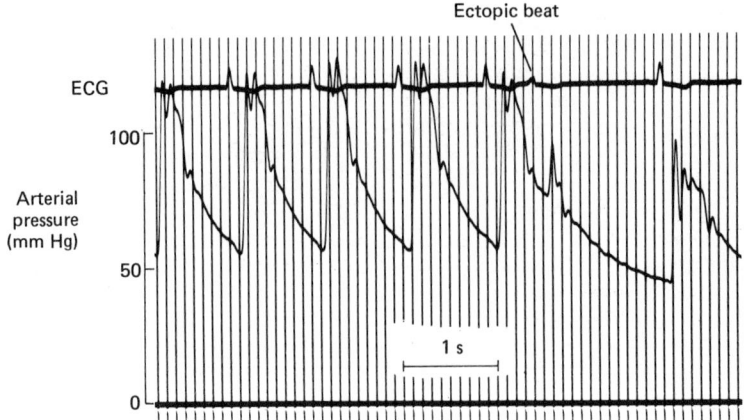

Figure 17–11. Bifid arterial pulse in a patient with hypertrophic obstructive cardiomyopathy showing Brockenbrough's sign, ie, decrease in systolic arterial pressure in a beat following an ectopic beat.

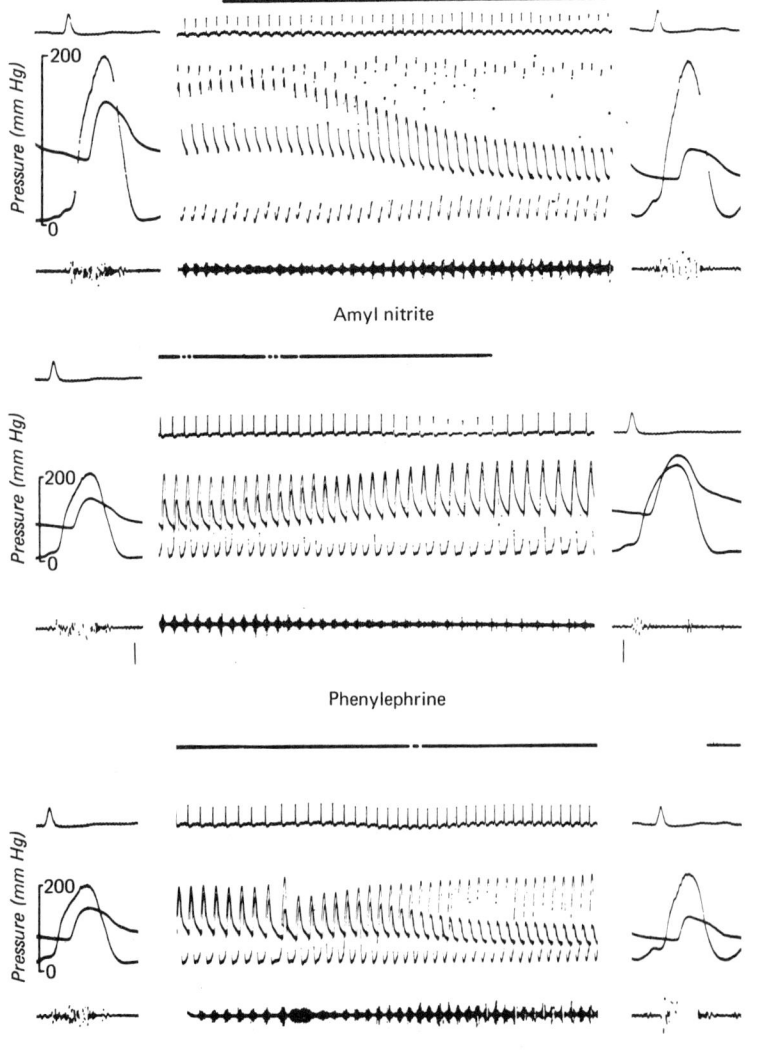

Figure 17–12. Simultaneous left ventricular and femoral artery pressure and phonocardiogram. *Top:* Increase of pressure gradient and systolic murmur with inhalation of amyl nitrite. *Middle:* Abolition of murmur and gradient with phenylephrine. *Bottom:* Increase of gradient and murmur with isoprenaline (isoproterenol). (Reproduced, with permission, from Nellen M in: *Hypertrophic Obstructive Cardiomyopathy.* Wolstenholme G, O'Connor M [editors]. Churchill Livingstone, 1971.)

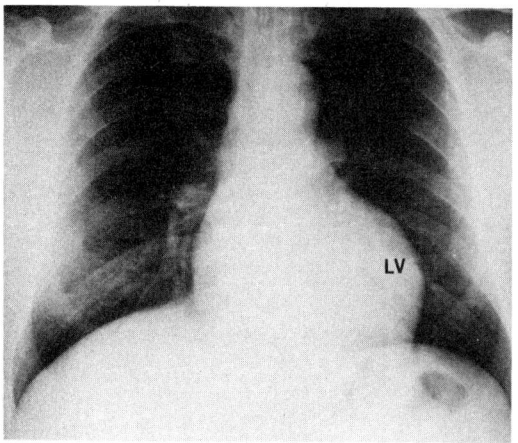

Figure 17-13. Chest x-ray of a patient with hypertrophic obstructive cardiomyopathy showing left ventricular predominance.

Parkinson-White forms of abnormality are sometimes seen.

D. X-Ray Findings: Left ventricular hypertrophy can usually be seen on chest x-ray (Fig 17-13), but the cardiac silhouette is often not much enlarged, because the hypertrophy takes place at the expense of the left ventricular cavity. The poststenotic dilatation seen in valvular aortic stenosis is absent, and calcification of the aortic valve is not seen on cinefluoroscopy. Left atrial enlargement is seldom marked, and pulmonary congestion may be present if left ventricular failure has occurred. Calcification in the mitral ring is found in about one-fourth of cases.

E. Special Investigations:

1. Noninvasive investigations–Echocardiography is the principal tool for clinical diagnosis. A normal aortic valve, asymmetric hypertrophy of the interventricular septum, and the characteristic systolic anterior motion of the anterior cusp of the mitral valve (Fig 17-14) strongly suggest the diagnosis. Sometimes in normal persons, systolic anterior motion of the mitral valve may be seen after amyl nitrite inhalation. Echocardiography can also provide noninvasive measurements of ventricular thickness. Indirect arterial pulse tracings, apexcardiograms, and diastolic time intervals show the nature of the bifid impulse and may demonstrate prolonged diastolic relaxation.

2. Invasive investigations–Left heart catheterization and left ventricular angiography are indicated in symptomatic cases in order to establish the diagnosis and severity of disease, especially if surgery is contemplated.

3. Pressure tracings–In patients with clear evidence of obstruction, there is a pressure difference between the body of the left ventricle and the subvalvular chamber. A closed-tip sidehole (Lehman) catheter should be used for studies in which the diagnosis is suspected. The outflow chamber distal to the obstruction can often be recognized by violent systolic oscillations of pressure. Withdrawal of the catheter from the body of the left ventricle to the outflow area ordinarily shows a pressure difference of 30–100 mm Hg in symptomatic cases, and no further pressure difference is seen on withdrawal across the aortic valve (Fig 17-15).

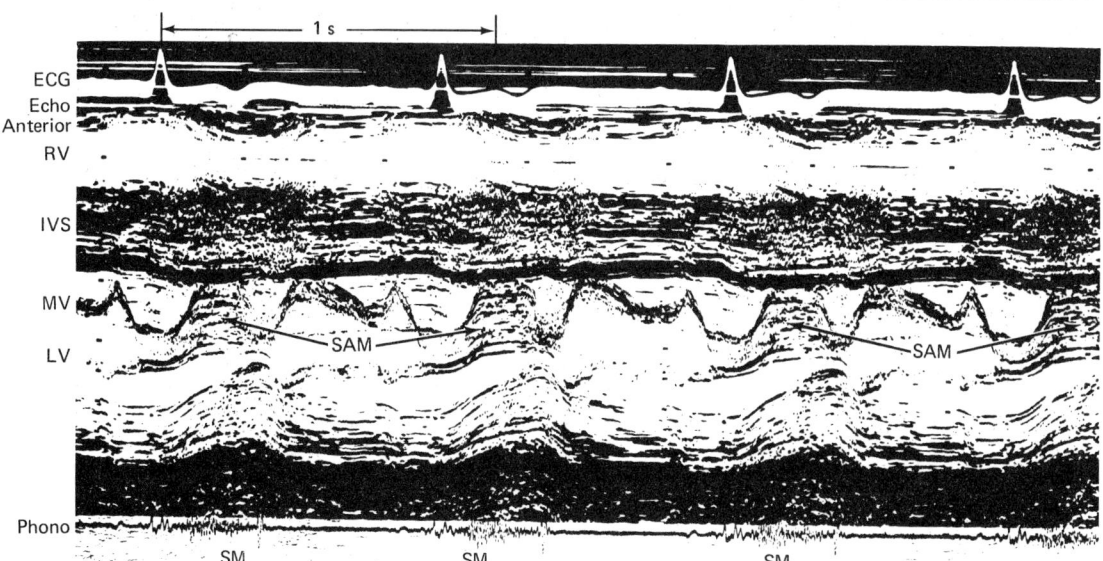

Figure 17-14. Echocardiogram showing systolic anterior motion (SAM) of mitral valve in a patient with hypertrophic obstructive cardiomyopathy. Septal (IVS) thickening and a long systolic murmur (SM) can also be seen. MV, mitral valve; RV, right ventricle; LV, left ventricle. (Courtesy of NB Schiller.)

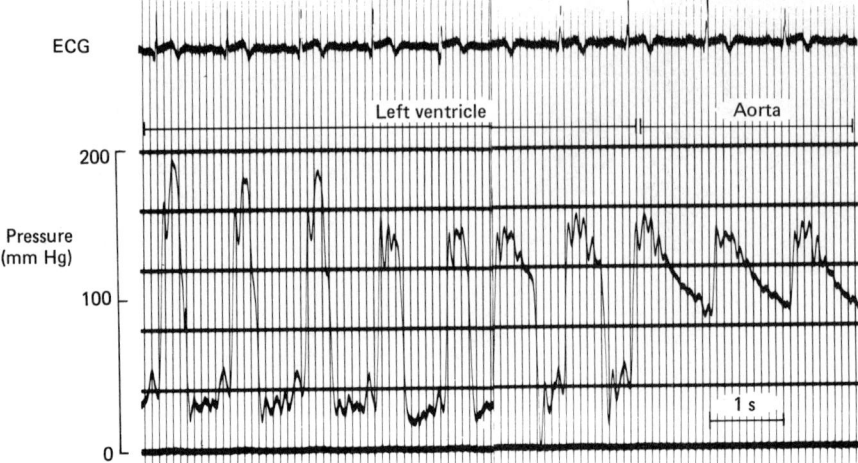

Figure 17–15. Withdrawal pressure tracing from left ventricle to aorta in a patient with hypertrophic obstructive cardiomyopathy. The pressure difference of 50 mm Hg is in the ventricle and not between the ventricle and the aorta.

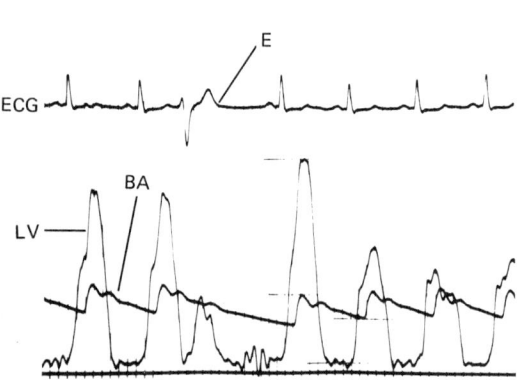

Figure 17–16. Pressure tracings in the left ventricle (LV) and brachial artery (BA) in a patient with hypertrophic obstructive cardiomyopathy. The pressure difference is greater after an ectopic beat (E).

4. Provocative tests–The hemodynamic findings can vary from moment to moment, even when provocative measures are not employed. The effects of ectopic beats on the pressure difference across the obstruction are shown in Fig 17–16. In cases in which there is little or no pressure difference within the ventricle, amyl nitrite inhalation can be used to reduce the peripheral resistance, encourage ventricular emptying, and induce obstruction. Similarly, an infusion of isoproterenol can be used to increase the force of cardiac contraction and bring about the physical signs, as shown in Fig 17–17. The Valsalva maneuver decreases venous return and increases or induces obstruction. Such provocative measures should only be used in patients with little or no obstruction, and simultaneous arterial and left ventricular pressure tracings should always be available.

5. Angiography–Left ventricular cineangiography is a useful confirmatory test. The hypertrophied left ventricular muscle mass can be seen to narrow the waist of the ventricle in early systole (Fig 17–18A). The subvalvular region during late systole takes on

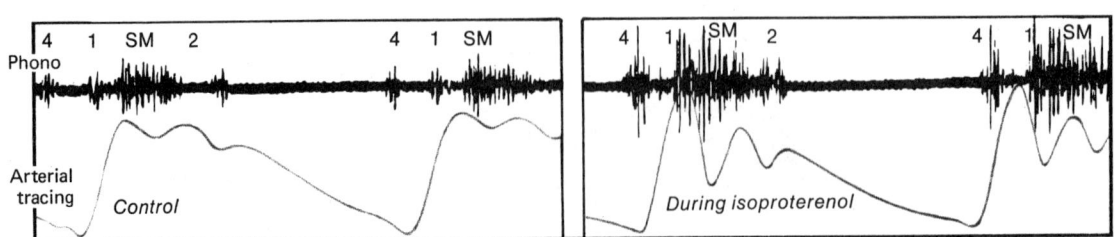

Figure 17–17. Phonocardiogram and external carotid pulse tracing in a patient with hypertrophic obstructive cardiomyopathy. During isoproterenol infusion, the atrial sound (4), the systolic murmur (SM), and the bifid nature of the arterial pulse are more obvious. (Courtesy of Roche Laboratories Division of Hoffman-La Roche, Inc.)

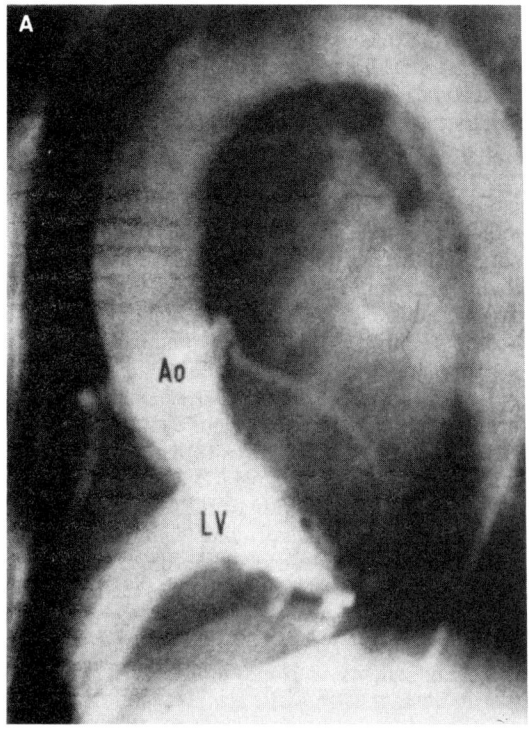 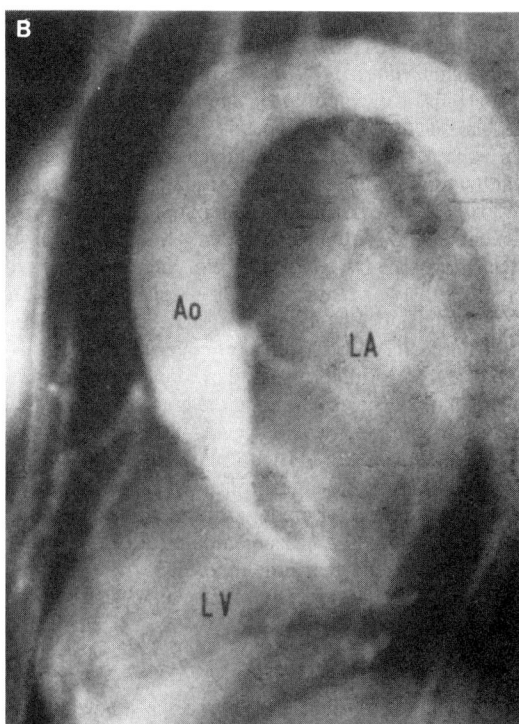

Figure 17–18. Angiographic features of hypertrophic obstructive cardiomyopathy. Single frame of angiogram following injection of contrast medium into the left ventricle in a patient with hypertrophic obstructive cardiomyopathy. In *A,* during early systole, the ventricular body is narrowed by hypertrophied muscle. In *B,* during late systole, the left ventricular body is empty and the cone-shaped shadow of the distal subvalvular chambers is seen. (Reproduced, with permission, from Cohen J et al: Hypertrophic obstructive cardiomyopathy. *Br Heart J* 1964;**26**:16.)

the appearance of an inverted cone filled with contrast material (Fig 17–18B). The body of the left ventricle is almost completely empty because of the exaggerated "muscle-bound" contraction that has expelled almost all of its contents. The base of the cone is the aortic valve; the posterior surface is the anterior cusp of the mitral valve; and the anterior surface is the hypertrophied interventricular septum. The tip of the cone is the site of the obstruction. Left ventricular angiography also shows mitral incompetence, but care must be taken to exclude spurious incompetence associated with ectopic beats. Angiography can also delineate rings and shelves of tissue which may be present in some cases and which are located below the aortic valve. Selective coronary angiography is seldom indicated, because the large coronary vessels in this disease fill well from aortic injections and are almost always normal.

6. Electrophysiologic studies–Because of the frequency of arrhythmias and conduction defects, intracardiac electrophysiologic studies have been performed and demonstrate prolongation of the HV interval (see Chapter 14) in the majority of patients (Ingham, 1978).

Differential Diagnosis

The physical signs of hypertrophic obstructive cardiomyopathy resemble those of mitral incompetence or ventricular septal defect more closely than those of aortic stenosis. There is, however, left ventricular outflow obstruction in both valvular and subvalvular lesions, and although the jerky, bifid pulse of obstructive cardiomyopathy is readily distinguished from the anacrotic, slow-rising pulse of aortic stenosis, this lesion does enter into the differential diagnosis in practice. Marked left ventricular hypertrophy is not seen in mitral incompetence or ventricular septal defect, and its presence in a patient with a long, harsh systolic murmur should suggest obstructive cardiomyopathy.

Complications

Atrial fibrillation and ventricular arrhythmias are important complications, and sudden death may occur. Young patients with familial disease seem most prone to these complications. Sudden death may be the first manifestation of hypertrophic cardiomyopathy, and it often occurs during or immediately after moderate or severe physical exertion (Maron, 1982). It may be related to ventricular arrhythmias or conduction defects. Left ventricular failure with pulmonary edema may follow the onset of atrial fibrillation. In other cases, left ventricular failure may actually relieve obstruction and help to improve the condition, because it leads to cardiac dilation. Mitral incompetence may be caused by long-term damage to the valve by turbulent flow in the outflow tract. Endocardial fibrosis and thickening are seen in this area and are thought to be due to mechanical trauma.

Treatment

In general, it is sound practice to reserve treatment for patients with symptoms and to follow all patients closely to determine whether their clinical status is stable or worsening.

A. Medical Treatment: Medical treatment may relieve symptoms, decrease the left ventricular outflow gradient, and prevent or decrease ventricular arrhythmias, but it has not unequivocally prevented progression of disease or affected survival rates (Anderson, 1984; Goodwin, 1982). Propranolol and other beta-adrenergic blocking drugs have been the mainstay of treatment for years. Sudden death can occur despite propranolol therapy. In some cases, the drug did not relieve the symptoms or left ventricular obstruction, and myomectomy was performed (see below). More recently, calcium entry–blocking agents have been employed before myotomy or myomectomy is attempted. Verapamil or nifedipine may benefit patients with hypertrophic cardiomyopathy by improving diastolic filling, increasing exercise capacity, and relieving symptoms, even when beta-blocking drugs have failed.

Verapamil, especially intravenously, may produce significant adverse effects, particularly hypotension, sinoatrial block with junctional rhythms, and atrioventricular block resulting from inhibition of atrioventricular nodal conduction (Epstein, 1981). Pulmonary edema has occurred but usually only in patients with left ventricular failure and pulmonary edema prior to therapy. Nifedipine lacks the sinoatrial and atrioventricular inhibitory effects of verapamil, but because it is a more potent vasodilator, it is more likely to produce hypotension.

Propranolol, the prototype of the beta blockers, is usually begun first because it decreases the force of left ventricular contraction to a level at which the ventricle no longer "obstructs its own outflow"; it also tends to prevent arrhythmias. The initial dose is 20–40 mg 3 times a day, and the dose is then increased until a satisfactory effect is obtained or side effects develop. Verapamil is usually begun at 40 mg orally every 8 hours, and this may be increased to tolerance. It should not be used if the patient has a history of pulmonary edema or if the left ventricular filling pressure is significantly elevated (> 20 mm Hg). Nifedipine has been used in a dose of 10 mg sublingually twice daily. Both verapamil and nifedipine increase the peak rate of left ventricular diastolic filling without affecting systolic function (Chatterjee, 1982; Lorell, 1982; Bonow, 1983). Amiodarone, 400–600 mg/d, abolishes ventricular tachycardia in most patients who have it and is significantly superior to verapamil; its important side effects are described in Chapter 15. It remains to be seen whether amiodarone decreases the incidence of sudden death thought to be due to the arrhythmia. McKenna (1985) believes it does.

B. Surgical Treatment: Surgical incision and resection of hypertrophied muscle bundles in the ventricular outflow tract is advocated in some centers, mitral valve replacement has been recommended in others, and even the production of bundle branch block has been suggested as a mode of therapy. It seems likely that the wide spectrum of cases accounts for the differences of opinion about treatment. Surgery is not advocated until medical treatment has been given a thorough trial. Muscular incision and resection are then recommended (Morrow, 1980; Beahrs, 1983). In one large series, improvement following surgery was only moderate, and the mortality rate was 8%; half of the postoperative deaths were sudden deaths. The overall annual mortality rate was 3.5% (Maron, 1978).

The question of whether to give digitalis often arises in patients with evidence of left ventricular failure. Digitalis has been thought to aggravate obstruction because it increases the force of cardiac contraction. The drug should obviously not be used unless left ventricular failure is present. In our experience, it is not harmful in patients with cardiac failure.

Prognosis

The long-term prognosis of hypertrophic obstructive cardiomyopathy is not fully established. The annual mortality rate is approximately 3% per year; most deaths are sudden deaths, especially in young patients. Most patients live for years; heart failure, systemic emboli, infective endocarditis, and arrhythmias occur gradually in older patients over a period of years (McKenna, 1981; Nishimura, 1983). The course is more benign when abnormal muscular hypertrophy develops later in life. In some patients, the characteristic murmur disappears with the onset of left ventricular failure, and the evidence of obstruction disappears as the failing ventricle dilates.

Pregnancy is well tolerated in young women with the disease unless cardiac failure is present.

3. RESTRICTIVE CARDIOMYOPATHY

This is the third general category of Goodwin's classification of cardiomyopathy and is the least common. It frequently overlaps the category of hypertrophic cardiomyopathy where hypertrophic changes decrease compliance of the ventricles and simulate some of the findings of restrictive cardiomyopathy. (See also Endomyocardial Fibrosis, p 562.) The term "restrictive" is used because a characteristic feature of the condition is a restriction in ventricular filling resulting from a noncompliant, less distensible ventricle. An infiltrative pathologic process is responsible for the decreased compliance and other clinical features.

Cause

Any infiltrative process of the myocardium that results in fibrosis or thickening, such as amyloid disease, hemochromatosis, glycogen storage disease, sarcoidosis, or endomyocardial fibrosis with or without the idiopathic hypereosinophilic (Löffler's) syndrome, may result in restriction in ventricular filling and the subsequent clinical picture of restrictive cardiomyopathy.

Pathology

The pathology is that of the underlying infiltrative process, occasionally of unknown cause but often due to one of the diseases mentioned below. The 2 ventricles may not be enlarged, but there is systemic venous congestion of the liver and peripheral tissues.

Criteria for Diagnosis

The diagnosis is usually made in a patient who has symptoms and signs of congestive heart failure and a raised venous pressure but in whom the heart is not significantly enlarged and who has echocardiographic findings of normal left and right ventricular dimensions, a relatively normal ejection fraction, and echoes representing fibrosis that do not correspond to vascular regions (Wahr, 1982; Acquatella, 1983). The absence of considerable hypertrophy of the left ventricle is in contrast to the clinical features of systemic congestive (right heart) failure.

The manifestations of the disease vary in the early and late stages; in full-blown cases, the disease may be indistinguishable from chronic constrictive pericarditis (see Chapter 18, p 581).

Clinical Findings

A. Symptoms: The earliest symptoms may be fatigue, peripheral edema, enlargement of the abdomen owing to ascites, and occasionally dyspnea resulting from pulmonary congestion but not acute pulmonary edema. The symptoms may be severe in the later stages.

B. Signs: The dominant features are raised venous pressure with prominent x and y descents and signs of systemic venous congestion, with enlarged, pulsating liver, slight or moderate ascites, and dependent edema. There may be a third heart sound later in the disease. Cardiac murmurs are usually minimal or absent. The carotid pulse is usually normal. Right or left ventricular heaves are usually absent, indicating no significant cardiac hypertrophy. Premature beats (usually ventricular) may occur, but cardiac arrhythmias (including ventricular tachycardia or fibrillation) or conduction defects may be late manifestations.

C. Laboratory Findings: The laboratory findings are those of the underlying disease. A striking eosinophilia characteristic of Löffler's syndrome should always be sought.

D. Electrocardiographic Findings: The electrocardiographic changes are usually nonspecific, with slight ST–T changes not characteristic of any particular condition. Considerable left ventricular hypertrophy is uncommon, but many different kinds of conduction defects or arrhythmias may occur.

E. X-Ray Findings: Left ventricular hypertrophy may be seen on the chest x-ray, but it is rarely dominant. Pulmonary venous congestion may occur, but it is usually not severe. Calcification of the pericardium is absent, but intracardiac calcification may occasionally be present.

F. Special Investigations:

1. Noninvasive investigations–Echocardiography provides one of the chief means of diagnosing the disease (see above, under criteria for diagnosis).

2. Invasive investigations–Cardiac catheterization and left ventricular angiography are helpful. The absence of segmental akinesia or of significant enlargement of one ventricular cavity is helpful in excluding congestive cardiomyopathy or old scars from myocardial infarction. Coronary arteriograms are usually normal. The characteristic hemodynamic feature of restrictive cardiomyopathy consists of elevation of the filling pressure of both ventricles, associated with a prominent x and rapid y descent, producing an M-shaped pattern. Left and right atrial pressures are also increased. The ventricles display the early diastolic dip and late plateau characteristic of restriction of ventricular filling, often indistinguishable from chronic constrictive pericarditis.

Differential Diagnosis

The main disease that must be ruled out is chronic constrictive pericarditis, which may produce identical clinical, radiologic, and hemodynamic findings (see Differential Diagnosis, p 582). Congestive cardiomyopathy must also be excluded. The ejection fraction is usually decreased below 30% and ventricular volumes are large in severe congestive cardiomyopathy, whereas these values are essentially normal in restrictive cardiomyopathy. Contractility of the left ventricle as seen in the left ventricular angiogram is essentially normal in restrictive cardiomyopathy but significantly reduced in congestive cardiomyopathy.

Treatment

There is no specific treatment for restrictive cardiomyopathy. Treatment of the underlying disease and of cardiac failure is indicated, and the patient should receive good general nutrition. If the patient has Löffler's syndrome, prednisone may lower the eosinophil count and decrease endocardial fibrosis. In a few patients, mitral valve replacement and resection of thrombotic and fibrosed areas of the endocardium proved useful, but the mortality rate was 10% (Graham, 1981).

Prognosis

The prognosis is that of the underlying disease, which may be slowly or rapidly progressive. Death usually occurs in a few years and is most commonly due to severe cardiac failure. Occasionally, sudden death may occur as a result of conduction defects or arrhythmias. Systemic emboli, especially those associated with endomyocardial fibrosis, may also cause death.

CHRONIC DISEASE OF THE MYOCARDIUM SECONDARY TO KNOWN METABOLIC DISEASE

THYROTOXIC HEART DISEASE

The increase in metabolic rate resulting from excess production of thyroid hormone requires that cardiac output and peripheral blood flow be increased, producing symptoms and signs that may be confused with heart disease. If there is underlying heart disease, the manifestations of cardiac failure in thyrotoxicosis are even more obvious. It may be difficult to distinguish the cardiac disease from the effects of circulatory hyperactivity produced by the increased metabolic rate. There is controversy in the literature about whether thyrotoxicosis per se can cause cardiac failure.

Clinical Findings

A. Symptoms: The predominant symptoms are those of the underlying thyrotoxicosis. Nervousness, agitation, sweating, palpitations, tremor, diarrhea, and weight loss are the usual symptoms. Dyspnea is usually not prominent.

There is a clear relationship between age and the prevalence of atrial fibrillation and cardiac failure; both are uncommon below age 40. The increase in frequency of both with age suggests that thyrotoxicosis unmasks subclinical coronary or hypertensive heart disease. Atrial fibrillation may induce cardiac failure in older patients with thyrotoxicosis.

B. Signs: Patients may have tachycardia, peripheral vasodilatation, sweating, systolic hypertension with increased pulse pressure, rapid upstroke of the carotid pulse, and flow murmurs in the heart. The signs may be less obvious in patients over 60 years of age. Eye signs are infrequent, and at least one-third have no palpable enlargement of the thyroid gland (Davis, 1974).

1. Predominant cardiac findings–Manifestations of hyperthyroidism are usually present in these patients but are often overlooked because cardiac symptoms are dominant. One can suspect the diagnosis by noting the warm, moist hands and relatively quick movements, which are surprising for a patient in heart failure.

2. Overlooked thyrotoxicosis–Thyrotoxicosis should always be suspected in patients with unexplained atrial fibrillation or congestive heart failure poorly responsive to digitalis therapy or in patients with systolic hypertension with a wide pulse pressure and a normal or short circulation time. This latter finding is in contrast to the delayed circulation time usually seen in patients with cardiac failure.

3. Absence of thyrotoxic symptoms–In so-called **apathetic thyrotoxicosis,** the patient is subdued and lacking in energy instead of excited and nervous. Patients with apathetic facies may have tremor, but hyperactive movements are more common. Increased peripheral blood flow with hyperemia often results in what has been called ''salmon skin.''

4. Cardiac symptoms and signs–Cardiac manifestations, mainly atrial fibrillation, may precede signs of thyrotoxicosis by months or years. Paroxysmal atrial tachycardia is infrequent, although atrial fibrillation is present in almost half of patients over age 60.

C. Laboratory Findings: Laboratory tests that help in the diagnosis of thyrotoxicosis are summarized in Table 17–6.

D. Electrocardiographic Findings: Except for sinus tachycardia, there are no abnormal signs on the ECG unless atrial fibrillation supervenes or independent cardiac disease is present.

E. X-Ray Findings: The chest x-ray is normal unless cardiac failure or pericardial effusion has developed, with cardiac enlargement or pulmonary congestion.

F. Special Investigations: The ejection fraction in hyperthyroidism is increased at rest but does not increase further and may fall with exercise. When patients are rendered euthyroid, the ejection fraction becomes less at rest but increases with exercise and may be greater during exercise than when the patient was hyperthyroid, suggesting abnormal left ventricular function with exercise (Forfar, 1982).

Differential Diagnosis

Overt thyrotoxicosis is usually obvious. Evidence of raised cardiac output, including vasodilatation and warm, moist skin, is important in differentiating thyrotoxic patients from those with anxiety states, in whom there may be increased sweating but cold, moist skin. Sleeping tachycardia is an important sign. Other causes of unexplained atrial fibrillation must be excluded if this is the presenting symptom or sign (eg, ''silent'' mitral stenosis, atrial septal defect, coronary heart disease, left atrial myxoma, or infective endocarditis). If weakness and weight loss are dominant findings, one must exclude neoplasms, various types of myopathies, liver disease, myasthenia, and depression. If cardiac failure due to no apparent cause is the presenting manifestation, one must exclude ischemic coronary cardiomyopathy, dilated cardiomyopathy, or cardiomyopathy associated with various systemic disorders (see below) as well as common varieties of cardiac failure that may have obscure features (valvular heart disease, atrial septal defect, ''burned-out'' hypertension, coronary disease, and cardiac failure resulting from untreated atrial fibrillation with a rapid ventricular rate).

Definitive diagnosis in these ''atypical'' cases is possible with the use of relatively specific biochem-

Table 17–6. Role of laboratory tests in diagnosis of thyrotoxicosis.*

Test	Normal Range†	Comment
Protein-bound iodine (PBI)	4–8 µg/dL	Classic test now largely supplanted by more specific T_4 test.
Serum thyroxine (T_4) concentration		
Total	4–11.5 µg/dL	Elevated values usually confirm hyperthyroidism unless T_4-binding globulin is also high.
Free	0.8–2.4 ng/dL	Independent of binding globulin.
Serum triiodothyronine (T_3) resin uptake	Female: 24–34% Male: 25–35%	A reflection of available binding sites in T_4-binding globulin. Should be used only in conjunction with measurement of serum T_4 to exclude possibility that increase in total serum T_4 results from increase in T_4-binding globulin.
Serum T_3 concentration	80–100 ng/dL	Considerable variability from laboratory to laboratory. Normal values decrease with advancing age. Absolute concentration of T_3 in serum is invariably elevated in hyperthyroidism and is elevated in association with normal serum T_4 in T_3 toxicosis.
Thyroid suppression	In 24-hour radioactive iodine uptake, decrease to less than 50% of initial value	Useful in some patients if serum measurements are borderline. Will not confirm hyperthyroidism, but a normal test excludes the diagnosis.
Serum thyroid-stimulating hormone concentration (TSH)	5–10 µU/mL	Basal values of no use in diagnosis of thyrotoxicosis. Lack of increase in response to thyrotropin-releasing hormone suggests hyperthyroidism.

*Reproduced, with permission, from Ingbar SH: When to hospitalize the patient with thyrotoxicosis. *Hosp Pract* (Jan) 1975;10:45.
†Values considered normal may differ from laboratory to laboratory.

ical studies, notably serum T_3, T_4, and, if necessary, radioiodine uptake. These tests may be interfered with by previous iodine intake, either as medication or during radiologic studies using iodine-containing contrast media.

Treatment

The treatment of thyrotoxic heart disease is similar to the treatment of thyrotoxicosis in the absence of cardiac disease, consisting usually of antithyroid drugs such as propylthiouracil or methimazole followed in several weeks by radioiodine. If the thyroid gland is very large, substernal, or multinodular, subtotal thyroidectomy may be the treatment of choice.

If the cardiovascular manifestations, especially tachycardia, are dominant and severe, beta-adrenergic blocking agents such as propranolol may be used to control the rapid heart rate and decrease the cardiac output with exercise. They do not affect the underlying excess thyroid secretion. Oral propranolol is usually adequate in doses of less than 160 mg/d; it can be given intravenously at a rate no faster than 1 mg/min if the clinical situation dictates rapid reversal of the cardiac symptoms—especially if thyroid storm is thought to be imminent. Younger individuals, however, require larger doses—up to 320 mg/d—and usually require more definitive treatment. Overall thyroid function is not affected by administration of propranolol, which should be considered an adjunct to other definitive therapeutic methods (Ingbar, 1981).

Prognosis

The early diagnosis of thyrotoxicosis may influence the subsequent therapeutic results. Twenty percent of the patients studied by Sandler (1959) died of congestive heart failure within 1–7 years after starting therapy; complete relief of symptoms occurred in only 40% and was directly related to the disappearance of atrial fibrillation after treatment. In patients in whom sinus rhythm followed treatment with radioiodine, no deaths occurred and all patients with cardiac failure were improved. In patients in whom atrial fibrillation persisted, 20% died. Electric cardioversion for the treatment of atrial fibrillation should improve these results if atrial fibrillation persists after treatment of thyrotoxicosis with radioiodine.

MYXEDEMA & MYXEDEMA HEART

Myxedema heart is a well-known entity described by Zondek in 1918. In most myxedema patients, pericardial effusion and not cardiac failure is responsible for the enlarged cardiac shadow seen radiologically. Investigations using echocardiography have shown that some patients have dilatation of the left ventricle without significant pericardial effusion, whereas others have dominant pericardial effusion with an essentially normal cardiac shadow, and a third group have a combination of both. The cause of the effusion is not clearly understood.

In one large series of cases of myxedema, the disease occurred spontaneously in 40% of patients, but in the remaining 60% it followed either ^{131}I therapy or thyroidectomy. At present, many more cases of myxedema are seen following successful ^{131}I therapy, and it is feared that with the passage of time the numbers will increase.

Clinical Findings

A. Symptoms: The symptoms of myxedema include weakness; fatigue; paresthesias; dry, puffy skin; hoarseness; thick tongue; and slow pulse. Patients with myxedema heart characteristically complain of exertional fatigue more than of dyspnea, angina, and periorbital and peripheral edema. The pulse volume has a small amplitude, with a weak carotid upstroke—in contrast to what would be expected in bradycardia. Paresthesias, deafness, and a husky hoarse voice may be prominent.

B. Signs: The cardiac findings in myxedema are summarized in Table 17–7. The cardiac manifestations of myxedema are usually due to pericardial effusion rather than cardiac failure. Orthopnea, raised venous pressure, enlargement of the liver, gallop rhythm, and pulmonary venous congestion are often absent. Following the removal of pericardial fluid, the cardiac size is often found to be normal.

The slow pulse may be *only relative* in patients with myxedema. For example, the heart rate may be only 60–70 beats/min, which would be an unusual finding in a patient with cardiomegaly and presumed congestive heart failure.

Patients may have effusions in the pericardial,

Table 17–7. Cardiac findings in myxedema.*

1. Exertional fatigue, dyspnea, or angina pectoris.
2. Periorbital and peripheral edema.
3. Relative bradycardia.
4. Low voltage of QRS complex, T and P waves on ECG.
5. Enlargement of cardiac shadow with:
   a. Weak and distant heart sounds
   b. Difficulty in finding apex beat
   c. Poor cardiac contraction to palpation and fluoroscopy
   d. Small pulse with slow carotid upstroke in face of bradycardia.
6. Effusions in pericardium, pleura, and peritoneum; tamponade rare.
7. Echocardiography may reveal cardiac enlargement, pericardial effusion, or both.
8. Hemodynamic findings:
   a. Decreased O_2 consumption
   b. Decreased cardiac output
   c. Decreased pulse rate
   d. Normal arteriovenous O_2 difference
   e. Normal response of cardiac output, systemic resistance, and right atrial pressure to exercise.

*Modified and reproduced, with permission, from Sokolow M: Heart disease in patients with thyroid dysfunction: Medical Staff Conference, University of California, San Francisco. *Calif Med* 1968;**109**:309.

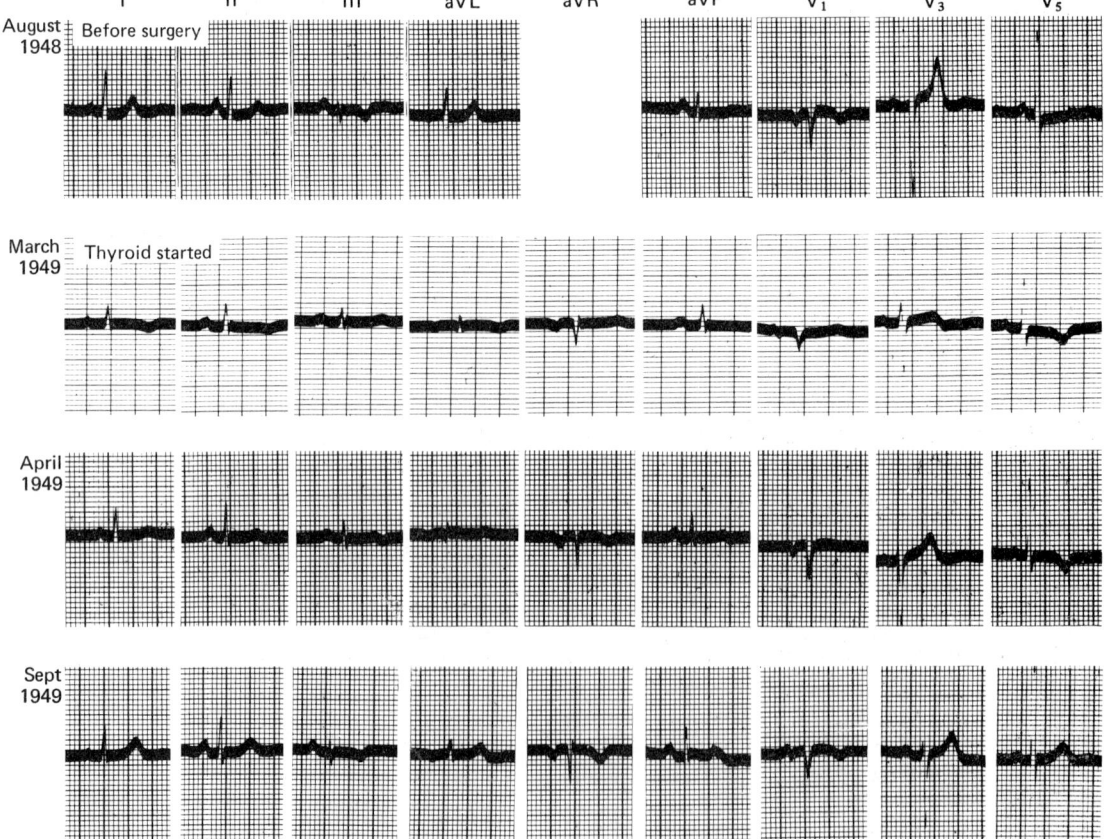

Figure 17–19. Hypothyroidism in a 47-year-old woman following thyroidectomy for hyperthyroidism in September 1948. BMR–51 in March 1949. Note progressive improvement in T waves after thyroid replacement was started in March 1949.

pleural, and peritoneal cavities; because of the slow development of effusion, large amounts of pericardial fluid may be found (2000–4000 mL).

C. Electrocardiographic Findings: Low voltage of the QRS complex as well as of the T and P waves suggests cardiac failure in patients with myxedema. A typical ECG showing the development and regression of T wave abnormalities in myxedema is presented in Fig 17–19.

D. X-Ray Findings: The cardiac shadow may be enlarged and may be due to cardiac failure, pericardial effusion, or a combination of the two (Fig 17–20).

E. Echocardiography: Echocardiograms can differentiate between enlarged cardiac shadows due to pericardial effusion and those due to left ventricular dilatation (Figs 17–20 and 17–21). Fig 17–20 shows a large pericardial effusion and decrease in the size of the heart following thyroxine therapy. Fig 17–21 presents an echocardiogram and serial chest films showing only minimal pericardial effusion but a dilated left ventricle, with a wide space between the anterior border of the mitral valve and the ventricular septum.

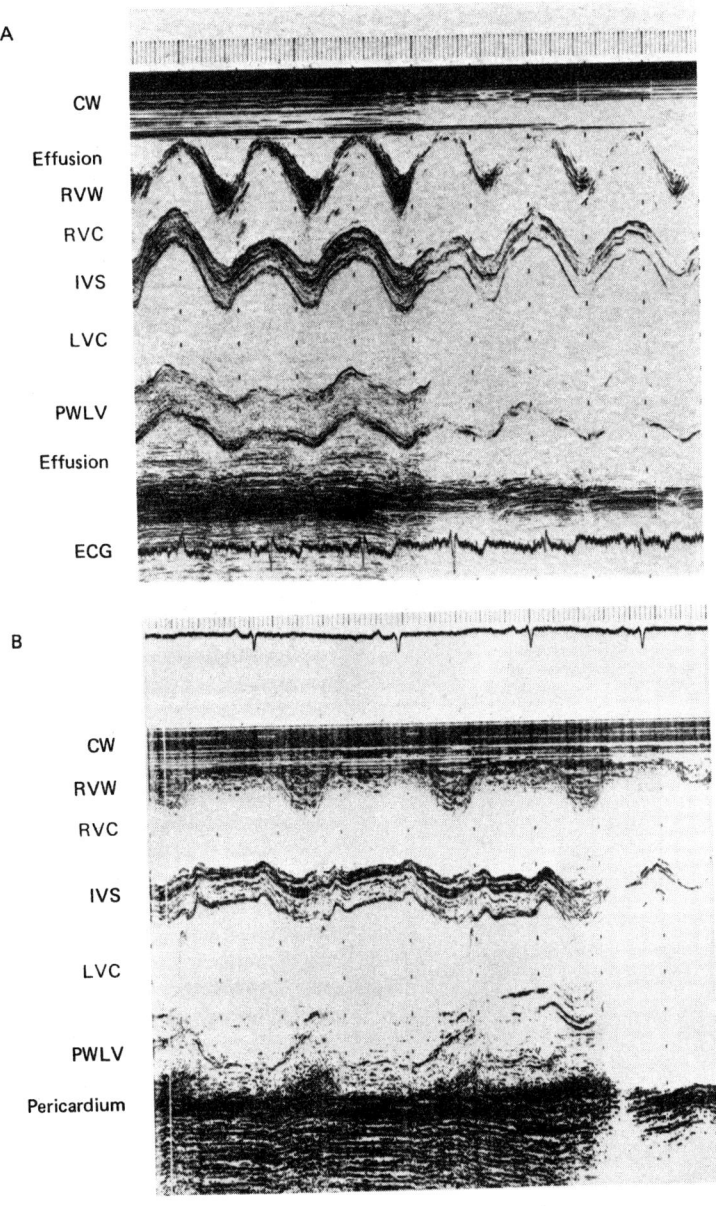

Figure 17–20. Echocardiogram of a 29-year-old woman with hypothyroidism (A) before and (B) after 2 months' treatment with levothyroxine sodium (Synthroid). CW, chest wall; RVW, right ventricular wall; RVC, right ventricular cavity; IVS, interventricular septum; LVC, left ventricular cavity; PWLV, posterior wall left ventricle.

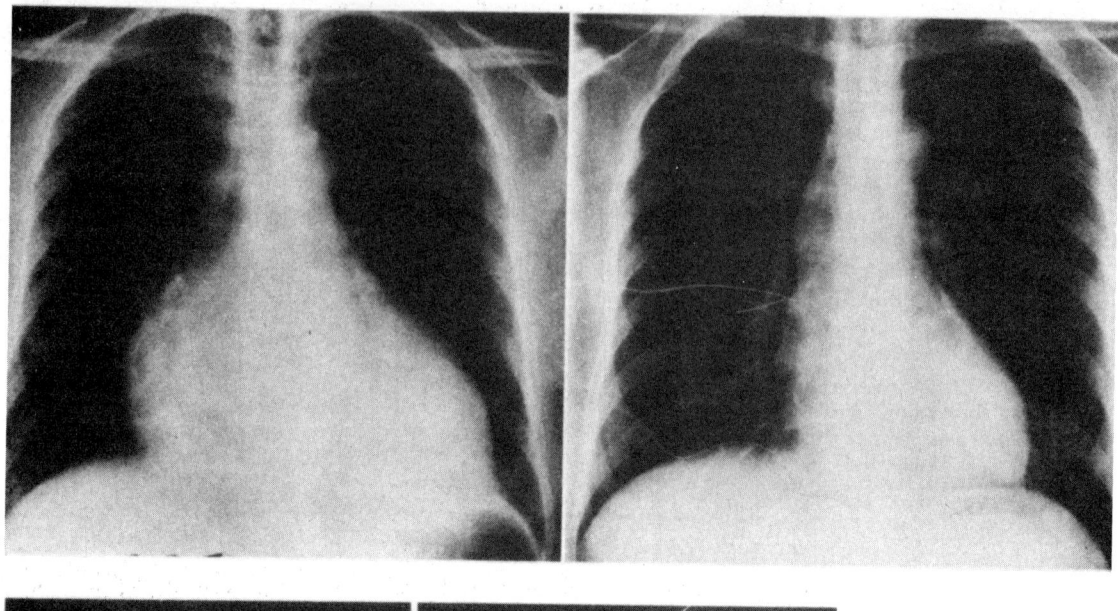

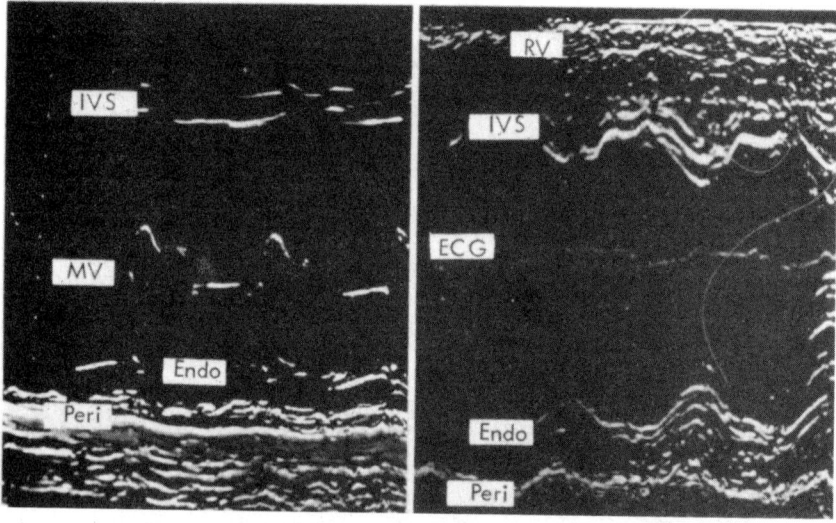

Figure 17–21. Top: Chest x-ray studies of patient with hypothyroid cardiomyopathy. **Left:** Before therapy, showing pronounced cardiomegaly. **Right:** Six months after institution of thyroxine therapy, the heart size has returned to normal. **Bottom:** Echocardiograms of patient with hypothyroid cardiomyopathy. **Left:** Before treatment, showing the dilated left ventricle (between IVS and Endo), with a short-axis diameter of 6.5 cm (normal: < 5.4 cm). Motion of interventricular septum and endocardial wall is notably reduced. A small posterior pericardial effusion is present. **Right:** After thyroxine replacement therapy. Left ventricular size is now normal (4.2 cm), and motion of the posterior left ventricular wall and interventricular septum is markedly improved. IVS, interventricular septum; MV, mitral valve; Endo, endocardium of posterior left ventricular wall; Peri, pericardium of posterior left ventricular wall; RV, anterior right ventricular wall. (Reproduced, with permission, from Reza MJ, Abbasi AS: Congestive cardiomyopathy in hypothyroidism. *West J Med* 1975;**123**:228.)

Following thyroxine therapy, left ventricular size becomes normal on chest films as well as echocardiograms.

F. Hemodynamic Data: Patients with myxedema heart do not require cardiac catheterization. The arteriovenous oxygen difference, response of cardiac output, peripheral resistance, and right atrial pressure to exercise are all normal. The cardiac index is low but increases normally with exercise. The cardiac index in myxedema is one-third that seen in patients with thyrotoxicosis.

Differential Diagnosis

The diagnosis of myxedema is frequently missed because the clinical manifestations occur slowly and subtly and may be attributed to aging, ie, as the patient tires more easily and becomes slower in thought and movement. Periorbital nonpitting edema, collections of serous fluid, and proteinuria may suggest nephritis. The diagnosis of cardiomyopathy is often made in myxedematous patients because of the presence of presumed cardiomegaly on radiologic examination.

Treatment

The response to treatment with thyroid hormone is dramatic, but severe angina, acute myocardial infarction, cardiac failure, psychotic reactions, and ventricular tachycardia may develop within 24–72 hours if the initial dose is too large. Treatment should be started with 12.5–25 μg of synthetic thyroxine and should be increased slowly by 12.5-μg increments over a period of weeks. Improvement may occur within days. If the patient has severe myxedema and develops angina pectoris following small-dose thyroid replacement therapy, a coronary bypass vein graft can be considered if a coronary arteriogram shows localized stenosis, in order to make thyroxine therapy feasible.

Prognosis

The enlarged heart shadow usually returns to normal after thyroid therapy with complete clinical resolution, often within a month, but relapses may occur rapidly if thyroid therapy is stopped.

ALCOHOLIC CARDIOMYOPATHY*

Excessive intake of alcohol may produce cardiomyopathy by a primary toxic effect on the heart, by associated nutritional deficiency (especially of thiamine, as in beriberi heart disease), or as a result of additives (cobalt in cobalt-beer cardiomyopathy). Chronic alcoholics may have intermittent thiamine deficiency or excessive requirements for thiamine, as when they develop fever owing to infections, or after a high-carbohydrate diet; therefore, a mixed picture of toxic alcoholic cardiomyopathy and nutritional beriberi heart disease may be found. Dietary deficiency of protein or calories infrequently causes chronic congestive cardiomyopathy. In populations afflicted by famine and in prisoners of war examined after a weight loss of about 20 kg, cardiac enlargement, hypoproteinemia, and cardiac failure are rarely seen; cardiac atrophy is much more common (Ramalingaswami, 1968). Endomyocardial fibrosis may be related to inadequate nutrition.

Involvement of the Liver

Alcohol not only affects the cells of the myocardium by direct toxic action; it also affects the cells of the liver, even in patients receiving good diets with adequate vitamins. As a result, patients may present with hepatic involvement as well as cardiac disease,

*See also beriberi heart disease and nutritional heart disease, pp 554 and 555.

although some patients tolerate large amounts of alcohol for many years without evident harm.

Relationship of Beriberi Heart Disease to Alcoholic Cardiomyopathy

In beriberi heart disease related to thiamine deficiency, high output failure is the predominant clinical feature. In contrast, the patient with alcoholic cardiomyopathy has signs of low cardiac output, weak pulses of small volume, and cold extremities. The heart is large and bulky, with a markedly decreased ejection fraction. Large doses of thiamine are ineffective in treatment of alcoholic cardiomyopathy, in contrast to beriberi heart disease.

Beriberi heart disease was formerly common in developing countries and found occasionally in the USA before it was known that thiamine supplements were necessary in patients receiving deficient diets. Alcoholic cardiomyopathy is common in persons who drink excessive alcohol daily, even though they may be receiving adequate nutrition and vitamins. Most cases of alcoholic cardiomyopathy in the USA are probably due to direct toxic action of alcohol on the myocardium.

Clinical Findings

The criteria for the diagnosis of alcoholic cardiomyopathy are similar to those of dilated or chronic congestive cardiomyopathy, with the exception of the history of excessive alcohol intake. The typical clinical picture is cardiac failure in a middle-aged person without coronary heart disease, hypertension, valvular heart disease, or congenital heart disease. There is a history of excessive alcohol intake over a period of many years; most patients have drunk more than 250 mL of whiskey or its equivalent every day for at least 10 years. Some believe that alcohol plays a role in at least half of all cases of chronic congestive cardiomyopathy.

A. Symptoms: The onset is usually insidious, with nonspecific fatigue, dyspnea, palpitations, and possibly edema.

B. Signs: There may be cardiac enlargement and left ventricular failure. When cardiac failure develops, it is low-output failure, with all its clinical features. The cardiac failure is chiefly left ventricular, but there may be right ventricular failure as well, with raised venous pressure, tricuspid insufficiency, a left or right ventricular heave, gallop rhythm, murmurs of functional mitral or tricuspid insufficiency and pulmonary rales, enlarged tender liver, and dependent edema. The arterial blood pressure may be elevated during severe failure; the pressure falls to normal when failure is improved with cardiac therapy.

C. Electrocardiographic Findings: Abnormalities, especially low voltage of QRS complexes, ST-T abnormalities, and left ventricular hypertrophy, may be present before the development of cardiac failure. Arrhythmias and conduction defects are common.

D. X-Ray Findings: Cardiac enlargement, cardiac failure, and pulmonary congestion may be present.

E. Special Investigations: In addition to left ventricular hypertrophy, patients have enlarged hearts with pulmonary venous engorgement; on coronary angiography and left ventricular cineangiography, the coronary arteries are normal and the ejection fraction is decreased, so that the heart is a large, boggy organ. Echocardiography can demonstrate the large left ventricle with decreased ejection fraction and the mitral valve floating within the left ventricular cavity (Fig 17–22).

Differential Diagnosis

Alcoholic cardiomyopathy must be distinguished from other congestive cardiomyopathies in patients with long-term excessive alcohol intake. Hypertension is excluded by normal blood pressure after restoration to the compensated state; coronary artery disease by the absence of angina pectoris or myocardial infarction; valvular heart disease by the decrease of murmurs when compensation is restored. Congenital heart disease is excluded by a negative history and no abnormalities on cineangiograms.

Treatment

If cardiomyopathy is discovered early, complete abstinence from alcohol may be beneficial, but later, abstinence may have only marginal benefit. Bed rest, intravenous thiamine (50 mg), and conventional treatment for heart failure are the mainstays of management. If this is not successful, vasodilatory or inotropic therapy is advised (see Chapter 10). If the disease is not too far advanced, improvement but not complete reversal may be achieved. Prolonged bed rest may be more effective in decreasing cardiac size in alcoholic cardiomyopathy than in ischemic cardiomyopathy, but relapse is common.

Prognosis

The heart may become much smaller and all cardiac symptoms may disappear following months of bed rest, but heart failure rapidly occurs when patients become ambulatory. Prolonged bed rest increases the hazard of multiple episodes of thromboembolism and has psychologic and economic consequences. With severe heart failure, the prognosis is poor—approximately a 50% mortality rate in 2 years (see Chapter 10).

BERIBERI HEART DISEASE

In the USA, beriberi heart disease is uncommon because thiamine deficiency severe enough to result in beriberi is rare. It is usually seen in malnourished chronic alcoholics, as described above. Beriberi is most common in populations and individuals (as in the Orient) who eat thiamine-deficient diets (Kawai, 1980).

Clinical Findings

Patients with beriberi have dyspnea, edema, and right heart failure in combination with warm extrem-

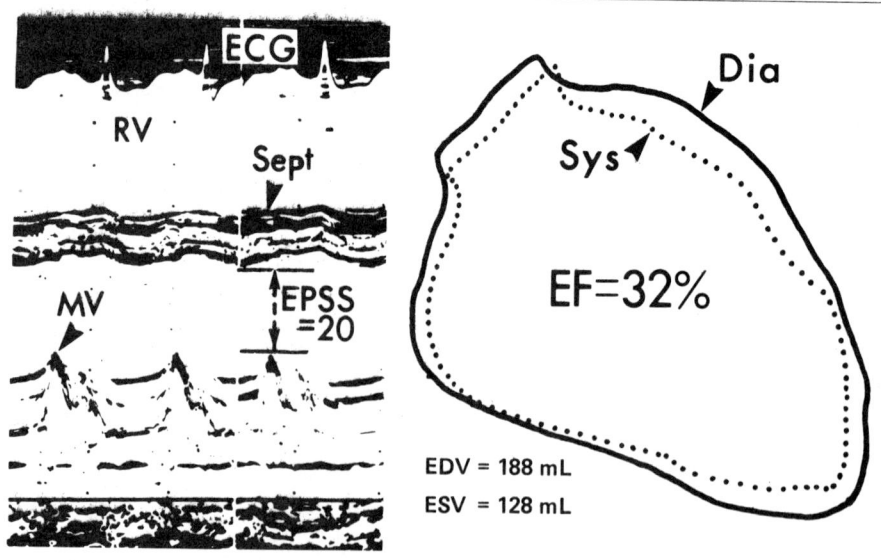

Figure 17–22. Echocardiogram of patient with alcoholic cardiomyopathy, demonstrating a decreased ejection fraction of 32%, a large end-diastolic volume, and a wide separation between the anterior portion of the mitral valve leaflet and the ventricular septum. EF, ejection fraction; EDV, end-diastolic volume; ESV, end-systolic volume; MV, mitral valve; RV, right ventricle; Sept, septum; EPSS, end (E) point of mitral valve separated from septum; Sys, systole; Dia, diastole. (Reproduced, with permission, from Massie BM et al: Mitral-septal separation: A new echocardiographic index of left ventricular function. *Am J Cardiol* 1977;39:1008.)

ities and bounding pulses characteristic of the high cardiac output state. When the low output phase of chronic alcoholic cardiomyopathy supervenes, consider the above descriptions.

Treatment & Prognosis

Beriberi heart disease improves rapidly when large doses (50 mg) of thiamine are given orally or parenterally. The skin temperature falls in hours after parenteral thiamine therapy. Enlargement of the heart and right heart failure subside within a matter of days to 1–2 weeks, and the syndrome does not occur when adequate thiamine supplements are given.

Beriberi heart disease is reversed by thiamine only when the process is relatively acute. Chronic alcoholic cardiomyopathy does not respond to thiamine.

NUTRITIONAL HEART DISEASE

As discussed above, malnutrition with selective deficiency of thiamine may cause beriberi heart disease and is in part responsible for the clinical features of alcoholic cardiomyopathy.

Deficiency of Calories, Proteins, Fats, & Vitamins (Total Malnutrition)

Under conditions of famine or semistarvation in which there are combined dietary deficiencies and not selective ones (as with thiamine), the heart responds with atrophy, interstitial edema, and disappearance of all pericardial fat, but the patient does not develop cardiac failure of either the beriberi type or the chronic alcoholic type (although the ECG may show nonspecific ST–T changes). Protein deficiency may cause kwashiorkor, a disease of children due to protein deficiency and characterized by hypoproteinemia and generalized edema. Cardiac failure due to protein starvation is uncommon both in children and (especially) in adults, although cardiac output may be decreased. When the diet is abruptly improved, as in liberated prisoners of war, generalized edema simulating cardiac failure may develop because of the abrupt increase in sodium intake associated with the normal diet; diuresis occurs spontaneously in weeks, aided by small amounts of diuretics. There have been no short-term cardiac sequelae.

The coincidence of chronic nutritional deficiency and endomyocardial fibrosis in developing tropical countries in Africa suggests that the latter may be due in part to malnutrition. However, in a famine in India in 1967, no mural thrombi or other abnormalities of the endocardial wall were found at autopsy (Ramalingaswami, 1968).

CHRONIC CARDIOMYOPATHY DUE TO SPECIFIC DISEASE ENTITIES, USUALLY OF UNKNOWN ORIGIN

SARCOIDOSIS

Sarcoidosis is a chronic granulomatous disease of unknown cause affecting chiefly young persons (average age about 25). Many organ systems are affected, but especially the lungs and the heart. The disease may cause cardiac failure, cor pulmonale, ventricular arrhythmias, heart block, and sudden death; autopsy studies show involvement of the heart in about 25% of fatal cases (Fig 17–23). Granulomas in patients with cardiac involvement are most commonly seen in the left ventricle, ventricular septum, and papillary muscles.

Clinical Findings

The most common cardiac feature is cor pulmonale secondary to fibrosis of the interstitial tissues of the lung and small pulmonary arteries resulting in pulmonary hypertension, right ventricular hypertrophy, and ultimately right ventricular failure (see Chapter 19).

A. Symptoms and Signs: The onset is with general symptoms of fatigue and malaise, acute uveitis, hilar adenopathy and nodular and fibrous pulmonary infiltrates on the chest film, and skin lesions, most characteristically erythema nodosum. Other systemic manifestations include hypercalcemia, hyperglobulinemia, and generalized adenopathy. Biopsy of the skin or lymph nodes shows extensive fibrosis and noncaseating granulomatous infiltration without organisms; the same process may affect the heart. Kveim-Siltzbach skin tests are positive in 80% of cases but are of limited value in diagnosis. The endocardium and valves are rarely involved. Cardiac failure is uncommon in sarcoidosis in general but occurs in a third of patients with cardiac sarcoidosis. There may be pericardial effusion, ventricular arrhythmias, syncope, or sudden death—especially upon exertion.

B. Serial Observations Leading to Treatment:

1. Pulmonary function studies and serial chest films demonstrate pulmonary fibrosis. If pulmonary function studies show progressive abnormalities, corticosteroid therapy may be tried, particularly if the patient has pulmonary hypertension, atrial gallop, a palpable pulmonary artery, or evidence on ECG of right ventricular hypertrophy.

2. Serial ECGs can detect progressive right ventricular hypertrophy, as well as involvement of the conduction system, in which case insertion of a pacemaker may prevent Stokes-Adams attacks and sudden death. Corticosteroids are usually ineffective when conduction defects and ventricular arrhythmias predominate in the clinical picture.

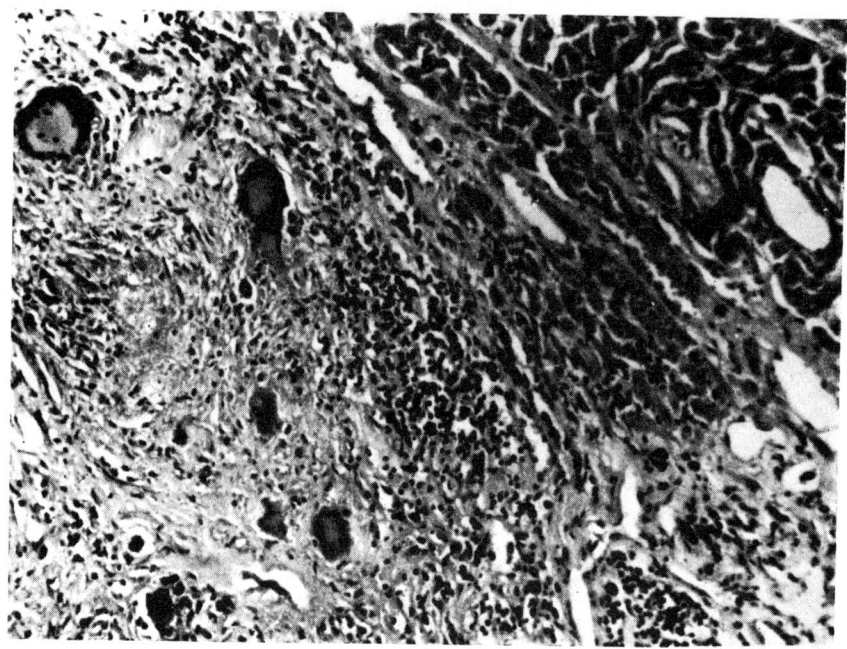

Figure 17–23. Sarcoid granuloma in myocardium with epithelioid cells, multinucleated giant cells, and lymphocytes. (× 350.) (Reproduced, with permission, from Fawcett FJ, Goldberg MJ: Heart block resulting from myocardial sarcoidosis. *Br Heart J* 1974;**36**:220.)

3. Thallium 201 scans may demonstrate perfusion defects due to granulomas; echocardiography may demonstrate impaired cardiac function even in asymptomatic patients (Kinney, 1980), but these findings do not influence treatment.

4. Endomyocardial biopsy may establish the diagnosis of myocardial sarcoma by demonstrating the typical granulomas.

C. Asymptomatic Features: Most patients, even with obvious sarcoid disease elsewhere, do not exhibit cardiac dysfunction, although electrocardiographic abnormalities (usually atrioventricular conduction delay, right ventricular hypertrophy, or ST–T changes) may be found. In proved sarcoidosis of the heart, complete atrioventricular block and atrioventricular and intraventricular conduction defects occur in approximately 25% of cases (Fig 17–24).

Prognosis

Once cardiac symptoms and signs appear, the prognosis is generally poor, but there are exceptions. Sudden death is responsible for most fatal cases. Early

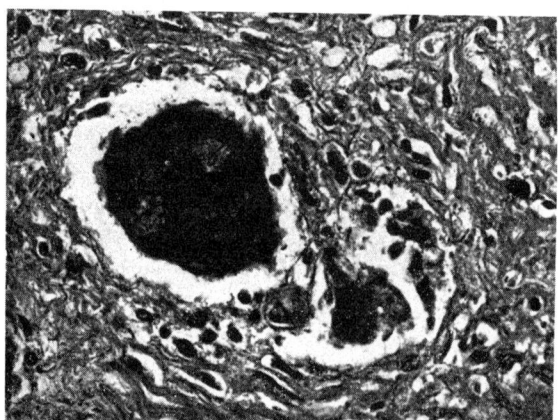

Figure 17–24. Atrioventricular bundle destroyed and replaced by dense fibrous tissue containing numerous giant cells in sarcoidosis. (Magnification × 365, H&E stain.) (Reproduced, with permission, from Porter GH: Sarcoid heart disease. *N Engl J Med* 1960;**263**:1350.)

recognition of conduction defects and treatment with pacemakers may improve the prognosis.

SYSTEMIC LUPUS ERYTHEMATOSUS

Lupus erythematosus is a systemic disease probably due to vasculitis secondary to autoimmunity and is characterized by deposition of immune complexes in the capillaries of visceral organs. The disorder affects the heart in 10–20% of cases, causing an inflammatory reaction that may be widespread or focal and involve the pericardium, the myocardium, and the valves. Chronic renal failure is most common, but patients may have pericardial effusion or cardiac failure. Systemic lupus erythematosus is one of the most common causes of pericardial effusion in tertiary care centers in the USA.

Clinical Findings

A. Symptoms and Signs: In serologic surveys designed to identify early manifestations of lupus erythematosus, the disease is often found to be chronic, mild, and characterized by a rash, slightly raised arterial pressure, arthritis, Raynaud's phenomenon, myopericarditis, and prompt response to corticosteroid therapy.

Cardiac involvement in active cases is suspected by enlargement of the heart, pericardial effusion, and changes on the ECG. A typical example of T wave inversions characteristic of myopericarditis in systemic lupus erythematosus is shown in Fig 17–25. Hypertension is common and may lead to left ventricular hypertrophy and left ventricular failure.

Other manifestations include a characteristic butterfly malar rash, photosensitivity reaction, Raynaud's phenomenon, arthritis resembling rheumatoid arthritis, and lupus nephritis (focal or diffuse proliferative glomerulitis, membranous glomerular nephropathy). The patient may have pleural effusion as well as central nervous system involvement, with seizures, chronic organic brain syndrome (dementia, confusion), aseptic meningitis, reversible psychosis, and peripheral neuritis. Libman-Sacks endocarditis may be found pathologically but is rarely a clinical problem.

B. Laboratory Findings: The diagnosis is confirmed by finding lupus erythematosus cells in the blood and pericardial fluid, a chronic false-positive serologic test for syphilis, antinuclear and other autoantibodies in the serum, hypergammaglobulinemia, an increased erythrocyte sedimentation rate, and reduced serum complement. Urinalysis reveals proteinuria and the characteristic "telescopic" findings (Krupp, 1943) in which all varieties of cells and casts are found simultaneously in the urinary sediment. Anemia, leukopenia, lymphopenia, and thrombocytopenia are common.

C. Special Investigations: Two-dimensional echocardiography may reveal left ventricular dysfunction or pericardial effusion.

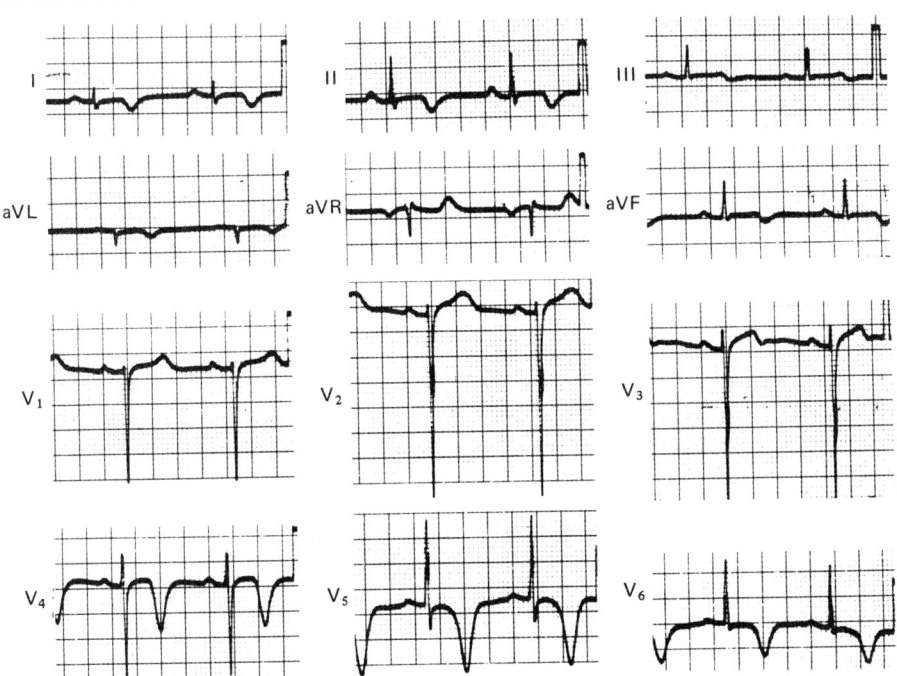

Figure 17–25. T wave inversions characteristic of myopericarditis in a 27-year-old woman with classic clinical lupus erythematosus.

Table 17–8. Causes of death in 36 patients with lupus erythematosus.*

Condition	Patients	
	Number	Percent
Sepsis	14	40
Cardiac disorders	8	20
Cerebrovascular accidents	4	11
Renal failure	4	11
Miscellaneous	6	18
Totals	36	100

*Reproduced, with permission, from the American Heart Association, Inc., Bulkley BH, Roberts WC: The heart in systemic lupus erythematosus and the changes induced in it by corticosteroid therapy: A study of 36 necropsy patients. Am J Med 1975;58:243.

Table 17–9. Drugs implicated (in descending order of importance) in the induction of a lupuslike syndrome.*

Procainamide	Penicillamine
Hydralazine	Oral contraceptive agents
Isoniazid	Phenothiazines
Sulfonamides	Quinidine
Penicillin	Ethosuximide
Tetracycline	Phenylbutazone
Streptomycin	Phenytoin
Aminosalicylic acid	Mephenytoin
Griseofulvin	Trimethadione

*Reproduced, with permission, from Bardana EJ, Pirofsky B: Recent advances in the immunopathogenesis of systemic lupus erythematosus. West J Med 1975;122:130.

Treatment

Although mild forms of systemic lupus erythematosus may be treated symptomatically, myocarditis and other serious complications of the disease require judicious use of corticosteroids. Prolonged careful clinical and laboratory follow-up may be necessary. Immunosuppressive drugs such as cyclophosphamide, azathioprine, or chlorambucil are used in resistant cases; most patients respond to corticosteroid therapy alone.

Prognosis

Sepsis is the most common cause of death in systemic lupus erythematosus and often occurs as a side effect of corticosteroid therapy. Other causes of death are heart disorders (myocardial infarction, arrhythmias, cardiac failure), progressive renal disease, and central nervous system involvement (see above and Table 17–8).

Early steroid therapy makes it less likely that the kidneys will become involved, so that much longer survival is now possible. The disease may be intermittently active but at times is fulminant. Large doses of cortisteroids are beneficial but also often cause adverse side effects.

DRUG-INDUCED CONNECTIVE TISSUE DISORDERS

Recently it has been recognized that a variety of drugs such as procainamide, hydralazine, phenytoin, and some of the phenothiazines may cause a syndrome indistinguishable from lupus erythematosus, with pericarditis, arteritis, and characteristic serologic changes (Table 17–9). In practically all instances, the syndrome subsides after withdrawal of the drug.

The worst offender is procainamide; at least half of all patients receiving it for about 6 months develop positive serologic changes and ultimately clinical signs of the lupuslike syndrome, which disappear slowly when the drug is stopped. The skin and kidneys are usually spared, and the first manifestations may be serologic and hematologic ones. The high frequency with which procainamide produces the syndrome prevents its use in chronic therapy of arrhythmias; however, since it may take months for the syndrome to appear, the drug may be used during the acute phase for short periods. Acetylprocainamide may be an effective antiarrhythmic agent and is less likely to produce the lupuslike syndrome.

The lupuslike syndrome occurs less commonly with hydralazine, particularly in the doses ordinarily prescribed. In patients receiving 200 mg/d or less, the syndrome is uncommon; it is much more common with doses of 600–800 mg/d.

SCLERODERMA

The diffuse fibrosis and vasculitis so obvious in the skin, gastrointestinal tract, and lungs in generalized scleroderma may also involve the heart. The clinical cardiac abnormalities in patients with scleroderma are tabulated in Table 17–10. Fig 17–26 shows the typical pathologic features of scleroderma involving the kidney. Similar changes are seen in the heart. Perivascular fibrosis is clearly shown. Congestive heart failure is rare in mild cases. In severe systemic scleroderma, cardiac failure, arrhythmia, and conduction defects are common.

The major cardiac lesion is fibrotic destruction of the conduction system and the small coronary arteries. The fibrotic lesions may also involve the myocardial cells, sometimes causing necrosis and angina pectoris. Despite the myocardial necrosis and fibrosis, the coronary arteries may be patent. Six of 8 patients studied postmortem by James (1974) died suddenly as a result of fibrous destruction of the sinoatrial and atrioventricular nodes. Cardiac arrhythmias were frequent in these patients. Electrocardiographic and clinical features of atrioventricular block, Stokes-Adams attacks, and sudden death are similar to those seen in cardiac sarcoidosis. Serial ECGs may determine when conduction defects have progressed, making it advisable to insert an artificial pacemaker to prevent sudden death.

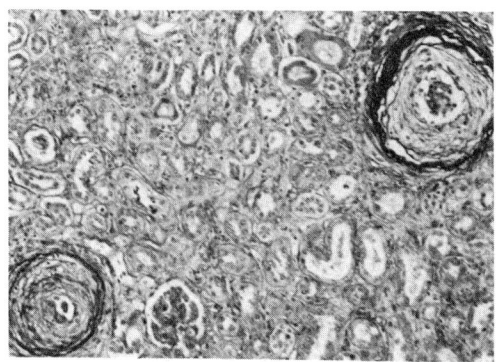

Figure 17-26. Pathologic features of scleroderma of the kidney (similar to myocardium). (Courtesy of O Rambo.)

Table 17-11. Frequency of cardiac symptoms and signs in 254 patients with rheumatoid arthritis and 254 controls.*

Cardiac Abnormality	Patients With Arthritis	Controls
Congestive heart failure	25	3
Angina pectoris	16	4
Enlargement of left ventricle	48	28
Enlargement of right ventricle	5	0
Atrial enlargement	6	1
Aortic systolic murmur	7	1
Aortic diastolic murmur	4	0
Mitral diastolic murmur	7	1
Totals	118	38

*Reproduced, with permission, from Cathcart ES, Spodick DH: Rheumatoid heart disease: A study of the incidence and nature of cardiac lesions in rheumatoid arthritis. *N Engl J Med* 1962; 266:959.

There is no specific treatment. Supportive treatment includes pacing for conduction defects and use of antiarrhythmic agents for complex ventricular arrhythmias and ventricular tachycardia, which may be documented by ambulatory electrocardiographic monitoring.

RHEUMATOID ARTHRITIS

Rheumatoid arthritis is a form of connective tissue disorder. Rheumatoid factor and other autoantibodies are present in the serum. The frequency of cardiac symptoms and signs in a large group of patients with rheumatoid arthritis is shown in Table 17-11. Rheumatoid arthritis may cause inflammatory changes in the pericardium, myocardium, and aortic valve, producing pericardial effusion and aortic insufficiency as the most common cardiac manifestations. The frequency with which pericarditis is detected is increased if echocardiograms are done on all patients with rheumatoid arthritis. A typical histologic example of rheumatoid vasculitis of the myocardium is shown in Fig 17-27. The process may involve the mitral valve and the myocardium. At autopsy, about a third of all patients with rheumatoid arthritis have evidences of pericarditis, conduction system abnormalities, or aortic valve disease. Clinically, however, only a small percentage of patients—probably less than 5%—have active cardiac disease. Rheumatoid arthritis may be a precursor of amyloid disease of the heart (see p 561).

Table 17-10. Clinical cardiac abnormalities in 47 patients with scleroderma.*†

Myocardial Lesion	Severe (13 patients)		Mild (10 patients)		Absent (24 patients)	
Congestive heart failure	11	(85%)	3	(30%)	8	(33%)
Congestive heart failure without renal or lung involvement	4	(31%)	0		0	
Angina pectoris	3	(23%)	0		0	
Ventricular irritability	8	(62%)	1	(10%)	1	(4%)
Conduction abnormality	8	(62%)	3	(30%)	6	(25%)
Right bundle branch block	5		1		3	
Left anterior hemiblock	2		2		5	
First-degree heart block	1		1		1	
Complete heart block	3		0		0	
Cardiac death	8	(62%)	2	(20%)	1	(4%)
Sudden death	5	(38%)	1	(10%)	0	
Congestive heart failure	3	(23%)	1	(10%)	1	(4%)
Constrictive pericarditis	0		0		1	(4%)
Total with clinical cardiac abnormalities	11	(79%)	4	(40%)	10	(42%)

*Five patients excluded because of coexisting severe epicardial coronary artery disease.
†Reproduced, with permission, from the American Heart Association, Inc., Bulkley BH et al: Myocardial lesions of progressive systemic sclerosis: A cause of cardiac dysfunction. *Circulation* 1976;53:483.

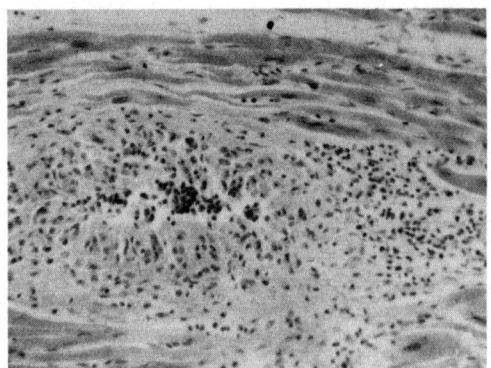

Figure 17–27. Inflammatory infiltrate of the myocardium in rheumatoid arthritis. (Courtesy of O Rambo.)

HEMOCHROMATOSIS

Hemochromatosis, an excess iron storage disease, can be classified as primary (idiopathic) or secondary (transfusion) hemosiderosis. Idiopathic hemochromatosis is genetic, transmitted as an autosomal dominant trait. Iron storage is increased because of enhanced intestinal absorption of iron from the normal 1 mg to 3 mg/d. The increased absorption ultimately leads to overloading of the body cells with iron (Finch, 1982).

Idiopathic genetic hemochromatosis is much commoner in men. Excessive amounts (10–40 g instead of the normal 1–2 g) of iron are retained and stored in the cells in the tissues, especially the liver cells, and provoke a variable fibrotic reaction that may involve the myocardium, interfering with left ventricular function. Iron deposition in the heart does not occur until the liver is first saturated with iron (Buja, 1971). A typical example is shown in Fig 17–28. Ordinary myocardial cells are affected more than the cells of the conductive system.

Secondary hemochromatosis is more common and usually due to multiple blood transfusions (100 or more) in chronic aplastic or hemolytic anemias or thalassemia. The 250 mg of iron in each unit of blood (500 mL) is stored in the body because excretion of iron cannot be increased. Iron is deposited as hemosiderin, leading to the alternative name **transfusion siderosis.** Rarely, iron loading results from excessive oral intake for many years or from congenital abnormalities of iron metabolism (eg, thalassemia major, transferrinemia, pyridoxine-responsive anemia) (Crosby, 1974, 1977).

Iron is deposited in the liver, pancreas, heart, spleen, thyroid, lymph nodes, adrenals, anterior pituitary, joints, gonads, lungs (to a lesser extent), and central nervous system (rarely). It presents clinically as "bronze" diabetes in association with cirrhosis, pituitary insufficiency, testicular atrophy, involvement of the heart, and arthropathy with chondrocalcinosis. Occasionally, chronic arthritis due to chondrocalcinosis suggests the possibility of the disease, especially in the relatives of patients with hemochromatosis.

The presenting symptoms and signs of cardiac

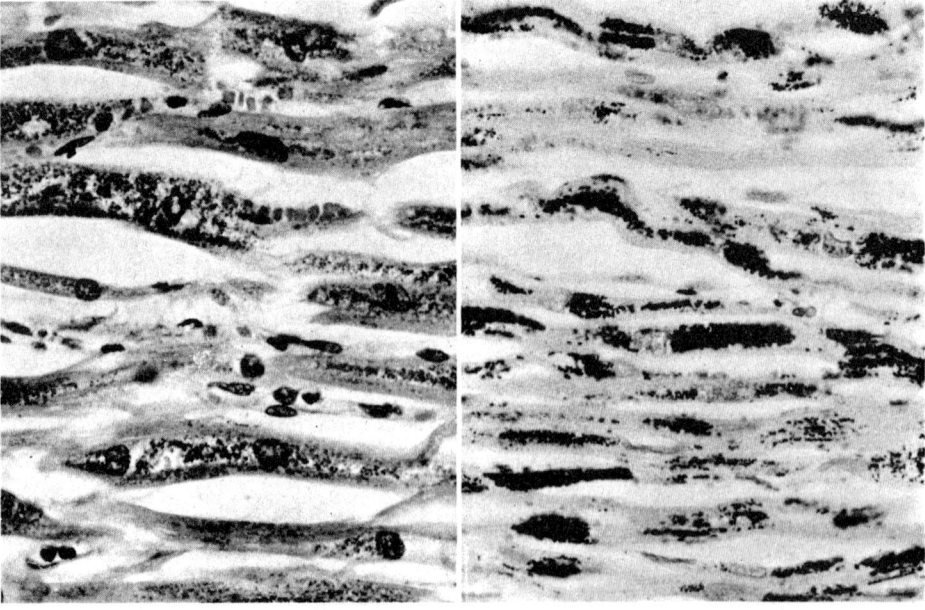

Figure 17–28. Histologic sections of left ventricular myocardium showing extensive iron depositions (dark areas). **Left:** H&E stain. **Right:** Iron stain. (Magnification, each × 560.) (Reproduced, with permission, from Arnett EN et al: Massive myocardial hemosiderosis: A structure-function conference at the National Heart and Lung Institute. *Am Heart J* 1975;**90**:777.)

deposition of iron may be similar to those of any infiltrative cardiac disease, with fatigue, dyspnea, gallop rhythm, ventricular arrhythmias, conduction defects, and signs of heart failure. The diagnosis can be established by biopsy of the liver, kidney, heart, or skin and the use of stains for stainable iron (hemosiderin) appropriate to the tissues obtained.

Screening Tests

Various screening tests have been used to detect preclinical disease. These have included determinations of serum ferritin, serum iron, transferrin saturation, or deferoxamine-chelatable iron. All are helpful, but direct demonstration of increased tissue iron is the definitive finding. Serum ferritin, the storage form of iron, was found to be increased in almost all relatives of patients with hemochromatosis who had increased iron stores, whereas it was rarely increased in relatives of those with normal iron stores (Halliday, 1977; Propper, 1977).

Cardiac involvement consists of atrial and ventricular arrhythmias, conduction defects, cardiac enlargement, and cardiac failure.

The course of the disease is usually unfavorable unless excess iron stores are removed early by frequent phlebotomies (see below). Early diagnosis can be made if the disease is suspected in every case of unexplained cardiomyopathy, cirrhosis, or diabetes, especially if the skin is an unusual bronze or a grayish tan color. Serum iron is usually normal, but iron-binding capacity is 60–70% (often more) saturated instead of the normal 20–40%.

Noninvasive radionuclide angiography has been used to determine the response of the ejection fraction to exercise in these patients. Changes in the ejection fraction may be the earliest manifestation of left ventricular dysfunction prior to the development of cardiac failure (Leon, 1979).

Treatment & Prognosis

Treatment consists of phlebotomy and, more recently, continuous subcutaneous administration of deferoxamine-B (see below) to decrease organ damage and prevent fibrosis (Weatherall, 1983). It has been estimated that 100 phlebotomies of 500 mL of blood once a week will eliminate the excess iron within 2 years. More rapid removal of blood may produce hypotension or cardiac arrhythmias. The condition can subsequently be controlled by intermittent phlebotomies that maintain the hemoglobin at about 11 g/dL.

In secondary hemochromatosis, phlebotomies are unsatisfactory. Deferoxamine, whether given subcutaneously or intravenously, has been shown to increase urinary iron excretion. A method for 12- to 24-hour subcutaneous infusion has been devised using a portable infusion pump and administration of the drug through a No. 27 needle placed in the subcutaneous tissues of the anterior abdominal wall (Propper, 1977; 1982). Although results are encouraging, the long-term effects are not known.

Serial determination of deferoxamine-chelatable iron is a safe and practical way of assessing the effect of phlebotomy as well as infusions of deferoxamine (Baldus, 1978). The results of regular blood transfusions in patients with beta-thalassemia are satisfactory for 2 or 3 decades, but most of the patients ultimately die of the effects of iron overload from the transfused blood (Pippard, 1977).

AMYLOID DISEASE

Amyloid disease of the heart is estimated to be responsible for about 5–10% of cases of cardiomyopathy due to causes other than coronary artery disease. It is usually primary in the heart but may be secondary to other conditions, eg, multiple myeloma, chronic infections, regional ileitis, chronic disorders of connective tissues such as rheumatoid arthritis, or periodic fever (familial Mediterranean fever). The cause is obscure, but a faulty immunologic response may be responsible for increased production by plasma cells and deposition of amyloid protein in the heart, kidney, and other organs of the body. The heart has a "glassy" appearance, and there may be generalized vasculitis involving the liver, spleen, and kidneys as well as the heart. The small vessels of the heart may have amyloid deposits in their walls that produce occlusive disease from the vasculitis as well as restrictive disease from the deposition of amyloid. A typical example is shown in Fig 17–29. Fig 17–30 is a typical Congo red stain preparation of amyloidosis from a rectal biopsy.

Clinical Findings

A. Symptoms and Signs: Amyloid disease of the heart is a restrictive cardiomyopathy and may be confused with constrictive pericarditis. Amyloid disease should be considered in all patients with plasma cell leukemia, multiple myeloma, chronic infections, and long-standing periodic fever. Definitive diagnosis is based on finding amyloid deposits in endomyocardial biopsies or in biopsies of the rectum, liver, or gums (Fig 17–29); of these sites, rectal biopsy is the most reliable of the simple and well-tolerated procedures and most likely to be positive. Subcutaneous fat biopsy may be diagnostic. The oral lesions, in addition to papules, may include macroglossia with a large, firm tongue resulting from amyloid deposition. The details of the present status of Bence Jones protein and the light chains of the immunoglobulins are discussed by Kyle (1983) and Glenner (1980).

Amyloid deposits consisting of fibrils of light chain immunoglobulins may be found anywhere in the myocardium; if large and extensive, they may produce restrictive cardiomyopathy; if small and scattered, especially in older individuals, they may not give rise to any cardiovascular symptoms or signs. If the amyloid deposits involve the conduction system (eg, the sinus node or the atrioventricular node), the patients may have ventricular arrhythmias or conduction defects,

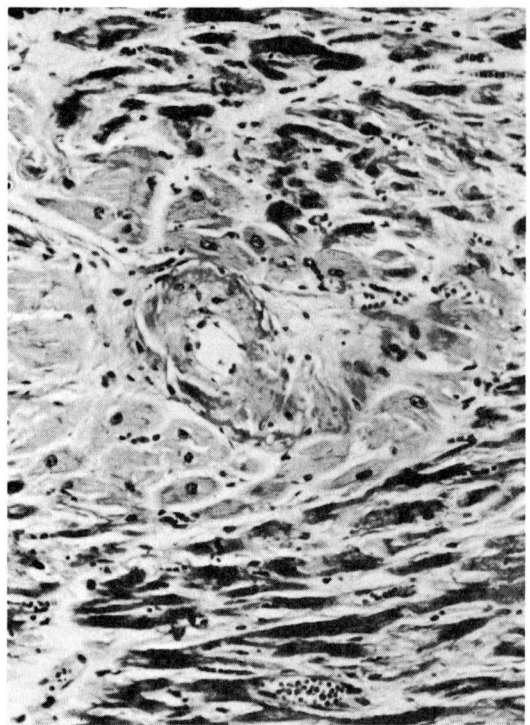

Figure 17–29. Amyloidosis involving the wall of a small artery and surrounding myocardium. Magnification × 150. The dark-staining areas are ischemic myocardial fibers. (Reproduced, with permission, from Castleman B [editor]: Case records of the Massachusetts General Hospital. N Engl J Med 1972;286:364.)

heart block, and syncope. The severity of amyloid involvement varies greatly.

Progressive renal failure may occur as excess protein is deposited in the basement membrane of the glomeruli.

B. Laboratory Findings: Bence Jones proteinuria is usually associated with multiple myeloma or secondary amyloidosis, although it occurs to a lesser

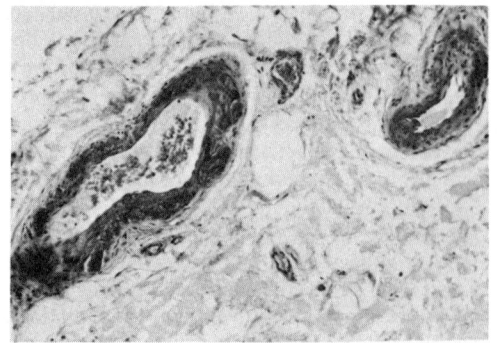

Figure 17–30. Rectal amyloidosis from rectal biopsy. Magnification × 40, Congo red stain. The dark areas are deposits of amyloid in the walls of blood vessels. (Courtesy of O Rambo.)

degree in primary amyloid disease, neoplastic diseases, and immunologic disorders such as Waldenström's macroglobulinemia. Bence Jones protein was discovered because it precipitates when heated to moderate temperatures (50–60 °C) but redissolves on further heating to 100 °C and then reprecipitates upon cooling. Other proteins (eg, albumin) precipitate upon heating but do not redissolve.

Bence Jones proteins are homogeneous light chain polypeptides of immunoglobulins that can be found in both urine and blood; the light chains can be found by electron microscopy or quantitative immunochemistry of the urinary sediment. The autoimmune nature of amyloid disease is supported by the finding that the characteristic protein represents the light chains of immunoglobulins (Glenner, 1980).

The distinction between primary and secondary amyloidosis has become blurred because of the lower incidence of chronic infections and the availability of more precise immunochemical methods (immunoelectrophoresis, immunoassay) of quantifying the light chain polypeptides in the urine and serum that characterize amyloid disease. Levels of light chain polypeptide immunoglobulins vary in different patients and at different times in the course of the disease.

C. Electrocardiography: The ECG sometimes arouses suspicion of an infiltrative process in the heart because of low voltage of the QRS complexes.

Treatment

The only treatment is that of the underlying condition causing the amyloidosis, eg, chronic infection. Attempts to treat primary amyloidosis with cytotoxic agents and corticosteroids have not been convincing. Two-year survival rates are 30–50% after the onset of cardiac symptoms.

ENDOMYOCARDIAL FIBROSIS & LÖFFLER'S ENDOCARDITIS
(See also Restrictive Cardiomyopathy, p 546.)

These uncommon conditions of unknown cause may be a single entity or different entities. Whether or not endomyocardial fibrosis and Löffler's endocarditis are identical or distinct pathologic processes, the cardiac lesion consists of endomyocardial fibrosis, myocarditis, endocardial thrombosis, and eosinophilic infiltration. Endomyocardial fibrosis and eosinophilic endocarditis are infrequent in the Western world but are common in developing countries. The cases with eosinophilia are often associated with leukemia and lymphoma, and these disorders should be sought. Endomyocardial fibrosis produces a plaque-like thickening of the endocardium that appears grossly as a white lining of the entire endocardium, frequently associated with mural thrombi and systemic or pulmonary emboli. The disease usually affects the endocardium and myocardium of the left more often than the right ventricle. There is interference with cardiac filling, and the patient may present with clinical features of restrictive cardiomyopathy and may be diagnosed as having chronic constrictive pericarditis (Parrillo, 1979; Cherian, 1983).

The onset of the disease is usually vague and insidious. It occurs in teenagers and young adults in developing countries and in older adults in developed ones. Some patients present with fever, suggesting a viral infection as the basic cause of the process.

Clinical Findings

When restriction of filling and emptying of the ventricles occurs because of the thick lining of endomyocardial fibrosis, the patient presents with cardiac failure of unknown cause. When the process affects predominantly the right ventricular endocardium, the patient may have pulmonary hypertension and right ventricular failure. This must be differentiated from mitral valve disease and chronic pulmonary disease—as well as from congenital heart disease in children and teenagers. Pericardial effusion followed by heart failure requires exclusion of tuberculous pericarditis. When the process involves the left ventricle, left ventricular failure may occur (see Chapter 10). In advanced cases, both right and left ventricular endocardiums are involved with both right and left ventricular failure and pulmonary hypertension. The diagnosis is suspected on the basis of the clinical features, including intracardiac calcification, but often cannot be distinguished from congestive cardiomyopathy.

Treatment & Prognosis

Treatment is generally only supportive, with conventional therapy for cardiac failure. Prednisone may be tried and occasionally produces a remission. In general, the prognosis is poor, and the patient usually lives only a few years.

SICKLE CELL DISEASE & CHRONIC ANEMIA

Sickle cell disease can cause cardiovascular manifestations. The anemia may increase the cardiac output (high-output failure), and the tendency of sickle cells to occlude small vessels may narrow the pulmonary or coronary arteries and produce cor pulmonale or angina. When the hemoglobin is less than 6 or 7 g/dL in any type of anemia, cardiac output is increased at rest (see Chapter 10), but the maximal cardiac output with exercise is still less than normal. The left ventricular ejection fraction is usually normal, and the systemic vascular resistance is decreased (Denenberg, 1983). Because of thrombotic obliteration of the pulmonary arteries that occurs in sickle cell disease, patients may develop right ventricular hypertrophy and pulmonary hypertension and ultimately right heart failure. The left ventricle is usually enlarged; this may be due to a combination of chronic anemia and the vascular occlusions that occur in sickle cell crises. If anemia is severe, there may be diastolic as well as systolic murmurs.

Treatment consists mainly of hydration with intravenous fluids and relief of pain by narcotics. There is no specific therapy of proved value.

CHAGAS' DISEASE
(American Trypanosomiasis)

Chagas' disease of the heart is an acute and chronic myocardial disease due to infection with the protozoan *Trypanosoma cruzi,* transmitted to humans in the feces of a *Triatoma* insect during blood feeding. The insect lives in the thatched roofs of adobe houses in South America, especially Brazil and Argentina, and bites its victims while they sleep. Chagas' disease is a major health problem in Central and South America, infecting one-third of the people and causing chronic cardiac disease in one-third of those infected. It is rare in the USA, although the insect vector has been found in Texas and some other southern states.

The organism does not multiply in the blood but can be isolated by culture in the acute phases. It penetrates cells of various organs and multiplies and spreads, ultimately involving the heart.

Clinical Findings

The disease has acute and chronic phases separated by a latent period of 10–20 years.

A. Acute Phase: The acute phase begins within days after the insect bite, with fever and a lesion of either the eye or the skin. The eye is swollen and discolored, with regional adenopathy (**Romaña's sign**). Skin inoculation results in a localized lesion called a **chagoma** (Fig 17–31), similar to a furuncle. During the acute phase, which lasts several months, electrocardiographic and radiologic signs of acute myocarditis or pericardial effusion can be demonstrated in approximately one-third of patients. Antibodies appear in the blood in about 2 months (Prata, 1968).

B. Late Chronic Phase: Many patients have no clinical signs in the acute phase, and the diagnosis is only made years later when they present with conduction defects, chronic congestive cardiomyopathy, dilatation of the esophagus, and serologic evidence of previous infection by *T cruzi,* plus a history of residence in an endemic area.

The chronic cardiac disease resembles idiopathic or chronic congestive cardiomyopathy, except that palpitations and conduction defects are more common and sudden death occurs in 20% of patients. In addition to dyspnea, palpitations, and syncope, patients have cardiac enlargement and aneurysms and thromboses of both ventricles and both atria. Systemic or pulmonary emboli are due to intracardiac thrombi. Coronary disease is uncommon.

When the pathologic lesion predominantly involves the conduction system, the ECG may show arrhythmia and atrioventricular or intraventricular conduction defects. Complete atrioventricular block may cause Stokes-Adams attacks, and artificial pacemakers may be required to prevent sudden death. Extensive chronic

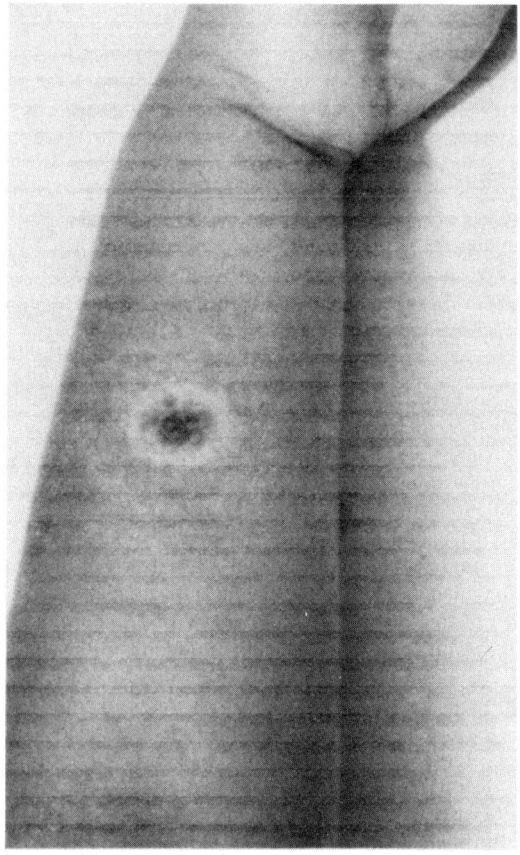

Figure 17-31. Inflammatory chagoma on the skin of the forearm in acute Chagas' disease. (Reproduced, with permission, from Prata A: Chagas' heart disease. *Cardiologia* 1968;52:79.)

---

inflammation and fibrosis are found on postmortem examination of patients with Chagas' myocarditis (Andrade, 1978).

Echocardiography

Distinctive M mode and 2-dimensional echocardiogram patterns have been found in Chagas' disease (Acquatella, 1980). These include left ventricular posterior wall hypokinesis and relatively preserved septal motion, apical aneurysms, or dyskinesias. The findings could be distinguished from congestive cardiomyopathy in most cases.

Treatment

Treatment is symptomatic, with pacemakers for syncope and conventional treatment of cardiac failure and systemic emboli when they occur. The only means of prevention is by improving housing and destroying the insect vector.

PERIPARTUM CARDIOMYOPATHY

Cardiac failure occurring just before, during, or within the first 2 months after delivery, in the absence of preexisting cardiac disease, is an uncommon disorder of unknown cause. The relationship to pregnancy is an essential part of the diagnosis, but the disease may be delayed for 1-3 months and the relationship to pregnancy may be overlooked. A high percentage (about 80%) of patients with idiopathic cardiomyopathy in the tropics give a history of onset in relationship to pregnancy (Burch, 1972).

It is not clear whether pregnancy is a precipitating cause of possible preexisting cardiomyopathy or whether this is a distinct clinical entity. A possible viral or immunologic disorder is supported by the consistency with which clinical reports describe the time of onset and the absence of any known preexisting cardiac disease prior to peripartum cardiac failure.

In some tropical countries, a high sodium intake is customary because of the native belief that it increases breast milk. It is also believed that the risk of puerpural sepsis can be diminished if patients remain in a hot room after delivery and if they are given 2 hot baths daily. The syndrome is more common in the humid, hot rainy season. It is postulated that the high sodium intake combined with the high environmental temperature greatly increases the cardiac output until cardiac failure occurs. Peripartum heart failure in this group of cases is therefore considered to be a form of high-output failure. There is rapid improvement in patients who are hospitalized and given a low-sodium diet and diuretics (Sanderson, 1979; Fillmore, 1977).

The clinical manifestations may be alarming, with the rapid development of cardiac failure and pericardial effusion shortly after delivery. Severe dyspnea, orthopnea, tachycardia, chest pain, cardiac enlargement, gallop rhythm, pulmonary rales, and pulmonary congestion on the chest film attest to the presence of severe left ventricular failure. Raised venous pressure indicates right ventricular failure as well. Systemic embolism may occur. Preeclampsia-eclampsia and acute glomerulonephritis must be excluded. The ECG shows primary T wave inversions (not secondary to conduction defects) in the left ventricular leads, suggesting acute myopericarditis, with which this disorder is frequently confused.

The clinical course usually lasts 3-6 months, and most patients recover following conventional treatment for cardiac failure, but some progress to dilated cardiomyopathy. Gilchrist (1963) found no evidence of residual cardiac symptoms or signs in 7 patients studied 1-10 years after congestive heart failure. Figs 17-32 and 17-33 illustrate the course in a 32-year-old woman who developed cardiac failure 4 months following delivery of a normal child. X-rays of the chest show decrease in size of the heart shadow, and ECGs show regression of electrocardiographic abnormalities.

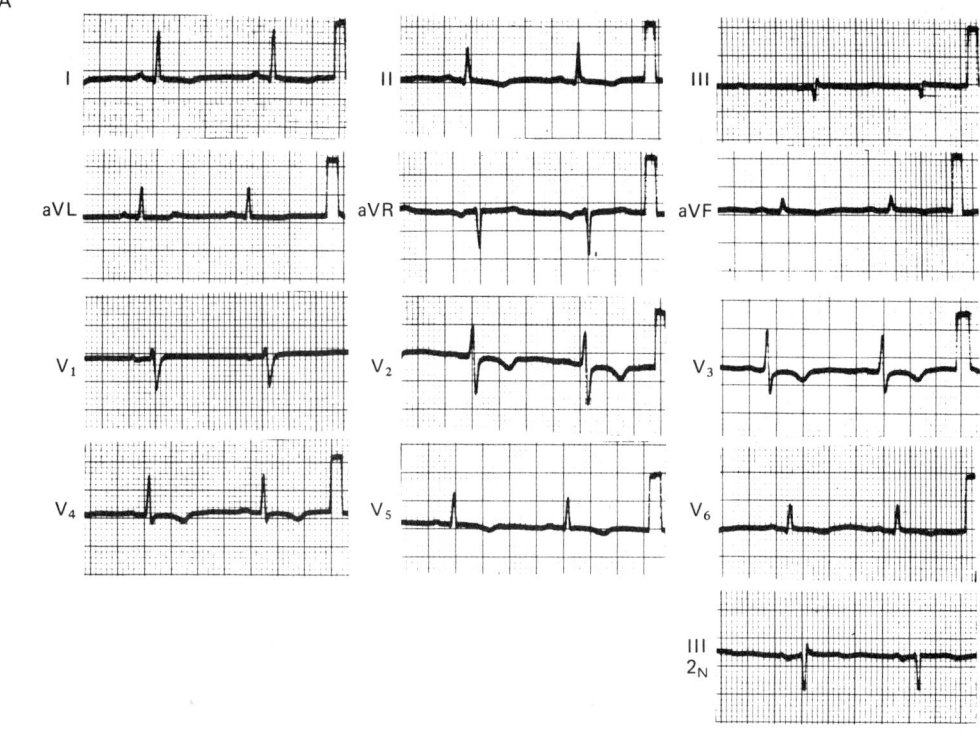
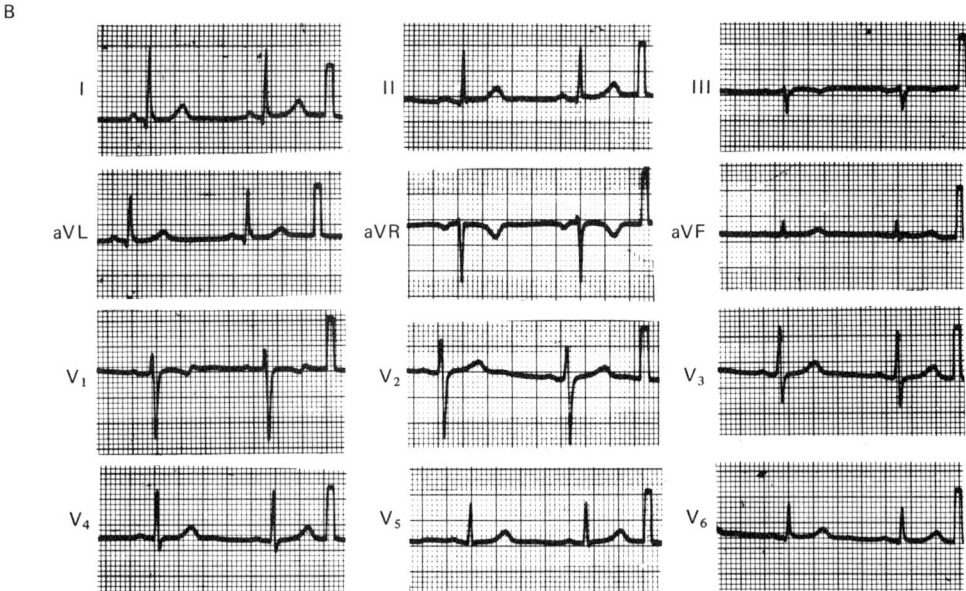

Figure 17–32. A: March 15, 1972. ECGs of same 32-year-old woman who developed cardiac failure 4 months following delivery of a normal child reveal regression of ECG abnormalities with diffuse T wave inversions on March 15, 1972. **B:** Completely gone by October 1, 1973.

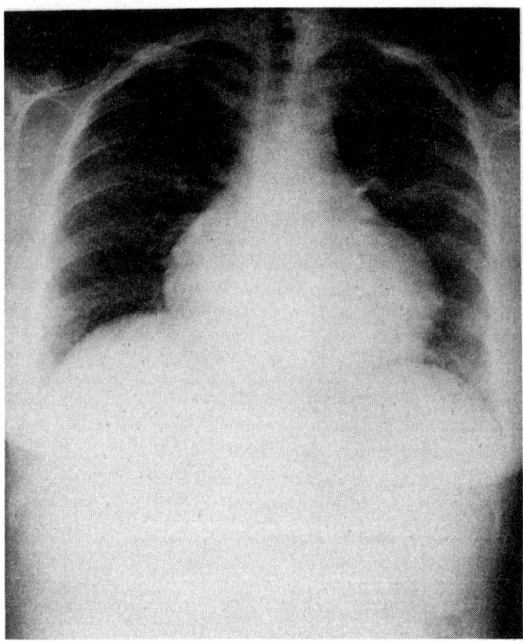 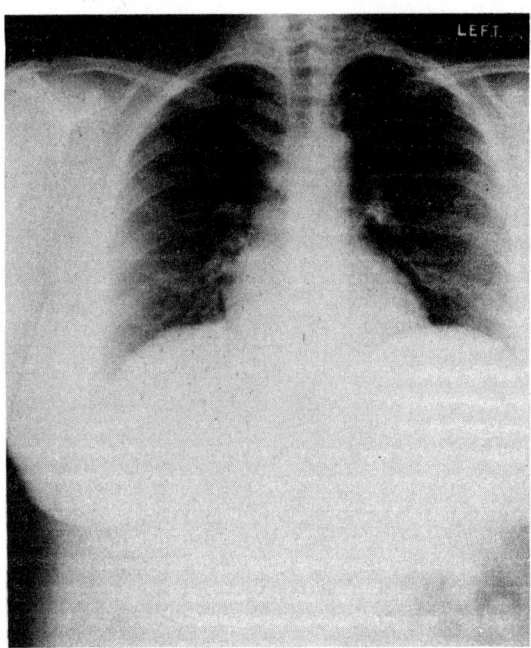

Figure 17-33. *A:* March 15, 1972. Chest film of a 32-year-old woman who developed cardiac failure 4 months following delivery of a normal child. Patient was perfectly well by October 1973. *B:* November 7, 1974. Films show decrease in size of cardiac shadow.

NEUROPATHIC DISORDERS & HEART DISEASE

Neuropathic disorders are a rare cause of heart disease. Patients with Friedreich's ataxia, dystrophia myotonica, and other neuropathic disorders may develop cardiac failure, arrhythmias, and conduction defects with Stokes-Adams attacks.

CARDIAC INVOLVEMENT IN INHERITED DISORDERS OF METABOLISM

These constitute a group of genetically determined enzymatic abnormalities and are only mentioned here for completeness. A comprehensive paper by Blieden (1974) classifies the inherited metabolic disorders and discusses them from the point of view of genetics, biochemistry, and clinical features. Attention is called to the fact that the cardiac manifestations may be the presenting features.

REFERENCES

General

Abelmann WH: Classification and natural history of primary myocardial disease. *Prog Cardiovasc Dis* 1984;**28**:73.

Fenoglio JJ et al: Diagnosis and classification of myocarditis by endomyocardial biopsy. *N Engl J Med* 1983;**308**:12.

Fowles RE, Mason JW: Endomyocardial biopsy. *Ann Intern Med* 1982;**97**:885.

Fowles RE, Mason JW: Role of cardiac biopsy in the diagnosis and management of cardiac disease. *Prog Cardiovasc Dis* 1984;**27**:153.

Goodwin JF: Congestive and hypertrophic cardiomyopathies: A decade of study. *Lancet* 1970;**1**:731.

Parrillo JE et al: The results of transvenous endomyocardial biopsy can frequently be used to diagnose myocardial diseases in patients with idiopathic heart failure. *Circulation* 1984;**69**:93.

Roberts WC, Ferrans VJ: Pathologic anatomy of the cardiomyopathies: Idiopathic dilated and hypertrophic types, infiltrative types and endomyocardial disease with and without eosinophilia. *Hum Pathol* 1975;**6**:287.

Wahr DW, Schiller NB: Evaluating myopericardial disease with echocardiography. *J Cardiovasc Med* 1982;**7**:799.

Acute Myocarditis Associated With Specific Diseases

Abelmann WH: Viral myocarditis and its sequelae. *Annu Rev Med* 1973;**24**:143.

Andy JJ et al: Trichinosis causing extensive ventricular mural endocarditis with superimposed thrombosis. *Am J Med* 1977;**63**:824.

Binak K et al: Circulatory changes in acute glomerulonephritis at rest and during exercise. *Br Heart J* 1975;**37**:833.

Boyer NH, Weinstein L: Diphtheritic myocarditis. *N Engl J Med* 1948;**239**:913.

El-Hagrassy MMO, Banatvala JE: Coxsackie-B-virus-specific IgM responses in patients with cardiac and other diseases. *Lancet* 1980;**2**:1160.

Fine I, Brainerd H, Sokolow M: Myocarditis in acute infectious diseases. *Circulation* 1959;**20**:859.

Gore I, Saphir O: Myocarditis: A classification of 1402 cases. *Am Heart J* 1947;**34**:827.

Grayston JT, Mordhorst CH, Wang San-Tin: Childhood myocarditis associated with *Chlamydia trachomatis* infection. *JAMA* 1981;**246**:2823.

Grist NR, Bell EJ: A 6-year study of coxsackievirus B infections in heart disease. *J Hyg (Camb)* 1974;**73**:165.

Heikkila J, Karjalainen J: Evaluation of mild acute infectious myocarditis. *Br Heart J* 1982;**47**:381.

Mason JW, Billingham ME, Ricci DR: Treatment of acute inflammatory myocarditis assisted by endomyocardial biopsy. *Am J Cardiol* 1980;**45**:1037.

Matsumori A et al: Treatment of viral myocarditis with ribavirin in an animal preparation. *Circulation* 1985;**71**:834.

Reyes MP, Lerner AM: Coxsackievirus myocarditis—with special reference to acute and chronic effects. *Prog Cardiovasc Dis* 1985;**27**:373.

Ruskin J, Remington JS: Toxoplasmosis in the compromised host. *Ann Intern Med* 1976;**84**:193.

Sainani GS, Dekate MP, Rao CP: Heart disease caused by coxsackie virus B infection. *Br Heart J* 1975;**37**:819.

Sokolow M, Garland LH: Cardiovascular disturbances in tsutsugamushi disease. *US Naval Medical Bulletin* 1945; page 1054.

Rheumatic Fever

Agarwal BL: Rheumatic heart disease unabated in developing countries. *Lancet* 1981;**2**:910.

Bland EF, Jones TD: Rheumatic fever and rheumatic heart disease: A twenty year report on 1000 patients followed since childhood. *Circulation* 1951;**4**:836.

Combined Rheumatic Fever Study Group: A comparison of short-term, intensive prednisone and acetylsalicylic acid therapy in the treatment of acute rheumatic fever. *N Engl J Med* 1965;**272**:63.

Disciascio G, Taranta A: Rheumatic fever in children. *Am Heart J* 1980;**99**:635.

Engleman EP, Hollister LE, Kolb FO: Sequelae of rheumatic fever in men: Four to eight year follow-up study. *JAMA* 1954;**155**:1134.

Feinstein AR, Stern EK: Clinical effects of recurrent attacks of acute rheumatic fever: A prospective epidemiologic study of 105 episodes. *J Chronic Dis* 1967;**20**:13.

Gordis L: The virtual disappearance of rheumatic fever in the United States: Lessons in the rise and fall of disease. (T. Duckett Jones Memorial Lecture.) *Circulation* 1985; **72**:1155.

Gotsman MS: Rheumatic fever in the 80s. (2 parts.) *Cardiovasc Rev Rep* 1985;**6**:861, 935.

Krause RM: The influence of infection on the geography of heart disease. *Circulation* 1979;**60**:972.

Schieken RM, Kerber RE: Echocardiographic abnormalities in acute rheumatic fever. *Am J Cardiol* 1976;**38**:458.

Sokolow M: Significance of electrocardiographic changes in rheumatic fever. *Am J Med* 1948;**5**:365.

Sokolow M, Snell A: Atypical features of rheumatic fever in young adults. *JAMA* 1947;**133**:981.

Stollerman GH: *Rheumatic Fever and Streptococcal Infections.* Grune & Stratton, 1975.

Svartman M et al: Immunoglobulins and complement components in synovial fluid of patients with acute rheumatic fever. *J Clin Invest* 1975;**56**:111.

UK and US Joint Report: The natural history of rheumatic fever and rheumatic heart disease: Ten-year report of a cooperative clinical trial of ACTH, cortisone and aspirin. *Circulation* 1965;**32**:457.

Yoshinoya S, Pope RM: Detection of immune complexes in acute rheumatic fever and their relationship to HLA-B5. *J Clin Invest* 1980;**65**:136.

Zabriskie JB: Rheumatic fever: The interplay between host, genetics, and microbe. *Circulation* 1985;**71**:1077.

Acute Myocardial Damage Due to Drug Toxicity

Alarcon-Segovia D: Drug-induced lupus syndromes. *Mayo Clin Proc* 1969;**44**:664.

Alexander J et al: Serial assessment of doxorubicin: Cardiotoxicity with quantitative radionuclide angiography. *N Engl J Med* 1979;**300**:278.

Appelbaum FR et al: Acute lethal carditis caused by high-dose combination chemotherapy: A unique clinical and pathological entity. *Lancet* 1976;**1**:58.

Blomgren SE, Condemi JJ, Vaughan JH: Procainamide-induced lupus erythematosus: Clinical and laboratory observations. *Am J Med* 1972;**52**:338.

Brennan FJ: Electrophysiologic effects of imipramine and doxepin on normal and depressed cardiac Purkinje fibers. *Am J Cardiol* 1980;**46**:599.

Bristow MR et al: Doxorubicin cardiomyopathy: Evaluation by phonocardiography, endomyocardial biopsy, and cardiac catheterization. *Ann Intern Med* 1978;**88**:168.

Elkayam U, Frishman W: Cardiovascular effects of phenothiazines. *Am Heart J* 1980;**100**:397.

Friedman MA et al: Doxorubicin cardiotoxicity: Serial endomyocardial biopsies and systolic time intervals. *JAMA* 1978;**240**:1603.

Goodwin JF, Oakley CM: The cardiomyopathies. *Br Heart J* 1972;**34**:545.

Kantrowitz NE, Bristow MR: Cardiotoxicity of antitumor agents. *Prog Cardiovasc Dis* 1984;**27**:194.

Langou RA et al: Cardiovascular manifestations of tricyclic antidepressant overdose. *Am Heart J* 1980;**100**:458.

Legha SS et al: Reduction of doxorubicin cardiotoxicity by prolonged continuous intravenous infusion. *Ann Intern Med* 1982;**96**:133.

Marshall JB, Forker AD: Cardiovascular effects of tricyclic antidepressant drugs: Therapeutic usage, overdose, and management of complications. *Am Heart J* 1982;**103**:401.

Torti FM et al: Reduced cardiotoxicity of doxorubicin delivered on a weekly schedule: Assessment by endomyocardial biopsy. *Ann Intern Med* 1983;**99**:745.

Von Hoff DD et al: Daunomycin-induced cardiotoxicity in children and adults: A review of 110 cases. *Am J Med* 1977;**62**:200.

Weinberger A et al: Endocardial fibrosis following busulfan treatment. *JAMA* 1975;**231**:495.

Congestive (Dilated or Primary) Cardiomyopathy

Beahrs MM et al: Hypertrophic obstructive cardiomyopathy: Ten- to 21-year follow-up after partial septal myectomy. *Am J Cardiol* 1983;**51**:1160.

Borer JS, Henry WL, Epstein SE: Echocardiographic observations in patients with systemic infiltrative disease involving the heart. *Am J Cardiol* 1977;**39**:184.

Brigden W: Cardiomyopathy. *Practitioner* 1963;**190**:222.

Brigden W: Uncommon myocardial diseases: The noncoronary cardiomyopathies. (2 parts.) *Lancet* 1957;**2**:1179, 1243.

Burch GE (editor): *Cardiomyopathy.* Vol 4 of: *Cardiovascular Clinics Series.* Davis, 1972.

Fuster V et al: The natural history of idiopathic dilated cardiomyopathy. *Am J Cardiol* 1981;**47**:525.

Goodwin JF: Hypertrophic diseases of the myocardium. *Prog Cardiovasc Dis* 1973;**16**:199.

Greenwood RD, Nadas AS, Fyler DC: The clinical course of primary myocardial disease in infants and children. *Am Heart J* 1976;**92**:549.

Hamby RI: Primary myocardial disease. *Medicine* 1970;**49**:55.

Harvey WP, Segal JP, Gurel T: The clinical spectrum of primary myocardial disease. *Prog Cardiovasc Dis* 1964;**7**:17.

Johnson RA, Palacios I: Dilated cardiomyopathies of the adult. (2 parts.) *N Engl J Med* 1982;**307**:1051, 1119.

Kawai C, Takatsu T: Clinical and experimental studies on cardiomyopathy. *N Engl J Med* 1975;**293**:592.

Massie BM et al: Mitral-septal separation: A new echocardiographic index of left ventricular function. *Am J Cardiol* 1977;**39**:1008.

Matsumori A, Kawai C: An animal model of congestive (dilated) cardiomyopathy: Dilatation and hypertrophy of the heart in the chronic stage in DBA/2 mice with myocarditis caused by encephalomyocarditis virus. *Circulation* 1982;**66**:355.

Olsen EGJ: Fundamentals of clinical cardiology: The pathology of cardiomyopathies: A critical analysis. *Am Heart J* 1979;**98**:385.

Parrillo JE et al: The results of transvenous endomyocardial biopsy can frequently be used to diagnose myocardial diseases in patients with idiopathic heart failure. *Circulation* 1984;**69**:93.

Report of the WHO/ISFC task force on the definition and classification of cardiomyopathies. *Br Heart J* 1980;**44**:672.

Shirey EK, Proudfit WL, Hawk WA: Primary myocardial disease: Correlation with clinical findings, angiographic and biopsy diagnosis. *Am Heart J* 1980;**99**:198.

Zee-Cheng C-S et al: High incidence of myocarditis by endomyocardial biopsy in patients with idiopathic congestive cardiomyopathy. *J Am Coll Cardiol* 1984;**3**:63.

Hypertrophic (Obstructive) Cardiomyopathy

Alvares RF et al: Isovolumic relaxation period in hypertrophic cardiomyopathy. *J Am Coll Cardiol* 1984;**3**:71.

Anderson DM et al: Hypertrophic obstructive cardiomyopathy: Effects of acute and chronic verapamil treatment on left ventricular systolic and diastolic function. *Br Heart J* 1984;**51**:523.

Beahrs MM et al: Hypertrophic obstructive cardiomyopathy: Ten- to 21-year follow-up after partial septal myectomy. *Am J Cardiol* 1983;**51**:1160.

Bonow RO et al: Atrial systole and left ventricular filling in hypertrophic cardiomyopathy: Effect of verapamil. *Am J Cardiol* 1983;**51**:1386.

Brock RC: Functional obstruction of the left ventricle. *Guys Hosp Rep* 1957;**106**:221.

Chatterjee K et al: Hypertrophic cardiomyopathy: Therapy with slow channel inhibiting agents. *Prog Cardiovasc Dis* 1982;**25**:193.

Epstein SE, Rosing DR: Verapamil: Its potential for causing serious complications in patients with hypertrophic cardiomyopathy. *Circulation* 1981;**64**:437.

Frank S, Braunwald E: Idiopathic hypertrophic subaortic stenosis: Clinical analysis of 126 patients with emphasis on the natural history. *Circulation* 1968;**37**:759.

Goodwin JF: The frontiers of cardiomyopathy. *Br Heart J* 1982;**48**:1.

Goodwin JF: Hypertrophic diseases of the myocardium. *Prog Cardiovasc Dis* 1973;**16**:199.

Henry WL et al: Mechanism of left ventricular outflow obstruction in patients with obstructive asymmetric septal hypertrophy (idiopathic hypertrophic subaortic stenosis). *Am J Cardiol* 1975;**35**:337.

Ingham RE et al: Electrophysiologic findings in patients with idiopathic hypertrophic subaortic stenosis. *Am J Cardiol* 1978;**41**:811.

Kaltenbach M et al: Treatment of hypertrophic obstructive cardiomyopathy with verapamil. *Br Heart J* 1979;**42**:35.

Lorell BH et al: Modification of abnormal left ventricular diastolic properties by nifedipine in patients with hypertrophic cardiomyopathy. *Circulation* 1982;**65**:499.

Maron BJ, Roberts WC, Epstein SE: Sudden death in hypertrophic cardiomyopathy: A profile of 78 patients. *Circulation* 1982;**65**:1388.

Maron BJ et al: Dynamic subaortic obstruction in hypertrophic cardiomyopathy: Analysis by pulsed Doppler echocardiography. *J Am Coll Cardiol* 1985;**6**:1.

Maron BJ et al: Long-term clinical course and symptomatic status of patients after operation for hypertrophic subaortic stenosis. *Circulation* 1978;**57**:1205.

Maron BJ et al: Prognostic significance of 24-hour ambulatory electrocardiographic monitoring in patients with hypertrophic cardiomyopathy: A prospective study. *Am J Cardiol* 1981;**48:**252.

Maron BJ et al: Results of surgery for idiopathic hypertrophic subaortic stenosis. *J Cardiovasc Med* 1980;**5:**145.

McKenna WJ et al: Improved survival with amiodarone in patients with hypertrophic cardiomyopathy and ventricular tachycardia. *Br Heart J* 1985;**53:**412.

McKenna WJ et al: The natural history of left ventricular hypertrophy in hypertrophic cardiomyopathy: An electrocardiographic study. *Circulation* 1982;**66:**1233.

McKenna WJ et al: Prognosis in hypertrophic cardiomyopathy: Role of age and clinical electrocardiographic and hemodynamic features. *Am J Cardiol* 1981;**47:**532.

Meinertz T et al: Significance of ventricular arrhythmias in idiopathic dilated cardiomyopathy. *Am J Cardiol* 1984;**53:**902.

Morrow AG et al: Left ventricular myotomy and myectomy in patients with obstructive hypertrophic cardiomyopathy and previous cardiac arrest. *Am J Cardiol* 1980;**46:**313.

Nishimura RA, Giuliani ER, Brandenburg RO: Hypertrophic cardiomyopathy. *Cardiovasc Rev Rep* 1983;**4:**931.

Popp RL, Harrison DC: Ultrasound in the diagnosis and evaluation of therapy of idiopathic hypertrophic subaortic stenosis. *Circulation* 1969;**40:**905.

St. John Sutton MG et al: Histopathological specificity of hypertrophic obstructive cardiomyopathy: Myocardial fibre disarray and myocardial fibrosis. *Br Heart J* 1980;**44:**433.

Steiner RE: Radiology of hypertrophic obstructive cardiomyopathy. *Proc R Soc Med* 1964;**57:**444.

Wigle ED et al: Hypertrophic cardiomyopathy: The importance of the site and the extent of hypertrophy. A review. *Prog Cardiovasc Dis* 1985;**28:**1.

Restrictive Cardiomyopathy

Acquatella H et al: Value of two-dimensional echocardiography in endomyocardial disease with and without eosinophilia: A clinical and pathologic study. *Circulation* 1983;**67:**1219.

Graham JM et al: Management of endomyocardial fibrosis: Successful surgical treatment of biventricular involvement and consideration of the superiority of operative intervention. *Am Heart J* 1981;**102:**771.

Resnekov L: Restrictive cardiomyopathy. *Primary Cardiol* (Sept) 1978;**4:**58.

Wahr DW, Schiller NB: Evaluating myopericardial disease with echocardiography. *J Cardiovasc Med* 1982;**7:**799.

Thyrotoxic Heart Disease & Myxedema

Brennan MD: Clinical pharmacology series on pharmacology in practice. 5. Thyroid hormones. *Mayo Clin Proc* 1980;**55:**33.

Davies CE, Mackinnon J, Platts MM: Renal circulation and cardiac output in low-output heart failure and in myxedema. *Br Med J* 1952;**2:**595.

Davis PJ, Davis FB: Hyperthyroidism in patients over the age of 60 years. *Medicine* 1974;**53:**161.

Ellis LB et al: Effect of myxedema on cardiovascular system. *Am Heart J* 1952;**43:**341.

Fahr G: Myxedema heart. *JAMA* 1925;**84:**345.

Forfar JC, Miller HC, Toft AD: Occult thyrotoxicosis: A correctable cause of "idiopathic" atrial fibrillation. *Am J Cardiol* 1979;**44:**9.

Forfar JC et al: Abnormal left ventricular function in hyperthyroidism. *N Engl J Med* 1982;**307:**1165.

Graettinger JS et al: Correlation of clinical and hemodynamic studies in patients with hyperthyroidism with and without congestive heart failure. *J Clin Invest* 1959;**38:**1316.

Graettinger JS et al: A correlation of clinical and hemodynamic studies in patients with hypothyroidism. *J Clin Invest* 1958;**37:**502.

Ingbar SH: The role of antiadrenergic agents in the management of thyrotoxicosis. *Cardiovasc Rev Rep* 1981;**2:**683.

Keating FR et al: Treatment of heart disease associated with myxedema. *Prog Cardiovasc Dis* 1960;**3:**364.

Kerber RE, Sherman B: Echocardiographic evaluation of pericardial effusion in myxedema: Incidence and biochemical and clinical correlations. *Circulation* 1975;**52:**823.

Nixon JV, Anderson RJ, Cohen ML: Alterations in left ventricular mass and performance in patients treated effectively for thyrotoxicosis. *Am J Med* 1979;**67:**268.

Pietras RJ et al: Cardiovascular response in hyperthyroidism: The influence of adrenergic-receptor blockade. *Arch Intern Med* 1972;**129:**426.

Reza MJ, Abbasi AS: Congestive cardiomyopathy in hypothyroidism. *West J Med* 1975;**123:**228.

Sandler IG, Wilson GM: The nature and prognosis of heart disease in thyrotoxicosis: A review of 150 patients treated with ^{131}I. *Q J Med* 1959;**28:**347.

Santos AD et al: Echocardiographic characterization of the reversible cardiomyopathy of hypothyroidism. *Am J Med* 1980;**68:**675.

Sokolow M: Heart disease in patients with thyroid dysfunction: Medical Staff Conference, University of California, San Francisco. *Calif Med* 1968;**109:**309.

Wayne EJ: Clinical and metabolic studies in thyroid disease. *Br Med J* 1960;**1:**78.

Zondek H: Das Myxödemherz. *München Med Wochenschr* 1918;**65:**1180.

Alcoholic Cardiomyopathy

Alexander CS: Cobalt-beer cardiomyopathy: A clinical and pathologic study of twenty-eight cases. *Am J Med* 1972;**53:**395.

Brigden W: Alcoholic cardiomyopathy. Page 203 in: *Cardiomyopathy*. Burch GE (editor). Davis, 1972.

Brigden W, Robinson J: Alcoholic heart disease. *Br Med J* 1964;**2:**1283.

Burch GE et al: Prolonged bed rest in the treatment of the dilated heart. *Circulation* 1965;**32:**852.

Massie BM et al: Mitral-septal separation: A new echocardiographic index of left ventricular function. *Am J Cardiol* 1977;**39:**1008.

Ramalingaswami V: Nutrition and the heart. *Cardiologia* 1968;**52:**57.

Regan TJ: Alcoholic cardiomyopathy. *Prog Cardiovasc Dis* 1984;**27:**141.

Symposium on alcohol. *Circulation* 1981;**64(3-Part 2).** [Entire issue.]

Beriberi & Nutritional Heart Disease

Kawai C et al: Reappearance of beriberi heart disease in Japan: A study of 23 cases. *Am J Med* 1980;**69:**383.

Ramalingaswami V: Nutrition and the heart. *Cardiologia* 1968;**52:**57.

Swanepoel A, Smythe PMJ, Campbell JAH: The heart in kwashiorkor. *Am Heart J* 1964;**67:**1.

Weiss S, Wilkins RW: The nature of the cardiovascular disturbances in nutritional deficiency states (beriberi). *Ann Intern Med* 1937;**11:**104.

Wenckebach KF: *Das Beriberi-Herz*. Springer, 1934.

Sarcoidosis

Fleming HA: Sarcoid heart disease. *Br Heart J* 1974;**36**:54.

Kinney EL et al: Thallium-scan myocardial defects and echocardiographic abnormalities in patients with sarcoidosis without clinical cardiac dysfunction. *Am J Med* 1980;**68**:497.

Longcope W, Freiman D: A study of sarcoidosis based on combined investigations of 160 cases, including 30 autopsies from the Johns Hopkins Hospital and Massachusetts General Hospital. *Medicine* 1952;**31**:1.

Roberts WC, McAllister HA Jr, Ferrans VJ: Sarcoidosis of the heart: A clinicopathologic study of 35 necropsy patients (group I) and review of 78 previously described necropsy patients (group II). *Am J Med* 1977;**63**:86.

Sarcoidosis: Medical Staff Conference, University of California, San Francisco. *West J Med* 1977;**126**:288.

Siltzbach LE et al: The course and prognosis of sarcoidosis around the world. *Am J Med* 1974;**57**:847.

Wheeler RC, Abelmann WH: Cardiomyopathy associated with systemic diseases. Page 284 in: *Cardiomyopathy*. Burch GE (editor). Davis, 1972.

Young JB, Kumpuris AG: Sarcoidosis: Cardiac complications. *Primary Cardiol* 1981;**7**:111.

Systemic Lupus Erythematosus

Ansari A, Larson PH, Bates HD: Cardiovascular manifestations of systemic lupus erythematosus: Current perspective. *Prog Cardiovasc Dis* 1985;**27**:421.

Bidani AK et al: Immunopathology of cardiac lesions in fatal systemic lupus erythematosus. *Am J Med* 1980;**69**:849.

Decker JL (moderator): Systemic lupus erythematosus: Evolving concepts. (NIH conference.) *Ann Intern Med* 1979;**91**:587.

Dubois EL (editor): *Lupus Erythematosus*, 2nd ed. Univ of Southern California Press, 1974.

Estes DE, Christian CL: The natural history of systemic lupus erythematosus by prospective analysis. *Medicine* 1971;**50**:85.

Grigor RR et al: Outcome of pregnancy in systemic lupus erythematosus. *Proc R Soc Med* 1977;**70**:99.

Harvey AM et al: Systemic lupus erythematosus: Review of the literature and clinical analysis of 138 cases. *Medicine* 1954;**33**:291.

Klemperer P, Pollack AD, Baehr G: Pathology of disseminated lupus erythematosus. *Arch Pathol* 1941;**32**:569.

Krupp MA: Urinary sediment in visceral angiitis (periarteritis nodosa, lupus erythematosus, Libman-Sachs disease): Quantitative study. *Arch Intern Med* 1943;**71**:54.

Moses S, Barland P: Laboratory criteria for a diagnosis of systemic lupus erythematosus. *JAMA* 1979;**242**:1039.

Scleroderma

Botstein GR, LeRoy EC: Primary heart disease in systemic sclerosis (scleroderma): Advances in clinical and pathologic features, pathogenesis, and new therapeutic approaches. *Am Heart J* 1981;**102**:913.

Bulkley BH, Klacsmann PG, Hutchins GM: Angina pectoris, myocardial infarction and sudden cardiac death with normal coronary arteries: A clinicopathologic study of 9 patients with progressive systemic sclerosis. *Am Heart J* 1978;**95**:563.

Clements PJ et al: The relationship of arrhythmias and conduction disturbances to other manifestations of cardiopulmonary disease in progressive systemic sclerosis (PSS). *Am J Med* 1981;**71**:38.

Gottdiener JS, Moutsopoulos HM, Decker JL: Echocardiographic identification of cardiac abnormality in scleroderma and related disorders. *Am J Med* 1979;**66**:391.

James TN: De subitaneis mortibus. 8. Coronary arteries and conduction system in scleroderma heart disease. *Circulation* 1974;**50**:844.

Norton WL, Nardo JM: Vascular disease in progressive systemic sclerosis (scleroderma). *Ann Intern Med* 1970;**73**:317.

Roberts NK et al: The prevalence of conduction defects and cardiac arrhythmias in progressive systemic sclerosis. *Ann Intern Med* 1981;**94**:38.

Smith JW et al: Echocardiographic features of progressive systemic sclerosis (PSS): Correlation with hemodynamic and postmortem studies. *Am J Med* 1979;**66**:28.

Ungerer RG et al: Prevalence and clinical correlates of pulmonary arterial hypertension in progressive systemic sclerosis. *Am J Med* 1983;**75**:65.

Rheumatoid Arthritis

Abel T et al: Rheumatoid vasculitis: Effect of cyclophosphamide on the clinical course and levels of circulating immune complexes. *Ann Intern Med* 1980;**93**:407.

Kirk J, Cosh J: The pericarditis of rheumatoid arthritis. *Q J Med* 1969;**38**:397.

Lie JT: Rheumatoid arthritis and heart disease. *Primary Cardiol* 1982; **8**:137.

Rapoport RJ et al: Cutaneous vascular immunofluorescence in rheumatoid arthritis: Correlation with circulating immune complexes and vasculitis. *Am J Med* 1980;**68**:325.

Yelin E et al: Work disability in rheumatoid arthritis: Effects of disease, social, and work factors. *Ann Intern Med* 1980;**93**:551.

Hemochromatosis

Arnett EN et al: Massive myocardial hemosiderosis: Structure-function conference at National Heart and Lung Institute. *Am Heart J* 1975;**90**:777.

Baldus WP et al: Deferoxamine-chelatable iron in hemochromatosis and other disorders of iron overload. *Mayo Clin Proc* 1978;**53**:157.

Bomford A, Williams R: Long term results of venesection therapy in idiopathic haemochromatosis. *Q J Med* 1976;**45**:611.

Buja LM, Roberts WC: Iron in the heart. *Am J Med* 1971;**51**:209.

Crosby WH: Current concepts in nutrition: Who needs iron? *N Engl J Med* 1977;**297**:543.

Crosby WH et al: Hemochromatosis (iron-storage disease). *JAMA* 1974;**228**:743.

Dabestani A et al: Primary hemochromatosis: Anatomic and physiologic characteristics of the cardiac ventricles and their response to phlebotomy. *Am J Cardiol* 1984;**54**:153.

Easley RM et al: Reversible cardiomyopathy associated with hemochromatosis. *N Engl J Med* 1972;**287**:866.

Edwards CQ et al: Homozygosity for hemochromatosis: Clinical manifestations. *Ann Intern Med* 1980;**93**:519.

Feller ER et al: Familial hemochromatosis: Physiologic studies in the precirrhotic stage of the disease. *N Engl J Med* 1977;**296**:1422.

Finch CA, Huebers H: Perspectives in iron metabolism. *N Engl J Med* 1982;**306**:1520.

Halliday JW et al: Serum-ferritin in diagnosis of haemochromatosis. *Lancet* 1977;**2**:621.

Hemochromatosis: Medical Staff Conference, University of California, San Francisco. *West J Med* 1978;**128**:133.

Leon MB et al: Detection of early cardiac dysfunction in patients with severe beta-thalassemia and chronic iron overload. *N Engl J Med* 1979;**301**:1143.

Milder MS et al: Idiopathic hemochromatosis: An interim

report. *Medicine (Baltimore)* 1980;**59**:34.

Niederau C et al: Survival and causes of death in cirrhotic and noncirrhotic patients with primary hemochromatosis. *N Engl J Med* 1985;**313**:1256.

Pippard MJ et al: Iron absorption in iron-loading anaemias: Effect of subcutaneous desferrioxamine infusions. *Lancet* 1977;**2**:737.

Propper R, Nathan D: Clinical removal of iron. *Annu Rev Med* 1982;**33**:509.

Propper RD et al: Continuous subcutaneous administration of deferoxamine in patients with iron overload. *N Engl J Med* 1977;**297**:418.

Rowe JW et al: Familial hemochromatosis: Characteristics of the precirrhotic stage of a large kindred. *Medicine* 1977;**56**:197.

Short EM, Winkle RA, Billingham ME: Myocardial involvement in idiopathic hemochromatosis. *Am J Med* 1981;**70**:1275.

Skinner C, Kensmure ACF: Haemochromatosis presenting as congestive cardiomyopathy and responding to venesection. *Br Heart J* 1973;**35**:466.

Vigorita VJ, Hutchins GM: Cardiac conduction system in hemochromatosis: Clinical and pathologic features of six patients. *Am J Cardiol* 1979;**44**:418.

Weatherall DJ, Pippard MJ, Callender ST: Iron loading and thalassemia: Experimental successes and practical realities. (Editorial.) *N Engl J Med* 1977;**297**:445.

Weatherall DJ, Pippard MJ, Callender ST: Iron loading in thalassemia: Five years with the pump. (Editorial retrospective.) *N Engl J Med* 1983;**308**:456.

Amyloid Disease

Brigden W: Cardiac amyloidosis. *Prog Cardiovasc Dis* 1964;**7**:142.

Cohen AS, Cathcart ES, Skinner M: Amyloidosis: Current trends in its investigation. *Arthritis Rheum* 1978;**21**:153.

Cueto-Garcia L et al: Serial echocardiographic observations in patients with primary systemic amyloidosis: An introduction to the concept of early (asymptomatic) amyloid infiltration of the heart. *Mayo Clin Proc* 1984;**59**:589.

Glenner GG: Amyloid deposits and amyloidosis: The β-fibrilloses. (2 parts.) *N Engl J Med* 1980;**302**:1283, 1333.

Isobe T, Osserman EF: Patterns of amyloidosis and their association with plasma-cell dyscrasia, monoclonal immunoglobulins and Bence-Jones proteins. *N Engl J Med* 1974;**290**:473.

Kyle RA, Greipp PR: Amyloidosis (AL): Clinical and laboratory features in 229 cases. *Mayo Clin Proc* 1983;**58**:665.

Kyle RA et al: Primary systemic amyloidosis: Comparison of melphalan/prednisone versus colchicine. *Am J Med* 1985;**79**:708.

Levisman JA et al: Echocardiographic findings in amyloid heart disease. *Circulation* 1975;**52(Suppl 2)**:II-208.

Lie JT: Amyloidosis and amyloid heart disease. *Primary Cardiol* 1982;**8**:75.

Ridolfi RL, Bulkley BH, Hutchins GM: The conduction system in cardiac amyloidosis: Clinical and pathologic features of 23 patients. *Am J Med* 1977;**62**:677.

Roberts WC, Waller BF: Cardiac amyloidosis causing cardiac dysfunction: Analysis of 54 necropsy patients. *Am J Cardiol* 1983;**52**:137.

Rukavina JG et al: Primary systemic amyloidosis: A review and an experimental, genetic, and clinical study of 29 cases with particular emphasis on the familial form. *Medicine* 1956;**35**:239.

St. John Sutton MG et al: Computerized M-mode echocardiographic analysis of left ventricular dysfunction in cardiac amyloid. *Circulation* 1982;**66**:790.

Solomon A: Bence Jones proteins and light chains of immunoglobulins. 15. Effect of corticosteroids on synthesis and excretion of Bence Jones protein. *J Clin Invest* 1978;**61**:97.

Wright JR et al: Relationship of amyloid to aging: Review of the literature and systematic study of 83 patients derived from a general hospital population. *Medicine* 1969;**48**:39.

Endomyocardial Fibrosis & Löffler's Endocarditis

Bell JA, Jenkins BS, Webb-Peploe MM: Clinical, haemodynamic, and angiographic findings in Löffler's eosinophilic endocarditis. *Br Heart J* 1976;**38**:541.

Brockington IF, Olsen EGJ: Löffler's endocarditis and Davies' endomyocardial fibrosis. *Am Heart J* 1973;**85**:308.

Cherian G et al: Endomyocardial fibrosis: Report on the hemodynamic data in 29 patients and review of the results of surgery. *Am Heart J* 1983;**105**:659.

Chew CYC et al: Primary restrictive cardiomyopathy: Nontropical endomyocardial fibrosis and hypereosinophilic heart disease. *Br Heart J* 1977;**39**:399.

Davies JNP: African endomyocardial fibrosis. Page 345 in: *Cardiomyopathy*. Burch GE (editor). Davis, 1972.

Falase AO, Kolawole TM, Lagundoye SB: Endomyocardial fibrosis: Problems in differential diagnosis. *Br Heart J* 1976;**38**:369.

Fauci et al: The idiopathic hypereosinophilic syndrome. *Ann Intern Med* 1982;**97**:78.

Hess OM et al: Pre- and postoperative findings in patients with endomyocardial fibrosis. *Br Heart J* 1978;**40**:406.

Löffler W: Endocarditis parietalis fibro-plastica mit Bluteosinophilie, ein eigenartiges Krankheitsbild. *Schweiz Med Wochenschr* 1936;**17**:817.

Olsen EGJ, Spry CJF: Relation between eosinophilia and endomyocardial disease. *Prog Cardiovasc Dis* 1985;**27**:241.

Parrillo JE et al: The cardiovascular manifestations of the hypereosinophilic syndrome: Prospective study of 26 patients, with review of the literature. *Am J Med* 1979;**67**:572.

Parry EHO, Abrahams DG: The natural history of endomyocardial fibrosis. *Q J Med* 1965;**34**:383.

Roberts WC, Buja LM, Ferrans VJ: Löffler's fibroplastic parietal endocarditis, eosinophilic leukaemia and Davies' endomyocardial fibrosis: The same disease at different stages? *Pathol Microbiol (Basel)* 1970;**35**:90.

Shaper AG: On the nature of some tropical cardiomyopathies. *Trans R Soc Trop Med Hyg* 1967;**61**:458.

Solley GO et al: Endomyocardiopathy with eosinophilia. *Mayo Clin Proc* 1976;**51**:697.

Somers K et al: Hemodynamic features of severe endomyocardial fibrosis of the right ventricle, including comparison with constrictive pericarditis. *Br Heart J* 1968;**30**:322.

Sickle Cell Disease & Chronic Anemia

Denenberg BS et al: Cardiac function in sickle cell anemia. *Am J Cardiol* 1983;**51**:1674.

Falk RH, Hood WB Jr: The heart in sickle cell anemia. *Arch Intern Med* 1982;**142**:1680.

Chagas' Disease

Acquatella H et al: M-mode and two-dimensional echocardiography in chronic Chagas' heart disease: A clinical and pathologic study. *Circulation* 1980;**62**:787.

Andrade ZA et al: Histopathology of the conducting tissue of the heart in Chagas' myocarditis. *Am Heart J* 1978;**95**:316.

Chagas C: Aspecto clinico da nova entidade morbida produzida pelo schizotrypanum cruzi. *Brasil-med* 1910; **24:**263.

Köberle F: Chagas' heart disease: Pathology. *Cardiologia* 1968;**52:**82.

Laranja FS et al: Chagas' disease: A clinical, epidemiologic and pathologic study. *Circulation* 1956;**14:**1035.

Oliveira JSM et al: Cardiac thrombosis and thromboembolism in chronic Chagas' heart disease. *Am J Cardiol* 1983;**52:**147.

Poltera AA, Cox JN, Owor R: Pancarditis affecting the conducting system and all valves in human African trypanosomiasis. *Br Heart J* 1976;**38:**827.

Prata A: Chagas' heart disease. *Cardiologia* 1968;**52:**79.

Rosenbaum MB: Chagasic myocardiopathy. *Prog Cardiovasc Dis* 1964;**7:**199.

Peripartum Cardiomyopathy

Brown AK et al: Cardiomyopathy and pregnancy. *Br Heart J* 1967;**29:**387.

Burch GE, Giles TD, Tsui CY: Postpartal cardiomyopathy. Page 269 in: *Cardiomyopathy*. Burch GE (editor). Davis, 1972.

Demakis JG et al: Natural course of peripartum cardiomyopathy. *Circulation* 1971;**44:**1053.

Fillmore SJ, Parry EHO: The evolution of peripartal heart failure in Zaria, Nigeria: Some etiologic factors. *Circulation* 1977;**56:**1058.

Gilchrist AR: Cardiological problems in younger women, including those of pregnancy and the puerperium. *Br Med J* 1963;**1:**209.

Julian DG, Szekely P: Peripartum cardiomyopathy. *Prog Cardiovasc Dis* 1985;**27:**223.

Melvin KR et al: Peripartum cardiomyopathy due to myocarditis. *N Engl J Med* 1982;**307:**731.

Sanderson JE et al: Postpartum cardiac failure: Heart failure due to volume overload? *Am Heart J* 1979;**97:**613.

Walsh JJ et al: Idiopathic myocardiopathy of the puerperium (postpartal heart disease). *Circulation* 1965;**32:**19.

Neuropathic Disorders & Inherited Disorders of Metabolism

Blieden LC, Moller JH: Cardiac involvement in inherited disorders of metabolism. *Prog Cardiovasc Dis* 1974;**16:**615.

Gottdiener JS et al: Characteristics of the cardiac hypertrophy in Friedreich's ataxia. *Am Heart J* 1982;**103:**525.

Perloff JK, DeLeon AC Jr, O'Doherty D: The cardiomyopathy of progressive muscular dystrophy. *Circulation* 1966;**33:**625.

Roberts WC, Honig HS: The spectrum of cardiovascular disease in the Marfan syndrome: A clinicomorphologic study of 18 necropsy patients and comparison to 151 previously reported necropsy patients. *Am Heart J* 1982;**104:**115.

Smith ER et al: Hypertrophic cardiomyopathy: The heart disease of Friedreich's ataxia. *Am Heart J* 1977;**94:**428.

Pericarditis 18

Pericardial disease usually involves the epicardium, often spreading to or from the myocardium. It almost always produces inflammatory changes, which include irritative and mechanical effects in addition to those caused by bacterial, viral, and fungal infections. Pericardial disease exhibits a wide spectrum of clinical manifestations and varies in importance from an inconsequential associated finding to a major cardiovascular problem, as in acute myopericarditis.

Causes of Pericardial Disease

The pericardium may be involved in acute bacterial or viral infections such as pneumonia, when infection spreads from the lungs or mediastinum, and in chronic infections such as tuberculosis. Other generalized conditions such as uremia, systemic lupus erythematosus, scleroderma, serum sickness, radiation therapy, rheumatoid arthritis, or different varieties of lymphoma or other malignant disorders, usually lung or breast cancer, may involve the pericardium. Although the involvement of the pericardium in these disorders is usually incidental, all of these conditions may occasionally cause significant hemodynamic changes (about 10% of cases). Uremia is coming to be an important factor in pericardial disease now that renal dialysis is widely used in the palliative treatment of chronic renal disease. The commonest primary pericardial infections are those due to viruses (eg, coxsackie B virus), but these infections usually also affect the myocardium. When myocarditis predominates, the clinical picture is as described in Chapter 17. Aseptic inflammatory changes are seen following acute myocardial infarction. They are especially noticeable in anteroseptal infarcts in which the necrosis of cardiac tissue involves the surface of the heart and causes changes that are indistinguishable from those due to inflammation. Another form of aseptic inflammation, postpericardiotomy syndrome, occurs both after myocardial infarction (3–6 weeks) and following cardiac surgery, with low-grade, probably autoimmune, self-limiting inflammation involving the pericardium and pleura. It was first seen after mitral commissurotomy and was originally thought to represent a recurrence of rheumatic fever. However, it is also seen after operations for congenital lesions.

Blunt or penetrating trauma such as that associated with stab wounds or rib fracture may damage the pericardium and lead to hemopericardium. Hemopericardium also occurs when vascular structures such as the heart or the aorta rupture into the pericardium.

Malignant disease also affects the pericardium, usually causing effusion. Neoplastic involvement of the pericardium may occur either by direct spread from the breast or lung or, more rarely, by bloodborne means, and the effusion is often large and recurrent. Tumor usually spreads directly by way of the mediastinum, but secondary deposits and even primary tumors of the pericardium (mesoendothelioma and sarcoma) can occur. The accumulation of fluid in the pericardial cavity seen in heart failure is due to transudation. In myxedema, enlargement of the cardiac silhouette is usually due to pericardial fluid but may be due to myocardial enlargement. In tuberculous cases, the infection is more chronic and effusion is relatively common. In some cases, other serous cavities (pleura or peritoneum) are also affected. The disease runs a chronic course, and pain, fever, and myocardial involvement are less prominent than in viral cases.

Clinical Findings

Pericarditis presents a spectrum of cases ranging from fibrinous (dry) pericarditis through pericardial effusion, with or without evidence of cardiac tamponade, to seroconstrictive and classic chronic pericardial constriction. These different manifestations are interrelated, as shown in Fig 18–1. Spread of the disease to involve the myocardium is not infrequent.

FIBRINOUS (DRY) PERICARDITIS

Clinical Findings

A. Symptoms: Fibrinous pericarditis most commonly occurs in the course of some other disease; thus, the symptoms depend on the cause, and pain is not necessarily a feature. In primary pericarditis caused by viral infection, pain, malaise, fever, and myalgia are the usual presenting symptoms. The pain is often worse with breathing, swallowing, or belching, and it may radiate to the shoulder. It is often substernal and associated with cough. The patient may obtain relief by sitting up and leaning forward or by kneeling on all fours. Pain characteristically decreases or disappears when effusion develops.

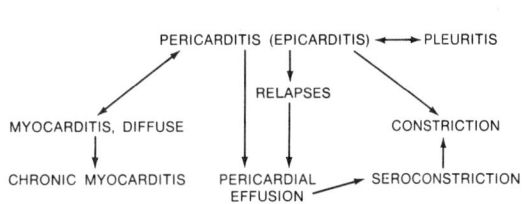

Figure 18–1. Spectrum of pericardial disease. (Reproduced, with permission, from Goldman MJ: Pericarditis. *West J Med* 1975;**123**:467.)

The pericarditis that occurs in about 15% of cases of acute myocardial infarction is not generally painful. It is noted about the third day after infarction, is usually transient, and is of little hemodynamic significance except when anticoagulants cause hemorrhage into the pericardial cavity. Postpericardiotomy syndrome, which occurs about 3–6 weeks after cardiac surgery or myocardial infarction, causes pericardial or pleural pain and may be associated with fever. It may be confused with hemorrhagic pericardial effusion due to anticoagulant therapy or postoperative infection.

B. Signs: The most important and often the only sign of fibrinous pericarditis is the development of a pericardial friction rub. In most cases in which pericarditis is secondary to a generalized disease, the only sign of pericardial involvement is a friction rub, which is often variable and transient. Pericardial friction produces a rough, scratchy 2- or 3-component superficial sound that is unrelated to other heart sounds. The components are associated with atrial systole, ventricular systole, and ventricular diastole. Friction can be confused with extraneous stethoscope sounds, with noise caused by hair on the chest, and with murmurs, especially to-and-fro murmurs. Both the bell and the diaphragm of the stethoscope are used to listen for friction rubs, and the patient should not breathe during auscultation.

C. Electrocardiographic Findings: Like the friction rub, electrocardiographic signs of pericarditis may be the only evidence indicative of pericardial involvement. Initially, electrocardiographic changes consist of ST–T segment elevation in all left ventricular leads (Fig 18–2), with preservation of the upward concavity, in contrast to the acute injury of acute myocardial infarction, in which the ST segment has upward convexity. Return of the ST segment (Fig 18–3) to the baseline in a few days is followed by symmetric T wave inversion. Reciprocal changes are absent except in aVR, and Q waves do not occur. It may be difficult to differentiate pericarditis from nontransmural myo-

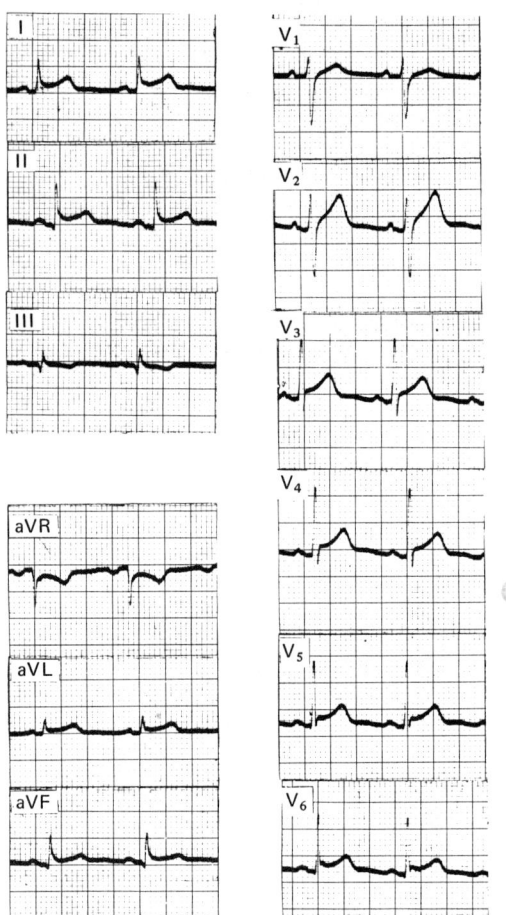

Figure 18–2. Acute pericarditis. ST segment elevation with concave upward curvature is seen in leads I, II, aVL, aVF, and V_{2-6}. Reciprocal ST segment depression is seen in cavity lead aVR. (Reproduced, with permission, from Goldschlager N, Goldman MJ: *Electrocardiography: Essentials of Interpretation.* Lange, 1984.)

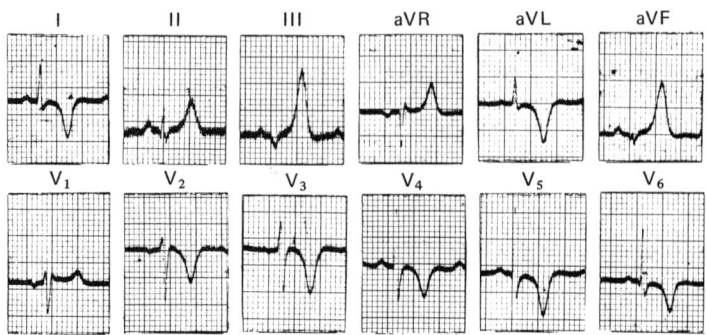

Figure 18–3. Pericarditis (late pattern). Deep, symmetrically inverted T waves in I, aVL, and V_{2-6}. The marked T wave abnormalities, unusual in pericarditis, may indicate concomitant myocarditis. (Reproduced, with permission, from Goldschlager N, Goldman MJ: *Electrocardiography: Essentials of Interpretation.* Lange, 1984.)

cardial infarction at the stage of T wave inversion because epicarditis is present, and the presence of other diagnostic features, especially elevated serum enzymes (myocardial band creatine phosphokinase), is required.

D. X-Ray Findings: The heart is not necessarily enlarged. Any radiologic changes should be attributed to the underlying disease.

E. Laboratory Findings: Leukocytosis of 10,000–20,000 is usually seen in viral pericarditis. A raised sedimentation rate is also found regardless of cause. Serologic abnormality due to generalized disease may be present (eg, positive LE cell preparation, presence of antinuclear antibody, or elevated serum creatinine).

F. Special Investigations: Fibrinous (dry) pericarditis has no hemodynamic effects per se. If and when effusion of more than about 15 mL develops, or when the inflammatory process heals, causing thickening of the pericardium, echocardiographic changes develop.

Differential Diagnosis

Acute viral pericarditis must be distinguished from acute myocardial infarction. In pericarditis, pain, fever, and electrocardiographic changes are present from the onset of illness. In myocardial infarction, pain comes first and is followed a few days later by fever and friction rub. Q waves are not seen in pericarditis. It is almost always possible to make the diagnosis by following the serial changes on the ECG, unless the patient is first seen after the third or fourth day and has nontransmural infarction. Serial examination of ECGs as well as specific myocardial enzyme studies (myocardial band creatine phosphokinase) should be used to decide whether the electrocardiographic changes seen in a patient who is suffering from some generalized disease are due to infarction. The diagnosis of associated myocarditis may prove difficult, and the distinction between pleural and pericardial inflammation is likewise difficult: The friction rub is related to inspiration in pleural inflammation and is heard during held respiration in pericardial inflammation, but in many cases the friction rub is pleuropericardial and shares the features of both entities.

Viral pericarditis is sometimes difficult to distinguish from tuberculous pericarditis. Viral cases tend to be more acute and are less likely to lead to effusion. Because tubercle bacilli are difficult to find, the fluid should be cultured. Diagnostic pericardiocentesis is indicated.

Complications

Myocardial involvement is almost inevitably present on microscopic examination. Clinical evidence of myocarditis is most frequently seen in viral pericarditis. Relapses and recurrences are also common, perhaps owing to autoimmune mechanisms. Progression of the disease, leading to effusion, seroconstriction, and classic chronic pericardial constriction, can occur in pericarditis due to any cause.

Treatment

The underlying disease should be treated and symptomatic therapy given for the pericarditis. In acute viral pericarditis, salicylates and expectant treatment are usually all that is needed, but corticosteroids may be helpful in severe cases. Corticosteroids are not indicated in tuberculous cases unless given with antituberculosis drugs. In postpericardiotomy syndrome, symptomatic treatment is also all that is necessary in most cases. If the pericarditis fails to clear in a week to 10 days, or if the infection is severe, corticosteroids are often utilized. Although there is no conclusive evidence that they are effective, a trial of treatment may be worthwhile. The development of pericarditis in a patient with uremia is an indication to start or increase the frequency of dialysis.

Prognosis

The prognosis in most cases of acute viral pericarditis is excellent, provided that myocardial involvement is minimal. Tuberculous cases respond to specific treatment, which must sometimes be administered without proof of the cause. The relative incidence of viral and tuberculous lesions varies in different areas, and viral lesions are now more common than tuberculous ones in the USA. In a few cases, the disease persists or recurs, and signs of pericardial constriction can develop in a period of weeks to months. This is rare, however. In most cases of fibrinous pericarditis, the prognosis depends more on the underlying disease, and pericardial involvement is only a minor part of the clinical picture. Relapses are common and may constitute a major problem.

PERICARDIAL EFFUSION WITHOUT TAMPONADE

If pericardial fluid accumulates slowly, the pericardium stretches, and there is little rise in pressure and little or no interference with cardiac filling.

Clinical Findings

A. Symptoms: Pericardial effusion per se causes no specific symptoms. The pain of pericarditis may disappear when effusion develops. On the other hand, pain may develop with hemopericardium as blood irritates the pericardium.

B. Signs: The physical signs of pericardial effusion depend on the amount of effusion. In the absence of evidence of tamponade, the pulse, pulse pressure, and blood pressure are normal, but the patient may appear anxious, and there is usually some tachycardia.

The heart appears enlarged in pericardial effusion. The cardiac impulse is usually difficult to detect but may be palpable. Heart sounds are often distant, and a friction rub may still be audible even though the pain has disappeared and significant effusion has occurred. Murmurs are usually absent.

C. Electrocardiographic Findings: The T waves are usually low, biphasic, inverted, or flat, and the

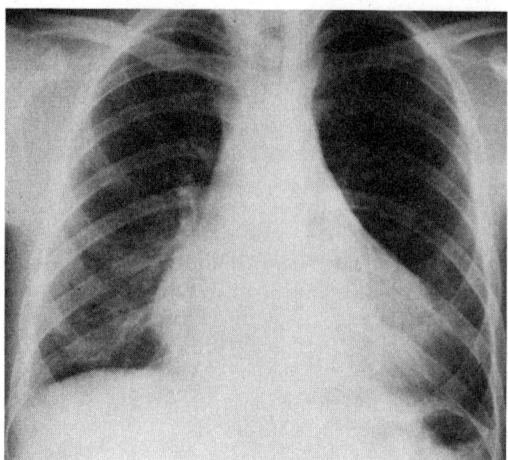

Figure 18–4. Chest x-ray of a patient with pericardial effusion.

overall voltage is low in the limb leads in pericardial effusion. There are no specific electrocardiographic changes, but electrical alternans is sometimes seen in pericardial effusion when the position of the heart changes as it beats.

D. X-Ray Findings: The cardiac silhouette is enlarged in pericardial effusion and may reach enormous proportions in chronic lesions without affecting cardiac function. The principal problem is to decide whether the heart itself is enlarged. The shape of the cardiac silhouette in pericardial effusion is triangular on posteroanterior view (Fig 18–4). An acute right cardiophrenic angle, clear lung fields, and associated pleural effusion are common. Left-sided pleural effusion is common in pericardial disease, whereas in heart failure effusion is usually bilateral. Serial examinations may be useful to determine changes in heart size. The lack of signs of specific chamber enlargement may be helpful. It is important not to confuse the massive cardiac enlargement seen in giant left atrium with pericardial effusion. Since the left atrium forms the right border of the heart in giant left atrium, right heart catheterization and right atrial angiography can produce misleading results and lead to an unnecessary and dangerous attempt at pericardiocentesis, with inadvertent puncture of the heart.

E. Special Investigations:

1. Noninvasive techniques–Specific diagnostic tests such as LE cell preparations, thyroid function tests, and renal function tests are indicated in some cases. Tuberculin testing and bacteriologic examination are required if an infective origin is suspected. Pericardial effusion is one of the conditions in which echocardiography is of particular help in diagnosis. The increase in the echo-free space between the posterior wall of the left ventricle and the pericardium is more reliable than the equivalent space at the front of the heart. Serial echocardiograms are thus particularly helpful in following the course of the disease. The development of adhesion and fibrosis with thickening of the pericardium as the effusion is absorbed is shown in Fig 18–5.

2. Invasive techniques–

a. Catheterization and angiography–Right heart catheterization and right atrial angiography were used in the past to help in the diagnosis of pericardial effusion, but they are less frequently employed now that echocardiography has become available. The finding of a significant—1 cm or more—gap between the catheter tip or the border of the contrast material in the atrium and the edge of the cardiac silhouette suggests the presence of fluid. Some physicians advocate coronary angiography, with injection of contrast medium into the left coronary artery to outline the anterior descending coronary artery on right anterior

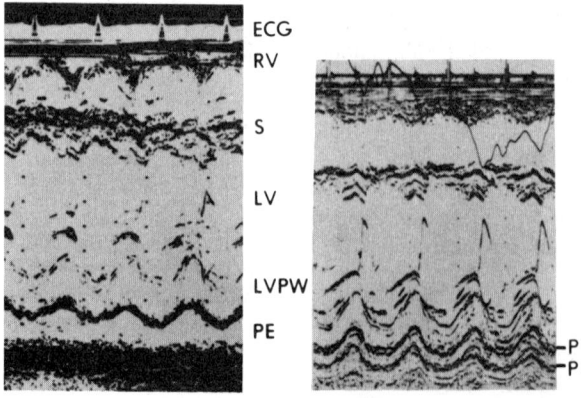

Figure 18–5. Serial echocardiograms 3 weeks apart in a patient with pericardial effusion showing development of pericardial thickening and fibrosis when the effusion is absorbed. RV, right ventricle; S, septum; LV, left ventricle; LVPW, left ventricular posterior wall; PE, pericardial effusion; P_1 and P_2, visceral and parietal pericardial layer. (Courtesy of NB Schiller.)

oblique view. If there is a significant shadow beyond the filled vessel, pericardial effusion is probably present. Intravenous injection of soluble gases (mainly CO_2) with the patient lying on the left side has also been used in the past for diagnosis. The gas accumulates as a bubble in the right atrium and outlines the right atrial wall to show the distortion due to the presence of fluid or pericardial thickening.

b. Pericardiocentesis—Although echocardiography is extremely valuable in indicating the presence and site of pericardial effusion, the ultimate diagnostic procedure is pericardiocentesis. The procedure is described on p 126. The data provided by echocardiography help the physician decide whether to tap the pericardium, and pericardiocentesis is seldom indicated if echocardiography is negative.

Differential Diagnosis

Enlargement of the heart due to dilatation or hypertrophy is virtually the only condition that must be distinguished from pericardial effusion, although primary tumor (angiosarcoma) may rarely enter into the differential diagnosis. In some cases there may be effusion in addition to cardiac enlargement. In these cases, the introduction of air into the pericardium at the time of pericardiocentesis serves to indicate heart size and the thickness of the pericardium. Echocardiographic examination has provided significant help in differentiating between pericardial effusion and cardiac enlargement.

Complications

Cardiac tamponade is the most important complication of pericardial effusion. It can occur with surprising speed, because the compliance of the pericardial cavity can be markedly nonlinear, and the accumulation of a small additional amount of fluid can cause a marked rise in intrapericardial pressure.

Treatment

The treatment of pericardial effusion depends on the cause and on the severity of the hemodynamic effects. If effusion is not great and there are no symptoms, supportive treatment is all that is needed, but if effusion is considerable or recurrent or if signs and symptoms of tamponade are developing, a pericardial tap should be performed. Purulent pericardial effusion should be drained and smear and culture of the fluid obtained for examination; thoracotomy is often necessary to achieve adequate drainage. Serous effusion that occurs in such diseases as tuberculosis, uremia, or cancer may need to be tapped repeatedly. This is especially true if malignant disease is the cause of the effusion. Chemotherapeutic agents may be instilled into the pericardial cavity after tapping to prevent recurrence of effusion. Tetracycline and nonabsorbable steroid compounds have also been used for this purpose. Dialysis may help to control effusions in patients with renal disease, but many kinds of effusion require no treatment other than measures treating the underlying cause.

Prognosis

The prognosis in pericardial effusion per se depends on the cause of the disease. Pericardial effusion is seldom a dangerous condition in the absence of tamponade, and repeated pericardiocentesis is seldom necessary for more than a few weeks except in malignant or other major systemic disease.

CARDIAC TAMPONADE

The time necessary for fluid to accumulate in the pericardial cavity can vary from seconds (in rupture of a major structure) to weeks or months in chronic infections. It is the *rate* of rise of intrapericardial pressure that is the most important factor in determining the development of the hemodynamic and clinical features of cardiac tamponade. When the fluid accumulates rapidly, or if effusion occurs into a pericardium thickened and noncompliant because of fibrosis, serious interference with cardiac filling can occur with remarkable speed. The compliance of the pericardial cavity is markedly nonlinear, so that although significant amounts of fluid can sometimes accumulate without much rise in pressure, a further slight increase in fluid may produce a considerable rise in pressure as well as symptoms and signs of cardiac tamponade.

Cardiac tamponade develops when the pressure in the pericardial cavity rises to a level equal to that in the heart during diastole. Because the right atrium and ventricle have the lowest diastolic pressures, they are the first structures to be compressed by the increasing pericardial pressure, and the compression is mainly diastolic. The venous pressure and the intracardiac and intrapericardial pressures rise together as pericardial tamponade progresses, and soon the diastolic pressures in both the left and right sides of the heart are raised. At this stage, respiration has a marked hemodynamic effect, and pulsus paradoxus develops. The increased negative intrathoracic pressure produced by inspiration stretches the right heart and opens up the compressed right ventricle, increasing its output and filling the lungs with blood. In severe cases, the interventricular septum may bulge to the left on inspiration. All these events interfere with left ventricular filling and cause an inspiratory fall in arterial pressure and left ventricular output. Conversely, on expiration, the right ventricular volume decreases and the blood stored in the lungs returns to the left heart, increasing its output. The reciprocal effects of inspiration and expiration on the right and left heart are not seen when there is an atrial septal defect, nor do they occur unless the diastolic pressures in both sides of the heart are equal. Thus, pulsus paradoxus is not seen when the left ventricle is hypertrophied and stiff, as occurs in some cases of chronic renal disease and hypertension; in these instances, left atrial pressure is higher than right atrial pressure, and the right ventricle is compressed before the left heart is.

Clinical Findings

A. Symptoms: Acute cardiac tamponade may cause symptoms ranging from anxiety, sweating, dyspnea, dizziness, and syncope to frank shock. The clinical picture ranges from slight circulatory and hemodynamic abnormalities to circulatory collapse.

B. Signs: Venous pressure is raised in cardiac tamponade except when severe dehydration has caused a reduction in circulating blood volume. The venous pressure does not usually show an increase with inspiration (Kussmaul's sign), probably because venous return is impaired throughout the cardiac cycle and not only in inspiration, as in pericardial effusion without tamponade. The rise in pericardial pressure interferes with cardiac filling throughout the whole of the cardiac cycle, and the rapid y descent seen in the jugular venous pulse in pericardial constriction is absent. The cardiac impulse is classically not palpable, the heart sounds are distant, and murmurs are absent. Since filling is impaired throughout diastole, the rapid filling phase of early diastole seen in pericardial constriction is not prominent, and a pericardial third sound ("knock") is seldom heard.

The pulse rate is rapid, and the blood pressure and pulse pressure are low. Pulsus paradoxus, defined as a fall of more than 10 mm Hg or 10% in systolic arterial blood pressure on normal inspiration, can be detected when the blood pressure is measured either indirectly or directly (Fig 18–6). The term pulsus paradoxus is a misnomer, because the condition is basically an exaggeration of the normal finding of a decrease in arterial pressure with inspiration and therefore is not actually "paradoxic" (see Chapter 3, p 44).

C. Electrocardiographic Findings: There are no specific electrocardiographic changes of cardiac tamponade, but the ECG is seldom normal. Low voltage and flat or inverted T waves are commonly seen.

D. X-Ray Findings: The heart is small in patients with acute tamponade, but since all combinations of effusion and constriction can occur, heart size is not of diagnostic value. The lung fields are usually clear, and the pulmonary vessels are not prominent.

E. Special Investigations:

1. Noninvasive techniques–The development of cardiac tamponade can be detected on the basis of narrowing of the outflow tract of the right ventricle seen on echocardiography. In the example shown in Fig 18–7, the right ventricular cavity is almost obliterated during expiration and only opens up on inspiration. Two-dimensional echocardiograms can also be used to demonstrate this important sign of cardiac tamponade. Fig 18–8 shows a sector scan in the long-axis view before and after pericardiocentesis. The change in size of the right ventricular outflow tract (RVOT) is clearly visible.

2. Invasive techniques–Management of cardiac tamponade is facilitated by monitoring systemic arterial, central venous, and pericardial pressures during pericardiocentesis. The procedure can be conveniently carried out in the cardiac catheterization laboratory. When intracardiac pressures are measured in tamponade, the diastolic pressures in the 2 ventricles and the pericardial cavity are equal. As fluid is withdrawn from the pericardium and tamponade is relieved (see Fig 18–9), these pressures at first fall together as cardiac output and arterial pressure increase and heart rate and pulsus paradoxus decrease. Ultimately, pericardial pressure falls below ventricular diastolic pressure, and at that point tamponade is relieved. Further withdrawal of fluid then leads to little or no hemodynamic improvement.

Differential Diagnosis

Cardiac tamponade must be distinguished from other acute cardiac emergencies such as hemorrhage,

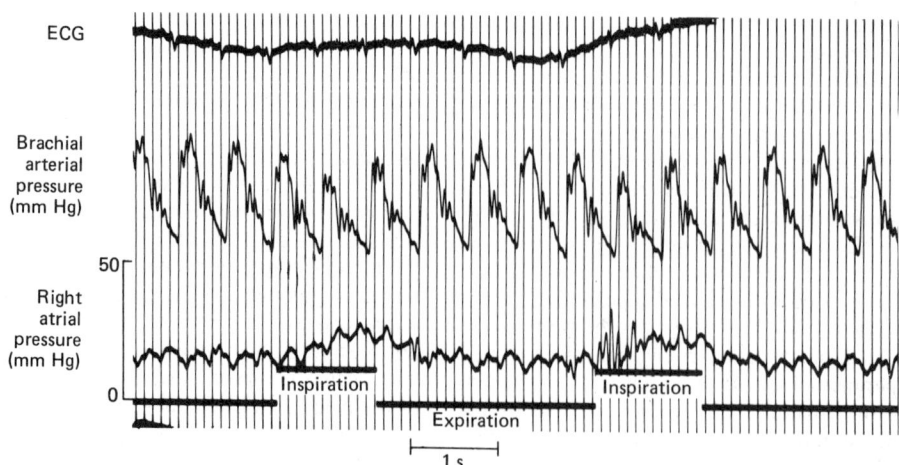

Figure 18–6. Brachial arterial and right atrial pressures showing pulsus paradoxus in a patient with constrictive pericarditis and an increase in right atrial pressure on inspiration (Kussmaul's sign). Both the systolic and diastolic atrial pressures rise with inspiration.

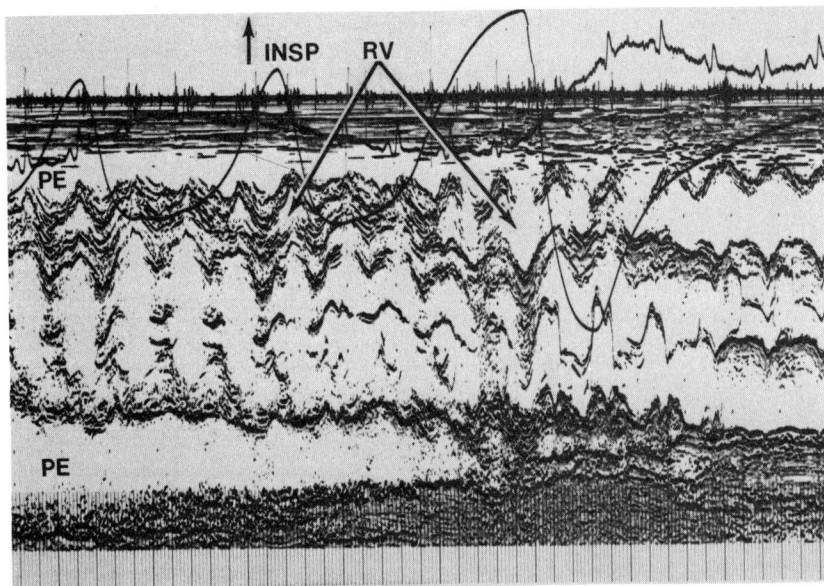

Figure 18–7. Echocardiogram showing cardiac tamponade in a patient with substantial pericardial effusion (PE). The right ventricular cavity (RV) is compressed and almost obliterated; it is seen to enlarge during inspiration. Inspiration (INSP) is upward. (Courtesy of NB Schiller.)

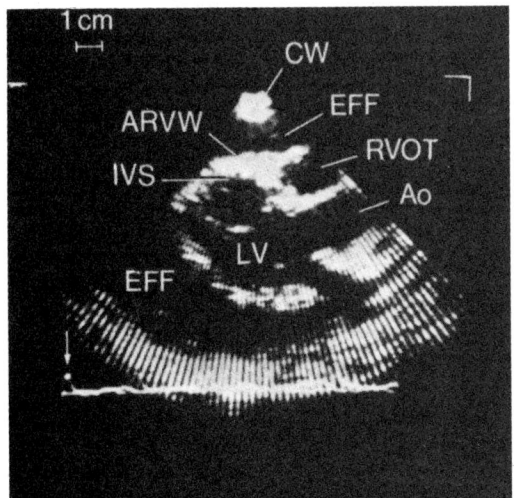
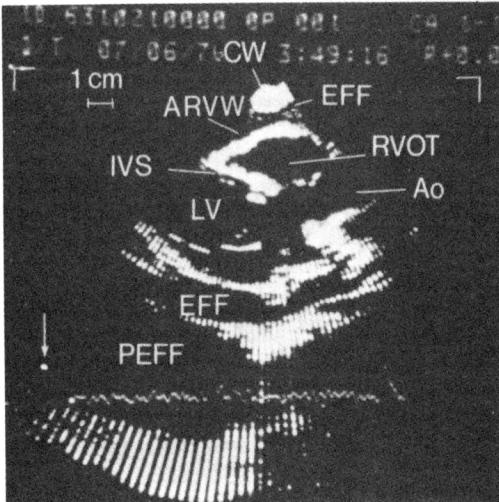

Figure 18–8. Two-dimensional echocardiograms before *(left)* and after *(right)* pericardiocentesis. These images, obtained in the long-axis view, encompass all portions of the heart seen in the standard M mode echocardiographic sweep. Before drainage, the right ventricular cavity is barely discernible below the aortoseptal junction, narrowing abruptly at this level. Following pericardiocentesis, the right ventricle expands and is well visualized to the midseptal level. Note diminished effusion size after drainage. Both studies were performed at end expiration and at end diastole (R + 0.00). The bright spot (arrow) represents the timing of camera gating at end diastole. The calibration factor is the same for the 2 studies. However, the posterior gain setting is reduced in the initial study, obscuring the pleural effusion (PEFF) seen later. LV, left ventricular cavity; CW, chest wall; ARVW, anterior right ventricular wall; EFF, effusion; IVS, interventricular septum; RVOT, right ventricular outflow tract; Ao, aorta. (Reproduced, with permission, from the American Heart Association, Inc., Schiller NB, Botvinick EH: Right ventricular compression as a sign of cardiac tamponade: Analysis of echocardiographic ventricular dimensions and their clinical implications. *Circulation* 1977;**56**:774.)

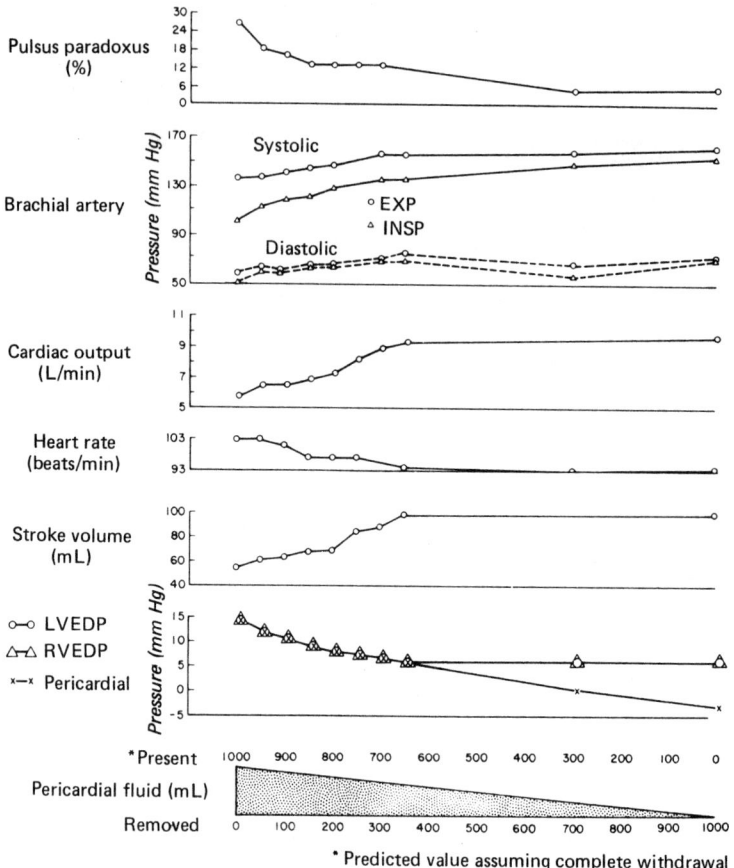

Figure 18-9. Hemodynamic changes during serial fluid withdrawals in a 22-year-old man with tamponade resulting from uremic pericarditis. Diagnostic levels of pulsus paradoxus persist as long as left ventricular end-diastolic pressure (LVEDP) remains equilibrated with pericardial pressure. RVEDP, right ventricular end-diastolic pressure; EXP, expiration; INSP, inspiration. (Reproduced, with permission, from the American Heart Association, Inc., Reddy PS et al: Cardiac tamponade: Hemodynamic observations in man. *Circulation* 1978;**58**:265.)

myocardial infarction, and pulmonary embolism. Signs of a falling arterial pressure and cardiac output and a rising venous pressure and heart rate should alert the physician to the possibility of cardiac tamponade, and pulsus paradoxus strongly suggests the diagnosis. Echocardiography is the most helpful diagnostic investigation.

Complications

The complications of cardiac tamponade include those of circulatory collapse, with inadequate perfusion of any organ system, but most commonly the brain and the kidneys. Early recognition and prompt treatment are essential, especially in acute cases.

Treatment

Acute cardiac tamponade is always an emergency, and the physician must always remain on the alert to prevent its recurrence. Pericardiocentesis is indicated as soon as the diagnosis is made. The procedure is described in Chapter 7 (p 126). The response to the removal of the first few milliliters of fluid is usually dramatic, but residual abnormalities in venous and pericardial pressures may be seen if both effusion and fibrosis were initially responsible for the tamponade.

Resection of a portion of the pericardium to allow free communication with the pleura may be needed if repeated pericardiocentesis fails to prevent recurrence. Instillation of chemotherapeutic agents into the pericardial cavity can also be used to prevent recurrence.

Prognosis

Acute cardiac tamponade is a life-threatening complication of pericardial disease, but the immediate prognosis is good with efficient treatment, provided that rupture of a major structure into the pericardium has not occurred. The long-term prognosis depends on the underlying cause of the pericardial disease.

PERICARDIAL CONSTRICTION

The term pericardial constriction is used to describe both the classic chronic disease (constrictive pericarditis) that mimics right heart failure, and the subacute condition, in which a rigid pericardium and pericardial fluid combine to compress the heart and interfere with its late diastolic filling (subacute effusive constrictive pericarditis). With the improved diagnostic techniques now available, more subacute cases are being recognized, especially since tuberculosis, the principal cause of chronic pericardial constriction, is no longer common in the Western world. Inflammatory (viral, associated with idiopathic mediastinal fibrosis, or sarcoidosis), uremic, neoplastic, and traumatic (including postcardiotomy and irradiation) pericardial diseases are more likely to cause the subacute form than classic chronic constrictive pericarditis, in which no evidence of effusion is ordinarily detectable.

The chronic inflammatory changes in the pericardial cavity surround the heart with a sheath of tough, unyielding fibrous tissue that interferes with cardiac filling. The actual, or effective, intrapericardial pressure rises, and the pressure in all heart chambers at the end of diastole rises. The heart is immobilized because it is encased in an unyielding fibrous cage that interferes with its excursion during contraction and relaxation. The more compliant chambers, the atria and the right ventricle, bear the brunt of the burden, but end-diastolic pressures in all cardiac chambers tend to be the same: about 15–25 mm Hg in severe cases. The encasement does not necessarily involve all chambers, but the effective intrapericardial pressure rises on both sides of the heart. Although the effects of the disease are more severe in the more distensible right heart, the left side is almost invariably involved also.

Clinical Findings

A. Symptoms: Swelling of the abdomen and legs is the symptom suggesting a diagnosis of constrictive pericarditis. Dyspnea is not generally prominent but is usually present in all cases to some degree. Anorexia, weakness, wasting, and dyspepsia are seen in advanced cases that have not been properly diagnosed. These symptoms are due to a combination of low cardiac output and marked hepatic congestion. A history of a previous attack of acute or subacute pericarditis is an important feature. The absence of a history of other forms of heart disease is also valuable. Pain is not a prominent feature of the disease. The patient is usually able to lie flat without any problem and does not suffer from paroxysmal nocturnal dyspnea.

B. Signs: The pulse is usually rapid and the blood pressure low. Pulsus paradoxus is present in classic cases of the disease, but in only about one-third of cases. The heartbeat is irregular in about 30% of cases because of atrial fibrillation. The onset of arrhythmia is related to the age of the patient and the severity of the disease.

The patient appears chronically ill in advanced cases. The neck veins are distended, the venous pressure is markedly raised, and there is a rapid y descent. Tamponade and constriction cannot be differentiated on the basis of a consistent difference in venous pulse. Venous pressure and the nature of the venous pulse are important in pericardial constriction. The neck veins usually show a major negative wave at the time of the y descent. This constitutes diastolic collapse of the veins and is caused by rapid filling of the right heart in early diastole at a time when intracardiac pressure is at its lowest after the end of systole. The sign is not specific for pericardial disease and can be seen in any form of severe right heart failure. Another nonspecific physical sign associated with pericardial disease is Kussmaul's sign, an inspiratory increase in venous pressure (Fig 18–6). When right heart filling is excessive, the increase in venous pressure occurring on inspiration cannot be accommodated in the restricted right atrium, and atrial pressure consequently rises. In pericardial constriction, cardiac filling stops abruptly when the heart meets the limits of the unyielding pericardial cavity. This shock is felt as a palpable diastolic impulse in some cases. It is associated with the pericardial "knock," or filling sound, that generally occurs after the time of the opening snap and before the time of the usual third sound (Fig 18–10). It can be the loudest sound in the cardiac cycle. There is usually no cardiac murmur, and the heart sounds are soft.

Rales may be present at the base of the lung, and the liver is usually markedly enlarged and tender but not pulsating. Ascites tends to be more prominent than ankle edema, and the combination of wasting and edema resembles that seen in advanced right heart failure or cirrhosis of the liver.

C. Electrocardiographic Findings: There are no specific electrocardiographic changes. The voltage in the limb and precordial leads tends to be low, and T wave inversion is common. The presence of significant right or left ventricular hypertrophy on the ECG contradicts a diagnosis of constrictive pericarditis.

D. X-Ray Findings: The heart is classically not significantly enlarged and shows no specific chamber enlargement. The pulmonary artery is not enlarged, and pulmonary congestion is seldom marked. Redistribution of pulmonary blood flow to the apexes speaks against the diagnosis. X-rays provide the most useful

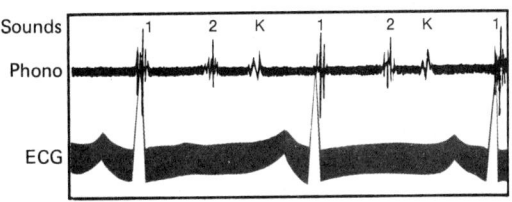

Figure 18–10. Phonocardiogram of typical sharp, early diastolic pericardial knock (K). (Courtesy of Roche Laboratories Division of Hoffman-La Roche, Inc.)

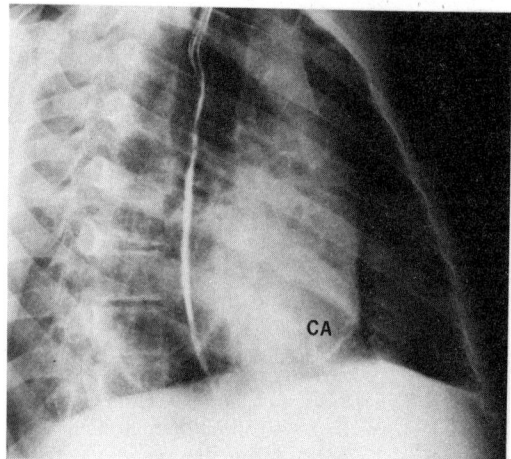

Figure 18–11. Chest x-ray of a patient with constrictive pericarditis showing calcification (CA) in the pericardium. Right anterior oblique view.

sign distinguishing myocardial disease from pericardial constriction, namely intrapericardial calcification, shown in Fig 18–11. This sign is most commonly seen in tuberculous cases, but it can occur in cases with viral origins. Signs of calcification on x-ray do not necessarily mean that constriction is always present, but if calcification is found, a primary myocardial cause for the patient's disease is unlikely except in tropical (African) endomyocardial fibrosis.

E. Special Investigations:

1. Noninvasive techniques–Venous pulse tracings, phonocardiography, and echocardiography are helpful in making the distinction between constrictive pericarditis and primary myocardial disease, but they are not absolutely diagnostic. The abrupt cessation of ventricular filling can be seen on echocardiography and contrasts with the ventricular dilatation and slowed ejection rate seen in cardiomyopathy. The thickness of the pericardium can be measured using computerized tomography. By this means, the thickened pericardium in patients with constriction can be distinguished from the normal pericardium in patients with restrictive cardiomyopathy.

2. Invasive techniques–Cardiac catheterization is often performed in an attempt to confirm the diagnosis. Unfortunately, there are no absolute diagnostic hemodynamic features that can help distinguish between constrictive pericarditis and restrictive cardiomyopathy, the principal condition with which constrictive pericarditis is confused. The problem of diagnosis is greatest when the level of diastolic pressure in all cardiac chambers is equal. There is little hemodynamic difference between interference with filling resulting from causes outside the heart, those in the heart wall, and those within the cardiac chambers. The hemodynamic features of impaired cardiac filling are shown in Fig 18–12 and include a marked diastolic dip and plateau in the right ventricular pressure tracing (square root sign), a marked diastolic drop in venous pressure, and equalization of end-diastolic pressure in all cardiac chambers. The square root sign is caused by limitation of cardiac filling, and the start of the plateau coincides with the audible filling sound. Pulsus paradoxus is not a specific sign of pericardial disease, and all the hemodynamic manifestations can be seen in patients with restrictive cardiomyopathy as well. These signs also occur in patients with endomyocardial fibrosis of the type seen in tropical Africa. In this condition, there is endocardial rather than pericardial calcification.

Although it is true that the distinction between pericardial and myocardial disease cannot be made with certainty, there are some features that strongly suggest primary myocardial disease. They are disproportionate increase in wedge pressure, low cardiac output, raised pulmonary vascular resistance, marked cardiac enlargement, raised pulmonary arterial pressure (systolic > 50 mm Hg), atrial gallop, marked pulmonary congestion, and a diastolic right ventricular pressure plateau less than 30% of systolic pressure.

The heart in constrictive pericarditis fills most rapidly in early diastole, and in some cases the distinction between pericardial and myocardial disease can be made from cineangiographic measurements of the rate of cardiac filling. In patients with myocardial disease, the heart fills more slowly than normally. Unfortunately, some patients with pericardial constriction also have myocardial disease, and the distinction based on the rate of ventricular filling is not clear-cut.

Differential Diagnosis

Superior vena caval obstruction, in which venous pulsation and evidence of inferior vena caval obstruction, with hepatic enlargement and ascites, are absent, should not be confused with constrictive pericarditis. Similarly, cirrhosis of the liver, in which the jugular venous pressure is not raised, should be readily distinguished. The principal entities with which constrictive pericarditis can be confused are restrictive cardiomyopathy (eg, due to amyloidosis) and endomyocardial fibrosis. The distinction is extremely difficult to make; furthermore, pericardial, myocardial, and endocardial fibrosis tend to influence one another because the fibrotic process tends to spread from one structure to the other. Pericardial fibrosis tends to involve the muscle of the thin-walled right ventricle; similarly, endocardial fibrosis tends to spread to the underlying cardiac muscle. Although exploratory thoracotomy may be indicated in difficult cases, it is harmful in patients with cardiomyopathy and should be avoided if possible.

The response to treatment with digitalis and its derivatives can be helpful in the diagnosis. The venous pressure may fall to normal in patients with right heart failure. In contrast, the venous pressure remains high in spite of medical therapy in constrictive pericarditis.

Complications

Involvement of the myocardium is such an inevi-

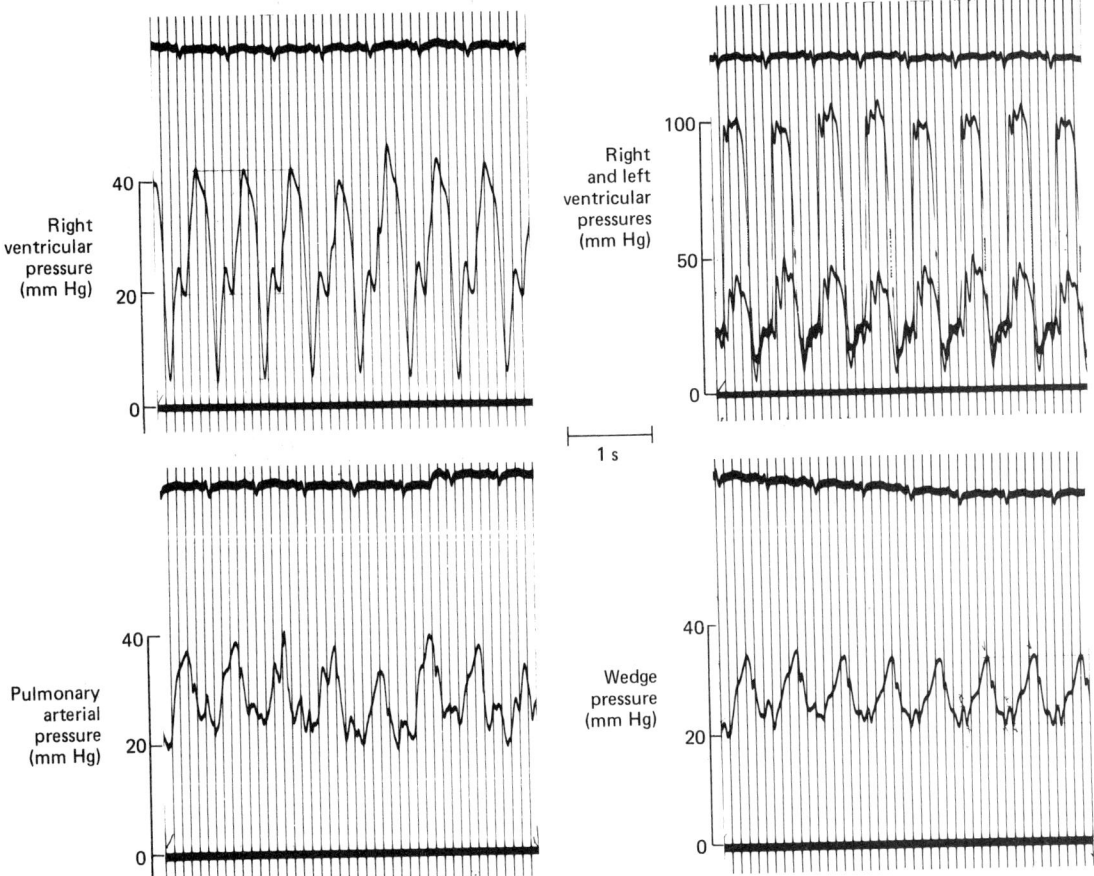

Figure 18-12. Intracardiac pressure tracings from a patient with constrictive pericarditis. The diastolic pressure is elevated to about 20 mm Hg in every chamber. The right ventricular pressure tracing shows a marked diastolic dip followed by a plateau (square root sign).

table consequence of pericardial constriction that it can hardly be called a complication. The effects are most clearly seen after surgery, when the heart (especially the right ventricle) may dilate when the constricting pericardium is removed, with subsequent cardiac dilatation and failure.

Treatment

Surgical resection of the shell of fibrous tissue around the heart is always indicated in symptomatic cases, preferably before marked hepatic enlargement has occurred. The operation is almost always palliative rather than curative, since some evidence of restricted motion of the heart is evident after operation, even though symptoms and signs may no longer be present. The operation can be either one of the easiest or one of the most difficult facing the cardiac surgeon. If there is a well-defined plane of cleavage between the fibrotic pericardium and the heart, or even a thin layer of fluid between the thickened pericardium and the heart, pericardial resection can be relatively simple. In most cases, however, especially when the disease is of long standing, the pericardium and the wall of the right ventricle form a single mass of dense fibrous tissue, and dissection is hazardous because of the danger of perforating the right ventricle. The left side of the heart may also be involved; if so, this side should be freed first to avoid pulmonary edema. Considerable judgment is necessary to decide when sufficient tissue has been resected to relieve the obstruction to filling. Intraoperative measurement of right atrial pressure is a help in determining the effects of surgery. If resection of the parietal pericardium does not result in a fall in venous pressure, epicardial resection is needed. The aim of the operation is to resect enough pericardial tissue to free the heart and lower the venous pressure significantly. If too much is removed, the right ventricle tends to dilate, and right heart failure results. Resection of fibrous tissue around the back of the heart is also often needed, and this may be technically difficult. The surgical mortality rate is about 5-10% and varies with the stage of the disease. It is higher in advanced cases. Any resected tissue should be examined histologically, and tubercle bacilli should be sought. If tuberculosis is not diagnosed by pathologic examination, specific diagnosis by other means is indicated, eg, tuberculin testing, sputum examination, or culture of gastric washings.

Restoration of sinus rhythm after operation is indicated in patients with atrial fibrillation or flutter.

Prognosis

The prognosis in constrictive pericarditis is reasonably good. The disease runs a chronic course. In patients in whom the disease is not diagnosed, the chronically raised venous pressure may be tolerated surprisingly well. Cardiac cirrhosis of the liver eventually develops. The principal determinant in prognosis is the success of the surgical treatment.

REFERENCES

General

Chandraratna PAN, Aronow WS: Detection of pericardial metastases by cross-sectional echocardiography. *Circulation* 1981;**63**:197.

Gottdiener JS et al: Late cardiac effects of therapeutic mediastinal radiation: Assessment by echocardiography and radionuclide angiography. *N Engl J Med* 1983;**308**:569.

Horowitz MS, Rossen R, Harrison DC: Echocardiographic diagnosis of pericardial disease. *Am Heart J* 1979;**97**:415.

John JT Jr, Hough A, Sergent JS: Pericardial disease in rheumatoid arthritis. *Am J Med* 1979;**66**:385.

Moncada R et al: Diagnostic role of computed tomography in pericardial heart disease: Congenital defects, thickening, neoplasms, and effusions. *Am Heart J* 1982;**103**:263.

Olson HG et al: Technetium-99m stannous pyrophosphate myocardial scintigrams in pericardial disease. *Am Heart J* 1980;**99**:459.

Pericarditis

Applefeld MM et al: Delayed pericardial disease after radiotherapy. *Am J Cardiol* 1981;**47**:210.

Applefeld MM et al: The late appearance of chronic pericardial disease in patients treated by radiotherapy for Hodgkin's disease. *Ann Intern Med* 1981;**94**:338.

Beaudry C: Uremic pericarditis and cardiac tamponade. *Ann Intern Med* 1966;**64**:990.

Comty CM, Cohen SL, Shapiro FL: Pericarditis in chronic uremia and its sequels. *Ann Intern Med* 1971;**75**:173.

Dressler W: The post-myocardial infarction syndrome: A report on 44 cases. *Arch Intern Med* 1959;**103**:28.

Engle MA et al: Viral illness and the post-pericardiotomy syndrome: A prospective study in children. *Circulation* 1980;**62**:1151.

Goldman MJ: Pericarditis. *West J Med* 1975;**123**:467.

Kumar S, Lesch M: Pericarditis in renal disease. *Prog Cardiovasc Dis* 1980;**22**:357.

Martin RG et al: Radiation-related pericarditis. *Am J Cardiol* 1975;**35**:216.

Montgomery JZ et al: Hemodynamic and diagnostic features of pericardial disease. *West J Med* 1975;**122**:295.

Ribot S et al: Treatment of uremic pericarditis. *Clin Nephrol* 1974;**2**:127.

Schrire V: Pericarditis (with particular reference to tuberculous pericarditis). *Australasian Ann Med* 1967;**16**:41.

Spodick DH: Differential diagnosis of acute pericarditis. *Prog Cardiovasc Dis* 1971;**14**:192.

Wheat LJ et al: A large urban outbreak of histoplasmosis: Clinical features. *Ann Intern Med* 1981;**94**:331.

Pericardial Effusion & Tamponade

Antman EM, Cargill V, Grossman W: Low pressure cardiac tamponade. *Ann Intern Med* 1979;**91**:403.

Davis S et al: Intrapericardial tetracycline for the management of cardiac tamponade secondary to malignant pericardial effusion. *N Engl J Med* 1978;**299**:1113.

Gabor GE, Winsberg F, Bloom HS: Electrical and mechanical alternation in pericardial effusion. *Chest* 1971;**59**:341.

Grose R et al: Left ventricular volume and function during relief of cardiac tamponade in man. *Circulation* 1982;**66**:149.

Guberman BA et al: Cardiac tamponade in medical patients. *Circulation* 1981;**64**:633.

Hancock EW: Cardiac tamponade. *Med Clin North Am* 1979;**63**:223.

Kleiman JH et al: Pericardial effusions in patients with end-stage renal disease. *Br Heart J* 1978;**40**:190.

Krikorian JG, Hancock EW: Pericardiocentesis. *Am J Med* 1978;**65**:808.

Kronzon I, Cohen ML, Winer HE: Diastolic atrial compression: A sensitive echocardiographic sign of cardiac tamponade. *J Am Coll Cardiol* 1983;**2**:770.

Lokich JJ: The management of malignant pericardial effusions. *JAMA* 1973;**224**:1401.

Martin RP et al: Localization of pericardial effusion with wide angle phased array echocardiography. *Am J Cardiol* 1978;**42**:904.

Ofori-Krayke SK et al: Late cardiac tamponade after open heart surgery: Incidence, role of anticoagulants in its pathogenesis and its relationship to the postpericardiotomy syndrome. *Circulation* 1981;**63**:1323.

Reddy PS et al: Cardiac tamponade: Hemodynamic observations in man. *Circulation* 1978;**58**:265.

Rinkenberger RL et al: Mechanism of electrical alternans in patients with pericardial effusion. *Cathet Cardiovasc Diagn* 1978;**4**:63.

Schiller NB, Botvinick EH: Right ventricular compression as a sign of cardiac tamponade: An analysis of echocardiographic ventricular dimensions and their clinical implications. *Circulation* 1977;**56**:774.

Shabetai R: Changing concepts of cardiac tamponade. *Mod Concepts Cardiovasc Dis* 1983;**52**:19.

Wei JY, Taylor GJ, Achuff SC: Recurrent cardiac tamponade and large pericardial effusions: Management with an indwelling pericardial catheter. *Am J Cardiol* 1978;**42**:281.

Weiss JM, Spodick DH: Laterality of pleural effusions in chronic congestive heart failure. *Am J Cardiol* 1984;**53**:651.

Wong B et al: The risk of pericardiocentesis. *Am J Cardiol* 1979;**44**:1110.

Constrictive Pericarditis

Candell-Riera J et al: Echocardiographic features of the interventricular septum in chronic constrictive endocarditis. *Circulation* 1978;**57**:1154.

Churchill ED: Decortication of the heart (Delorme) for adhesive pericarditis. *Arch Surg* 1929;**19:**1457.

Garrett J, O'Neill H, Blake S: Constrictive pericarditis associated with sarcoidosis. *Am Heart J* 1984;**107:**394.

Hancock EW: Subacute effusive constrictive pericarditis. *Circulation* 1971;**43:**183.

Hanley PC, Shub C, Lie JT: Constrictive pericarditis associated with combined retroperitoneal and mediastinal fibrosis. *Mayo Clin Proc* 1984;**59:**300.

Hirschmann JV: Pericardial constriction. *Am Heart J* 1978;**96:**110.

Isner JM et al: Differentiation of constrictive pericarditis from restrictive cardiomyopathy by computed tomographic imaging. *Am Heart J* 1983;**105:**1019.

Kutcher MA et al: Constrictive pericarditis as a complication of cardiac surgery: Recognition of an entity. *Am J Cardiol* 1982;**50:**742.

Mann T et al: Effusive-constrictive hemodynamic pattern due to neoplastic involvement of the pericardium. *Am J Cardiol* 1978;**41:**781.

Ribiero P et al: Constrictive pericarditis as a complication of coronary artery bypass surgery. *Br Heart J* 1984;**51:**205.

Schnittger I et al: Echocardiography: Pericardial thickening and constrictive pericarditis. *Am J Cardiol* 1978;**42:**388.

Somers K et al: Hemodynamic features of severe endomyocardial fibrosis of the right ventricle, including comparison with constrictive pericarditis. *Br Heart J* 1968;**30:**322.

Tyberg TI, Goodyer AVN, Langou RA: Genesis of pericardial knock in constrictive pericarditis. *Am J Cardiol* 1980;**46;**570.

Tyberg TI et al: Left ventricular filling in differentiating restrictive amyloid cardiomyopathy and constrictive pericarditis. *Am J Cardiol* 1981;**47:**791.

Veerasamy KG et al: Subacute constrictive uremic pericarditis: Survival after pericardiectomy. *JAMA* 1976;**235:**1351.

White PD: Chronic constrictive pericarditis (Pick's disease) treated by pericardial resection. *Lancet* 1935;**2:**597.

Wood P: Chronic constrictive pericarditis. *Am J Cardiol* 1961;**7:**48.

19 Pulmonary Heart Disease

The principal site of involvement in pulmonary heart disease is the pulmonary vascular bed. The pulmonary blood vessels, arterioles, capillaries, and veins may be affected by heart disease, leading to pulmonary parenchymal involvement, or by pulmonary disease, leading to cardiac involvement, mainly affecting the right heart.

PULMONARY HYPERTENSION

The development of increased pulmonary arterial pressure (pulmonary hypertension) represents the most important response of pulmonary blood vessels to disease. Pulmonary hypertension may result from primary parenchymal disease of the lungs, from changes in the walls of the blood vessels, or from obstruction to the lumen caused by thrombosis or embolization. The term "cor pulmonale" is used to describe right heart involvement, and cor pulmonale is said to be present when any right-sided abnormality can be demonstrated; frank right heart failure does not have to be present.

Pulmonary circulation in the adult seems to be almost completely passive when compared to the systemic circulation. It behaves as an unreactive, low-pressure, low-resistance, short, high-flow pathway from the heart via the pulmonary arteries to the pulmonary capillary bed, which constitutes the large (100 m^2) site of gas exchange.

Mechanism of Production of Pulmonary Hypertension

The principal stimuli evoking a response in the pulmonary arterioles are (1) alveolar hypoxia, as occurs with exposure to high altitude, and (2) pulmonary venous hypertension. The site of reaction in both cases is the smooth muscle of the pulmonary arterioles. Both stimuli cause arteriolar vasoconstriction that is at first functional, spasmodic, and reversible; with time, however, the vasoconstriction develops into organic muscular hypertrophy, which is ultimately irreversible. The age at which the patient is first exposed to these stimuli and their magnitude and duration play an important role in determining the response of the pulmonary circulation. Since responsiveness decreases with age, stimuli that have been present since birth or infancy cause more severe and less readily reversible changes. Hypoxia and raised pulmonary venous pressure interact; consequently, pulmonary hypertension is more severe in patients living at higher altitudes who have disorders causing raised pulmonary venous pressure. Similarly, patients with diseased pulmonary vessels are prone to pulmonary embolism, thrombosis, and infarction, all of which aggravate the development of pulmonary hypertension.

Effects of Loss of Lung Tissue

The normal pulmonary circulation is capable of handling increased blood flow without much concomitant rise in pressure. The pressure/flow characteristics of pulmonary circulation are thus highly nonlinear, and the use of a single value (in mm Hg/L/min) to describe its resistance is overly simplistic. Increasing flow without increasing pressure implies the opening up of parallel circulatory pathways. It follows that loss of lung tissue, eg, following pneumonectomy, decreases the reserve capacity of the pulmonary vascular bed and increases the tendency for pulmonary hypertension to develop. As progressively larger amounts of lung tissue are removed, the capacity of the pulmonary vascular bed is ultimately reduced to a level at which the normal cardiac output cannot be accommodated without an increase in pulmonary arterial pressure. In chronic lung disease, alveolar hypoxia, the effects of which are potentiated by hypercapnia and acidosis, causes an additional potentially reversible element of pulmonary hypertension.

Effects of Increased Left Atrial Pressure

Pulmonary arterial vasoconstriction in response to a rise in left atrial pressure is the most important cause of pulmonary hypertension and right heart failure in patients with heart disease. The mechanism of this reaction is unknown. The magnitude of the response varies considerably in different patients, but younger persons usually show greater changes. Although mitral stenosis is the classic example of a lesion causing raised pulmonary vascular resistance in adults, any long-standing moderate or severe increase in left atrial pressure—eg, left atrial myxoma, aortic valve disease, systemic hypertension, cardiomyopathy, or any combination of causes—can result in raised pulmonary vascular resistance. Pulmonary hypertension does not inevitably follow raised left atrial pressure. In some cases, chronic left atrial hypertension causes marked dyspnea and recurrent pulmonary edema without provoking any vasoconstrictive reaction in the pulmonary arterioles.

Pulmonary Hypertension in Patients With Lung Disease

Patients with parenchymal lung disease tend to develop pulmonary hypertension during acute exacerbations of their disease. Thus, during acute episodes of asthma, bronchitis, or pneumonia, the combination of lung disease and alveolar hypoxia leads to an acute rise in pulmonary arterial pressure. The pulmonary arterial pressure may fall to normal when the acute illness subsides, but with time some permanent changes occur, and ultimately the pulmonary hypertension becomes permanent.

Pulmonary Hypertension in Schistosomiasis (Bilharziasis)

Bilharzial heart disease is due to the deposition of ova of *Schistosoma (Schistosoma japonicum, Schistosoma mansoni,* or *Schistosoma haematobium)* in the lung. The condition arises from urinary or intestinal tract infection, and the disease is common in Egypt in agricultural workers in the Nile delta. The ova lodge in the pulmonary arterioles during their migration through the body and produce an inflammatory change that on healing leaves a nodule. The change leads to pulmonary hypertension, right ventricular hypertrophy, and right heart failure. The classic radiologic signs include a large pulmonary artery and diffuse mottling of the lung parenchyma. Beaded nodules in the arterioles have been called bilharzial tubercles (Bedford, 1946).

The clinical picture is one of right heart failure without lung disease and is similar to that in primary pulmonary hypertension. It is not uncommon to see aneurysmal dilatation of the pulmonary artery and marked enlargement of the right ventricle.

There is no satisfactory treatment when cor pulmonale develops. Prevention of bilharziasis consists of avoiding wading or swimming in stagnant fresh water in which the snail vector *(Planorbis)* lives.

Primary Pulmonary Hypertension

In rare cases, pulmonary arterial vasoconstriction occurs without a rise in left atrial pressure, giving rise to a disease known as primary, or idiopathic, pulmonary hypertension. The condition is commonest in premenopausal women but can occur at any age. The onset is insidious and the course usually relentlessly progressive, leading to death in 2–8 years from intractable right heart failure. A familial incidence has been reported, and the condition is more prevalent in persons living at high altitude.

Thromboembolic pulmonary hypertension can occur as a separate identifiable disease in patients who have such frequent episodes of pulmonary embolism that complete resolution between attacks is impossible. It is difficult to differentiate between vasospasm and thromboembolism in the genesis of primary pulmonary hypertension because multiple small pulmonary emboli can trigger reflex changes and may also produce pulmonary vasoconstriction.

PULMONARY ARTERIOVENOUS FISTULA

Pulmonary arteriovenous fistula is a rare but specific form of pulmonary vascular disease. This condition, which is often associated with hereditary hemorrhagic telangiectasia (Osler's disease), consists of congenital arteriovenous malformations in the lungs that give rise to cyanosis, clubbing of the fingers, and a high output state. Venous blood passing through the abnormal channels often causes a bruit; in addition, the blood is not exposed to oxygen in the lungs, so that arterial desaturation occurs that is exaggerated on exercise. Cardiac output is increased, and polycythemia and increased blood volume follow. The condition is most frequently seen in young adults and tends to mimic congenital heart disease. Hemoptysis is a common complication. Resection of the lobe of the lung that is the malformation site is the principal treatment. Unfortunately, the lesions are often multiple, and if this is not detected preoperatively, a second lesion may sometimes enlarge and cause a recurrence of the condition after operation. The lesions usually show up on plain chest x-rays, as shown in Fig 19–1, and their vascular nature can be readily determined by pulmonary angiography (Fig 19–2).

PULMONARY EMBOLISM

Pulmonary embolism is an important complication of heart disease. Its incidence and significance are extremely difficult to determine. Data based on autopsy findings indicate that pulmonary embolism is extremely common, some studies having found thrombus in pulmonary vessels in over half of patients. The distinction between antemortem and postmortem thrombus may be difficult to make. Agonal embolism and thrombosis in situ in the slow-moving blood in the lungs of moribund patients almost certainly account for many of the thrombi seen at autopsy.

The significance of the thrombotic material found at autopsy is difficult to determine. In massive pulmonary embolism in which a large mass of red cells, fibrin, and platelets impacts in a main pulmonary artery and causes a sudden fatal obstruction to the circulation, the importance of the event is plainly

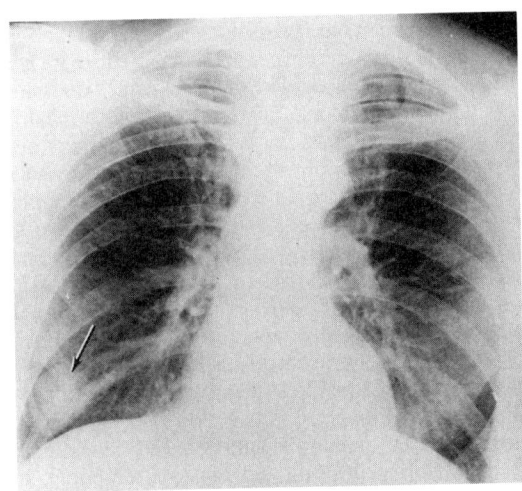

Figure 19–1. Chest x-ray showing a pulmonary arteriovenous fistula in the lower lobe of the right lung.

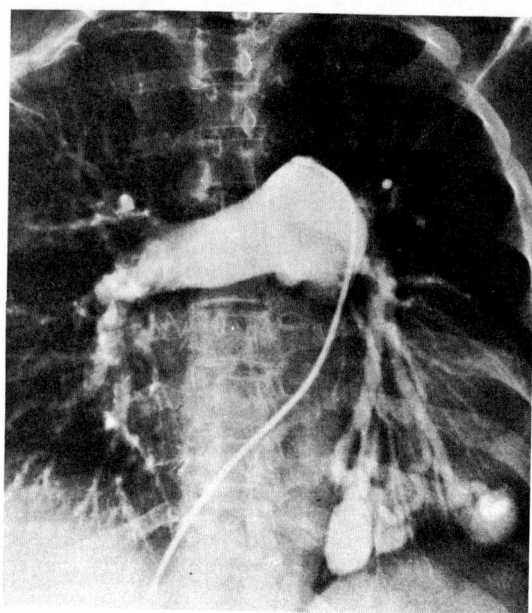

Figure 19-2. Angiogram showing 3 large arteriovenous fistulas in left lower lobe of the lung. (Reproduced, with permission, from Dines DE et al: Pulmonary arteriovenous fistulas. *Mayo Clin Proc* 1974;**49**:460.)

evident. However, in chronically ill patients with wasting diseases who are comatose for several days, the episode is likely to be masked.

These considerations are not intended to underestimate the importance of pulmonary embolism as a complication, but only to show that autopsy studies may not provide a realistic view of the incidence and clinical picture. Pulmonary embolism is insidious, often missed on physical examination, and often misdiagnosed as pneumonia, atelectasis, pleurisy, pulmonary congestion, or edema.

Obstruction of the pulmonary vascular bed involving the lumen of blood vessels—pulmonary embolism or thrombosis—is more common in patients with heart disease than in those with lung disease. The nature and amount of embolic material, the site of obstruction, and the rate of removal of embolic material all play a part in determining the clinical picture, and the previous state of the pulmonary circulation determines whether the lung undergoes infarction or not. Normal lungs obtain their blood supply from both pulmonary and bronchial arteries. When the lungs are congested, as occurs in heart failure or in prolonged immobilization of comatose patients, bronchial blood flow is not ordinarily sufficient to maintain the viability of lung tissue that has been deprived of its pulmonary arterial blood supply. In such cases of congestion, the affected area of lung is infarcted and consolidated, which deprives it of air and causes a temporary loss of function.

The manifestations of pulmonary embolism vary greatly. Acute massive impaction of several hundred grams of thrombus in the main pulmonary artery can cause acute circulatory collapse or shock, with almost instantaneous death. There can also be repeated showers of multiple microscopic emboli, eg, schistosome ova in bilharziasis. Small emboli lodge in the pulmonary arterioles far out in the lungs and cause much more insidious pulmonary changes; in rare cases, right heart failure is the first clinical manifestation. The site of origin of the embolic material is commonly the veins of the legs and pelvis, but fat emboli from the bone marrow following fracture of the long bones also occur. Soft, recently formed thrombus is much more readily lysed than well-organized old thrombus or fat. Thus, the ability of the thrombolytic processes of the body to dispose of embolic material by breaking it up into smaller pieces that lodge in more peripheral parts of the lung constitutes an important and highly variable factor in the clinical course of pulmonary embolism.

The cross-sectional area of the pulmonary arterial bed increases with each division of the pulmonary artery. Consequently, as embolic material moves farther out in the lungs, pulmonary blood flow progressively increases, pulmonary arterial pressure progressively falls, and right ventricular overload is relieved. Acute overload of the right heart, like acute overload of the left heart, tends to produce a different clinical picture from that observed in chronic obstruction of pulmonary blood flow. The magnitude of the overload can also vary because the pulmonary embolism may be massive or only moderate. There is thus a wide variation in severity of the clinical effects of pulmonary embolism, further complicated by variations in the state of the preexisting pulmonary circulation and the efficiency of the thrombolytic mechanisms. It may be several weeks before hypertrophy occurs in the right heart in response to sudden severe pulmonary vascular obstruction. A sudden acute rise in systemic venous pressure, without marked increase in pulmonary arterial or right ventricular pressure, is thus the principal effect of an acute lesion on the right side of the heart. Inadequate left-sided venous return, with an acute fall in left ventricular output, tachycardia, hypotension, shock, and circulatory collapse, dominates the clinical picture, and it may be difficult to determine whether the basic lesion is right-sided or left-sided. In more chronic, less rapidly developing, less severe lesions, right ventricular output can be maintained and the compensatory changes—right ventricular hypertrophy and dilatation—are more obvious.

Massive Pulmonary Embolism; Acute Right Heart Failure (Acute Cor Pulmonale)

Acute cor pulmonale is seen almost exclusively in association with massive pulmonary embolism. Massive pulmonary embolism usually occurs in apparently healthy persons who may be of any age. The disease affects females more often than males. Patients have usually been recently subject to some minor trauma. Recent normal delivery, hernia operation, minor gynecologic or urologic surgery, varicose vein operation, or some other procedure involving the legs or pelvis is ordinarily the precipitating factor. Loosely adherent, soft, friable thrombus forms undetected in the veins of the legs or pelvis (phlebothrombosis). The thrombus suddenly breaks loose (in classic cases during straining at stool) and lodges at or near the bifurcation of the main pulmonary artery. The patient complains of sudden, severe central chest pain and collapses, often with loss of consciousness. Death can occur within a few minutes if the thrombus is large and does not dislodge. If the thrombus is smaller or moves more peripherally, either spontaneously or in response to pounding on the chest or chest compression, acute cor pulmonale rather than sudden death is seen, and the condition may run a subacute course.

Dyspnea, cyanosis, anxiety, impaired consciousness, and all the manifestations of an acute circulatory catastrophe are present. The diagnosis is difficult to confirm in the face of simultaneous emergency and supportive treatment and the general hectic activity involved in managing an acute life-threatening situation. Physical examination may not reveal any specific diagnostic signs. The ECG and chest x-ray may not be diagnostic in the earliest stages. The ECG will not necessarily show the changes of acute myocardial infarction, the disorder that must be considered most frequently in the differential diagnosis. The electrocardiographic changes of acute right ventricular overload can mimic myocardial infarction. Evidence of oligemic lungs, perhaps with an asymmetric increase in translucency, may be seen on chest radiographs in patients who survive the initial episode by 30 minutes or more. Evidence of arterial hypoxia ($P_{O_2} < 70$ mm Hg) is nonspecific.

The place of surgical removal of embolic material in the treatment of massive pulmonary embolism has been the subject of controversy in recent years. A confirmed diagnosis of massive pulmonary embolism with accessible thrombus in the main pulmonary artery or its branches is required before surgery is performed. This necessitates emergency pulmonary angiocardiography, preferably done in an operating room in a center equipped to perform cardiopulmonary bypass. Since such facilities are not widely available, less drastic measures must also be instituted. Anticoagulation with heparin (5000–10,000 units intravenously, repeated every 3 hours) can help to break up the thrombus, move it to a more peripheral part of the lung, and prevent extension. Any factor that moves the obstructing thrombus farther down the pulmonary artery may promote the patient's recovery. Even a small increase in the flow of blood to the lungs will sometimes help to provide a venous return to the left heart and will also avoid the development of secondary thrombosis around the embolus. Manipulation of a cardiac catheter in the pulmonary artery may serve to move the thrombus farther down the vessel; turning the patient into various positions and striking forceful blows to the precordium may also help.

Streptokinase and urokinase are enzymes that have been extensively tested as therapeutic agents for the lysis rather than the prevention of thrombi. Both are now approved for clinical use in the USA. Extreme care is needed in their use, because they may induce hemorrhage in patients who have wounds that are healing. They are contraindicated in all patients in whom surgery, childbirth, liver or kidney biopsy, or arterial puncture has occurred in the previous 10 days. Recent cerebrovascular accidents, any bleeding tendency, and severe hypertension also contraindicate their use. Both enzymes are expensive, and it seems doubtful that either will find an important place in the treatment of pulmonary embolism.

Prevention of massive pulmonary embolism is clearly preferable to treatment. Patients with a history of pulmonary embolism, deep venous thrombosis, cerebral thrombosis, or thrombophlebitis should not use oral contraceptives. The morbidity and mortality rate from pulmonary embolism is 4–8 times higher in women who take oral contraceptive drugs. Encouraging patients to move about in bed and allowing them to walk about in their rooms as soon as possible after minor surgery or childbirth have helped to reduce the incidence of massive pulmonary embolism. Subcutaneous heparin injections in low doses (2500–3000 units every 6–8 hours) in the postoperative period or intravenous dextran 70 administered with intravenous fluids after surgery has reportedly been effective in reducing the incidence of fatal massive pulmonary embolism in double-blind studies. The results have been best in patients undergoing abdominal surgery. Low-dose heparin has not proved to be valuable in hip replacement or prostatic surgery, mainly because of the prevalence of postoperative hemorrhage. Fat embolism, following fractures of the long bones, is an indication for steroid therapy. In thrombophlebitis (which is a much more common condition), smaller, more adherent thrombi that provoke local pain, swelling, and signs of inflammation occur. These seldom if ever break loose, and prophylactic measures other than avoiding oral contraceptives are of doubtful value.

Moderate Pulmonary Embolism

The description of massive pulmonary embolism given above concerns cases in which no prior heart or lung disease is present, cardiopulmonary reserve is large, and bronchial arterial blood supply is good. In most cardiac patients, however, these conditions do not exist. The clinical picture in such patients is different. Relatively small emboli that would pass unnoticed in a healthy person cause serious problems, with exacerbation of congestive heart failure or pulmonary infarction, with pain, pleural irritation, hemoptysis, and effusion. The venous stasis and congestion seen in heart failure predispose to thrombus formation not only in the legs but also in the right heart and even in the lungs themselves, so that pulmonary thromboembolic complications are especially common in cardiologic practice. Pulmonary embolism in which a moderate-sized embolus lodges in the lungs and is sufficiently large to occlude the artery leading to a lobe or a lobule is an insidious condition that is often overlooked. Data obtained at autopsy indicate a surprisingly high incidence of thrombi in the lungs (> 50% of cases), and this suggests that agonal lesions may be common.

Clinical Findings

A. Symptoms: The classic symptoms of a chest pain that is often worse on inspiration, dyspnea, cough, and hemoptysis in susceptible patients such as those with congestive heart failure, mitral valve disease, or myocardial infarction should strongly suggest a diagnosis of pulmonary embolism. Not infrequently, unexplained dyspnea, fever, tachycardia, increase in venous pressure, or worsening of venous congestion provides a clue to the diagnosis, but in many cases the acute episode passes unnoticed.

B. Signs: Physical signs in the lungs depend on the development of consolidation or pleural involvement. Pleural friction rub, impaired movement, dullness to percussion, diminished air entry, and bronchial breathing can be heard, and signs of pleural effusion may develop. Signs of increased pulmonary arterial pressure such as increased right ventricular impulse, increased intensity of the pulmonary valve closure sound, or palpable pulmonary artery pulsation should be sought.

C. Electrocardiographic Findings: The signs of pulmonary embolism on the ECG are variable. A peaked right atrial P wave may be seen, and atrial arrhythmias, especially fibrillation or flutter, can occur. A change in electrical axis toward the right; right bundle branch block, either complete or incomplete (Fig 19–3); and T wave inversions in the anterior chest leads (V_{1-3}) are seen in about 10–15% of patients. In some cases, Q waves in leads II, III, and aVF mimic posterior myocardial infarction. In most cases, nonspecific ST changes and slight right axis deviation are seen. Patients with associated coronary disease may show changes indicative of myocardial ischemia.

D. X-Ray Findings: The patient may be too ill for anything except a bedside x-ray, which is often unsatisfactory. Significant pulmonary embolism can occur even with completely clear lung fields, and radiologic evidence of consolidation following pulmonary infarction takes up to 12 hours to develop. The diaphragm tends to be high on the side of the lesion, which is commonly at the base of the lung. A wedge-shaped shadow extending out to the pleural surface

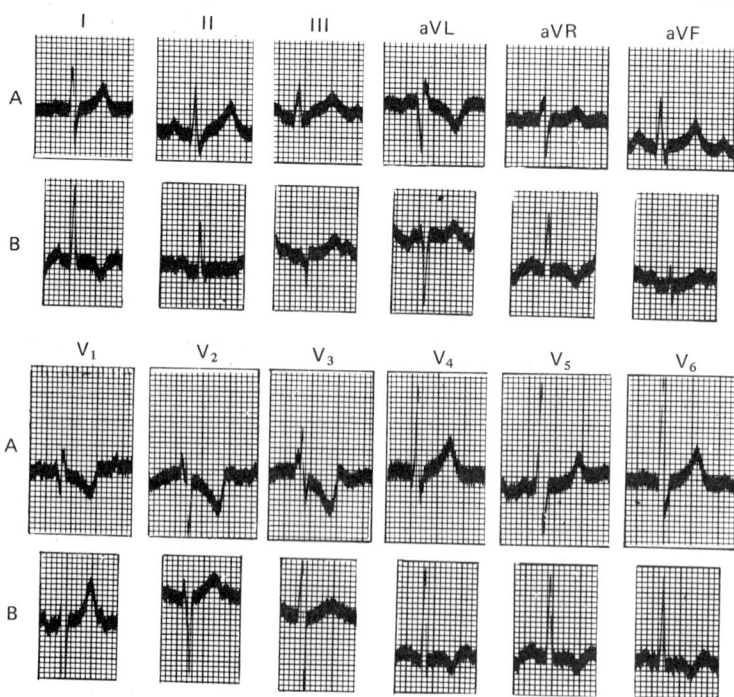

Figure 19–3. Incomplete right bundle branch block as a manifestation of acute right ventricular strain. **A:** The pattern is that of an incomplete right bundle branch block (rsR' complexes with depressed ST segments and inverted T waves in V_{1-3}). **B:** Five days after **(A):** There has been a marked change. The incomplete right bundle branch block is no longer present. In the interval the T waves have become inverted in leads I, aVR, and V_{4-6}. *Clinical status:* At **(A)** the patient had an episode of acute pulmonary infarction. Five days later he had markedly improved. The ECG in **(A)** was a reflection of acute right ventricular strain. The pulmonary hypertension had clinically subsided by **(B)**, and the second ECG demonstrated the abnormalities associated with the basic heart disease, beriberi. (Reproduced, with permission, from Goldman MJ: *Principles of Clinical Electrocardiography,* 12th ed. Lange, 1986.)

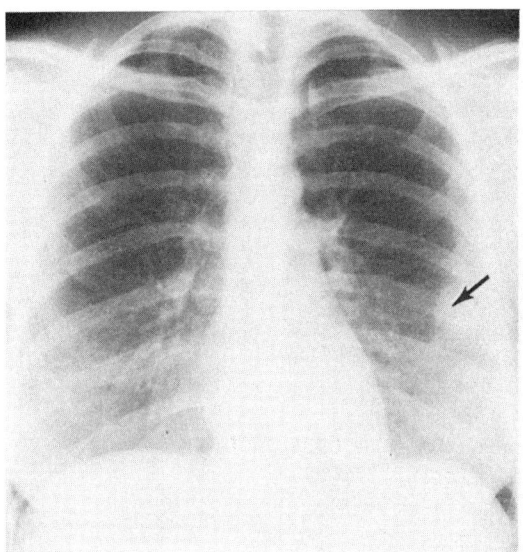 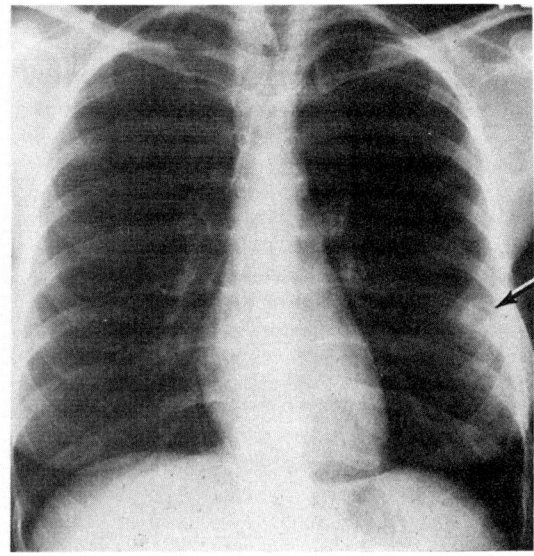

Figure 19–4. Serial chest x-rays of a woman patient with pulmonary infarction. The infarct has formed a cavity in the second (right-hand) x-ray. (Courtesy of G Gamsu.)

is a classic manifestation, as shown in Fig 19–4. The lesion may cavitate later, and pleural effusion at the costophrenic angles or in the interlobular fissures is not uncommon.

E. Special Investigations: Leukocytosis, increased sedimentation rate, increased serum enzymes (lactate dehydrogenase and serum glutamic-oxaloacetic transaminase), and slight increase in indirect bilirubin concentration are seen in many cases. Arterial P_{O_2} is often reduced (< 70 mm Hg), but the finding is nonspecific. External radioactive scanning following injection of radionuclides such as radioiodinated or ^{99m}Tc-labeled human serum albumin has proved valuable in patients who have no history of prior lung disease. The results of lung scans must be interpreted together with simultaneous or near-simultaneous chest x-rays and ventilation scans using ^{133}Xe. Pulmonary lesions other than emboli can give rise to clear, unperfused areas on the lung scan, and only the finding of an unperfused area in a segment of lung that is clear on the chest x-ray is significant. Pulmonary emboli can clear so rapidly and can move to the periphery of the lungs so readily that confusion may occur when the radioactive scan and chest x-ray are obtained even a few hours apart. Newer scintigraphic methods using ^{15}O-labeled CO_2 may be more sensitive and specific, but the necessity of having to be near a cyclotron for the preparation of the isotope makes their general use unlikely.

Pulmonary angiography can be used to demonstrate blockage of the pulmonary vasculature, which may be present although it does not appear on a chest radiogram, as shown in Fig 19–5. It provides the clearest, most definitive evidence for the diagnosis of pulmonary embolism. While it is mandatory before any form of surgical treatment, angiography carries a definite risk of death or morbidity and is expensive in terms of manpower and equipment. Protagonists of angiography point out that unnecessary anticoagulant therapy probably carries an equal or greater risk because of hemorrhagic complications. It is logical, therefore, to restrict angiography to patients with significant symptoms in whom lung scans give equivocal results. A normal lung scan effectively excludes serious pulmonary embolism, and a clearly positive perfusion scan with a normal chest x-ray and a normal ventilation scan provides adequate evidence on which to base anticoagulant therapy. With this approach, pulmonary angiography can probably be restricted to fewer than 20% of patients in whom the diagnosis is seriously in question.

Complications

Secondary thrombus with further blockage of pulmonary vessels, inadequate recanalization, and secondary infection of infarcted lung tissue are the principal complications of pulmonary embolism. Recurrence of pulmonary embolism is always possible. However, complete recovery with full recanalization is the usual outcome, and the complication of chronic thromboembolic pulmonary hypertension is rare. Such chronic hypertension develops only after a long period of several months or years of repeated embolization, possibly with some associated impairment of the thrombolytic mechanisms.

Differential Diagnosis

The diagnosis of pulmonary embolism can be extremely difficult, especially in patients who are ill from other causes and in postoperative patients. The

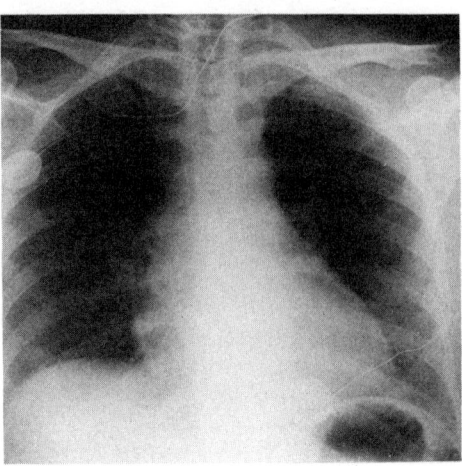 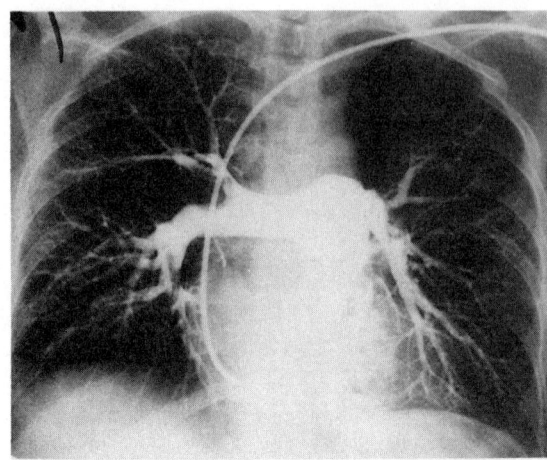

Figure 19-5. Normal chest x-ray *(left)* obtained on the same day as a pulmonary angiogram *(right).* The angiogram shows significant obstruction to the right and left upper lobes, even though the chest x-ray was normal. (Courtesy of G Gamsu.)

condition is so insidious that it should be suspected in any sick patient in whom unexplained deterioration or failure to thrive is detected. The physician must maintain a high index of suspicion in order to make the correct diagnosis. In many cases the diagnosis can be made in retrospect from careful examination of the chart of the vital signs. A sudden increase in heart rate or respiratory rate, followed by an unexplained rise in temperature on the following day, may have occurred in a patient with an obvious pulmonary infarct that was not previously apparent. Intercurrent lower respiratory tract infections can be readily mistaken for pulmonary emboli and vice versa. Likewise, minor, short-lived episodes of acute pulmonary congestion may cause a similar clinical picture. Repeated episodes of embolism tend to differ slightly in their manifestations, whereas recurrent pulmonary congestion tends to produce a series of similar episodes.

Pulmonary embolism enters into the differential diagnosis of almost all forms of lung disease and many varieties of heart disease. It occurs during the course of these diseases and may also be confused with the diseases themselves. Thus, pneumonia and atelectasis (especially if they occur postoperatively) and pleurisy with or without effusion may all be confused with pulmonary infarction. Hemorrhage into the lung is an important feature of pulmonary infarction that is also seen in other conditions such as bronchial carcinoma, tuberculosis, or any disease causing hemoptysis. Acute chest pain in pulmonary embolism can be confused with that occurring in myocardial infarction, spontaneous pneumothorax, pericarditis, aortic dissection, and even upper abdominal disease such as cholecystitis or perforated peptic ulcer.

Treatment

The principal decision in treatment is whether to use anticoagulant therapy. Anticoagulant therapy is more generally accepted in pulmonary embolism than in any other disorder. Intravenous heparin (5000–10,000 units intravenously, followed by 5000 units intravenously every 4–6 hours) has become almost standard treatment, followed by warfarin (Coumadin), 30–50 mg on the first day, 10–15 mg on the second day, and a maintenance dose of 5–15 mg, depending on the prothrombin time, on subsequent days. Anticoagulant therapy is generally maintained for 6 weeks to 3 months after an episode of pulmonary embolism.

There are no measures that absolutely prevent the development of pulmonary embolism in cardiac patients, but initiating active leg exercises and breathing exercises, avoiding long periods of bed rest (especially with pressure on the popliteal fossa), and discontinuing the use of oral contraceptives are useful. The physician must exercise care in treating cardiac patients who are in a sitting position. Excessive flexing of the knee and sitting in cramped positions in automobiles and on airplanes predispose to venous stasis. In patients with embolism that recurs in spite of anticoagulant treatment, inferior vena caval ligation, either partial or complete, has been advocated. However, this procedure does not necessarily prevent embolism, and it may even provide another site for thrombus formation; it also often leads to edema of the legs. The thrombolytic process is generally so effective that the long-term (6- to 12-week) prognosis depends on the underlying cardiac condition rather than on the embolism. No specific treatment is needed for pulmonary infarction. Control of pain and antibiotics for the treatment of secondary lung infection may be required. If infarction results in severe hemoptysis, anticoagulant therapy may have to be withdrawn.

There is a place for surgical treatment late in the course of pulmonary thromboembolic disease. In rare cases, the patient is left with severe and disabling dyspnea due to pulmonary hypertension resulting from blockage of large pulmonary arteries. Exploring the pulmonary arteries, with cardiopulmonary bypass and hypothermia, in an attempt to extract old endothelialized embolic material has proved valuable in some cases (Moser, 1983). The mortality rate of the operation is about 15%, and the principal complication is reperfusion pulmonary edema. This problem can persist for up to 3 months postoperatively. While surgery is palliative rather than curative, the pulmonary vascular resistance can fall dramatically, and symptomatic improvement can be gratifying.

Prognosis

Pulmonary embolism seldom leads to chronic lung disease. If the patient survives the acute episode, whether it is a massive embolism or a moderate-sized one involving pulmonary infarction, the lesion almost invariably heals completely without leaving a scar. The prognosis in acute massive embolism improves with the passage of time; however, most patients die within the first hour. This important cause of death in previously healthy people accounts for over 40,000 fatalities per year in the USA. In those who survive the first hour, the prognosis improves, partly because of the opportunity for treatment and partly because the embolic material may have broken up and moved to a more peripheral area of the lungs. Chronic pulmonary hypertension occurs when there are frequent recurrent episodes of embolism with inadequate time between episodes for resolution of the disease process or when there are inadequate thrombolytic mechanisms.

RIGHT HEART FAILURE SECONDARY TO CHRONIC LUNG DISEASE

Chronic cor pulmonale is defined as heart *disease* (rather than heart *failure*) that is secondary to disease of the respiratory system. Right ventricular enlargement secondary to chronic disease of the respiratory system is most commonly due to parenchymal lung diseases such as fibrosis, emphysema, or pneumonia. The clinical picture is little influenced by the underlying cause, which may be pulmonary granuloma, sarcoidosis, scleroderma, pneumoconiosis, or any form of fibrosis, including idiopathic lesions (Hamman-Rich disease). Usually, one of recurrent episodes of pulmonary infection or bronchial obstruction leading to temporary increases in the load on the right heart and right heart failure. Any lesion producing alveolar hypoxia causes a vicious circle because of increased pulmonary arterial pressure due to pulmonary vasoconstriction. This mechanism is involved in alveolar hypoventilation due to weakness or paralysis of the respiratory muscles and also in central nervous system disease leading to inadequate pulmonary ventilation. Both can cause chronic cor pulmonale even when the lungs themselves are normal. Massive obesity, as in the Pickwickian syndrome, can also cause right heart failure; it is another cause of alveolar hypoventilation in which the lungs are normal. Chest wall disorders such as kyphosis and scoliosis may occasionally lead to heart failure but usually only when chest infection is present. Arterial hypoxia increases cardiac output by causing systemic vasodilation and especially by increasing the heart rate. These factors tend to aggravate right heart failure. Since patients with chronic lung disease are often middle-aged and have smoked cigarettes for many years, associated atherosclerotic heart disease is common, and an element of left heart failure is frequently present in addition to right heart failure. Some feel that right heart failure can lead to left heart failure as the enlarging right ventricle displaces the left ventricle backward, but this is difficult to prove.

Clinical Findings

A. Symptoms: Dyspnea is the primary symptom in patients with chronic cor pulmonale. Coexisting pulmonary and cardiac disease may make it difficult to determine the cause of dyspnea. In the usual case of chronic cor pulmonale, dyspnea is most commonly due to the increased work of breathing resulting from the mechanical effects of the lung disease causing the right heart overload.

However, dyspnea is also seen in the rarest form of chronic cor pulmonale—primary pulmonary hypertension. In this condition, the mechanical properties of the lungs are normal, and some other explanation must be sought to explain the dyspnea. An inadequate systemic cardiac output is thought to cause alveolar hyperventilation, and excessive ventilation, especially during exercise, is thought to be responsible for the dyspnea. Edema of the ankles, abdominal swelling, and right upper quadrant pain due to hepatic congestion are often seen. Palpitations, weakness, syncope, and coldness of the hands and feet with Raynaud's phenomenon also occur in primary pulmonary hypertension.

B. Signs:

1. Noncardiac signs–Patients with arterial hypoxia due to bronchitis tend to exhibit hypervolemia and vasodilatation rather than the vasoconstriction and low output state seen in patients with emphysema and primary pulmonary hypertension. Patients with chronic lung disease have been divided into "blue bloaters," in whom hypoxia, hypervolemia, recurrent bronchitis, and cor pulmonale are prominent, and "pink puffers," in whom hypoxia is absent, hypovolemia and emphysema are common, and cor pulmonale is rare. Similarly, cor pulmonale has been classified as either hypoxic or pulmonary hypertensive, depending on whether a high output or a low output state predominates. Such generalizations are useful in delineating the different mechanisms involved but must not be taken as definitive, mutually exclusive categories.

Cyanosis and clubbing of the fingers are often seen. The cyanosis may be peripheral, due to the low cardiac output in patients with pulmonary hypertension, or central and associated with significant arterial hypoxemia ($P_{O_2} < 60$ mm Hg) and hypercapnia ($P_{CO_2} > 50$ mm Hg) in patients with chronic lung disease or alveolar hypoventilation. Clubbing of the fingers is most frequently seen in patients with chronic pulmonary infections or bronchial carcinoma. Tachycardia and a raised jugular venous pressure with a and v waves occur. Hepatomegaly, ascites, and edema of the ankles are seen if the patient is in right heart failure.

2. Cardiac signs–Cardiac manifestations depend on the nature of the lung disease. In patients with emphysema, bronchitis, or bronchial obstruction, the cardiac impulse may be difficult to palpate because of overlying lung tissue. The sounds may be distant and murmurs absent. Conversely, in primary pulmonary hypertension, a prominent right ventricular heave below the sternum, a loud pulmonary valve closure component of a closely split second heart sound and ejection click, and a short pulmonary systolic murmur are noted, often with a pulmonary diastolic (Graham Steell) murmur due to pulmonary incompetence. In later stages, a pansystolic high-pitched murmur of tricuspid incompetence is often easily detected.

C. Electrocardiographic Findings: Sinus rhythm is the rule, and the ECG shows evidence of right atrial or ventricular predominance. In patients with severe obstructive lung disease, right atrial hypertrophy may be all that is apparent. Electrocardiographic changes of right ventricular hypertrophy (Fig 19–6), like the physical signs, are sometimes masked. In patients with marked pulmonary hypertension, the reverse is true, and clear evidence of right ventricular hypertrophy, with P pulmonale, tall R waves, and ST depression with T wave inversion in the right-sided chest leads, is prominent, as shown in Fig 19–7.

D. X-Ray Findings: Enlargement of the main pulmonary artery is the most reliable radiologic indication of chronic cor pulmonale. The degree of cardiac enlargement, although obvious in serial radiograms, may be unimpressive, especially in emphysema. Right ventricular and right atrial enlargement are seen in primary pulmonary hypertension, as shown in Fig 19–8. Pulmonary congestion is not seen unless associated left-sided disease is present. In practice, many patients with chronic lung disease have associated left ventricular disease, and it may be difficult to ascertain how much damage has been done by cardiac disease and how much by pulmonary disease. Superimposed pulmonary congestion and intercurrent pulmonary infections further complicate the differentiation of the effects of heart disease from those of lung disease.

E. Special Investigations: Polycythemia with hematocrit levels above 50% is usually present in hypoxic patients. Measurement of arterial blood gas tensions and pH is necessary in acutely ill patients in order to assess the severity of pulmonary failure. Right heart catheterization is indicated in patients with pulmonary hypertension in order to confirm the diagnosis by determining wedge pressure. Such investigations are extremely important, because lesions repairable by surgery, such as mitral stenosis and left atrial myxoma, can easily be overlooked during examina-

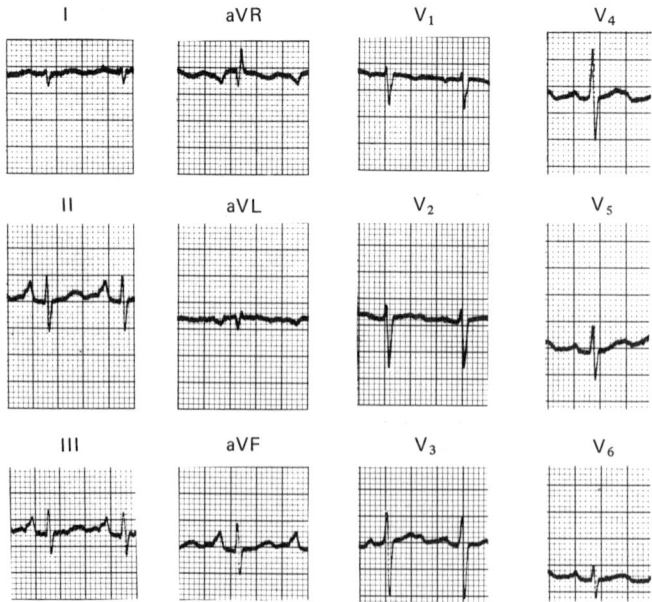

Figure 19–6. Pulmonary emphysema and cor pulmonale. The tall peaked P waves in leads II, III, and aVF are consistent with right atrial hypertrophy. There are small initial QRS forces to the left (r in lead I) with greater terminal forces to the right (S in I). These terminal forces are directed superiorly (S in II, III, and aVF). This is an example of the S_1, S_2, S_3 syndrome. The tracing is consistent with pulmonary emphysema. The prominent P waves are the only positive evidence of right heart overload. (Reproduced, with permission, from Goldman MJ: *Principles of Clinical Electrocardiography*, 12th ed. Lange, 1986.)

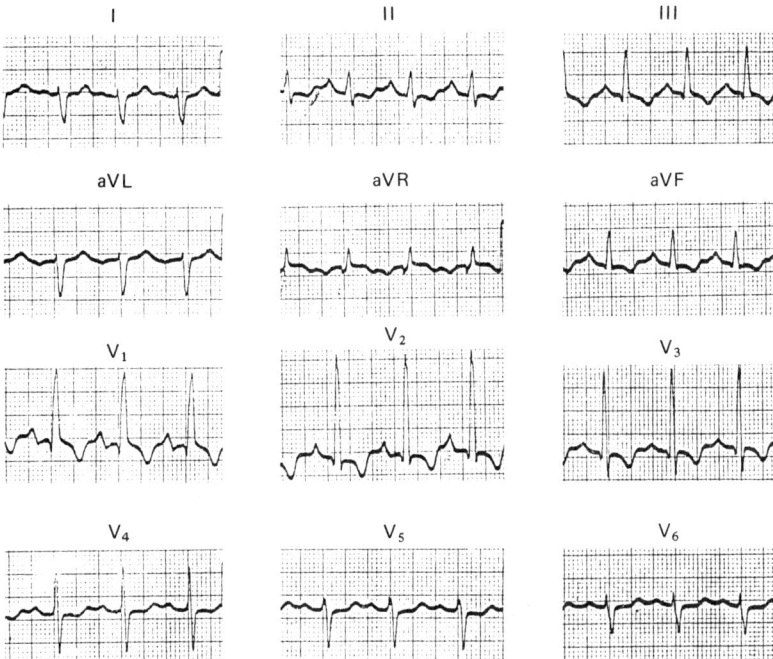

Figure 19–7. ECG from a patient with primary pulmonary hypertension, showing severe right ventricular hypertrophy. Note the monophasic tall R preceded by a small Q in V_1 and the small R and deep S in V_6. The P wave in V_1 is upright and directed anteriorly, indicating right atrial hypertrophy, and there is also right axis deviation with a deep S in lead I and a tall R in lead III.

tion. Pulmonary hypertension in association with congenital heart lesions (Eisenmenger's syndrome) may enter into the differential diagnosis, but the presence of right-to-left shunting causing arterial desaturation does not necessarily indicate congenital heart disease, since a foramen ovale can open up in chronic cor pulmonale when right atrial pressure rises above left atrial pressure.

Differential Diagnosis

Disorders to be differentiated from right heart failure due to lung disease include mitral stenosis, thromboembolic pulmonary hypertension, and Eisenmenger's syndrome. When coincidental pulmonary disease is present, the differential diagnosis can be extremely difficult. Cardiac catheterization is indicated when clear evidence of pulmonary hypertension is found. This diagnosis is suspected more commonly than it is proved, and clinical signs of right heart failure (palpable pulmonary arterial pulsation and loud pulmonary valve closure) tend to be unreliable signs of pulmonary hypertension.

Complications

Right heart failure is such an integral part of chronic cor pulmonale that it is hardly a complication. Similarily, chest infection, pulmonary thrombosis, embolism, and alveolar hypoxia occur so frequently in the course of the disease that they are not really consid-

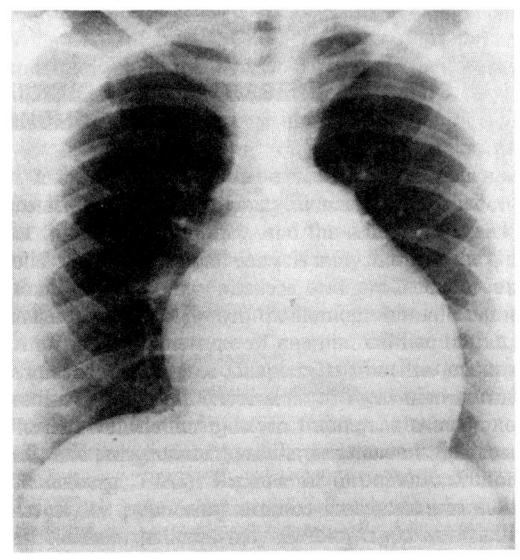

Figure 19–8. Chest x-ray cardiac enlargement, with prominence of the pulmonary artery, right atrium, and right ventricle, in a patient with primary pulmonary hypertension. The lung fields are abnormally translucent in association with reduced pulmonary blood flow.

ered complications. Atrial arrhythmias are relatively common in acute exacerbations of pulmonary infection, but chronic atrial fibrillation is rare. Pulmonary valvular incompetence causing an immediate diastolic (Graham Steell) murmur over the pulmonary artery is more a part of the disease than a complication.

Treatment

The prevention of heart failure is of the utmost importance in patients with lung disease. Prevention involves early and vigorous treatment of chest infections, vaccination against influenza, and avoidance of contact with persons who have upper respiratory tract infections. Cigarette smoking is extremely likely to have a serious effect on cardiopulmonary function in patients with cor pulmonale. Every effort should be made to persuade the patient to stop smoking.

The most important principles of therapy are to improve respiratory function, relieve arterial hypoxemia, reduce pulmonary hypertension, and improve right ventricular function.

The patient must first be treated vigorously and effectively for any intercurrent chest infection that is clearly present, or such infection must be carefully ruled out if there are no apparent symptoms. Relief of arterial hypoxia by oxygen therapy with a mask or nasal catheter as described in Chapter 7 is of great help. The dangers of oxygen therapy—abolition of the patient's hypoxic ventilatory drive and hypoventilation with serious CO_2 retention—have been exaggerated. Any tendency toward hypoventilation with oxygen should be remedied by the use of assisted or artificial ventilation via an endotracheal tube, with clearing of the air passages. Opinions differ about the indications for intensive artificial ventilation in patients in pulmonary failure (which is defined as a P_{CO_2} level > the P_{O_2} level). Tracheostomy and artificial ventilation with frequent endotracheal suction and fiberoptic bronchoscopy are readily performed in some centers.

The present trend is toward long-term intubation rather than tracheostomy. Improvements in the design of endotracheal tubes and low pressure cuff inflation have made it possible to continue intubation for as long as 2 or 3 months, with hoarseness as the only long-term complication. Intubation is less likely than tracheostomy to result in infection, hemorrhage, mediastinal emphysema, and tracheal stenosis.

The treatment of right heart failure with digitalis and diuretics is of secondary importance and is seldom effective as a sole treatment regimen. Digitalis has a reputation for ineffectiveness in patients with cor pulmonale, but there is no evidence that it is harmful except when excessive doses are administered in the hope of slowing the heart rate. In older patients in whom there is associated left ventricular disease, digitalis is often of value and should always be tried. Chronic anticoagulant therapy may be of value for patients with obvious thromboembolic complications. Such therapy is also used in patients with primary pulmonary hypertension but without evidence of benefit. The treatment of primary pulmonary hypertension is particularly unsatisfactory, and the patient develops increasingly severe right heart failure in spite of all measures, including corticosteroid therapy, which is often given as a last resort in the hope that some form of collagen disease is responsible for the pulmonary hypertension. Diazoxide in doses starting at 200 mg 3 times a day has been advocated. It can sharply reduce pulmonary vascular resistance and must be used with caution because it also lowers systemic vascular resistance. Care must be exercised in giving vasodilator drugs to patients with primary pulmonary hypertension, as fatalities have occurred during pharmacologic studies undertaken in the course of cardiac catheterization. Vasodilator drugs other than diazoxide have been tried (eg, hydralazine, phentolamine, isoproterenol) with varying results. Other agents such as indomethacin, epoprostenol (prostacyclin, PGI_2), and verapamil or nifedipine may also prove beneficial in some cases. Corticosteroids may be of value in the treatment of chronic cor pulmonale associated with connective tissue disorders (eg, scleroderma), but they do not generally help patients who are in right heart failure.

End-stage pulmonary hypertension is becoming a prime indication for heart-lung transplantation. The patients are generally young, and the prognosis with conventional treatment is gloomy and reasonably predictable. The initial results are encouraging, but this form of therapy is clearly still experimental.

Prognosis

Cor pulmonale is such a late manifestation of pulmonary disease that the prognosis is poor. Pulmonary reserve has been severely compromised by the time a patient develops either hypercapnia secondary to inadequate ventilation or right ventricular enlargement. The prognosis is best in patients who have a severe pulmonary infection but little or no chronic underlying lung disease. Because such patients cannot be positively identified until after the acute infection has been treated, intensive measures are indicated in emergency situations for patients who have not previously been under the care of a physician. The prognosis in primary pulmonary hypertension is poor. Death in 2–8 years is the rule. Patients with thromboembolic disease live longer because favorable factors such as lysis and organization of thrombi may influence the clinical picture.

The prognosis in patients with pulmonary hypertension who develop the disease while taking birth control pills is better than in those in whom this possible etiologic factor is absent, since stopping oral contraceptives may prevent further progress of the disease and improve the prognosis.

DIFFERENTIATION OF HEART DISEASE & LUNG DISEASE

Lung disease and heart disease often coexist. The harmful effects of cigarette smoking predispose to chronic bronchitis and emphysema and also to carcinoma of the bronchus. They also increase the risk of premature coronary artery disease. In consequence, many patients suffer from both cardiac and pulmonary disease, and the 2 compound each other. Whereas the distinction between pure lung disease and pure heart disease is relatively easy, separating the pulmonary and cardiac elements in mixed lesions is extremely difficult.

Clinical Findings

A. Symptoms: Dyspnea is an important symptom in both heart and lung disease. The dyspnea of lung disease tends to be episodic, being worse at some times than others. It is not infrequently present at rest, when attacks of asthma, bronchospasm, or acute bronchitis occur. It may also be worse on exercise, especially when asthma or bronchospasm is induced by effort. The dyspnea of emphysema produces a basic, permanent, irreversible level of dyspnea. Although the patient's dyspnea may be worse at times, it never remits completely. It is thus important in obtaining a history of dyspnea to find out how much the patient's breathlessness varies from day to day and to concentrate on the level of dyspnea on the patient's "best day." If significant emphysema is present, dyspnea will be present even on the "best day." Conversely, if the patient has a normal exercise tolerance on the best day, then emphysema is not present.

Chest pain occurs in both heart and lung disease. The patient with lung disease complains of a tight constricting feeling across the chest on exertion or at rest when bronchitis or bronchospasm is present. This can usually be distinguished from anginal pain, because it is discomfort rather than pain and usually neither radiates like angina nor is so quantitatively related to exertion. Pleural pain suggests lung disease but can occur in heart disease when pulmonary embolism leads to pulmonary infarction.

Cough occurs both in heart disease and lung disease. Its presence is much more common in lung disease, but pulmonary congestion secondary to raised left atrial pressure can also cause cough. The cough in heart disease is dry and unproductive unless pulmonary edema develops, when profuse watery sputum occurs. The cough of pulmonary congestion often comes on with exercise. Cough with purulent, mucopurulent, rusty, or tenacious sputum is indicative of lung disease. Hemoptysis occurs in both heart and lung disease, and its presence is not often of value in distinguishing heart and lung disease.

B. Signs: In comparison with symptoms, there is much less overlap in physical signs between heart and lung disease. Pleural friction rubs and rales and rhonchi can occur in both. The pulmonary signs associated with pulmonary congestion and edema can be mistaken for those of asthma or bronchospasm, but "cardiac asthma" is not often confused with asthma or bronchitis because of the history of previous attacks in asthma and the presence of obvious signs of mitral or left ventricular disease in patients with pulmonary congestion.

C. Electrocardiographic Findings: The ECG is particularly helpful in distinguishing between heart and lung disease in cigarette smokers. The presence of evidence of left ventricular predominance with ST–T wave changes in the left-sided leads indicates that there is at least some heart disease. Atrial arrhythmias occur in both varieties of disease, but chronic atrial fibrillation is more common in heart disease.

D. X-Ray Findings: Cardiac enlargement is difficult to interpret. The heart is often smaller than normal in patients with emphysema, and hearts of apparently normal size may in fact be enlarged for those particular patients.

E. Special Investigations: One of the principal uses of pulmonary function tests is to distinguish between heart and lung disease. Whereas the vital capacity is reduced in patients with pulmonary congestion, the maximum expiratory flow rates are relatively normal, and the flow-volume curves do not indicate significant obstruction. The percentage of the vital capacity expelled in the first second is greater than 70 in heart disease but is less than 70 in patients with significant obstruction due to lung disease. In difficult cases, the measurements of lung compliance, lung and airway resistance, and lung volume may be required to detect the large lung volumes, high resistance, and normal or increased compliance in emphysema. The variation in the values of compliance and resistance with the respiratory rate, characteristic of chronic lung disease, is also helpful in diagnosis. Air trapping on expiration and large closing volumes are also characteristic of obstructive lung disease.

Arterial blood gas measurements should be made if there is any doubt. The hypoxia and hypercapnia (P_{O_2} < 70 mm Hg, P_{CO_2} > 45 mm Hg) often seen in lung disease are rare in heart disease except when pulmonary edema is present. In difficult cases, cardiac catheterization with measurement of pulmonary vascular resistance and full pulmonary function studies are likely to be needed to separate the effects of lung disease from those of heart disease.

REFERENCES

Adams WR, Veith I (editors): *Pulmonary Circulation.* Grune & Stratton, 1958.

Bedford DE et al: Bilharzial heart disease in Egypt: Cor pulmonale due to bilharzial pulmonary endarteritis. *Br Heart J* 1946;**8**:87.

Bell WR, Simon TL: A comparative analysis of pulmonary perfusion scans with pulmonary angiograms. *Am Heart J* 1976;**92**:700.

Bell WR, Simon TL: Current status of pulmonary thromboembolic disease: Pathophysiology, diagnosis, prevention, and treatment. *Am Heart J* 1982;**103**:239.

Bergofsky EH et al: Cardiorespiratory failure in kyphoscoliosis. *Medicine* 1959;**38**:263.

Burwell CS et al: Extreme obesity associated with alveolar hypoventilation: A Pickwickian syndrome. *Am J Med* 1956;**21**:811.

Camerini F et al: Primary pulmonary hypertension: Effects of nifedipine. *Br Heart J* 1980;**44**:352.

Cheely R et al: The role of noninvasive tests versus pulmonary angiography in the diagnosis of pulmonary embolism. *Am J Med* 1981;**70**:17.

Christie RV: Emphysema of the lungs. *Br Med J* 1944;**1**:143.

Comroe JH Jr: *Physiology of Respiration*, 2nd ed. Year Book, 1974.

Davis HH et al: Alveolar-capillary oxygen disequilibrium in hepatic cirrhosis. *Chest* 1978;**73**:507.

Dexter L: Thromboemboli as a cause of cor pulmonale. *Bull NY Acad Med* 1965;**41**:981.

Dines DE et al: Pulmonary arteriovenous fistulas. *Mayo Clin Proc* 1974;**49**:460.

Edwards WD, Edwards JE: Clinical primary pulmonary hypertension: Three pathologic types. *Circulation* 1977;**56**:884.

Elkayam U et al: Unfavorable hemodynamic and clinical effects of isoproterenol in primary pulmonary hypertension. *Cardiovasc Med* 1978;**3**:1177.

Filley GF et al: Chronic obstructive bronchopulmonary disease. 2. Oxygen transport in two clinical types. *Am J Med* 1968;**44**:26.

Fleming HA, Bailey SM: Massive pulmonary embolism in healthy people. *Br Med J* 1966;**1**:1322.

Fletcher CM et al: The diagnosis of pulmonary emphysema in the presence of chronic bronchitis. *Q J Med* 1963;**32**:33.

Goldsmith RS: Infectious diseases: Helminthic. Chapter 26 in: *Current Medical Diagnosis & Treatment 1986.* Krupp MA, Chatton MJ, Tierney LM Jr (editors). Lange, 1986.

Groote Schuur Hospital Thromboembolus Study Group: Failure of low-dose heparin to prevent significant thromboembolic complications in high-risk surgical patients: Interim report of prospective trial. *Br Med J* 1979;**1**:1447.

Gross NJ: Pulmonary effects of radiation therapy. *Ann Intern Med* 1977;**86**:81.

Hall RJC et al: Subacute massive pulmonary embolism. *Br Heart J* 1981;**45**:681.

Harris P, Heath D: *The Human Pulmonary Circulation*, 2nd ed. Churchill Livingstone, 1977.

Haworth SG: Primary pulmonary hypertension. *Br Heart J* 1983;**49**:517.

Kiil J et al: Prophylaxis against postoperative pulmonary embolism and deep-vein thrombosis by low-dose heparin. *Lancet* 1978;**1**:1115.

Klinke WP: Treatment for primary pulmonary hypertension. *Am Heart J* 1980;**100**:587.

Lie JT: Nosology of pulmonary vasculitides. (Editorial.) *Mayo Clin Proc* 1977;**52**:520.

Mahmoud AA: Schistosomiasis. *N Engl J Med* 1977;**297**:1329.

McDonald IG et al: Major pulmonary embolism: A correlation of clinical findings, haemodynamics, pulmonary angiography, and pathological physiology. *Br Heart J* 1972;**34**:356.

McGoon MD, Edwards WD: Primary pulmonary hypertension: Current status. *Mod Concept Cardiovasc Dis* 1985;**545**:29.

McIlroy MB, Apthorp GH: Pulmonary function in pulmonary hypertension. *Br Heart J* 1958;**20**:397.

Mitchell JRA: Can we really prevent postoperative pulmonary emboli? *Br Med J* 1979;**1**:1523.

Moser KM: Pulmonary embolism. *Am Rev Respir Dis* 1977;**115**:829.

Moser KM et al: Chronic thrombotic obstruction of major pulmonary arteries: Results of thromboendarterectomy in 15 patients. *Ann Intern Med* 1983;**99**:299.

Nichols AB et al: Scintigraphic detection of pulmonary emboli by serial positron imaging of inhaled ^{15}O-labeled carbon dioxide. *N Engl J Med* 1978;**299**:279.

Oakley C, Somerville J: Oral contraceptives and progressive pulmonary vascular disease. *Lancet* 1968;**1**:890.

Packer M: Vasodilator therapy for primary pulmonary hypertension: Limitations and hazards. *Ann Intern Med* 1985;**103**:258.

Reitz BA et al: Heart-lung transplantation: Successful therapy for patients with pulmonary vascular disease. *N Engl J Med* 1982;**306**:557.

Rich S, Brundage BH, Levy PS: The effect of vasodilator therapy on the clinical outcome of patients with primary pulmonary hypertension. *Circulation* 1985;**71**:1191.

Rosenow EC III, Osmundson PJ, Brown ML: Pulmonary embolism. *Mayo Clin Proc* 1981;**56**:161.

Rubin LJ, Peter RH: Oral hydralazine therapy for primary pulmonary hypertension. *N Engl J Med* 1980;**302**:69.

Rudolph A et al: Effects of tolazoline hydrochloride (Priscoline) on circulatory dynamics of patients with pulmonary hypertension. *Am Heart J* 1958;**55**:424.

Shepherd JT et al: Clinical physiological and pathological considerations in patients with idiopathic pulmonary hypertension. *Br Heart J* 1957;**19**:70.

Short DS, Bedford DE: Solitary pulmonary hypertension. *Br Heart J* 1957;**19**:93.

Sokolow M, Katz LN, Muscovitz AN: The electrocardiogram in pulmonary embolism. *Am Heart J* 1940;**19**:166.

Stauffer JL, Olson DE, Petty TL: Complications and consequences of endotracheal intubation and tracheotomy: A prospective study of 150 critically ill adult patients. *Am J Med* 1981;**70**:65.

Stein PD, Willis PW III, DeMets DL: History and physical examination in acute pulmonary embolism in patients without preexisting cardiac or pulmonary disease. *Am J Cardiol* 1981;**47**:218.

Sutton GC, Hall RJC, Kerr IH: Clinical course and late prognosis of treated subacute massive, acute minor and chronic pulmonary thromboembolism. *Br Heart J* 1977;**39**:1135.

Tibbutt DA et al: Comparison by controlled trial of streptokinase and heparin in treatment of life-threatening pulmonary embolism. *Br Med J* 1974;**1**:343.

Via-Reque E, Rattenborg CC: Prolonged oro- or nasotracheal intubation. *Crit Care Med* 1981;**9**:637.

Wagenvoort CA, Wagenvoort N: *Pathology of Pulmonary Hypertension.* Wiley, 1977.

Wang SWS et al: Diazoxide in treatment of primary pulmonary hypertension. *Br Heart J* 1978;**40**:572.

Watkins WD et al: Prostacyclin and prostaglandin E_1 for severe idiopathic pulmonary artery hypertension. *Lancet* 1980;**1**:183.

Weisman IM, Rinaldo JE, Rogers RM: Positive end-expiratory pressure in adult respiratory failure. *N Engl J Med* 1982;**307**:1381.

Westlake EK et al: Carbon dioxide narcosis in emphysema. *Q J Med* 1955;**24**:155.

Wood P: Pulmonary hypertension. *Br Med Bull* 1952;**8**:348.

Diseases of the Aorta & Systemic Arteries

20

The diseases described under this heading include syphilitic aortitis and aneurysm, arteritis involving arteries of different sizes, systemic embolism, and systemic arteriovenous fistula. Arteritis and systemic embolism occur in a wide variety of diseases, and the accounts in this chapter deal mainly with the cardiologic aspects.

SYPHILITIC CARDIOVASCULAR DISEASE

Pathology

The basic lesion in the tertiary form of syphilis that affects the cardiovascular system is endarteritis obliterans. The primary site of disease is the thoracic aorta, and endarteritis of the vasa vasorum weakens the media and causes swelling and scarring of the intima, giving rise to the characteristic "crow's foot" or "tree bark" markings seen at autopsy. The changes in the intima can narrow the ostia of the coronary vessels and also affect the aortic valve cusps. The weakening of the media leads to dilation of the aorta that, in addition to causing fusiform or saccular aneurysms in the thoracic aorta, leads to aortic valve ring dilation and progressive aortic incompetence.

Clinical Findings

Syphilitic heart disease has become much rarer in the past 50 years since effective treatment of primary syphilis has been widely available. When it does occur, the disease is less florid, and instead of causing symptoms in persons 40–60 years of age, cardiovascular syphilis now affects older persons. Consequently, atherosclerotic lesions almost always coexist with syphilitic lesions. Atherosclerotic aneurysms are described in Chapter 9. In contrast to syphilitic aneurysms, they are usually fusiform rather than saccular and are much more likely to involve the descending aorta. Syphilitic aneurysms of the thoracic aorta act as space-occupying, expanding, cardiovascular "tumors" that compress and erode surrounding structures. They occur more commonly in men by a factor of 3:1. Their clinical manifestations vary with the site of the aneurysm. Aneurysms of the ascending aorta classically produce physical signs; aneurysms of the arch of the aorta cause symptoms; and aneurysms of the descending aorta cause pain or are asymptomatic.

A. Symptoms: Symptoms appear late in cardiovascular syphilis, and significant abnormalities may be found in asymptomatic patients. Pain in the chest is the most important symptom of aortic aneurysm. In descending thoracic aortic lesions, pain is caused by erosion of the vertebral column, and it is constant, boring, severe, and worse at night. Ascending aortic lesions involving coronary ostia may cause angina pectoris, with pain at rest or during exercise. The angina occurs as the result of interference with coronary blood flow. Ascending aortic lesions may occur with or without aortic incompetence. Pain may also arise from aortic lesions that do not involve the coronary vessels; this pain is attributed to stretching of aortic tissue. The symptoms associated with aneurysms of the arch of the aorta stem from pressure on surrounding structures and include cough due to pressure on the trachea or left bronchus, hoarseness due to pressure on the left recurrent laryngeal nerve, dysphagia due to pressure on the esophagus, swelling of the neck and face due to superior vena caval compression, and hemoptysis. This last manifestation may be the final symptom when the aneurysm ruptures into the bronchial tree.

B. Signs: The signs of aortic aneurysm may be attributable to the lesion, as in visible or palpable pulsation localized to the right of the sternum, which is more specific than the pulsation in the suprasternal notch seen with minor aortic dilatation. Signs caused indirectly by involvement of neighboring structures include the wide pulse pressure and water-hammer pulse of aortic incompetence, jugular venous distention and facial edema due to superior vena caval obstruction, Horner's syndrome (enophthalmos, miosis, and ptosis) due to sympathetic nerve compression, and tracheal tug. This latter sign is elicited by standing behind the patient and pulling the larynx upward; the "tug" of the aneurysm pulls the cervical structures down with each heartbeat. Cardiac enlargement, which is often massive, results from aortic incompetence. The immediate diastolic murmur of aortic incompetence is heard to the right of the sternum. The aortic valve closure sound is often high-pitched and has a tambour drumbeat quality even in the absence of an aneurysm or aortic incompetence. Aortic systolic murmurs are commonly heard, both with and without aortic incompetence, and they should not be taken as evidence of aortic stenosis. Signs of left ventricular failure may be present in patients with aortic incompetence. Associated neurologic signs of central nervous system syphilis are common and help point out the syphilitic cause of the aortic aneurysm.

C. Electrocardiographic Findings: There are no specific syphilitic changes on the ECG. Left ventricular hypertrophy occurs in response to aortic incompetence. Left bundle branch block and ischemic ST and T wave changes can occur in older persons.

D. X-Ray Findings: Aortic dilatation is often visible in patients with aortitis without aneurysm formation. Aortic aneurysms give rise to abnormal shadows on the chest x-ray that vary enormously from case to case. An example of an aneurysm of the arch of the aorta is shown in Fig 20–1. To distinguish between aneurysms and other tumors is difficult. Transmitted pulsations are not readily distinguished from the direct expansile pulsation of an aneurysm. Lack of pulsation does not exclude the possibility of an aneurysm, because thrombus formation may obliterate the cavity and leave a solid tumor. Calcification should be sought in the wall at the origin of the ascending aorta, where it is virtually pathognomonic of a syphilitic lesion. Calcification in the aortic arch and knuckle is much more common and is indicative of atherosclerosis. Syphilitic calcification is thin, beaded, and eggshell-like. It is usually seen best on the left anterior oblique or lateral view, as shown in Fig 20–2. When the descending aorta is involved, erosion of the thoracic vertebral column should be sought on the lateral view. Syphilis virtually never involves the abdominal aorta.

E. Special Investigations: Positive serologic tests for syphilis, either past or present, are most helpful in the diagnosis, but negative tests do not exclude the possibility of syphilitic disease any more than a positive test indicates that a given lesion is syphilitic. An elevated blood sedimentation rate is almost always seen when syphilitic cardiovascular disease is active and untreated. Echocardiography may help in the diagnosis, and cardiac catheterization and angiography are indicated if surgical treatment is contemplated. Angiography may be needed to distinguish aneurysms from other intrathoracic tumors; the procedure is generally well tolerated. The possibility of associated neurosyphilis should not be overlooked. Lumbar puncture should be performed in order to detect cerebrospinal fluid abnormalities associated with tertiary syphilis, tabes, or general paresis.

Differential Diagnosis

The differential diagnosis of syphilitic lesions is often difficult. Syphilitic aneurysms can be confused with intrathoracic tumors and cysts, and their luetic origin cannot always be proved. Atherosclerotic aneurysms can also occur; these are more likely to dissect than syphilitic aneurysms. Although positive serologic tests are of great value, they do not always indicate the true cause of the lesion. Furthermore, mixed lesions also occur.

Treatment

If syphilitic disease is active or progressive and especially if serologic tests are positive, antisyphilitic treatment with penicillin is indicated before any surgical measures are undertaken. Older remedies such as potassium iodide by mouth may be helpful in the control of pain and pressure symptoms. Penicillin treatment for syphilitic cardiovascular disease should be undertaken in the hospital, if possible, because of the possibility of a Jarisch-Herxheimer reaction. This involves a sudden acute allergic response attributed to massive death of spirochetes. It causes swelling of the aortic endothelium and may occlude the coronary ostia. Initial treatment should use a small (10,000 units) test dose of penicillin combined with corticosteroids (eg, prednisone, 10–20 mg every 6 hours) for the first few doses. The treatment of choice for cardiovascular syphilis is benzathine penicillin G, 7.2

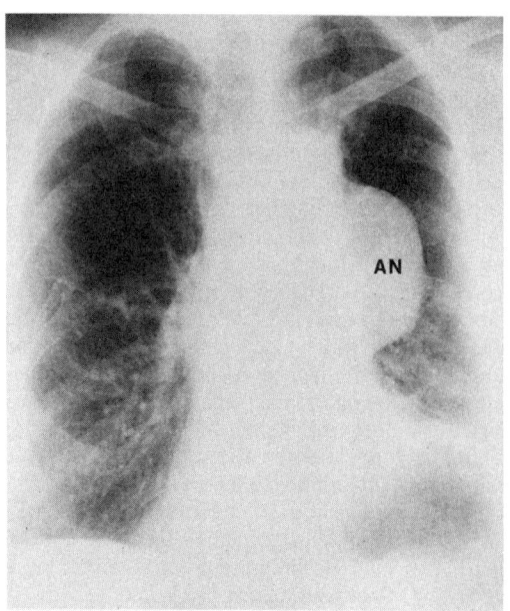

Figure 20–1. Chest x-ray showing a syphilitic aneurysm of the arch of the aorta (AN).

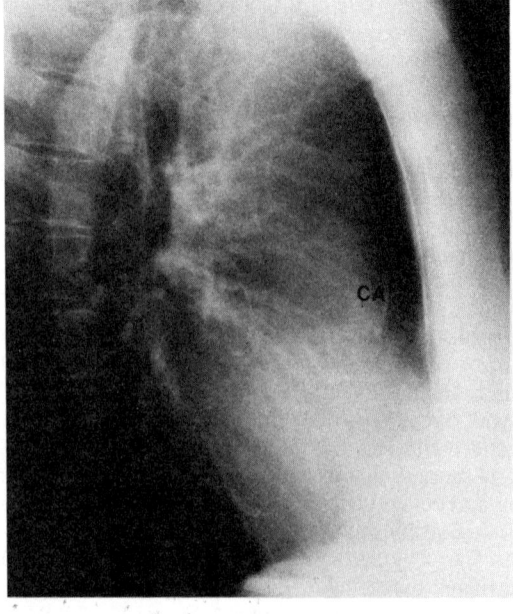

Figure 20–2. Lateral chest x-ray showing linear calcification (CA) of the ascending aorta in a patient with syphilitic aortitis.

million units total, divided into weekly doses of 2.4 million units by intramuscular injection for 3 successive weeks. Alternative treatment consists of aqueous procaine penicillin G, 9 million units total, administered as 600,000 units a day by intramuscular injection for 15 days. In patients who are allergic to penicillin, tetracycline, 500 mg orally 4 times a day for 30 days, is recommended, or erythromycin, 500 mg orally 4 times a day for 30 days.

Surgical resection of syphilitic aneurysms and aortic valve replacement for aortic incompetence should always be considered. Direct surgery for ostial coronary lesions may be necessary. If the patient is asymptomatic and the disease shows no evidence of progression, the patient's progress should be monitored. The results of valve replacement in syphilitic lesions are similar to those obtained in operation on lesions due to other causes. The aorta in patients with syphilis holds sutures securely, and the tissues tend to be less friable than in Marfan's syndrome.

Complications

Almost all of the manifestations of syphilitic cardiovascular disease can be regarded as complications, since endarteritis obliterans of the vasa vasorum, which is the basic lesion, has no direct effects, and expansion of the aorta is a secondary effect. Rupture of the aorta into any hollow thoracic structure is a late complication that is inevitably fatal. Thrombosis in association with stasis is common, but secondary embolism is rarer than in atherosclerotic lesions. Cardiac arrhythmias, complete atrioventricular block, infective endocarditis, and acute aortic dissection seldom occur. It should be remembered that the primary lesion is aortic and that cardiac involvement is almost always secondary, although gummatous myocarditis may be seen at autopsy.

Prognosis

The prognosis in syphilitic cardiovascular disease has greatly improved with better treatment of primary and secondary syphilis. Inadequately treated patients rather than untreated ones form the majority of cases. In partially arrested syphilitic disease, the patient develops a lesion in later life that progresses more slowly and carries a better prognosis. When the aortic valve is diseased, with significant aortic incompetence, the prognosis is worse. It is also worse when the aortic arch is involved in aneurysm formation because of the large number of vital structures that can be readily affected. The cause of death in patients with cardiovascular syphilis is now usually atherosclerotic in origin, and death in middle age (age 40–60) is rare.

ARTERITIS

Arteries of various sizes may be involved in an inflammatory process that can be either idiopathic or part of some generalized systemic disease. A clinical classification of the various vasculitis syndromes is presented in Table 20–1. The 3 types of lesions that produce arteritis as their main manifestation are temporal arteritis, aortic arch arteritis (Takayasu's disease), and polyarteritis nodosa. In the other diseases, either the other manifestations predominate or the arteritis is a pathologic feature found on histologic examination.

The term temporal arteritis is not specific but refers to a form of arteritis that is usually associated with giant cell formation and involves the cranial arteries of older persons, usually Caucasian women in the age group from 65 to 75. Although the temporal arteries are a readily accessible site of lesions, their involvement is not inevitable, and the clinical picture overlaps that of Takayasu's disease.

Takayasu's disease (pulseless disease) is a form of arteritis that classically affects the aorta and its major branches, especially those leading to the head and upper limbs in young Oriental women. In some cases other vessels such as the descending aorta and renal arteries may be involved (Fig 20–3). Giant cell formation may be seen histologically, and smaller arteries can also be involved. Thrombosis of major vessels and embolization are the major manifestations. After several major aortic branches have been occluded, the pressure in the remaining vessels rises, because the heart pumps into a restricted vascular bed. This leads to cardiac hypertrophy and ultimately to left ventricular failure.

Polyarteritis nodosa is a multisystem disease of

Table 20–1. Clinical classification of vasculitis syndromes, indicating the wide variety of conditions in which the syndromes may occur.*

Usually characterized by necrotizing vasculitis	
Temporal arteritis	Henoch-Schönlein purpura
Wegener's granulomatosis	"Classic" polyarteritis
Aortic arch arteritis	nodosa
Occasionally complicated by necrotizing vasculitis	
Rheumatic diseases	**Respiratory diseases**
Rheumatoid arthritis	Löffler's syndrome
Systemic lupus	Asthma
erythematosus	Serous otitis media
Dermatomyositis	**Hypersensitivity**
Ankylosing	Serum sickness
spondylitis	Drug allergy
Rheumatic fever	Amphetamine abuse
Infections	**Paraproteinemias**
Hepatitis B	Essential cryoglobulinemia
Acute respiratory	Multiple myeloma
infections	Macroglobulinemia
Streptococcal	**Others**
infections	Dermal vasculitis
Poststreptococcal	Ulcerative colitis
glomerulonephritis	Cogan's syndrome
Infective endocarditis	Colon carcinoma

*Modified and reproduced, with permission, from Christian CL, Sergent JS: Vasculitis syndromes: Clinical and experimental models. *Am J Med* 1976;**61**:385.

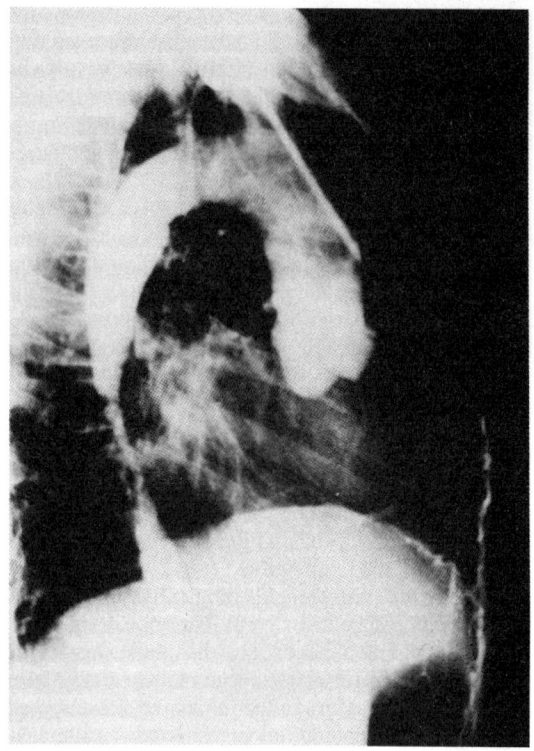

Figure 20–3. Aortogram showing narrowing of the descending aorta due to Takayasu's disease in a child. (Courtesy of Dr Dai Ru-ping.)

unknown cause that is usually considered one of the connective tissue disorders but is primarily a diffuse vasculitis with aneurysm formation involving the small arteries throughout the body. Diffuse vasculitis may occur as a variant of polyarteritis nodosa. James (1966, 1977) has noted that small coronary arteries varying from 0.1 to 1 mm in diameter may be involved, producing angina pectoris, myocardial infarction, and left ventricular failure with ventricular arrhythmias. The lesions in polyarteritis nodosa can occur anywhere in the body. The kidney, heart, gastrointestinal tract, lungs, and central nervous system are commonly affected. Because of the variability of the site and severity of the individual lesions, the clinical features can mimic almost any disease.

Clinical Findings

A. Symptoms: The symptoms of arteritis vary widely with the site of the lesion. In temporal arteritis, the principal presenting symptom is headache with a throbbing swelling over the affected artery. Pain on mastication (jaw claudication), fever, malaise, visual disturbance—blurring of vision or even sudden blindness—or neurologic disturbances are commonly seen. In other cases, the disease is more general, and arthralgia, abdominal pain, or chest pain may be the presenting symptom. In Takayasu's disease, the effects of sudden occlusion of a major vessel may be the first manifestation, eg, limb pain, hemiplegia, or sudden blindness. The presenting symptoms of polyarteritis nodosa are extremely variable.

B. Signs: The signs of arteritis, like the symptoms, vary widely. Loss of the pulse of a major vessel and a bruit over a vessel are the commonest signs, and systemic hypertension, which may be secondary to renal ischemia, is also a prominent feature. Systemic hypertension is also common in polyarteritis nodosa; in consequence, cardiac enlargement, fundal changes, and proteinuria are often seen. The age of the patient varies in the different forms of arteritis. Temporal arteritis commonly occurs in women over age 65, whereas Takayasu's disease is most frequently seen in women 20–30 years of age. Polyarteritis nodosa is more common in men than in women and occurs at any age.

C. Electrocardiographic Findings: Electrocardiographic changes resulting from hypertension, with left ventricular hypertrophy and ST–T wave changes, may be seen. In some cases, actual myocardial infarction occurs, with consequent changes on the ECG.

D. X-Ray Findings: The heart is not infrequently enlarged, and signs of pulmonary congestion or infarction may develop.

E. Laboratory Findings and Special Investigations: Leukocytosis, perhaps with eosinophilia, is not uncommon. The sedimentation rate is raised, and tests of renal function often show impairment. Biopsy of an easily accessible lesion constitutes the most important means of establishing the diagnosis, and if giant cell arteritis is suspected it is worthwhile to biopsy the temporal artery even if it is not clinically involved. The classic picture of arteritis may be found in any organ, and biopsy of a small sensory nerve (eg, the sural nerve at the ankle) may provide diagnostic information, especially in polyarteritis nodosa. Skin, muscle, and renal biopsy are often used. In difficult cases, help can sometimes be obtained from selective angiography. For example, mesenteric angiography may demonstrate multiple small aneurysms on the arteries to the gut.

Differential Diagnosis

The differential diagnosis of arteritis covers almost the entire range of medicine. The possibility of arteritis must be borne in mind with any patient in whom more than one organ system is involved.

Complications

Blindness, hemiplegia, myocardial infarction, left heart failure, renal failure, and systemic embolization are some of the more severe complications of arteritis. Almost any complication can occur, and the diseases generally run a steadily progressive course.

Treatment

The treatment of arteritis is unsatisfactory. Corticosteroids are commonly used, and there is evidence that they can prevent and even reverse blindness in some cases. If hypertension is a feature, the blood pressure should be reduced with antihypertensive drugs (see Chapter 9), and surgery to relieve renal arterial obstruction should be considered. Immunosupressive drugs (eg, cyclophosphamide or azathioprine) have been used, particularly in polyarteritis nodosa, but their effectiveness is not established.

Prognosis

The prognosis is poor, especially when renal or left heart failure occurs. Most patients die within 5 years.

SYSTEMIC EMBOLISM

Systemic embolism is an important complication of a number of heart diseases, including valvular and congenital heart disease, infective endocarditis, and myocardial infarction, which have been discussed elsewhere in this book. This section deals with embolism that is apparently unrelated to heart disease as well as embolism that has an established cardiac cause. It also deals more extensively with the manifestations and treatment of systemic embolism affecting particular parts of the systemic arterial bed.

Factors Promoting Thrombosis

The 3 factors promoting thrombosis in the left side of the heart and great vessels are stasis, changes in composition of the blood, and endothelial damage. Stasis is associated both with dilatation of such chambers as the left atrium, left ventricle, and aorta and with ineffective contraction, as occurs in atrial fibrillation and myocardial infarction. Changes in composition of the blood may be due to hemoconcentration, polycythemia, or an increase in the number or stickiness of platelets, as occurs in certain blood diseases. Endothelial damage is usually the result of inflammation (using the term in its widest sense to include trauma, ischemic necrosis, mechanical damage, and infections). The role of drugs, especially oral contraceptive agents, is also important in the development of thrombosis. Such drugs increase blood lipids and platelet stickiness and have been demonstrated to increase the chances of thromboembolism.

The Nature of Embolic Material

Not all embolism is due to the accumulation of thrombotic material. Emboli composed of microorganisms, especially fungi from exuberant vegetations, can cause important damage. Valve tissue, artificial valve material, pieces of tumor (as in left atrial myxoma), foreign bodies (eg, in drug addicts), calcium, and aggregates of platelets and fibrin from heart valves or atheromatous lesions may cause embolism.

The clinical consequences of embolism vary, widely. This fact is explained by the great variety of materials that form the emboli and by the differences in the age and size of the thrombus that breaks off. Fresh red thrombus is the commonest form of embolic material. Because it is often readily lysed by the defense mechanisms of the body, in many cases the clinical effects of embolism, although severe and dramatic at onset, are relatively short-lived and are followed by complete or almost complete recovery. In contrast, if organized thrombus, calcium, tumor material, or a large mass of *Candida* organisms constitutes the embolus, the obstruction to the blood vessel will be permanent.

The State of the Arterial Bed

The state of the arterial bed where the embolus lodges is an important variable in the clinical picture. Healthy young persons with normal blood vessels and a well-marked capacity to develop good collateral circulation withstand embolism better than do older, more atherosclerotic persons in whom degenerative changes have already occurred. Thus, age and age-related disease influence the clinical effects of embolism. Local spasm of the embolized vessel can also suddenly occur in response to the impact of the embolus, and such spasms aggravate the acute manifestations of an embolism. The role played by secondary thrombosis in exacerbating the damage also varies, and in some cases thrombosis of the vein accompanying the embolized artery leads to secondary pulmonary embolism. If the embolus contains viable virulent organisms, abscesses may occur. If the organisms are less virulent, they may simply weaken the wall of the artery, and a mycotic aneurysm may form, as in infective endocarditis.

Specific Sites of Embolism

Many emboli lodge in sites where they provoke no clinical manifestations. Skeletal muscles harbor emboli without any signs of disease. The kidneys are also capable of accommodating emboli, and scars from infarcts that have occurred at various times are occasionally seen at autopsy in patients who have died of congestive heart failure. The liver with its double arterial blood supply is seldom if ever the site of infarction except in polyarteritis nodosa. The visceral manifestations of embolism generally occur as infarction, with death and necrosis of tissue, which is clinically recognizable only when the infarction is large or strategically placed or when it interferes with organ function. The central nervous system is the prime site for embolism that is likely to cause symptoms and signs. Even here, however, areas of infarction are found at autopsy in patients who had no clinical manifestations of any lesion.

A. Cerebral Embolism:

1. In patients with heart disease—Embolic material lodged in the brain produces the most serious and dramatic clinical manifestations of embolism. The onset is instantaneous, often with loss of consciousness or convulsions. Neurologic damage is most severe at onset. Hemiplegia, aphasia, and loss of vision are the commonest acute severe manifestations. Almost any clinical neurologic picture can occur, but an instantaneous, dramatic onset is the most characteristic feature. Spasm of the cerebral vessels and cerebral edema tend to make initial damage seem greater than it is, and recovery of function, although variable, is frequently remarkably rapid and surprisingly complete.

The physician's course of action in treating a patient who has just suffered a cerebral embolism depends on the certainty of the diagnosis of cerebral embolism. If the physician has not seen the patient before, the heart should be examined carefully for evidence of valvular disease, and a history of possible heart disease should be elicited from relatives. Head injury, subarachnoid hemorrhage, cerebral thrombosis, and intracerebral hemorrhage must be ruled out, and the patient must be closely watched for evidence of clinical deterioration or recovery. The foot of the bed should be raised and oxygen administered by face mask. The addition of CO_2 to act as a cerebral vasodilator has been advocated, but there is little or no evidence that this procedure is beneficial. Systemic vasodilators should be avoided because they tend to reduce cerebral perfusion pressure. Lumbar puncture is indicated if there is any doubt about the diagnosis. The cerebrospinal fluid is seldom if ever hemorrhagic in cases of embolism. Cerebral angiography is not indicated, since embolectomy is never performed in cases of spontaneous cerebral embolism involving intracranial vessels. The place of anticoagulant therapy in the treatment of cerebral embolism is not clear. Hemorrhage into the area of infarction and secondary thrombosis around the site of embolism can occur and exacerbate neurologic damage. The most logical course is to continue anticoagulant therapy if the patient has already been given anticoagulants and to withhold it in all other cases. In comparison with the prognosis in cerebral hemorrhage or cerebral thrombosis, the prognosis in cerebral embolism without anticoagulant therapy is sufficiently good that striking evidence of therapeutic benefit would be necessary to justify the use of anticoagulants in all patients.

Rehabilitation of the patient should be started as soon as possible. Improvement in nervous system function tends to occur at an exponentially decreasing rate over a 2-year period after the episode of embolism. Complete or almost complete recovery occurs in over 80% of patients with mitral valve disease who suffer cerebral embolism from left atrial thrombus. However, recovery seldom occurs if endocarditis is the cause of the embolus. The management of patients with mitral disease in whom cerebral embolism has occurred is not altered by the embolus. Mitral valve surgery is performed if indicated but not solely because of the embolus. The indications for restoration of sinus rhythm by cardioversion are similar to those in patients without embolism.

Embolism is, if anything, more common after valve replacement than before the operation, and restoration of sinus rhythm is likely to be only temporary unless the atrial fibrillation is of recent onset. Another embolism may well occur when atrial fibrillation recurs. Anticoagulant therapy is recommended by many, but it does not always prevent embolism.

2. In patients without heart disease—A different form of cerebral embolism frequently occurs in patients with atherosclerotic lesions involving the vessels of the head. In this case, the clinical picture is different from that seen in patients with heart lesions. The emboli are smaller and much more likely to be multiple, and the entire clinical picture is much more insidious, causing symptoms that have been labeled as transient ischemic attacks. Small aggregations of platelets and thrombi form on ulcerative atherosclerotic lesions in moderate-sized arteries such as the internal carotid or vertebral artery. Pieces of these thrombi dislodge and move to other areas, giving rise to repeated episodes that resemble one another and always involve vessels distal to the lesion. Dizziness, sudden vertigo, weakness or paralysis, faintness, loss of speech, and sudden blindness are the common presenting features. A systolic bruit should be listened for in the neck and a full neurologic examination performed. Every attempt should be made to see the patient during an attack, when central nervous system abnormalities are more likely to be detected. The clinical picture is likely to be confused with that of arrhythmia, aortic stenosis, senile dementia, or central nervous system disease rather than that associated with embolism from thrombotic material accumulated in the heart.

Doppler blood velocity measurements and ultrasonic imaging of the vessels in the neck are helpful in diagnosis, and cerebral angiography is required for diagnostic purposes if surgical treatment of extracranial lesions is contemplated.

B. Coronary Embolism: (See also Chapter 8.) Coronary embolism presents a clinical picture that is indistinguishable from that of myocardial infarction due to atherosclerosis. Embolism presumably can occur without infarction and pass unnoticed in young patients and persons with excellent collateral blood supply. The onset of coronary embolism is instantaneous, and syndromes in which there is a gradual onset of chest pain are not seen. Electrocardiographic changes develop in the usual manner, and the clinical course is usually benign if the source of the embolus is left atrial thrombus. The reason is that in such cases, the embolic material (fresh red thrombus) is readily lysed. Embolism with calcific material in patients with aortic valve disease carries a much poorer prognosis. The treatment is similar to that in patients with lesions due to an atherosclerotic cause; in most instances, a period of rest under observation is the only thing that is required.

C. Peripheral Embolism Involving the Extremities: It is rare for embolism involving the arms to cause symptoms sufficient to warrant treatment. Exceptions occur when the embolic material is not thrombus. In such cases embolectomy may be indicated. The commonest sites of embolization requiring urgent treatment are the external iliac and femoral arteries. If the embolus lodges farther down the leg, collateral circulation through the profunda femoris artery is usually sufficient to maintain adequate circulation unless significant atherosclerosis is also present. Femoral arterial occlusion usually causes an acute, severe pain in the leg, with loss of sensation, pallor, and a cold, pulseless limb.

The severe ischemic pain provides the most important indication for surgical treatment. The femoral artery is readily accessible in the groin, and the dangers of damaging distal tissues are negligible. It is not necessary to localize the site of the embolus accurately by means of angiography because balloon-tipped (Fogarty) catheters can be passed up and down the vessel and used to extract thrombus from areas not directly accessible through the incision. Any embolic material should always be saved for bacteriologic and histologic examination. The diagnosis of atrial myxoma has occasionally been accomplished by this means, and the nature of the infecting organism in endocarditis has been established by analysis of embolic material.

Surgical exploration should be undertaken as soon as possible after diagnosis. It can be conveniently carried out under local anesthesia. In the period before operation the limb should be kept cool in order to slow the metabolic processes. Meperidine (50–150 mg intramuscularly) should be given for relief of pain. Problems may arise if the patient is not seen until some time after an acute episode. Embolectomy can be beneficial even as long as a week after an acute episode, and the length of time that has elapsed since the embolism should not necessarily be taken as a contraindication to surgical exploration. In cases seen shortly after the acute episode, anticoagulation can be delayed until after operation. If surgery is not to be undertaken, anticoagulation with heparin should be given (5000–10,000 units intravenously every 4–6 hours), followed by warfarin (Coumadin), 30–50 mg on the first day, 10–15 mg on the second day, and a maintenance dose of 5–15 mg, depending on the prothrombin time, on later days. The heparin should be stopped on the third day when the prothrombin time is prolonged.

The prognosis following embolism in the leg depends mainly on the degree of atherosclerosis and consequently on the age of the patient. The prognosis is worse in patients with mural thrombi following myocardial infarction and in those with endocarditis. Intermittent claudication following the acute episode occurs occasionally, but in younger patients in whom the source of embolus is left atrial thrombus, recovery is usually complete.

D. Other Sites of Embolism: Mesenteric embolism causes severe epigastric pain of acute onset, with or without acute circulatory collapse. Mesenteric embolism must be differentiated from other acute abdominal emergencies. Melena occurs within a few hours, followed by paralytic ileus with vomiting and abdominal distention. Surgical exploration with bowel resection is often performed, but the results are not uniformly good. As with all other forms of systemic embolism, expectant treatment can sometimes give good results, especially if the embolus moves to a more distal site and blood flow is thereby restored. Anticoagulant therapy is contraindicated because hemorrhage into the gut is almost always present.

Renal embolism seldom causes significant difficulties. The commonest manifestations are hematuria and renal colic associated with the passage of blood clots or dull flank pain due to the embolus itself. Acute renal failure is rarely seen. Renal embolism may be followed by hypertension (see Chapter 9). Studies of renal function and renal angiography in patients with mitral stenosis and systemic hypertension have shown evidence of segmental renal ischemia, and embolism should be considered when systemic hypertension is seen in association with mitral valve disease—especially when atrial fibrillation is present.

Splenic embolism may cause left upper quadrant pain and tenderness and may be associated with perisplenitis, a friction rub, and pain that is worse on inspiration. Mild analgesics are usually all that is required.

Investigation of Causes of Embolism

It is not uncommon for the patient to present with one or more acute episodes and symptoms highly suggestive of embolism. There may be no obvious signs of heart disease to account for the episodes. Careful examination of the heart reveals no evidence of valvular disease. The heart is not enlarged, and the ECG is within normal limits. In such cases, echocardiography, cardiac catheterization, pulmonary angiography, and complete examination of the left heart chambers are often performed, especially in order to rule out a lesion that is amenable to surgery, such as left atrial myxoma.

Ulcerative atheromatous lesions in the aorta or in the carotid artery should also be considered as possible causes. If the lesions are confined to some specific part of the circulation, a lesion in the artery supplying that area (eg, a vessel in the head) may be suspected as the cause. In most cases in which the cause is not immediately obvious and emboli involve more than one area, an explanation is not found. Paradoxic embolism via a patent foramen ovale is sometimes suggested as a cause, but this is difficult to prove or disprove until autopsy. Embolism has always been a common postmortem finding in both the systemic and the pulmonary circulations. In dying patients circulation is often extremely sluggish in the period just before death. Small nodular thrombotic (marantic) lesions are not uncommonly found on the heart valves at autopsy, particularly in patients dying of malignant disease.

SYSTEMIC ARTERIOVENOUS FISTULA

A systemic arteriovenous fistula provides a low-resistance pathway through which blood can flow from the high-pressure arterial bed into the low-pressure venous system. The volume flow rate through the fistula depends on the size of the communication and on the height of the arterial pressure above the venous pressure. If a normal blood flow is to be maintained to perfuse the body in the presence of a fistula, the cardiac output must be increased by an amount equal to the fistula flow. The fistula flow thus constitutes a constant unremitting load on the heart, and if the fistula is large or if cardiac function is impaired, heart failure is likely to develop.

Systemic arteriovenous fistulas may be congenital, as in hemangiomatous lesions, or traumatic. The trauma may be due to stab or gunshot wounds that establish a communication between an artery and its adjacent vein, often in a limb. In some cases the trauma is surgical, and a fistula forms after an operation. Nephrectomy, cholecystectomy, and laminectomy are among the more common operations in which this complication occurs. In other cases, the systemic arteriovenous fistula is purposely created to provide ready access to a blood vessel with high flow for the treatment of renal failure by hemodialysis.

Pathophysiology

A systemic arteriovenous fistula is a prime cause of a high-output state (see Chapter 10). The extra load on the heart resulting from a high-output state gives rise to a number of secondary effects that become more important as the patient becomes older or cardiac function deteriorates.

When there is a systemic arteriovenous fistula, the baroreceptor mechanisms act to maintain a normal arterial blood pressure. The tendency for the arterial pressure to fall as blood leaks out of the arterial bed leads to tachycardia, increased cardiac output, and vasoconstriction in other beds that, unlike the fistula, are capable of responding to sympathetically mediated peripheral vasoconstriction. The increased cardiac output constitutes a constant extra load on the heart that varies with the size of the fistula. Although the load is well tolerated if the fistula is small and the patient is young, problems arise when the fistula is large (30% increase in resting output) or when age-related changes such as atherosclerosis or hypertension are present. When the load on the heart is so great that adequate perfusion of the body—especially the kidneys—cannot be maintained, a form of heart failure called high-output failure develops.

High-output failure. Some increase in blood volume occurs in any arteriovenous fistula that is large enough to increase the resting cardiac output significantly. When renal perfusion is inadequate, further increase in blood volume with salt retention and edema occurs. This increases the load on the heart. The left ventricular and later the right ventricular end-diastolic pressures rise, and the patient develops heart failure. The picture that results is remarkable in that the peripheral vasoconstriction, weak pulse, and hypodynamic cardiac impulse with cool extremities and peripheral cyanosis seen in low-output failure are replaced by a bounding pulse, warm moist palms, a hyperdynamic cardiac impulse, warm limbs, and pink skin. The acuteness of the onset of the load, its magnitude, and its duration are important variables determining the clinical picture.

Clinical Findings

A. Symptoms: The patient is sometimes aware of the flow through the fistula, which gives rise to a buzzing sensation localized to the affected area. Palpitations, fatigue, and dyspnea are seen, but, in general, exercise tolerance is well maintained, because the fall in systemic resistance with exercise tends to decrease the fistula flow. The patient may notice that the skin near the fistula is warmer than normal and notice overgrowth of blood vessels around the site of the lesion.

B. Signs: The pulse is bounding and the heart rate increased. The pulse pressure is increased and the skin warm and moist. If the fistula is in a limb, that limb often grows to be longer than the opposite one, and tortuous varicose veins develop near the site of the fistula. Increased venous pressure occurs late in the disease. The heart is often enlarged, with a hyperdynamic cardiac impulse and a loud first sound. Third and fourth heart sounds may be heard, and a systolic murmur not infrequently develops in association with the increased stroke volume. A palpable and audible bruit is also detectable over the site of the fistula. This sign is of most help when the fistula is in the abdomen or back. If the fistula is accessible and can be occluded by manual compression, its clinical significance can be assessed. If the fistula is significant, its occlusion raises the systemic vascular resistance and provokes a baroreceptor response. This consists of bradycardia and peripheral vasodilation. The fall in heart rate on occlusion and the increase on release (Branham's sign) constitute the best means of assessing a fistula at the bedside. In older patients and those with renal failure, this simple test is less reliable, and a significant fistula can be present in a patient in whom Branham's sign is negative.

C. Electrocardiographic Findings: Tachycardia and minor changes indicative of left ventricular overload (high-voltage QRS complexes and ST–T wave changes in the left ventricular leads) are seen. Significant hypertensive changes may be present in patients undergoing dialysis.

D. X-Ray Findings: The heart is usually enlarged, with a left ventricular configuration, and serial chest x-rays are valuable in demonstrating progressive enlargement. Pulmonary congestion is only seen in the late stages, when heart failure is present.

E. Special Investigations: Blood volume is increased in most cases of fistula of significant degree, and mild anemia is seen because it is the plasma volume that is raised. Echocardiography shows the left ventricle to be dilated and overactive, with evidence of excessive wall motion. Doppler blood velocity measurements can be used to determine the hemodynamic significance of the fistula. Cardiac catheterization is not indicated for diagnosis, but if it is performed, the intracardiac pressures are found to be relatively normal and the cardiac output raised.

Differential Diagnosis

Systemic arteriovenous fistula must be distinguished from other forms of high-output state, eg, pregnancy, thyrotoxicosis, beriberi, anemia, and Paget's disease. Heart failure due to hypertensive or atherosclerotic disease or cardiomyopathy may be confused with or associated with the effects of a fistula, especially in patients undergoing hemodialysis. The possibility that the fistula is playing a part in cardiac problems must always be kept in mind in such patients, especially when the stress of anemia is added. In addition, the development of heart failure after a surgical operation should raise the possibility that an arteriovenous fistula has been accidentally created.

Complications

A fistula may become infected, leading to endarteritis with subsequent hemorrhage or embolism. The fistula may progressively increase in size as the abnormal blood vessels grow in response to increased flow through them, or spontaneous thrombosis of the fistula may occur. Heart failure is the most important complication, and the purpose of treatment is to prevent its development.

Treatment

Any arteriovenous fistula that is of clinical significance—one causing bradycardia on occlusion or one large enough to increase heart size—should be closed if possible. Traumatic fistulas and those accidentally created at surgery are usually readily dealt with surgically, but hemorrhage may be difficult to control at operation. Congenital malformations with arteriovenous fistulas often recur after surgical attempts to eradicate them. Fistulas that are created to facilitate hemodialysis may have to be reduced in size if they cause too large a cardiac load; if they become thrombosed, another fistula may have to be created.

Digitalis and diuretics are generally less effective in the treatment of high-output failure than in the treatment of low-output failure, and elimination of the fistula or at least reduction of its size is the treatment of choice.

Prognosis

The prognosis of systemic arteriovenous fistula depends on the ease with which its cardiovascular effects can be eliminated. The results are worst in patients with large congenital malformations. The prognosis of patients with renal failure undergoing hemodialysis should not be influenced by the fistula. A fistula large enough to provide an adequate route for dialysis can be achieved without compromising cardiac function in almost every case.

REFERENCES

Bron KM, Gajaraj A: Demonstration of hepatic aneurysms in polyarteritis nodosa by arteriography. *N Engl J Med* 1970;**282**:1024.

Christian CL, Sergent JS: Vasculitis syndromes: Clinical and experimental models. *Am J Med* 1976;**61**:385.

Chumbley LC: Allergic granulomatosis and angiitis (Churg-Strauss syndrome): Report and analysis of 30 cases. *Mayo Clin Proc* 1977;**52**:477.

Cohen RD, Corn DL, Ilstrup DM: Clinical features, prognosis, and response to treatment in polyarteritis. *Mayo Clin Proc* 1980;**55**:146.

Cohen SM et al: Cardiac output and peripheral bloodflow in arteriovenous aneurysm. *Clin Sci* 1948;**7**:35.

Conn DL et al: Immunologic mechanisms in systemic vasculitis. *Mayo Clin Proc* 1976;**51**:511.

Crane C: Atheromatous embolism to lower extremities in arteriosclerosis. *Arch Surg* 1967;**94**:96.

Cryer PE, Kissane J (editors): Multiple arterial occlusions in a young woman. *Am J Med* 1975;**59**:837.

Dale WA (editor): *Management of Arterial Occlusive Disease.* Year Book, 1971.

Dalen JE, Howe JP III: Dissection of the aorta: Current diagnostic and therapeutic approaches. *JAMA* 1979;**242**:32.

Dalen JE et al: Dissection of the aorta: Pathogenesis, diagnosis, and treatment. *Prog Cardiovasc Dis* 1980;**23**:237.

Ehrenfeld WK, Hoyt WF, Wylie EJ: Embolization and transient blindness from carotid atheroma. *Arch Surg* 1966;**93**:787.

Fauci AS: Vasculitis: New insights amid old enigmas. *Am J Med* 1979;**67**:916.

Fauci AS et al: Cyclophosphamide therapy of severe systemic necrotizing vasculitis. *N Engl J Med* 1979;**301**:235.

Fogarty TJ, Cranley JJ: Catheter technic for arterial embolectomy. *Ann Surg* 1965;**161**:325.

Fogarty TJ et al: A method for extraction of arterial emboli and thrombi. *Surg Gynecol Obstet* 1963;**116**:241.

Ghose MK, Shensa S, Lerner PI: Arteritis of the aged (giant cell arteritis) and fever of unexplained origin. *Am J Med* 1976;**60**:429.

Hamilton CR Jr, Shelly WM, Tumulty PA: Giant cell arteritis: Including temporal arteritis and polymyalgia rheumatica. *Medicine* 1971;**50**:1.

Holman E: *Arteriovenous Aneurysms.* Macmillan, 1937.

Holsinger DR, Osmundson PJ, Edwards JE: The heart in periarteritis nodosa. *Circulation* 1962;**25**:610.

Hull RG, Asherson RA, Rennie JAN: Ankylosing spondylitis and an aortic arch syndrome. *Br Heart J* 1984;**51**:663.

Hunder GG et al: Daily and alternate-day corticosteroid regimens in treatment of giant cell arteritis: Comparison in a prospective study. *Ann Intern Med* 1975;**82**:613.

Huston KA, Hunder GG: Giant cell (cranial) arteritis: A clinical review. *Am Heart J* 1980;**100**:99.

Huston KA et al: Temporal arteritis: A 25-year epidemiologic, clinical and pathologic study. *Ann Intern Med* 1978;**88**:162.

Ishikawa K: Natural history and classification of occlusive thromboaortopathy (Takayasu's disease). *Circulation* 1978;**57**:27.

Ishikawa K: Survival and morbidity after diagnosis of occlusive thromboaortopathy (Takayasu's disease). *Am J Cardiol* 1981;**47:**1026.

Jaffe HW: The laboratory diagnosis of syphilis: New concepts. *Ann Intern Med* 1975;**83:**846.

James TN: Small arteries of the heart. *Circulation* 1977;**56:**2.

James TN, Birk RE: Pathology of the cardiac conduction system in polyarteritis nodosa. *Arch Intern Med* 1966;**117:**561.

Jones E, Bedford DE: Syphilitic angina pectoris. *Br Heart J* 1943;**5:**107.

Klein RG et al: Large artery involvement in giant cell (temporal) arteritis. *Ann Intern Med* 1975;**83:**806.

Love WS, Werner CG: Observations upon syphilis of the heart, coronary ostia and coronary arteries: With special reference to the myocardial lesions noted in stenosis of the coronary ostia. *Am J Syphilis* 1934;**18:**154.

Lupi-Herrera E et al: Takayasu's arteritis: Clinical study of 107 cases. *Am Heart J* 1977;**93:**94.

Moore P, Fauci AS: Neurologic manifestations of systemic vasculitis: A retrospective and prospective study of the clinicopathologic features and responses to therapy in 25 patients. *Am J Med* 1981;**71:**517.

Parrillo JE, Fauci AS: Necrotizing vasculitis, coronary angiitis, and the cardiologist. *Am Heart J* 1980;**99:**547.

Pyeritz RE, McKusick VA: The Marfan syndrome: Diagnosis and management. *N Engl J Med* 1979;**300:**771.

Roberts WC, Wibin EA: Idiopathic panaortitis, supra-aortic arteritis, granulomatous myocarditis and pericarditis. *Am J Med* 1966;**41:**453.

Rose GA, Spencer H: Polyarteritis nodosa. *Q J Med* 1957;**26:**43.

Schrire V: Arteritis of the aorta and its major branches. *Australas Ann Med* 1967;**16:**33.

Shelhamer JH et al: Takayasu's arteritis and its therapy. *Ann Intern Med* 1985;**103:**121.

Steiner I, Hlava A, Prochaska J: Calcific coronary embolization associated with cardiac valve replacement: Necropsy x-ray study. *Br Heart J* 1976;**38:**816.

Strachan RW, How J, Bewsher PD: Masked giant-cell arteritis. *Lancet* 1980;**1:**194.

Szilagyi DE et al: Peripheral congenital arteriovenous fistulas. *Surgery* 1965;**57:**61.

Thompson JE et al: Arterial embolectomy: A 20-year experience with 163 cases. *Surgery* 1970;**67:**212.

Vecht RJ et al: Acute dissection of the aorta: Long-term review and management. *Lancet* 1980;**1:**109.

Walker DH, Mattern WD: Rickettsial vasculitis. *Am Heart J* 1980;**100:**896.

Wees SJ, Sunwoo IN, Oh SJ: Sural nerve biopsy in systemic necrotizing vasculitis. *Am J Med* 1981;**71:**525.

Wylie EJ, Ehrenfeld WK: *Extracranial Occlusive Cerebrovascular Disease: Diagnosis and Management.* Saunders, 1970.

Miscellaneous Forms of Heart Disease: Cardiac Tumors, Hypotension, Neurocirculatory Asthenia, & Traumatic Heart Disease

CARDIAC TUMORS

Cardiac tumors are more frequently metastatic than primary. Although pathologic evidence of cardiac or pericardial involvement can be found in about 10% of autopsies in patients with malignant disease, the incidence of clinical manifestations is less. The site of the primary tumor is most often in the lung or the breast, indicating that the tumor is likely to spread locally to involve the heart or pericardium. Various types of lymphoma also tend to involve the heart, again mainly by spread from the mediastinum. Metastases seldom affect left ventricular function, although when pericardial effusion occurs, the patient may show manifestations of pericardial tamponade. The most common primary malignant tumors involving the heart are sarcomas. The most common benign tumor is a myxoma—usually left atrial myxoma—although the right atrium may be involved and, more rarely, the ventricle.

Clinical Findings

A. Symptoms: The presenting symptoms in patients with cardiac tumors are often bizarre and confusing. Posturally variable dyspnea, cough, and syncope can occur. Chest pain is not infrequent, and evidence of systemic or pulmonary congestion, with dyspnea or edema, is sometimes seen. In patients with metastases, there is often no clinical clue to involvement of the heart in the patient's history.

B. Signs: Evidence of pericardial involvement may be found with pericardial friction or increased venous pressure. In myxoma there are often changing murmurs, perhaps influenced by posture. The tumor is often pedunculated and mobile, and the degree of obstruction to blood flow varies with posture and varying hemodynamic events. The patient may thus have a diastolic murmur in one body position but not in another. There may be a filling sound resembling a third heart sound that occurs when a mobile tumor hits the mitral valve in early diastole ("tumor plop"). Careful search for evidence of embolism is always important, and the recovery of embolic material for histologic examination is sometimes of diagnostic value. In some cases of myxoma, systemic signs such as fever, tachycardia, and clubbing of the fingers are seen.

C. Electrocardiographic Findings: There are no specific electrocardiographic changes in cardiac tumors. High-voltage P waves have been reported in rare cases of myxoma, and P mitrale is sometimes seen. If pulmonary hypertension develops, there may be right ventricular hypertrophy on the ECG.

D. X-Ray Findings: Bizarre outlines of the cardiac shadow and enlargement of the heart shadow due to pericardial effusion should be sought. Left atrial enlargement is seen in left atrial myxoma in many cases (see Chapter 12).

E. Laboratory Findings and Special Investigations: A raised sedimentation rate, anemia, and raised serum globulin are sometimes seen in myxomas. Echocardiography can be helpful in showing dense multiple echoes posterior to the anterior mitral valve leaflet in diastole. Pre- and postoperative echocardiograms in a patient with left atrial myxoma are shown in Fig 21–1. The results of echocardiography are not always so dramatic, and the tumor can be missed. Two-dimensional echocardiography is more likely to provide a correct diagnosis. Full studies with right and left heart catheterization and angiography are always needed before exploration is undertaken. Raised atrial or venous pressures on the right or left side are usually found, and in left atrial myxoma pulmonary congestion with perhaps a raised pulmonary vascular resistance is common. The tumors are usually slow-growing, and the disease is therefore insidious. CT scan and magnetic resonance imaging are helpful in establishing the diagnosis. Angiography is most useful in diagnosis. Left atrial myxoma can often be seen on left ventricular angiography. The small amount of mitral incompetence that often accompanies left ventricular injections of contrast material may outline the tumor, and the motion of the myxoma as it moves up and down with the heartbeat can sometimes be seen. An angiogram in a patient with right atrial (Fig 21–2) myxoma shows how a filling defect can be demonstrated. In patients with other forms of primary or secondary tumors, pericardiocentesis is often responsible for the establishment of the diagnosis when malignant cells are demonstrated in the fluid.

Differential Diagnosis

Left atrial myxoma is most likely to be confused with rheumatic disease of the mitral valve. The episodic nature of the symptoms and signs and the presence of systemic manifestations are the most useful features in diagnosis. Other primary or secondary

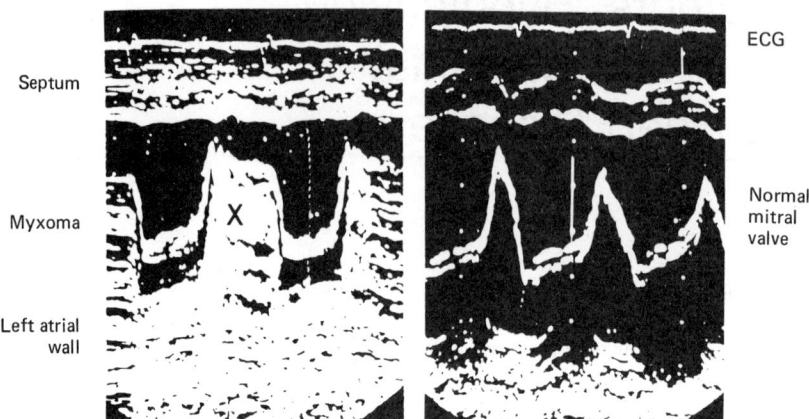

Figure 21–1. *Left:* Preoperative echocardiogram showing mass of echoes (X) posterior to the anterior mitral valve cusp and continuous with the left atrial wall in diastole. In systole, no such echoes are present. Posterior descent of anterior mitral cusp is restricted. *Right:* In postoperative echocardiogram, mass of echoes posterior to the anterior mitral valve cusp is no longer present, and descent of the cusp in diastole is normal. Atrial fibrillation is present. (Reproduced, with permission, from Srivastava TN, Fletcher E: The echocardiogram in left atrial myxoma. *Am J Med* 1973;**54**:136.)

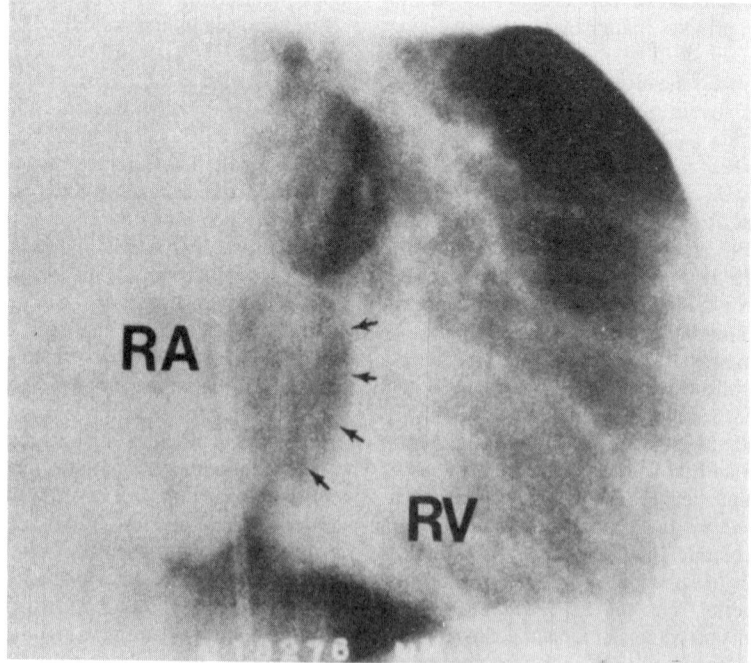

Figure 21–2. Right atrial angiocardiogram in 30-degree right anterior oblique view. Arrows indicate edge of filling defect. RA, right atrium; RV, right ventricle. (Reproduced, with permission, from Berman ND et al: Angiographic demonstration of blood supply of right atrial myxoma. *Br Heart J* 1976;**38**:764.)

tumors involving the heart can be confused with pericardial disease, with myocarditis or cardiomyopathy, or with valvular heart disease in some instances. The systemic manifestations of myxoma bring to mind many differential diagnoses, eg, infective endocarditis, connective tissue disorders, occult malignant disease, and chronic infections.

Treatment

Surgical removal of a right or left atrial myxoma is usually curative, although the tumor may rarely recur. Malignant cardiac tumors are usually fatal whether they are metastatic or primary angiosarcomas. Malignant pericardial effusion from metastatic disease usually requires systemic chemotherapy combined with local instillation of chemicals or radiotherapy (or both) to the pericardium.

Prognosis

Without treatment, patients with atrial myxoma may gradually develop worsening symptoms of pulmonary or systemic venous congestion as the tumor grows. Sudden death may occur if the mitral valve becomes totally obstructed. Pulmonary emboli in right atrial myxoma may lead to severe pulmonary symptoms and, if repeated, to pulmonary hypertension and right heart failure. Systemic emboli from left atrial myxoma may lead to hemiplegia, loss of a limb, or other severe vascular occlusions. Systemic symptoms of fever, arthralgia, and fatigue may cause chronic invalidism until one of the major cardiac or embolic catastrophes occurs.

HYPOTENSION

Hypotension should be regarded as a symptom rather than a disease.

Hypotension cannot be defined in terms of a specific level of arterial blood pressure—systolic or diastolic. The adequacy of the level of blood pressure is indicated by the patient's symptoms and in particular by the response to changes in posture. Remarkably low pressures can be tolerated in the supine position; and, conversely, when patients who have been hypertensive suffer a fall in pressure, symptoms may occur at surprisingly high pressure levels.

Causes of Hypotension

Hypotension results from inadequate cardiac output, as in myocardial infarction; from inadequate circulating blood volume; or from failure of the normal reflex mechanisms that maintain a constant arterial pressure. All these factors operate in a number of disorders, and several may combine in a given patient to cause the primary symptom of hypotension—dizziness or faintness—that is made worse when the patient suddenly stands up.

Disturbances of blood volume are clinically more common than disturbances of reflex control of the circulation, and they stem from 2 factors. One is a decrease in plasma or red cell volume due to hemorrhage, fluid loss, diarrhea, vomiting, unrecognized internal hemorrhage, dehydration, excessive diuresis, or excessive sweating; the other is a change in capacity of a blood-filled compartment (heart, arteries, capillaries, or veins).

Decreased blood volume as a cause of hypotension is particularly striking in adrenal insufficiency disorders, eg, Addison's disease and hypopituitarism. Wasting disorders of the bowel associated with diarrhea and anemia are also commonly associated with hypotension, and a sudden episode of faintness with hypotension is often the first manifestation of gastrointestinal hemorrhage.

Abnormalities of reflex control of arterial pressure usually result from disease of the central nervous system and its autonomic pathways. Disease may also affect the peripheral parts of the autonomic nervous system via innervation of blood vessels that are particularly susceptible to the effect of drugs.

Clinical Features

The clinical picture of hypotension associated with an inadequate blood volume is dominated by the effects of the compensatory mechanisms that are mediated by the autonomic nervous system. These effects cause anxiety, weakness, palpitations, tachycardia, restlessness, vasoconstriction, sweating, pallor, and cold extremities. In contrast, in hypotension associated with autonomic nervous system disease, the patient faints, with few or no accompanying symptoms. Dizziness and dimness of vision usually give little warning of impending loss of consciousness. Recovery is rapid when cerebral blood flow is restored with the patient in the recumbent position.

Hypotension Associated With Inadequate Blood Volume

A. Vasovagal Attacks and Fainting: The commonest form of hypotension is that seen in simple fainting. A sudden muscular vasodilation mediated by cholinergic sympathetic nerves results in an acute fall in effective blood volume owing to sudden pooling of blood in peripheral areas of the body (normally the legs). Simple fainting occurs in normal subjects and may also be provoked by disease, especially myocardial infarction with or without pain. Fainting may also occur during cardiologic investigations. The vagus nerve plays an important part in the mechanism of fainting, and simple faints are sometimes called vasovagal attacks. The primary stimulus to simple fainting may be physical or psychic. Trauma, pain, or stimulation of vagal afferents—especially in the ascending aorta near the right coronary ostium—may cause hypotension, even in recumbent subjects. Fear, the sight of blood, observing trauma to others, or seeing other people faint may all cause hypotension. Premonitory symptoms include feeling alternately hot and cold, yawning, sweating, and an uneasy or sinking feeling in the epigastrium. The patient looks pale and develops bradycardia before the ultimate sudden acute muscular vasodilation occurs.

B. Prevention and Treatment of Fainting Attacks: Fainting attacks can be aborted by lying down or raising the legs or by administering intravenous atropine (0.4–0.8 mg). A tendency to faint is aggravated by all the factors causing low blood volume and also by a hot environment, prolonged standing, an empty stomach, pregnancy, suddenly standing up, nervousness, and novel surroundings. Fainting seldom occurs spontaneously in supine subjects, but it can readily be provoked during arterial puncture or coronary artery catheterization. If the patient has lost consciousness, recovery may take 15–45 minutes. The earlier restorative measures are instituted, the sooner recovery occurs. Raising the legs and administering atropine are specific remedies. Vasoconstrictive drugs such as norepinephrine and angiotensin have no place in treatment.

Bradycardia is the most important indication that reflex factors are involved in syncope in patients with hypotension. Dramatic improvement occurs after the administration of atropine in patients with myocardial infarction in whom reflex hypotension has occurred. A short period of cerebral and cardiac hypoperfusion is relatively harmless in healthy young subjects, but disastrous consequences may result in older atherosclerotic patients with cerebral or coronary arterial disease and in those with aortic or pulmonary stenosis. Cerebral and myocardial infarction may result, and ventricular arrhythmia may occur during periods of marked vagal bradycardia. The role of simple vasovagal attacks in causing sudden death in patients with heart disease is not known.

Hypotension Associated With Abnormal Reflex Control Mechanisms

A. Autonomic Insufficiency: Postural (orthostatic) hypotension due to disturbances of autonomic nervous system control is seldom seen in patients under age 50. It occurs in patients with diabetes mellitus or uremia associated with peripheral neuropathy, in tabes dorsalis, and in various types of degenerative central nervous system disease involving the basal ganglia. It also causes Shy-Drager syndrome, which resembles parkinsonism. At least 2 of the classic triad of symptoms—postural hypotension, impaired sweating, and loss of sexual function, with impotence in men—are usually present. No associated disease is found in about one-third of cases. The diagnostic physical finding is a progressive fall in arterial pressure when the patient is standing or when the lower body is subjected to suction, as shown in Fig 21–3. There is little or no accompanying increase in heart rate. In the lower body suction procedure, the subject lies flat, with the legs and pelvis enclosed in an airtight box. Pressure in the box is reduced by sucking air out of the system at a rate sufficient to maintain a desired level of pressure around the legs.

A lack of overshoot in arterial pressure also occurs after Valsalva's maneuver, as shown in Fig 21–4. This finding should be sought in direct arterial pressure tracings because it cannot always be accurately assessed in noninvasive bedside studies using indirect methods. Sympatholytic (antihypertensive) drugs, diuretics, tranquilizers, potassium depletion, and primary aldosteronism also impair circulatory reflex reactivity. In some cases, myocardial infarction causes unexplained loss of autonomic nervous system function; in rare cases, autonomic insufficiency is seen in acute viral infections.

B. Treatment of Autonomic Insufficiency: The treatment of postural hypotension due to autonomic insufficiency consists of eliminating any factors that tend to reduce blood volume or impair circulatory reactivity. In addition, active measures to expand blood volume should be instituted. Such simple remedies as increasing salt intake and raising the head of the bed to provide a constant stimulus to the autonomic nervous system control mechanisms during sleep often

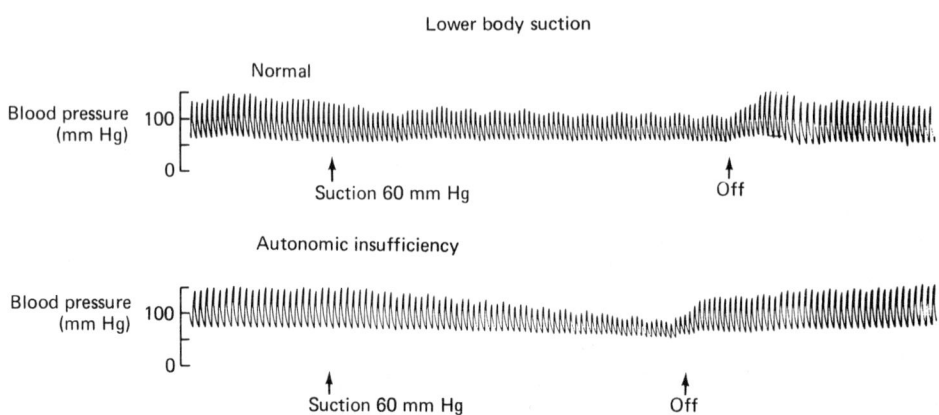

Figure 21–3. Arterial pressure tracings from a normal subject and a patient with autonomic insufficiency showing the effects of negative pressure applied to the lower body. There is a progressive fall in blood pressure and no overshoot when the pressure is released in the patient with autonomic insufficiency.

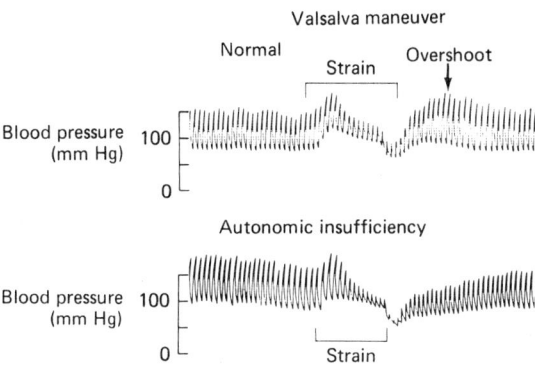

Figure 21–4. Arterial pressure tracings from a normal subject and a patient with tabes dorsalis and autonomic nervous system insufficiency. There is a greater fall in pressure during the period of strain and no overshoot on release of pressure in the patient with autonomic nervous system insufficiency.

help. Avoiding sudden changes in posture and stopping or decreasing medication such as antihypertensive drugs, sedatives, tricyclic antidepressants, and alcohol, which impair circulatory reactivity, may also improve symptoms. Blood volume expansion by means of fludrocortisone acetate and prevention of the shifting of large volumes of blood to the legs by means of elastic lower-body stockings should be reserved for patients in whom simple measures have failed. It should be remembered that the primary function of autonomic nervous system reflex control is to limit rises in arterial pressure and that patients with autonomic insufficiency are frequently hypertensive in the supine or head-down position. The measures taken to prevent hypotension in the standing position often result in hypertension in the supine position. When autonomic insufficiency is due to central nervous system disease, paralysis of the nervous control system is almost inevitably irreversible. Treatment is basically palliative, but indomethacin (75–150 mg/d) is worth trying. Alpha-adrenergic agonists, eg, dihydroergotamine and midodrine, can help but are likely to cause supine hypertension. The prognosis depends on the underlying pathologic process. Patients whose heart rates change in response to posture, exercise, and other stimuli live longer than those with fixed heart rates.

NEUROCIRCULATORY ASTHENIA
(Cardiac Neurosis)

The functional cardiac disorder known as neurocirculatory asthenia is also called effort syndrome, disordered action of the heart, soldier's heart, and Da Costa's syndrome. This condition causes the most difficulty during wartime, when conscription mobilizes apparently healthy men who develop symptoms either during military training or during actual combat that make them entirely unfit for military service. Da Costa first described the condition in the American Civil War; Thomas Lewis in World War I and Paul Wood in World War II were both involved in defining and diagnosing the condition. A similar clinical picture is seen in civilian life, but in that context the symptoms vary from patient to patient, and the 4 classic symptoms of dyspnea, palpitations, chest pain, and fatigue seen in wartime are supplemented by other complaints.

Clinical Findings

The spectrum of cases is wide, with incapacity varying from mild to severe. The condition has usually been present before military service and is found in men, women, and children. Wood stressed the psychologic aspects of the disorder and considered the condition to be a form of anxiety neurosis. Physicians sometimes unwittingly contribute to the patient's neurotic tendency by stressing the need for rest in patients with heart disease. The patient becomes fearful of exercise, and the combination of anxiety and inactivity is particularly likely to produce the clinical picture of cardiac neurosis. Occasionally, prolonged enforced bed rest in suspected cases of rheumatic fever may lead to cardiac neurosis. The physician must guard against the possibility of causing or aggravating neurotic tendencies, especially in young persons.

A. Symptoms: Dyspnea on exertion or on exposure to threatening situations is the predominant symptom, and all symptoms are aggravated by mental or physical stress. The breathlessness often involves an inability to get a deep enough or satisfying breath. The patient takes deep sighing breaths that reduce alveolar and arterial CO_2, resulting in respiratory alkalosis. This provokes cerebral arterial vasoconstriction. Increased anxiety, headaches, dizziness, faintness, and even loss of consciousness can result. In addition, the ionized calcium level decreases with respiratory alkalosis; this can provoke numbness and tingling in fingers and lips, tetany, carpopedal spasm, and convulsions (hyperventilation syndrome). The vicious cycle of anxiety, hyperventilation, and cerebral symptoms that in turn increase anxiety is extremely common and can be broken by the old-fashioned remedy of having the patient rebreathe expired air from a bag. Other symptoms, in the order of frequency, are weakness, palpitations, noncardiac pain in the left chest, fatigue, cold sweating (especially of the palms), nervousness, dizziness, headache, tremulousness, sighing, flushing, cramps, paresthesias, dryness of the mouth, vasovagal fainting, insomnia, increased frequency of micturition, diarrhea, and anorexia. Although some of these symptoms may be indicative of organic cardiac disease in certain circumstances, they are also readily recognized as symptoms of an anxiety state.

B. Signs: The patient is often thin and of asthenic build. A distaste for physical activity and a rapid resting heart rate are usually present. Blood pressure may be increased if the patient is excited when examined, but persistent hypertension is not found. The heart rate increases readily with exercise or when the patient stands up after lying down or squatting. Return of the heart rate to normal after exercise is delayed. Hyperventilation and tachypnea are common, particularly with stress, but no abnormal physical signs other than occasional systolic ejection or late systolic murmurs or clicks are found on examination. The presence of hemodynamically insignificant organic heart disease, a trivial "functional" murmur, or insignificant electrocardiographic changes may complicate the picture, and it may be extremely difficult to decide which problems are functional.

C. Electrocardiographic Findings: The ECG is usually normal apart from sinus tachycardia, although ST segment changes simulating ischemia may be seen.

D. X-Ray Findings: Chest x-ray shows a normal or reduced heart size.

E. Special Investigations: An exercise test may be useful in demonstrating disproportionate tachycardia, hyperventilation, and tachypnea. Cardiac catheterization reveals normal pressures and a cardiac output that is often raised.

Differential Diagnosis

Active rheumatic fever, rheumatic carditis, anemia, thyrotoxicosis, systemic arteriovenous fistula, tuberculosis, pleurisy, influenza, or any high-output state must be differentiated from neurocirculatory asthenia. The diagnosis of effort syndrome probably includes more than one condition; with time, various different syndromes will probably be identified. There is almost certainly a relationship between effort syndrome and poor physical conditioning. Modern life in the Western world has meant a low average level of physical activity for the general population. Physical inactivity tends to produce a physiologic state resembling that seen in effort syndrome. Prolonged bed rest, debilitating illness, or simple inactivity all reduce exercise tolerance, cause disproportionate tachycardia, and result in marked tiredness after effort. Physical training programs are capable of altering the response to exercise.

The physiologic "defect" in untrained persons is a failure in the mechanisms distributing cardiac output to different parts of the systemic circulation. Muscular exercise involves a marked increase in muscle blood flow. As a compensatory mechanism, perfusion of nonessential parts of the systemic circulation (skin, kidneys, other viscera, and nonexercising muscles) is ordinarily reduced. If nonessential perfusion is maintained, the total cardiac output for a given work load is greater than normal; a higher pulse rate and limited exercise tolerance result. Training programs can reduce both cardiac output and heart rate at submaximal loads and increase the subject's maximal exercise performance. The arteriovenous oxygen difference at a given work load consequently increases. The statement that training increases the amount of oxygen extracted by the muscles is not correct. The arteriovenous oxygen difference is increased because a larger proportion of cardiac output perfuses the exercising muscles, and blood draining exercising muscles is low in oxygen content.

Treatment

Like patients with any form of neurosis, those with cardiac neurosis respond poorly to treatment such as exercise training programs, and they are not generally treated sympathetically by physicians. It is possible that some patients will be shown to have enzymatic defects in their muscles and that the present consensus that the condition is entirely psychologic will be proved false. The clinical manifestations so closely resemble those of sympathetic nervous system overactivity that propranolol should be given a trial in gradually increasing doses up to 200 mg/d.

Prognosis

Patients with cardiac neurosis can usually lead relatively normal lives if they are not subject to stress. There is no evidence that cardiac neurosis shortens life. Patients who develop symptoms while in the armed forces usually recover when they return to civilian life. However, some patients persist in self-imposed chronic invalidism.

TRAUMATIC HEART DISEASE

Many of the ways in which trauma can affect the heart have been mentioned in the chapters dealing with coronary disease, hypertension, congenital heart disease, valvular disease, arrhythmias, and pericarditis.

The most important cause of cardiac trauma in peacetime is automobile accidents. Injury to the heart is not usually foremost in the minds of physicians dealing with acutely injured persons, and the manifestations of cardiac trauma can be easily overlooked when other more obvious injuries are present. The anterior aspect of the right ventricle is subject to damage in sudden deceleration injuries. Thus, when a person is thrown forward onto the steering wheel of an automobile, the myocardium may be bruised, the anterior descending coronary artery may be damaged, or hemopericardium may result.

Damage to the mitral, aortic, and tricuspid valves may give rise to acute valvular incompetence. In the case of the mitral valve, rupture of the chordae tendineae or acute disruption of an already abnormal (prolapsing) valve may cause or aggravate mitral incompetence. Falling and hitting the anterior chest against a sharp edge, such as a table, may also cause mitral valve damage.

A particularly important insidious injury is localized rupture of the aorta in motorcyclists who are thrown from their machines. The aorta tends to rupture at its weakest point—at the aortic isthmus, just distal to the origin of the left subclavian artery. A small tear in the intima can result in hemorrhage that is confined to the adventitia and does not spread to the pleural space or mediastinum. Rising pressure around the vessel can occlude the aorta and produce a false aneurysm, shutting off the blood flow to the lower body. Renal ischemia, acute hypertension, and renal failure can occur insidiously, and the lesion is easily missed.

Stabbings and gunshot wounds of the heart may result in hemopericardium, ventricular perforation, or late cardiac rupture at the site of a myocardial contusion. Not all direct cardiac trauma is immediately fatal, and the fall in arterial pressure associated with shock may limit hemorrhage.

Systemic arteriovenous fistula is an important cause of problems in the weeks following trauma. The close relationship between arteries and veins in different areas of the body makes fistula formation an important complication of stab and gunshot wounds. Surgical trauma may also cause similar lesions. Fistulas have developed after cholecystectomy, nephrectomy, and laminectomy; and fistulas at the elbow and groin have been seen following cardiac catheterization. If the fistula is due to a wound and is close to the surface, the diagnosis is relatively easy, but more deeply situated fistulas may not be detected until high-output cardiac failure develops (see Chapter 10).

Minor forms of trauma associated with straining or lifting heavy objects may be the precipitating cause of acute cardiac events such as mitral valve disruption (see Chapter 12) or aortic dissection.

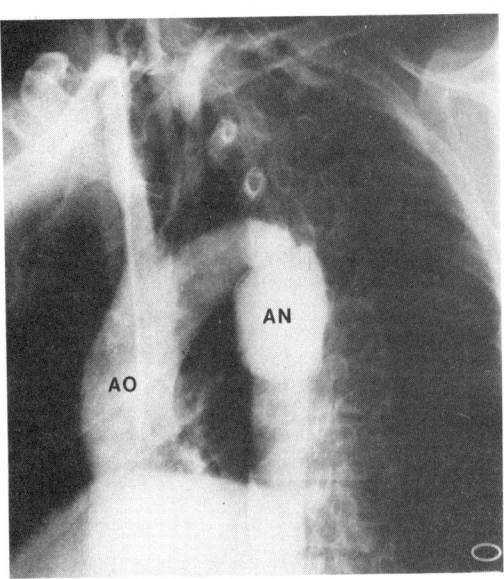

Figure 21-5. Angiogram showing a left anterior oblique view of the aorta. A traumatic false aneurysm (AN) is shown at the isthmus of the aorta (AO). The lesion resulted from an automobile accident and caused acquired coarctation.

Clinical Findings

A. Symptoms: Symptoms of cardiac damage are often absent, either because the patient is unconscious or because trauma to other areas dominates the picture. Chest pain can be due to myocardial ischemia or pericardial involvement, and dyspnea and pulmonary edema can occur with acute valvular incompetence. In arteriovenous fistula formation, the patient often notices local warmth and a buzzing sensation in the neighborhood of the fistula.

B. Signs: Examination of the cardiovascular system in injured persons is always important. The jugular venous pressure will be raised if there is tamponade. The pulses in the legs will be diminished or absent and urinary output decreased or absent if there is a ruptured aorta, and murmurs will be present if valvular damage has occurred. Listening for bruits in the abdomen or back may disclose deep-seated fistulas.

C. Electrocardiographic Findings: Electrocardiographic changes are often the first indication that cardiac damage has occurred. ST-T wave changes due to pericardial involvement or even indications of myocardial infarction can be seen, and all patients with chest injuries should have an ECG recorded as soon as possible after injury.

D. X-Ray Findings: Chest x-ray can demonstrate pericardial effusion and rib fractures that may have caused cardiac damage. Localized aortic rupture does not show up on chest x-ray, but hemothorax, mediastinal hemorrhage, and emphysema can be detected.

E. Special Investigations: Angiography is the only effective means of diagnosing localized aortic rupture. An angiogram of a traumatic false aneurysm of the aorta is shown in Fig 21-5.

Differential Diagnosis

A high index of suspicion and an awareness of the possibility of cardiac trauma in injured persons are the most important factors in diagnosis. The longer the interval between injury and the development of cardiac symptoms, the more difficult the recognition of a traumatic cause.

Treatment

Emergency surgical treatment, with exploration of the injured area, must always be considered after emergency measures have stabilized the patient's condition sufficiently to permit operation. Pericardiocentesis may be needed to treat cardiac tamponade, and operative treatment of direct cardiac trauma can be remarkably successful.

Prognosis

The prognosis following cardiac trauma is surprisingly good if the patient survives the first few hours. Trauma usually involves healthy young persons who can withstand injury well and have great powers of recuperation. The long-term prognosis for specific lesions is similar to that when more usual causes are responsible.

REFERENCES

Cardiac Tumors
Berman ND et al: Angiographic demonstration of blood supply of right atrial myxoma. *Br Heart J* 1976;**38**:764.
Bulkley BH, Hutchins GM: Atrial myxomas: A fifty year review. *Am Heart J* 1979;**99**:639.
Depace NL et al: Two dimensional echocardiographic detection of intraatrial masses. *Am J Cardiol* 1981;**48**:954.
Fenoglio JJ Jr, McAllister HA Jr, Ferrans VJ: Cardiac rhabdomyoma: A clinicopathologic and electron microscopic study. *Am J Cardiol* 1976;**38**:241.
Fyke FE et al: Primary cardiac tumors: Experience with 30 consecutive cases since the introduction of two-dimensional echocardiography. *J Am Coll Cardiol* 1985;**5**:1465.
Godwin JD et al: Computed tomography: A new method for diagnosing tumor of the heart. *Circulation* 1981;**63**:448.
Goodwin JF: The spectrum of cardiac tumors. *Am J Cardiol* 1968;**21**:307.
Harvey WP: Clinical aspects of cardiac tumors. *Am J Cardiol* 1968;**21**:328.
Heath D: Pathology of cardiac tumors. *Am J Cardiol* 1968;**21**:315.
Hedfors E, Mogensen L: Atrial myxoma: 12 cases operated in Stockholm 1954–1973. *Eur J Cardiol* (Aug) 1974;**2**:101.
Lokich JJ: The management of malignant pericardial effusions. *JAMA* 1973;**224**:1401.
Perry LS et al: Two-dimensional echocardiography in the diagnosis of left atrial myxoma. *Br Heart J* 1981;**45**:667.
Peters MN et al: The clinical syndrome of atrial myxoma. *JAMA* 1974;**230**:695.
Petsas AA et al: Echocardiographic diagnosis of left atrial myxoma: Usefulness of suprasternal approach. *Br Heart J* 1976;**38**:627.
Pitcher D et al: Cardiac tumours: Non-invasive detection and assessment by gated cardiac blood pool radionuclide imaging. *Br Heart J* 1980;**44**:143.
St. John Sutton MG et al: Atrial myxomas: A review of clinical experience in 40 patients. *Mayo Clin Proc* 1980;**55**:371.
Steiner RE: Radiologic aspects of cardiac tumors. *Am J Cardiol* 1968;**21**:344.
Strohl KP: Angiosarcoma of the heart: A case study. *Arch Intern Med* 1976;**136**:928.
Waxler EB, Kawai N, Kasparian H: Right atrial myxoma: Echocardiographic, phonocardiographic, and hemodynamic signs. *Am Heart J* 1972;**83**:251.

Hypotension
Bannister R: Chronic autonomic failure with postural hypotension. *Lancet* 1979;**2**:404.
Biglieri EG, McIlroy MB: Abnormalities of renal function and circulatory reflexes in primary aldosteronism. *Circulation* 1966;**33**:78.
Bradbury S, Eggleston C: Postural hypotension: A report of three cases. *Am Heart J* 1925;**1**:73.
Brigden W, Sharpey-Schafer EP: Postural changes in peripheral blood flow in cases with left heart failure. *Clin Sci* 1950;**9**:93.
Chobanian AV et al: Mineralocorticoid-induced hypertension in patients with orthostatic hypotension. *N Engl J Med* 1979;**301**:68.
Edmonds ME, Sturrock RD: Autonomic neuropathy in the Guillain-Barré syndrome. *Br Med J* 1979;**2**:668.
Hilsted J et al: Hemodynamics in diabetic orthostatic hypotension. *J Clin Invest* 1981;**68**:1427.
Hopkins A, Neville B, Bannister R: Autonomic neuropathy of acute onset. *Lancet* 1974;**1**:769.
Jennings G, Esler M, Holmes R: Treatment of orthostatic hypotension with dihydroergotamine. *Br Med J* 1979;**2**:307.
Kochar MS, Itskovitz H: Treatment of idiopathic orthostatic hypotension (Shy-Drager syndrome) with indomethacin. *Lancet* 1978;**1**:1011.
Kroenke K: Orthostatic hypotension. *West J Med* 1985;**143**:253.
Schirger A et al: Midodrine: A new agent in the management of idiopathic orthostatic hypotension and Shy-Drager syndrome. *Mayo Clin Proc* 1981;**56**:419.
Sharpey-Schafer EP: Circulatory reflexes in chronic disease of the afferent nervous system. *J Physiol (Lond)* 1956;**134**:1.
Shy GM, Drager GA: A neurological syndrome associated with orthostatic hypotension. *Arch Neurol* 1960;**2**:511.
Valsalva AM: *De Aure Humana: Traj ad Rhenum.* Utrecht. G. Vand Water 84, 1707.
Wagner HN Jr: Orthostatic hypotension. *Bull Johns Hopkins Hosp* 1959;**105**:322.

Neurocirculatory Asthenia
Cohen ME, White PD: Neurocirculatory asthenia: 1972 concept. *Milit Med* 1972;**137**:142.
DaCosta JM: On irritable heart: A clinical study of a form of functional cardiac disorder and its consequences. *Am J Med Sci* 1871;**61**:17.
Grant RT: Observations on the after-histories of men suffering from the effort syndrome. *Heart* 1925;**12**:121.
Lewis T: *The Soldier's Heart and the Effort Syndrome.* Hoeber, 1919.
Wood PH: DaCosta's syndrome. (3 parts.) *Br Med J* 1941;**1**:767, 805, 845.

Traumatic Heart Disease
Barber H: The effects of trauma, direct or indirect, on the heart. *Q J Med* 1944;**13**:137.
Liedke AJ, DeMuth WE: Non-penetrating cardiac injuries: A collective review. *Am Heart J* 1973;**86**:687.
Mackintosh AF, Fleming HA: Cardiac damage presenting late after road accidents. *Thorax* 1981;**36**:813.
Parmley LF et al: Non-penetrating traumatic injury of the aorta. *Circulation* 1958;**17**:1086.
Symbas PN: Cardiac trauma. *Am Heart J* 1976;**92**:387.

Heart Disease in Pregnancy   22

Heart disease in pregnancy has become less important in developed countries because valvular and congenital heart diseases are now recognized and treated prior to childbearing age. Rheumatic heart disease, especially mitral stenosis, accounts for about 90% of cases of heart disease in pregnant women but is usually mild because those with more severe disease have had surgical treatment. Acute rheumatic fever, the precursor of rheumatic valvular heart disease, is much less common today than was the case 20–30 years ago, in part because of prompt treatment of streptococcal infections. In developing countries, cardiac surgery is less frequently performed and the clinical problems of pregnancy in women with severe mitral stenosis still arise.

Congenital heart disease is now recognized at a much earlier age as a result of greater availability of neonatal and pediatric cardiac care units. With the exception of the infrequent Eisenmenger syndrome, in which shunt defects are associated with severe pulmonary hypertension, severe congenital heart disease is treated surgically before childbearing age. Immunization against rubella before pregnancy occurs has resulted in a marked decrease in the incidence of rubella in early pregnancy, one of the important causes of congenital heart disease. The prevalence of congenital heart disease has not decreased in recent years, but even before the advent of open heart surgery, untreated congenital heart disease was responsible for only 3–5% of all cases of heart disease in pregnancy.

CLASSIFICATION

Pregnant women with heart disease can be divided into 2 general categories. The first category consists of women with preexisting heart disease in whom the physiologic load imposed by pregnancy increases the work of the heart. In such cases, if the reserve capacity of the heart is compromised, the heart may fail. Preexisting heart disease is usually valvular or congenital, but hypertensive heart disease, mitral valve prolapse, and hypertrophic cardiomyopathy may also occur in women of childbearing age. Coronary heart disease is very rare at this age except in women with severe type I (insulin-dependent) diabetes mellitus or homozygous genetic hypercholesterolemia.

The second category is made up of women with disease induced by pregnancy, eg, preeclampsia-eclampsia, peripartum cardiomyopathy, thromboembolic disease causing multiple pulmonary emboli and pulmonary hypertension, and dissection of the aorta or of a coronary artery.

PHYSIOLOGIC CHANGES DURING PREGNANCY, LABOR, & THE PUERPERIUM

Pregnancy

The most striking cardiovascular change in pregnancy is an increase in the cardiac output of about 30% by the third or fourth month, usually owing to increased stroke volume. The heart rate increases only slightly (Table 22–1), as does oxygen consumption. Systemic vascular resistance decreases despite the raised cardiac output because of the arteriovenous fistula–like pregnant placenta and possibly as a result of increased prostaglandin production. There is a marked increase in total body water, of which 75% is extracellular, reaching a maximum in the second trimester. Plasma volume and red cell volume also increase in normal pregnancy (Table 22–1). The increased extracellular fluid is in part the result of increased aldosterone secretion, as well as increased deoxycorticosterone (DOC) (Ehrlich, 1980). Plasma renin and angiotensin are substantially increased, yet blood pressure in most normal pregnancies actually falls, especially in the first 2 trimesters. Body weight increases

Table 22–1. Effect of pregnancy on maternal circulatory and respiratory functions.*

Function	Change
Heart rate	Slow increase of 10 beats/min from 14 to 30 weeks. Rate maintained at this level to 40 weeks.
Arterial blood pressure	Systolic unchanged until the 30th week. Diastolic slightly reduced (period of maximal pulse pressure).
Venous blood pressure	Arms: No change. Legs: Gradual marked increase between 8 and 40 weeks.
Cardiac output	Increase of 30–50% by the 32nd week; decline to 20% increase at 40 weeks.
Total body water	Increased between 10 and 40 weeks.
Plasma and blood volume	Rise of 15% between 12 and 32 weeks; slight decline to 40 weeks.
Red cell mass	Increased 15% between 16 and 40 weeks.
Vital capacity	Rises 15% by the 20th week; decline of 5% by 40 weeks.
Oxygen consumption	Increased 10–15% between 8 and 40 weeks.
Circulation time	Decreases from 13 to 11 s by 32nd week, then returns to 13 s by 40th week.
Glomerular filtration rate	Increases 30–50% by second trimester.

*Modified and reproduced, with permission, from Benson RC: *Handbook of Obstetrics & Gynecology*, 8th ed. Lange, 1983.

an average of 10 kg. The increased renin secretion in the first trimester may be due to prostaglandins or changes in sodium and water balance, or both.

The glomerular filtration rate increases in normal pregnancy but decreases in preeclampsia. This results in a greatly increased filtered load of sodium, all of which is reabsorbed or excreted except for a small amount that is progressively retained, so that by the end of pregnancy approximately 500 meq of sodium is retained in the extracellular fluid volume and in the developing fetus.

The relative increase in plasma and blood volume in comparison to red cell mass accounts for the hemodilution and fall in hemoglobin during pregnancy; this is often confused with true anemia.

Patients with cardiac disease may develop symptoms of cardiac failure early in pregnancy if their cardiac reserve is severely limited. In such cases, therapeutic abortion can still be performed vaginally. Some patients may tolerate pregnancy well until the last 1–2 months, despite the fact that the load has been present all through pregnancy.

In the latter part of pregnancy, the position of the mother is quite important in influencing cardiac output, which is reduced in the supine position (by mechanical obstruction of the inferior vena cava and decreasing venous return) and increased in the lateral position.

Oxygen consumption at rest increases progressively during pregnancy, whereas cardiac output increases in the first and second trimesters and for unknown reasons falls in the last several weeks of pregnancy. This may be due to the arteriovenous fistula–like function of the placenta. The high output state resembles that seen in arteriovenous fistulas, and the patient has a hyperdynamic cardiac impulse, raised venous pressure, dilated and pulsating digital arteries, warm skin, and decreased systemic vascular resistance.

Labor & the Puerperium

In addition to marked changes in arterial and pulse pressure and in pulse rate with uterine contractions during labor, cardiac output increases with each contraction, especially in the supine position. Strong uterine and cardiac contractions and decreased preload due to blood loss may enhance left ventricular obstruction in hypertrophic cardiomyopathy. These factors may produce chest pain or dyspnea.

Most of the hemodynamic changes return to normal by 10 days after delivery. With the exception of peripartum cardiomyopathy, cardiac complications of pregnancy are rare after that time.

CARDIAC DISEASE IN PREGNANCY

The cardiovascular load of normal pregnancy is large, but most normal women and women with mild valvular or congenital heart disease or hypertension tolerate pregnancy without difficulty. If cardiac function is impaired in the prepregnant state or worsens in the first few weeks of pregnancy, cardiac complications progressively increase. Patients who have had cardiac failure in a previous pregnancy are more apt to develop cardiac failure in the current pregnancy. The most serious varieties of heart disease complicating pregnancy are severe mitral or aortic stenosis, Eisenmenger's syndrome, cyanotic congenital heart disease (especially if not corrected by previous surgery) (see Chapter 11), primary pulmonary hypertension, and severe coarctation of the aorta. In the presence of these varieties of cardiac disease, cardiac failure or arrhythmias may be anticipated as pregnancy continues and may cause serious problems at the time of delivery.

Diagnosis

The recognition of cardiac disease or of early cardiac failure may be difficult in pregnant women, especially if they have not been seen prior to pregnancy. The increased blood volume, cardiac output, and hyperdynamic cardiac state may cause cardiac ejection murmurs, raised venous pressure, hyperdynamic cardiac impulse, physiologic S_3, symptoms of dyspnea, and, especially later in pregnancy, edema resulting from sodium retention or venous obstruction by the large uterus. These normal physiologic changes of pregnancy must be recognized as such and not attributed to cardiac failure. Vital capacity does not normally change during pregnancy, and a decrease indicates developing pulmonary venous congestion. Basal vital capacity should be determined early in pregnancy so that changes can be assessed; a single test is not useful.

Treatment

If possible, the presence and severity of cardiac disease should be determined before a woman becomes pregnant, in order to evaluate the risks of pregnancy and to initiate therapeutic measures. Cardiac failure is uncommon in patients who, before pregnancy, had minimal symptoms and good cardiac reserve, with class I or II impairment (New York Heart Association criteria). If the limitation was more severe prior to pregnancy and patients were in class III or IV, if they had a history of cardiac failure in a previous pregnancy, or if they had one of the severe varieties of cardiac disease mentioned above (and on p 620)—and especially if symptoms increase in the first trimester of pregnancy and are not controlled by medical therapy—therapeutic abortion should be recommended.

A. General Measures: Pregnant women with heart disease should have adequate rest and a nutritious diet. It is important to correct anemia and thyrotoxicosis. Patients should give up alcohol and stop smoking and avoid excessive sodium intake or weight gain. If cardiac symptoms are not severe or if they appear late in pregnancy, treatment consists of bed rest, restriction of sodium intake, digitalis, and antihypertensive agents if indicated. Bed rest throughout the remainder of pregnancy may allow a woman to maintain the pregnancy and avoid the development of cardiac failure. The fetal mortality rate is increased in patients who develop cardiac symptoms during pregnancy, possibly because of impaired uterine and placental perfusion, and management of the pregnant cardiac patient should also include careful examination of the fetal heart sounds and fetal movements.

Mitral valve prolapse, which occurs in 5–10% of women, requires no special treatment during pregnancy. In one prospective study, there were no cardiac complications in the mother or abnormalities in the infants. Prophylactic antibiotics are advised during delivery (Rayburn, 1981).

The factors that increase obstruction in hypertrophic cardiomyopathy, such as vasodilatation, hypotension, or greatly increased cardiac contractions, should be avoided. The use of diuretic agents is controversial in patients who gain excessive weight or develop edema, because thiazides decrease plasma volume, which may decrease plasma and uterine blood flow. In general, it is best for patients to avoid drugs and rely on diet and a low sodium intake to prevent excessive weight gain and edema (see below).

Iron therapy should not be given for the hemodilution of pregnancy unless the hemoglobin is less than 10–11 g/dL. In patients who have valvular or congenital heart disease, antibiotic prophylaxis to prevent infective endocarditis should be given before delivery. In older pregnant patients with mitral stenosis, adequate treatment of atrial fibrillation with digitalis may prevent pulmonary venous congestion.

B. Surgical Treatment: In patients with surgically curable cardiac lesions such as severe mitral stenosis or severe coarctation, it is preferable to delay definitive surgery until after delivery or, even better, to perform it before pregnancy. When the patient is first seen during pregnancy with severe cardiac failure, surgery may be undertaken then. Because medical treatment of cardiac failure has improved, the need for cardiac surgery in pregnancy has become considerably less.

C. Hypertension: (See p 620.) The management of hypertension due to hypertensive disease of pregnancy (preeclampsia), preexisting hypertension, or the hypertension of coarctation is important because of the hazard of aortic dissection and cardiac failure. It is estimated that half of all cases of dissection of the aorta in women occur during pregnancy, not all of them in women with hypertension.

D. Management of Delivery: It is controversial whether cardiac patients should be delivered by cesarean section or vaginal delivery. Physiologic studies are difficult during labor because of the rapid fluctuations of cardiac output, blood pressure, pulse rate, and adrenergic impulses associated with anxiety. In most patients with cardiac disease, the vaginal delivery, with deliberate rupture of the membranes if the cervix is dilated, combined with the use of low forceps, causes less physiologic disturbance and is tolerated better than cesarean section. Although the physiologic and circulatory changes of cesarean section are often relatively slight with skilled anesthesia and surgery, it is better to avoid an abdominal operation if possible.

Sterilization is advisable for the patient with an inoperable underlying disease and cardiac failure during pregnancy. If the patient has a cardiac condition that is amenable to cardiac surgery and operation can be performed after delivery, or if the cardiac symptoms have been precipitated by reversible and perhaps nonrecurrent situations, sterilization should not be performed, because many women deliver normal infants after the underlying cardiac condition has been corrected surgically.

E. Management of Patients With Cardiac Prostheses: Patients with valvular prostheses may tolerate pregnancy well. The decision whether to stop anticoagulant therapy may be difficult. If anticoagulants are stopped, systemic emboli may develop, even with cloth-covered prostheses. If anticoagulants are continued, there is a greater risk of spontaneous abortion, stillborn fetuses, central nervous system abnormalities in live-born infants, and maternal hemorrhage following spinal or epidural block or during delivery. Despite the risks, some women have continued to receive oral anticoagulants throughout pregnancy. The proper treatment is not agreed on.

F. Management of Cardiac Arrhythmias: The incidence of cardiac arrhythmias during pregnancy has been increasing, because women who had corrective surgery for heart disease as children are now surviving to reproductive age and more women are delaying pregnancy until age 30 or older. If the underlying cardiac disease does not cause hemodynamic abnormalities and cardiac function is good, most arrhythmias are well tolerated and can be treated as outlined in Chapter 15. Most conventional drugs can be given without damage to the fetus. Digitalis, quinidine, beta-adrenergic blockers, lidocaine, and verapamil can be considered relatively safe, but phenytoin has caused birth defects. Table 22–2 (Rotmensch, 1983) summarizes antiarrhythmic drug therapy during pregnancy.

Prognosis

Most patients with cardiac disease tolerate pregnancy surprisingly well if modern methods of treating cardiac failure and arrhythmias are available. Women with residual cyanotic congenital heart disease not corrected by previous surgery whose prepregnancy cardiac function was only fair or poor have a substantial incidence of cardiac failure or arrhythmias and deliver fewer live infants (Whittemore, 1982). The exceptions are severe mitral or aortic stenosis, severe coarctation of the aorta, primary pulmonary hypertension, Eisenmenger's syndrome, and cyanotic congenital heart disease. Good prenatal care, awareness of the cardiac functional capacity of the patient prior to pregnancy, and appropriate surgical treatment may prevent cardiac problems during pregnancy. Unpredictable factors such as respiratory infections, atrial fibrillation, and other arrhythmias may complicate a straightforward clinical situation. These complica-

Table 22–2. Guide to the use of antiarrhythmic drugs in pregnancy.*

Drug	Route of Administration	Clinical Application	Therapeutic Concentration	Comments
Digoxin	Oral, IV	Paroxysmal supraventricular tachyarrhythmias; rate control in chronic atrial fibrillation and flutter	1–2 µg/mL	Adjust dosage when quinidine or verapamil are given concomitantly.
Quinidine	Oral	Prophylaxis in atrial and ventricular tachyarrhythmias	2–5 µg/mL	Excessive doses may lead to premature labor.
Procainamide	Oral, IV	Termination and prophylaxis in atrial and ventricular tachyarrhythmias	4–8 µg/mL	High incidence of maternal antinuclear antibodies and lupuslike syndrome with chronic use.
Disopyramide	Oral, IV	Atrial and ventricular tachyarrhythmias	3–7 µg/mL	One report documents uterine contractions.
Beta-adrenergic blocking agents	Oral, IV	Termination and prophylaxis in atrial and ventricular tachyarrhythmias; rate control in chronic atrial fibrillation	Variable	Chronic administration may be associated with intrauterine growth retardation.
Phenytoin	Oral, IV	Digitalis toxicity; refractory ventricular tachyarrhythmias	10–18 µg/mL	High risk of malformations ("fetal hydantoin syndrome").
Verapamil	Oral, IV	Paroxysmal supraventricular tachycardia; rate control in chronic atrial fibrillation	15–30 ng/mL	Rapid intravenous injection may occasionally cause maternal hypotension and fetal distress.
Lidocaine	IV	Drug of choice in ventricular tachyarrhythmias; digitalis toxicity	2–4 µg/mL	Toxic doses and fetal acidosis may cause central nervous system and cardiovascular depression in newborns.

*Modified and reproduced, with permission, from Rotmensch HH, Elkayam U, Frishman W: Antiarrhythmic drug therapy during pregnancy. Ann Intern Med 1983;98:487.

tions should be treated promptly and appropriately. Severe cardiac complications are uncommon today and probably will become even less so.

The prognosis for pregnancy in patients with hypertrophic cardiomyopathy is good. No deaths occurred in mothers or infants in a large series reported by Oakley (1979).

HYPERTENSIVE DISORDERS OF PREGNANCY

Hypertension during pregnancy may occur independently of pregnancy, as in essential hypertension, pheochromocytoma, or coarctation of the aorta, or it may be a complication of pregnancy, as in preeclampsia or eclampsia. In essential hypertension, raised arterial pressure either precedes pregnancy or occurs early in pregnancy, whereas preeclampsia is characterized by normal blood pressure prior to pregnancy or early in pregnancy but a rise in pressure in the last trimester. Preeclampsia may complicate essential hypertension, in which case the blood pressure is raised early in pregnancy, and later the pressure increases substantially and is associated with proteinuria and edema. Pheochromocytoma and coarctation of the aorta are independent processes diagnosed and treated as discussed in Chapters 9 and 11.

ESSENTIAL HYPERTENSION

Essential hypertension is relatively uncommon (about 5%) in the USA and elsewhere in the Western world in young women, as contrasted with a prevalence of about 20% for individuals in their 40s and 50s. Repeated blood pressures exceeding 140/90 mm Hg before the 20th week or a history of chronic hypertension prior to pregnancy distinguishes essential hypertension from preeclampsia. Multiple readings are required for diagnosis of hypertension, because pressures frequently vary over a period of time (Chapter 9). Diagnosis may be complicated in pregnant women because vasodilatation produces a fall in pressure in the second trimester. Individuals seen for the first time in the second trimester may be considered to be normotensive even though observations before and after pregnancy indicate that the individual is indeed hypertensive. The diagnosis of essential hypertension must be based only on the arterial pressure, because in the age range of the usual pregnant patient, vascular complications are uncommon, and the ECG and examination of the ocular fundi and heart usually show no abnormalities. If the hypertension is severe, and if vascular complications are present during the first few months of pregnancy, the likelihood of preeclampsia and an increased probability of fetal death may be an indication for therapeutic abortion.

Essential hypertension in pregnancy does not differ greatly from essential hypertension in nonpregnant women, and the decision regarding treatment depends on the severity of the hypertensive disorder. Slight elevations of pressure in the absence of vascular abnormalities require observation, but the decision regarding drug treatment can be delayed until after delivery. Fetal death is more frequent in patients with more severe hypertension, but it is possible to control the elevated blood pressure and improve maternal and fetal prognosis.

Treatment

The medical treatment of hypertension in pregnant women is similar to that in nonpregnant women (see Chapter 9). Treatment must begin at an early stage. Rest and sodium restriction may be sufficient to lower the pressures to normal in mild to moderate hypertension. If the hypertension is more severe, methyldopa, beta-adrenergic blocking drugs, and hydralazine can be used. Methyldopa has been used extensively during pregnancy, with excellent control of blood pressure and with only a 10% fetal mortality rate in severely hypertensive women. Hydralazine can be used orally or parenterally; in the latter instance, the blood pressure falls in 15–30 minutes. Hydralazine can be combined with methyldopa and beta-adrenergic blocking drugs. Oxprenolol, a beta-adrenergic blocking drug, may be superior to methyldopa (Gallery, 1979). Atenolol has also been used with good results (Rubin, 1983). Preeclampsia occurs in 10–20% of cases. Unless the hypertension is severe, it is advisable to discontinue or decrease antihypertensive drugs 2–3 days before delivery. Data on the effects of treatment of hypertension on the newborn infant are limited, but adverse effects are uncommon.

Induction of labor and management of delivery should be similar to techniques used in cardiac disease in pregnancy. Vaginal delivery is usually satisfactory, with early rupture of the membranes and the use of low forceps to shorten the duration of labor. A few patients first develop raised arterial pressure in the postpartum period. The course of the condition is usually benign, and treatment should be withheld for 3–6 months unless complications occur or the diastolic pressure rises alarmingly (to about 110–120 mm Hg).

Prognosis

The prognosis of essential hypertension in pregnancy is usually good unless preeclampsia is severe or eclampsia with convulsions develops. Control of blood pressure with modern antihypertensive drugs has made therapeutic abortion unnecessary in most cases, although cesarean section late in pregnancy is preferable to drug therapy if severe preeclampsia or convulsions occur. Malignant hypertension or cardiac or renal failure discovered early in pregnancy may warrant therapeutic abortion, especially if the patient has preexisting renal disease. The differentiation of renal disease due to chronic glomerulonephritis or chronic pyelonephritis from essential hypertension is difficult if renal impairment is present when the patient is first seen. In addition to benefit to the mother, antihypertensive therapy with methyldopa or oxprenolol (see above) results in a significantly improved fetal outcome. In terms of both birth weight and general health, the surviving infants of mothers treated with antihypertensive agents were similar to those of untreated mothers. Diuretics are usually avoided because of the possible decrease in plasma volume and uterine and placental blood flow. Some authorities disagree and use diuretics as basic treatment (Finnerty, 1980).

PREECLAMPSIA-ECLAMPSIA

Preeclampsia, the clinical syndrome of hypertension, edema, and proteinuria developing in the last trimester of pregnancy, progresses as a continuum at various rates and extends from mild preeclampsia to severe eclampsia with convulsions. Preeclampsia occurs in about 5% of pregnancies. The disorder has gradually declined in incidence in the past several decades (see Prognosis), possibly as a consequence of better prenatal care. Eclampsia is much less frequent, occurring in about 0.1% of pregnant women.

Pathophysiology

The cause of preeclampsia is unknown, and many theories have been offered. The condition is more frequent in the first pregnancy, in patients with preexisting hypertension, in twin pregnancies, in patients with a history of preeclampsia, in patients with hydatidiform mole, and in some populations of black women. Preeclampsia may result from impaired uteroplacental perfusion; this is supported by the observation that during preeclampsia, plasma volume, glomerular filtration rate, and uterine and placental blood flow decrease about 25% in recumbency. The gravid uterus has a poorer arterial blood supply in preeclampsia as compared to the nongravid or normal pregnant uterus. Preeclampsia has been produced in animals by constricting the uterine arteries to reduce the uterine blood flow.

Elevated blood pressure is not the only manifestation of preeclampsia; at autopsy and renal biopsy, thromboses and immunoglobulin deposits have been found in the kidney, liver, and elsewhere (see below).

A. Hemodynamic and Volume Changes: In preeclampsia, as compared to normal pregnancy, systemic vascular resistance is increased; plasma and red cell volume, glomerular filtration rate, and renal blood flow are decreased; sodium retention is enhanced; and uric acid clearance falls (Lindheimer, 1981).

B. Role of Prostaglandins and the Renin-Angiotensin System: Prostaglandin E (PGE) can be synthesized by the uterus. The reduced uteroplacental blood flow may decrease PGE synthesis and increase the secretion of renin, setting in motion the sequence of events leading to increased production of angiotensin and hypertension (Fig 22–1).

Renin is produced by the uterus and chorion as well as by the kidney; plasma renin and aldosterone

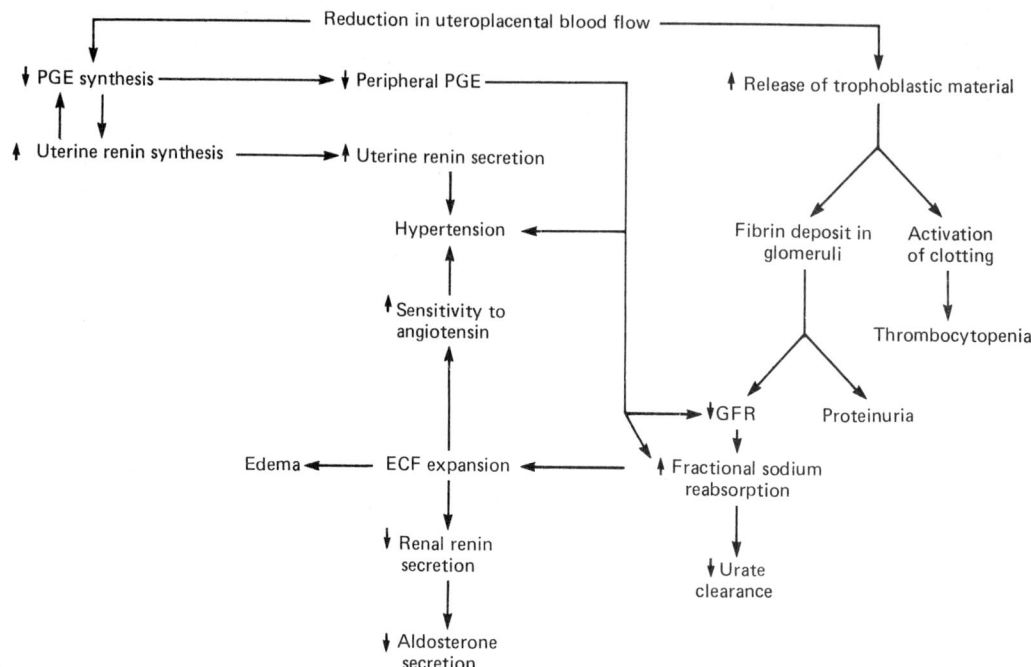

Figure 22–1. Hypothesis for the pathophysiology of preeclampsia-eclampsia. Diminished uteroplacental blood flow leads to a possible decrease in uterine synthesis of PGE but an increase in renin synthesis. In addition, fibrin deposits in the glomeruli cause a reduction in GFR and an increase in sodium retention. PGE, prostaglandin E; GFR, glomerular filtration rate; ECF, extracellular fluid. (Reproduced, with permission, from Ferris TF: Toxemia of pregnancy: A model of human hypertension. *Cardiovasc Med* 1977;**2**:877.)

are lower in pregnancy associated with hypertension than in normal pregnancy (Pedersen, 1983).

C. Renal and Hepatic Changes in Preeclampsia; Possible Immunologic Mechanisms: The proteinuria that occurs as part of the characteristic triad of hypertension, edema, and proteinuria in preeclampsia is considered to be of glomerular origin. Renal biopsies have shown endothelial swelling, narrowing of the lumen of the capillaries, deposits of fibrin in the glomeruli, evidences of intravascular coagulation, and "glomerular endotheliosis" (Lindheimer, 1981). About one-fourth of patients with preeclampsia show evidence of chronic renal disease (nephrosclerosis, chronic glomerulonephritis, or chronic pyelonephritis). There may be a correlation between the clinical severity of preeclampsia and the density and pattern of IgM and IgG deposits in the glomeruli of the kidney. The typical electron microscopic appearance of renal biopsy specimens in preeclampsia is fibrin and immunoglobulin deposition in the capillary loops, especially deposition of IgM and complement. Complement deposits occur within the walls of afferent and efferent arterioles (Petrucco, 1974). Similar deposits of fibrin, immunoglobulins, and complement were found in the livers of preeclamptic but not normal pregnant women by means of immunofluorescence (Fig 22–2).

Thus, an immunologic mechanism may be responsible for the renal and hepatic lesions of preeclampsia, with a primary vascular disorder similar to the transplant rejection mechanism involving the antibody system. Antiplacental antibodies may be produced that result in deposition of immunoglobulins and complement in the kidney. Because of the familial occurrence of preeclampsia, genetic factors are being actively investigated.

The severity of preeclampsia and eclampsia may be related to the magnitude of the deposition of the immunoglobulins, but the mechanism by which this is accomplished is at present obscure.

Clinical Findings

Preeclampsia is defined as a syndrome encountered in the second half of pregnancy that is characterized by at least 2 of 3 cardinal manifestations (Page, 1953):

1. A rather abrupt increase of blood pressure amounting to 30 mm Hg or more systolic and 15 mm Hg or more diastolic after the 26th week of pregnancy.
2. The appearance (or sudden increase) of proteinuria of at least 0.5 g/d; and
3. Edema in the upper half of the body.

Any 2 of these must be manifest on 2 occasions at least 6 hours apart. If convulsions occur in addition to the above criteria, the case is classified as eclampsia.

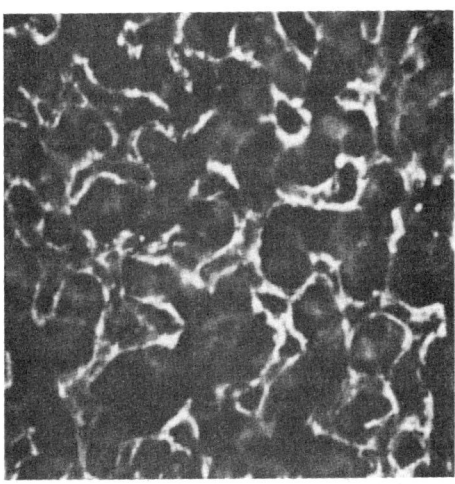

Figure 22-2. Diffuse staining of hepatic sinusoids with fluorescent antiserum to fibrinogen. (Reproduced, with permission, from Arias F, Mancilla-Jimenez R: Hepatic fibrinogen deposits in preeclampsia: Immunofluorescent evidence. N Engl J Med 1976;295:578.)

Generalized edema is common in pregnancy and when present in the lower half of the body is not considered diagnostic of heart failure. The increased tubular reabsorption of sodium and water causes edema in the upper half of the body that may precede the appearance of proteinuria and hypertension. About 6% of all pregnant women in the USA develop preeclampsia, and one in 20 of this total group develops convulsions with eclampsia. Approximately 5% of patients with eclampsia die of the disease. There are about 1500 maternal deaths each year and about 15,000 fetal deaths. Deaths from preeclampsia are rare.

Apart from weight gain, edema in the upper half of the body, proteinuria, and hypertension, patients with preeclampsia may develop headache, drowsiness, visual disturbances, dyspnea, and, if the hypertension is severe, pulmonary edema and cardiac failure. Cerebral hemorrhage causes 10% of deaths in eclampsia. Acute tubular necrosis rarely causes death but may occur in severe eclampsia. Hypotension may develop in severe eclampsia with hemorrhage and necrosis in the adrenal glands.

Clinical Course

The onset of preeclampsia may be gradual or sudden, and the diagnosis may be difficult to establish in the early stages because the pathophysiologic changes may be present before clinical symptoms or signs appear. Women who later develop preeclampsia may show differences in their response to angiotensin before proteinuria and a rise in blood pressure occur. Patients may develop edema similar to the edema of normal pregnancy. The proteinuria may be slight, and the elevation of blood pressure may be slight and variable.

In mild cases, restriction of activity and sodium intake may be sufficient to reverse the process by increasing uterine, renal, and placental blood flow. If proteinuria increases, if blood pressure rises, or if symptoms such as blurred vision, decreased urine output, or rapid gain in weight develop, the patient should be hospitalized. Papilledema, hemorrhages, and exudates are rare. The development of a generalized boring headache signals an impending convulsion and should be the immediate indication for more intensive hospital therapy, including termination of pregnancy.

Prevention

Prevention depends on good prenatal care, good nutrition, education so that patients recognize the earliest development of preeclampsia, bed rest and sodium restriction when manifestations first appear, recommendations against subsequent pregnancies in patients who have had severe preeclampsia, and antihypertensive drugs to control preexisting hypertension in patients who become pregnant.

When signs of impending convulsions (see above) appear, delivery is the best preventive treatment for eclampsia. Eclampsia does not occur after the uterus is emptied.

Treatment

A. Preeclampsia: Bed rest and sodium restriction usually reverse the process in mild preeclampsia. Thiazides should not be used because they may exaggerate the diminished plasma volume in patients with preeclampsia. Pharmacologic agents lower blood pressure but do not affect the pathophysiology of the condition and do not decrease the fetal mortality rate. If preeclampsia does not subside after a few days of hospital care, the pregnancy should be interrupted by cesarean section or, if the patient is near term, labor should be induced. The infant mortality rate is greater the longer preeclampsia persists. In severe preeclampsia, the infant mortality rate is 5 times the normal rate. The transition from severe preeclampsia to eclampsia with convulsions is one of degree rather than of kind. It is preferable to interrupt the pregnancy by cesarean section if convulsions, muscular twitching, severe headache, epigastric pain (vascular crisis), or visual disturbances are imminent. Interruption of pregnancy is the most reliable means of preventing the transition from preeclampsia to eclampsia.

B. Eclampsia: If convulsions occur, the clinical situation is much worse; the maternal mortality rate is 5% and the fetal mortality rate about 20–25%. Prevention of convulsions is a cardinal goal of therapy. Convulsions should be managed by use of intravenous magnesium sulfate, absolute rest in bed, constant nursing care, and avoidance of anything that disturbs the patient and may precipitate a convulsion. Delivery should be postponed until the convulsions can be stopped. Magnesium toxicity (blood levels >6 meq/L) may occur when use is prolonged. Magnesium toxicity is suggested clinically by absent patellar reflexes and low urine output (< 30–40 mL/h). Both urine output and patellar reflexes should be monitored before each dose of magnesium sulfate is given. In a consecutive series of 154 cases managed by this method, there were no maternal deaths and all infants weighing more than 4 lb survived (Pritchard, 1975). Antihypertensive drugs should be used if the diastolic blood pressure is elevated to 110 mm Hg or more. Some patients with eclampsia have cerebral edema rather than hypertension as the mechanism of their convulsions, and magnesium sulfate therapy is therefore preferred. For reasons that are not clear, eclampsia is less frequent today. If the patient is oliguric, intravenous fluids should be used with caution. Pregnancy should not be terminated unless the patient has had no convulsions for 24–48 hours.

Prognosis

Maternal deaths are now rare in preeclampsia. Preeclampsia is more frequent in patients with preexisting essential hypertension or renal disease than in patients who were normotensive before pregnancy. About 25% of patients who develop hypertension in late pregnancy have unsuspected chronic renal disease on renal biopsy and not preeclampsia.

Infants of mothers with preeclampsia have a mortality rate 3–5 times as high as those of normal mothers. About half of cases of eclampsia that occur in multiparous women are preceded by hypertension. When eclampsia complicates previous hypertension, the fetal mortality rate approximates 50%.

The prognosis of mild preeclampsia is good with bed rest and sodium restriction, but if the condition progresses with increase of weight, edema, proteinuria, and hypertension, termination of pregnancy should be instituted promptly before convulsions occur. In primiparous women with eclampsia, there is no increased incidence of permanent hypertension (Chesley, *Clin Exp Hypertens,* 1980).

Multiparous women who survive eclampsia have a worse prognosis and an incidence of cardiovascular deaths almost 3 times the expected number. Perhaps "gestational" hypertension (without proteinuria) is a sign of latent essential hypertension. Convulsions may lead to cerebral hemorrhage, pulmonary edema, aortic dissection, and adrenal hemorrhage or necrosis. Interruption of pregnancy in severe preeclampsia usually prevents convulsive eclampsia. Treatment of convulsions permits cesarean section, reducing the maternal and fetal mortality rate. Patients with a history of severe preeclampsia or eclampsia should be discouraged from becoming pregnant again.

REFERENCES

Arias F, Mancilla-Jimenez R: Hepatic fibrinogen in preeclampsia: Immunofluorescent evidence. *N Engl J Med* 1976;**295:**578.

Bay WH, Ferris TR: Factors controlling plasma renin and aldosterone during pregnancy. *Hypertension* 1979;**1:**410.

Benson RC: *Handbook of Obstetrics & Gynecology,* 8th ed. Lange, 1983.

Birkeland SA, Kristofferson K: Pre-eclampsia: A state of mother-fetus immune imbalance. *Lancet* 1979;**2:**720.

Bodzenta A, Thomson JM, Poller L: Prostacyclin activity in amniotic fluid in pre-eclampsia. *Lancet* 1980;**2:**650.

Bortolotti U et al: Pregnancy in patients with a porcine valve bioprosthesis. *Am J Cardiol* 1982;**50:**1051.

Burwell CS: The management of heart disease in pregnant women. *Bull Johns Hopkins Hosp* 1954;**95:**130.

Chesley LC: The remote prognostic significance of the level of blood pressure in pregnancy. *Clin Exp Hypertens* 1980;**2:**777.

Chesley LC: Severe rheumatic cardiac disease and pregnancy: The ultimate prognosis. *Am J Obstet Gynecol* 1980;**136:**552.

Chesley LC, Annitto JE, Cosgrove RA: The remote prognosis of eclamptic women: Sixth period report. *Am J Obstet Gynecol* 1976;**124:**446.

Cockburn J et al: Final report of study on hypertension during pregnancy: The effects of specific treatment of the growth and development of the children. *Lancet* 1982;**1:**647.

Davison JM: The kidney in pregnancy: A review. *J R Soc Med* 1983;**76:**485.

Ehrlich EN, Nolten WE, Lindheimer MD: Mineralocorticoids and the regulation of sodium metabolism in normal and hypertensive pregnancy: A review. *Clin Exp Hypertens* 1980;**2:**803.

Elkayam U, Gleicher N: Cardiac problems in pregnancy: 1. Maternal aspects: The approach to the pregnant patient with heart disease. *JAMA* 1984;**251:**2838.

Elliott DL et al: Medical illness and pregnancy: An annotated bibliography of recent literature. *Ann Intern Med* 1983;**99:**83.

Ferris TF: Toxemia of pregnancy: A model of human hypertension. *Cardiovasc Med* 1977;**2:**877.

Fillmore SJ, Parry EHO: The evolution of peripartal heart failure in Zaria, Nigeria: Some etiologic factors. *Circulation* 1977;**56:**1058.

Fine LG (moderator): Systemic lupus erythematosus in pregnancy. (UCLA Conference.) *Ann Intern Med* 1981;**94:**667.

Finnerty FA Jr: Hypertension and pregnancy. *J Cardiovasc Med* 1980;**5:**559.

Gallery EDM et al: Randomised comparison of methyldopa and oxprenolol for treatment of hypertension in pregnancy. *Br Med J* 1979;**1:**1591.

Gant NF Jr, Worley RJ: *Hypertension in Pregnancy: Concepts and Management.* Appleton-Century-Crofts, 1980.

Gilchrist AR: Cardiological problems in younger women, including those of pregnancy and the puerperium. *Br Med J* 1963;**1:**209.

Gray MJ: Use and abuse of thiazides in pregnancy. *Clin Obstet Gynecol* 1968;**11:**568.

Hall JG, Pauli RM, Wilson KM: Maternal and fetal sequelae of anticoagulation during pregnancy. *Am J Med* 1980;**68:**122.

Handin RI: Thromboembolic complications of pregnancy and oral contraceptives. *Prog Cardiovasc Dis* 1974;**16:**395.

Homans DC: Peripartum cardiomyopathy. *N Engl J Med* 1985;**312:**1432.

Ibarra-Perez C et al: The course of pregnancy in patients with artificial heart valves. *Am J Med* 1976;**61:**504.

Kotchen TA et al: Plasma renin activity, reactivity, concentration and substrate following hypertension during pregnancy: Effect of oral contraceptive agents. *Hypertension* 1979;**1:**355.

Ladner E et al: Dynamics of uterine circulation in pregnant and nonpregnant sheep. *Am J Physiol* 1970;**218:**257.

Lindheimer MD, Katz AI: Hypertension in pregnancy. *N Engl J Med* 1985;**313:**675.

Lindheimer MD, Katz AI: Pathophysiology of preeclampsia. *Annu Rev Med* 1981;**32:**273.

Lindheimer MD, Katz AI, Zuspan FP (editors): *Hypertension in Pregnancy*. Wiley, 1976.

Lutz DJ et al: Pregnancy and its complications following cardiac valve prostheses. *Am J Obstet Gynecol* 1978;**131:**460.

MacGillivray I, Campbell DM: The relevance of hypertension and oedema in pregnancy. *Clin Exp Hypertens* 1980;**2:**897.

McAnulty JH, Metcalfe J, Ueland K: General guidelines in the management of cardiac disease. *Clin Obstet Gynecol* 1981;**24:**773.

Mendelson CL: The management of delivery in pregnancy complicated by serious rheumatic heart disease. *Am J Obstet Gynecol* 1944;**48:**329.

Metcalfe J, Ueland K: Maternal cardiovascular adjustments to pregnancy. *Prog Cardiovasc Dis* 1974;**16:**363.

Oakley GDG et al: Management of pregnancy in patients with hypertrophic cardiomyopathy. *Br Med J* 1979;**1:**1749.

Page EW: *The Hypertensive Disorders of Pregnancy*. Thomas, 1953.

Pedersen EB et al: Preeclampsia: A state of prostaglandin deficiency? Urinary prostaglandin excretion, the renin-aldosterone system, and circulating catecholamines in preeclampsia. *Hypertension* 1983;**5:**105.

Petrucco OM et al: Immunofluorescent studies in renal biopsies in pre-eclampsia. *Br Med J* 1974;**1:**473.

Pettifor JM, Benson R: Congenital malformations associated with the administration of oral anticoagulants during pregnancy. *J Pediatr* 1975;**86:**459.

Pitts JA, Crosby WM, Basta LL: Eisenmenger's syndrome in pregnancy: Does heparin prophylaxis improve the maternal mortality rate? *Am Heart J* 1977;**93:**321.

Pollak VE, Nettles JB: The kidney in toxemia of pregnancy: A clinical and pathologic study based on renal biopsies. *Medicine* 1960;**39:**469.

Pritchard JA, Pritchard SA: Standardized treatment of 154 consecutive cases of eclampsia. *Am J Obstet Gynecol* 1975;**123:**543.

Rayburn WF, Fontana ME: Mitral valve prolapse and pregnancy. *Am J Obstet Gynecol* 1981;**141:**9.

Romney B: Hypertension in pregnancy. *Cardiovasc Rev Rep* 1980;**1:**632.

Rotmensch HH, Elkayam U, Frishman W: Antiarrhythmic drug therapy during pregnancy. *Ann Intern Med* 1983;**98:**487.

Rubin PC et al: Placebo-controlled trial of atenolol in treatment of pregnancy-associated hypertension. *Lancet* 1983;**1:**431.

Salazar E et al: The problem of cardiac valve prostheses, anticoagulants, and pregnancy. *Circulation* 1984;**70(Suppl):**1.

Scott JS, Jenkins DM, Need JA: Immunology of pre-eclampsia. *Lancet* 1978;**1:**704.

Selzer A: Management of pregnant patients with valvular heart disease. *Primary Cardiol* (Feb) 1981;**7:**127.

Sullivan JM, Ramanathan KB: Management of medical problems in pregnancy: Severe cardiac disease. *N Engl J Med* 1985;**313:**304.

Tamari I et al: Medical treatment of cardiovascular disorders during pregnancy. *Am Heart J* 1982;**104:**1357.

Whittemore R, Hobbins JC, Engle MA: Pregnancy and its outcome in women with and without surgical treatment of congenital heart disease. *Am J Cardiol* 1982;**50:**641.

Wilson M et al: Blood pressure, the renin-aldosterone system and sex steroids throughout normal pregnancy. *Am J Med* 1980;**68:**97.

23 | Cardiac Disease & the Surgical Patient

INTRODUCTION

Anesthesia and general surgery are a hazard to all patients, especially infants and young children, but the risk in patients in good preoperative physical condition is low in contrast to that with serious cardiac disease. With modern anesthesia, sophisticated techniques of electrocardiographic, echocardiographic, and blood pressure monitoring, and the ready availability of potent therapeutic agents in the event of untoward developments, cardiac problems are usually minimal unless the preoperative cardiac state was precarious because of known cardiac disease. As a result, middle-aged and elderly individuals with or without known cardiac disease are often referred for preoperative assessment in order to estimate the added risk of anesthesia and surgery and the need for special prophylactic or preoperative treatment.

RISKS OF ANESTHESIA & SURGERY

The risks to any surgical patient include both anesthetic and surgical complications, many of which are preventable. Unexpected hemorrhage, acidosis, impaired ventilation, hypercapnia, decreased systemic vascular resistance, decreased cardiac contractility and conduction, cardiac arrhythmias (with or without increased release of catecholamines), and hypotension with or without a decreased blood volume (such as may occur from hemorrhage)—all interfere with cardiovascular function. Some anesthetic agents such as cyclopropane increase adrenergic activity to the cardiovascular system, whereas others such as halothane reduce cardiovascular sympathetic tone. Anesthetic agents decrease the force of cardiac contraction and may decrease cardiac output. Release of catecholamines may induce arrhythmia or hypertension. Drugs that inhibit the sympathetic nervous system may induce hypotension and reduced systemic flow that impair coronary perfusion, especially in patients with preexisting coronary atherosclerotic lesions. Muscle-relaxing drugs may induce bradycardia and release large amounts of potassium from injured muscles following trauma.

Each hazard producing respiratory or cardiac problems poses a greater risk in patients who have underlying cardiac disease. Cardiac arrest with ventricular fibrillation is the most feared event and is principally due to excessive blood loss, hypotension, accidental administration of potassium or its release by muscle-relaxing drugs, airway obstruction as a result of laryngeal spasm or aspiration of gastric contents, difficulty in intubation at the onset of the surgical procedure, or hypoxemia and acidosis secondary to impaired ventilation. These complications can be minimized by preoperative evaluation and by prophylactic continuous monitoring of cardiovascular variables, eg, arterial pressure, ECG, and intermittent evaluation of blood gases. Preoperative placement of an endocardial right ventricular pacemaker should be done in patients who have sick sinus syndrome with bradycardia, Stokes-Adams attacks, or bifascicular block with episodes of dizziness or syncope. Meticulous anesthetic and surgical technique combined with prompt recognition and treatment of any complication that may arise decreases the hazard to the patient. Postoperative sodium and water retention may occur, causing disturbances in fluid and electrolyte balance.

URGENT VERSUS ELECTIVE SURGERY

Because of the increased hazard of general surgery in the cardiac patient, especially in those with coronary heart disease, the physician must answer certain questions to ascertain when the risks of surgery exceed the risks of the underlying disease and when the reverse is true. Key questions that must be answered are the following: (1) Is the operation urgent or elective? (2) If elective, does the patient have cardiac disease? (3) What is the risk of the underlying surgical disease if surgery is not performed? (4) What additional risk does the heart disease impose on the surgical procedure? (5) Is the surgical diagnosis correct, or could the symptoms, such as abdominal pain, be a manifestation of cardiac disease and not a surgical disease?

URGENT SURGERY

Urgent operations must be done regardless of the underlying cardiac disease and include conditions that threaten life or limb, eg, gross hemorrhage, strangulated hernia, perforation of the bowel or gallbladder, acute bowel obstruction, proximal aortic dissection, ruptured aortic aneurysm, and arterial embolism. The presence of heart disease does not mean that the patient will not tolerate the surgical procedure; one should not withhold a lifesaving procedure merely because of the presence of heart disease.

CARDIAC CONDITIONS MASQUERADING AS SURGICAL ILLNESSES

Gastrointestinal symptoms, including acute abdominal pain, may so dominate the clinical picture that heart disease is not recognized or, if recognized, is not thought to be responsible for the symptoms. Early evidence of cardiac failure is often overlooked because it is overshadowed by the gastrointestinal symptoms. The most common causes of diagnostic confusion are the following:

(1) Angina pectoris or myocardial infarction presenting with predominant epigastric pain.

(2) Fairly abrupt right heart failure presenting with right upper quadrant pain simulating gallbladder disease. This is particularly apt to occur in patients with tight mitral valve disease who develop atrial fibrillation or in patients with mild right heart failure following exercise.

(3) Slowly developing right heart failure, which may present with nonspecific gastrointestinal symptoms of anorexia, nausea, a sensation of heaviness and fullness after meals, and perhaps vomiting. These lead to weight loss and may seem to justify a diagnosis of carcinoma of the upper gastrointestinal tract. If there are no murmurs, the diagnosis of heart disease is often missed.

(4) Pulmonary infarction presenting as jaundice, leading to a diagnosis of biliary tract disease.

(5) Right heart failure or constrictive pericarditis presenting as ascites.

(6) Dysphagia, which may be the presenting symptom in a variety of heart diseases, eg, mitral stenosis with large left atrium, pericarditis, aortic aneurysm, aortic dissection, or anomalies of the aortic arch.

(7) Acute rheumatic fever, which may present with acute abdominal pain, especially in children.

(8) Acute abdominal pain, which may result from acute myocardial infarction or emboli to the splenic, renal, or mesenteric arteries in infective endocarditis or atrial fibrillation. Surgical treatment may be required secondarily if gangrene of the bowel occurs.

(9) Nausea and vomiting, which may occur in cardiac failure, especially as a result of digitalis therapy.

Space does not permit a discussion of the differential diagnosis of these conditions, but one should search for positive diagnostic evidence of heart disease: (1) A history of angina pectoris, dyspnea on effort, orthopnea, or previous ventricular arrhythmias or atrial fibrillation or flutter. (2) Cardiac enlargement with a left or right ventricular heave, with or without characteristic murmurs. (3) Evidence of right heart failure, with increased venous pressure, enlarged and tender liver, and edema or ascites. Orthopnea, decreased vital capacity, and rales and gallop rhythm may be present in left ventricular failure. (4) Signs of myocardial necrosis with fever, tachycardia, or enzyme changes. (5) Typical serial electrocardiographic changes of ischemia, infarction, hypertrophy, pericarditis, etc. (6) Echocardiographic evidence of cardiac abnormality, as in (5). (7) Radiologic evidence of cardiac enlargement or pulmonary venous congestion.

Considering the possibility of heart disease during the diagnostic process often leads to a better examination and appropriate therapy.

PREOPERATIVE EVALUATION OF THE SURGICAL PATIENT WITH KNOWN OR SUSPECTED CARDIOVASCULAR DISEASE

A thorough history and physical examination combined with a resting ECG, a 2-dimensional echocardiogram, chest x-ray, and noninvasive procedures such as nuclear angiography are usually sufficient to diagnose obvious cardiac disease. Twelve- to 24-hour monitoring of the ECG may be required if the patient has unexplained symptoms of dizziness, syncope, weakness, chest pain, or palpitations in order to determine the presence of cardiac arrhythmias, heart block, or ischemic ST depression.

See p 630 for discussion of drugs that the patient might be taking and that might influence the general state of health or the outcome of operation.

RECOGNITION OF HEART DISEASE

The presence of heart disease is recognized on the basis of symptoms, significant murmurs, an enlarged heart, electrocardiographic or echocardiographic abnormality, evidence of cardiac failure, hypertension, conduction defects, atrial fibrillation or flutter, or ventricular arrhythmias. A history of angina pectoris or previous myocardial infarction, Stokes-Adams attacks, cardiac failure, intermittent claudication, or cerebral ischemic attacks may alert the physician to the possibility of cardiac disease. A history of antihypertensive treatment or treatment for cardiac failure may be obtained.

Preoperative ECGs are often valuable but may be difficult to interpret. A patient with known previous myocardial infarction may have a normal ECG; even more importantly, a patient with "unstable angina" may have a normal ECG. Conversely, grossly abnormal changes may be due to an old healed infarct and are therefore of lesser importance in deciding whether or not elective surgery should be performed. A baseline ECG is advisable to interpret postoperative changes. An ECG may also show evidence of digitalis therapy, electrolyte disturbances, conduction defects, or arrhythmias. In general, a stable abnormality on the ECG in the absence of cardiac failure or a change in the pattern of angina pectoris indicates that the patient will probably tolerate surgery almost as well as a normal individual. Such a patient with a healed previous myocardial infarction has an added mortality risk of about 3–5%.

Echocardiography may reveal unexpected findings. In selected cases, nuclear angiography and perfusion studies may be indicated.

The most important contraindications to elective surgery are recent angina pectoris, a crescendo change in the pattern of angina pectoris in recent weeks or months, unstable angina, acute myocardial infarction, myocardial infarction within the preceding 3 months, severe aortic stenosis, a high degree of atrioventricular block, untreated cardiac failure, and severe hypertension.

A multifactorial index providing point scores for various predictors of cardiac risk has been used to estimate the additional risk following major noncardiac surgery. These include age over 70 years, recent myocardial infarction, raised venous pressure, S_3 gallop, multiple premature beats, hypoxemia, hypokalemia, elevated serum creatinine, and aortic stenosis. The weighted index serves as a basis for predicting the probability of postoperative cardiac complications and for fashioning guidelines for managing and assessing patients requiring major surgery (Goldman, 1983).

SPECIFIC DISEASE PROBLEMS

1. CORONARY HEART DISEASE

The usual patient seen for preoperative evaluation is an older individual with possible coronary heart disease. The physician should search for a history of recent change in the character of the anginal pain, pain at rest, unstable angina, or the possibility of recent myocardial infarction. If known coronary disease is stable, without change in the pattern of pain or in serial ECGs; if there are no symptoms or signs of cardiac failure; and if at least 3–6 months have elapsed since myocardial infarction, the surgeon can proceed if the indications for surgery are clear and definite, but the additional cardiac mortality rate is about 3–5%.

Emergency surgery must often be done despite a recent myocardial infarction, but the mortality rate is high. Important but not lifesaving surgery is best delayed at least 3 weeks if possible. Purely elective surgery should be postponed for 3–6 months whenever possible.

In patients with known coronary heart disease, the added risk of a new myocardial infarction, as indicated previously, decreases as the time interval following the previous myocardial infarction lengthens. It averages about 10–20% if surgery is performed within the first 3 months after an acute myocardial infarction and decreases to 3–5% if it is delayed for at least 6 months. The diagnosis of a new myocardial infarction during or following operations is often difficult because of medication for postsurgical pain and the relative diagnostic unreliability of postoperative serum enzymes except for MB (myocardial band) creatine phosphokinase isoenzymes. The mortality rate is about 30% if a new infarct occurs during or after surgery. A new myocardial infarction is more common with operations on the chest and upper abdomen than in those involving the pelvis or lower abdomen and is more apt to occur on the second or third postoperative day than on the day of operation. For this reason, postoperative patients with known or suspected coronary heart disease should be monitored by daily ECGs and MB creatine phosphokinase isoenzyme determinations in order to determine whether a new infarction has occurred. Older individuals without known coronary heart disease may have flattening of the T waves in the left ventricular leads postoperatively but rarely have deep inversions of the T wave, ischemic ST depression, or new Q waves. Development of the last 3 suggests myocardial ischemia or infarction. Ventricular arrhythmias (see below) are more common during and following surgery when coronary heart disease is present; if the patient is known to have angina pectoris, continuous monitoring of the ECG is recommended, and the physician should pay careful attention to the possible development of hypoxia, hypotension, and acidosis. If the patient has severe atherosclerosis elsewhere (eg, aortoiliac) and borderline left ventricular function, a flow-directed catheter should be introduced preoperatively to allow intermittent measurements of pulmonary artery diastolic, or "wedge," pressure, cardiac output, and blood gases. As noted previously, any indication of an acute change in the preoperative condition, such as unstable angina, means that elective surgery should be postponed, usually for at least 3 months.

2. HYPERTENSION

Patients with uncomplicated chronic hypertension, even with left ventricular hypertrophy and an abnormal ECG, tolerate surgery without a significantly increased mortality rate if there are no evidences of coronary heart disease or cardiac failure and if renal function is normal. Antihypertensive medication can be decreased during the week before surgery but should be continued until the night before surgery, and the anesthesiologist should be alerted to the medications used and informed about any difficulties noted in preoperative control of blood pressure. If medications are stopped earlier, there may be wide fluctuations in blood pressure during surgery (Pickering, 1983). If diuretics have been given, the body potassium must be replenished preoperatively.

3. ARRHYTHMIAS

Chronic atrial fibrillation with a well-controlled ventricular rate does not increase the risk of surgery, nor does an asymptomatic isolated right or left bundle branch block. Bifascicular block in asymptomatic patients does not require prophylactic pacing but does require close observation. Second- or third-degree atrioventricular block is a warning sign, especially if associated with left or right ventricular conduction defects; a transvenous electrode catheter should be inserted into the right ventricle before the surgical procedure and the patient monitored, with a pacemaker available in case ventricular standstill occurs. Infrequent atrial or ventricular premature beats usually do not require special treatment, can often be relieved with simple sedatives such as phenobarbital, and may disappear while anesthesia is being given. Monitoring of the ECG during anesthesia and surgery has shown that ventricular arrhythmias are infrequent unless there is underlying left ventricular disease or unless catecholamine release is excessive as a result of ventilatory problems.

If ventricular premature beats preoperatively are frequent and from multiple foci, or if they occur in salvos, surgery can be delayed and the ectopic ventricular beats suppressed with drugs such as quinidine, 200–400 mg orally 2–4 times daily, or procainamide, 250–500 mg orally 3 or 4 times daily. If the clinical situation is more urgent, or if it is considered unsatisfactory to delay surgery for 2–3 days to obtain the effect from oral drugs, lidocaine, 2% solution (20 mg/mL), 50–100 mg intravenously, followed by an intravenous infusion of 1–2 mg/min, will usually quickly abolish the premature beats.

If the premature beats are unifocal and infrequent, they should not be treated with antiarrhythmic drugs but monitored by continuous electrocardiography. If salvos of ventricular beats or complex arrhythmias develop, intravenous lidocaine should be used.

4. VALVULAR HEART DISEASE

Severe aortic stenosis, tight mitral stenosis, and severe coronary ostial involvement due to syphilitic aortitis are the 3 major "valvular" conditions in which general surgery presents a considerably increased hazard. An aortic systolic murmur not associated with evidence of severe aortic valvular disease or significant left ventricular hypertrophy does not increase the mortality rate. Mitral insufficiency is usually tolerated well, but tight mitral stenosis, especially if the patient has sinus rhythm, may result in acute pulmonary edema if the patient abruptly develops atrial fibrillation during surgery.

5. CONGENITAL HEART DISEASE

In the absence of cardiac failure, ventricular septal defect and atrial septal defect usually pose no particular problems or extra hazard. Pulmonary hypertension with Eisenmenger's syndrome carries a significantly increased mortality risk, and surgery should be performed only upon urgent indications. Patients with coarctation of the aorta and patent ductus arteriosus should have their congenital lesions repaired before undergoing elective general surgical procedures. Mild pulmonary stenosis is not a contraindication to elective surgery, but severe pulmonary stenosis is a contraindication because of the hazard of acute right heart failure and a reversed shunt through the foramen ovale or a small atrial septal defect. Patients with tetralogy of Fallot or other cyanotic congenital cardiac lesions are relatively poor surgical risks because of the polycythemia and because of the possibility of contraction of the infundibulum of the right ventricle, with resulting decrease in pulmonary blood flow.

6. CARDIAC FAILURE

Patients with mild cardiac failure whose symptoms and signs are controlled with digitalis and diuretics have only a slightly increased risk from general surgery provided ordinary activity does not cause symptoms. Patients who have dyspnea even when walking on level ground; orthopnea or nocturnal dyspnea; and signs of cardiac failure such as gallop rhythm, increased venous pressure, and rales are at a significantly increased risk, and surgery should be delayed if possible. Cardiac failure should be treated adequately before surgery. It is desirable to have the patient's condition stabilized for at least a month before surgery and to avoid digitalis toxicity and potassium depletion by diuretics. Diuretics and digitalis can then be withheld for a few days before surgery. Digitalization of a patient with cardiac hypertrophy but no heart failure is unwise because of the hazard of digitalis toxicity, including arrhythmias. Although digitalis has a positive inotropic action even in normal hearts, clinical evidence of benefit from the drug has not been demonstrated when it has been given to patients with hypertrophy but no failure. If there is a question about whether or not heart failure is present preoperatively, a period of bed rest and restricted dietary sodium may be adequate treatment.

MANAGEMENT OF KNOWN CARDIAC DISEASE PRIOR TO GENERAL SURGERY

If the preoperative assessment reveals known cardiac disease or severe hypertension, especially in the presence of acute symptoms, anemia, an unstable state, serious ventricular arrhythmias, heart block, or cardiac failure, these conditions should be managed before the surgical procedure is undertaken. The treatment of any cardiac condition discovered in the preoperative evaluation should be along the lines of treatment discussed elsewhere in this book and should not differ substantially in the patient with an elective surgical condition from treatment of a nonsurgical patient. Careful judgment is required in patients with more urgent surgical conditions, and delay in surgery for as long as possible may be indicated until the cardiac status is somewhat improved. If the surgical condition is urgent, the ability of the physician to treat the cardiac problem may be limited, and surgical treatment must take precedence even though the risk is considerably enhanced.

If the patient has severe valvular or coronary heart disease correctable by cardiac surgery, or if there are transient cerebral ischemic attacks proved by aortogram to be due to significant carotid stenosis, surgical treatment of the correctable lesion should precede elective general surgery in order to avoid pulmonary edema, cardiac arrest, or hemiplegia, which may follow the increased demands and variable blood pressure resulting from anesthesia and surgery. In such cases, carotid occlusive disease should usually be treated first unless the cardiac lesion is life-threatening. Fortunately, unexpected severe cardiac disease is uncommon in the patient scheduled for elective surgery, so the psychologic and other disturbances incident to cancellation of scheduled operations are reduced. Middle-aged or elderly patients suspected of having heart disease should be admitted to the hospital for a few days before scheduled surgery to allow effective diagnosis and management of any cardiac problem that is unexpectedly elicited. Alternatively, this preoperative evaluation can be done on an outpatient basis if there are no symptoms or important physical findings of cardiovascular disease.

SPECIAL PRECAUTIONS

In addition to conducting a preoperative surgical evaluation for any heart condition that should be managed before elective cardiac or other surgery, the physician should take special precautions if patients are receiving general treatment that may require modification because of the intended surgery. As a rule, anticoagulants should be stopped 2–3 days before surgery and resumed about 3 days postoperatively. Patients who have had intensive or prolonged corticosteroid treatment, even if it has been stopped for several months, should be identified, and supplementary corticosteroids should be administered (up to the equivalent of 200–300 mg of hydrocortisone per day preoperatively and for several days postoperatively). Patients receiving long-acting insulin for diabetes mellitus should be given regular insulin, and frequent analyses of urine, blood sugar, and ketones should be performed. Any hypersensitivity to drugs, especially antibiotics, should be determined so that patients will not receive them inadvertently. The administration of sodium-containing fluids should be carefully controlled during the preoperative, intraoperative, and postoperative periods because of the known sodium and water retention that follows general surgical operations. Sodium retention is probably due to hemodynamic and perhaps hormonal influences on the nephron. Water retention is due to increased secretion of ADH and not to increased aldosterone levels or decreased glomerular filtration rate. Sodium retention occurring postoperatively or arising from the use of intravenous sodium-containing fluids may precipitate pulmonary edema, and the speed and volume of the infused fluid should be regulated with this hazard in mind. If there is preoperative anemia or extensive blood loss during surgery, red cell mass rather than whole blood should be given slowly, and the patient should be supine and closely watched. If dyspnea, rales, or raised jugular venous pressure appears, the patient should be placed in the Fowler position to decrease the pulmonary blood volume and the infusion slowed or stopped.

MONITORING IN THE PRESENCE OF SEVERE CARDIAC DISEASE

If urgent surgery is required in the patient with severe coronary disease, aortic stenosis, mitral stenosis, or atrioventricular block; if extensive surgery is required in patients with borderline cardiac reserve; or if the multifactorial risk index is high, the patient should be monitored directly by a Swan-Ganz catheter. If it is difficult to evaluate the physiologic status in elderly patients thought to be at high risk, preoperative invasive assessment should be considered (Del Guercio, 1980), but this should not be a routine practice. Noninvasive clinical, echocardiographic, and radionuclide studies usually suffice. The intra-arterial blood pressure and pulmonary artery pressure (or, preferably, the pulmonary wedge pressure) should be intermittently recorded and blood gas measurements periodically determined. A temporary transvenous right ventricular pacemaker should be inserted when indicated to allow prompt institution of pacing in the event complete heart block develops. Emergency cardiac drugs and facilities for defibrillation should be readily available.

The choice and details of anesthesia are best left to the anesthesiologist, who must be alerted to any possible problems that might occur and informed of any medications the patient has taken even if they have recently been discontinued, such as digitalis, diuretics, antihypertensive agents, corticosteroids, insulin, propranolol, anticoagulants, or tricyclic antidepressants.

REFERENCES

Angelini P et al: Cardiac arrhythmias during and after heart surgery. *Prog Cardiovasc Dis* 1974;**16:**469.

Ayres SN, Grace WJ: Inappropriate ventilation and hypoxemia as causes of cardiac arrhythmias: The control of arrhythmias without antiarrhythmic drugs. *Am J Med* 1969;**46:**495.

Del Guercio LRM, Cohn JD: Monitoring operative risk in the elderly. *JAMA* 1980;**243:**1350.

Driscoll A et al: Post-operative myocardial infarction. *N Engl J Med* 1961;**264:**633.

Gazes PC: Noncardiac surgery and dentistry in cardiac patients. *Primary Cardiol* 1983;**9:**52.

Giardina EG, Heissenbuttel RH, Bigger JT Jr: Intermittent intravenous procaine amide to treat ventricular arrhythmias: Correlation of plasma concentration with effect on arrhythmia, electrocardiogram, and blood pressure. *Ann Intern Med* 1973;**78:**183.

Goldman L: Cardiac risks and complications of non-cardiac surgery. *Ann Intern Med* 1983;**98:**504.

Hahnemann Symposium on Cardiovascular Pulmonary Problems Before and After Surgery. 3. Shock and electrolyte disturbances. *Am J Cardiol* 1963;**12:**587.

Kaplan JA et al: The role of the intra-aortic balloon in cardiac anesthesia and surgery. *Am Heart J* 1979;**98:**580.

Katholi RE, Nolan SP, McGuire LB: The management of anticoagulation during noncardiac operations in patients with prosthetic heart valves: A prospective study. *Am Heart J* 1978;**96:**163.

Katz JD et al: Pulmonary artery flow-guided catheters in the perioperative period: Indications and complications. *JAMA* 1977;**237:**2832.

Katz RL: Hazardous effects of drugs in hypertensive patients scheduled for elective surgery. *Cardiovasc Med* 1978;**3:**1185.

Katz RL, Bigger JT Jr: Cardiac arrhythmias during anesthesia and operation. *Anesthesiology* 1970;**33:**193.

Marriott HJL: Differential diagnosis of supraventricular and ventricular tachycardia. *Geriatrics* 1970;**25:**91.

Mason DT: What the experts think: Antihypertensives and surgery. (Part 2.) *Primary Cardiol* (April) 1980;**6:**91.

Mauney FM Jr et al: Post-operative myocardial infarction. *Ann Surg* 1970;**172:**497.

Michaels L: Incidence of thromboembolism after stopping anticoagulant therapy: Relationship to hemorrhage at the time of termination. *JAMA* 1971;**215:**595.

Moore ED: Common patterns of water and electrolyte change in injury, surgery and disease. (4 parts.) *N Engl J Med* 1958; **258:**277, 325, 377, 427.

Mundth ED, Austen WG: Postoperative intensive care in the cardiac surgical patient. *Prog Cardiovasc Dis* 1968;**11:**229.

Nattel S, Rangno RE, Van Loon G: Mechanism of propranolol withdrawal phenomena. *Circulation* 1979;**59:**1158.

Oaks WW, Moyer JH (editors): *Pre- and Postoperative Management of the Cardiopulmonary Patient.* Grune & Stratton, 1970.

Pastore JO et al: The risk of advanced heart block in surgical patients with right bundle branch block and left axis deviation. *Circulation* 1978;**57:**677.

Perlroth MG, Hultgren HN: The cardiac patient and general surgery. *JAMA* 1975;**232:**1279.

Pickering TG: Anesthesia and surgery for the hypertensive patient. *Cardiovasc Rev Rep* 1983;**4:**1569.

Price HL: *Circulation During Anesthesia and Operation.* Thomas, 1967.

Raftery EB: Diagnosis and management of myocardial infarction during anesthesia. *Proc R Soc Med* 1973;**66:**1209.

Reitemeier RJ: Electrolytic imbalance: Problems associated with gastrointestinal surgery. *Med Clin North Am* 1962;**46:**1001.

Rogers MC: Anesthetic management of patients with heart disease. *Mod Concepts Cardiovasc Dis* 1983;**52:**29.

Salem MR et al: Cardiac arrest related to anesthesia: Contributing factors in infants and children. *JAMA* 1975;**233:**238.

Steen PA, Tinker JH, Tarhan S: Myocardial reinfarction after anesthesia and surgery. *JAMA* 1978;**239:**2566.

Thibault GE et al: Medical intensive care: Indications, interventions, and outcomes. *N Engl J Med* 1980;**302:**938.

Tinker JH, Tarhan S: Discontinuing anticoagulant therapy in surgical patients with cardiac valve prostheses. *JAMA* 1978; **239:**738.

Tinker JH et al: Management of patients with heart disease for noncardiac surgery. *JAMA* 1981;**246:**1348.

Wells PH, Kaplan JA: Optimal management of patients with ischemic heart disease for noncardiac surgery by complementary anesthesiologist and cardiologist interaction. *Am Heart J* 1981;**102:**1029.

Williams JF Jr, Morrow AG, Braunwald E: The incidence and management of "medical" complications following cardiac operations. *Circulation* 1965;**32:**608.

Index

A bands, 7
A mode echocardiography, 84
"A" point, 86
A_2, 54
  loud, in systemic hypertension, phonocardiogram of, 55
a waves, 47
  giant, 48
  as indication of ventricular compliance, 75
Abdomen
  examination of, 50
  pain in, 38
    as symptom of arteritis, 602
Abscesses, septic, 512
Absolute refractory period, 432
Accelerated conduction syndrome, 454
Accelerated idioventricular rhythm, 173
  ECG of, 495
  treatment of, 181
Accessory pathway, lateral, 454
Acetylcholine, 586, 595
ACG, 56
Acid-base balance
  alterations in, and premature ventricular beats, 487
  assessment of, 65
  disturbances of, 65
Acidosis, 123, 476, 586
  metabolic, 35, 65, 78, 501
  respiratory, 65
Acromegaly, 253
ACTH, 246
Action potential, 13
Activation, retrograde, 486
Activity, physical, in hypertension, 258
Adenomas, parathyroid, 249
Adrenal gland, adenoma of, 244
Adrenal hyperplasia, 244
  associated with virilism, 11-hydroxylase deficiency in, 248
  congenital, 248
Adrenal scan, in aldosteronism, 245
Adrenal vein catheterization, in aldosteronism, 245
Adrenergic beta-blockers, 216
Adrenergic inhibitors, adverse effects of, 261
Adrenocortical hormones, and hypertension, 218, 247
Adriamycin
  and acute myocardial damage, 537
  cardiotoxic effect of, 313
Afterload, 19, 23
  reduction of, 125

Age, and rise in blood pressure, 218
Aging, degenerative changes due to, 29
Agonal embolism, 587
Air embolism, as complication of bedside catheterization, 106
Airway, in cardiopulmonary resuscitation, 121
Albumin
  human serum, radioiodinated, 591
  iodine-labeled, 69
Alcohol
  and hypertension, 258
  ventricular premature beats due to, 487
Alcoholic cardiomyopathy, **553–555**
  echocardiogram of, 554
Aldactone, 259
Aldomet, 260
Aldosterone, 26
  antagonists of, sites of action of, 301
  plasma, in aldosteronism, 245
Aldosteronism
  primary, 227, **243**
  secondary, 246
Alkali ingestion, 65
Alkalosis, 476
  metabolic, 65
    in diuretic therapy, 302
  and premature ventricular beats, 487
  respiratory, 65
Alpha-adrenergic agonists, centrally acting, in hypertension, 259
Alpha-adrenergic blocking agents, 250
  in cardiac failure, 316
  and hypertension, 267
Alveolar collapse, 124
Alveolar hypoventilation, 593
Alveolar hypoxia, 586, 593
Ambulation, after myocardial infarction, 180, 188
Ambulatory blood pressure readings, 221, 223
Ambulatory monitoring of ECG, 484
Amiloride, in hypertension, 259
Amines, sympathetic, 183
  autonomic, and renin release, 215
Aminoglycosides, in infective endocarditis, 518
Aminophylline, 51, 320
  in chronic angina pectoris, 158
Amiodarone, 490
  in hypertrophic cardiomyopathy, 546
  and preexcitation syndromes, 460
Amoxicillin, in genitourinary and gastrointestinal tract surgery, 518

Amphetamines, and acute myocardial damage, 537
Ampicillin
  in genitourinary and gastrointestinal tract surgery, 518
  in prevention of endocarditis, 517
Amplitude of pulse, 42
Amrinone, in heart failure, 319
Amyl nitrite, 25, 541
  in acute angina pectoris, 156
  in hypertrophic obstructive cardiomyopathy, 542
  inhalation of, 62
Amyloid deposits, 561
Amyloid disease, 561
Anacrotic pulse, 405
Anastomotic vessels, 26
Anemia, 64, 289, 476
  chronic, 563
  in heart failure, 312
  in subacute infective endocarditis, 513
  and systolic ejection murmur, 59
Anesthesia
  and premature ventricular beats, 487
  and surgery in heart disease, risks of, 626
Aneurysm
  aortic, syphilitic, 599
  atherosclerotic, 599
    chest x-ray of, 600
    resection of, 601
  false, 187
  left ventricular, 176, **185**
    echocardiograms of, 186
    paradoxic rocking impulses in, 51
    resection of, **187,** 502
  of sinus of Valsalva, 421
  traumatic false, 615
  ventricular, 176, 499
    left, 185, 187
      echocardiograms of, 186
    resection of, 502
Angina
  decubitus, 37
  pectoris, 36, 37, **144–163,** 599
    acute, treatment of, 156
    character and duration of, 37
    and chronic coronary disease, 190
    chronic, treatment of, 157
    coronary arteriography in, 151
    and coronary artery anatomy, 160
    diagnosis of, 94
    education as part of treatment for, 159

Angina (cont'd)
  pectoris (cont'd)
    of effort (stable), **144–161**
      causes of death in, 160
      and exercise testing, 148
      fourth heart sound in, 56
      invasive investigation of, 151
      and myocardial infarction
        prevention of, 156
        relationship to, 160
      noninvasive investigation of, 148
      pain in, 147
      provocation and relief of, 37
      at rest, 37
      site and radiation of, 37
      social and psychologic factors in, 158
      surgical relief of, 192
      treatment of, 155
    preinfarction, 161
    Prinzmetal's, 37, 146
    unstable, 37, **161–163**
      pathophysiology of, 161
    walk-through, 37
    variant, 37, **144**, 146
Angiocardiography, 111
  pulmonary, 589
Angiogram(s)
  coronary, interpretation of, 112
  pulmonary, 592
  quality of, 111
  renal, in renal artery stenosis, 230, 240
  single-pass nucleotide, 172
Angiography
  cerebral, 604
  coronary, 112
    complications of, 118, 145
    in mitral stenosis, 376
    digital, computer-enhanced, 95
    digital subtraction, 151
  left ventricular, 110
    in angina pectoris, 154
    in measurement of chamber volumes, 70
    in mitral stenosis, 376
  pulmonary, 298, 591
  radionuclide, 98
    in angina pectoris, first-pass technique, 99
    gated equilibrium technique, 99
    temporal subtraction, 95
Angioplasty, percutaneous transluminal
  coronary, 114, 194
  renal, 242
Angiosarcoma, 577
Angiotensin, 26
Angiotensin I, 215, 216
Angiotensin II, 215, 216, 217
Angor animi, 38
Ankylosing spondylitis, and aortic incompetence, 414
Anomalous left coronary artery, ECG of, 362
Anomalous pulmonary venous drainage, total, 360
Anorexia
  and chronic constrictive pericarditis, 581
  and digitalis toxicity, 308
  and right ventricular failure, 292
Anterior chest wall syndrome, 155
Anterior infarction, conduction defects in, 174

Antiarrhythmic agents, 191, 488
  administration of
    long-term oral, 489
    rapid, 488
  clinical characteristics of, 490
  in myocardial infarction, 191
  in pregnancy, 620
Antibiotics
  in infective endocarditis, 510, 518
  in renal failure, 521
Antibody
  antimyosin, 171
  antinuclear, 575
    procainamide-induced, 491
Anticoagulant therapy, 159
  in acute myocardial infarction, 179, 192
  in cerebral embolism, 603
  in mixed mitral stenosis and incompetence, 384
  during pregnancy, 620
  in pulmonary embolism, 592
Anticoagulation
  in massive pulmonary embolism, 588
  prior to cardioversion, 482
Antidepressants, tricyclic, in heart failure, 313
Antihypertensive drugs, 209, **259–269**
  adverse effects of, 261
  sequential regimen of, 264
Antileukemic agents, in heart failure, 313
Antimicrobial regimens, in infective endocarditis, 520
Antimony, and acute myocardial damage, 537
Antimyosin antibody, 171
Antinuclear antibody, 575
  procainamide-induced, 491
Anti–platelet-aggregating agents, in myocardial infarction, 191
Antistreptolysin O titer, 535
Anturane, in myocardial infarction, 191
Anxiety, 36, 589
  pain associated with, 36
Aorta, 4
  aneurysms of, 599
  ascending, eggshell calcification of, 418
  coarctation of. *See* Coarctation of aorta.
  dissection of, 38, 43, 234, 235
    in aortic incompetence, 414
    classification of, 234
    as complication of cardiac catheterization, 118
    length of survival of patients with, 237
    pathogenesis of, 236
    roentgenographic findings in, 234
  examination of, in heart failure, 296
  hemodynamics of, 23
  overriding, 342
  rupture of, in cardiovascular syphilis, 601
  and systemic arteries, diseases of, **599–608**
Aortic acceleration, measurement of, 77
Aortic arch(es), 11
  arteritis of, 601
Aortic balloon counterpulsation, 184
  and vasodilator therapy, 184
Aortic dilatation, in aortitis, 599
Aortic ejection click, schematic diagram of, 52

Aortic ejection murmur, systolic, schematic diagram of, 58
Aortic incompetence, 38, 43, 60, 599
  acute, 400, 412
    dyspnea of, 415
  anatomic features of, 413
  causes of, 414
  chronic, 400, 412
  echocardiogram of, 419
  hemodynamically significant, 412
  and left heart failure, chest x-ray of, 418
  left ventricular and wedge pressure tracings in, 419
  phonocardiogram of, 416
  predominant, **412–432**
    cardiac catheterization data in, 421
    withdrawal pressure tracing of, 420
Aortic insufficiency, in infective endocarditis, 519
Aortic pressure
  in circulatory system, 26
  effect in coronary perfusion, 25
  and left ventricular pressure, 17
Aortic regurgitation, rheumatic, diastolic murmur in, phonocardiogram of, 57
Aortic runoff, in aortic incompetence, 416, 421
Aortic second sound, loud, in systemic hypertension, 55
Aortic sinuses, 6
Aortic stenosis. *See* Stenosis, aortic.
Aortic systolic murmurs, as signs of cardiovascular syphilis, 600
Aortic valve(s), 6
  area of, 74
  calcification in, 404
  closure of, sound of, 55
  disease of, **400–431**, 586
    anatomic features of, 402
    assessment of, carotid arterial pulse in, 43
    classification of, 400
  lesions of
    causes of, 400
    hemodynamically insignificant, 401
  and mitral valve
    disease of, combined, 423
    lesions of, combined, clinical course of, 424
  normal and stenotic, echocardiograms of, 409
  replacement of, 411, 422
    in cardiovascular syphilis, 601
  ring dilatation of, 599
Aortitis
  and ejection murmur, 59
  syphilitic, 600
    calcification in, x-ray of, 600
    sound of aortic valve closure in, 55
Aortocoronary grafts, 69
Aortopulmonary defects, anatomic sites of, 347
Aortopulmonary fistulas, and continuous murmurs, 61
Aortopulmonary window, 346
Apathetic thyrotoxicosis, 548
Apex, of heart, 1
Apex beat, of heart, 51
Apexcardiogram, 56
Apexcardiography, 101

Apnea, 50
Apprehension, in acute myocardial infarction, 165
Apresoline, 259, 260
Arachnodactyly, 49
Arcus senilis, 46
Arfonad, 260, 267
Argyll-Robertson pupil, 46
Arm(s)
  embolism of, 604
  examination of, in patients with heart disease, 48
  measurement of blood pressure in, 43
Arrest, cardiac. *See* Cardiac arrest.
Arrhythmias, 172
  in acute myocardial infarction, 172, 491
  atrial, 181, **466–484**
    in atrial septal defect, 332
    in chronic cor pulmonale, 595
    in preexcitation syndromes, prevention of, 460
    in pulmonary embolism, 590
  atrial paroxysmal, in Wolff-Parkinson-White syndrome, management of, 459
  cardiac, **466–509**
    effectiveness of drugs in, 487
    management of, in pregnancy, 620
    and cardiac disease, 310
    as complication of catheterization, 116, 478
    correction of, in heart failure, 299
    digitalis-induced, frequency of, 309
    drugs in management of, 492
    in Fallot's tetralogy, 338
    in rheumatic fever, 535, 536
  supraventricular, **466–484**
    in acute myocardial infarction, frequency of, 174
    and surgery, 628
  ventricular, 140, 172, 173, **484–503**
    and aortic incompetence, 415
    and click-murmur syndrome, 389
    and hypertrophic cardiovascular hypertrophy, 545
    incidence of, 485
    treatment of, 180, 181
Arsenic, and acute myocardial damage, 537
Arterial bed
  hemodynamics of, 23
  in systemic embolism, 603
Arterial blood
  pulmonary, 66
  sampling of, 105
Arterial blood pressure, 44
  control of, 26
  diastolic, 43
    increased, 211
    drop in, 210
  mean, 72, 73
  systolic, 74
  measurement of, direct, and sphygmomanometry, 43
  normal values, 78
  peak, 72
  pulmonary, increased, 586
  systemic, 72
  systolic, 42, 43
    increased, 211
Arterial catheterization, retrograde, 110

Arterial CO_2 tension, 65
Arterial embolism, 177
Arterial hypoxia, 593
Arterial pH, 65, 501
Arterial P_{O_2}, normal, 78
Arterial pulse, in aortic stenosis, 405
Arterial puncture, 105
Arterial vasoconstriction, pulmonary, 586
Arterial wave form, normal, pressure tracing of, 72
Arter(ies). *See also specific arteries.*
  coronary
    anatomy of, 6
    and distribution of, 153
    in relation to angina pectoris, 160
    spasm of, 25, 37
  cranial, 601
  femoral, occlusion of, 605
  great, transposition of, **357–358**
    anatomic features of, 359
    corrected, 358
  in hypertension, 225
  larger, changes in, 225
  normal, structure of, 133
  pulmonary
    entry into, in cardiac catheterization, 108
    idiopathic dilatation of, 330
    large, as sign of schistosomiasis, 587
    pressure in, recordings of, 108
    main, 2
    vasoconstriction of, 586
  systemic, and aorta, diseases of, **599–608**
  wall of, thickness of, as indication of atherosclerosis, 42
Arteriogram, using Judkins technique, 112
Arteriography
  clinical indications for, 152, 240
  coronary, 134, 145
  in angina pectoris, 152
Arteriolar caliber, decreased, 211
Arteriolar vasoconstriction, 586
Arterioles, pulmonary, 586
Arteriosclerosis, coronary, 226
Arteriotomy, 112
Arteriovenous fistula(s)
  in cardiac catheterization, 118
  continuous murmur in, 61
  high-output failure due to, 295
  pulmonary, 587
    x-ray of, 588
  systemic, 599, **605–607**
Arteriovenous oxygen difference, 289
Arteritis, 599, **601–603**
  aortic arch, 601
  Takayasu's, 601
  temporal, 601
Arthralgia, as symptom of arteritis, 602
Arthritis, 534
  in rheumatic fever, 534
  rheumatoid, 559
    cardiac symptoms and signs in, 559
    inflammatory infiltrate of, 560
Artifacts, in indirect measurement, 43
Artificial valve(s)
  as embolic material, 603
  patients with, 426
Aschoff nodule, 533

Ascites
  in chronic constrictive pericarditis, 581
  in chronic lung disease, 593
  in congestive heart failure, 50
  and effusions, in heart failure, 313
  in right heart failure, 294
Aspirin
  in angina pectoris, 159
  in myocardial infarction, 191
  in rheumatic fever, 536
Asthenia, neurocirculatory, 40, 291, **613–614**
Asthma, 35, 586, 597
  cardiac, 291, 597
Asymmetric left ventricular hypertrophy, 539
Asymptomatic coronary heart disease, 141
Asynchrony, of atria and ventricles, 486
  in ventricular tachycardia, 495
Atelectasis, 124, 588, 592
Atenolol, in hypertension, 263, 621
Atheroma(s)
  defined, 133
  mechanisms of production of, 133
Atherosclerosis, 132, 225
  clinical manifestations of, 232
  coronary, 164
    treatment of, 114
  defined, 133
  and ejection murmur, 59
  lesion of, 133
  pathogenesis of, 134
  risk factors in, **134–139**
Atherosclerotic aneurysms, 599
Atherosclerotic changes, premature, and earlobe sign, 46
Atherosclerotic coronary heart disease, pathogenesis of, 133
Atherosclerotic plaques, 133, 211
Atresia, tricuspid, 359
Atrial anatomy, 22
Atrial bigeminal rhythm, ECG of, 468
Atrial contraction
  and fourth heart sound, 56
  in ventricular tachycardia, 495
Atrial depolarization, ectopic (P'), 467
Atrial electrode catheters, right, 467
Atrial extrasystoles, 466
Atrial fibrillation. *See* Fibrillation, atrial.
Atrial flutter. *See* Flutter, atrial.
Atrial flutter-fibrillation, 480
Atrial gallop
  right, as sign of right ventricular failure, 293
  schematic diagram of, 52
Atrial hypertrophy, left, ECG of, 295
Atrial kick, 289
Atrial myxoma, 605, 610
  in differential diagnosis of infective endocarditis, 517
  left, 110, 376, 586, 609
    clubbing of fingers and nail beds in, 49
Atrial natriuretic factors, 470
  in hypertension, 217
Atrial P wave, peaked right, as sign of pulmonary embolism, 590
Atrial pacemaker, 478
Atrial pacing
  in paroxysmal atrial arrhythmia, 460
  rapid, 478, 482

Atrial premature beats, 181, 467
  concealed, 467
  ECG of, 468
  treatment of, 468
Atrial pressure, indirect left, 106
Atrial rate and ventricular response, 480
Atrial septal defect, 49, **325–333**, 479, 480
  anatomic features of, 326
  at birth, 325
  chest x-rays of, 326, 331
  clinical findings in, 325
  closure of, 332
  complications of, 330
  diastolic murmur due to, 60
  in differential diagnosis of pulmonary stenosis, 336
  ECG of, 327, 331
  echocardiogram in, 329
  and ejection murmur, 59
  ostium secundum, wide splitting of second heart sound in, phonocardiogram of, 54
  phonocardiogram in, 59, 327
  sinus venosus, chest x-ray of, 328
  square wave response in, pressure tracing of, 76
  and systolic ejection murmur, 59
  treatment and prognosis in, 332, 333
Atrial systole, 289
Atrial systolic murmur, 60
Atrial tachycardia. See Tachycardia, atrial.
Atrioventricular block, 310, 470
  in aortic incompetence, 421
  in aortic stenosis, 411
  causes of, 440
  first-degree (partial), 440
    conduction defect in, 443
  increased by digitalis, 480
  partial progressive, with Wenckebach phenomenon, 470
  second-degree, 444
    conduction defects in, 444
    defined, 440
    Mobitz type I (Wenckebach), 185, 187, 441, 444
    Mobitz type II, 185, 187, 444
      diagram of, 444
      prophylactic demand pacemakers in, 185
  third-degree (complete), 52, 311, 440, 442, 445, 497
    with atrioventricular dissociation, 48
    ECG of, 446
    treatment of, 447
    two-to-one, 441, 470
    transition to complete block, 445
Atrioventricular canal, 11
Atrioventricular conduction
  decrease of, in supraventricular tachycardia, 476
  defects in, 440
    acute, 442
    in acute myocardial infarction, 174
    chronic, 443
    ECG of, **509–515**
  degree of, in paroxysmal atrial tachycardia, 470

Atrioventricular conduction (cont'd)
  increased by drugs, 476
  two-to-one, 480
Atrioventricular defects, 141
Atrioventricular dissociation, 310, 472, 497
  complete heart block with, 48
  junctional rhythms with, treatment of, 478
Atrioventricular node, 7
Atrium
  left, 4
  right, 4
  and ventricle, asynchrony of, 486
Atropine, 116, 185, 492, 493
  for bradycardia, 124
  in fainting, 612
  and refractory period, 458
Atropine test, 438
Auscultation of heart, **51–62**
  technique of, 51
Auscultatory gap, defined, 44
Austin Flint murmur, 60, 417, 424, 515
  phonocardiogram, echocardiogram, and ECG of, 417
Automaticity, 432
  increased, ventricular premature beats due to, 486, 487
Autonomic insufficiency, 612
  arterial pressure tracings of, 612
Autonomic sympathetic amines, 195
  and renin release, 215
Autoregulation, 25, 139
AVA, 74
Axis, of heart, 1
Azathioprine, 603

B mode echocardiography, 84
Back, examination of, in patients with heart disease, 50
Bacteremia, in differential diagnosis of infective endocarditis, 517
Bacteria, gram-negative, as cause of endocarditis, 511, 521
Bactericidal activity, testing for, 518
Baffes procedure, for transposition of great arteries, 358
Ballistocardiography, 101
Balloon catheter, 182
Balloon counterpulsation, aortic, 184
  and vasodilator therapy, 184
Balloon-tipped catheters, 106, 176, 605
Balloon valvuloplasty, percutaneous, 338
Barometric pressure, 64
Baroreceptors
  areas of, 27
  in hypertension, 214
  mechanisms of, 26, 606
  reflex arc of, 77
  responses to change in arterial pressure, 76
Bat's wing densities, in hypertension, 230
Bat's wing infiltrates, 175, 418
  x-ray of, 83
Beats
  apex, of heart, 51
  capture, 494, 496

Beats (cont'd)
  Dressler, 496
  dropped, 445
  ectopic, 70
    during injection of contrast material, pressure tracing of, 71
    effect on arterial pressure, 73
    junctional, 47
    ventricular, during catheterization, 117
  fusion, 494, 496
  premature, 445, **466–469**
    atrial, 181, 467
      concealed, 467
      ECG of, 468
      treatment of, 468
    junctional, 467
    supraventricular, 467
    ventricular. See Premature beats.
Bed rest, 319
  following myocardial infarction, 188
  prolonged, risk of, 299
Bedside care, 179
Bedside versus laboratory procedures, 105
Bence Jones proteinuria, in amyloidosis, 562
Bendroflumethiazide, 259
Benzathine penicillin G, in syphilitic cardiovascular disease, 600
Beriberi heart disease, 312, 553, 554
  and alcoholic cardiomyopathy, 553
  ECG of, 590
Beta-adrenergic blocking agents, 143, 157, 191, 216, 289
  approved by FDA for hypertension, 263
  and atrial fibrillation, 481
  in chronic angina pectoris, 157
  and chronic coronary disease, 191
  in heart failure, 313
  and hypertension, 263, 267, 270
  in hypertrophic cardiomyopathy, 546
  and myocardial infarction, 157, 178, 179, 191
  in pregnancy, 620
  in supraventricular tachycardia, 476, 477
Beta-sitosterol, 156
Bezold reflex, 27
Bicarbonate, 65
  sodium, in ventricular fibrillation or tachycardia, 123
Bidirectional shunts, 67
Bifascicular block, 175, 452
  chronic, causes of syncope in, 453
Bifid pulse in hypertrophic obstructive cardiomyopathy, 540, 542
Bigeminal rhythm, atrial, ECG of, 468
Bilateral bundle branch block, 175, 451
Bilharzial tubercles, 587
Bilharziasis, pulmonary hypertension in, 587
Biofeedback, in hypertension, 259
Bipolar Lewis lead, 467
Björk-Shiley prosthetic aortic valve, 378
Blalock-Hanlon operation, for transposition of great arteries, 358
Blalock-Taussig operation, for tetralogy of Fallot, 61, 342

Blindness
  as complication of arteritis, 602
  sudden, 604
    as symptom of arteritis, 602
Bloating, as sign of right ventricular failure, 293
Block
  atrioventricular. See Atrioventricular block.
  bifascicular, 175, 452
  bundle branch. See Bundle branch block.
  infranodal, complete, 175
  sinoatrial, 310
  trifascicular, 443
  unifascicular, 451
Blocking agents, beta-adrenergic. See Beta-adrenergic blocking agents.
Blood
  arterial, pulmonary, 66
  bubbles in, detection of, 92
  buffering system of, 65
  composition of, changes in, 603
  oxygen-carrying capacity of, 64
  pH of, 65
  sampling of, in cardiac catheterization, 109
  sedimentation rate of, elevated, 600
  supply to brain, acute interruption of, 221
  transfusion of
    in cardiac patients, 125
    hemochromatosis due to, 560
  venous, mixed, 66
Blood chemistry findings, in hypertension, 227
Blood cultures, in diagnosis of endocarditis, 513
Blood flow
  coronary, pathophysiology of, 139
  effective (Q_{eff}), 67
  measurement of, 69
  pulmonary, 67, 68
  systemic, 67, 68
  visceral, 29
Blood gases, arterial, 319
Blood pool scans, radioisotope gated, 172
Blood pressure, 42, **43–45**
  brachial arterial, normal, 28
  and circadian rhythm, 211
  emotional factors influencing, 218
  evaluation of, 256
  in hypertension, 221
  measurement of, **72–74**
    in arm, 43
    in legs, 44
    patient position in, 43
    variations in, 222
  and morbid events, 233
  normal, factors in, 210
  normal values, 78
  number of readings required, 257
  recording of, 221, 222
  rise of
    with age, 218
    factors opposing, 210
  systolic and diastolic, increases in, 211
  transient elevations of, 210
Blood pressure cuff, 43

Blood vessels
  examination of, in hypertension, 224
  types of, in humans, 27
Blood volume, **69–72**
  circulating, as controlled variable in circulatory system, 26
  control of, 27
  effective
    central, 76
    indirect indications of, 28
  effects of posture on, 28
  inadequate, and hypotension, 611
  measurement of, 28
  normal, 79
  total, 69
Blubbering murmur, 61
Blue bloaters, 593
Blue hemoglobin, 64
Blurring of vision, as symptom of arteritis, 602
Body surface area, 66
Borderline hypertension, 256
Bounding pulse, as sign of arteriovenous fistula, 606
Brachial arterial blood pressure, normal, 28
Brachial arterial cutdown technique, 110
Brachial artery pressure curve, 42
Brachial pulse, 42
  in hypertrophic obstructive cardiomyopathy, 540
Bradyarrhythmias, in acute myocardial infarction, 174, 175
Bradycardia, 116, 434
  in arteriovenous fistula, 607
  in hypotension, 612
  and myocardial infarction, 435
  reflex, 76
  sinus, 173, 185
Bradycardia-tachycardia syndrome, 437
Brain
  circulation to, 29
  and hypertension, 226
Branham's sign, 295, 606
Breath, shortness of, 34
Breathing
  Cheyne-Stokes, 51
  periodic, 50
  in ventricular failure, 51
  work of, 35
Brockenbrough's sign, 541
Bronchial carcinoma, 592
  clubbing of fingers and nail beds in, 49
Bronchial collateral flow, 60
Bronchitis, 35
  and mitral stenosis, 377
  in winter, 291
Bronchospasm, 291, 597
Bruce protocol, and stress ECGs, 94, 148
Bruit(s)
  over blood vessel, as sign of arteritis, 602
  palpable and audible, as sign of arteriovenous fistula, 606
  systolic
    in neck, 604
    in peripheral vessels, 60
Bubbles, in blood, detection of, 92

Buffering system of blood, 65
Bulbus cordis, 4, 11
Bulge, left parasternal, as sign of ventricular septal defect, 50
Bumetanide, in cardiac failure, 302
Bundle
  of His. See His bundle.
  of Kent, 454
Bundle branch(es)
  conduction in, defects in, 141
  left and right, 7
Bundle branch block, 448
  in acute myocardial infarction, 174
  bilateral, 175, 451
  left, 53, 54, 448
    intermittent, ECG of, 450
  right, 448, 473
    incomplete, in pulmonary embolism, ECG of, 590
    intermittent, ECG of, 449
    as sign of pulmonary embolism, 591
    widely split second heart sound in, phonocardiogram of, 53, 54
Buried P waves, 473
Bypass, coronary, 163, **192–194**, 502
  benefits and adverse effects of, 193
  complications of, 194
  late consequences of, 194
  relief of symptoms with, 194

c wave, **47**
C8 to T4 segmental dermatomes, and anginal pain, 146
Cachexia, cardiac, 41
Café coronary, 122, 142
Calcification
  in aortic valves, 404
  coronary, 160
  intrapericardial, 582
  of mitral valve ring, 386
  syphilitic, 600
  as x-ray sign in heart failure, 296
Calcium
  as embolic material, 603
  in muscle contraction, 21
Calcium chloride, as cardiac stimulant, 123
Calcium entry–blocking agents, 157
  in cardiac failure, 313
  in chronic angina pectoris, 157
  and hypertension, 269, 271
  in hypertrophic cardiomyopathy, 546
  in supraventricular tachycardia, 476
Calf tenderness, as sign of venous thrombosis, 50
Candida, 603
Cannon waves, 48, 486
  defined, 474
  irregular, 48
Capacitance, as analog of compliance, 75
Capacitance vessels, 210
Capacity, oxygen-carrying, 65
Capillary pressure, pulmonary, 107
Capoten, in hypertension, 259
Captopril, 242, 268
  adverse effects of, 265
  in afterload reduction, 126
  in heart failure, 317
  in hypertension, 259, 268, 271

Capture beats, 494, 496
Carbamino compound, 65
Carbon dioxide
  arterial, tension of, 65
  for periodic breathing, 51
  retention of, 124
  transport of, 65
Carbon dioxide narcosis, 124
Carbon dioxide–oxygen exchange in tissues, 64
Carbonic anhydrase inhibitors, sites of action of, 301
Carcinoid valvular heart disease, 424
Carcinoma, bronchial, 592
  clubbing of fingers and nail beds in, 49
Cardiac. *See also* Heart.
Cardiac arrest, 121, 500
  in unstable angina, ECG after, 162
Cardiac arrhythmias, **466–509**. *See also* Arrhythmias.
Cardiac asthma, 291, 597
Cardiac cachexia, 41
Cardiac catheterization. *See* Catheterization.
Cardiac cells, electrical properties of, 432
Cardiac conditions masquerading as surgical illnesses, 626
Cardiac contraction
  effects of sympathetic nervous system on, 27
  force and velocity of, 305
  mechanism of, 12
  molecular basis of, 12
Cardiac cycle, **14–21**
  blood flow in, **23–26**
  events of, 14, 16
Cardiac failure. *See* Heart failure.
Cardiac function, assessment of, **75–77**
Cardiac glycoside preparations, 304
Cardiac hypertrophy, 178
  and cardiac failure, 225
  and compliance, 287
Cardiac impulse
  hyperdynamic, as sign of arteriovenous fistula, 606
  in hypertrophic obstructive cardiomyopathy, 541
  tapping, 51
Cardiac index, 66, 78
Cardiac loop, 10
  formation of, 9
Cardiac lymph node, 7
Cardiac massage, 122
  external, 501
Cardiac measurements and electrical analogs, **74–75**
Cardiac muscle
  diagram of, 8
  and skeletal muscle, differences between, 19
Cardiac muscle fiber, phases of action potential in, 15
Cardiac nerves, 7
Cardiac neurosis, 613
Cardiac output, 320
  and age, 218
  computer calculation of, 66
  decreased, 165
  determination of
    by Doppler ultrasound, 85
    by indicator (dye) dilution, 66

Cardiac output (cont'd)
  distribution of, 30
  increased, 211
  low, 76, 581
  measurement of, **65**, 109
  normal resting, 78
Cardiac pain
  and aortic stenosis, 405
  ischemic. *See* Angina pectoris.
Cardiac performance, limitation of, 31
Cardiac prostheses, management of patients with, 619
Cardiac rupture, 177, 187
Cardiac shunts, measurement of, **66–69**
Cardiac standstill, 117
Cardiac syncope, 39
Cardiac tamponade, 44, **577–580**
  in pericardial effusion, echocardiogram of, 579
Cardiac transplantation, 320
Cardiac trauma, 614
Cardiac tumors, **609–611**
Cardiac values, normal, 78
Cardiac valves, 6
Cardiogenic shock, 172, 176
  and intra-aortic balloon pumping, 130
  treatment of, 181
Cardiologic investigations
  invasive, **105–120**
  noninvasive, **80–104**
  routine, 80
  special, 80
Cardiomyopathy, 586
  alcoholic, **553–555**
  echocardiogram of, 554
  chronic, **537–548**
    classification of, 538
    due to specific disease entities, **555–564**
  congestive, 288, **538**
  dilated, **538–539**
  hypertrophic obstructive, 59, 60, 91, 411, **539**
    long pansystolic ejection murmur in, 60
    provocative tests in, 544
  hypothyroid, chest x-ray in, 552
  ischemic, 538
  pathology of, 527
  peripartum, **564**, 617
  primary, 538
  restrictive, **546**, 582
Cardiophrenic angle, right, acute, 576
Cardiopulmonary function, 64
  testing of, 100
Cardiopulmonary resuscitation, **121–124**
Cardiopulmonary system
  and muscular exercise, 11
  ranges of normality in, 29
  and stresses, 11
Cardiovascular disease, average annual incidence of, 220
Cardioversion, 123, 181, 477, 498
  anticoagulation prior to, 482
  elective, 126
  electric, in digitalis toxicity, 311
  in paroxysmal atrial flutter, 483
Carditis, in rheumatic fever, 534, 535

Cardizem, in supraventricular tachycardia, 476
Carey-Coombs murmur, 535
Carotid arterial stenotic lesions, murmurs due to, 60
Carotid pulse, 43, 46
Carotid sinus
  massage of, 148, 157
  effect on murmurs, 62
  syncope of, 39
Catapres, 259
Catecholamines, normal ranges of, 250
Catheter(s)
  balloon, 182
  balloon-tipped, 106, 176, 605
  broken, as complication of cardiac catheterization, 118
  electrode, right atrial, 467
  fling, 72
  Fogarty, 605
  Gensini, 110
  His bundle, 113
  Judkins, 110
  Lehman, 111
  multiple-hole, 111
  NIH, 111
  pigtail, 109
  Swan-Ganz, 66, 105, 106, 175, 178, 476
  thermodilution, 106, 178
  triple-lumen Swan-Ganz, 182
Catheter ablation, of His bundle, in atrial tachycardia, 460
Catheter recanalization, 115
Catheterization
  adrenal vein, in aldosteronism, 245
  arterial, 105
  bedside, **105–106**
    complications of, 106
    indications for, 106
  cardiac, 375, 582, 600
    arrhythmias during, 478
    in cardiomyopathy, 529
    complications of, **116–119**
    diagnostic
      elective, **106–111**
      indications for, 107
    exercise during, 113
    in mitral stenosis, 375
    morbidity and mortality rates of, 119
    in predominant aortic incompetence, 421
    in predominant aortic stenosis, 410
    in pulmonary stenosis, 336
    in ventricular septal defect, 345
    complications common to all forms of, **116–118**
    coronary sinus, and atrial pacing, 113
  left heart, **109–111**
    complications of, 118
    measurements during, 110
    transseptal, 109, 110
  percutaneous
    femoral, 118
    subclavian, 129
  retrograde
    arterial, 110
      brachial, 109, 110
      percutaneous femoral artery, 109

Catheterization (cont'd)
  right heart, **107–108**
    complications of, 118
    and percutaneous venous catheterization, **109–110**
    therapeutic procedures involving, 114
    transseptal, 111
    venous, 105
Catheter-tip manometers, 72, 77
Cedilanid-D, 307
  dosages and routes of administration, 304
Central blood volume, effective, 76
Central nervous system
  in hypertension, **214,** 220, 227
  in ventricular premature beats, 486
Cephalosporin, in prevention of endocarditis, 517
Cerebral angiography, 604
Cerebral circulation, dominance of, 26
Cerebral embolism, 221, 603, 604
Cerebral hemorrhage, 221
Cerebral infarction, 177
  thrombotic, 221
Cerebral ischemia, 39
Cerebral vessels, spasm of, in cerebral embolism, 603
Cerebrovascular accidents, 39
Cervical spine disease, degenerative, 155
Cesarean section, in heart disease, 619
Chagas' disease, **563–564**
  acute, myocarditis due to, 532
Chagoma, inflammatory, 563
Chamber volumes, cardiac, angiographic measurements of, 70
Charcot-Bouchard microaneurysms, 221, 226
Chest
  compression of, mechanism of action of, 122
  deformities of, and heart disease, 50
  infection of, in chronic cor pulmonale, 595
  pain in. *See* Pain, chest.
  x-ray of, in hypertension, 230
Chest wall syndrome, anterior, 155
Cheyne-Stokes breathing, **51,** 292
Chlorine, dyspnea due to, 35
Chlorothiazide, 259
Chlorthalidone, 259
Choking, on food, 121, 122
Cholecystectomy, 606
Cholecystitis, 592
Cholesterol, 135
  and HDL and estrogens, 137
Cholestyramine, to lower serum lipids, 135
Chorea, Sydenham's, in rheumatic fever, 534
Cigarette smoking, 298, 596
  in atherosclerosis, 137
  and hypertension, 291
  and sudden death, 143, 502
Cineangiograms, 70
  left ventricular, in angina pectoris, 154
Cineangiography, 112
Cinefluoroscopy, 95

Circadian rhythm and blood pressure, 211
Circulating blood volume, 69
Circulation(s)
  cerebral, dominance of, 26
  component parts of, 11
  control of, **26–28**
  coronary, 6, 23
    anomalies of, 361
    diagram of, 26
    pressure-flow relationships in, 25
  heart as servant of, 31
  physiologic function of, **11–30**
  pulmonary, 30, 586
    pressure/flow characteristics of, 586
  special, 29
Circulatory collapse, 580, 588
Circulatory control mechanisms, 12, 21
Circulatory reflex reactivity, factors affecting, 612
Circulatory system, physiology of, **1–33**
Circus movement, 434, 472, 480
Cirrhosis of liver, 582
Claudication
  in hypertension, 221
  jaw, as symptom of arteritis, 602
Clearance methods, of blood flow measurement, 69
Click(s)
  aortic, schematic diagram of, 52
  ejection, schematic diagram of, 58
  midsystolic, schematic diagram of, 52
  pulmonary systolic ejection, schematic diagram of, 52
  systolic, 56
Click-murmur syndrome, 57, **386**
  systolic, 513
Clofibrate, 156
Clonidine, 259, 265, 271
  adverse effects of, 261
Closure
  aortic valve (A_2), 55, 56
  of mitral and tricuspid valves, 52
  pulmonary valve (P_2), 52
Closure sound
  drumbeat quality of, as sign of cardiovascular syphilis, 599
  drumlike aortic valve, 55
  loud pulmonary valve, in pulmonary hypertension, 55
  tambour aortic valve, 55
Clubbing
  of fingers, 49, 513, 587
    in chronic lung disease, 593
  of nail beds, 49
  of toes, as sign of cyanotic congenital heart disease, 50
CO_2. *See* Carbon dioxide.
Coarctation of aorta, 43, 60, 251, 290, **352–355,** 619
  anatomic features of, 353
  chest x-ray of, 353
  in hypertension, 226
  pressure tracings of, 354
  systemic collateral vessels in, 50
Cobalt, 553
Cobalt-beer cardiomyopathy, 553
Coeur en sabot, 341

Coffee, and hypertension, 258
Cold pressor test, effect on murmurs, 62
Cold spots, 169
Colestipol, to lower serum lipids, 156
Collateral circulation, 241
Collateral flow, bronchial, 60
Collateral vessels, systemic, in coarctation of aorta, 50
Commissurotomy, mitral, 573
Compensatory mechanisms, 289
  in hypotension, 611
Compensatory pause, 467, 487
Complement, deposition of, in pre-eclampsia, 622
  and congestive heart failure, 485
Compliance
  defined, 75
  vascular, 75
  ventricular, *a* wave as indication of, 75
Computer-based x-ray tomography, 96
Computer-enhanced digital angiography, 95
Computerized tomography, in pericarditis, 582
Concealed atrial premature beats, 467
Concealed conduction, 433, 443, 467
Concealed Wolff-Parkinson-White syndrome, 460, 472
Concentric hypertrophy, 288
Conductance, 74
Conduction. *See specific types.*
  failure of, 433
  velocity of, 433
Conduction defects, 168, **432–465.** *See also specific types.*
  in acute myocardial infarction, 174, 442
  congenital, 361
  intermittent, 453
  pacemaker therapy in, 453
  rate-dependent, 453
Conduction syndrome, accelerated, 454
Conduction system, 7, 13
  in myocardial disease, pathology of, 528
Conductivity, 433
Congestion
  pulmonary, 588
    acute, 35
  as x-ray sign in heart failure, 296
Congestive cardiomyopathy, 288, **538**
  dilated, 538
Congestive heart failure, 76, 589
  and complex ventricular premature beats, 484
  diagnosis of, 290
  in Fallot's tetralogy, 338
  in rheumatic fever, 536
  right-sided, 290
Connective tissue disorders, 253
  in differential diagnosis of infective endocarditis, 517
  in heart failure, 311
Consciousness
  impaired, 589
  loss of, in cerebral embolism, 603
Consolidation, 590
Constriction, pericardial, 46, 48, **581**

Constrictive pericarditis, 294, 581
  calcification in, chest x-ray of, 582
  pressure tracings in, 49, 583
Continuous murmur(s), 61
  and patent ductus arteriosus, phonocardiogram of, 61
Contraceptives, oral, 603
  and atherosclerosis, 137
  hypertension due to, 252
  and pulmonary embolism, 589
  and pulmonary hypertension, 596
Contractility, 75–77
  myocardial, 19
Contraction
  atrial, and fourth heart sound, 56
  cardiac
    effects of sympathetic nervous system on, 27
    mechanism of, 12
    molecular basis of, 12
  isovolumetric, 15
  muscular, 13
  ventricular, 495
Contrast material, effects of, 111
Converting enzyme(s), inhibitors of, 268, 317
Convulsions
  in cerebral embolism, 603
  due to eclampsia, 623
Cor pulmonale, 49, 124, 292
  acute, 588
  chronic, defined, 593
  defined, 586
  hypoxic, 593
  and pulmonary emphysema, 594
  pulmonary hypertensive, 593
Cor triatriatum, 377
Coronary, café, 122, 142
Coronary arter(ies)
  anatomy of, 153
  and angina pectoris, 160
  disease of
    and click-murmur syndrome, 389
    and mitral incompetence, 396
    and mixed mitral stenosis and incompetence, 384
  premature, 597
  probability of, 149
  three-vessel, 176
  and ventricular premature beats, 493
  embolism of, 134
  involvement in disease in relation to survival, 160
  left, 6
  mural obstruction of, 140
  right, 6
  spasm of, 25, 37
  thrombosis of, 134, 164
  variability in anatomic pattern of, 6
Coronary atherosclerosis, 164
  treatment of, 114
Coronary bypass, 163, **192–194**, 502
  benefits and adverse effects of, 193
  complications of, 194
  late consequences of, 194
  relief of symptoms with, 194
Coronary care unit, 178
  resuscitation in, 121

Coronary circulation, 6, 23
  anomalies of, 361
  diagram of, 26
  pressure-flow relationships in, 25
Coronary embolism, 604
Coronary heart disease, **132–208**, 501
  atherosclerotic, pathogenesis, of, 133
  chronic (established), 190
  classification of, 132
  death rates due to, 192
  effect of hypertension in, 232
  latent, 141
  management of, prior to surgery, 629
  manifestations of, 133
  and nonfatal myocardial infarction, 256
  pathogenesis of, 133, 139
  and pregnant patient, **617–625**
  presenting clinical manifestations of, 132, 133
  risk of, and high-density lipoproteins, 136
  specific types of, **144–192**
  subclinical, 34
  in surgical patients, 628
  surgically modified, 324
  and ventricular premature beats, 493
Coronary insufficiency, acute, 161
Coronary perfusion, aortic pressure in, 25
Coronary sinus, 7
Coronary spasm, 113, 133, **144**, 146, 157
  and decreased myocardial supply, 145
Coronary steal syndrome, 194
Coronary stenosis, diagnosis of, 134
Coronary sulcus, 1
Coronary thrombosis, 164
Corrigan pulse, 416
Corrigan waves, venous, 486
Corticosteroid(s), 575, 600, 602
  in heart failure, 313
  in rheumatic fever, 536
Costochondritis, pain of, 38
Cotton wool exudates, 223
Cough, 590, 597
  chronic, history of, 298
  on exercise, 39
  exertional, 289
  and hemoptysis, as symptoms of heart disease, 39
  long-standing, 291
  as symptom of cardiovascular syphilis, 599
  syncope, 39
Coumadin, 592
Counterpulsation
  external, 130
  intra-aortic balloon, 130, 184
Countershock, 481
  DC, 123
  electrical, 127
  external, 498
Coxsackie B myocarditis, 529
Coxsackie B pericarditis, 573
CPK, 95, 166, 172
Cranial arteries, 601
Crease in ear, as sign of premature atherosclerotic changes, 46
Creatine phosphokinase, 95, 166, 172
  myocardial band, 575
  isoenzymes of, 172

Creatinine, serum, elevated, 575
Creatinine clearance and digoxin clearance, relationship of, 306
Crepitations, as signs of heart disease, 50
Crista supraventricularis, 4
Critical coupling interval, 468
Crow's foot markings, 599
Cryosurgical ablation, in preexcitation syndromes, 460
Cryotherapy, in supraventricular tachycardia, 478
Cushing's disease, **246–248**
Cushing's syndrome, 227, **246–248**
  diagnosis of, 247
  effect on ECG, 85
Cutdown technique, brachial arterial, 110
Cuvette densitometer, 66
Cuvier, ducts of, 8
Cyanosis, 45, 589
  at birth, in Fallot's tetralogy, 338
  differential, 351
  of fingers, in chronic lung disease, 593
  as symptom of heart disease, 41
Cyanotic congenital heart disease, 35, 49, 64
Cycle ergometer, 94, 113, 148
Cyclophosphamide, and rheumatic fever, 537
Cyclosporine, 320
Cyproheptadine, in Cushing's syndrome, 248
Cytomel, 639
Cytotoxic agents, and rheumatic fever, 537
Cytoxan, and rheumatic fever, 537

"D" point, 90
Da Costa's syndrome, 38, 40, 613
Dalmane, 247, 476
Damping systems, 72
Daunorubicin, cardiotoxic effect of, 313
DC countershock, 123, 475
  restoration of sinus rhythm by, in mitral stenosis, 377
DC defibrillator, 123
Death
  impending, feeling of, 38
  sudden, **141–144**, 190, 485, 493, 500, 502, 503
  age-adjusted incidence of, 142
  causes of, 142
  and cigarette smoking, 143
  click-murmur syndrome, 389
  and hypertrophic obstructive cardiomyopathy, 545
  prevention of, 142, 191
  prodromal symptoms in, 141
  reversibility of, in primary ventricular fibrillation, 144
  in sarcoidosis, 555
  and ventricular arrhythmias, 390
Decompensation, cardiac, 287
  pathophysiology of, 289
Decremental conduction, 433
Defibrillation, 181, 500, 501
  emergency, 123
  follow-up data on, 501

Defibrillation (cont'd)
  in ventricular fibrillation, 144
Defibrillator, automatic implantable, in prevention of sudden death, 143
Degenerative changes, cardiac, 29
Degenerative disease
  of cervical spine, 155
  of disks, 155
  of thoracic spine, 155
Dehydration, fatigue due to, 40
Delayed diastolic murmur, 60
  schematic diagram of, 58
Delivery
  management of, in heart disease, 619
  normal, in acute cor pulmonale, 588
Delta wave, in Wolff-Parkinson-White syndrome, 457
Demand pacemaker(s), 127
  prophylactic, in Mobitz II block, 185
Demerol, 179
Deoxycorticosterone excess syndromes, 247
Depolarization(s), 13
  atrial, ectopic, 467
  P', 467
Deslanoside, 307
  dosages and routes of administration, 304
Desoxycorticosterone, 245
Development and aging, 28
Dextrocardia, 362
Diabetes mellitus, 155, 502
  in atherosclerosis, 136
Dialysis, 607
  in pericardial effusion, 577
  renal, 573
  and renal failure, 274
Diastole, ventricular, 18
Diastolic collapse of neck veins, 581
Diastolic gallop, phonocardiogram of, 57
Diastolic murmur(s), 60
  delayed, schematic diagram of, 58
  immediate
    in chronic cor pulmonale, 596
    schematic diagram of, 58
    as sign of cardiovascular syphilis, 599
  inflow, schematic diagram of, 58
  in rheumatic aortic regurgitation, phonocardiogram of, 57
Diastolic pressure, 43
  factors leading to increases in, 211
Diazepam, 179, 476, 498
Diazoxide, 260, **267**, 596
  adverse effects of, 261, 265
  in cardiac failure, 317
Dibenzyline, 251
Dicrotic notch, 54, 72
Differential cyanosis, 351
Diffusion, 101
Digital subtraction angiography, 151
Digitalis, 184, **304–311**, 481, 596
  and acute myocardial damage, 537
  administration of, ST-T changes resulting from, 308
  antibodies to, 311
  bioavailability of, 305
  in congestive heart failure due to rheumatic fever, 536

Digitalis (cont'd)
  dosages and routes of administration, 304, 305
  effect on ECG, 81
  and elective cardioversion, 126
  electrophysiologic action of, 305
  in heart failure, 313
  and hypokalemia, 292
  mechanism of action of, 305
  nonparoxysmal supraventricular (junctional) tachycardia due to, 472
  pathophysiologic and hemodynamic effects of, 305
  pharmacokinetics of, 305
  and premature ventricular beats, 492
  recurrent cardiac failure in, prevention of, 305
  and refractory period, 458
  in supraventricular tachycardia, 476, 477
  toxicity of, 308
    in paroxysmal atrial tachycardia, 470
    prevention of, 311
    treatment of, 311
    in Wolff-Parkinson-White syndrome, 459
Digitalis-induced increased atrioventricular block, 480
Digitalization
  adequate, criteria of, 308
  and heart rate, in treatment of mixed mitral stenosis and incompetence, 385
Digitoxin
  dosages and routes of administration, 304, 305
  serum levels of, 307
Digoxin, 488, 492
  administration of, 307
  clearance of, and blood urea nitrogen, relationship of, 306
  dosages and routes of administration, 304
  half-life of, 306
  levels of, affected by dosage, 306
  in pregnancy, 620
  serum levels of, 306, 307
  in supraventricular tachycardia, 477
Dilated cardiomyopathy, **538–539**
Diltiazem, 157, 158
  in cardiac failure, 313
  in supraventricular tachycardia, 476
Diphtheritic myocarditis, 532
Dipyridamole, in myocardial infarction, 192
Direct arterial pressure measurement and sphygmomanometry, correlation between, 43
Disk disease, degenerative, 155
Disopyramide, 490, 492
  in heart failure, 313
  in pregnancy, 620
Dissection
  aortic, 38, 43, 234, 235
    in aortic incompetence, 414
    classification of, 234
    length of survival of patients with, 237
    pathogenesis of, 236
    prognosis of, 237

Dissection (cont'd)
  aortic (cont'd)
    roentgenographic findings in, 234
  arterial, as complication of cardiac catheterization, 118
Dissociation, atrioventricular, 472, 497
  complete block with, 48
  junctional rhythms with, treatment of, 478
Diuresis
  excessive sodium loss with, 300
  in treatment of cardiac failure, 182, 183
Diuretic(s)
  adverse effects of, 261
  clinical use of, 302
  and hypertension, 258
  loop, 300
    in cardiac failure, 302
  mercurial, in heart failure, 300
  oral, 260
    indications for, 302
    sites of action of, 301
  therapy with
    caution with, 303
    in heart failure, 300
    rational use of, 300
  thiazide
    dosages of, 302
    introduction of, 300
    toxicity of, 302
Diuril, 259
Dizziness, 604
  and aortic stenosis, 405
  in cardiac arrhythmia, 540
  Holter monitoring findings in, 436
  in hypertrophic obstructive cardiomyopathy, 540
  in hypotension, 611
  in pulmonary stenosis, 333
  and syncope, 39
Dobutamine, 183, 316, 318
Dobutrex, in cardiac failure, 318
Dopamine, 183, 184
  in heart failure, 318
Doppler blood velocity measurement, 604
Doppler echocardiography, 82
Doppler equation, 85
Doppler transducer, 84
Doppler ultrasound, 85
Dorsal root pain, 38
Doxorubicin
  cardiotoxic effect of, 313
  and rheumatic fever, 537
dp/dt, 77
dp/dt$_{max}$, 77
Dressler beats, 496
Dressler's syndrome, 187
Dropped beats, 445
Drug(s)
  and acute myocardial damage, 537
  antiarrhythmic, administration of
    long-term oral, 489
    rapid, 488
  effect on murmurs, 62
  effect on ECG, in hypertension, 230
  in heart failure, withdrawal of, 313
  for hypertension, **259–272**
  in management of arrhythmias, 492
  psychotropic, 488

Dry pericarditis, 573
Ductus arteriosus, 4, 11
  patent, 290, **346–349**
    and aortopulmonary window, 347
    chest x-ray of, 348
    and continuous murmur, phonocardiogram of, 61
    diastolic murmur due to, 60
    murmur of, schematic diagram of, 58
Duroziez's sign, 416
dv/dt, 20
Dyrenium, 259
Dyspepsia, as symptom of chronic constrictive pericarditis, 581
Dysphagia, as symptom of cardiovascular syphilis, 599
Dyspnea, **34–36,** 289, 479, 586, 589, 590
  in acute myocardial infarction, 165
  in acute pulmonary edema, 35
  due to anxiety, 36
  and aortic incompetence, 414
  cardiac versus pulmonary, 35
  chemical stimuli as cause of, 35
  in chronic constrictive pericarditis, 581
  diagnostic value of, 36
  episodic, 35
  on exertion, and aortic stenosis, 405
  in Fallot's tetralogy, 338
  in heart disease, 34
  in heart failure, 290
  at high altitude, 36
  in hypertrophic obstructive cardiomyopathy, 540
  and low cardiac output, 35
  mechanism of, 34
  and mitral incompetence, 381, 393
  and mitral stenosis, 369
  in normal subjects, 34
  paroxysmal, 35
    nocturnal, 289
      and mitral stenosis, 371
    as symptom of heart failure, 291
  pulmonary congestion as cause of, 35
  in pulmonary stenosis, 333
  at rest, 36
Dysrhythmias, in acute myocardial infarction, incidence of, 173
Dystrophia myotonica, 566

"E" point, 86
E point separation, 176
Ear, examination of, in patients with heart disease, 46
Ear crease, as sign of premature atherosclerotic changes, 46
Ear oximeter, 101
Earlobe sign, 46
Ebstein's malformation, 119, **355–357**
  anatomic features of, 356
  chest x-ray of, 356
  ECG and pressure tracing of, 357
ECG, 13
  in acute myocardial infarction, 167
  and angina pectoris, 148
  effect of drugs on, in hypertension, 230
  in hypertrophic obstructive cardiomyopathy, 541

ECG (cont'd)
  in hypertrophy, 291
  intracardiac, 113
  investigations using, special, **93–95**
  monitoring of
    ambulatory, 484
    continuous, 93
  recording of, **81–82**
Echocardiogram
  A mode, 84
  aortic root, 236
  aortic valve, 86
  B mode, 84
  in cardiomyopathy, 91
  in left atrial myxoma, 609
  M mode, 84, 89
    normal findings in, 86, 87
    showing aortic valve and aorta, 89
    showing normal mitral valve, 88
    showing right and left ventricles, 89
  normal, 292
Echocardiography, **82–92,** 328, 582
  in atrial septal defect, 328
  bedside, 176
  in cardiac tamponade, 579
  clinical uses of, 88
  Doppler, 82
  in heart failure, 292
  left ventricle, 89, 228
  limitations of, 90
  in mitral stenosis, 374
  mitral valve, 86
  motion, 84
  in pulmonary stenosis, 336
  two-dimensional, 84, 90
    in angina pectoris, 151
  in ventricular septal defect, 345
Echovirus myocarditis, 531
Ectopic atrial depolarization, 467
Ectopic beats, 70
  during injection of contrast material, pressure tracing of, 71
  effect on arterial pressure, 73
  heart rate in, 42
  in hypertrophic obstructive cardiomyopathy, 541
  junctional, 47
  ventricular, 117
Ectopic P wave, 467
Edecrin, 260
Edema, 588
  of ankles, 289
    in chronic lung disease, 594
    and right heart failure, 593
  cerebral, in cerebral embolism, 603
  dependent, as sign of right ventricular failure, 293
  facial, as sign of cardiovascular syphilis, 599
  idiopathic, 41
  mild, treatment of, 302
  pitting
    as evidence of congestive heart failure, 50
    as sign of right heart failure, 294
  in preeclampsia-eclampsia, 621
  pulmonary. See Pulmonary edema.
  sacral, 289
  as symptom of heart disease, 40
Edrophonium, in supraventricular tachycardia, 477

Edwards procedure, for transposition of great arteries, 358
Effort syncope, 39
Effort syndrome, 38, 613
Effusions, 573
  and ascites, in heart failure, 313
  pericardial, 44, 126, **575–577**
    acute, 303
    cardiac tamponade in, echocardiogram of, 579
    chest x-ray of, 576
    in heart failure, 312
    without tamponade, 575
  pleural, 579
Effusive constrictive pericarditis, 581
Ehlers-Danlos syndrome, 325
Eisenmenger's reaction, 349
Eisenmenger's syndrome, 125, **349–352,** 595
  acquired, 330
  chest x-ray of, 350
  ECG of, 351
Ejection click
  phonocardiogram of, 55
  pulmonary systolic or aortic, schematic diagram of, 52
  schematic diagram of, 58
  systolic, 56
Ejection fraction, 70
Ejection murmurs, 59
  pansystolic, long, in hypertrophic obstructive cardiomyopathy, 60
  systolic, 58
    aortic, 58
    pulmonary, 58
Electric blankets, as source of electrical interference in recording of ECG, 81
Electrical alternans, 576
Electrical analogs and cardiac measurements, **74–75**
Electrical countershock, 127
Electrical impulse, propagation of, 13
Electrocardiography, **81–82.** *For items concerning electrocardiogram and electrocardiographic, see* ECG.
  exercise, **93–95**
  stress
    and angina pectoris, 148
    precautions during, 149
  treadmill, 94
Electrocution, risk of, in recording of ECG, 81
Electrode catheters, right atrial, 467
Electrode paste, 81
Electrode, platinum, 69
Electrophysiologic studies, 113
Electrophysiology, 432
Embolectomy, 604
Emboli
  cerebral, 221
  in infective endocarditis, 516
  renal, 513
  in subacute infective endocarditis, 512
  systemic, 482
  risk of, 480
Embolic material, nature of, 603
Embolism
  agonal, 587
  arterial, 177
  causes of, 605

Embolism (cont'd)
  cerebral, 221, 603, 604
  in chronic cor pulmonale, 595
  coronary, 604
  coronary artery, 134
  following cardiac catheterization, 118
  mesenteric, 605
  paradoxic, 605
  peripheral, of extremities, 604
  pulmonary. See Pulmonary embolism.
  renal, 605
  sites of, 603
  splenic, 605
  systemic, 599, **603–605**
    and mitral incompetence, 395
    and mitral stenosis, 371
    and mixed mitral stenosis and incompetence, 379, 384
Embolization, systemic, as complication of arteritis, 602
Emergency room procedures, in acute myocardial infarction, 178
Emetine
  and acute myocardial damage, 537
  in heart failure, 313
Emotional factors influencing blood pressure, 218
Emphysema, 35, 593, 597
Enalapril, in hypertension, 268, 269
Encainide, 490
  and preexcitation syndromes, 460
Encephalopathy, hypertensive, 234
Endarteritis, 607
  obliterans, 599
End-diastolic pressure, left ventricular, 71
Endocardial cushion defect, complete, 325
Endocarditis
  bacterial, prevention of, 517
  as complication of bedside catheterization, 106
  echocardiograms in, 514
  fungal, 516, 521
  due to gram-negative bacteria, 521
  infective, 49, 292, **510–526**
    acute differentiated from subacute, 510
    antibiotic prophylaxis in, 510, 517
    in aortic stenosis, 411
    in atrial septal defect, 332
    cardiac failure in, 523
    chemotherapeutic agents for, 518, 520, 521
    clinical features of, **512–518**
    complexity of management of, 510
    differential diagnosis of, bacteremia in, 517
    hosts likely to develop, 511
    microorganisms causing, 511
    and mitral incompetence, 387, 396
    and mixed mitral stenosis and incompetence, 384
    pathogenesis and pathology of, 511
    persistent and resistant, 523
    prognosis of, 523
    and prosthetic valves, 522
    in pulmonary stenosis, 336
    treatment of, 518
  Libman-Sacks, 557

Endocarditis (cont'd)
  Löffler's, 562
  prevention of, 517
    in mixed mitral stenosis and incompetence, 384
  prosthetic valve, 522
  rheumatic, and valvular disease, 368
  splinter hemorrhages as sign of, 49
  due to staphylococci, 516, 520
  due to *Streptococcus faecalis*, 520
  due to *Streptococcus viridans*, 520
  subacute, in patients with negative blood cultures, 523
Endocrine dysfunction, in hypertension, 227
Endomyocardial biopsy, 114, 531
Endomyocardial fibrosis, 553, 562, 582
Endothelial damage, 603
  theory of, 134
End-pulmonary capillary oxygen saturation, 68
Enophthalmos, as sign of cardiovascular syphilis, 599
Entry flow, 16
Enzyme inhibitors, angiotensin-converting, 268
Enzymes, myocardial, 166
  determinations of, 95
Eosinophilia, in arteritis, 602
Epicardial mapping, 458
Epidemic typhus fever, myocarditis due to, 617
Epigastric pulsations, 51
Epileptic seizures, 39, 121, 123
Epinephrine, 123
  in ventricular fibrillation or tachycardia, 123
Ergometer, cycle, 94, 113, 148
Ergonovine test, 113
Erythema
  annulare, in rheumatic fever, 535
  marginatum, in rheumatic fever, 535
  nodosum, 45
Erythromycin, 601
  in prevention of endocarditis, 517
Escape pacemaker(s), 446
Escape rhythms, 173, 432, 497
  passive, 472
Esidrix, 259
Esophageal leads, 467, 474
Esophageal spasm, pain of, 38
Essential hypertension. See Hypertension, essential.
Estrogens, and atherosclerosis, 137
Ethacrynate sodium, 260
Ethacrynic acid, 259, 300
  in cardiac failure, 302
  dosages of, 302
  effect on serum electrolytes, 261
  sites of action of, 301
Ethmozin, 490
Excitability and refractoriness, 432
Excitable gap, 434
Excitation, of heart, 14
Excitation-contraction coupling, 21
  mechanism of, 73
Exercise
  and circulatory physiology, 30
  and dyspnea, 34
  effect on normal values, 78
  in electrocardiography, **93–94**

Exercise (cont'd)
  first heart sound in, 52
  graded, 159, 188
    electrocardiographic studies of, 148
  programs of, 159
Exercise testing, 101
  and angina pectoris, 148
  in myocardial infarction, 180
Exertional fatigue, 291
Expiration, 52
  effect on murmurs, 62
External counterpulsation, 130
Extracardiac factors, in heart failure, 303
Extrasystoles, atrial, 466
Extremities, peripheral embolism of, 604
Eyes, examination of, in patients with heart disease, 46

"F" point, 86
F waves, 480
Facial edema, as sign of cardiovascular syphilis, 599
Fainting
  in Fallot's tetralogy, 39, 340
  in hypotension, 611
  in pulmonary stenosis, 333
  in systemic embolism, 604
  vasovagal, 39
Fallot's tetralogy, 40, 43, 61, **338**
  anatomic features of, 339
  chest x-ray of, 339, 341
  differential diagnosis of, 336, 342
  ECG of, 340
  fainting attacks in, 39, 340
  indicator dilution curve of, 68
False aneurysm, traumatic, 615
Family history, as risk factor in atherosclerosis, 137
Fat emboli, 588
Fatigue
  exertional, 291
  in heart disease, 40
  in heart failure, 291
  in hypertrophic obstructive cardiomyopathy, 540
  in right ventricular failure, 293
Femoral arterial occlusion, 605
Femoral catheterization, percutaneous, 118
Femoral pulse, 43, 48
  and radial pulse, simultaneous palpation of, 43
Fetal hydantoin syndrome, 620
Fever
  familial Mediterranean, 561
  in rheumatic fever, 534
  in subacute infective endocarditis, 512
  as symptom of arteritis, 602
Fibrillation
  atrial, 181, 289, **479**
    chronic, 480
    conditions associated with, 480
    effect on arterial pressure, 73
    effect of quinidine on, 483
    heart rate in, 42
    in mitral stenosis, 372, 376, 480

Fibrillation (cont'd)
  atrial (cont'd)
    and mitral valve disease, pressure tracing of, 73
    and mixed mitral stenosis and mitral incompetence, 383
    onset of, 369
    premature beats in, 466, 467
    pressure tracing in, 49
    recurrence of, prevention of, 482
    in Wolff-Parkinson-White syndrome, 457
    treatment of, 459
  ventricular, 118, 140, 141, 142, 181, 487, 493, **500–502**
    in acute myocardial infarction, 173
    defibrillation in, 144
    ECG of, 494
    emergency measures in, 143
    late, 181
    patient education in, 143
    prehospital follow-up data on, 502
    prevention of, 493
    prophylactic drugs to prevent recurrences, 502
    resuscitation in, 143
    risk factors in, control of, 502
    treatment of, 123, 181
    in ventricular premature beats, 486
Fibrinous pericarditis, 573
Fibromuscular hyperplasia, of renal arteries, 239
Fibrosis, 593
  endomyocardial, 553, 562, 582
Fibrous tissue, resection of, 583
Fick principle, 65
  in estimation of intracardiac and intrapulmonary shunts, 66
Filling pressures, 288
Filling sound, 581
Fingers
  examination of, in patients with heart disease, 49
  and nail beds, clubbing of, 49
First-degree (partial) atrioventricular block, 440
  atrioventricular conduction defect in, 443
  treatment of, 447
First heart sound, 52
  loudness of, and length of PR interval, 52
  and mitral stenosis, 372
  phonocardiogram and ECG of, 52
  in relation to fourth heart sound, 56
  split, schematic diagram of, 52
First-pass technique of angiography, 99
Fixed-rate pacemaker, 127
Flecainide, 491
Floppy valve, 388
Floppy valve syndrome, 386
Flowmeter techniques, of blood flow measurement, 69
Flurazepam, 247, 476
Flutter, atrial, 479, 480
  effect of quinidine on, 483
  recurrence of, prevention of, 482
Flutter-fibrillation, atrial, 480
Fogarty balloon catheter, 118, 605
Fontan's procedure, 360
Foramen ovale, 11, 595

Foreign bodies, as embolic material, 603
Fourth heart sound, 56
Fraction, regurgitant, 72
Framingham Study, 142
Frank lead system, 93
Frank-Starling curve(s), 288
Frank-Starling law of heart, 19
Frank-Starling mechanism, 52
Friction rubs
  pericardial, 62, 177, 574
  pleural, 597
Friedreich's ataxia, 566
Fundal changes, in hypertension, 224
Fungi, endocarditis due to, 521
Furosemide, 183, 259, 260, 300
  dosages of, 302
  in cardiac failure, 302
  sites of action of, 301
Fusion ventricular beats, 494, 496

Gallbladder disease, pain of, 38
Gallop(s)
  atrial, 293
  diastolic, phonocardiogram of, 57
  palpable, 51
  presystolic, 55, 56
    or atrial, schematic diagram of, 52
    phonocardiogram of, 57
  S_3, 290
  summation, 56
Gallop rhythm, 56
Gamma counting camera, 97
Ganglionic blocking agents, 209, 267
Gas exchange, 66
Gas tension, 64
Gastrointestinal disorders, and chest pain, 155
Gated blood pool scanning, 172
Gated equilibrium technique of angiography, 99
Gensini catheter, 110
Gentamicin
  in genitourinary and gastrointestinal tract surgery, 518
  in prevention of endocarditis, 517
Giant *a* wave, 48
Giant cell formation, 601
Giant left atrium, 576
Giant *v* wave, 48
Girdle pain, 38
Gitaligin, dosages and routes of administration, 304
Glenn's operation, for tricuspid atresia, 360
Glomerular endotheliosis, in preeclampsia, 622
Glomerular nephritis, 513
Glucagon, in heart failure, 319
Glutamic-oxaloacetic transaminase, serum, 95, 166, 591
Goiter, 46
Goldblatt disease, 214
Gooseneck deformity, in ostium primum defect, 330
Gorlin formula, 74, 408
Graded exercise, 159, 188
  electrocardiographic studies of, 148
Gradients, pressure, 74
Grafts, aortocoronary, 69

Graham Steell murmur, 351, 372, 424, 594
  in cor pulmonale, 596
Gram-negative bacteria, endocarditis due to, 511, 521
Granuloma, pulmonary, 593
Gravity, and circulatory system, 12
Great arteries, transposition of, **357–358**
  anatomic features of, 359
  corrected, 358
Great vessels, 2
Ground loops, 81
Growing pains, in rheumatic fever, 534
Growth, and aging, 28
Growth hormone, excessive production of, 253
Guanabenz, in hypertension, 259, 265
Guanethidine, 259, **265**, 271
  adverse effects of, 261
  side effects in, 265

H^+ ion concentration, 65
Hamman-Rich disease, 593
HDL, 135, 137
Headaches
  in hypertension, 219
  as symptom of arteritis, 602
Heart. *See also* Cardiac.
  abnormal position of, 362
  anatomy of, **1–11**
    functional, **18–23**
    microscopic, **7–8**
  anterior view of, 1
    with anterior wall removed to show right ventricular cavity, 5
  apex of, 1
  apex beat of, 51
  axis of, 1
  boot-shaped, 341
  chambers of, **4–6**
    volumes of, angiographic measurements of, 70
  clinical physiology of, **64–79**
  cross section of, showing positions of left and right ventricles, 22
  diseases of
    atherosclerotic coronary, pathogenesis of, 133
    and chest deformities, 50
    congenital, **324–367**
      cyanotic, 35, 49, 64
      and mitral incompetence, 387
      and surgery, 629
    coronary, **132–208**. *See also* Coronary heart disease.
      classification of, 132
      pathogenesis of, 139
    dyspnea in, 34
    functional and therapeutic classification of, 41
    hypertensive, **209–286**
    ischemic, 133
    and lung disease, differentiation of, 596
    and neuropathic disorders, 566
    nutritional, 555
    physical examination of patient with, **42–63**

Heart (cont'd)
  diseases of (cont'd)
    in pregnancy, classification of, 617
    psychologic, 613
    pulmonary, **586–598**
    recognition of, 627
    rheumatic, and valvular disease, 368
    in surgical patients, **626–631**
    thyrotoxic, 548
    traumatic, **614–615**
    and mitral incompetence, 386
    visible pulsation as sign of, 50
  disordered action of, 613
  disorders of, miscellaneous, **609–616**
  displacement of, due to abnormalities of thoracic cage, 362
  electrical activity of, 13
  embryology of, **8–11**
  enlargement of, 288, 577
    in cardiovascular syphilis, 599
    in heart failure, 291
    in heart and lung disease, 597
    in pulmonary hypertension, 596
  examination of, **50–62**
    in hypertension, 224
  excitation in, sequence of, 14
  external appearance of, **1–4**
  inspection of, 50
  left
    catheterization of, 70
      complications of, 118
      different approaches to, 109
    failure of, 593
      as complication of arteritis, 602
    from left side with left ventricular free wall and mitral valve cut away, 5
    with left ventricular wall turned back to show mitral valve, 6
  left-sided aspect of, 2
  lesions of, congenital, complex and combined, **357–361**
  lymphatics of, 7
  mural thrombosis of, 134
  muscle cell of, 7
  palpation of, 51
  physiology of, 12
  position within pericardial sac, 1
  posterior aspect of, 2
  radiologic examination of, 295
  revascularization of, 192
  right, with right wall reflected to show right atrium, 4
  right-sided aspect of, 2
  rupture of, 177, 187
  as servant of circulation, 31
  shadow of
    abnormal, as sign of heart failure, 295
    size of, 82
  soldier's, 613
  systemic diseases affecting, 311
  transplantation of, 320
  tumors of, 577, **609**
  valves of, 6. See also specific types.
    artificial, multiple involvement, 423
Heart failure, 48, 65, **287–323**, 607
  acute, 295
    in infective endocarditis, 516, 519

Heart failure (cont'd)
  in acute myocardial infarction, 165, 175
  and atrial septal defect, 330
  causes of, 287
  clinical findings in, **289–295**
  compensatory mechanisms in, 287
  congestive, 76, 589
    and complex ventricular premature beats, 484
    diagnosis of, 290
    in Fallot's tetralogy, 338
    in rheumatic fever, 536
    right-sided, 290
  definitions of, 287
  differential diagnosis of, 297
  diuretic therapy in, 300
  factors precipitating, 287
  hemodynamic and pathophysiologic features of, **287–289**
  high-output, **289**, 294
  and hypertension, 219, **232**, 291
  in infective endocarditis, 523
  laboratory findings in, 297
  left, 288, 593
    as complication of arteritis, 602
    periodic breathing in, 51
    pulsus alternans in, 44
  with low-output state, inotropic agents for, 318
  in lung disease, prevention of, 596
  mechanisms of, 32
  mild or moderate, treatment of, 182
  peripartum, 564
  prognosis in, 321
  radiologic examination in, **295–297**
  response, 76
  right, 40, 289, 292
    acute, 588
    in chronic cor pulmonale, 593
    secondary to chronic lung disease, 587, **593**
  severe, emergency treatment of, 182, **319–320**
  simulation of, by noncardiac and nonthoracic conditions, 297
  "snowman," 361
  sodium reabsorption in, 300
  and surgery, 629
  treatment of, 182, **298–321**
    vasodilators in, 315
  and ventricular premature beats, 494
Heart-lung transplantation, in Eisenmenger's syndrome, 352
Heart murmurs, 59
  effects of posture on, 62
  heard in back, 50
  in hypertrophic obstructive cardiomyopathy, 540
  timing of, 58
Heart sounds. See Sound(s), heart.
Heart surgery, 192
  factors influencing, 193
Heberden, William, 37
Heimlich maneuver, 122
Hematocrit, 69
Hematuria, 50, 605
  microscopic, as sign of embolism, 512
Hemiblock, 451, 452

Hemiplegia
  in cerebral embolism, 603
  as complication of arteritis, 602
  as symptom of arteritis, 602
Hemochromatosis, **560–561**
Hemoconcentration, 603
Hemodialysis, 607
Hemodynamic factors influencing murmurs, 61
Hemodynamic findings in Fallot's tetralogy, 338
Hemodynamic indices, normal values, 78
Hemodynamic interaction between stenosis and incompetence, in mixed mitral valve lesions, 381
Hemodynamic monitoring
  bedside, 175
  in myocardial infarction, 184
Hemodynamic and volume changes, in pregnancy, 621
Hemodynamically insignificant aortic valve disease, anatomic features of, 402
Hemodynamically insignificant mitral incompetence, 386
  click and murmurs in, phonocardiogram of, 58
  late systolic murmur of, 58
Hemodynamically significant mitral incompetence, 390
Hemodynamics, of aorta and arterial bed, 23
Hemoglobin, 64
  blue (reduced), 64
    dissociation curve of, 64
  red (oxygenated), 64
Hemopericardium, 177, 573, 575
Hemoptysis, 177, 221, 587, 592, 597
  and cough, as symptoms of heart disease, 39
  and mitral stenosis, 371
  as symptom of cardiovascular syphilis, 599
Hemorrhages
  cerebral, 221
  as complication of cardiac catheterization, 118
  into lung, 592
  splinter, as sign of endocarditis, 49
Hemorrhagic telangiectasia, hereditary, 587
Hemosiderin, 561
Hemosiderosis, 560
Henle, loop of, 300
Heparin, 589, 592
Hepatic congestion, 581
Hepatic distention, 38
Hepatic and renal changes in preeclampsia, 622
Hepatojugular reflux, 47
  as sign of right heart failure, 293
Hereditary hemorrhagic telangiectasia, 587
  lesions of, 45
Hernia
  hiatal, 155
  pain of, 38
  operation for, in acute cor pulmonale, 588
Heroin addicts
  overdose in, dyspnea due to, 35

Heroin addicts (cont'd)
 and pulmonary edema, 291
Herpes zoster, 155
 pain associated with, 38
Hexamethonium, 209, 254, 267
Hiatal hernia, 155
 pain of, 38
High-altitude pulmonary edema, 124
High-density lipoproteins, 135, 137
 and risk of coronary heart disease, 136
High-output failure, 289, 294, 606
High-output state, 606
 and systolic ejection murmur, 59
High-voltage P waves, 609
High-voltage QRS complexes, 606
Hill's sign, 416
His bundle, 7
 catheter ablation of
  in atrial tachycardia, 460
  in supraventricular tachycardia, 478
His bundle catheter, 113
His bundle recordings, 472, 497
 in bradycardia-tachycardia syndrome, 438
 diagrammatic illustration of, 435
 in first-degree (partial) atrioventricular block, 443
 indications for, 453
 in second-degree atrioventricular block, 445
 in third-degree (complete) atrioventricular block, 446
 in Wolff-Parkinson-White syndrome, 457
Histamine, in pheochromocytoma, 250
History taking, **34–41**
HLA-B5, in rheumatic fever, 533
Hoarseness
 in cardiovascular syphilis, 599
 in heart disease, 40
Holosystolic murmurs, 59
Holter monitor, 188
Holter monitoring, 148, 436, 502
Homans' sign, 50
Homeostatic mechanisms, and blood pressure, 210
Horner's syndrome, as sign of cardiovascular syphilis, 599
Hot spots, 170
Howard test, 241
Hum, venous, 61
Hydralazine, 184, 259, 260, **264,** 271, 316
 adverse effects of, 261, 265
 in afterload reduction, 125
 in cardiac failure, 317
 dosage and route of administration of, 315
 during pregnancy, 621
 in heart failure, 316
 and nitrates, 316
 systemic lupus erythematosuslike syndrome due to, 558
 as vasodilator, 125
Hydrochlorothiazide, 259
 effect on serum electrolytes, 264
Hydrodiuril, 259
Hydrogen, 69
Hydrothorax, 290
 as sign of right heart failure, 294

17-Hydroxycorticosteroids, 247
5-Hydroxyindoleacetic acid, 425
11β-Hydroxylase deficiency, 248
17α-Hydroxylase deficiency, 248
21-Hydroxylase deficiency, 248
Hygroton, 259
Hyperaldosteronism, 243, 246, 248
Hyperbaric chambers, 124
Hypercapnia, 35, 586
 and premature ventricular beats, 487
Hypercholesterolemia, 134, 135, 501
 familial, 136
 type II, 135
Hypercortisolism, 246
Hyperdynamic cardiac impulse, as sign of arteriovenous fistula, 606
Hyperemia, reactive, 25
Hyperglycemia, asymptomatic, 136
Hyperkalemia, ECG in, 82
Hyperlipidemia
 primary, nondietary treatment of, 156
 as risk factor in atherosclerosis, 134
 and sudden death, 502
 type IV, 156
Hyperosmolarity, 71
Hyperplasia
 cellular intimal, 225
 fibromuscular, of renal arteries, 239
Hyperpnea, 34
Hyperstat, 260
Hypertension, 43, 45, **209–286,** 501
 and age, 218
 atrial natriuretic factors in, 217
 baroreceptors in, 214
 in black population, 218
 borderline, 256
 and brain, 226
 central nervous system in, 214
 clinical findings in, **219–230**
 complications of, **233–237**
 and coronary disease, 232
 course and prognosis in, 230
 differentiation of, from myocardial infarction, 230
 and ejection murmur, 59
 electrocardiographic findings in, 227
 epidemiologic studies of, **218–237**
 essential
  pathophysiology of, 214
  in pregnancy, **620–621**
  treatment of, **254–277**
 established, 212
 etiology and classification of, 209
 follow-up of
  evaluation in, 274
  therapy for, 275
 general measures in, **258–259**
 intravenous urograms in, 230
 kidney in, 226
 labile, defined, 211
 malignant, 231
  ECG of, 229
  hexamethonium treatment of, 272
  symptoms marking onset of, 232
 mild, 230, 256
 and mortality rates, 219
 oral contraceptives causing, 252
 pathophysiology of, **210–218**

Hypertension (cont'd)
 phases in, 211
 physical signs in, 221
 in preeclampsia-eclampsia, 621
 prognosis of, 233
 psychologic factors in, 217
 pulmonary. *See* Pulmonary hypertension.
 renal angiogram in, 240
 renal artery stenosis with, 244
 renin-angiotensin system in, 215
 as risk factor in atherosclerosis, 136
 secondary, 209, **237**
  diseases and disorders associated with, **237–254**
  pathophysiology of, 217
 prevalence of, 238
 severe, in children, 268
 social and psychologic factors in, 217
 and sodium intake, 214
 and sudden death, 502
 and surgery, 628
 sympathetic nervous system in, 214
 systemic, 26, 586
  loud aortic second sound in, 55
  phonocardiogram of, 55
  or pulmonary, fourth heart sound due to, 56
  as sign of arteritis, 602
 systolic, 213
 treatment of, 255
  according to severity of, 257
  effect on prognosis, 233
 vascular complications of, 256
 x-ray findings in, 230
Hypertensive disorders of pregnancy, **620–624**
Hypertensive encephalopathy, 234
Hypertensive heart disease, **209–286**
Hypertensive heart failure, 232, 291
Hypertensive retinopathy, 223, 224
Hyperthyroidism, in heart failure, 311
Hypertrophic cardiomyopathy, 467
 obstructive, 59, 60, 91, 411, 539
  long pansystolic ejection murmur in, 60
Hypertrophic subaortic stenosis, idiopathic, 539
Hypertrophy, 51
 asymmetric, 539
 cardiac, 178
  and cardiac failure, 225
  and compliance, 287
 concentric, 288
 left atrial, ECG of, 295
 left ventricular, 227
  diagnosis of, 228
  and drugs, 230
  ECG of, 288
  in hypertension, 228
  mortality rate and initial degree of, 231
 right ventricular, 587
  ECG of, 295, 336
  as sign of right ventricular failure, 293
Hyperventilation, 35, 50, 65
Hypokalemia, 260, 300
 effect on ECG, 83
 and premature ventricular beats, 492

Hyponatremia
  depletional, 303
  dilutional, 289
  in diuretic therapy, 303
Hypotension, 43, 116, **611–613**
  in acute myocardial infarction, 165
  postural, 300
  and premature ventricular beats, 487
Hypotensive therapy, object of, 269
Hypothermia, 124
Hypothyroid cardiomyopathy, chest x-ray in, 552
Hypoventilation, 51, 65
  alveolar, 593
Hypovolemia, 300
Hypoxia, 35, 68, 124, 476
  alveolar, 586, 593
  in chronic cor pulmonale, 593
  arterial, 593
  at high altitude, 36
  nonparoxysmal supraventricular (junctional) tachycardia due to, 472
  and premature ventricular beats, 487

I bands, 7
^{131}I hippurate, 242
Idiopathic hypertrophic subaortic stenosis, 539
Idiopathic long QT syndrome, 460
Idioventricular rhythm, accelerated, 173, 497
  ECG of, 495
  treatment of, 181
IHSS, 539
Ileitis, regional, 561
Image defects, 171
Image intensifiers, 111
Immediate diastolic murmur, 60
  in chronic cor pulmonale, 596
  schematic diagram of, 58
Immune complex nephritis, 513
Immunologic hypothesis of preeclampsia-eclampsia, 622
Immunosuppressive drugs, 603
Impending death, feeling of, 38
Impulses
  palpable, 51
  rocking, paradoxic, 51
  tapping, in mitral valve disease, 51
Inactivity, as risk factor in atherosclerosis, 138
Inderal, 259, 260
Indigestion, in acute myocardial infarction, 165
Indocyanine green, in measurement of cardiac output, 66
Infarct(s)
  anterior and inferior, atrioventricular conduction defects in, 442
  myocardial, size of, 171
Infarction
  anterior
    atrioventricular conduction defects in, 442
    conduction defects in, 174
  cerebral, 177
    thrombotic, 221
  inferior
    atrioventricular conduction defects in, 442

Infarction (cont'd)
  inferior (cont'd)
    conduction defects in, 174
  myocardial. See Myocardial infarction.
  nontransmural, 164, 170
  pulmonary, 35, 586
    and mitral stenosis, 377
  right ventricular, 166, 182
  subendocardial, 164
  topography of, 153
  transmural, 164, 170
Infective endocarditis, 49, **510–526**
  acute
    clinical features of, **516–518**
    differentiated from subacute, 510
  antibiotics in, 510, 517
  in aortic incompetence, 421
  in aortic stenosis, 411
  cardiac failure in, 523
  in click-murmur syndrome, 389
  complexity of management of, 510
  differential diagnosis of, 517
  in hemodynamically insignificant aortic valve disease, 401
  hosts likely to develop, 511
  microorganisms causing, 511
  and mitral incompetence, 389, 396
  in mitral stenosis, prevention of, 377
  and mixed mitral stenosis and incompetence, 384
  pathogenesis and pathology of, 511
  persistent and resistant, 523
  and prosthetic valves, 522
  in pulmonary stenosis, 337
  subacute, clinical features of, **512–516**
Inflammation, aseptic, 573
Inflow murmur, diastolic, schematic diagram of, 58
Infranodal block, complete, 175
Infundibular muscular spasm, 340
Infundibular stenosis, 59
Inhibitors, angiotensin-converting enzyme, 268
Inotropic agents, 318
Inspiration
  effect on murmurs, 62
  effect on pressure tracings, 49
Intensive care unit, resuscitation in, 121
Intercostal neuritis, 155
Intermittent capture of ventricles, 472
Interval
  AH, 435
  critical coupling, 468
  HV, 435, 442
  PR, 435
  length of, effect on loudness of first heart sound, 52
  QT, prolongation of, 482
  S_2–OS, and mitral stenosis, 371
Interventricular septum, perforation of, 185
Intra-aortic balloon counterpulsation, 320
Intra-aortic balloon pumping, 130
Intracardiac electrograms, 113
Intracardiac and intrapulmonary shunts
  effect on blood flow, 66, 67
  estimation by Fick principle, 67

Intracardiac pressure
  measurements of, in atrial septal defect, 330
  rise in, rate of, 577
Intracardiac recording, in Wolff-Parkinson-White syndrome, 457
Intracardiac sounds, extra, 56
Intracoronary thrombolytic therapy, for myocardial infarction, 114
Intrapericardial calcification, 582
Intrathoracic pressure, 101
  negative, 44
Intropin, in heart failure, 318
Intubation, and premature ventricular beats, 487
Invasive investigations, **105–120**
Inversine, 259, 267
Iodine, protein-bound, 549
Iodine-labeled albumin, 69
Iron, and hemochromatosis, 560
Ischemia, 476
  cerebral, 39
  myocardial, 140, 299
    ECG of, 451
    noninvasive investigation of, 141
  in myocardial infarction, 164
  nonparoxysmal supraventricular (junctional) tachycardia due to, 472
  and premature ventricular beats, 486
Ischemic attacks, transient, 604
Ischemic cardiac pain. See Angina pectoris.
Ischemic cardiomyopathy, 538
Ischemic heart disease, and mitral incompetence, 386
Ischemic zone of excitability, 499
Ismelin, 259
Isometric exercise, and circulatory physiology, 30
Isometric handgrip, effect on murmurs, 62
Isoproterenol, 492
  for bradycardia, 124
  effect in hypertrophic obstructive cardiomyopathy, 542
  in heart failure, 318
Isoptin, 476
Isosorbide dinitrate, 179, 315
  in afterload reduction, 125
  dosage and route of administration, 316
  in heart failure, 182, 315
  as vasodilator, 125
Isotopes
  in myocardial infarction, 170, 171
  radioactive, for measuring cardiac output, 66
Isovolumetric contraction, 15

Janeway's lesion, 512
Jarisch-Herxheimer reaction, 600
Jarisch-von Bezold reflex, vagal, 174
Jaw claudication, as symptom of arteritis, 602
Joint pains, in rheumatic fever, 534
Jones criteria, for diagnosis of rheumatic disease, 534
Judkins catheter, 110
Judkins technique, 109, 112

Jugular vein
  internal and external, 46
    distention of, as sign of cardiovascular syphilis, 599
    pulse of
      examination of, 46
      in paroxysmal atrial tachycardia, 470
      in right ventricular failure, 293
Junctional ectopic beats, 47
Junctional pacemakers, secondary, escape of, 472
Junctional premature beats, 467
Junctional reciprocating tachycardia
  paroxysmal, 469
  treatment of, 478
Junctional rhythms, with atrioventricular dissociation, 478
Junctional (supraventricular) tachycardia, nonparoxysmal, 469, **472–478**
  defined, 472

Keith-Wagener (KW) changes, and blood pressure readings, 223
Kerley's B lines, 166, 296, 373
  as x-ray signs in heart failure, 296
Kidney(s). See also Renal.
  circulation in, 29
  in hypertension, 226
  symptoms of, 220
Knock, pericardial, 56, 581
Krypton, radioactive, 69
Kussmaul's sign, 48, 578, 581
  ECG of, 578
Kveim-Siltzbach skin tests, 555
Kyphoscoliosis, 110, 362, 363
  chest x-ray of, 363
Kyphosis, 50, 593

Labetalol, and hypertension, 267
Labile hypertension, 211
Labor and puerperium, physiologic changes during, 618
Laboratory tests, standard, 80
Lactate dehydrogenase, 95, 591
  serum, 166
Laminar flow, diagram of, 17
Laminectomy, 606
Lanatoside C, dosages and routes of administration, 304
Lanoxin, dosages and routes of administration, 304
Laplace, law of, 20, 288
Lasix, 259, 260
Lateral accessory pathway, 454
LDH, 95
LDL, 135
LE cell, 489
LE cell preparation, positive, 575
Leads
  esophageal, 467
  Lewis, 496
    bipolar, 467
Left anterior hemiblock, 452
Left atrial hypertrophy, ECG of, 295
Left atrial myxoma, 376, 586, 609
Left atrial pressure, indirect, 106
Left bundle branch block, 53, 54, 448
  intermittent, ECG of, 450

Left heart
  catheterization of, 70
    complications of, 118
    different approaches to, 109
  failure of, 593
    as complication of arteritis, 602
Left posterior hemiblock, 452
Left ventricle
  aneurysm of, 185
  decompensation in, mechanisms leading to, 225
  disease of, associated with mitral incompetence, 393
  echocardiography of, 186, 227
  ejection time, 102
  end-diastolic pressure in, 71, 288
  failure of, 51, 288, 290, 411
    acute, 175
    in acute myocardial infarction, 165
    in aortic incompetence, 415, 421
    in aortic stenosis, 411
    in cardiovascular syphilis, 599
    pulsus alternans in, 44
  function of, 102
    assessment of, 70
    effect of contrast material on, 71
  hypertrophy of
    asymmetric, 539
    diagnosis of, 228
    and dilatation of, 414
    ECG of, 288
    in hypertension, 228
  overload of, 606
  volume of, 70, 288
  wall of, dysfunction or rupture of, 185
Left ventricular ejection, 15
Left ventricular function, assessment of, 77
Left ventricular pressure
  and aortic pressure, 17
  rate of change of, 77
Left ventricular stroke work index, 288
Left-to-right shunts, 67
  first heart sound in, 52
  fixed split of second heart sound in, 53
  indicator dilution curve of, 68
  and systolic ejection murmur, 59
Legs
  blood pressure in, measurement of, 44
  embolism of, 605
Lehman catheter, 110, 111, 543
Lenegre's disease, 440
Length-tension relationships, and ventricular pressure, 20
Leukocytosis, 591
  in arteritis, 602
Lev's disease, 440
Lewis leads, 496
  bipolar, 467
Libman-Sacks endocarditis, 557
Lidocaine, 123, 181, 311, 475, 477, 488, 492, 498
  in cardiac arrhythmias, 487
  in pregnancy, 620
  and refractory period, 458
  in ventricular fibrillation or tachycardia, 123
Ligamentum arteriosum, 4
Light-headedness, in acute myocardial infarction, 165

Lipoproteins, 135, 139
Lipoprotein-cholesterol distributions, 135
Liver
  in alcoholic cardiomyopathy, 553
  cirrhosis of, 582
    clubbing of fingers and nail beds in, 49
  engorgement of, as sign of right ventricular failure, 293
  and spleen, enlargement and tenderness of, as sign of systemic venous congestion, 50
Long QT syndrome, idiopathic, 460
Long-term exercise, in circulatory physiology, 31
Loop diuretics, 300
  in cardiac failure, 302
Loop of Henle, 300
Lorcainide, 460, 492
Low-density lipoproteins, 135
Lower extremities, examination of, in patient with heart disease, 50
Lown-Ganong-Levine syndrome, 455
Lumbar puncture, 600
Lung(s). See also Pulmonary.
  compliance of, 75, 101
  disease of
    and acute respiratory tract infections, 298
    chronic, right heart failure secondary to, 593
    and heart disease, differentiation of, 596
    obstructive, 44
  examination of, in patients with heart disease, 50
  hemorrhage into, 592
  parenchyma of, mottling of, as sign of schistosomiasis, 587
  resection of, 587
  scanning of, 97
  stiffness of, 101, 290
  tissue of, loss of, 586
Lung fields on x-ray, 82
Lung-to-brain circulation time, 51
Lupus erythematosus, 253, 573
  causes of death in, 558
  cell preparation, positive, 575
  ECG in, 557
  systemic, **557–558**
Lupus nephritis, 557
Lupuslike connective tissue disorder, 489
Lutembacher's syndrome, 330
LVET, 102
Lymph node, cardiac, 7
Lymphatics, of heart, 7
Lymphedema, 41
Lymphoma, 573, 609

M mode (motion) echocardiography, 84, 88
M zone, 8
Machinery murmur, 61, 346
Macroglossia, 561
Magnesium sulfate, in preeclampsia-eclampsia, 623
Magnetic resonance imaging, 100, 151
Maladie de Roger, 343
Malaise, as symptom of arteritis, 602

Malignant hypertension. *See* Hypertension, malignant.
Malnutrition, total, 555
Manometers, catheter-tip, 72
Mapping, myocardial ST segment, 95
Marantic lesions, 605
Marfan's syndrome, 49, 89, 91, 325, 601
   and aortic incompetence, 414
   echocardiogram in, 89, 91
MB CPK, 172
MB fraction of creatine phosphokinase, 95
Mean arterial pressure, 72, 73
Mean systolic pressure, 73
Mecamylamine, 259, 267
   adverse effects of, 261
Meditation therapy for hypertension, 259
Mediterranean fever, familial, 561
Melena, 605
Mellaril, 488
Menopause, and coronary disease, 137
Meperidine, 179
Mercurial diuretics
   in heart failure, 300
   sites of action of, 301
Mercury-203, radioactive, 242
Mesenteric embolism, 605
Mesoendothelioma, 573
Metabolic acidosis, 35, 65, 78, 501
Metabolic alkalosis, 65
Metabolic energy equivalents, 188
Metabolic rate, normal resting, 11
Metabolism, 65
   inherited disorders of, cardiac involvement in, 566
Metanephrine, 250
Methimazole, 549
Methyldopa, 259, 260, 270
   adverse effects of, 261
   during pregnancy, 621
   and hydrochlorothiazide, antihypertensive effect of, 262
Metolazone, 259
Metoprolol
   and atrial fibrillation, 481
   and hypertension, 263, 270
Metyrapone, in Cushing's syndrome, 248
Mexiletine, 490
Microaneurysms, Charcot-Bouchard, 221, 226
Microangiopathy, 136
Microthrombi, 133
Middiastolic murmur, 60
Midsystolic click, schematic diagram of, 52
Milrinone, in cardiac failure, 319
Mineralocorticoids, and hypertension, 218
Minipress, 259, **264**
Minoxidil, 259, **265**, 271, 315
   adverse effects of, 261
   in afterload reduction, 126
   in cardiac failure, 317
   dosage and route of administration, 316
Miosis, as sign of cardiovascular syphilis, 599
Mitotane, in Cushing's syndrome, 248

Mitral insufficie
   in infective en
Mitral regurgitatio
Mitral valve, 6
   area of, 74
      normal, 78
   closure of, 52
   cusp of, prolapse of,
   disease of, 332, 368,
      and aortic valve disea
         423
      and atrial fibrillation, p
         tracing of, 73
      cause of, 369
      classification of, 369
      tapping cardiac impulse in,
      and tricuspid valve disease, c
         bined, 424
   disruption of, 389
   incompetence of, **386–397**
      anatomic features of, 391
      causes of, 386
      chest x-ray of, 394
      hemodynamically insignificant, 386
         click and murmurs in, phonocardiogram of, 58
         late systolic murmur of, 58
         phonocardiogram, apexcardiogram, and ECG of, 388
      hemodynamically significant, 390
      large and jerky pulse of, 42
      late systolic murmurs due to, 59
      and left ventricular disease, 393
      and palpable impulses, 51
      pansystolic murmur of, 58, 59
      phonocardiogram of, 393
      pressure tracings in, 392
      prognosis in, 397
      pulmonary capillary and pulmonary artery pressure tracings, 395
      and ring calcification, 386
      treatment of, surgical, 332, 396
      valvuloplasty in, 396
   prolapse of, 388
      in pregnancy, 619
   replacement of, 378
      and cerebral embolism, 603
      in mitral incompetence, 397
   rheumatic lesion of, phonocardiogram in, 59
   slope of, 374
   stenosis of. *See* Stenosis, mitral valve.
Mitral valvotomy, 377, **425**
Mobilization program following myocardial infarction, 188
Mobitz type I (Wenckebach) atrioventricular block, 174, 444
   second-degree, 185
   treatment of, 447
Mobitz type II atrioventricular block, 174, 444
   prophylactic demand pacemakers in, 185
   second-degree, 185
   treatment of, 447
Moduretic, in hypertension, 259
Morphine sulfate, 179, 319
Motion echocardiography, 84, 88
Mouth-to-mouth breathing, 501
Mouth-to-mouth resuscitation, 122

                diagram of,
         mediate
      in chronic cor pulmonale, 596
      schematic diagram of, 58
      as sign of cardiovascular syphilis, 599
      and mitral stenosis, with presystolic accentuation, 371
      in rheumatic aortic regurgitation, phonocardiogram of, 57
   effect of posture on, 62, 609
   ejection, 59
   Graham Steell, 351, 372, 424, 594
      in cor pulmonale, 596
   heard in back, 50
   holosystolic, 59
   in hypertrophic obstructive cardiomyopathy, 540
   inflow, diastolic, schematic diagram of, 58
   innocent, 59
   machinery, 61, 346
   middiastolic, 60
   pansystolic, 59
      ejection, long, in hypertrophic obstructive cardiomyopathy, 60
      schematic diagram of, 58
   of patent ductus arteriosus, schematic diagram of, 58
   presystolic, in mitral stenosis, 60
      phonocardiogram of, 57
      schematic diagram of, 58
   in right heart failure, 293
   seagull cry, 423
   sound content of, 93
   systolic, 59
      aortic, as sign of cardiovascular syphilis, 599
      atrial, 60
      ejection, 59
         schematic diagram of, 58
      late, 59, 386, 388
         of hemodynamically insignificant mitral incompetence, 58
      phonocardiogram of, 55
      pulmonary ejection, schematic diagram of, 58
   timing of, diagram of, 58
   to-and-fro, 61, 574
   transmission of, 61
   of tricuspid incompetence, 594

...ses of
..., 15
...ascular system, 11
...ulatory physiology, 30
...skeletal pain, 38
...sset's sign, 416
Mustard's operation, for transposition of great arteries, 358
MVA, 74
Myeloma, multiple, 561
Myocardial band creatine phosphokinase, 166, 575
  fraction of, 95
  isoenzymes of, 172
Myocardial contractility, 19
Myocardial damage, acute, due to drug toxicity, 537
Myocardial disease, **527–572**
  acute, unsuspected or unrecognized, in heart failure, 303
  effect on valvular lesions, 368
  and pericardial disease, distinction between, 582
Myocardial enzymes, 166
  determinations of, 95
Myocardial imaging, 97
Myocardial infarct, size of, 171
Myocardial infarction, 119, 140, 590
  acute, **163–190**, 503
    activity after, 180
    and acute conduction defects, 442
    anticoagulant therapy in, 179
    arrhythmias in, 172
      management of, 491
    atrioventricular conduction defects in, 174
    bradyarrhythmias in, 174
    cardiac failure in, 175
    complications in, 172
      treatment of, 180, 185
    conduction defects in, 442
    convalescent activity in, 188
    differentiated from acute viral pericarditis, 574
    dysrythmias in, incidence of, 173
    ECG of, 167, 168, 169
      in presence of old infarct, 167
    emergency room procedures in, 178
    home care of, 178
    hospital care of, 178
    immediate treatment measures in, 178
    laboratory findings in, 166
    overall mortality rate in, 189
    oxygen therapy in, 179
    pain in, 164
      relief of, 179
    prodromal symptoms in, 165
    prognosis of, 191
    rehabilitation in, 188
    rest in, 179
    return to normal ECG in, 168
    serial ECG changes in, 167

..dial infarction (cont'd)
..cute (cont'd)
    sexual activity after, 191
    shock and cardiac failure in, 166
    signs in, 165
    supraventricular arrhythmias in, frequency of, 174
    systemic manifestations of, 165
    tachyarrhythmias in, 172
    therapeutic measures in, relation to hemodynamic indices, 181
    ventricular fibrillation in, 173
    ventricular premature beats in, 484
    ventricular tachycardia in, 493
  in angina pectoris, prevention of, 156
  anterior, atrioventricular conduction defects in, 442
  and bradycardia, 435
  as complication of arteritis, 602
  differentiation of
    from hypertension, 228
    from unstable angina, 161
  electrocardiographic changes in, 167
  evaluation following, 190
  inferior, atrioventricular conduction defects in, 442
  intracoronary thrombolytic therapy for, 114
  isotopes in, 170, 171
  late prognosis of, 190
  with left ventricular aneurysm, 185
  life adjustment after, 190
  minor, 172
  mobilization program following, 188
  nonfatal, and death from coronary heart disease, 256
  pain of, 38
  previous, relationship to angina pectoris, 160
  radioisotope studies of, 168
  rehabilitation after, 192
  with rupture, 177
  secondary prevention of, 191
  streptokinase in, 115
  uncomplicated, activity following, 180
Myocardial ischemia, 140, 147, 299
  ECG of, 451
  noninvasive investigation of, 141
  and unusual demands, 140
Myocardial oxygen consumption, 78
Myocardial ST segment mapping, 95
Myocardial tissue
  biopsy of, 114
  ischemic necrosis of, 163
Myocardial toxicity, 481
  and quinidine concentration, relationship between, 481
Myocardial work, and oxygen consumption, 18
Myocardiopathy, cobalt-beer, 553
Myocarditis
  and cardiomyopathy, **527–529**
  due to Chagas' disease, 532
  diphtheritic, 532
  poliovirus, 531
  and specific diseases, **529–533**
  viral, 527
Myocardium
  biopsy of, 527

Myocardium (cont'd)
  diseases of, **527–572**
    chronic, secondary to known metabolic disease, 548
    classification of, 528
    and pericardial disease, in differential diagnosis of heart failure, 298
Myxedema, 40, 573
  cardiac findings in, 550
  in heart failure, 311
  and myxedema heart, **549–553**
Myxoma, 609
  atrial, 605, 609, 610
    in differential diagnosis of infective endocarditis, 517
  left, 376, 586, 609
    chest x-ray in, 376
    clubbing of fingers and nail beds in, 49
    as contraindication to left heart catheterization, 110

Nadolol, in hypertension, 263
Nail beds and fingers, clubbing of, 49
Na^+-K^+ exchange site, 302
Natriuretic factor, atrial, 470
Naturetin, 259
Nausea
  in acute myocardial infarction, 165
  and digitalis toxicity, 308
Neck
  examination of, in patients with heart disease, **46–48**
  mechanical stimulation of, 39
  prominent pulse in, 43
Necrosis, fibrinoid, 226
Negative waves, in neck veins, 581
Nephrectomy, 606
Nephritis
  glomerular, 513
  immune complex, 513
Nephron, physiology of, 300
Nephrosclerosis, 225
  in hypertension, 220
Nephrosis, in hypertension, 227
Nephrotic syndrome, 41
Nerves, cardiac, 7
Nervous system, regulation of renin release by, 216
Neuritis, intracostal, 155
Neurocirculatory asthenia, 40, 291, **613–614**
Neurofibromatosis, 249, 253
Neuropathic disorders, and heart disease, 566
Neurosis, cardiac, 613
New York Heart Association's criteria for functional capacity and therapeutic class, 41
Nicotinic acid, to lower serum lipids, 156
Nifedipine, 157, 158, 259
  in heart failure, 182, 313, 317
  in hypertrophic cardiomyopathy, 546
  in supraventricular tachycardia, 476
NIH catheter, 110, 111
Nipride, 260
  dosage and routes of administration, 315

Nitrates
  in angina pectoris
    acute, 156
    chronic, 157
  in cardiac failure, 317
  and hydralazine
    combination of, 316
  in heart failure, 316
  oral, in heart failure, 315
  topical, 316
  transdermal, 316
  in unstable angina, 162
Nitroglycerin, 25, 164, 179, 183
  in afterload reduction, 125
  in cardiac failure, 317
  hemodynamic effects of, 183
  intravenous, 316
  transdermal, 182
  in unstable angina, 162
  as vasodilator, 125
Nitroglycerin ointment, 316
  dosage and route of administration, 316
  in heart failure, 182, 315
Nitrol, dosage and route of administration, 316
Nitroprusside, sodium, 183, 184, 260, 261, **268,** 315
  adverse effects of, 261
  in afterload reduction, 125
  in cardiac failure, 183, 317
  dosage and routes of administration, 315
  hemodynamic effects of, 184
  as vasodilator, 125
Nitrous oxide, 69
Nocturia
  in edema, 291
  in heart disease, 40
Node(s)
  Aschoff, 533
  atrioventricular, 7, 434
  sinoatrial, 7, 432
  of skin, in heart disease, 45
Nodules, subcutaneous, in rheumatic fever, 534, 535
Nonconducted atrial premature beat, ECG of, 468
Noninvasive investigations, **80–104,** 151
Nonparoxysmal supraventricular (junctional) tachycardia, 469, 472
  defined, 472
Nonparoxysmal ventricular tachycardia, treatment of, 181
Nontransmural myocardial infarction, 164, 170
Norepinephrine, 183
  in heart failure, 318
  plasma, and age, 218
Normality, ranges of, in cardiovascular system, 29
Normetanephrine, 250
Nosebleeds, recurrent, in rheumatic fever, 535
Noxious gases, dyspnea due to, 35
Nuclear medical investigations, 96
Nutritional heart disease, 555

Obesity, massive, 593
Obstructive cardiomyopathy, hypertrophic, 59, 60, 91, 411, 467, 539
  long pansystolic ejection murmur in, 60
Obstructive lung disease, 44
17-OHCS, 247
Ohm's law, 74
Opening snap, 56
  in mitral stenosis, 371
    phonocardiogram of, 57
  schematic diagram of, 52
Opiates, 179
Oral contraceptive agents, 603
  and atherosclerosis, 137
  hypertension due to, 252
  and pulmonary embolism, 589
  and pulmonary hypertension, 596
Oral diuretics, indications for, 302
Oretic, 259
Organomercurials, sites of action of, 301
Orthopnea, 35, 289
  as symptom of heart failure, 291
Osler's disease, 587
  lesions of, 45
Osler's nodes, 45, 512
Osmolality, 26
Ostium primum defect, 326, 327
  ECG of, 327
  gooseneck deformity of, 330
  left ventricular angiogram of, 330
Ostium secundum defect, 325
  atrial septal, wide splitting of second heart sound in, phonocardiogram of, 54
Overdrive suppression, 478
  of rapid pacing, 499
Overload, acute, of right heart, 588
Oximeter, ear, 101
Oxprenolol, and hypertension, 621
Oxygen, 51
  capacity for, 64
  consumption of, 66
    and myocardial work, 18
    normal, 11
  effect of, 68
  in emergency treatment of heart failure, 319
  saturation with, 64
    end-pulmonary capillary, 68
    and oxygen content, distinction between, 65
  therapy with, **124–125,** 596
    in acute myocardial infarction, 179
    in specific conditions, 124
  transport of, 11, **64–65**
  uptake of, in lungs, 64
Oxygen content, 64, 65
Oxygen hemoglobin dissociation curve, 64
Oxygen tension, 64
Oxygenated hemoglobin, 64
Oxygen-carrying capacity of blood, 64
Oxygen-CO_2 exchange, in tissues, 64

P mitrale, 609
P pulmonale, as sign of chronic cor pulmonale, 594
P waves, 13
  atrial, peaked right, as sign of pulmonary embolism, 590
  buried, 473
  ectopic, 467
  high-voltage, 609
  premature, 467
  in right ventricular failure, 294
P_2, 52
  loud, in pulmonary hypertension, phonocardiogram of, 55
P', 467
Pacemaker(s), 127
  artificial, 81
  checking operation of, 129
  complications of, 130
  components of, 127
  in conduction disease, 453
  demand, 127, 185
  endocardial, 300
  escape, 446
    junctional, secondary, 472
  external, 123
  fixed-rate, 127
  implantation of, 439
  insertion of, indications for, 129
  permanent, 184
  proper functioning of, 448
  prophylactic, 174
  R wave–inhibited, 127
  in supraventricular tachycardia, 478
  temporary, 129, 311
    transvenous, 124
  in ventricular fibrillation, 502
  in ventricular tachycardia, 500
Pacing
  atrial
    in paroxysmal atrial arrhythmia, 460
    rapid, 478, 482, 499
  atrioventricular, atrial and sequential, 127
  modes of, international code of, 127, 128
  paired, 74
  prophylactic, 175
Packed red cells, 125
Pain
  abdominal, 38
  in acute myocardial infarction, 38, 164
  relief of, 179
  in acute thoracic disease, 38
  in angina pectoris, 145
  cardiac
    and aortic stenosis, 405
    ischemic. *See* Angina pectoris.
    mechanism of, 36
  chest, **36–38,** 590, 597
    acute, 592
    in cardiovascular syphilis, 599
    in Fallot's tetralogy, 336, 338
    and gastrointestinal disorders, 155
    in hypertension, 221
    in hypertrophic obstructive cardiomyopathy, 539, 540
    in pulmonary stenosis, 333
  of costochondritis, 38

Pain (cont'd)
  dorsal root, 38
  of esophageal spasm, 38
  of gallbladder disease, 38
  girdle, 38
  of hiatal hernia, 38
  limb, as symptom of arteritis, 602
  musculoskeletal, 38
  pleural, 597
  of Tietze's syndrome, 38
  visceral, 36
Palpable gallops, 51
Palpable impulses, 51
Palpation
  of heart, 51
  of pulse, 42
Palpitations, 88
  examination and ECG during, 39
  and mitral stenosis, 371
  and mixed mitral stenosis and incompetence, 381
  in pulmonary stenosis, 333
Pansystolic murmur, 59
  ejection, long, in hypertrophic obstructive cardiomyopathy, 60, 541
  schematic diagram of, 58
Papilledema, 224, 272
Paracentesis, abdominal, 313
Paradoxic embolism, 605
Paradoxic rocking impulses, 51
Paradoxic splitting of second sound, 53
  phonocardiogram of, 54
Paralysis, 604
Paralytic ileus, 605
Parathyroid adenomas, 249
Paresis, 600
Paroxysmal atrial arrhythmia, in Wolff-Parkinson-White syndrome, management of, 459
Paroxysmal atrial tachycardia, 470
Paroxysmal junctional reciprocating tachycardia (PJRT), 469
Paroxysmal nocturnal dyspnea, 291
Paroxysmal supraventricular (atrial) tachycardia, 469, 470
  ECG of, 475
  with block, 308, 478
Paroxysmal tachycardia, initiation of, 467
Partial atrioventricular block, 440
Partial pressure, 64
Passive escape rhythms, 472
Patent ductus arteriosus, 290, **346–349**
  and aortopulmonary window, 347
  chest x-ray of, 347, 348
  murmur due to, 60
    phonocardiogram of, 61
    schematic diagram of, 58
Patient-cycled respirators, 125
PBI, 549
PC pressure, 107
P_{CO_2}
  normal, 65
  and pH, relationship between, 65
Peak arterial pressure, 72
Peaked right atrial P wave, as sign of pulmonary embolism, 590
Pectus excavatum, 50, 330, 362
  chest x-ray of, 362

Pediatric cardiology, 324
PEEP, 125
Penicillin, 600
  hypersensitivity to, 523
  in prevention of endocarditis, 517
  prophylaxis with
    in mitral stenosis, 377
    in mixed mitral stenosis and incompetence, 384
    in rheumatic fever, 536
Penicillin G, in infective endocarditis, 517
Pentazocine, 179
Pentolinium, 267
PEP, 102
PEP/LVET ratio, 102
Peptic ulcer, perforated, 592
Percussion of heart, 51
Percutaneous balloon valvuloplasty, 338
Percutaneous transluminal angioplasty
  coronary, 114, 194
  renal, 242
Percutaneous transvenous endomyocardial biopsy, 527
Perforated peptic ulcer, 592
Perforation, of interventricular septum, 185
Perfusion, myocardial, radioisotope studies of, 168
Pericardial constriction, 48, **581**
Pericardial disease, 44, **573–585**
  causes of, 573
  and myocardial disease, distinction between, 582
  pulsus paradoxus in, 44
  spectrum of, 573
Pericardial effusion, 44, 126, **575–580**
  acute, 303
  cardiac tamponade in, echocardiogram of, 579
  chest x-ray of, 576
  in heart failure, 312
  without tamponade, 575
Pericardial friction rubs, 62, 177, 298, 574
Pericardial knock, 56, 581
  phonocardiogram of, 581
Pericardial sac, 1, 10
Pericardial tamponade, 45
Pericardial tap, 126, 577
Pericardiocentesis, 126, 577, 580
Pericarditis, 177, 187, **573–585**
  acute, ECG of, 574
  constrictive, 294, 581
    calcification in, chest x-ray of, 582
    pressure tracing in, 49, 583
  coxsackie B, 573
  late pattern, ECG of, 574
  in rheumatic fever, 534, 536
  tuberculous, 575
Pericardium and myocardium, diseases of, in differential diagnosis of heart failure, 298
Periodic breathing, 50
Periodic fever, 561
Peripartum cardiomyopathy, 564, 617
  ECG of, 565
Peripheral embolism of extremities, 604
Peripheral vascular disease, 43

Peripheral vasodilatation, as sign of arteriovenous fistula, 606
Personality factors, as risk factors in atherosclerosis, 138
Petechiae, as sign of embolism, 45, 512
Pethidine, 179
PGE, 621
PGI_2, in atherosclerosis, 137
pH
  arterial, 65, 501
  blood, 65
  normal, 78
  and P_{CO_2}, relationship between, 65
Phase image analysis, 99
Phenobarbital, 247
Phenothiazines, 488
  in heart failure, 313
  systemic lupus erythematosus–like syndrome due to, 558
Phenoxybenzamine, 251
  in pheochromocytoma, 251
Phentolamine, 183
  in afterload reduction, 125
  in heart failure, 183, 317, 319
  in pheochromocytoma, 249, 251
  as vasodilator, 125
Phenylephrine, 477
  effect in hypertrophic obstructive cardiomyopathy, 541
Phenytoin, 144, 311, 477, 488, 489
  in cardiac arrhythmias, 487
  in pregnancy, 620
  and refractory period, 458
  systemic lupus erythematosus–like syndrome due to, 558
Pheochromocytoma, 227, **249–251**
  histamine test in, 250
  sites of, 249
  symptoms in, 280
  treatment of acute episodes of, 251
Phlebitis, as complication of bedside catheterization, 106
Phlebograms, external, 93
Phlebothrombosis, 177, 299, 589
Phlebotomy, in hemochromatosis, 561
Phonocardiogram, 406
Phonocardiography, 93, 582
Phosgene, dyspnea due to, 35
Pickwickian syndrome, 593
Pigtail catheter, 109
Pindolol, in hypertension, 263
Pink puffers, 593
Pituitary, transsphenoidal microresection of, 248
PJRT (paroxysmal junctional reciprocating tachycardia), 469
Planimetry, 73
Planorbis, 587
Plaques, elevated fibrous, 133
Plasma cholesterol levels
  age-adjusted, 135
  sex-adjusted, 135
Plasma skimming, 23
Plasma volume, 69
Plateau pulse, 405
Pleural effusion, 44, 50, 290, 579
  as sign of right heart failure, 294, 296
Pleural fluid, as sign of heart disease, 50
Pleural friction rub, 590, 597

Stenosis (cont'd)
  mitral valve (cont'd)
    with pulmonary hypertension, chest x-ray of, 373
    small pulse of, 42
    pressure reduction across and flow through, 140
  pulmonary, 48, 55, **333–338**
    anatomic features of, 334
    chest x-ray of, 334
    clinical findings in, 333
    fourth heart sound due to, 56
    peripheral arterial, 60
    phonocardiograms of, 335
    pulmonary thrombosis and embolism in, 337
    systolic ejection murmur due to, 59
    treatment of, 337
  pulmonary arterial, peripheral, 60
  tricuspid, diastolic murmur due to, 60
Stenotic lesions
  carotid arterial, murmurs due to, 60
  renal arterial, murmurs due to, 60
Stenotic valves, pressure difference across, 74
Sternum, depression of, 50, 362
Stethoscope, in heart auscultation, 51
Stokes-Adams attacks, 141, 175, 446, 493, 528
  with artificial pacing, 54
  ECGs of, 452
  with heart block, 185
Strain, postural, 155
Strain-gauge electromanometers, 72
Strain-gauge pressure transducer, 106
Streptococcal sore throat, treatment of, 536
Streptococci, in rheumatic fever, 533
Streptococcus
  and infective endocarditis, 511
  faecalis, endocarditis due to, 520
  viridans, endocarditis due to, 520
Streptokinase, 589
  in acute myocardial infarction, 115, 179
Stress, and cardiovascular system, 11
Stress electrocardiographic tests, 148
Striated muscle, mechanism of contraction of, 14
Stroke, 221
Stroke volume, 19, 42, 70, 78, 288
  defined, 70
  high, and ejection murmur, 59
  increased, and heart failure, 288
  ratio of, to end-diastolic volume, 70
ST-T wave, 13
  in arteriovenous fistula, 606
  changes in, 606
Subendocardial infarction, 164
Sudden death, **141–144**, 190, 485, 493, 500, 502, 503
  age-adjusted incidence of, 142
  in aortic stenosis, 411
  causes of, 142
  and cigarette smoking, relationship between, 143
  and click-murmur syndrome, 389
  emergency treatment for, 143
  and hypertrophic obstructive cardiomyopathy, 545

Sudden death (cont'd)
  prevention of, 142, 191
  prodromal symptoms in, 141
  reversibility of, in primary ventricular fibrillation, 144
  in sarcoidosis, 555
  and ventricular arrhythmias, 390
  in Wolff-Parkinson-White syndrome, 459
Sulfinpyrazone, in myocardial infarction, 191
Sulfonamides, in rheumatic fever, 536
Summation gallop, 56
  phonocardiogram of, 57
Superior vena cava, 4
Supernormal phase of excitability, 432
Supraventricular arrhythmias, **466–484**
  in acute myocardial infarction, frequency of, 174
  QRS complex in, widening of, 496
Supraventricular premature beats, 466
Supraventricular rhythms, and ventricular rhythm, differentiation on ECG, 473
Supraventricular tachycardia, **469–472**
  atrial paroxysmal, 469
    ECG of, 475
  ECG of, 469
  junctional nonparoxysmal, 469, 472
  recurrent, prevention of, 478
  treatment of, 475
Surgery
  coronary heart, 192
    factors influencing, 193
  in heart disease
    risks of, 626
    special precautions in, 630
    urgent, 626
    versus elective, 626
SVR, defined, 74
Swan-Ganz catheter, 66, 105, 106, 175, 178, 476
  bedside monitoring with, 320
Sweating
  in acute myocardial infarction, 165
  and aortic incompetence, 416
Swelling
  of abdomen and legs, in chronic constrictive pericarditis, 581
  of neck and face, in cardiovascular syphilis, 599
Sydenham's chorea, in rheumatic fever, 534
Sympathetic amines, 183
Sympathetic nervous system
  in hypertension, 214
  stimulation of, in heart failure, 289
Sympathomimetic drugs, and acute myocardial damage, 537
Syncope, 39
  cardiac, 39
  carotid sinus, 39
  in chronic bifascicular block, 453
  cough, 39
  effort, 39
  in hypertrophic obstructive cardiomyopathy, 540
  in myocardial infarction, 165
  unexplained, 448

Syncytium of heart muscle cells, 7, 12
Syphilis
  and aortic incompetence, 414
  and ejection murmur, 59
  serologic tests for, 600
  tertiary, 599, 600
Syphilitic aneurysm, 599
  chest x-ray of, 600
  resection of, 601
Syphilitic aortitis, 599
  calcification in, 600
  sound of aortic valve closure in, 55
Syphilitic cardiovascular disease, 599
Systemic arterial pressure, 72
Systemic arteries and aorta, diseases of, **599–608**
Systemic arteriovenous fistula, 599, **605–607**
Systemic blood flow, 67, 68
  measurement in atrial septal defect, 329
Systemic emboli, 482, 599, **603**
  and mitral incompetence, 396
  risk of, 480
Systemic embolization, and arteritis, 602
Systemic hypertension, 26, 586
  loud aortic second sound in, 55
  phonocardiogram of, 55
  or pulmonary hypertension, fourth heart sound due to, 56
  as sign of arteritis, 602
Systemic resistance
  normal, 78
  vascular, 74, 78
Systole, ventricular, 15
Systolic bruits, in peripheral vessels, 60
Systolic clicks, 56
  ejection, 56
  pulmonary or aortic, schematic diagram of, 52
Systolic hypertension, 213
Systolic murmurs, 59
  aortic, in cardiovascular syphilis, 599
  aortic ejection, schematic diagram of, 58
  atrial, 60
  ejection, 59
  in hypertrophic obstructive cardiomyopathy, 541
  late, 59, 386, 388
    schematic diagram of, 58
  phonocardiogram of, 55
  pulmonary ejection, schematic diagram of, 58
Systolic pressure, 42, 43
  factors leading to increases in, 211
  mean, 73
  normal, 78
Systolic time intervals, 102

T system, 7
T waves, 13, 72
  inversion of, 581
    in chronic cor pulmonale, 594
    in fibrinous pericarditis, 574
    in pericardial constriction, 581
    in pulmonary embolism, 590
T_3, serum, 549

INDEX / 657

Shunts (cont'd)
  right-to-left, 67
  small, detection of, 68
Shy-Drager syndrome, 612
Sick sinus syndrome, 437
Sickle cell disease, and chronic anemia, 563
Sighing respirations, 36, 291, 613
Single-pass nucleotide angiogram, 172
Sinoatrial block, 310
Sinoatrial disease, chronic, precautions in investigations of, 438
Sinoatrial node, 7, 432
  function of, depression of, 472
Sinus, aortic, 6
Sinus arrest, 437
Sinus arrhythmia, heart rate in, 42
Sinus bradycardia, 173, 185, 437
Sinus node
  action potential of, 15
  function of, evaluation of, 436
Sinus rhythm, restoration of, 126, 480, 483
  by DC conversion in mixed mitral stenosis and incompetence, 384
Sinus standstill, 174
Sinus tachycardia, 472
Sinus of Valsalva, 61
  aneurysm of
    and aortic stenosis, 421
    rupture of, 61
Sinus venosus, 9
  defect of, 325
Sipple's disease, 249
Skeletal muscle and cardiac muscle, differences between, 19
Skin
  circulation to, 29
  examination of, in heart disease, 45
  lesions of
    in heart disease, 45
    in rheumatic fever, 534
Sliding filament hypothesis, 15, 19
Slow ventricular tachycardia, 497
Smoking, cigarette, 291, 596
  in atherosclerosis, 137
  and hypertension, 258
Snap, opening, schematic diagram of, 52
"Snowman heart," 361
Social factors, in hypertension, 217
Sodium
  depletion of, 302
  inadvertent rapid administration of, in heart failure, 312
  infusions containing, 312
  intake of
    in heart failure, 289, 299
    and hypertension, 214
  reabsorption of
    in cardiac failure, 300
    sites of, in nephron, 301
Sodium bicarbonate, 501
Sodium nitroprusside, 183, 184, 260, 261, **268**, 315
  adverse effects of, 261
  in afterload reduction, 125
  dosage and routes of administration, 315
  in heart failure, 315
  hemodynamic effects of, 184
  as vasodilator, 125

Sodium-potassium exchange site, 300, 301
Soldier's heart, 613
Sones catheter, 110
Sones method, 112
Sones technique, 109
Sore throat, streptococcal, 536
Sound(s)
  aortic valve closure, 55
  heart, 51
    disappearance or muffling of, as indication of diastolic pressure, 43
    first, 52
      phonocardiogram and ECG of, 52
      in relation to fourth heart sound, 56
      split, schematic diagram of, 52
    fourth, 56
      in relation to first heart sound, 56
      as sign of heart failure, 292
    second, 52
      in atrial septal defect, 327
      loud, aortic, in systemic hypertension, 55
      pulmonary, 294
      splitting of
        paradoxic, 53
        phonocardiogram of, 53, 54
        physiologic, 53
        reversed, 53
        schematic diagram of, 52
    third, 56
      phonocardiogram of, 55
      schematic diagram of, 52
    timing of, 51, 52
  intracardiac, extra, 56
  pulmonary valve closure, loud, 55
Spasm, coronary, 113, 144
  arterial, 25
Specificity, defined, 80
Speech, loss of, 604
Sphygmomanometer, 43
Sphygmomanometry, 42
  and direct arterial pressure measurement, correlation between, 43
Spider nevi, 45
Spironolactone, 259
  dosages of, 302
  in heart failure, 314
  in hypokalemia, 302
Spleen and liver, enlargement and tenderness of, as sign of systemic venous congestion, 50
Splenic embolism, 605
Splenomegaly, 513
Splinter hemorrhages, as sign of endocarditis, 49
Split, fixed, 53
Square root sign, 583
  pressure tracing of, 583
Square wave, in Valsalva's maneuver, 76
Squatting
  and exertional dyspnea, as symptoms of heart disease, 40
  in Fallot's tetralogy, 338
ST segment
  depression of
    in chronic cor pulmonale, 594
    of myocardial ischemia, 147

ST segment (cont'd)
  elevation of, in fibrinous pericarditis, 574
  mapping of, 95
Stable angina, **144–160**
Stamey test, 241
Standstill
  sinus, 174
  ventricular, 144
Staphylococci, endocarditis due to, 511, 521
Starling mechanism, 73
Starling's law, 19, 42
Starr-Edwards ball and cage valve, 412
Stasis, 603
Static exercise, and circulatory physiology, 30
Stenosis
  aortic, 53
    anatomic features of, 403
    arterial pulse in, 405
    calcific, 110
    cause of, 404
    chest x-ray of, 408
    congenital, 404
    ECG of, 406, 407
    fourth heart sound due to, 56
    importance of, 401
    and incompetence
      interaction of, 400
      mixed murmur in, 61
    and insufficiency, 406
    phonocardiogram in, 406
    predominant, 401
      cardiac catheterization data in, 410
    prognosis in, 412
    progression of, 404
    and sinus of Valsalva aneurysm, 421
    subvalvular and supravalvular, 400
    systolic ejection murmur due to, 59
    wedge pressure tracings in, 108
  coronary, diagnosis of, 134
  idiopathic hypertrophic subaortic, 539
  infundibular, 59
  mitral valve, 39, **369–379**, 586, 594
    anatomic features of, 370
    atrial fibrillation in, control of, 483
    cardiac catheterization data in patients with, 375, 376
    course of, 377
    diastolic murmur due to, 60
    echocardiogram of, 374
    first heart sound in, 52
    and incompetence
      mixed, **379–385**
        anatomic features of, 380
        phonocardiogram of, 382
        wedge and left ventricular tracings of, 383
    mitral opening snap in, phonocardiogram of, 57
    phonocardiogram of, 371
    presystolic murmur in, 57, 58
    prognosis in, 378

Restrictive cardiomyopathy, 546
Resuscitation, 501
　cardiopulmonary, **121–124**
　　in a hospital setting, 123
　　in a public place, 121
　　in ventricular fibrillation, 144, 501
Reticulum, sarcoplasmic, 7
Retinas, examination of, in hypertension, 223
Retinopathy, hypertensive, 224
Retrograde activation, 486
Retrograde arterial catheterization, 110
Retrograde conduction, 486
Rheumatic aortic regurgitation, diastolic murmur in, phonocardiogram of, 57
Rheumatic aortic valve, 511
Rheumatic endocarditis, and valvular disease, 368
Rheumatic fever, **533–537**
　in aortic incompetence, 414
　and aortic valvular lesions, 400
　in differential diagnosis of infective endocarditis, 517
　electrocardiographic abnormalities in, 535
　and mitral incompetence, 386, 387
　recurrent, prevention of, 536
Rheumatic heart disease, and pregnancy, 617
Rheumatic mitral lesions
　development of, 369
　phonocardiogram in, 59
Rheumatic myocarditis
　and mitral incompetence, 396
　and mixed mitral stenosis and incompetence, 384
Rheumatic nodules, 45
Rheumatoid arthritis, **559**, 573
　and amyloidosis, 561
　cardiac symptoms and signs in, 559
　inflammatory infiltrate of myocardium in, 560
Rhonchi, 597
Rhythms
　accelerated idioventricular, 173, 495
　　ECG of, 495
　　treatment of, 181
　atrial bigeminal, ECG of, 468
　escape, 173, 432, 497
　gallop, 56
　passive, 472
　reentry, ventricular, premature beats due to, 486
　sinus, normal, restoration of, 126, 480, 483
　　by DC conversion, in mixed mitral stenosis and incompetence, 384
　tictac, in acute myocarditis, 529
　triple, 56
　ventricular, differentiation on ECG, 473
Rib notching, as x-ray sign of heart failure, 297
Rickettsial diseases, acute myocarditis in, 532
Right atrial electrode catheters, 467
Right axis deviation, as sign of pulmonary embolism, 590
Right bundle branch block, 448, 473
　incomplete, in pulmonary embolism, ECG of, 590

Right bundle branch block (cont'd)
　intermittent, ECG of, 449
　as sign of pulmonary embolism, 590
　widely split second heart sound in, phonocardiogram of, 53
Right heart
　catheterization of
　　complications of, 118
　　in mitral stenosis, 375
　failure of, 40, 587
　　acute, 588
　　in chronic cor pulmonale, 595
　　in pulmonary stenosis, 335, 337
　　secondary to chronic lung disease, **593–596**
　overload of, acute, 588
Right ventricle, 18
　enlargement of, secondary to chronic respiratory disease, 593
　failure of, 289
　hypertrophy of, 587
　　ECG in, 295, 336
　infarction of, 166, 182
　pressure recordings of, 108
Right-to-left shunts, 66
　indicator dilution curve of, 68
Romana's sign, 563
Roth spots, 512
　as evidence of infective endocarditis, 46
rt-PA, in myocardial infarction, 180
Rubella, congenital heart disease due to, 617
Rupture
　of aorta in cardiovascular syphilis, 601
　of heart, 177, 187
　of left ventricular wall, 185
　of sinus of Valsalva aneurysm, 61

S_1, 52
S_2, 54
S_2–OS interval, and mitral stenosis, 371
S_3, 56
　schematic diagram of, 52
S_3 gallop, 290
S_4, 56, 225
　schematic diagram of, 52
Salicylates, 575
　in rheumatic fever, 536
Salmon skin, in thyrotoxicosis, 548
Salt intake, in heart failure, 289
Salt retention, pathophysiologic mechanisms of, 289
Saralasin, 268
Sarcoid granuloma, in myocardium, 556
Sarcoidosis, **555–556**, 593
　giant cells in, 556
Sarcolemma, 7
Sarcoma, 573, 609
Sarcomere, 7
Sarcoplasmic reticulum, 7, 21
Saturation, oxygen, 64
　end-pulmonary, capillary, 68
Scalenus anticus syndrome, 155
Scavenger effect, 135
Schistosoma
　haematobium, 587
　japonicum, 587
　mansoni, 587

Schistosomiasis, pulmonary hypertension in, 587
Scimitar vein syndrome, 325
Scleroderma, **558**, 573, 593
　clinical cardiac abnormalities in, 559
　of kidney, pathologic features of, 559
Scoliosis, 50, 593
Seagull cry murmur, 423
Seconal, 476
Second heart sound, 52
　in atrial septal defect, 327
　loud, aortic, in systemic hypertension, 55
　pulmonary, 294
　splitting of
　　paradoxic, 53
　　phonocardiogram of, 53, 54
　　physiologic, 53
　　reversed, 53
　　schematic diagram of, 52
Second wind phenomenon, 146
Second-degree atrioventricular block, 444
　conduction defects in, 444
　defined, 440
　treatment of, 447
　Wenckebach-type, 441, 444
Sedation, 179, 476
Sedimentation rate, elevated, 600
　in arteritis, 602
Segmental wall motion, 177
Seizures, epileptic, 39, 121, 123
Sensitivity, defined, 80
Septation, 10
Septic abscesses, 517
Septum
　primum, 11
　secundum, 11
Serologic tests for syphilis, 600
Serpasil, 259, 260
Severinghaus slide rule, 65
Sexual activity, after acute myocardial infarction, 191
SGOT, 95
Shock, 43, 588
　and cardiac failure, in acute myocardial infarction, 166
　cardiogenic, 172, 176
　　and intra-aortic balloon pumping, 130
　treatment of, 181
Short-term exercise, and circulatory physiology, 30
Shoulder-hand syndrome, 188
Shunts
　bidirectional, 67
　cardiac, measurement of, **66–69**
　estimations of
　　accuracy of, 67
　　by indicator dilution methods, 68
　intracardiac, and intrapulmonary, estimation of, by Fick principle, 66
　left-to-right, 67
　　first heart sound in, 52
　　fixed split of second heart sound in, 53
　　indicator dilution curve of, 68
　　and systolic ejection murmur, 59

Pulsus
  alternans, 44, 75, 409
  bigeminus, 42
  bisferiens, 405
  paradoxus, 44, 578
  tardus, 42, 405
Pump, failure of, 176
Puncture
  arterial, 105
  left ventricular, 110
    direct percutaneous, 109
    transthoracic, 110
  venous, 105
Purkinje fibers, 7
  action potential of, 15
PVR, 74

Q waves, abnormal, 168
  in acute myocardial infarction, 168
  as signs of pulmonary embolism, 590
QA$_2$ interval, 102
Q$_{eff}$, 67
QRS, 13
QRS complexes, 174, 185
  aberrant, 467
  high-voltage, 606
  narrow, 472
  wide, in supraventricular rhythms, 496
QRS wave, 13
QS complexes, 167
QT interval, prolongation of, 482
QT syndrome, long, 460
Quincke's pulse, 416
Quinidine
  atrial flutter due to, 480
  for cardiac arrhythmias, 492
    long-term oral administration of, 489
    rapid administration of, 488
  in cardioversion, 127
  concentration of, and myocardial toxicity, relationship between, 481
  in digitalis toxicity, 311
  effects on atrial arrhythmias, 482
  effects on ECG, 82
  effects on ventricular tachycardia, 497
  in heart failure, 313
  in pregnancy, 620
  and refractory period, 458
  in sudden death, 144
  in ventricular fibrillation, 502
Quinidine gluconate, 181

R on T phenomenon, 432, 488, 494
R wave, tall, as sign of chronic cor pulmonale, 594
Radial pulse, 42, 43
  and femoral pulse, simultaneous palpation of, 43
Radiation therapy, 573
Radioactive chromium–labeled red cells, 69
Radioactive isotopes, for measuring cardiac output, 66
Radioactive krypton, 69
Radioiodinated human serum albumin, 591
Radioiodine, 549

Radioisotope gated blood pool scans, 172
Radioisotope scan, pulmonary, 298
Radioisotope studies
  in angina pectoris, 150
  in coronary disease, 150
  of kidney, 242
  of myocardial perfusion, 168
Radioisotopes, 100
Radiologic investigations, special, 95
Radionuclear studies, 328
Radionuclide angiography, 98
  in angina pectoris, 151
Radionuclide studies, in asymptomatic myocardial ischemia, 141
Rales, 290, 597
  in chronic constrictive pericarditis, 581
  in heart disease, 50, 292
Rashkind procedure, for transposition of great arteries, 358
Rastelli procedure, for truncus arteriosus, 359
Rate-dependent conduction defects, 453
Raynaud's phenomenon, 557
Recanalization, catheter, 115
Reciprocating tachycardia, paroxysmal junctional, 469
  treatment of, 478
Recirculation of dye, in determination of cardiac output, 66
Recklinghausen's disease, 249, **253**
Red cell volume, 69
Red cells, radioactive chromium–labeled, 69
Red hemoglobin, 64
Reentrant pathway, schematic diagram of, 434
Reentry, 433
  causes and occurrence of, 434
  requirements for, 433
Reentry circuits, 468
Reentry pathways, 478
  random, 500
Reentry rhythms, ventricular premature beats due to, 486
Reflex bradycardia, 76
Reflex control mechanisms, abnormal, and hypotension, 612
Refractoriness, and excitability, 432
Refractory period, 432
  absolute, 432
  effective, of accessory pathway, 457
  relative, 432
Regitine, in pheochromocytoma, 251
Regurgitant fraction, 72
Rehabilitation programs, after myocardial infarction, 192
Reiter's syndrome, and aortic incompetence, 414
Relative refractory period, 432
Relaxation therapy, in hypertension, 259
Renal. *See also* Kidney.
Renal angiogram, in renal artery stenosis, 230, 240
Renal arteries
  fibromuscular hyperplasia of, 239
  stenosis of, **238–243**
    with hypertension, 244
    prognosis of, 242

Renal arteries (cont'd)
  stenosis of (cont'd)
    surgical and medical treatment of, compared, 244
  stenotic lesions of, murmurs due to, 60
Renal biopsies, in preeclampsia, 622
Renal colic, 605
Renal dialysis, 573
Renal embolism, 605
Renal failure, 177, 185
  antibiotic dosage in, 521
  as complication of arteritis, 602
  and dialysis, 274
  in hypertension, 220
Renal function
  differential assessment of, 241
  in digitalis administration, 305
Renal ischemia, segmental, 605
Renal parenchymal lesions, 252
Renal percutaneous transluminal angioplasty, 242
Renal studies, radioisotopic, 242
Renal vein renin levels, differential, 241
Renin, 26, 215
  in hypertension, 238
  levels of, factors affecting, 215
  plasma
    and age, 218
    in aldosteronism, 245
  release of
    and autonomic sympathetic amines, 215
    feedback regulation of, 216
  renal, 217
  renal vein, 241
Renin-angiotensin system, 28
  in hypertension, **215–218**
  inhibitors of, 242, 268
  and prostaglandins, in preeclampsia-eclampsia, 621
Renin-angiotensin-aldosterone system, 210
Repolarization, 13
Reproductive organs, circulation to, 30
Reserpine, 259, 260, **262**, 270
  adverse effects of, 261
Resin, in treatment of hyperlipidemias, 156
Resin uptake test, 549
Resistance, vascular, 74
  pulmonary, 74
    normal, 78
  systemic, 74
    and age, 218
    normal, 78
Respiration, 42
  sighing, 291, 613
Respirators, 125
Respiratory acidosis, 65
Respiratory alkalosis, 65
Respiratory depression, 124
Respiratory tract, infections of, acute, and lung disease, 298
Rest
  in acute myocardial infarction, 179
  bed, 319
    prolonged, risk of, 299
  in heart failure, 299
Resting cardiac output, normal, 78
Resting ventilation, normal, 78

Propranolol (cont'd)
  effectiveness in cardiac arrhythmias, 487
  in hypertension, 263, 270
  in hypertrophic obstructive cardiomyopathy, 546
  and refractory period, 458
  in supraventricular tachycardia, 476
Propylthiouracil, 549
Prorenin, 216
Prostacyclins, in atherosclerosis, 137
Prostaglandins, 210
  in atherosclerosis, 137
  biosynthesis of, pathway of, 138
  and blood pressure, 210
  and renin-angiotensin system, in preeclampsia-eclampsia, 621
  and thrombosis, 137
Prosthetic heart valves, endocarditis on, 522
Protein-bound iodine, 549
Proteinuria, 50
  in hypertension, 227
  in preeclampsia-eclampsia, 621
Psychologic factors in hypertension, 217
Psychologic heart disorders, 613
Psychologic stress, acute, 142
Psychophysiologic reactions, cardiovascular, 155
Psychotherapy, in hypertension, 259
Psychotropic drugs, 488
Ptosis, as sign of cardiovascular syphilis, 599
Puerperium, physiologic changes during, 618
Pulmonary angiocardiography, 589
Pulmonary angiogram, 592
Pulmonary angiography, 591
Pulmonary arterial blood, 65
Pulmonary arterial pressure, increased, 586
Pulmonary arterial stenosis, peripheral, 60
Pulmonary arterial vasoconstriction, 586
Pulmonary arterioles, 586
Pulmonary arteriovenous fistula, 587
Pulmonary artery
  entry into, in cardiac catheterization, 108
  idiopathic dilatation of, 330
  large, as sign of schistosomiasis, 587
  main, 2
  pressure in, recordings of, 108
  vasoconstriction of, 586
Pulmonary blood flow, 66, 67, 68, 100
Pulmonary capillary pressure, 107
Pulmonary circulation, 30, 586
Pulmonary congestion, 588
  acute, 35
  as x-ray sign in heart failure, 296
Pulmonary edema, 50, 289, 479
  acute
    emergency treatment of, 319–320
    as symptom of heart failure, 291
    x-ray of, 296
  in acute myocardial infarction, 165

Pulmonary edema (cont'd)
  as complication of catheterization, 116
  and heroin, 291
  high-altitude, dyspnea associated with, 36
  interstitial, 35
  oxygen therapy in, 124
  recurrent, 586
  x-ray of, 83
Pulmonary ejection murmur, systolic, schematic diagram of, 58
Pulmonary embolism, 35, 177, **587–593**
  acute, 38
  anticoagulant therapy in, 592
  as complication of bedside catheterization, 106
  in heart failure, 312
  massive, 588
    in differential diagnosis of heart failure, 298
  moderate, 589
Pulmonary emphysema and cor pulmonale, ECG of, 594
Pulmonary flow measurement, in atrial septal defect, 329
Pulmonary function tests, 100
  in differentiation of heart and lung disease, 597
Pulmonary granuloma, 593
Pulmonary heart disease, **586–598**
Pulmonary hypertension, 155, 290, 373, **586–587**
  acquired, 349
  in bilharziasis, 587
  in differential diagnosis of pulmonary stenosis, 336
  effects of increased left atrial pressure in, 586
  fourth heart sound due to, 56
  idiopathic, 587
  loud pulmonary valve closure sound in, 55
  mechanism of production of, 586
  and mitral stenosis, 373
  mortality rate in, 378
  signs of, 372
  and oral contraceptives, 596
  primary, 587
  in schistosomiasis, 587
  thromboembolic, 587, 595
    chronic, 591
  venous, 586
Pulmonary hypertensive cor pulmonale, 593
Pulmonary incompetence, 372, 420
  and mitral stenosis, 372
Pulmonary infarction, 35, 586
  and mitral stenosis, 377
Pulmonary plethora, in atrial septal defect, 327
Pulmonary second sound, 294
Pulmonary stenosis, 48, 56, **333–338**
  anatomic features, 334
  chest x-ray of, 334
  clinical findings in, 333
  fourth heart sound due to, 56
  phonocardiogram of, 334, 335
  pulmonary thrombosis and embolism in, 337

Pulmonary stenosis (cont'd)
  systolic ejection murmur due to, 59
  treatment of, 337
Pulmonary systolic ejection click, schematic diagram of, 52
Pulmonary thrombosis in chronic cor pulmonale, 595
Pulmonary trunk, 2
Pulmonary valve, 6
  stenotic, pressure tracing of, 337
Pulmonary valve closure, 55
  sound of, delayed, phonocardiogram of, 55
Pulmonary vascular bed, 586
Pulmonary vascular resistance, 74
  in atrial septal defect, 330
  normal, 78
  raised, in mitral stenosis, 371
Pulmonary veins
  congestion of, 479
  drainage of, anomalous, total, 360
  relocation of, 332
Pulmonary ventilation, 65
Pulmonic. See Pulmonary.
Pulsations
  epigastric, 51
  palpable, to right of sternum, 599
  visible, as sign of heart disease, 50
Pulse(s), **42–45**
  amplitude of, 42
  anacrotic, 405
  bifid, in hypertrophic obstructive cardiomyopathy, 541, 542
  bounding, as sign of arteriovenous fistula, 606
  femoral, 43
  in hypertrophic obstructive cardiomyopathy, 540
  jugular
    as sign of right heart failure, 293
    venous
      examination of, 46
      in paroxysmal atrial tachycardia, 470
  large and jerky, of mitral incompetence, 42
  of major vessel, loss of, as sign of arteritis, 602
  palpation of, 42
  plateau, 405
  popliteal, 43
  prominent, in neck, 43
  Quincke's, 416
  radial, 42, 43
    and femoral, simultaneous palpation of, 43
  rate of, 43
  small, of mitral stenosis, 42
  venous, 46
    normal, 47
  water-hammer, 416
    as sign of cardiovascular syphilis, 599
  wave velocity of, 42
Pulse deficit, 480
Pulse pressure, 42, 72, 213
  wide, as sign of cardiovascular syphilis, 599
Pulseless disease, 601
Pulseless patient, 121

Pleural pain, 597
Pleurisy, 588, 592
Pneumoconiosis, 593
Pneumonectomy, 586
Pneumonia, 35, 586, 588, 592, 593
Pneumothorax, 35, 44, 118
  spontaneous, 155
PO_2, 64
  arterial, normal, 65, 78
Poliovirus myocarditis, 531
Polyarteritis nodosa, 253, 602
  incidence of, at necropsy, 253
Polyarthralgia, in rheumatic fever, 534
Polycythemia, 64, 297, 587, 594, 603
  vera, in heart failure, 312
Polyuria, as symptom of heart disease, 40
Popliteal pulse, 43
Positive airway pressure, 125
Positive end-expiratory pressure, 125
Positive pressure breathing, in emergency treatment of heart failure, 319
Positive waves, 47
Positron emission tomography, 100, 151
Postectopic potentiation, 73
Postpericardiotomy syndrome, 573, 574
Postural strain, 155
Posture
  during blood pressure measurement, 43
  effects on heart murmurs, 62
Potassium
  depletion of, fatigue due to, 40
  foods high in, 262
  intake of, dietary, 262
  loss of, in diuretic therapy, 300
  salts of, 181
  serum, low, 245
  supplements of, 301
Potassium chloride, 478
Potassium iodide, 600
Potassium-sparing diuretics, adverse effects of, 261
Potential, action, 13
Potentiation, postectopic, 73
Potts operation, 342
PR interval, length of, effect on loudness of first heart sound, 52
Prazosin, 259, 264, 270, 315
  adverse effects of, 261
  in afterload reduction, 126
  in cardiac failure, 317
  dosage and routes of administration, 316
Precoronary care, 178
Prednisone, 562, 600
  in rheumatic fever, 536
Preeclampsia
  defined, 621
  renal and hepatic changes in, 622
Preeclampsia-eclampsia, **621–624**
  pathophysiology of, hypothesis for, 622
Preejection period, 102
Preexcitation
  type A, 456
  type B, 456
  ventricular, 454

Preexcitation syndrome, prevention of atrial arrhythmias in, 460
Pregnancy
  cardiac disease in, 618
  and cardiomyopathy, 564
  and circulation, 30
  effect on maternal circulatory and respiratory functions, 617
  heart disease in, **617–625**
  hypertensive disorders of, 619, **620–624**
  in patients with cardiac prostheses, 619
  physiologic changes in, **617–618**
  surgical treatment during, 619
  and systolic ejection murmur, 59
Preinfarction angina, 161
Preload, 19
Premature beats, 445
  atrial, 181, 467
    concealed, 467
    ECG of, 468
    nonconducted, ECG of, 468
    treatment of, 468
  complex, 485
  junctional, 467
  supraventricular, 467
  ventricular, 141, 144, 180, 308, **484–493**
    in acute myocardial infarction, 484
    in bigeminy and trigeminy, ECG of, 484
    complex, and congestive heart failure, 485
    ECG of, 494
    grading system for, 485
    induced by graded exercise, 487
    and mortality rates, 191
    multifocal, 144
    role of central nervous system in, 486
    significance of, 486
    treatment of, 487
Premonitory symptoms, in myocardial infarction, 164
Pressor agents, 477
Pressoreceptors, 214
Pressure
  aortic
    in circulatory system, 26
    effect in coronary perfusion, 25
    and left ventricular pressure, 17
  arterial
    diastolic, 43
    mean, 72, 73
    peak, 72
    systemic, 72
    systolic, 42, 43
    mean, 73
  barometric, 64
  blood, **43–45**
    measurement of, **72–74**
      in arm, 43
      cuff for, 43
      direct arterial, and sphygmomanometry, correlation between, 43
      in legs, 44
      patient position in, 43
  changes in
    and blood flow, 210

Pressure (cont'd)
  changes in (cont'd)
    in systemic circulation, 12
  difference in, across stenotic valves, 74
  end-diastolic, left ventricular, 71
  and flow wave transmission, 23
  gradients of, 74
    measurement of, 86
  intracardiac
    measurements of, in atrial septal defect, 330
    rise in, rate of, 577
  intrathoracic, 101
    negative, 44
  partial, 64
  positive airway, 125
  positive end-expiratory, 125
  pulmonary capillary, 107
  pulse, 42, 72, 213
    wide, as sign of cardiovascular syphilis, 599
  recording of, 106, **108–109**
  tracings of
    damped and control, 72
    in hypertrophic obstructive cardiomyopathy, 542
  venous, 46
  ventricular
    left, rate of change of, 77
    and length-tension relationships, 20
    recording of, 109.
  wedge, 106
    measurement of, 111
      in Eisenmenger's syndrome, 351
    validity of, 107
Pressure curve, brachial artery, 42
Pressure load, 287
Pressure-flow relationships, 23, 74
Presystolic gallop, 55, 56, 225
  phonocardiogram of, 56, 57
  schematic diagram of, 52
Presystolic murmur, in mitral stenosis, 60
  phonocardiogram of, 57
  schematic diagram of, 58
Prinzmetal's variant angina, 37, **144**
Procainamide, 144, 181, 477, 481, 488, 489, 492, 497, 502
  in cardiac arrhythmias, 489
  in cardioversion, 127
  in pregnancy, 620
  and refractory period, 458
  systemic lupus erythematosus–like syndrome due to, 558
Procaine penicillin G, 601
Procardia, in hypertension, 259
Prodromal symptoms
  in acute myocardial infarction, 165
  in sudden death, 141
Profunda femoris artery, 604
Prominent pulse in neck, 43
Propafenone, 492
Prophylactic pacemaker, 174
  demand, in Mobitz II block, 185
Prophylaxis, antibiotic, in infective endocarditis, 517
Propranolol, 144, 259, 260, 311, 477, 488, 489, 492
  adverse effects of, 261
  and atrial fibrillation, 481

Tabes dorsalis, 600
  arterial pressure tracings of, 612
Tachyarrhythmia, in acute myocardial infarction, 172
Tachycardia, 289, 292, 436
  atrial, ECG of, 471
  ECG of, 473
  junctional, ECG of, 474
  junctional reciprocating paroxysmal, 469
    treatment of, 478
  nonparoxysmal supraventricular (junctional), 469, 472
    defined, 472
    treatment of, 181
  paroxysmal supraventricular (atrial), 469, 470
    with block, 478
    ECG of, 474
    initiation of, 467
  sinus, 472
  supraventricular, 469
    causes of, 470
    ECG of, 473, 474, 475
    treatment of, 475
  ventricular, 118, 144, 181, 485, **493**
    ablation of site of, 499
    in acute myocardial infarction, 493
    in coronary angiography, 118
    defined, 493
    diagnosis of, 493
    ECG of, 494
    effects of quinidine on, ECG of, 498
    recurrent, 499
    slow, 497
    treatment of, 123, 181
    in ventricular premature beats, 485
Takayasu's arteritis, 601
Tamponade, 118, 126, 177
  cardiac
    in pericardial effusion, ECG of, 579
    with pulsus paradoxus, 44
  pericardial, 45
Tea, and hypertension, 258
Technetium ^{99m}Tc, 97, 99, 242
Technetium ^{99m}Tc pyrophosphate, 169
Technetium ^{99m}Tc sodium pertechnetate, 99
Technetium-labeled pyrophosphate, 97
Telangiectasia, hereditary hemorrhagic, 587
Temperature, effects on cardiac pain, 37
Temporal arteritis, 601
Temporal subtraction angiography, 95
Tensilon, in supraventricular tachycardia, 477
Teprotide, 242
Tetracycline, 601
Tetralogy of Fallot. See Fallot's tetralogy.
Thallium-201, 97, 169
Thallium-201 stress scintigrams, 97
Thallium-201 studies, in angina pectoris, 151
Therapeutic procedures
  in cardiac disorders, **121–131**
  involving catheterization, 114

Thermistor, 66
Thermistor bead, 106
Thermodilution, 66
Thermodilution catheters, 106, 182
Thermodilution method, of blood flow measurement, 69
Thiamine, deficiency of
  in alcoholic cardiomyopathy, 553
  in beriberi heart disease, 312, 554
Thiazide diuretics, 260, 300, 302
  sites of action of, 301
Thiocyanate, 316
Thioridazine, 488
Third heart sound, 56
  phonocardiogram of, 55
  schematic diagram of, 52
Third-degree (complete) atrioventricular block, 440, 445
  treatment of, 447
Thoracic cage, and heart displacement, 362
Thoracic disease, acute, pain in, 38
Thoracic spine disease, 155
Thoracocentesis, 313
Thoracotomy, 577
"Three" sign, 353, 354
Thrills, 51
Thromboembolic phenomena, 185
Thromboembolic pulmonary hypertension, 587, 595
Thromboembolism, 587
Thrombolytic therapy, in myocardial infarction, 179
  intracoronary, 114
Thrombophlebitis, 41, 589
  as complication of bedside catheterization, 106
Thrombosis
  in cardiovascular syphilis, 601
  coronary, 164
  coronary artery, 134
  factors promoting, 603
  mural, 134
    and myocardial infarction, 139
  and prostaglandins, 137
  pulmonary, in chronic cor pulmonale, 595
  venous, 50
Thromboxanes
  in atherosclerosis, 137
  in hypertension, 210
Thyroid suppression test, 549
Thyroidectomy, subtotal, 549
Thyroid-stimulating hormone, serum, 549
Thyrotoxic heart disease, 548
Thyrotoxicosis, 480, 548
  and ejection murmur, 59
  laboratory tests for, 549
Thyroxine, serum, 549
Tibial pulse, posterior, 43
Tictac rhythm, 529
  in acute myocarditis, 529
  in rheumatic fever, 535
Tietze's syndrome, 155
  pain of, 38
Time constant, 75
Timing of heart sounds, 52
Timolol, in hypertension, 263
To-and-fro murmur, 61, 574
Tocainide, 490

Tomography, 96
  computerized, in pericarditis, 582
  positron emission, 100, 151
  x-ray, computer-based, 96
Total blood volume, 69, 70
Tourniquets, in rotation, 125, 320
Torsade de points, 497
Tracheostomy, emergency, 123
Training, physical, and circulatory physiology, 31
Transcendental meditation, in hypertension, 259
Transfusion, blood, in cardiac patients, 125
Transient ischemic attacks, dizziness and syncope, in 39
Transluminal angioplasty
  coronary, 114, 194
  renal percutaneous, 242
Transmural infarction, 164, 170
Transplantation
  cardiac, 320
  heart-lung, in Eisenmenger's syndrome, 352
Transposition of great arteries, 357
  anatomic features of, 358
  corrected, 358
    anatomic features of, 359
Transsphenoidal microresection of pituitary, 248
Transthoracic left ventricular puncture, percutaneous, 110
Traumatic false aneurysm, 615
Traumatic heart disease, **614–615**
  and mitral incompetence, 386
Treadmill electrocardiography, 94
Triamterene, 259
  dosages of, 302
  in hypokalemia, 302
Triatoma, 563
Trichinella spiralis, 532
Trichinosis, myocarditis due to, 532
Tricuspid atresia, 360
Tricuspid regurgitation, 290
Tricuspid valve, 6
  atresia of, 290, **359**
  closure of, 52
  disease of, and mitral valve disease, combined, 424
  incompetence of, 48, 327
    and mitral stenosis, 372
    pansystolic murmur due to, 58, 59, 594
    pressure tracing of, 49
  insufficiency of, 293
    in acute endocarditis, 519
  stenosis of, diastolic murmur due to, 60
Tricyclic antidepressants, 488
  and acute myocardial damage, 537
  in heart failure, 313
Trifascicular block, and atrioventricular block, 443
Triiodothyronine, serum, 549
Trimazosin, in heart failure, 316
Trimethaphan, 183, 260, 267
  adverse effects of, 261
  in cardiac failure, 317
Triple-lumen Swan-Ganz catheter, 182
Triple rhythm, 56
"Tripple ripple," 541

Troughs x_1, x_2, and y, 47
Truncus arteriosus, 11, **359**
  anatomic features of, 360
Trunk, pulmonary, 4
Trypanosoma
  cruzi, 532, 563
  gambiense, 532
Trypanosomiasis
  acute myocarditis in, 532
  African, 532
  American, 563
TSH, serum, 549
Tubercles, bilharzial, 587
Tuberculosis, 592
Tuberculous pericarditis, 575
Tubular system, 7
Tumor plop, 56
Tumors. See also specific types.
  as embolic material, 603
Turner's syndrome, 335
Two-dimensional echocardiography, 84, 90
  in angina pectoris, 151
Two-to-one block, 441, 467, 470
TXA_2, in atherosclerosis, 137
Type A personality, 138
Type B personality, 138

Ulcer, peptic, perforated, 592
Ulcerative atheromatous lesions, 605
Ultrasonic examination, 82
Ultrasonic flowmeter, 69
Ultrasonic imaging, 604
Ultrasonic information, modes of display of, 84
Ultrasonography, 82
Ultrasound, Doppler, 85
Ungerleider tables, 82
Unifascicular block, 451
Unstable angina, 37, **161–163**
Uremia, pericardial disease due to, 573
Urinalysis
  in hypertension, 227
  in systemic lupus erythematosus, 557
Urogram, intravenous, in renal artery stenosis, 239
Urokinase, 589
Urologic surgery, in acute cor pulmonale, 589
Uteroplacental perfusion, impaired, preeclampsia due to, 621

v waves, 48, 176
  giant, 48
Vagal reflex, Jarisch–von Bezold, 174
Vaginal delivery, in heart disease, 619
Vagus nerve, stimulation of, in supraventricular tachycardia, 476
Valium, 179, 476
Valsalva, sinuses of, 6
  aneurysm of
    and aortic stenosis, 421
    rupture of, 61
Valsalva's maneuver, 76, 541, 612
  effect on murmurs, 62
  pressure tracing of, 76
Valve(s). See also specific types.
  calcification of, in pulmonary stenosis, 337

Valve(s) (cont'd)
  disease of, **368–431**
    carcinoid, 424
    etiology of, 368
    iatrogenically modified, 425
    multiple, 423
    and surgery, 629
    triple, 424
  diseased, and infective endocarditis, 512
  incompetence of
    measurement of, 71
    in pulmonary stenosis, 337
  lesions of
    acute, natural history of, 368
    chronic, natural history of, 368
    prosthetic, endocarditis on, 522
  replacement of, double, 424
  stenotic, pressure difference across, 74
  tissue of, as embolic material, 603
  normal, and infective endocarditis, 512
Valvotomy, mitral, 377, 425
Valvuloplasty
  in acute mitral incompetence, 396
  percutaneous balloon, 389
Vancomycin
  in genitourinary and gastrointestinal tract surgery, 518
  in prevention of endocarditis, 517
Vanillylmandelic acid, 250
Variant angina, 37, **144**
Varicose veins
  in arteriovenous fistula, 606
  surgery for, in acute cor pulmonale, 589
Vascular bed, pulmonary, 586
Vascular compliance, 75
Vascular disease, peripheral, 43
Vascular lesions, in stroke, 221
Vascular resistance, 74
  pulmonary, 74
    in atrial septal defect, 330
    normal, 78
    raised, in mitral stenosis, 371
  systemic, 74
    and age, 218
    normal, 78
Vasculitis, diffuse, 602
Vasculitis syndromes, clinical classification of, 601
Vasoconstriction
  arteriolar, 586
  pulmonary arterial, 586
Vasodilatation, peripheral, as sign of arteriovenous fistula, 606
Vasodilators, 25
  adverse effects of, 261, 265
  in afterload reduction therapy, 125
  and aortic balloon counterpulsation, 184
  in cardiac failure, 182, 183, **314**, 317
Vasopressin, 26
Vasopressors, 183
Vasospasm, 587
Vasovagal attacks, 116, 611
Vasovagal fainting, 39
Vectorcardiography, 93
Veins. See also specific veins.
  diastolic collapse of, 581

Veins (cont'd)
  in hypertension, 225
  jugular
    distention of, as sign of cardiovascular syphilis, 599
    internal and external, 46
    pulse in, in paroxysmal atrial tachycardia, 470
  of neck, examination of, 46
  pulmonary
    congestion of, 479
    drainage of, anomalous, total, 360
    relocation of, 332
  varicose
    in arteriovenous fistula, 606
    surgery for, in acute cor pulmonale, 589
Vena cava
  inferior, ligation of, 592
  superior, 4
    obstruction of, 582
Venesection, 125, 319
  bloodless, 125
Venous blood, mixed, 66
Venous catheterization, 105
Venous Corrigan waves, 474, 486
Venous hum, 61
Venous pressure, 46
Venous pulse, 46
  normal, 47
Venous puncture, 105
Venous stasis, 41
Venous thrombosis, 50
Ventilation, 65, 100
  pulmonary, 65
Ventilation-perfusion mismatching, 124
Ventilatory assistance, 125
Ventilatory disorders, 476
Ventricle
  and atria, asynchrony of, 486
  left, 5. See also Left ventricle.
    echocardiograms of, 186
  right, 4, 18. See also Right ventricle.
Ventricular aneurysms, 176, 499
  left, 185, 187
  echocardiograms of, 186
  resection of, 502
Ventricular arrhythmias, 140, 172, 482, **484–503**
  and aortic incompetence, 415
  and click-murmur syndrome, 389
  and hypertrophic obstructive cardiomyopathy, 545
  incidence of, 485
  treatment of, 180, 181
Ventricular beats, ectopic, during catheterization, 117
Ventricular compliance, 75
Ventricular conduction defects, 448
Ventricular contraction, asynchrony with atrial contraction, in ventricular tachycardia, 495
Ventricular diastole, 18
Ventricular ejection, 23
  left, 15
  pattern of, and ventricular shape, 23
Ventricular enlargement, 23
  right, secondary to chronic respiratory disease, 593

Ventricular failure
  left, 51, 288, **290**, 410
    acute, 175
    in aortic incompetence, 421
    pulsus alternans in, 44
    as sign of cardiovascular syphilis, 599
    periodic breathing in, 51
  right, 289
Ventricular fibrillation. *See* Fibrillation, ventricular.
Ventricular filling
  abrupt cessation of, 582
  and third heart sound, 56
Ventricular function
  assessment of, 75
  impaired, evidence of, 75
  left
    assessment of, 70, 77
    effect of contrast material on, 71
Ventricular heave, 291
  right, 293
Ventricular hypertrophy
  left, 227
    diagnosis of, 228
    and drugs, 230
    ECG of, 288
    in hypertension, 228
    mortality rate and initial degree of, 231
  right, 587
    ECG of, 295, 336
    as sign of right ventricular failure, 293
Ventricular infarction, right, 166
Ventricular preexcitation, 454
Ventricular premature beats, 141, 144, 180, 308, **484–493**
  in acute myocardial infarction, 484
  in bigeminy and trigeminy, ECG of, 484
  and central nervous system, 486
  complex, and congestive heart failure, 485
  ECG of, 494
  grading system for, 485
  hazards of, 486
  induced by graded exercise, 487
  and mortality rates, 191
  multifocal, 144
  significance of, 486
  treatment of, 487
Ventricular pressure
  left, rate of change of, 77
  and length-tension relationships, 20
  recording of, 109
Ventricular rate, and digitalis, 480
Ventricular response, in atrial fibrillation, 480
Ventricular rhythms, differentiation on ECG, 473
Ventricular septal defect, 60, 177, 290, **343**
  anatomic features of, 344
  in differential diagnosis of pulmonary stenosis, 336
  ECG of, 345
  left parasternal bulge as sign of, 50
  murmurs in, 61
    pansystolic, 58, 59
  x-ray of, 344

Ventricular septum, perforated, 177
Ventricular shape, and pattern of ventricular ejection, 23
Ventricular standstill, 144
Ventricular systole, 15
Ventricular tachycardia. *See* Tachycardia, ventricular.
Ventricular volume, 20
  left, 70, 78
Ventricular wall, left, dysfunction or rupture of, 185
Ventriculoatrial conduction, 496
Verapamil, 157, 158, 490
  in cardiac failure, 182, 313.
  in hypertrophic cardiomyopathy, 546
  in pregnancy, 620
  and refractory period, 458
  in supraventricular tachycardia, 476
Vertigo, 39
  sudden, 604
Vessels
  great, 2
  peripheral, systolic bruits in, 60
  spasm of, 116
Visceral blood flow, 29
Vision
  disturbance of, in arteritis, 602
  loss of, in cerebral embolism, 603
Vitamin K, 592
VMA, 250
Volume
  of radial pulse, 42
  ventricular, 20
Volume load, 287
Volume replacement, 182
Vomiting, in acute myocardial infarction, 165
Vulnerable phase, 432

Wall motion
  abnormalities of, 70, 172
  segmental, 177
Warfarin, 592
Water intake, in heart failure, 290
Water retention, pathophysiologic mechanisms of, 289
Water-hammer pulse, 416
  as sign of cardiovascular syphilis, 599
Waves
  a, 47
    giant, 48
    in ventricular compliance, 75
    abnormal or exaggerated, 48
  c, 47
    cannon, 48, 486
    defined, 474
    irregular, 48
  Corrigan, venous, 474, 486
  delta, in Wolff-Parkinson-White syndrome, 457
  F, 480
  negative, in neck veins, 581
  P
    atrial, in pulmonary embolism, 590
    buried, 473
    ectopic, 467
    high-voltage, 609
    premature, 467
    in right ventricular failure, 294

Waves (cont'd)
  positive, 47
  pulse, velocity of, 42
  Q
    abnormal, 168
    in acute myocardial infarction, 168
    as sign of pulmonary embolism, 590
  R, tall, as sign of chronic cor pulmonale, 594
  square, in Valsalva's maneuver, 76
  ST–T, in arteriovenous fistula, 606
  T, 72
    inversion of, 581
      in chronic cor pulmonale, 594
      in fibrinous pericarditis, 574
      in pericardial constriction, 581
      in pulmonary embolism, 590
  v, 47
    giant, 48
Weakness
  in acute myocardial infarction, 165
  in chronic constrictive pericarditis, 581
  in systemic embolism, 604
Wedge pressure, 106
  measurement of, 111
  in Eisenmenger's syndrome, 351
  validity of, 107
Weight
  loss of, in heart disease, 41
  reduction of, in hypertension, 258
Wenckebach (Mobitz type I) atrioventricular block
  diagram of, 444
  second-degree, 441, 444
Wenckebach pauses, 185, 445
Wenckebach phenomenon, 174
  partial progressive atrioventricular block with, 470
Wide pulse pressure, in cardiovascular syphilis, 599
Willis, circle of, 29
Wolff-Parkinson-White conduction, 496
Wolff-Parkinson-White syndrome, 454, 456
  atrial fibrillation in, treatment of, 459
  concealed, 460, 472
  effect of drugs in, 455
Wytensin, in hypertension, 259

x **descent, 47**
x_1 trough, 47
x_2 trough, 47
Xanthoma tuberosum, 45
X-ray, chest, 82
  in hypertension, 230
X-ray tomography, computer-based, 96

y **descent, 48**
  rapid, 581
y trough, 47, 48
Yoga, in hypertension, 259

Z lines, 7
Zaroxolyn, 259
Zone, M, 8
Zuckerkandl, organ of, 249

Lange Medical Publications titles are available at all medical bookstores within the USA. If you wish to order directly from the publisher, please complete and mail the attached postage-paid card. Where applicable, availability is indicated in parentheses.

1. **Current Medical Diagnosis & Treatment 1986,** Krupp et al (A1413-2) **$29.50**
2. **Current Pediatric Diagnosis & Treatment, 9th ed.,** Kempe et al (A1414-0) **$29.00** (9/86)
3. **Current Obstetric & Gynecologic Diagnosis & Treatment, 6th ed.,** Benson (A1412-4) **$30.50** (9/86)
4. **Current Emergency Diagnosis & Treatment, 2nd.,** Mills et al (A0027) **$28.00**
5. **Current Surgical Diagnosis & Treatment, 7th ed.,** Way (A0019) **$31.50**
6. **Basic & Clinical Pharmacology, 3rd ed.,** Katzung (A0553-6) **$28.00** (6/86)
7. **Pharmacology: A Review,** Katzung & Trevor (A0031) **$13.00**
8. **Review of General Psychiatry,** Goldman (A0030) **$24.00**
9. **Basic & Clinical Endocrinology, 2nd ed.,** Greenspan & Forsham (A0547-8) **$27.00** (6/86)
10. **Basic & Clinical Immunology, 6th ed.,** Sites et al (A0548-6) **$27.50** (7/86)
11. **Harper's Review of Biochemistry, 20th ed.,** Martin et al (A0003) **$24.50**
12. **Biochemistry: A Synopsis,** Colby (A0033) **$13.00**
13. **Basic Histology, 5th ed.,** Junqueira et al (A0570-0) **$21.50**
14. **Review of Medical Physiology, 12th ed.,** Ganong (A0013) **$22.50**
15. **Physiology: A Study Guide,** Ganong (A0032) **$12.00**
16. **Review of Medical Microbiology, 17th ed.,** Jawetz et al (A8432-5) **$20.00** (6/86)
17. **Correlative Neuroanatomy & Functional Neurology, 19th ed.,** Chusid (A0001) **$19.50**
18. **General Urology, 11th ed.,** Smith (A0009) **$24.00**
19. **General Ophthalmology, 11th ed.,** Vaughan & Asbury (A3108-6) **$21.00**
20. **Principles of Clinical Electrocardiography, 12th ed.,** Goldman (A0008) **$19.00**
21. **Clinical Cardiology, 4th ed.,** Sokolow & McIlroy (A0023) **$26.50** (5/86)
22. **Electrocardiography: Essentials of Interpretation,** Goldschlager & Goldman (A0029) **$13.00**
23. **Physician's Handbook, 21st ed.,** Krupp et al (A0002) **$16.50**
24. **Handbook of Pediatrics, 15th ed.,** Silver et al (A3635-8) **$16.50** (7/86)
25. **Handbook of Poisoning, 12th ed.,** Dreisbach & Robertson (A3643-2) **$16.50** (9/86)
26. **Handbook of Obstetrics & Gynecology, 9th ed.,** Benson (A3627-5) **$16.50** (9/86)

ORDER CARD

Please send me the following books. If I wish, I may return the book(s) within 30 days and receive a full credit/refund.

1. Krupp (A1413-2) $29.50
2. Kempe (A1414-0) $29.00
3. Benson (A1412-4) $30.50
4. Mills (A0027-1) $28.00
5. Way (A0019-8) $31.50
6. Katzung (A0553-6) $28.00
7. Katzung (A0031-3) $13.00
8. Goldman (A0030-5) $24.00
9. Greenspan (A0547-8) $27.00
10. Stites (A0548-6) $27.50
11. Martin (A0003-2) $24.50
12. Colby (A0033-9) $13.00
13. Junqueira (A0570-0) $21.50
14. Ganong (A0013-1) $22.50
15. Ganong (A0032-1) $12.00
16. Jawetz (A8432-5) $20.00
17. Chusid (A0001-6) $19.50
18. Smith (A0009-9) $24.00
19. Vaughan (A3108-6) $21.00
20. Goldman (A0008-1) $19.00
21. Sokolow (A0023-0) $26.50
22. Goldschlager (A0029-7) $13.00
23. Krupp (A0002-4) $16.50
24. Silver (A3635-8) $16.50
25. Dreisbach (A3643-2) $16.50
26. Benson (A3627-5) $16.50

☐ Payment enclosed, including handling charge.
☐ Charge to my   ☐ VISA   ☐ Mastercard

Name _____
Address _____
City/State/Zip _____
Signature _____
Affiliation _____

Card Number _____
Expiration Date _____

Amount $ _____
State Tax $ _____
Handling $ _____
TOTAL $ _____

Mail and make check payable to:

Appleton-Century-Crofts
25 Van Zant St.
E. Norwalk, CT 06855

Prices are subject to change without notice. Prices advertised are applicable in the U.S., its territories and possessions only. For orders outside the U.S. and Canada contact: Prentice-Hall Intl., Englewood Cliffs, NJ 07632. In Canada, contact: Prentice-Hall Canada, Scarborough, Ontario, M1P 2J7.

BUSINESS REPLY MAIL
FIRST CLASS PERMIT NO. 150 E. NORWALK, CT

POSTAGE WILL BE PAID BY ADDRESSEE

NO POSTAGE
NECESSARY
IF MAILED
IN THE
UNITED STATES

APPLETON-CENTURY-CROFTS
LANGE MEDICAL PUBLICATIONS

DEPARTMENT B
25 VAN ZANT STREET
EAST NORWALK, CT 06855